a LANGE medical book

CURRENT
Diagnosis & Treatment: Rheumatology

Fourth Edition

Editor

John H. Stone, MD, MPH
Professor of Medicine
Harvard Medical School
The Edward A. Fox Chair in Medicine
Massachusetts General Hospital

New York   Chicago   San Francisco   Athens   London   Madrid   Mexico City
New Delhi   Milan   Singapore   Sydney   Toronto

Current Diagnosis & Treatment: Rheumatology, Fourth Edition

2 3 4 5 6 7 8 9   LCR   26 25 24 23 22

ISBN 978-1-259-64464-1
MHID 1-259-64464-2
ISSN 1547-8998

Notice

Medicine is an ever-changing science. As new research and clinical experience broaden our knowledge, changes in treatment and drug therapy are required. The authors and the publisher of this work have checked with sources believed to be reliable in their efforts to provide information that is complete and generally in accord with the standards accepted at the time of publication. However, in view of the possibility of human error or changes in medical sciences, neither the authors nor the publisher nor any other party who has been involved in the preparation or publication of this work warrants that the information contained herein is in every respect accurate or complete, and they disclaim all responsibility for any errors or omissions or for the results obtained from use of the information contained in this work. Readers are encouraged to confirm the information contained herein with other sources. For example and in particular, readers are advised to check the product information sheet included in the package of each drug they plan to administer to be certain that the information contained in this work is accurate and that changes have not been made in the recommended dose or in the contraindications for administration. This recommendation is of particular importance in connection with new or infrequently used drugs.

This book was set in Minion by KnowledgeWorks Global Ltd.
The editors were Kay Conerly and Kim J. Davis.
The production supervisor was Catherine Saggese.
Project management was provided by Sarika Gupta, KnowledgeWorks Global Ltd.

This book is printed on acid-free paper.

McGraw Hill books are available at special quantity discounts to use as premiums and sales promotions, or for use in corporate training programs. To contact a representative, please visit the Contact Us pages at www.mhprofessional.com.

With love and gratitude and in memory of "Yiayia":

Bessie D. Nikitas
1926–2019
She played a larger-than-life role in my family.
She graced and inspired our lives.
Her hands grace the cover of this book.

Contents

*Deceased.

Section VIII. Disorders of Bone

Section IX. Imaging & Genetics

Color insert appears between pages 300 and 301.

Contributors

A. O. Adebajo, MBChB, FWACP,
 MSc (Cambridge) FRCP, FACP, FAcMed
Faculty of Medicine, Dentistry and Health
University of Sheffield
Sheffield, United Kingdom
Chapter 44 The Rheumatic Manifestations of Acute &
 Chronic Viral Infections

Tochi Adizie, MBChB, MRCP
Department of Rheumatology
The Royal Wolverhampton NHS Trust
Wolverhampton, United Kingdom
Chapter 44 The Rheumatic Manifestations of Acute &
 Chronic Viral Infections

Brittany Adler, MD
Department of Medicine, Division of Rheumatology
Johns Hopkins University School of Medicine
Baltimore, Maryland
Chapter 25 Autoimmune Myopathies, Immune-Mediated
 Necrotizing Myopathies, & Their Mimickers

Sheila L. Arvikar, MD
Division of Rheumatology, Allergy, and Immunology
Massachusetts General Hospital
Instructor, Harvard Medical School
Boston, Massachusetts
Chapter 16 Reactive Arthritis

Alexia A. Belperron, PhD
Research Scientist
Section of Rheumatology, Department of Internal Medicine
Yale University School of Medicine
New Haven, Connecticut
Chapter 43 Lyme Disease

Johnathan A. Bernard, MD
Department of Orthopaedic Surgery
Johns Hopkins University School of Medicine
Baltimore, Maryland
Chapter 6 Approach to the Patient with Shoulder Pain

Linda K. Bockenstedt, MD
Harold W. Jockers Professor of Medicine
Section of Rheumatology, Department of Internal Medicine
Yale University School of Medicine
New Haven, Connecticut
Chapter 43 Lyme Disease

Francesco Boin, MD
Professor of Medicine
Director, Division of Rheumatology
Director, Scleroderma Center
Cedars Sinai Medical Center
Los Angeles, California
Chapter 23 Scleroderma (Systemic Sclerosis)

Marcy B. Bolster, MD
Director, Rheumatology Fellowship
 Training Program
Massachusetts General Hospital
Associate Professor of Medicine
Harvard Medical School
Boston, Massachusetts
Chapter 52 Paget Disease of Bone

David Borenstein, MD
Clinical Professor (Emeritus)
The George Washington University
 Medical Center
Washington, D.C.
Chapter 7 Approach to the Patient with Neck Pain

Pilar Brito-Zerón, MD, PhD
Chapter 24 Primary Sjögren Syndrome

Edward S. Chen, MD
Assistant Professor, Division of Pulmonary
 & Critical Care Medicine
Johns Hopkins Hospital
Co-Director, Sarcoidosis Clinic
Johns Hopkins Bayview
Medical Director, Respiratory
 Care Services
Johns Hopkins University
 School of Medicine
Baltimore, Maryland
Chapter 46 Sarcoidosis

Neal Chen, MD
Assistant Professor of Orthopaedic Surgery
Harvard Medical School
Hand & Arm Center
Massachusetts General Hospital
Boston, Massachusetts
Chapter 4 Hand & Wrist Pain:
 A Systematic Approach

Hyon K. Choi, MD, DrPH
Professor of Medicine, Harvard Medical School
Director, Gout and Crystal Arthropathy Center
Director, Clinical Epidemiology and Health Outcomes
Division of Rheumatology, Allergy, and Immunology
Department of Medicine, Massachusetts General Hospital
Boston, Massachusetts
Chapter 40 Gout

Lisa Christopher-Stine, MD, MPH
Department of Medicine, Division of Rheumatology
Johns Hopkins University School of Medicine
Baltimore, Maryland
Chapter 25 Autoimmune Myopathies, Immune-Mediated Necrotizing Myopathies, & Their Mimickers

Sharon A. Chung, MD, MAS
University of California San Francisco
San Francisco, California
Chapter 55 Genetics & Genetic Testing in Rheumatology

Jill C. Costello, MD
Assistant Clinical Professor of Medicine
Division of Rheumatology
Clement J. Zablocki VA Medical Center
Medical College of Wisconsin
The Hub for Collaborative Medicine
Milwaukee, Wisconsin
Chapter 41 Calcium Pyrophosphate Deposition Disease

Courtney B. Crayne, MD, MSPH
Instructor of Pediatrics
Division of Pediatric Rheumatology
Children's Hospital of Alabama
University of Alabama at Birmingham
Birmingham, Alabama
Chapter 18 Juvenile Idiopathic Arthritis

Lindsey A. Criswell, MD, MPH, DSc
University of California San Francisco
San Francisco, California
Chapter 55 Genetics & Genetic Testing in Rheumatology

Randy Q. Cron, MD, PhD
Professor of Pediatrics
Arthritis Foundation, Alabama Chapter, Endowed Chair
Director, Division of Pediatric Rheumatology
Children's Hospital of Alabama
University of Alabama at Birmingham
Birmingham, Alabama
Chapter 18 Juvenile Idiopathic Arthritis

Gaye Cunnane, PhD, MB, FRCPI
Clinical Professor of Rheumatology
Trinity College Dublin
Consultant Rheumatologist
St James's Hospital
Dublin, Ireland
Chapter 45 Whipple Disease

Maria Dall'Era, MD
Professor and Chief, UCSF Division of Rheumatology
Jean S. Engleman Distinguished Professorship in Rheumatology
Director, UCSF Lupus Clinic and Rheumatology Clinical Research Center
Department of Medicine
University of California San Francisco
San Francisco, California
Chapter 19 Systemic Lupus Erythematosus

Rajiv K. Dixit, MD
Clinical Professor of Medicine
University of California San Francisco
Director, Northern California Arthritis Center
Walnut Creek, California
Chapter 2 Joint Aspiration & Injection; Chapter 8 Approach to the Patient with Low Back Pain

Geetha Duvuru, MD, MRCP
Division of Nephrology and Rheumatology
Department of Medicine
Johns Hopkins University School of Medicine
Baltimore, Maryland
Chapter 35 IgA Vasculitis (Henoch-Schönlein Purpura)

Doruk Erkan, MD, MPH
Associate Attending Rheumatologist
Hospital for Special Surgery
Associate Physician-Scientist
Barbara Volcker Center for Women and Rheumatic Disease
Associate Professor of Medicine
Weill Cornell Medicine
New York, New York
Chapter 21 Antiphospholipid Syndrome

Ursula Fearon, PhD
Consultant Rheumatologist
St. Vincent's University Hospital
Dublin, Ireland
Chapter 13 Rheumatoid Arthritis

Erin G. Floyd, MD
PGY1 Internal Medicine Intern, Primary Care
University of Wisconsin, Madison
Madison, Wisconsin
Chapter 11 Fibromyalgia

Howard W. Francis, MD, MBA, FACS
Richard Hall Chaney, Sr. Professor of Otolaryngology
Chair, Department of Head and Neck Surgery &
    Communication Sciences
Duke University Health System
Durham, North Carolina
*Chapter 50 Sensorineural Hearing Loss (Immune-Mediated
    Inner Ear Disease)*

Michael T. Freehill, MD
Department of Orthopaedic Surgery
Johns Hopkins University School of Medicine
Baltimore, Maryland
Chapter 6 Approach to the Patient with Shoulder Pain

Allan C. Gelber, MD, MPH, PhD
Professor of Medicine
Deputy Director for Education and
    Faculty Development
Division of Rheumatology
Johns Hopkins University School of Medicine
Baltimore, Maryland
Chapter 39 Osteoarthritis

Lianne S. Gensler, MD
Associate Professor of Medicine,
    Division of Rheumatology
University of California San Francisco
San Francisco, California
*Chapter 15 Axial Spondyloarthritis & Arthritis Associated
    with Inflammatory Bowel Disease*

Elena Gkrouzman, MD
Hospital for Special Surgery,
    Rheumatology Fellow
New York, New York
Chapter 21 Antiphospholipid Syndrome

Andrew Gross, MD
Professor of Medicine
Medical Director, Rheumatology
University of California San Francisco
San Francisco, California
*Chapter 10 Approach to the Patient with Knee Pain;
    Chapter 11 Fibromyalgia*

Philippe Guilpain, MD, PhD
University of Montpellier Medical School
University of Montpellier
Department of Internal Medicine,
    Multi-Organic Diseases
Saint-Eloi Hospital
Montpellier, France
Chapter 14 Adult Onset Still Disease (AOSD)

Ahmet Gül, MD
Division of Rheumatology,
    Department of Internal Medicine
Istanbul Faculty of Medicine
Istanbul University
Istanbul, Turkey
Chapter 34 Behçet Disease

Daniel Guss, MD, MBA
Assistant Professor, Harvard Medical School
Foot and Ankle Service
Department of Orthopaedic Surgery
Massachusetts General Hospital
Boston, Massachusetts
Newton-Wellesley Hospital
Newton, Massachusetts
*Chapter 5 Approach to the Patient
    with Foot & Ankle Pain*

Janice He, MD
Orthopedics Fellow, Hand Surgery
Hand & Arm Center
Massachusetts General Hospital
Boston, Massachusetts
*Chapter 4 Hand & Wrist Pain:
    A Systematic Approach*

Ambrose J. Huang, MD
Assistant Professor of Radiology
Harvard Medical School
Division of Musculoskeletal Imaging
    and Intervention
Department of Radiology
Massachusetts General Hospital
Boston, Massachusetts
Chapter 53 Musculoskeletal Magnetic Resonance Imaging

Mary Beth Humphrey, MD, PhD, FACP
Professor of Medicine
Associate Dean for Research, College of Medicine
Division Chief of Rheumatology, Immunology, and Allergy
University of Oklahoma Health Sciences Center
Oklahoma City, Oklahoma
Chapter 51 Osteoporosis & Glucocorticoid-Induced Osteoporosis

M. Elaine Husni, MD, MPH
Cleveland Clinic Foundation
Orthopaedic and Rheumatologic Institute
Department of Rheumatic and Immunologic Diseases
Vice Chair, Arthritis Center
Director, Arthritis & Musculoskeletal Treatment Center
Cleveland, Ohio
Chapter 17 Psoriatic Arthritis

Ravi S. Kamath, MD, PhD
Musculoskeletal Radiologist
Fairfax Radiological Consultants, PC
Fairfax, Virginia
Chapter 53 Musculoskeletal Magnetic Resonance Imaging

Sarah F. Keller, MD, MA
Staff Rheumatologist
Orthopaedic and Rheumatology Institute
Department of Rheumatic & Immunologic Diseases
The Cleveland Clinic
Cleveland, Ohio
Chapter 52 Paget Disease of Bone

Arezou Khosroshahi, MD
Associate Professor of Medicine
Emory University School of Medicine
Rheumatology Division
Atlanta, Georgia
Chapter 20 Treatment of Systemic Lupus Erythematosus

Minna J. Kohler, MD, RhMSUS
Director, Rheumatology Musculoskeletal Ultrasound
    Program
Division of Rheumatology, Allergy and Immunology
Massachusetts General Hospital
Instructor in Medicine
Harvard Medical School
Boston, Massachusetts
*Chapter 54 Musculoskeletal Ultrasound
    in Rheumatology*

Cristina M. Lanata, MD
University of California San Francisco
San Francisco, California
*Chapter 55 Genetics & Genetic Testing
    in Rheumatology*

Craig Lareau, MD
Assistant Professor
University of Massachusetts Medical School
Boston, Massachusetts
Orthopaedic Foot & Ankle Surgeon
New England Orthopaedic Surgeons
Springfield, Massachusetts
*Chapter 5 Approach to the Patient with
    Foot & Ankle Pain*

Jean W. Liew, MD
University of Washington
Seattle, Washington
*Chapter 15 Axial Spondyloarthritis & Arthritis Associated
    with Inflammatory Bowel Disease*

S. Sam Lim, MD, MPH
Professor of Medicine and Epidemiology
Clinical Director, Division of Rheumatology
Emory University
Chief of Rheumatology
Grady Health System
Atlanta, Georgia
Chapter 20 Treatment of Systemic Lupus Erythematosus

Candice Low, MD
St. Vincent's Hospital
Dublin, Ireland
Chapter 13 Rheumatoid Arthritis

C. Benjamin Ma, MD
Professor in Residence
Sports Medicine and Shoulder Surgery
Vice Chair, Adult Clinical Operations
Department of Orthopaedic Surgery
University of California San Francisco
San Francisco, California
Chapter 10 Approach to the Patient with Knee Pain

Andrew L. Mammen, MD, PhD
Muscle Disease Unit, Laboratory of Muscle Stem Cells and
    Gene Regulation
National Institute of Arthritis and Musculoskeletal
    and Skin Diseases
National Institutes of Health
Bethesda, Maryland
Departments of Neurology and Medicine
Johns Hopkins University School of Medicine
Baltimore, Maryland
*Chapter 25 Autoimmune Myopathies, Immune-Mediated
    Necrotizing Myopathies, & Their Mimickers*

Jennifer Mandal, MD
Assistant Professor of Medicine
UCSF Division of Rheumatology
Zuckerberg San Francisco General Hospital
San Francisco, California
Chapter 23 Scleroderma (Systemic Sclerosis)

Alexandre Maria, MD, PhD
Department of Internal Medicine, Multi-Organic Diseases
University of Montpellier Medical School
Saint-Eloi Hospital
Montpellier, France
Chapter 14 Adult Onset Still Disease (AOSD)

Kavitha Mattaparthi, MD
Department of Medicine
University of Oklahoma Health Sciences Center
Oklahoma City, Oklahoma
Chapter 51 Osteoporosis & Glucocorticoid-Induced Osteoporosis

Simon C. Mears, MD, PhD
Professor
Department of Orthopaedic Surgery
University of Arkansas for Medical Sciences
Little Rock, Arkansas
Chapter 9 Approach to the Patient with Hip Pain

Lester D. Miller, MD
Associate Clinical Professor of Medicine
Rheumatology Division
University of California San Francisco Medical Center
San Francisco, California
Chapter 13 Rheumatoid Arthritis

John A. Mills, MD
Chapter 1 Physical Examination of the Musculoskeletal System

David R. Moller, MD
Professor Emeritus, Medicine
Johns Hopkins University
Ellicott City, Maryland
Chapter 46 Sarcoidosis

Nadia D. Morgan,* MD, MHS
Instructor of Medicine
Division of Rheumatology
Johns Hopkins University School of Medicine
Baltimore, Maryland
Chapter 22 Raynaud Phenomenon

Sandra B. Nelson, MD
Massachusetts General Hospital
Harvard Medical School
Boston, Massachusetts
Chapter 42 Septic Arthritis

Anne Louise Oaklander, MD, PhD
Department of Neurology
Massachusetts General Hospital
Harvard Medical School
Department of Pathology (Neuropathology)
Massachusetts General Hospital
Boston, Massachusetts
Chapter 12 Complex Regional Pain Syndrome (Reflex Sympathetic Dystrophy) & Posttraumatic Neuralgia

Lawrence K. O'Malley, MD
Assistant Professor
Department of Orthopaedic Surgery
University of Arkansas for Medical Sciences
Little Rock, Arkansas
Chapter 9 Approach to the Patient with Hip Pain

George N. Papaliodis, MD
Director of the Ocular Immunology
and Uveitis Service
Massachusetts Eye and Ear Infirmary
Harvard Medical School
Boston, Massachusetts
Chapter 49 Ocular Inflammatory Diseases for Rheumatologists

Manuel Ramos-Casals, MD, PhD
Sjögren Syndrome Research Group (AGAUR)
Laboratory of Autoimmune Diseases Josep Font, IDIBAPS-CELLEX
Department of Medicine, University of Barcelona
Department of Autoimmune Diseases
ICMiD, Hospital Clínic, C/Villarroel
Barcelona, Spain
Chapter 24 Primary Sjögren Syndrome

James T. Rosenbaum, MD
Professor of Medicine, Ophthalmology, and Cell Biology
Chair, Division of Arthritis and Rheumatic Diseases
Edward E. Rosenbaum Professor of Inflammation Research
Oregon Health & Science University
Chair Emeritus
Legacy Devers Eye Institute
Legacy Health System
Portland, Oregon
Chapter 49 Ocular Inflammatory Diseases for Rheumatologists

Ann K. Rosenthal, MD
Will and Cava Ross Professor of Medicine and Chief of Rheumatology
Medical College of Wisconsin/Clement J. Zablocki VA Medical Center
The Hub for Collaborative Medicine
Milwaukee, Wisconsin
Chapter 41 Calcium Pyrophosphate Deposition Disease

Philip Seo, MD, MHS
Director, The Johns Hopkins Vasculitis Center
Associate Professor of Medicine
Johns Hopkins University School of Medicine
Baltimore, Maryland
Chapter 30 Eosinophilic Granulomatosis with Polyangiitis (Churg-Strauss Syndrome)

*Deceased

Naomi Serling-Boyd, MD
Division of Rheumatology, Allergy
   and Immunology
Massachusetts General Hospital
Boston, Massachusetts

Chapter 31 Polyarteritis Nodosa; Chapter 32 Cryoglobulinemia;
   Chapter 36 Primary Angiitis of the Central Nervous System;
   Chapter 38 Miscellaneous Forms of Vasculitis; Chapter 47
   Relapsing Polychondritis

Antoni Sisó-Almirall, MD, PhD
Department of Medicine
University of Barcelona Department of
   Autoimmune Diseases
ICMiD, Hospital Clínic, C/Villarroel
Barcelona, Spain

Chapter 24 Primary Sjögren Syndrome

Umasuthan Srikumaran, MD
Department of Orthopaedic Surgery
Johns Hopkins University School of Medicine
Baltimore, Maryland

Chapter 6 Approach to the Patient with
   Shoulder Pain

John H. Stone, MD, MPH
Professor of Medicine
Harvard Medical School
Director, Clinical Rheumatology
Massachusetts General Hospital
Boston, Massachusetts

Chapter 28 Granulomatosis with Polyangiitis; Chapter 29
   Microscopic Polyangiitis; Chapter 30 Eosinophilic
   Granulomatosis with Polyangiitis (Churg-Strauss
   Syndrome); Chapter 31 Polyarteritis Nodosa; Chapter 32
   Cryoglobulinemia; Chapter 33 Hypersensitivity
   Vasculitis; Chapter 35 IgA Vasculitis (Henoch-Schönlein
   Purpura); Chapter 36 Primary Angiitis of the Central
   Nervous System; Chapter 37 Thromboangiitis Obliterans
   (Buerger Disease); Chapter 38 Miscellaneous Forms of
   Vasculitis; Chapter 47 Relapsing Polychondritis;
   Chapter 48 IgG4-Related Disease; Chapter 50 Sensorineural
   Hearing Loss (Immune-Mediated Inner Ear Disease)

Alex Truong, MD
Department of Medicine
Emory Midtown Hospital
Atlanta, Georgia

Chapter 25 Autoimmune Myopathies,
   Immune-Mediated Necrotizing Myopathies,
   & Their Mimickers

Sebastian Unizony, MD
Co-Director, Vasculitis and Glomerulonephritis Center
Rheumatology, Allergy and Immunology Division
Massachusetts General Hospital
Assistant Professor of Medicine,
Harvard Medical School
Boston, Massachusetts

Chapter 26 Giant Cell Arteritis & Polymyalgia Rheumatica;
   Chapter 27 Takayasu Arteritis

Douglas J. Veale, MD, FRCPI, FRCP(Lon)
Head of The EULAR Centre of Excellence Dublin
The Centre for Arthritis and Rheumatic Disease
Director of Translational Research & Adjunct Professor of
   Medicine, University College Dublin
Fellow of The Conway Institute of Biomedical &
   Biomolecular Research
Consultant Rheumatologist
St. Vincent's University Hospital
Dublin, Ireland

Chapter 13 Rheumatoid Arthritis

Scott Weiner, DO
Department of Orthopaedic Surgery
Johns Hopkins University School of Medicine
Baltimore, Maryland

Chapter 6 Approach to the Patient with Shoulder Pain

Mark H. Wener, MD
Professor
Immunology Division, Department of Laboratory Medicine
Adjunct Professor, Rheumatology Division,
   Department of Medicine
University of Washington
Seattle, Washington

Chapter 3 Laboratory Testing

Fredrick M. Wigley, MD
Professor of Medicine
Associate Director, Division of Rheumatology
Johns Hopkins University School of Medicine
Baltimore, Maryland

Chapter 22 Raynaud Phenomenon

John H. Wilckens, MD
Associate Professor, Orthopaedic Surgery
Orthopaedic Medical Director
Johns Hopkins at White Marsh
Director, White Marsh Ambulatory Surgery Center
Chief, Orthopaedic Surgery Sports Medicine Division
Johns Hopkins University School of Medicine
Baltimore, Maryland

Chapter 6 Approach to the Patient with Shoulder Pain

David W. Wu, MD
Assistant Clinical Professor of Medicine
University of California San Francisco
Northern California Arthritis Center
John Muir Medical Center
Walnut Creek, California
Chapter 2 Joint Aspiration & Injection

Mark Yakavonis, MD
Clinical Fellow, Harvard Medical School
Foot and Ankle Service
Department of Orthopaedic Surgery
Massachusetts General Hospital
Boston, Massachusetts
Newton-Wellesley Hospital
Newton, Massachusetts
Chapter 5 Approach to the Patient with Foot & Ankle Pain

Chio Yokose, MD
Division of Rheumatology, Allergy, and Immunology
Massachusetts General Hospital
Harvard Medical School
Boston, Massachusetts
Chapter 40 Gout

Muhammad Zaheer, MD
Department of Medicine
University of Oklahoma Health Sciences Center
Oklahoma City, Oklahoma
Chapter 51 Osteoporosis & Glucocorticoid-Induced Osteoporosis

Preface

There is no field of medicine more broad and fascinating than rheumatology. Our field is, after all, the *in vivo* expression of immunology. Rheumatology is the sum of all symptoms, the accumulation of all physical findings, the full expression of all laboratory abnormalities, the library of all radiological manifestations, and the catalogue of all pathological features that can occur when the immune system goes awry – whatever the cause. Rheumatology is also the litany of local insults to joints, muscles, bones, and tendons that develop either acutely or as the result of wear, tear, overuse, aging, and other processes of life. Finally, rheumatology is the emotional impact of these disorders on the lives of human beings.

There is no field of medicine in which the "hands-on" approach to the patient is more vital to making the correct diagnosis than in rheumatology. The time devoted to a careful history and an insightful physical examination is immensely reassuring to the patient – *"Someone is listening. Someone knows what this is!"*. Time spent with the patient guides the remainder of the evaluation, if indeed more is needed, and dictates treatment.

Finally, there is no field of medicine in which therapies have advanced more dramatically since the start of this century than in rheumatology. Our growing ability to treat rheumatological problems and transform patients' lives is a gift to patients, and a privilege for those who love this field.

John H. Stone, MD, MPH

Physical Examination of the Musculoskeletal System

1

John A. Mills, MD

The musculoskeletal system constitutes a demanding part of the physical examination in terms of both knowledge and time. The most important insight with regard to the physical examination is that the skillful examiner focuses this critical task through information obtained in a careful history. The second critical realization is that a thorough knowledge of musculoskeletal anatomy is essential to the performance of an accurate and meaningful examination. An atlas should be at hand (or only a few computer strokes away) as a quick reference.

OBTAINING A HISTORY

The clinician may begin the patient interview by asking the following two questions: (1) Are the patient's symptoms articular in nature? and (2) do they derive from a musculotendinous location? If the answer to either of these questions is yes, then the examiner can begin to focus his or her efforts on the specific anatomic parts referred to by the patient in the history, bearing in mind two points:

- Referred pain and an incomplete understanding of the anatomy may affect the patient's localization of the complaint. For example, "hip pain" perceived over the lateral side while rolling over in bed at night is more likely to be trochanteric bursitis than pathology of the true hip joint.
- Musculoskeletal complaints are sometimes part of overarching, systemic disorders that affect the joints, muscles, bones, and tendons.

Pain present at rest usually indicates an acute inflammatory, neurologic, or neoplastic process. In addition to determining which musculoskeletal structures are the source of the patient's symptoms, the overall objectives of the examination should be kept in mind. These are outlined in Table 1–1.

SPECIFIC EXAMINATION TECHNIQUES

▶ Observation

The examiner should take the opportunity to observe the patient's posture and mobility when he or she first enters the examination room. Alternatively, if the patient is already in the examining room or on the examination table when first encountered, the examiner should request at some point during the assessment that the patient stand, walk a few yards, and sit again. Gait analysis (for limp) can help separate a primary joint issue from extra-articular manifestations of an underlying condition, such as weakness. This exercise also facilitates the identification of certain deformities. Genu varum or pes planus, for example, become more evident with weight bearing.

▶ Palpation

A bilateral comparison may be helpful in evaluating a swollen area. The anatomic extent of swelling should be verified by palpation, keeping in mind the anatomy of the part. The presence of free fluid is determined by ballottement alternatively at two positions over the swollen area. Joint effusions are most easily detected over their extensor surfaces, where they are not covered by a flexor retinaculum, nerves, and blood vessels. The bony margins of the normal joint can usually be felt on the extensor surface. The inability to feel the joint margins is evidence of synovial swelling or joint effusion. Comparing the metacarpophalangeal (MCP) or metatarsophalangeal (MTP) joints in this way is a sensitive test for rheumatoid arthritis.

The presence of local warmth or erythema as signs of inflammation should be noted. The knee, ankle, and wrist joints should all be cooler than the skin over their adjoining long bones. This is gauged most effectively by placing the dorsum of the examiner's hand over the portion of the

Table 1–1. Overall objectives of the physical examination.

A. Define the anatomic distribution of the problem.
  • Is the process monoarticular?
  • Is it polyarticular? If so, is it symmetric or asymmetric?
  • Does it involve only one extremity?
  • Is it axial?
  • Is it complex?

B. Ascertain whether or not there are local signs of an inflammatory process.

C. Determine if anatomic disruption is present, ie, joint instability, tendon rupture, bone fracture, or deformity.

D. Distinguish between true muscle weakness as opposed to fatigue or disuse atrophy.

E. Establish if constitutional symptoms, such as fever or weight loss, implicate a systemic process, or other symptoms are present that direct attention to other organs.

limb adjacent to the joint in question and then placing the dorsum of the hand over the joint itself. A warmer temperature over these joints strongly suggests the presence of inflammation.

Pain on Motion

Almost all causes of joint pain, including rheumatoid arthritis, permit some relatively painless passive range of motion. Pain elicited by the slightest movement suggests a septic joint, gout, rheumatic fever, intra-articular hemorrhage, tumor, or joint fracture. Both passive and active range of motion should be tested. Pain caused by active but not passive motion often implicates an extra-articular source of the problem, such as a tenosynovitis. A good example of this is the assessment of shoulder pain in patients with polymyalgia rheumatica (PMR). PMR patients are often unable to raise their arms above their heads by themselves because of the intensity of the pain caused by active motion. Yet with passive motion, they are generally able to raise their arms completely over their heads and have substantially less pain compared to active motion while doing so.

Range of Motion

Measuring the range of motion in joints is useful for documenting the course of arthritis and the degree of disability. Several measurements systems are in use. A simple one is to use a positive sign before the measurement in degrees for flexion, abduction, internal rotation, or pronation, and a negative sign for the opposite motion, all measured from the "anatomic position." For example: Shoulder flexion −45 + 160, abduction −30 + 90. A prepared form or template saves time.

THE PHYSICAL EXAMINATION

Hands

Observe for full finger joint extension. The volar surfaces of the palms and fingers should make full contact when placed together. In making a fist, each fingertip should touch the MCP crease.

Synovial swelling of the proximal interphalangeal (PIP) and MCP joints can be detected readily by the presence of soft tissue swelling on either side of the dorsal aspects. The examiner supports the palm in individual fingers with both hands and palpates the joint margins using the thumbs of both hands or the thumb and index finger of one. When synovial fluid swelling is present, the joint margins will be less distinct compared to the same joint on the opposite hand. Inflammation of the distal interphalangeal (DIP) joints has a limited differential diagnosis that includes osteoarthritis (typically characterized by Heberden nodes), gout (with tophi often occurring at sites of Heberden nodes), and psoriatic arthritis. Septic arthritis, trauma, sarcoidosis, and syphilis are also in the differential diagnosis. Classic rheumatoid arthritis rarely involves the PIP joint alone. Psoriatic arthritis of the PIP joints commonly stimulates the juxta-articular periosteum, giving them a fusiform, erythematous appearance called a sausage digit. Pain caused by lateral compression of the MCP joints as a group is a good screening test for small joint polyarthritis.

Secondary contracture of the intrinsic muscles of the hand in patient with rheumatoid arthritis leads to the swan-neck deformity characterized by fixed hyperextension of the PIP and flexion of the DIP joints. Ulnar deviation and inability to extend the MCP joints of the fingers are the result of the rheumatoid disruption of the soft tissue tethers. These erosive changes permit the long extensor tendons to slip off the metacarpal heads. Inability to fully extend the PIP joints is a result of separation of the two slips of the long extensor tendon and their subluxation to either side of the joint. This leads to what is known as the boutonniere deformity. Extensive inflammation of finger joint capsules and ligaments in patients with systemic lupus erythematosus can result in joint laxity and diverse deformities in the absence of bone erosion.

Bony enlargements of the DIP joints (Heberden nodes) are a feature of hereditary osteoarthrosis and are often accompanied by similar changes in the PIP joints (Bouchard nodes). That process commonly affects the thumb carpometacarpal joint also, producing a squared appearance to the base of the joint and inability to extend it fully. The MCP joints are rarely affected by osteoarthritis but a similar appearance of the second and third MCP joints may be seen in patients with hemochromatosis. Careful palpation of the palm near the distal palmar crease also permits the identification of a major local source of patients' discomfort: trigger finger. The localized swellings of tendons that restrict finger motion within the tendon sheath can be felt by palpating the tendon at the distal palmar crease as the finger is flexed or extended. The patient is generally able to identify the most tender area, often precisely the site for a highly effective glucocorticoid injection.

Wrists

Arthritis of the wrists is usually caused by an inflammatory process. The exceptions are wrist pain related to carpal subluxation or fracture that can be reliably detected only by radiography. Synovitis of either the true radiocarpal or intercarpal joints is common among patients with rheumatic disorders. The absence of pain at the wrist on pronation or supination of the forearm suggests that the process is restricted to the carpus. When swelling is prominent on the dorsal or volar aspects of the joint, tenosynovitis of the extensor or flexor tendons respectively should be suspected. This can be confirmed by observing the axial movement of the swelling when the fingers are moved. Swelling and tenderness over the ulnar styloid is common in rheumatoid arthritis and may be followed by dorsal subluxation of the ulnar head.

Pain and tenderness at the radial styloid is often caused by irritation of the extensor pollicis longus tendon where it crosses the radial head. This disorder, known as de Quervain tenosynovitis, is caused by repeated lifting with the palm oriented vertically. The diagnosis of de Quervain tenosynovitis can be confirmed by Finkelstein test. de Quervain tenosynovitis is discussed further in Chapter 4.

Elbow

The causes of inflammation of the elbow joint include rheumatoid arthritis, seronegative arthritides, septic arthritis, and gout. Swelling and effusions in the joints present at the radial head on the lateral aspect of the radiohumeral joint. Pronation and supination of the forearm is often painful and restricted. Synovial swelling in the olecranon fossa prevents full extension of the joint by limiting entry of the olecranon process. Acute inflammation of the olecranon bursa over the tip of the elbow is usually caused by gout or infection, but more chronic benign swelling can also be caused merely by direct trauma. The extensor surface of the ulna just below the olecranon is a common site for a rheumatoid nodule.

Epicondylitis is an enthesopathy of the common wrist flexor origin at the medial epicondyle (golfer's elbow) or that of the extensors at the lateral epicondyles (tennis elbow). Tenderness is present over or immediately below the epicondyle and pain is elicited by resisted wrist flexion or extension, respectively. Tenderness to palpation over the medial part of the elbow is also the most commonly identified tender point in patients with fibromyalgia.

Shoulder

The motion of the shoulder is the most complex of any joint. Consequently, it is often difficult to determine the exact cause of shoulder pain. With most activities, the glenohumeral joint moves in several planes simultaneously. Scapulothoracic translocation can increase its apparent range misleadingly. The joint should be examined while scapular motion is observed or restricted by placing a hand over the shoulder on the trapezius ridge. The range of motion of the glenohumeral joint precludes ligamentous stabilization, which is replaced by dynamic control provided by the concerted action of the four rotator cuff muscles. Painful contractions of the shoulder tend to induce rotator cuff muscle dyssynergia, which is itself painful and can obscure the primary cause of the problem. Passive or active motions that minimize rotator cuff function include rotation of the humerus while the arm is hanging vertically oriented for flexion and extension in the sagittal plane. If those movements produce pain, true glenohumeral joint disease is present.

Shoulder joint pain is felt in the area of the deltoid muscle. Pain proximal to the olecranon is more often of cervical or thoracic apex origin. The capsule of the glenohumeral joint extends medially to the coracoid process. Tenderness at that site is the only place where it can be confidently assigned to the glenohumeral joint because the rest of the area is covered by the rotator cuff apparatus. Swelling of the glenohumeral joint is best appreciated at the anterior margin of the deltoid muscle just below the acromion, where an effusion, if present, can be balloted.

The shoulder drop sign is a good test for rotator cuff pathology. The shoulder should be passively flexed in the sagittal plane to 90 degrees, preferably with the elbow also flexed to reduce leverage. The humerus is supported while being rotated to the coronal plane and the forearm is extended and pronated. Support of the arm is then gently withdrawn while the patient is instructed to maintain the arm in this abducted position. The onset of pain and dropping of the arm is a positive sign. Tenderness over the lateral tip of the shoulder just below the acromion is often attributed to subacromial bursitis but in fact this is almost always due to pathology in the supraspinatous tendon. Inflammation of the long head of the biceps tendon at the groove where it crosses the humerus may cause widespread shoulder pain. In addition to tenderness immediately over the bicipital groove, the diagnosis can be confirmed by Yergason sign. The patient should sit with the elbow flexed and the forearm pronated, resting on the thigh. The examiner grasps the wrist and asks the patient to supinate the forearm against resistance, which will cause pain in the bicipital groove.

Restricted and painful active or passive motion of the shoulder in all directions is diagnostic of a frozen shoulder caused by generalized capsular inflammation and constriction. This is frequently idiopathic but may also result from traumatic injury. The patient may be able to move the arm only by scapulothoracic motion. Inflammation of the acromioclavicular or sternoclavicular joints can occur in rheumatoid arthritis or septic arthritis, the latter being especially common in injection drug users. Tenderness and swelling is easily appreciated at the site. Shrugging of the shoulder while lying on the affected side is painful.

Hip

Gait analysis can help define the nature of hip disease. Dwell time on the affected hip is limited compared to its opposite. Forward lurching as the leg is extended with each step indicates either fixed hip flexion or pain caused by tensing a swollen or inflamed hip capsule. Movement of the upper trunk over the weight-bearing hip suggests either adductor (gluteus maximus) weakness or its inhibition. Joint loading, by increasing intra-articular pressure, aggravates many different causes of hip pain. A positive Trendelenburg sign will be detected. This sign is demonstrated by having the examiner place his or her hands on both iliac crests and asking the patient to raise one leg or the other. Weight bearing on the painful side cause the opposite iliac crest to drop.

Restricted hip motion can be masked by compensatory movement of the pelvis. Children with very mobile lumbar spines, for example, can nearly completely conceal a fused hip. In order to restrict pelvic motion during examination, the patient should hold the opposite hip fully flexed. Any pelvic motion will be revealed by movement of the flexed knee. Loss of motion caused by hip disease first restricts full extension followed by inversion, eversion, and then abduction. Inability to keep the extended leg on the table while fully flexing the opposite indicates some loss of full extension as a result of either hip disease or a periarticular problem, such as iliopsoas tendinitis. Passive log rolling of the extended leg while the patient is supine can detect early guarding and restricted motion. Performing the FABER maneuver (flexion, abduction, and external rotation) is a test for painful—as well as limited—motion. Because the hip joint is supplied by the femoral nerve, pain emanating from the true hip joint is perceived in the groin, anteromedial thigh, and often in the knee. In some cases, hip pain is felt only in the knee. Pain in the buttock is more often caused by a sciatic nerve problem.

Groin or anterior thigh pain when the hip is actively flexed against resistance or passively extended may be caused by iliopsoas tendinitis or bursitis. Local tenderness is usually present. Iliopsoas lesions must be distinguished from femoral hernias and enthesopathy of the thigh adductors. In the latter case, the tenderness is located at the pubic tubercle more medially. Pain located in the buttock, on passive internal rotation and adduction of the hip (as an initiating a golf swing) is symptomatic of piriformis tendinitis or bursitis. When felt deep inside the pelvis it may be a symptom of obturator bursitis, which can be confirmed by palpating the margin of the lesser sciatic foramen per rectum.

Apparent and true leg length discrepancy may reflect either fixed hip abduction, abduction, or lumbar spine scoliosis. It can be distinguished from true leg shortening by measuring each side from the anterior/superior iliac spine to the medial tibial plateau or medial malleolus. True leg length shortening occurs in superior subluxation of the hip or severe destructive disease of the joint.

Pain over the greater trochanter points to trochanteric bursitis or, equally commonly, gluteus enthesopathy (usually of the gluteus medius) or a tear of the gluteus muscle. Because the gluteus tendons insert into the trochanter, it can be difficult to differentiate these problems by palpation. Pain felt while rolling over in bed is most likely due to bursitis. In contrast, trochanteric pain aggravated by prolonged standing or stair climbing typically indicates gluteus medius tendinitis.

Knee

The knee is the most commonly painful joint because it is subject to almost all causes of articular pathology. The alignment of the knee should be observed while the patient is standing. Varus or valgus malalignment may be congenital or acquired. Erosion of articular cartilage from either the medial or lateral tibiofemoral compartment is a common cause. Valgus alignment results in abnormal compression of the lateral opposing surfaces of the patellofemoral articulation. In individuals who are symptomatic, manual displacement of the patella on an extended knee produces discomfort. This is known as the **apprehension sign**. The lateral angle at the extended knee, the acute angle, is measured along the axis of the femur and through the midpoint of the patella to the tibial tubercle. The valgus angles in young women of less than 20 degrees can be ignored and corrects as the skeleton matures. Activities that involve excessive weight bearing on partially flexed knees cause chondromalacia of the undersurface of the patella. This condition is associated with a feeling of crepitus when the hand is placed over the patella as the knees are extended against gravity. When severe, it can be a cause of the pain. Crepitus can also indicate the presence of loose bodies within the joint.

Most knee disorders are accompanied by a synovial effusion that is best detected by eliciting the bulge sign. The knee must be as fully extended as possible. The effusion is demonstrated by first directing the fluid entered into the suprapatellar synovial recess by stroking upward over the medial patellofemoral articulation. Fingers are then immediately drawn downward from above the lateral patellofemoral groove while carefully observing the hollow between the patella and a medial condyle for a bulge. Chronic and relatively painless effusions may also protrude posteriorly into the popliteal space to produce a Baker cyst. Although such cysts can be sizable and track down beneath the gastrocnemius muscle, they are more often felt as a firm lump in the popliteal space. The knee must be fully extended since even slight flexion increases the capacity of the joint and a small effusion will diminish. Chronic synovial swelling, as in patients with rheumatoid arthritis, will produce a collar-like thickening immediately above the patella where the suprapatellar recess creates a double layer of the joint lining. It is frequently tender to palpation.

Because the tibial plateau is almost flat, translocation of the femoral condyles (rolling across the examination table) during flexion and extension is prevented by the menisci, which form a shallow cup, and the cruciate ligaments. A tendency within knee to give way while bearing weight or to lock suggests the presence of damage to the structures or a loose soft tissue fragment in the joint. Displaced menisci may be palpated along the margin of the tibial plateau but can be more reliably detected by the McMurray test. The McMurray test is performed by flexing the knee as far as possible, grasping the foot holding the thigh with the other hand and either internally or externally rotating the tibia while exerting either a varus or valgus strain. During knee extension, a torn meniscal fragment may become caught in the joint, producing pain and arrested motion.

Classically, the torn meniscus is opposite to the direction of tibial rotation, although that is not invariable. An injured infrapatellar synovial fold (plica), which is attached to the intracondylar notch, can result in symptoms that are similar to those of a torn meniscus, especially in young athletes.

Traumatic elongation or rupture of the cruciate ligaments allows abnormal anteroposterior translocation of the femoral condyles onto the tibial plateau. The anterior cruciate ligament limits posterior condylar translocation (ie, it prevents the tibia from sliding anteriorly) and the posterior cruciate ligament limits anterior displacement of the femur. The drawer test demonstrates increased anteroposterior instability of the joint by attempting to move the proximal tibia back and forth over the femoral condyles. Because the anterior cruciate ligament is normally relaxed by flexion of the knee, any abnormal laxity of that structure should be tested within knee and no more than 20–30 degrees of flexion. When the posterior cruciate ligament has been damaged, hamstring spasm may draw the tibia posteriorly. This must be minimized by flexing the knee to 90 degrees when testing for the integrity of the posterior cruciate ligament.

Pain caused by medial or collateral ligament injury or insufficiency is listed by supporting the knee in a fully extended position and abruptly applying a valgus or varus strain to the tibia. Some slight laxity is usually observed, especially in young or loose-jointed individuals. Comparison of the two sides is necessary.

There are several bursae around the knee. Inflammation in these bursae can cause pain upon weight bearing. The prepatellar bursa can be injured by prolonged kneeling. Another bursa under the patellar tendon is subject to both direct pressure and excessive quadriceps tension. The anserine bursa, which is located below the medial tibial plateau between the tibia and the biceps femoris tendon, becomes painful and swollen in individuals who are overweight and have valgus knee alignment.

Ankle

Careful examination is required to distinguish between true talotibial and subtalar joint pathology as well as injury to the complex ligamentous support of those joints. In addition, the tendons to the foot may be injured where they turn sharply behind the malleolae. Examination by sequential active, passive, and resisted isometric maneuvers can usually distinguish between those possible sources of pain. Synovial swelling and effusions of the talotibial joint are appreciated best over the anterior joint line, on either side of the tibialis anterior tendon and over the synovial fold below the flexor retinaculum over the neck of the talus. Swelling in relation to the malleolae is usually present also but is difficult to distinguish from that caused by injury to a ligament or tendon in the area.

Pain and limitation of motion related to the subtalar joint is detected by grasping the heel and applying a varus or valgus strain while holding the tibia. A normal range of motion is variable. The ankle and foot should also be examined while the patient is standing in order to detect eversion of the hindfoot, manifested as valgus deviation of the calcaneus and Achilles tendon. This may reflect either deltoid ligament insufficiency or weakness of the tibialis posterior muscle. Pes planus is also best seen on standing.

Inflammation of the joints or tendon sheaths in the compartment below the medial malleolus can compress the posterior tibial nerve and cause chronic pain in the foot and ankle.

Foot

Pain around the heel has several possible causes. It is a common manifestation of reactive arthritis. Tenderness near the insertion of the Achilles tendon reflects either enthesopathy or inflammation of the bursa that lies immediately above the upper corner of the calcaneus and the tendon insertion. Plantar surface heel pain and tenderness is usually caused by so-called plantar fasciitis, which includes enthesopathy of the plantar ligament or the origin of the flexor digitorum brevis at its attachment to the calcaneus just anterior to the heel pad. The heel pad itself may become painful by prolonged standing on hard surface without adequate heel cushioning. Pain elicited by lateral compression of the heel distinguishes talalgia from plantar enthesopathy.

Inflammation of the intertarsal and tarsometatarsal joints is often difficult to localize. There is variable intraconnectivity of the synovial cavities in the midfoot, and this region may become diffusely swollen. In patients with rheumatoid arthritis or its seronegative variants, the MTP and PIP joints are affected as much as the hands, and they should be examined in the same way. Chronic inflammation that results from damage to the transverse metatarsal ligaments leads to cockup deformities of the toes and prolapse of the metatarsal heads. The metatarsal arch is flattened and the metatarsal heads can be felt as tender, pebble-like structures on the plantar service at the base of the toes. Transverse compression of the metatarsals is a good sign for arthritis of any of the MTP joints. This maneuver can also identify pain from a Morton neuroma in one of the intraosseous nerves.

Stiffness of the first MTP joint (hallux rigidus) or valgus toe deviation that may be associated with varus positioning of the metacarpal can cause chronic foot pain.

Spine

For the detection of scoliotic or kyphotic deformities, the patient should be observed standing, preferably barefoot. The range of normal lumbar lordosis is considerable but a curve of more than 30 degrees or none at all is usually abnormal. Have the patient bend forward as far as possible. A rotational deformity will be revealed by twisting of the thorax. The Schober index, a measure of a loss of flexibility of the lumbar spine, is useful in the longitudinal evaluation of patients with ankylosing spondylitis. The Schober index is measured by marking the lumbosacral junction (the first "valley" detected while probing up toward the midline over the sacrum), measuring up a distance of 10–15 cm, and making a second mark. The patient is then asked to flex forward as far as possible. The line should separate by a distance about 50% greater than that originally measured. The index is more useful for following disease progression than for initial diagnosis. Measuring the distance between the fingertips and the floor when fully flexed is also useful; however, it can be limited by reduced hip flexion.

Observe neck rotation, flexion, and extension. Patients with normal neck flexion and extension can touch the tip of the jaw to the sternum and to extend the neck to form a straight line from the surface of the sternum to the horizontal ramus of the mandible. The ability to bend the neck in the coronal plane (ie, tilt the head) is variable but is often the most painful motion with intravertebral disk disease or the presence of nerve root compression. Measuring the distance between the occiput and the wall while the patient is standing with his heels against it is a good way to document flexion deformity of the upper trunk and neck.

Lateral bending of the thoracolumbar spine is assessed with the patient standing. The spine should form a smooth curve from the lower lumbar to midthoracic levels. A straight segment indicates either an abnormality of that level or paraspinous muscle spasm. This can be an early manifestation of ankylosing spondylitis.

The spondyloarthropathies often affect the costovertebral joints, thus limiting chest expansion. Measuring chest expansion helps identify and follow those disorders. Inflammation of the sacroiliac joints is a common early manifestation of the spondyloarthropathies. It is often asymmetric in psoriatic or reactive arthritis. Local tenderness may be detected over the joints at the "dimples of Venus." A sensitive test for sacroiliac inflammation is the McConnell maneuver. This is performed by having the patient lie on the side of the less painful joint and grasp and hold the dependent leg fully flexed while the examiner supports and extends the other leg with one hand. The examiner restricts pelvic motion during leg extension by placing the other hand on the iliac crest. The McConnell maneuver, which causes a twisting strain through the joints, should be performed gently because it can be quite painful in the presence of sacroiliitis.

Joint Aspiration & Injection

2

David W. Wu, MD

Rajiv K. Dixit, MD

ESSENTIALS OF DIAGNOSIS

▶ The major components of synovial fluid analysis are assessing fluid clarity and color, determining the cell count, examining for crystals, and obtaining culture.

▶ Joint aspiration should be performed promptly whenever septic arthritis is suspected because synovial fluid cell count, Gram stain, and culture are necessary to establish or exclude joint space infection.

▶ Synovial fluid analysis can be diagnostic in cases of crystalline arthritis.

▶ The synovial fluid white cell count is the most reliable means of distinguishing noninflammatory (<2000 cells/mm³) from inflammatory (>2000 cells/mm³) forms of arthritis.

▶ Joint injections with corticosteroid are often the swiftest means of providing relief to patients with inflamed joints.

Joint aspiration (arthrocentesis) is a simple and important diagnostic and therapeutic procedure that can be performed in a rheumatologist's office. Analysis of synovial fluid obtained from arthrocentesis is an integral component for the diagnosis of many rheumatologic conditions. Joint injections are safe and effective in the treatment of a variety of rheumatologic conditions. A fundamental knowledge of musculoskeletal anatomy, coupled with experienced supervision, are important in improving outcomes and minimizing complications.

▶ Indications for Joint Aspiration

The most important indication for joint aspiration is removal of fluid from a swollen, inflamed joint for synovial fluid analysis. Joint aspiration should be performed promptly when septic arthritis is suspected, such as the presence of an unexplained, acute monoarticular arthritis. Synovial fluid cell count, Gram stain, and culture are necessary to establish or exclude joint space infection, while the presence of crystals can be diagnostic of a crystalline arthropathy.

Removal of fluid from a tense, inflamed joint provides significant therapeutic benefit, often with immediate pain relief that allows weight bearing and movement of the affected joint. Aspiration of fluid from an infected joint decreases intra-articular pressure, the number of activated inflammatory cells, and the concentration of destructive enzymes and cytokines that can damage articular and periarticular structures. Although septic joints can be aspirated daily to prevent reaccumulation of inflammatory synovial fluid, current practice has moved to arthroscopic lavage, debridement, and drain insertion rather than repeated arthrocentesis. Removal of blood from a hemarthrosis may be beneficial by reducing intra-articular pressure and preventing the development of adhesions. Furthermore, untreated recurrent hemarthrosis may lead to joint damage.

▶ Synovial Fluid Analysis

Synovial fluid is normally present in a small volume in each joint. For example, even in a large joint such as the knee, the amount of synovial fluid is estimated to be less than 5 mL. Synovial fluid is an ultrafiltrate of plasma supplemented with protein and proteoglycans produced by fibroblast-like synoviocytes. The fluid forms a thin interface between surfaces of articular cartilage allowing for friction-free movement. The major proteoglycan found in synovial fluid is the high-molecular-weight molecule hyaluronan which gives the fluid its characteristic viscosity while the glycoprotein lubricin imparts the lubricating capacity of synovial fluid. Excess synovial fluid can accumulate as a result of noninflammatory, inflammatory, and septic processes. The major components of synovial fluid analysis are assessing fluid clarity and color, determining the cell count, examining for crystals, and obtaining Gram stain and culture.

Determination of synovial fluid glucose and protein have little diagnostic value and should not be ordered. The viscosity of synovial fluid can be informally assessed by the "string test." Normal synovial fluid is highly viscous due to its hyaluronan content. When a drop is expressed from the end of the needle, normal synovial fluid forms a long string. Increasing levels of inflammation are associated with digestion of hyaluronan, decreased viscosity, and decreased "stringiness" of the fluid.

A. Clarity and Color

The first step of synovial fluid analysis is gross inspection of the fluid and visual determination of clarity and color. The major determinant of clarity and color is the cell count. Noninflammatory fluid, such as that associated with osteoarthritis, has a low cell count and is clear. Synovial fluid from inflammatory forms of arthritis, such as systemic lupus erythematosus or rheumatoid arthritis, has higher cell counts and is translucent and yellow. Fluid from highly inflammatory processes, such as septic joints or crystal-induced arthropathies, has very high cell counts and is opaque and white to yellow. Hemarthrosis, caused by bleeding into a joint, is characterized by opaque, red synovial fluid. Gross inspection of synovial fluid can also lead to the detection of rice bodies. These tissue particles can consist of fibrin and a collagen core and are associated with rheumatoid arthritis, lupus, and septic arthritis. Milk of urate can also be detected grossly. This milky white or chalky synovial fluid is associated with massive quantities of urate crystals, occurring in the setting of acute gout.

B. Cell Count

Analysis of synovial fluid white cell count can provide important diagnostic information regarding the potential cause of the underlying inflammatory arthritis (see section "Classes of Synovial Fluid"). Normal synovial fluid has less than 200 white cells/mm^3, most of which are mononuclear. In pathologic effusions, the synovial fluid leukocyte count is generally less than 2000 white cells/mm^3 in noninflammatory forms of arthritis and greater than 2000 white cells/mm^3 in inflammatory arthritis. White cell counts greater than 50,000 white cells/mm^3 (mostly polymorphonuclear), in the absence of a crystalline arthropathy (particularly gout and pseudogout) should prompt the clinician to search for and empirically treat a diagnosis of septic arthritis until infection has been excluded. In general, inflammatory arthritis is associated with a polymorphonuclear leukocyte predominance, though synovial fluid of patients with viral arthritis, lupus, and other connective tissue disease can be associated with monocyte and lymphocyte predominance.

C. Crystals

Crystal analysis is performed on a wet mount of the synovial fluid. This can be prepared by placing a single drop of fluid on a clear glass slide and then covering it with a cover slip. Crystal analysis is best performed under polarized light. Using the first-order red compensator, birefringent material in the specimen appears as yellow or blue. Crystals that are yellow when oriented parallel, and blue when perpendicular, to the slow axis of vibration of the red compensator are negatively birefringent by convention. Conversely, crystals that are blue when oriented parallel, and yellow when perpendicular, to the slow axis of vibration of the red compensator are positively birefringent. The strength of birefringence, color, and shape of the crystals are helpful distinguishing characteristics (Table 2–1).

Monosodium urate (MSU) crystals are needle-shaped and strongly negatively birefringent. They are often found intracellular as a result of synovial fluid leukocyte phagocytosis. They are the easiest to identify with a polarized light microscope because of their strong birefringence and the typically high crystal load during an acute gout attack. The sensitivity of an examination for urate crystals in acute gout is greater than 90%.

Calcium pyrophosphate dihydrate (CPPD) crystals are rhomboid-shaped and positively birefringent. CPPD crystals are weakly birefringent and thus dim and difficult to detect even with a polarized light microscope. Concordance between labs in identification of CPPD crystals is lower than with identification of MSU crystals.

Hydroxyapatite or basic calcium phosphate (BCP) crystals are associated with osteoarthritis and are present within the joint and in periarticular locations. These crystals are also associated with "Milwaukee shoulder," a destructive syndrome characterized by large but noninflammatory effusions, pain, and loss of function. Hydroxyapatite crystals are not birefringent and form amorphous clumps that stain red with alizarin red S. They may appear as refractile "shiny coins" on light microscopy.

Calcium oxalate crystals can be seen in patients with primary oxalosis or in renal failure. These crystals are rod or tetrahedron-shaped and either positively birefringent or have indeterminate birefringence.

Synovial fluid lipid abnormalities can be seen in various states. Cholesterol crystals are large, flat plates with notched corners and are strongly birefringent. These crystals are associated with chronic inflammation such as uncontrolled rheumatoid arthritis, chronic gout and CPPD, and chronic infection. The chronic inflammation seen in these conditions is associated with cell breakdown with accumulation of membrane cholesterol. Lipids that enter the synovial fluid in inflammatory joint disease, hemarthrosis, and trauma to subsynovial fat can form spherules with birefringence in the shape of a Maltese cross. The arms of the cross that parallel the slow axis of vibration of the red compensator are blue and thus, these spherules are positively birefringent. Clinical associations of lipid spherules include trauma and pancreatitis. The presence of gross or microscopic lipid droplets is usually associated with significant intra-articular injury such as fracture. As is the case with lipid spherules, lipid droplets have also been described in association with hemorrhagic effusions and nontraumatic inflammatory effusion.

Table 2–1. Crystalline arthropathies.

	Shape	Birefringence	Misc.	Clinical Associations	
Monosodium urate	Needle	Strong, negative		Gout	
CPPD	Rhomboid	Weak, positive		Pseudogout	
BCP	Refractile "shiny coins" on light microscopy	No	Stain red w/ alizarin red S	OA, Milwaukee shoulder	
Calcium oxalate	Rod or tetrahedron	Positive or indeterminate	Stain red w/ alizarin red S	Oxalosis, renal failure	
Cholesterol	Large, flat plates with notched corners	Strong, no axis		Chronic inflammation (eg, RA, chronic gout, chronic infection)	
Lipid spherules	Maltese cross	Positive		Inflammatory joint disease, hemarthrosis, trauma, pancreatitis	
Lipid droplets	Refractile globules	No	Stain w/Sudan dye	Fracture	
Glucocorticoids		Yes, positive or negative		Prior joint injection with glucocorticoids	

BCP, basic calcium phosphate; CPPD, calcium pyrophosphate dihydrate; OA, osteoarthritis; RA, rheumatoid arthritis.

Glucocorticoids from previous joint injections, talc from gloves, and debris can form birefringent crystals which mimic crystalline arthritis.

The presence of intracellular crystals in synovial fluid inflammatory cells is diagnostic of a crystal-induced arthropathy. However, this diagnosis does not rule out infection, so it is always wise to culture the fluid from an acute monoarticular arthritis even when crystals are identified. In addition, a patient may have more than one crystal-induced arthropathy.

D. Culture and Gram Stain

Gram stain and culture should be performed on synovial fluid from any patient in whom infection is suspected. While a wide range of pathogens can cause septic arthritis, the most common bacteria implicated in septic arthritis are the gram-positive cocci, *Staphylococcus aureus*, *Streptococcus pyogenes*, and *Streptococcus pneumoniae*. Other bacteria associated with septic arthritis include the gram-negative coccus, *Neisseria gonorrhoeae*, and the gram-negative bacilli, *Pseudomonas aeruginosa* and *Escherichia coli*. The sensitivity of synovial fluid cultures for nongonococcal septic arthritis is approximately 90%. Gram stain of synovial fluid has lower sensitivity, ranging from 50% to 75%, but high specificity. Microbiologic analysis is usually performed on fluid collected in a sterile tube. However, if the aspiration is difficult, material within the needle may be expressed onto a sterile swab and sent for culture and sensitivity studies. Synovial fluid cultures are usually negative in the early phases of gonococcal arthritis. About half the patients with purulent gonococcal arthritis have a positive synovial fluid culture. Nucleic acid amplification testing is more sensitive than synovial fluid culture in patients with gonococcal arthritis. In cases of mycobacterial infection, cultures may require several weeks of incubation to isolate the causative agent. PCR is highly sensitive and specific for the detection of microorganisms, including mycobacteria in synovial fluid and tissue, and allows for earlier identification of mycobacteria. Due to the rapid joint destruction, morbidity, and mortality associated with septic arthritis, a rapid and specific diagnosis is crucial, and empiric antibiotics should be initiated in the appropriate clinical setting until a diagnosis of septic arthritis is confirmed or ruled out (see Chapter 42, Septic Arthritis).

E. Classes of Synovial Fluid

Four classes of synovial fluid have been defined and can serve as a guide to differential diagnosis (Table 2–2). It is important to recognize, however, that synovial fluid associated with a particular diagnosis is not always confined to one of these classes.

Class I (noninflammatory) synovial fluid is defined by a synovial fluid white cell count of less than 2000/mm^3. Class I fluid is transparent with a color ranging from clear to yellow. Osteoarthritis is the most common cause of class I synovial fluid. Other causes include posttrauma, chondromalacia patella, osteonecrosis, hypothyroidism (often with especially viscous fluid), Charcot arthropathy, amyloidosis, and sarcoidosis (which also can cause inflammatory synovial fluid).

Class II (inflammatory) synovial fluid has white cell counts from 2000/mm^3 to 50,000/mm^3. Polymorphonuclear leukocytes predominate. The appearance of class II synovial fluid ranges from translucent to opaque and is yellow or white; it is characteristic of noninfected, inflammatory forms of arthritis. In systemic lupus erythematosus, white cell counts are usually between 2000/mm^3 and 30,000/mm^3. The cell counts in rheumatoid arthritis and the spondyloarthropathies are typically 5000–50,000/mm^3; however, the pseudoseptic presentations of these disorders can generate higher counts (but rarely >100,000/mm^3). In crystal-induced arthropathies, cell counts of 30,000–50,000/mm^3 are typical, but greater than 100,000/mm^3 are sometimes observed. Less common causes of class II fluid include systemic rheumatic diseases such as dermatomyositis and mixed connective tissue disease, Still disease, relapsing polychondritis, postinfectious arthritis, and the systemic vasculitides.

Class III (septic) synovial fluid has white cell counts greater than 50,000/mm^3, often greater than 100,000/mm^3, with a polymorphonuclear leukocyte predominance, and the

Table 2–2. Classes of synovial fluid.

Characteristic	Normal	I Noninflammatory	II Inflammatory	III Septic	IV Hemorrhagic
WBC count	<200/mm^3	<2000/mm^3	2000–50,000/mm^3	>50,000/mm^3	Variable
PMN leukocyte percentage	<25	<25	>50	>75	50–75
Clarity	Transparent	Transparent	Transparent to opaque	Opaque	Bloody
Color	Clear to yellow	Clear to yellow	Yellow or white	Yellow or white	Red
Clinical associations (examples)		Osteoarthritis Trauma Osteonecrosis	RA SLE Crystalline	Septic arthritis	Trauma TB Coagulopathy Neoplasia PVNS

PMN, polymorphonuclear; PVNS, pigmented villonodular synovitis; RA, rheumatoid arthritis; SLE, systemic lupus erythematosus; TB, tuberculosis; WBC, white blood cell.

appearance is opaque and yellow (sometimes white). Class III synovial fluid is typical of septic arthritis caused by infection with *S. aureus*, streptococci, and gram-negative organisms. Although these infections classically cause very inflammatory fluid (>100,000 white cells/mm^3), synovial fluid cell counts can be considerably lower early in the course of infection, in partially treated infection, or in cases of overwhelming sepsis. Counts less than 50,000 white cells/mm^3 are common in gonococcal arthritis and in chronic infections, such as those caused by mycobacteria or fungi.

Class IV (hemorrhagic) fluid is red and opaque. In contrast to blood return due to a traumatic aspiration, class IV fluid is "defibrinated" and does not clot ex vivo. Class IV synovial fluid is typically seen in trauma, tuberculosis, pigmented villonodular synovitis, neoplasia, coagulopathies, and Charcot arthropathy.

▶ Therapeutic Aspiration and Injection

A. Equipment

The specific procedure and size of the joint determine the size of the syringe needed for aspiration. Syringes 3 mL and smaller are usually adequate for injecting lidocaine and corticosteroids into a peripheral target. Three- to 10-mL syringes are preferred for aspiration of small joints, and 10- to 20-mL syringes are best for intermediate and large joints, such as the elbow, ankle, glenohumeral joint, or knee. For aspiration of large synovial fluid effusions in large joints, a 60-mL syringe may be more appropriate. For facilitation of aspiration, when using a large syringe, it is important to break the vacuum in the syringe before introducing it into the joint. To aspirate more than 100 mL from an arthritic joint, several large syringes or a stopcock on the end of a syringe may be used. If using several syringes, or if an aspiration is to be followed by an injection, a Kelly clamp can stabilize the needle (which should be left in place) while the syringes are changed.

The size of the needle depends on the procedure. Needles as small as 25 or 30 gauge are most appropriate for injecting lidocaine into articular or periarticular structures before aspiration or for injecting glucocorticoids into small joints. A 25-gauge needle can also be used to aspirate synovial fluid or periarticular interstitial fluid from small, acutely inflamed joints, such as the first metatarsophalangeal joint in acute gout. A 1.5-inch, 22-gauge needle is useful for injecting large joints, such as the knee, or deep structures, such as the trochanteric bursa. These 22-gauge needles can also be used to aspirate small joints, but 19- or 20-gauge needles are indicated for the aspiration of large joints, joints with large amounts of synovial fluid, or joints or cysts with inspissated synovial fluid.

Other equipment needed includes povidone-iodine swabsticks, alcohol swabs, adhesive bandages ("Band-Aids"), and nonsterile gloves.

B. Medications

Some clinicians use a 10- to 15-second stream of ethyl chloride to numb the skin before a joint injection, while others choose not to use local anesthesia and rely on a quick, sure puncture using the smallest possible needle. Lidocaine (1–2%, without epinephrine) is a safe and effective local anesthetic that can be injected into the capsule and periarticular structures after raising a subcutaneous wheal and before aspiration is attempted, as aspiration without benefit of anesthesia can be quite painful. For therapeutic injections, lidocaine is generally drawn with the corticosteroid to be given to reduce postinjection flares, especially with extra-articular injections. The lidocaine also provides a degree of immediate relief of symptoms. This can help identify the accurate placement of the injection and can also impart diagnostic information. When injecting a small joint, there is a volume restriction and as such, the lidocaine may be omitted from the corticosteroid injection. Single-dose vials of lidocaine, although more costly, are less likely to be contaminated.

A number of locally injected pharmacologic agents have been used in the treatment of rheumatic disorders. Local corticosteroids in conjunction with lidocaine are valuable in the treatment of the rheumatic diseases. Joints, tenosynovium, bursae, and even the epidural space can be injected with a reasonable expectation of benefit. Although most target tissues can be injected without radiographic guidance, hip and epidural space injections are performed under radiographic guidance. Local injections are an efficient way to administer high concentrations of corticosteroids directly into target tissues, maximizing the desired anti-inflammatory effects of the medication, and minimizing the many unpleasant side effects associated with systemic corticosteroids. Patients should be aware that injection of local corticosteroids, although frequently helpful, generally only offers temporary symptomatic relief. The long-term efficacy of the procedure depends in large part on the nature of the underlying problem.

Several preparations of corticosteroids are commercially available and differ in their characteristics. Long-acting crystalline suspensions of injectable corticosteroids have been used for decades and remain the mainstay. These less soluble compounds are more potent and longer acting and thus may be more effective in the treatment of chronic inflammatory processes. However, they are more likely to lead to subcutaneous fat atrophy and cutaneous pigment change when injected into superficial structures such as the lateral epicondyle in the treatment of lateral epicondylitis. The most commonly used crystalline corticosteroids in adults are triamcinolone (acetonide and hexacetonide) and methylprednisolone. Dexamethasone and hydrocortisone are more soluble and shorter acting and may be less effective. These however, may be less likely to cause subcutaneous atrophy and pigment changes. In the 2019 American College of Rheumatology/Arthritis Foundation Guideline for the Treatment of Juvenile Idiopathic Arthritis, triamcinolone hexacetonide was strongly recommended over triamcinolone acetonide for intra-articular injections. The recommendation was based on observations of more complete and longer duration of clinical response without increased adverse effects in children.

Corticosteroid injections should be administered judiciously. Repeated injections may lead to laxity of the periarticular supporting structures and soft-tissue atrophy. No solid data provide guidance on which to base definitive recommendations. However, in most instances, a single joint or soft-tissue target probably should not be injected more than three times a year.

C. General Considerations, Contraindications, and Potential Complications

By achieving a local anti-inflammatory effect, corticosteroid injections can help treat persistent synovitis and recurrent effusions in rheumatoid arthritis, seronegative spondyloarthropathy, gout, and other forms of inflammatory arthritis as well as osteoarthritis, bursitis, and tendinitis. They can be effective in cases where systemic treatments are not indicated, have failed, or as an adjunct to systemic treatment. Corticosteroid injections can help to decrease pain, stiffness, and inflammation, and improve range of motion and function. There are few contraindications to joint and soft-tissue injections. Joint injections should be avoided in cases of systemic infections, when cellulitis or ulcers exist on the same limb, and when psoriasis, eczema, or infection is present at the injection site. An INR of greater than 2.5 from warfarin or bleeding disorder is also a contraindication. Injection of prosthetic joints should be performed by an orthopedic surgeon. Side effects of steroid injections include local bleeding, postinjection flare, skin atrophy and pigment changes, fat atrophy, flushing and/or palpitations, and transient hyperglycemia. Septic arthritis is rare and the risk can be minimized by adhering to strict aseptic technique.

▶ Description of Procedures

The optimal approach to joint and soft-tissue injections of the upper and lower extremities are described and illustrated in the following pages in a systematic order from distal to proximal. Clinicians should perform joint aspiration and injections using safe and fundamentally sound technique to achieve accurate needle placement while minimizing the risk of complications. If a joint effusion is present, the effusion should be aspirated prior to injection. Aspiration should be performed slowly to avoid generating significant negative pressure that can draw synovial tissue into the opening of the needle and actually prevent adequate withdrawal of fluid. Difficulty in aspiration of synovial fluid may also be secondary to increased viscosity, presence of debris such as rice bodies, and loculation of fluid. Manipulation and redirection of needle placement is often helpful. Regardless, it is a good, safe practice to pull back the plunger before injecting a joint or soft tissue. The risk of tendon rupture can be minimized by avoiding

intratendinous injections by not injecting against resistance. Joint infection after aspiration or injection is extremely rare, but the possibility of complications must always be minimized. The injection or aspiration target is first carefully identified. It is then marked with a circular impression on the skin using the tip of a ballpoint pen or the proximal tip of a povidone-iodine swabstick. Povidone-iodine is then applied to the identified arthrocentesis site and allowed to dry. An alcohol swab is then used to wipe off the dried povidone-iodine to prevent skin irritation. The injection site may then be anesthetized with a spray of ethyl chloride. A lidocaine injection, as discussed earlier, is often used if a joint aspiration is to be carried out since this usually necessitates the use of a larger bore needle. The use of nonsterile gloves is recommended to protect the clinician from the patient's body fluids.

Technique, approach, and the corticosteroid preparation used may differ amongst clinicians. While these descriptions reflect the authors' own practices and preferences to some extent, these approaches have been selected and illustrated to serve as a general guide for the clinician to achieve a safe and effective procedure.

A. Upper Extremity Joint Injections

1. Proximal interphalangeal (PIP) joint injection (Figure 2–1)

Materials: 25-gauge needle or insulin syringe, 5–10 mg triamcinolone or methylprednisolone.

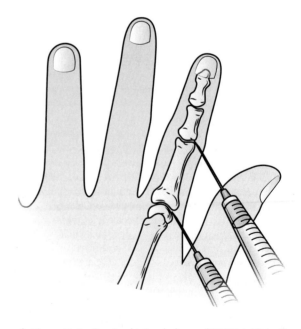

▲ **Figure 2–1.** Proximal interphalangeal (PIP) joint injection and metacarpophalnageal (MCP) joint injection.

Procedure:

1. With the digit slightly flexed, palpate and mark the PIP joint space medial or lateral to the extensor tendon at the dorsal aspect of the digit.

2. Insert the needle at an approximately 45-degree angle, passing the tip of the needle under the extensor tendon.

3. The goal of the injection is to place the needle tip within the joint capsule and not necessarily in the joint space between the bones.

2. Metacarpophalangeal (MCP) joint injection (Figures 2–1 and 2–2)

Materials: 25-gauge needle or insulin syringe, 10 mg triamcinolone or methylprednisolone.

Procedure:

1. With the digit slightly flexed, palpate and mark the MCP joint space medial or lateral to the extensor tendon at the dorsal aspect of the digit. For second MCP joint injections, a radial approach is preferred.

2. Insert the needle at an approximately 45-degree angle, passing the tip of the needle under the extensor tendon.

3. First carpometacarpal (CMC) joint injection (Figure 2–3)

Materials: 25-gauge needle, 10–20 mg triamcinolone or methylprednisolone.

Procedure:

1. Palpate and mark the first CMC joint proximal to the first metacarpal at the anatomical snuff box while flexing the thumb across the palm.

2. Insert the needle obliquely, avoiding the radial artery as it traverses the anatomical snuff box.

CMC (basal) Joint Arthritis

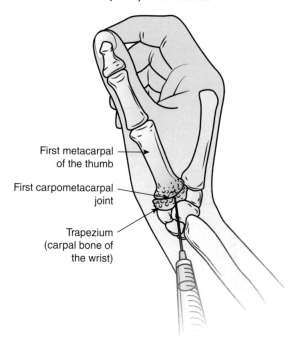

First metacarpal of the thumb

First carpometacarpal joint

Trapezium (carpal bone of the wrist)

▲ **Figure 2–3.** First carpometacarpal (CMC) joint injection.

4. Wrist joint injection (Figure 2–4)

Materials: 25-gauge needle, 20–30 mg triamcinolone or methylprednisolone. For aspiration, use a 21-gauge needle or larger gauge needle.

Procedure:

1. Palpate and mark the radiocarpal joint by flexing and extending the wrist. The joint space can be palpated

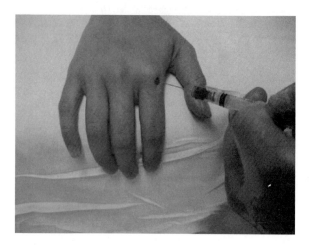

▲ **Figure 2–2.** Metacarpophalangeal (MCP) joint injection.

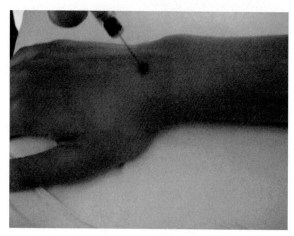

▲ **Figure 2–4.** Wrist joint injection.

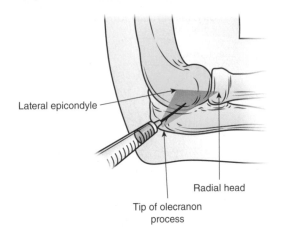

▲ **Figure 2–5.** Elbow joint injection.

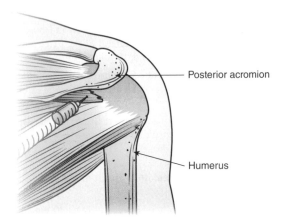

▲ **Figure 2–6.** Shoulder joint injection.

just distal to Lister tubercle (bony prominence at the dorsal aspect of the distal radius).

2. Insert the needle perpendicular to the skin at the joint line.

5. Elbow joint injection (Figure 2–5)

Materials: 23-gauge needle, 20–40 mg triamcinolone or methylprednisolone. For aspiration, use a 21-gauge or larger needle.

Procedure:

1. A lateral approach is recommended to avoid the ulnar nerve.

2. With the elbow flexed at 90 degrees, identify the lateral epicondyle, radial head, and the tip of the olecranon process. These landmarks form a triangle.

3. Mark the point of entry at the center of the triangle where a cleft is palpable.

4. Insert the needle perpendicular to the skin, aiming for the center of the joint.

6. Shoulder joint injection (Figure 2–6)

Materials: 21-gauge needle, 40 mg triamcinolone or methylprednisolone.

Procedure:

1. A posterior approach is recommended to avoid neurovascular structures.

2. With the patient seated, palpate and mark the point of entry 1 cm inferior and 1 cm medial to the posterior tip of the acromion.

3. Insert the needle in an anterior direction aiming for the coracoid process until bone is encountered at the joint space.

7. Acromioclavicular joint injection (Figure 2–7)

Materials: 25-gauge needle, 10 mg triamcinolone or methylprednisolone.

Procedure:

1. Palpate and mark the acromioclavicular joint.

2. Insert the needle perpendicular to the skin directing it inferiorly and posteriorly, aiming for the center of the joint space.

B. Upper Extremity Soft-Tissue Injections

1. Trigger finger injection (Figure 2–8)

Materials: 25-gauge needle or insulin syringe, 5–10 mg triamcinolone or methylprednisolone.

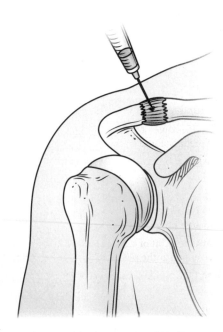

▲ **Figure 2–7.** Acromioclavicular joint injection.

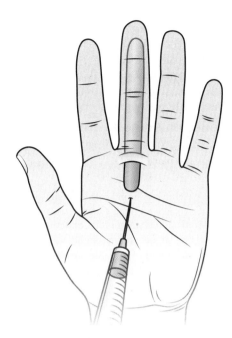

▲ **Figure 2–8.** Trigger finger injection.

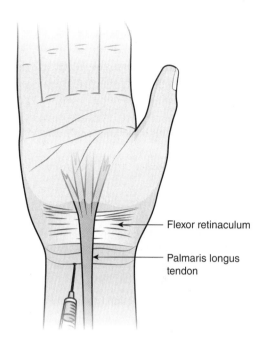

▲ **Figure 2–9.** Carpal tunnel injection.

Procedure:

1. The patient's palm should face upwards.

2. Mark the point of entry. For the index finger, just distal to the proximal palmar crease. For the long finger, in between the proximal and distal creases, for the ring and little fingers, just distal to the distal crease, for the thumb, just proximal to the digital crease and sesamoid bones of the thumb. The thickened tendon sheath is often palpable.

3. Insert the needle at a 30-degree distal inclination and inject the tendon heath.

2. Carpal tunnel injection (Figure 2–9)

Materials: 25-gauge needle, 20 mg triamcinolone or methylprednisolone.

Procedure:

1. The patient's palm should face upward.

2. Palpate the palmaris longus tendon by asking the patient to flex at the wrist while opposing the thumb and little finger.

3. Mark the point of entry just ulnar to the palmaris longus tendon at the proximal wrist crease.

4. Insert the needle at a 45-degree angle toward the index finger.

3. de Quervain tendonitis injection (Figure 2–10)

Materials: 25-gauge needle, 20 mg triamcinolone or methylprednisolone.

Procedure:

1. The patient's wrist should be in neutral position and turned on the side with radial side up.

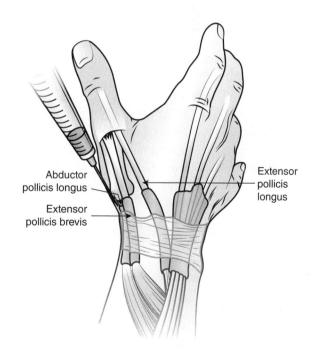

▲ **Figure 2–10.** de Quervain tendonitis injection.

2. Identify the abductor pollicis longus (APL) and extensor pollicis brevis (EPB) tendons by asking the patient to extend the thumb.

3. Mark the point of entry between the APL and the EPB tendons just distal to the radial styloid.

4. Insert the needle at a 45-degree angle aiming proximally toward the radial styloid.

4. Lateral epicondylitis injection (tennis elbow) (Figure 2–11)

Materials: 23-gauge needle, 20–30 mg triamcinolone or methylprednisolone.

Procedure:

1. The patient's elbow should be flexed to 90 degrees.

2. Identify and mark the most tender point at the junction of the common extensor tendon and lateral epicondyle.

3. Insert the needle until the periosteum is reached, withdraw slightly, then inject.

5. Medial epicondylitis injection (golfer's elbow)

Materials: 23-gauge needle, 20–30 mg triamcinolone or methylprednisolone.

Procedure:

1. Identify and mark the most tender point at the junction of the common flexor tendon and medial epicondyle.

2. Insert the needle until the periosteum is reached, withdraw slightly, then inject.

3. Avoid the posterior surface of the medial epicondyle to avoid the ulnar nerve.

6. Olecranon bursa injection

Materials: 23-gauge needle, 20 mg triamcinolone or methylprednisolone.

Procedure:

1. Aspirate the bursa prior to injection.

2. Approach from the lateral aspect of the bursa and aim for the center of the bursa.

3. Approach from the tip of the bursa may cause a chronic leak. Also avoid approach from the medial aspect of the bursa to avoid encountering the ulnar nerve.

7. Subacromial bursa injection (Figure 2–12)

Materials: 23-gauge needle, 20–40 mg triamcinolone or methylprednisolone.

Procedure:

1. This injection may be indicated not only for subacromial bursitis but also for impingement syndrome, rotator cuff tendonitis, adhesive capsulitis, and calcific tendonitis.

2. With the patient seated and the arm in internal rotation, palpate and mark the depression just inferior to the posterior and lateral aspect of the acromion.

3. Insert the needle aiming anteromedially toward the coracoid process.

C. Lower Extremity Joint Injections

1. Metatarsophalangeal (MTP) joint injection

Materials: 25-gauge needle or insulin syringe, 10–20 mg triamcinolone or methylprednisolone.

Procedure:

1. With the digit slightly flexed, palpate and mark the MTP joint space medial or lateral to the extensor tendon at the dorsal aspect of the digit. For first MTP injection, a medial approach is preferred.

2. Insert the needle at an approximately 45-degree angle, passing the tip of the needle under the extensor tendon.

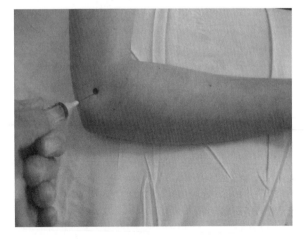

▲ **Figure 2–11.** Lateral epicondylitis injection (tennis elbow).

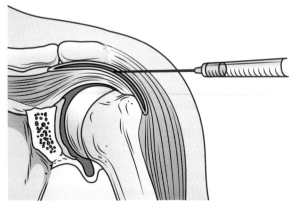

▲ **Figure 2–12.** Subacromial bursa injection.

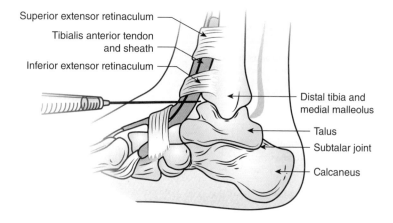

Superior extensor retinaculum
Tibialis anterior tendon and sheath
Inferior extensor retinaculum
Distal tibia and medial malleolus
Talus
Subtalar joint
Calcaneus

▲ **Figure 2–13.** Ankle joint injection, tibiotalar joint.

2. Ankle joint injection

a. Tibiotalar joint (Figure 2–13)

Materials: 23-gauge needle, 20–40 mg triamcinolone or methylprednisolone. For aspiration, use a 21-gauge or larger needle.

Procedure:

1. The patient should be in a supine position with the ankle slightly plantar flexed.

2. Identify the space between the anterior border of the medial malleolus and the medial border of the tibialis anterior tendon and palpate this space for the articulation of the talus and tibia.

3. Mark the site of injection medial to the tibialis anterior tendon. Insert the needle in a posterolateral direction.

4. Inserting the needle medial to the tibialis anterior tendon avoids the dorsalis pedis artery and deep peroneal nerve.

b. Subtalar joint (Figure 2–14)

Materials: 23-gauge needle, 20–30 mg triamcinolone or methylprednisolone.

Procedure:

1. The patient should be in a supine position with ankle in inversion.

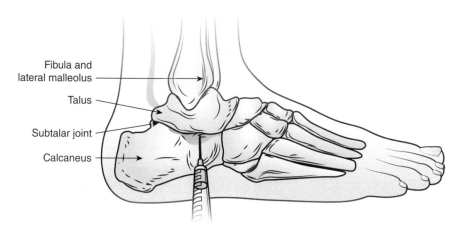

Fibula and lateral malleolus
Talus
Subtalar joint
Calcaneus

▲ **Figure 2–14.** Subtalar joint.

2. Identify the subtalar joint by palpating a cleft between the talus and calcaneus just anterior and inferior to the lateral malleolus while gently inverting and everting the foot.

3. Mark the site of injection just anterior and inferior to the lateral malleolus.

4. Insert the needle perpendicularly directing toward the medial malleolus.

3. Knee joint injection (Figure 2–15)

Materials: 21-gauge needle, 40–80 mg triamcinolone or methylprednisolone. For aspiration, use a 21-gauge or larger needle.

Procedure:

1. The patient should be in a supine position with the knee slightly flexed.

2. Palpate and mark the point of entry at the lateral or medial border of the patella just under the patella at the point where the proximal one-third meets the distal two-thirds.

3. Insert the needle under the patella directing in a slightly cephalad direction toward the suprapatellar pouch.

4. Hip joint injection—The hip joint should only be aspirated and injected under imaging guidance due to the depth of the joint and proximity of the neurovascular bundle.

D. Lower Extremity Soft-Tissue Injections

1. Morton's neuroma injection

Materials: 25-gauge needle, 10–20 mg triamcinolone or methylprednisolone.

Procedure:

1. Palpate and mark the point of entry halfway between the third and fourth MTP heads and ½ inch proximal to the web space on the dorsal side.

2. Insert the needle perpendicular to the skin.

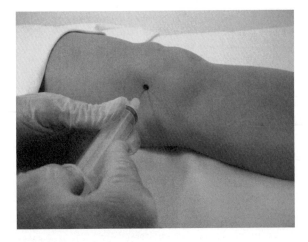

▲ **Figure 2–15.** Knee joint injection.

2. Plantar fascia injection

Materials: 23-gauge needle, 20–30 mg triamcinolone or methylprednisolone.

Procedure:

1. The patient should be in a lateral decubitus position on the affected leg.

2. Palpate and mark the point of maximal tenderness at the medial calcaneal tuberosity.

3. Using a medial approach, insert the needle perpendicular to the skin slightly distal to the medial calcaneal tuberosity and advance the needle to the bony surface.

4. Avoid re-injection to decrease risk of plantar fascia rupture and fat pad atrophy.

3. Retrocalcaneal bursa injection

Materials: 23-gauge needle, 20 mg triamcinolone or methylprednisolone.

Procedure:

1. Palpate and mark the point of entry just anterior to the Achilles tendon and just proximal to the calcaneus.

2. From the medial or lateral side, insert the needle perpendicular to the skin.

3. It is critical to avoid intratendinous Achilles injection by not injecting against resistance.

4. As such, if available, ultrasound-guided injection is preferred.

5. Avoid re-injection to decrease risk of Achilles tendon rupture.

4. Tibialis posterior tendon sheath injection

Materials: 25-gauge needle, 10–20 mg triamcinolone or methylprednisolone.

Procedure:

1. Identify the posterior tibial artery posterior to the medial malleolus. Mark the posterior tibial artery to avoid it.

2. Insert the needle at a 45-degree angle just posterior to the distal end of the medial malleolus. The first structure posterior to the medial malleolus is the tibialis posterior tendon.

3. If available, it is best to perform the injection under ultrasound guidance to avoid intratendinous injection that increases the risk of rupture and consequent loss of the longitudinal arch resulting in pes planus.

5. Tarsal tunnel injection

Materials: 25-gauge needle, 10–20 mg triamcinolone or methylprednisolone.

Procedure:

1. Indicated for tarsal tunnel syndrome secondary to entrapment of the posterior tibial nerve.

2. Identify the posterior tibial artery posterior to the medial malleolus. Mark the posterior tibial artery to avoid it.

3. Mark the point of entry posterior to the medial malleolus and anterior to the posterior tibial artery.

4. Insert the needle at a 45-degree angle.

6. Pes anserine bursa injection

Materials: 23-gauge needle, 20–40 mg triamcinolone or methylprednisolone.

1. The patient should be in a supine position.

2. Palpate and mark the pes anserine bursa located about 5 cm below the medial joint line of the knee and between the tibia and insertions of the sartorius, gracilis, and semi-tendinosis muscles.

3. Advance the needle and inject adjacent to the periosteum.

7. Trochanteric bursa injection (Figure 2–16)

Materials: 23-gauge needle, 40 mg triamcinolone or methylprednisolone.

1. The patient should lie on the side, with the affected leg facing upwards.

2. Palpate and mark the most tender point over the greater trochanter, the bony prominence at the proximal, lateral femur.

3. Insert the needle perpendicular to the skin until the bone of the greater trochanter is reached, withdraw slightly, and inject.

▶ Extended-Release Corticosteroid

Triamcinolone acetonide extended-release (ER) injectable suspension was recently approved by the Food and Drug Administration (FDA) as an extended-release corticosteroid to treat osteoarthritis knee pain. It consists of microspheres of poly(lactic-co-glycolic acid) (PLGA) containing triamcinolone acetonide. A pharmacokinetic study demonstrated prolonged intra-articular residence time for the ER formulation compared to standard triamcinolone while peak plasma concentrations were much lower with the ER formulation. Approval was based on a randomized, double-blind trial which demonstrated significant reduction in active daily pain intensity scores at week 12 compared to placebo, but not compared to the significantly less expensive standard crystalline suspension triamcinolone acetonide. A recent study demonstrated a smaller increase in serum glucose levels in diabetic patients following injection with triamcinolone acetonide ER compared to standard triamcinolone acetonide.

▶ Viscosupplementation

The viscoelasticity of synovial fluid is reduced in osteoarthritis in part related to a decrease in the molecular weight and concentration of hyaluronic acid. A number of hyaluronic acid preparations are commercially available for intra-articular knee injection and claim to increase the viscoelasticity of synovial fluid and provide symptomatic relief. There is, however, a lack of convincing evidence based on controlled trial data indicating a clinically meaningful benefit over intra-articular placebo of this expensive product. Its routine use is not recommended.

▶ Platelet-Rich Plasma

Platelet-rich plasma (PRP) is an autologous blood product produced by centrifugation of whole blood that yields a concentration of platelets above the baseline value. The mechanism of action of PRP is not well understood. It is thought to provide high concentrations of growth factors, including tissue growth factor and platelet-derived growth factors, that can mediate the proliferation of mesenchymal stem cells (MSCs) and increase matrix synthesis and collagen formation. It may also have anti-inflammatory properties.

PRP has predominantly been used to treat tendon-related pathologies (tennis elbow, patellar tendinopathy, Achilles tendinopathy, and rotator cuff tears) and osteoarthritis (mostly knees). At present, there is a lack of convincing evidence about the efficacy of PRP injections for symptomatic relief in patients with osteoarthritis or tendon-related pathologies. No trials have examined the structural effects of PRP in osteoarthritis joints.

▶ Stem Cell Therapy

An increasing number of orthopedic clinics in the United States are marketing intra-articular "stem cell" treatments for osteoarthritis. The term "mesenchymal stem cell" can

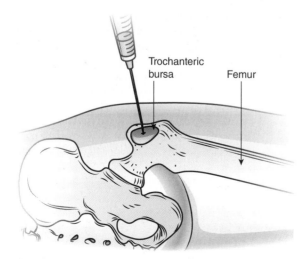

Trochanteric bursa

Femur

▲ **Figure 2–16.** Trochanteric bursa injection.

be misleading as it refers to a heterogeneous population of cells from diverse tissues with varying levels of multipotency. The biologic plausibility for their use is based on their self-renewable properties, multilineage differentiation potential, and immunomodulatory capacity. Many human tissues, including bone marrow, adipose tissue, umbilical cord blood, and synovium, are sources of MSCs. These cells, autologous or allogeneic, may be injected directly or with arthroscopic guidance, with or without culture expansion. Sometimes, concomitant treatment such as PRP injection or hyaluronic acid injection is used.

To date, there is very limited preliminary data on clinical outcomes and cartilage repair. At present, its use in clinical practice cannot be recommended.

▶ Ultrasound

By convention and as described in this chapter, joint and soft-tissue aspirations and injections are generally performed with a strong working knowledge of the anatomy and important landmarks and without imaging guidance. However, with the increased availability of musculoskeletal ultrasound, the use of ultrasound guidance for aspiration and injection has increased. Prior to the procedure, ultrasound can provide diagnostic information, such as the presence of inflammation, an effusion, and synovial hypertrophy. Furthermore, ultrasound allows real-time visualization of accurate needle placement and delivery of medication while avoiding anatomic structures such as nerves and vessels that can be identified on ultrasound. While several studies have demonstrated improved accuracy of needle placement when comparing ultrasound-guided injections to landmark-guided injections, the evidence demonstrating improved efficacy and safety of ultrasound-guided injections is limited.

In the indirect approach of ultrasound guidance, ultrasound is used to better define the anatomic region to be aspirated or injected and a mark is made to indicate the site of needle insertion. In the direct approach, the needle is introduced and aspiration or injection is performed under direct sonographic visualization. The direct approach allows for continuous monitoring of the procedure but requires more experience and hand-eye coordination. Other general factors that may limit the use of ultrasound include the time and cost of training, the cost of equipment, the added time required to utilize ultrasound, and cost to the patient. Ultrasound guidance is highly desirable in certain situations such as aspiration and injection of deep-seated joints such as the hip and sacroiliac joint or where there is a high risk of inadvertently damaging adjacent anatomic structures such as nerves and vessels. An ultrasound-guided procedure can also be helpful following either the unsuccessful aspiration of a distended joint (dry tap) or an ineffective conventional corticosteroid injection. In the majority of cases, however, it is reasonable to aspirate and inject without ultrasound guidance.

▶ Synovial Biopsy

Sometimes, joint pathology cannot be identified by synovial fluid analysis. Sampling of synovial tissue may then help to define the pathological process particularly in the evaluation of an undiagnosed monoarthritis. Biopsy material may be obtained percutaneously (with or without ultrasound guidance) or arthroscopically. Visual guidance of arthroscopic biopsy allows sampling of the most severely involved areas of pathology.

Diagnoses of indolent infections such as tuberculosis and nontubercular granulomatous infection or noninfectious forms of granulomatous arthritis such as sarcoidosis may require synovial biopsy. Although synovial fluid cytological studies can sometimes reveal the presence of malignant cells, neoplastic arthritis conditions are usually diagnosed by histologic analysis of synovial biopsy material. Pigmented villonodular synovitis should be considered in a chronic monoarthritis especially of the knee or hip. It has a characteristic MRI appearance related to hemosiderin deposition in the synovium in association with large cystic lesions in bone, but histopathologic confirmation is generally required. Finally, several rare infiltrative or metabolic disorders such as amyloidosis, ochronosis, hemochromatosis, and Wilson disease that can affect the joints have characteristic biopsy features.

Laboratory Testing

3

Mark H. Wener, MD

Laboratory tests for rheumatic disease are performed for various reasons: to diagnose, to clarify whether a condition is inflammatory or noninflammatory, to establish a prognosis, to monitor disease activity, to assess the extent or severity of organ involvement, to predict efficacy and toxicity of therapies, and to monitor treatment side effects. In addition, there may be administrative indications for laboratory testing, for example, to qualify for a specialty medication, to qualify a patient for a clinical trial, to determine if a patient satisfies classification criteria for a disease, and to include a patient in data registries and repositories. To support a clinical diagnostic impression, laboratory tests are most effective when used in conjunction with data from the history and physical examination. Laboratory tests for autoimmune rheumatic diseases nearly always lack sufficient sensitivity and specificity to establish diagnoses independently and therefore should be considered "probabilistic" rather than diagnostic tests. Table 3–1 summarizes laboratory and other tests commonly used to help clarify the diagnosis in typical presentations of patients with rheumatic diseases.

PROBALISTIC LABORATORY TESTING & STATISTICS

Because many rheumatologic conditions in which serologic tests play a prominent role in diagnosis are relatively rare in the general population, positive tests obtained from an unselected population are much more likely to be false-positive than true-positive results. Testing should not be ordered to screen a general population or in patients with low probability of having the disease being tested, since the **positive predictive value** (probability of having a disease after a positive test result) is strongly influenced by the pre-test probability that the tested individual has the disease under consideration. A variety of statistics are used to describe laboratory tests, as shown in Table 3–2. Tests with **positive likelihood ratios** (LR) over 10 (such as anticitrullinated peptide antibody tests for rheumatoid arthritis, with LR+ = 12.5) are considered excellent tests

for confirmation of a clinical diagnosis when the test result is positive. However, even the best tests available can be misleading in subjects who are not likely to have the disease being evaluated.

Most laboratory tests of rheumatic disease are reported in quantitative units. Statistics about sensitivity and specificity of a test are often provided at a single cutoff or threshold, the upper limit of the reference or normal range. Clinical reasoning and diagnostic considerations also take into account the degree of abnormality of a test result; a highly abnormal result is more likely to be clinically significant compared to one that is barely abnormal.

For many autoimmune laboratory tests, the same test may be abnormal in a number of different conditions. Figure 3–1 illustrates some important principles for the number of antinuclear antibody (ANA) tests in the diagnosis of systemic lupus erythematosus (SLE). The different colored curves (labeled black for normal individuals, dark blue for SLE patients, and light blue for a disease control population such as rheumatoid arthritis) show the relative proportions within each population with a positive ANA at a given titer (the x-axis). The distribution of ANA results in normal individuals is much lower than that in SLE patients. The SLE curve is shifted to the right; that is, it includes high ANA titers. Another disease population, however, lies in between the normal and SLE populations. As the graph depicts, an ANA with a titer of 1:640 has a high likelihood of being present in an SLE population, is rare in the normal population, and can occur in other disorders. The ratio of the heights of the curves at any given ANA titer (x-axis) illustrates the positive likelihood ratio for ANA titers at that point. Whereas an ANA of titer 1:40 does not help distinguish between diagnostic possibilities, an ANA of titer 1:640 has a high positive likelihood of being associated with SLE or another rheumatologic condition.

Figure 3–1 also demonstrates some of the challenges with calculating the specificity of a laboratory test, since the specificity depends on the comparison/reference population. A test with a specificity of 95% with respect to a healthy

Table 3–1. Laboratory tests frequently ordered for typical clinical presentations.

Presentation	Priority Lab Tests	Secondary Tests to Consider
Acute monoarthritis	Synovial fluid exam: white blood count and differential, crystal exam, gram stain, culture	Serum uric acid, consider CRP or ESR, consider chlamydia/GC nucleic acid test or culture, CBC with differential, PT/PTT
Chronic monoarthritis	Synovial fluid exam: WBC and differential, crystals, Gram stain, culture including AFB and fungus, joint imaging	HLA-B27, Lyme serology (depending on geographic history), consider synovial biopsy, consider chlamydia/GC nucleic acid test, consider inflammatory bowel disease tests, consider HIV
Chronic polyarthritis	ESR and/or CRP, rheumatoid factor, ACPA (anti-CCP), ANA	ANA subsets if appropriate, CK if myopathy, consider hepatitis virus antibodies, CBC, metabolic panel, urinalysis
Inflammatory back pain, enthesitis	HLA-B27	CRP and/or ESR, consider HIV
Diffuse arthralgias or myalgias	ESR, CRP, TSH, CBC	If indicative findings: ANA, CK, metabolic panel, hepatitis virus antibodies, consider HIV
Vasculitis syndromes	Urinalysis, CBC, metabolic panel (creatinine, liver tests), ESR, CRP, ANCA panel, cryoglobulins, hepatitis virus serologies, ANA if SLE features, C3 and/or C4 complement	Possibly antiglomerular basement membrane (pulmonary-renal syndromes), possibly antiphospholipid panel, blood cultures, biopsies as appropriate, imaging/angiogram as appropriate
Thrombosis syndromes, recurrent miscarriage	Antiphospholipid panel, lupus anticoagulant, ANA, CBC with platelets and peripheral smear	Hematology thrombosis tests, serum protein electrophoresis (for hyperviscosity), cold agglutinins, cryoglobulins
Fever of unknown origin, fever with rash	CBC with differential and peripheral smear, metabolic panel, ferritin, CRP, blood and other cultures, Tb γ-interferon release assay, HIV, viral studies	Bone marrow biopsy, flow cytometry, consider fungal serologies, consider syphilis serology, thick/thin smear, echocardiogram, imaging as appropriate, skin biopsy as appropriate, serum protein electrophoresis

ACPA, antibodies to citrullinated peptide antigens; AFB, acid fast bacteria; ANA, antibodies to nuclear antigens; ANCA, antibodies to neutrophil cytoplasmic antigens; CBC, complete blood count; CCP, cyclic citrullinated peptides; CK, creatine kinase; CRP, C-reactive protein; ESR, erythrocyte sedimentation rate; GC, gonococcal; HIV, human immunodeficiency virus; PT, prothrombin time; PTT, prothrombin time; SLE, systemic lupus erythematosus; Tb, tuberculosis; TSH, thyroid-stimulating hormone (thyrotropin); WBC, white blood cell count.

Table 3–2. Commonly used laboratory statistics.

Sensitivity = percentage of diseased population with positive tests results
  = (positive tests in those with disease)/(total with disease). Ideal is 100%.

Specificity = percentage of nondiseased (reference or normal) population with negative test results.
  = (negative tests in those without disease)/(total without disease). Ideal is 100%.

Likelihood ratio of a positive test (LR+) = sensitivity/(100% − specificity)
  = ratio of the proportion of positive tests in those with the disease to the proportion of positive tests in those without disease, ie, (percent true positive)/(percent false positives)
  Ideal is infinity. Excellent test is >10, moderate test is 5–10.

Likelihood ratio of a negative test (LR−) = (100% − sensitivity)/specificity
  = ratio of the proportion of negative test results among diseased to the proportion of negative results in those without disease, ie, (percent false negative/percent true negative).
  Ideal is 0. Excellent test is <0.1. Moderate test is 0.1–0.2.

Note that likelihood ratios do not depend on pretest probability. The posttest odds of having disease can be calculated by multiplying the pretest odds times the likelihood ratio, choosing LR+ vs LR− based on the test result.

Positive predictive value (posttest likelihood of having the disease)
  Probability that a subject has the disease after a positive test result. Ideal is 100%.

Negative predictive value (posttest likelihood of NOT having the disease)
  Probability that a subject does not have the disease after a negative test result. Ideal is 100%.

Positive and negative predictive values depend very much on the pretest probability (the prevalence of disease in the population tested), as well as sensitivity and specificity of the test.

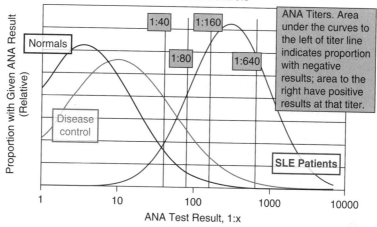

Theoretical Distribution of ANA in SLE, Normal Subjects, and Disease Controls

▲ Figure 3–1. Theoretical distribution of results of test for antibodies to nuclear antigens (ANA). Theoretical distributions of immunofluorescence ANA results in a population of normal individuals (shown in black), systemic lupus erythematosus (SLE) patients (shown in dark blue), and a rheumatic disease control group (shown in light blue). The ANA titer is shown on the x-axis, in a log scale. Approximately 5% of normal individuals have a positive ANA at or above a 1:80 titer, versus about 80% of patients presenting with lupus and 20% of the disease control group. The relative heights of the curves along the x-axis provide a likelihood ratio that a given ANA value will be associated with that condition. The ANA test can be thought of as a probabilistic test, rather than a diagnostic result. Clinicians use this probabilistic reasoning informally in evaluating quantitative test results.

population may be only 70% specific with respect to a population of patients with other rheumatic disorders.

SOME PRINCIPLES OF BASIC IMMUNOLOGY AS APPLIED TO CLINICAL IMMUNOLOGY TESTING

False-positive tests for autoantibodies detract from their clinical utility. Some basic immunology factors have an impact on the presence of false-positive results.

▶ Factors Contributing to False-Positive Autoantibody Tests

Antibodies are encoded by **immunoglobulin genes** involving combinations of heavy-chain constant region genes splicing with heavy-chain variable region genes and light-chain constant region genes splicing with light chain variable region genes. This is followed by transcription and the assembly of the heavy and light chains within B cells and plasma cells. The heavy- and light-chain variable region genes encode the amino acid sequences responsible for binding to the target antigen epitopes (binding sites). In contrast, the constant regions, particularly those in the Fc regions of the heavy chains, influence the function of the immunoglobulin proteins. Differences in the Fc regions provide the basis for typing immunoglobulins as belonging to the IgG subclasses, IgM, IgA, IgE, or IgD.

B cells, which express immunoglobulin-like cell surface receptors, may undergo **negative selection** (ie, B cells are eliminated or silenced) to avoid binding to self-antigens, allowing **self-tolerance**. They also undergo **positive selection** for binding to some antigens. When exposed to antigens under appropriate conditions such as following immunization with adjuvants, B cells expand in number and undergo further immunoglobulin gene mutation to select immunoglobulins that bind more tightly or avidly to the target. This process is termed **affinity maturation**. The recognition of a broader range of epitopes on a given antigen by B cells as they mature is a phenomenon termed **epitope spreading**.

The selection process occurs partly on the basis of the expression by B cells of unmutated germline genes that are inherited. For affinity maturation to occur as part of a mature immune response, however, the immunoglobulin gene DNA in B cells undergoes **recombination and somatic mutation**, that is, alterations in the inherited DNA sequences. The processes of recombination and somatic mutation are influenced profoundly by **helper T cells** and **regulatory T cells**, and various cytokines. These processes occur within the germinal centers of lymph nodes or in extranodal germinal centers, where maturing B cells interact with the relevant T cells.

Autoantibodies arise because of a loss of self-tolerance, leading to reactivity of immunoglobulins against self-antigens. Understanding of the mechanisms of tolerance loss and the reasons for autoantibody production remain incompletely understood, but certain autoantibody targets are characteristic of distinct autoimmune rheumatic diseases and are therefore helpful in diagnosis. The autoantibody response in autoimmune disease patients typically reflects **affinity maturation and B-cell expansion**, leading to high titers of autoantibodies measured in patient sera. Sometimes low-avidity and germ-line encoded immunoglobulins have autoantibody reactivity in the absence of disease. In such individuals harboring these benign autoantibodies, disease never develops. In virtually all autoimmune diseases studied, however, the **presence of autoantibodies precedes the diagnosis** of the autoimmune disease, sometimes by up to a decade. Over the months and years prior to the onset of symptoms sufficient to establish a diagnosis, epitope spreading occurs and the levels of autoantibodies rise, likely as a result of increases in both the avidity of immunoglobulin molecules and their concentrations.

The phenomenon **benign autoimmunity** remains incompletely understood but is clinically important because it can cause **false-positive autoantibody results** in subjects without disease. In any individual at a single time point, it can be difficult to determine if the presence of an autoantibody portends development of autoimmune disease. Over time, rising titers of autoantibodies and development of other autoantibodies associated with the same diagnosis suggest progression toward the clinical expression of an autoimmune disease.

INFLAMMATORY MARKERS

Certain changes in plasma protein concentrations occur in a stereotypical fashion during systemic inflammation. These changes, termed **the acute phase response**, largely reflect the influence of proinflammatory cytokines such as interleukin-1, interleukin-6, and tumor necrosis factor-alpha (TNF-α) on the liver and other organs. In acute inflammation, the production of proteins such as fibrinogen, haptoglobin, ferritin, and C-reactive protein (CRP) increases. In contrast, the synthesis of other proteins such as albumin and transferrin decreases. In chronic inflammation, erythrocyte production falls as immunoglobulin and complement protein levels rise.

Daniels LM, Tosh PK, Fiala JA, et al. Extremely elevated erythrocyte sedimentation rates: associations with patients' diagnoses, demographic characteristics, and comorbidities. *Mayo Clin Proc.* 2017;92:1636-1643. [PMID: 29101933]

Kermani TA, Schmidt J, Crowson CS, et al. Utility of erythrocyte sedimentation rate and C-reactive protein for the diagnosis of giant cell arteritis. *Semin Arthritis Rheum.* 2012;41:866-871. [PMID: 22119103]

Schaffner M, Rosenstein L, Ballas Z, Suneja M. Significance of hyperferritinemia in hospitalized adults. *Am J Med Sci.* 2017;354:152-158. [PMID: 28864373]

Smolen JS, Aletaha D. Interleukin-6 receptor inhibition with tocilizumab and attainment of disease remission in rheumatoid arthritis: the role of acute-phase reactants. *Arthritis Rheum.* 2011;63(1):43-52. [PMID: 21204103]

Wener MH, Daum PR, McQuillan GM. The influence of age, sex, and race on the upper reference limit of serum C-reactive protein concentration. *J Rheumatol.* 2000;27:2351-2359. [PMID: 11036829]

▶ Erythrocyte Sedimentation Rate

The erythrocyte sedimentation rate (ESR) test performed by the traditional Westergren method involves placing diluted whole blood in a graduated test tube under standardized conditions and allowing the red cells to settle under the influence of gravity. The rate of settling is reported as the ESR in millimeters per hour. The rate is governed in part by the electrical charges on the red blood cell (RBC) membranes that exert a weak repulsive force between cells, leading to a lowering of the ESR. The ESR is accelerated by most forms of anemia because fewer RBCs are available to repel each other. The erythrocyte membrane repulsion is also counteracted in the presence of higher plasma concentrations of asymmetric charged proteins such as fibrinogen and immunoglobulins, conditions found during inflammation. The increased presence of such proteins also leads to an elevation in the ESR. The ESR thus **reflects both acute and chronic inflammation** and is increased to varying degrees in most inflammatory states, particularly those associated with hypergammaglobulinemia (eg, SLE). However, ESR elevation is not universal in inflammation. Among the seronegative spondyloarthropathies, for example, the ESR is often low to normal despite obvious and highly symptomatic joint inflammation.

The ESR test is influenced by the handling of the patient specimen, for example, by allowing a specimen to remain at room temperature for more than a few hours. The ESR is affected by abnormal RBC shape and size. Sickle cell anemia, for example, tends to lower the ESR because sickled cells settle more slowly. Factors that can increase the ESR even in the absence of inflammation include the presence of monoclonal immunoglobulins and hypoalbuminemia, by increasing the contribution of asymmetric proteins relative to symmetric albumin. Extreme elevations of ESR greater than 100 mm/h (Westergren method) are likely due to infection, malignancy, or autoimmune rheumatic diseases. Giant cell arteritis (GCA) is one of the conditions often associated with extreme elevations of ESR. Otherwise, unexplained extreme elevation in ESR can be a clue to that diagnosis in an appropriate clinical setting.

Virtually all laboratories use a reference (normal) range for ESR that is different for men and women, but most do not have an age-adjusted reference range. The 95th percentile value is usually considered the upper limit of normal for a given reference population. As the population ages, various mildly inflammatory conditions develop that increase 95th percentile value even in apparently healthy ambulatory individuals, such that the "normal" ESR value tends to increase with age. Convenient formulas for calculating the age- and gender-adjusted upper limit of the reference range of ESR are available (Table 3–3).

Table 3–3. "Bed-side" estimated upper limit of reference ranges of ESR and CRP.

	ESR (mm/h, Westergren)	CRP (mg/L)
Women	$\dfrac{(Age + 10)}{2}$	$\dfrac{(Age + 30)}{5}$
Men	$\dfrac{Age}{2}$	$\dfrac{Age}{5}$

Estimates of upper limit of reference range (upper limit of normal) for ESR and CRP, with adjustments for age and sex. The increases above the conventional upper limit of normal (not adjusted for age) may be due to degenerative processes with low-grade inflammation, such as osteoarthritis, atherosclerosis, etc.

▶ C-Reactive Protein

CRP is produced rapidly by the liver in response to inflammatory cytokines. CRP has a biological role in clearing pathogenic microbes, nucleic acids, and other substances from the circulation, and can activate complement. It is generally a reliable marker of inflammation in rheumatoid arthritis and most other rheumatic diseases. However, it is less reliable as an index of inflammation in SLE patients; in fact, very elevated concentrations of CRP (>100 mg/L) in SLE patients suggest the presence of infection, rather than active SLE. A similar ESR/CRP dissociation is also observed in IgG4-related disease, which is often associated with a strikingly high ESR owing to hypergammaglobulinemia but a relatively low or normal CRP concentration.

Confusion in the interpretation of CRP results can arise because laboratories differ in how they report CRP. Whereas some labs report CRP values in units of mg/L, others report in units of mg/dL, with 10-fold different numeric results. Furthermore, labs differ in the cutoff concentration used for an abnormal result. CRP results are sometimes used to assess minor degrees of inflammation as a risk factor for coronary artery disease, using a cutoff to alert for increased risk at 2 or 3 mg/L, and values above those thresholds might be flagged. Alternatively, CRP results are sometimes used to assess active inflammatory disease, using a threshold for flagging at the 95th percentile in a population, typically in the range of 8–12 mg/L. Caution must be used to interpret the units and flags on reported results.

CRP concentrations are higher on average in women and in obesity and are somewhat higher in African Americans compared to Caucasians. CRP concentrations also increase with age. A "bedside" formula can be used to estimate the upper limit adjusted by age and gender (see Table 3–3).

▶ Ferritin

Serum ferritin is measured most commonly in the assessment of potential iron deficiency, associated with low ferritin concentrations, or iron overload conditions such as hereditary hemochromatosis, associated with elevated ferritin concentrations that are often in the range of 1000 ng/mL (upper limit of the reference normal range in most laboratories is approximately 200 ng/mL in women and 300 ng/mL in men). Serum ferritin can be elevated also because of hepatic damage or hepatic necrosis, or with renal disease. In addition, ferritin is a positive acute phase reactant, released from the liver and mononuclear phagocytes during inflammation. Elevations in ferritin are characteristic of systemic-onset juvenile idiopathic arthritis (JIA), that is, Still disease. Extreme elevations (>5000 ng/mL) are a hallmark of macrophage activation syndrome (MAS), particularly as a complication of Still disease or adult Still disease, and also can be observed in patients with other causes of extreme macrophage activation, such as hemophagocytic syndrome or hemophagocytic lymphohistiocytosis. Such dramatic elevations of ferritin are not required for the diagnosis of MAS, however. In children with systemic-onset JIA, a ferritin concentration over 684 ng/mL is one of the classification criteria for MAS.

Rarely, the serum concentration of ferritin exceeds the limits that clinical laboratory instruments measure accurately, which could lead to a reported ferritin concentration that is much lower than the actual concentration. Clinicians should feel comfortable contacting clinical laboratories to discuss discrepant or unexpected laboratory values.

A. Nephelometry, the Precipitin Curve, and the High-Dose Hook Effect

Nephelometers, instruments that quantify light scatter, are common immunoassay platforms in clinical laboratories. Reagent antibodies directed against the analyte (the substance being measured or analyzed) bind the analyte, and together they form immune complex aggregates, which scatter more light as more analyte is added.

When these aggregates are large enough, they form visible precipitates. Immunoprecipitation response is described by the precipitin curve (Figure 3–2). In Figure 3–2, each oval depicts an antigen molecule, and each Y represents an IgG antibody molecule. On the left side of the curve, the zone of

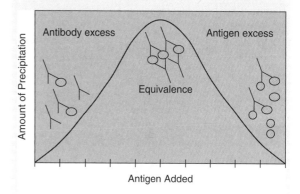

▲ **Figure 3–2.** Precipitin curve.

antibody excess, adding more antigen leads to more precipitation. Precipitation peaks at the zone of equivalence, where antigen and antibody binding sites are equimolar, and an extended lattice or network of large immune complexes forms. On the right side of the curve, the zone of antigen excess, increasing antigen leads to smaller immune complexes and less precipitation as antibody binding sites are saturated by epitopes on individual antigen molecules, preventing lattice formation. At extremely high levels of added antigen, there is no precipitate. The term "prozone" has been used to describe a falsely negative or normal immunoprecipitation result when there is an extreme excess.

Nephelometers operate under the same principles, with a similar response curve (Figure 3–3). On the left side of the curve (the light blue dashed line), increasing analyte (antigen) leads to increased light scatter. Analytes present in that range of the curve are correctly quantified (as depicted for analyte concentration "a"). Automated nephelometers typically flag as "out of range" values with excessive light scatter (the dark blue dashed line at analyte concentration "b"). The right side of the curve shows that at extreme elevations, more analytes lead to less light scatter (the gray dashed line). Since the shape of the curve reverses and aims downward after the expected increase, this phenomenon is known to clinical chemists as a "high dose hook effect," based on the reversed "hook" shape of the response curve. Very high concentrations of analyte (depicted as "c" analyte added) produce the same light scatter as "x" analyte added and would be reported incorrectly as a low value, despite the very high concentration. Nephelometric assays are optimized to perform in the typical range of analyte concentration and are usually very accurate. However, if an analyte is extremely elevated (eg, 100 times the upper limit of the reference range, as can occur for serum ferritin), the assay could report incorrect values.

Among the assays performed by nephelometry and of importance in rheumatology are ferritin; IgG subclasses; rheumatoid factor (RF); complement proteins C3 and C4; and immunoglobulins IgG, IgA, and IgM. High-dose hook effects leading to erroneous results have been reported for ferritin and IgG4, because in extreme pathologic conditions, the concentrations of these analytes can far exceed the expected concentrations, and therefore the assays may operate on the

antigen excess (right side) of the response curve. If this is suspected, the specimen can be prediluted and reassayed. If the result does not dilute as expected, the possibility of a high-dose hook effect could be the explanation.

▶ Clinical Utility of Inflammatory Marker Measurement: Adjuncts for Classification, Diagnosis, & Monitoring

The ESR and CRP are adjuncts in the diagnosis of rheumatoid arthritis, and inflammatory markers are frequently ordered to monitor rheumatoid arthritis. Control of inflammation as assessed by normalization of CRP correlates with lack of radiographic progression in rheumatoid arthritis patients and with other measures of inflammation. Utility in disease monitoring with these tests is less clear for other rheumatic diseases. While many clinicians measure both ESR and CRP, in rheumatoid arthritis patients they usually correlate well and either is likely to be sufficient. CRP is generally preferred as an inflammation marker because it is less influenced by factors other than inflammation. To assess acute infection, CRP also has the advantage of increasing more rapidly at the onset of infection and resolving more rapidly as patients improve. In addition, CRP is a protein that is stable in serum, whereas the ESR is subject to change because of specimen handling. However, neither the ESR nor the CRP is specific for any particular cause of inflammation, and they may be elevated in inflammatory arthritis, vasculitis, acute or chronic infection, malignancy, after surgery or trauma, or after other causes of inflammation or tissue destruction. Either the ESR or the CRP can be mildly to moderately elevated at times without any clear cause, and therefore neither is an unequivocal indication of inflammation or another cause for concern. The level of concern depends, to some degree, on the height of acute phase reactant elevation but also understanding of the clinical context in which the laboratory abnormality is found. Ordering these tests should be individualized, since clinical assessments of diagnosis or disease activity often do not require laboratory test corroboration.

The ESR and CRP are the major laboratory tests used in the diagnostic evaluation of GCA and polymyalgia rheumatica. The great majority of patients with these conditions have acute phase reactant elevations. Moreover, the degree of elevation of the ESR and CRP measurements in these conditions is often extremely high. However, up to 5% of patients with biopsy-proven GCA do not have elevations in either ESR or CRP, even when the laboratory tests are obtained before initiation of corticosteroid treatment. Either the ESR or CRP may be used as part of the monitoring strategy for GCA and polymyalgia rheumatica, but it is seldom appropriate to base treatment decisions entirely on the results of these tests alone. Careful clinical-laboratory correlation is always required because the results of acute phase reactant testing—whether elevated or normal—can be misleading.

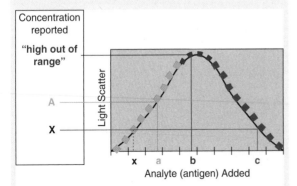

▲ **Figure 3–3.** Nephelometer result curve (with high-dose hook).

Table 3–4. Sensitivity, specificity, and likelihood ratios for IgM RF and ACPA tests for RA.

Test	Sensitivity	Specificity	Positive Likelihood Ratio	Negative Likelihood Ratio
IgM RF	69%	85%	4.9 CI 4.0–6.0	0.38 CI 0.31–0.42
Anti-CCP	67%	95%	12.5 CI 9.7–16.0	0.36 CI 0.33–0.44

ACPA, antibodies to citrullinated peptide/protein antigen; anti-CCP, antibodies to cyclic citrullinated peptides; CI, confidence interval; IgM, immunoglobulin M; RA, rheumatoid arthritis; RF, rheumatoid factor. Data from Nishimura K, Sugiyama D, Kogata Y, et al. Meta-analysis: diagnostic accuracy of anti-cyclic citrullinated peptide antibody and rheumatoid factor for rheumatoid arthritis. Ann Intern Med. 2007;146(11):797-808.

RHEUMATOID ARTHRITIS TESTS (Table 3–4)

▶ Rheumatoid Factor: Diagnostic & Prognostic, but Marginal Specificity

RF is an autoantibody directed against the Fc portion of IgG, the main immunoglobulin in normal serum (Figure 3–4). The term "rheumatoid factor" reflects the historical fact that RFs were recognized originally in patients with rheumatoid arthritis and are most tightly linked with that diagnosis, but the presence of RF is not specific for rheumatoid arthritis. Clinical laboratories usually measure serum IgM RF, that is, an IgM antibody directed against the Fc portion of IgG (Figure 3–4). Although IgA RF and IgG RF also exist, tests for those variants are rarely used in the United States. The RF test can be performed by visually examining the agglutination (clumping) of IgG-coated latex particles or RBCs induced by RF. Laboratories that assay for RF by agglutination typically quantify the amount of RF by serial serum dilution to find the highest dilution (titer) at which agglutination is visible. Dilutions are typically performed in twofold titer increases

Antigen = normal IgG

Antibody = IgM RF

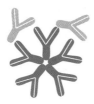

IgM RF binding to normal IgG

▲ **Figure 3–4. Rheumatoid factor.** Normal IgG, IgM rheumatoid factor (RF), and IgM RF shown bound to the Fc region of two IgG molecules.

Table 3–5. Causes of positive rheumatoid factor tests.

Clinical Conditions Associated with Rheumatoid Factor
• Rheumatoid arthritis
• Other rheumatic diseases
– Sjögren syndrome (~90%)
– Systemic lupus erythematosus (15–20%)
– Mixed cryoglobulinemia syndrome (95%)
– Sarcoidosis (~15%)
– Parvovirus arthropathy (~15%, transient)
• Chronic infection
– Chronic hepatitis C infection (~50%)
– Chronic osteomyelitis
– Bacterial endocarditis
• Monoclonal IgM paraproteins (Waldenstrom macroglobulinemia, lymphoma)
• Normal aging (RF present at low titers)

IgM, immunoglobulin M; RF, rheumatoid factor.

(eg, 1:80, 1:160, 1:320, and so on, with the highest serum dilution yielding a positive result ultimately reported). The test results of manual methods can vary substantially, depending on reagent and other technical issues. In large clinical laboratories, tests for RF are performed on automated analyzers, with results reported in international units, based on international calibration standards.

Positive tests for IgM RF are present in about 50–60% of patients with rheumatoid arthritis at their initial presentation, and in about 70–80% of patients with chronic rheumatoid arthritis in tertiary referral clinics. In reference normal populations, the prevalence of RF is about 5%, with somewhat higher prevalence (approximately 10%) in healthy older subjects. The likelihood of a positive RF in healthy populations is somewhat higher in women than in men. RF may also be present in the serum of patients with other rheumatic diseases or with chronic infections (Table 3–5). Therefore, the presence of RF should not be considered diagnostic, but its presence substantially increases the likelihood that a patient with polyarthritis has rheumatoid arthritis. The presence of RF also has important prognostic value. The finding of high levels of RF (generally >50 international units) in a patient with rheumatoid arthritis predicts that the patient will have more severe joint disease and will be more likely to develop extra-articular disease if not treated appropriately. Therefore, the presence of high-titer RF also influences clinical decisions regarding treatment; disease associated with risk factors for a poor prognosis should be considered for more aggressive treatment.

▶ Antibodies to Citrullinated Peptide/Protein Antigens/Anti-CCP: Diagnostic & Prognostic, More Specific than RF

Antibodies to citrullinated peptide/protein antigen (ACPA) tests are used to establish the diagnosis of rheumatoid arthritis and to help understand prognosis. Citrulline is an amino acid produced by posttranslational modification of arginine, converting an amino group of arginine into a carboxyl group. ACPAs are often measured using a reagent that is a circular peptide containing citrulline. Therefore, the test for ACPA is frequently called "antibodies to cyclic citrullinated peptides" (anti-CCP). ACPA may be measured using alternative citrullinated antigens, including citrullinated vimentin, different forms of cyclic citrullinated peptides, and others. Differences in the clinical tests used to measure ACPA are relatively minor, and for practical purposes the available ACPA tests are nearly equivalent in their clinical performance.

The sensitivity of ACPA for rheumatoid arthritis is similar to that of RF for this disease. That is, approximately 75–80% of patients with rheumatoid arthritis develop ACPA over the course of their disease. The specificity of ACPA is significantly higher than RF, because ACPA are rare in autoimmune conditions such as primary Sjögren syndrome and chronic infections such as hepatitis C. A large majority of patients with rheumatoid arthritis who have serum RF also have ACPA. Thus, identification of a patient who has a highly positive assay for RF test but a negative ACPA test is a clue that the positive RF may be the result of another condition, such as chronic viral hepatitis, sarcoidosis, vasculitis associated with antineutrophil cytoplasmic antibodies (ANCA), or another immune-mediated autoimmune disease.

Moderate to high titers of ACPA are prognostic in that they are associated with a greater risk of severe disease compared to the situation in which the patient is ANCA negative. Borderline and low levels of ACPA do not have the same diagnostic and prognostic significance as high concentrations, and caution should be used when interpreting them. As an example, some patients with psoriatic arthritis have significant serum ACPA titers, and positive ACPAs are found occasionally in a variety of other conditions.

Indications for testing RF and ACPA are similar: diagnosis and prognostication. They are used to confirm that a patient with inflammatory arthritis has rheumatoid arthritis and to help establish the prognosis of these patients. According to American College of Rheumatology/European League Against Rheumatism ACR/EULAR classification criteria for rheumatoid arthritis, low positive tests are results between the upper limit of normal and three times the upper limit of normal. High positive results are those more than three times the upper limit of normal. High-titer RF and ACPA results indicate a more severe prognosis of rheumatoid arthritis. ACPA tests have a greater positive predictive value than RF; if only one of the two tests is to be ordered, ACPA is preferred because of greater specificity and positive likelihood ratio, leading to higher positive predictive value. However, once a diagnosis of rheumatoid arthritis has been established, there is usually no need to measure these tests again since they are not reliable disease activity markers.

Aggarwal R, Liao K, Nair R, Ringold S, Costenbader KH. Anti-citrullinated peptide antibody assays and their role in the diagnosis of rheumatoid arthritis. *Arthritis Rheum.* 2009;15:1472-1483. [PMID: 19877103]

Bossuyt X. Anticitrullinated protein antibodies: taking into account antibody levels improves interpretation. *Ann Rheum Dis.* 2017;76:e33. [PMID: 28119288]

Nishimura K, Sugiyama D, Kogata Y, et al. Meta-analysis: diagnostic accuracy of anti-cyclic citrullinated peptide antibody and rheumatoid factor for rheumatoid arthritis. *Ann Intern Med.* 2007;146:797-808. [PMID: 17548411]

Wener MH, Hutchinson K, Morishima C, Gretch DR. Absence of antibodies to cyclic citrullinated peptide in sera of patients with hepatitis C virus infection and cryoglobulinemia. *Arthritis Rheum.* 2004;50:2305-2308. [PMID: 15248231]

SYSTEMIC LUPUS ERYTHEMATOSUS

Virtually all patients with systemic lupus erythematosus (SLE) develop autoantibodies over the course of their illness. Most make more than one autoantibody that can be identified using clinical laboratory tests.

▶ Autoantibodies to Nuclear Antigens: The Hallmark of SLE

Autoantibodies to nuclear antigens (ANA) are present in more than 95% of SLE cases at some point in the course of their illness, and most patients are consistently ANA positive. Although ANA-negative SLE does exist, the persistent absence of ANA and lack of at least one lupus-associated autoantibody should lead one to question the diagnosis. The presence of a positive ANA at a clinically significant titer is a key criterion for epidemiologic classification of a patient as having SLE. Positive ANAs and antibodies to closely related antigens are also commonly detected in other autoimmune rheumatic diseases such as systemic sclerosis (both diffuse and limited cutaneous disease), Sjögren syndrome, dermatomyositis, and overlap syndromes (Table 3–6).

A. Immunofluorescence

The traditional assay for ANA involves immunofluorescence microscopy, in which fluorescent-labeled antibodies to human IgG are used to detect the presence, amount (titer), and pattern of IgG from the patient's serum that binds to structures within the cells. The substrate to which the patient's serum and then the fluorescent-labeled antibodies to IgG are applied is a HEp-2 cell line (a squamous cell carcinoma cell line grown on glass microscope slides). The labeled antibodies that bind to antibodies from patient's serum are detected by fluorescence microscopy.

The common ANA nuclear immunofluorescence staining patterns reported include the speckled, homogenous,

Table 3–6. Characteristic ANA test positive rates (sensitivity) in various rheumatic diseases.

Antibody	NI	SLE	Drug LE	MCTD	Sjögren Syndrome	dc Systemic Sclerosis	CREST/lc Systemic Sclerosis	DM/PM	RA
ANA	1–20	95–99	100	95	70–90	90	95	80	30
dsDNA	0.5	60–80			30				
Histones		60	70						
Sm/RNP		40		90		10	10	15	
Sm		30							
Ro (SSA)	0.5	40			50–90				5
La (SSB)		15			60				
Scl-70		—				25	10		
RNA polymerase 3						10			
Centromere						50	85		
Jo-1 (cytoplasmic)								30	
Ribosomal P (cytoplasmic)	1	20							
RF (not an ANA)	<5	10			80				60

Sensitivity of various autoantibody laboratory tests in different autoimmune rheumatic diseases.
CREST/lc systemic sclerosis, syndrome of calcinosis, Raynaud phenomenon, esophageal dysmotility, sclerodactyly, telangiectasia, or limited cutaneous systemic sclerosis; dc systemic sclerosis, diffuse cutaneous systemic sclerosis (scleroderma); DM/PM, dermatomyositis, polymyositis (including synthetase syndrome); MCTD, mixed connective tissue disease; NI, normal reference population; SLE, drug SLE, spontaneous or drug-induced SLE; RA, rheumatoid arthritis; RF, rheumatoid factor; RNP, ribonucleoprotein.

nucleolar pattern, and centromere patterns (Figure 3–5). Those different staining patterns are caused by antibodies reacting with specific antigens whose distributions within the nucleus are reflected by the patterns. The importance of this is that antibodies directed against specific antigens tend to be associated with particular autoimmune rheumatic diseases. The centromere pattern, for example, is strongly associated with antibodies to the centromere B protein. These antibodies, in turn, are closely associated with limited cutaneous systemic sclerosis (the CREST syndrome). Antibodies to DNA, to histone, or to DNA-histone complexes typically are associated with a homogeneous staining pattern. In contrast, antibodies to various RNA-protein complexes are usually associated with a speckled staining pattern.

The correspondence between staining patterns and antibodies to specific antigens is imperfect. Therefore, detection of a positive ANA by immunofluorescence should be followed by tests for antibodies to specific nuclear antigens ("ANA subsets") that would provide evidence supporting a particular clinical diagnosis. Table 3–7 shows common ANA immunofluorescence patterns and the specific antibodies characteristically associated with those patterns.

Not all of the autoantigens associated with lupus and related autoimmune rheumatic disease are located within the nucleus. The upshot of this is that a patient may be ANA negative by immunofluorescence but still have an autoantibody that provides important insight into diagnosis. The first example of this described was the SSA/Ro antigen.

Antibodies to the SSA/Ro antigen may be present in the absence of a positive ANA measured by immunofluorescence. Another example is antiribosomal P antibodies, which are associated with cytoplasmic as opposed to nuclear staining by immunofluorescence. Finally, some of the myositis-associated autoantibodies (MAA), including antisynthetase antibodies (which are variably ANA positive), antimelanoma differentiation-associated 5 (MDA5), and antisignal recognition peptide (SRP), are not associated with nuclear staining.

Immunofluorescence testing is often inconsistent between laboratories, unfortunately. This depends in part on how the HEp-2 cells used as substrate for testing are generated by the laboratory performing the test itself or by the reagent manufacturer. Factors such as the reagents used, the microscope and lighting used, and the training of personnel also have substantial impacts on interpretations emerging from a particular laboratory. Approaches to improve automation and standardization of ANA immunofluorescence testing are under way.

B. Alternatives to ANA Immunofluorescence

Alternatives to ANA immunofluorescence testing are available. One approach uses enzyme-linked immunosorbent assays (ELISA), in which nuclear extracts containing various antigens coat plastic wells. IgG from the patient's serum is allowed to react with the antigens. The presence of bound IgG is detected with enzyme-linked antihuman IgG followed by an enzyme

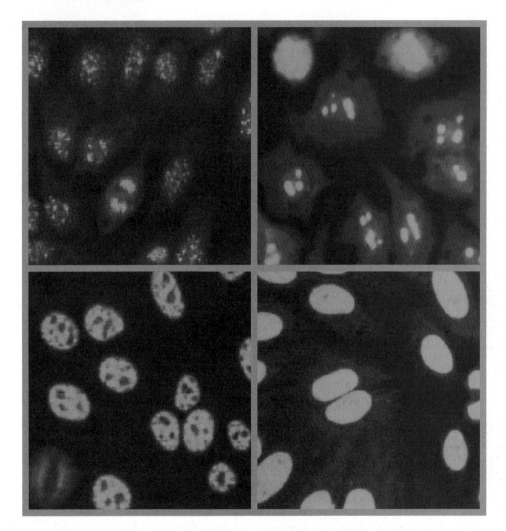

▲ **Figure 3–5. Patterns of antibodies to nuclear antigen (ANA) performed by immunofluorescence microscopy.** Representative appearance of ANA tests performed by immunofluorescence microscopy on HEp-2 cells. Top left: anticentromere pattern. Top right: nucleolar pattern. Lower left: speckled pattern. Lower right: diffuse/homogeneous pattern. **(See color insert.)** (Used with permission from Kathleen Hutchinson.)

Table 3–7. Immunofluorescence IFA ANA patterns typically associated with rheumatic disease autoantibodies.

Pattern	Antigens Recognized
Centromere	Centromere antigens (centromere proteins A and B)
Homogeneous	DNA, chromatin, histones, others
Speckled	Extractable nuclear antigens (Sm, RNP, SS-A, SS-B), Scl70, RNA polymerase III, others. Uncommon antibodies: Ku, Mi-2, TIF1γ, NXP2
Nucleolar	Scleroderma-related (fibrillarin, Th/To, PM/Scl, Scl70), others
Cytoplasmic	Ribosomal P, Jo-1, and other antisynthetase antibodies Uncommon antibodies: signal recognition peptide, MDA5 (may also be negative by immunofluorescence microscopy)

MDA5, melanoma differentiation factor 5; NXP2, nuclear matrix protein-2; TIF1γ, transcription intermediary factor 1-γ.

substrate that allows quantitative color development. This approach allows reproducible quantitation by an automated colorimetric read-out but does not permit reporting of an ANA pattern that is possible with immunofluorescence. However, if individual autoantigens are used to coat the plastic wells without adding other antigens, antibodies to single, specific antigens can be detected by ELISA. This approach is commonly used to detect and quantify individual antibodies, including autoantibodies to ANA subset antigens.

Another approach involves measuring several (typically about 6–12) distinct autoantibodies simultaneously. This **multiplex bead immunoassay** (MBIA) approach typically uses antigen-coated fluorescent microbeads with distinct colors (wavelengths), with each color used to detect antibodies to a different antigen. The assay is considered positive if at least one of the individual antibodies tests positive. The MBIA is equivalent to performing several simultaneous ELISA tests. In many laboratories, the ANA immunofluorescence has been replaced by the MBIA even though although not all nuclear antigens are tested in the MBIA. MBIA testing is performed on automated platforms, does not require as much technical expertise or time as ANA immunofluorescence, and is therefore viewed as cost-effective and efficient. A major shortcoming of this approach, however, is that it does not detect autoantibodies to antigens that are not specifically tested as part of the multiplex panel.

CHARACTERISTIC AUTOANTIBODIES ASSOCIATED WITH SLE

▶ Antibodies to Double-Stranded DNA (Anti-dsDNA): Diagnosis & Monitoring

Double-stranded DNA is the characteristic autoantigen associated with SLE. When anti-dsDNA antibodies are present in high titer, they are very specific for SLE. The measured levels of anti-dsDNA typically fluctuate and correlate with disease activity, particularly in patients with significant kidney involvement due to diffuse proliferative lupus nephritis. Measurement of anti-dsDNA helps to confirm a diagnosis of SLE and can help assess disease activity in SLE. Substantial evidence indicates that they are not only biomarker antibodies, but also that they play a role in the pathogenesis of lupus, combining with DNA as antigen and forming immune complexes associated with tissue damage. In addition, nucleic acid-antibody complexes activate immune cells, leading to more autoimmunity.

Positive tests for anti-dsDNA can be seen occasionally in patients without SLE. For example, patients treated with TNFα antagonists for rheumatoid arthritis, psoriatic arthritis, Crohn disease, or other indications may develop drug-induced anti-dsDNA and positive ANAs, but few of those develop drug-induced lupus. In those who develop drug-induced lupus, the autoantibodies and symptoms typically resolve after stopping the medication. dsDNA antibodies are also detected in some patients with ANA-positive autoimmune hepatitis.

▶ Extractable Nuclear Antigens: Sm & RNP

SLE patients also make antibodies to RNA-protein complexes. Two antigens commonly associated with the formation of such antibodies are the Sm and RNP antigens, both of which are nuclear antigens. Unlike some other nuclear antigens, Sm and RNP antigens are soluble in typical saline solutions, and thus can be solubilized or extracted from nuclei of cells. For this reason, they are sometimes called "extractable nuclear antigens" (ENA). Antibodies to the Sm antigen were identified first in a lupus patient named Smith, hence the Sm designation. Anti-RNP (ribonuclear protein) antibodies are also known as U1-RNP antibodies.

Anti-Sm antibodies have a high specificity for SLE. In contrast, antibodies to U1-RNP can occur in a number of other conditions in addition to SLE. Some patients also make antibodies to a macromolecular particle in which the Sm and U1-RNP antigen complexes are combined. High titers of antibodies to this Sm/RNP complex in the absence of antibodies to the Sm antigen are characteristic of the rheumatologic overlap syndrome known as mixed connective tissue syndrome (MCTD). Such patients would be reported to have anti-RNP antibodies. The clinical features of these patients typically represent an overlap between those of SLE and systemic sclerosis patients.

▶ Antiribosomal P Antibodies

The sera from SLE patients also may contain antibodies to various antigens located within the cell cytoplasm rather than the nucleus. The most prominent and clinically useful of these antibodies are directed against ribosomal antigens, particularly proteins within the ribosome known as ribosomal-P. Antiribosomal antibodies demonstrate diffuse cytoplasmic fluorescence staining on HEp2 cells and can be detected by specific tests, as well. Antiribosomal P antibodies, which have a high specificity for SLE, tend to be observed in lupus patients with neuropsychiatric lupus.

▶ Anti-SSA/Ro & Anti-SSB/La

The SSA and SSB antibodies were described in patients with primary Sjögren syndrome, leading to their designations as "SS" antibodies. There are also often found in patients with SLE and occasionally in other autoimmune rheumatic conditions, for example, systemic sclerosis and inflammatory myopathies. They are also called Ro and La antibodies, respectively.

The Ro and La antibodies are particularly associated with a form of lupus called subacute cutaneous lupus, characterized by prominent chronic nonscarring photosensitive rashes. Furthermore, the Ro antibody is strongly associated with the neonatal lupus syndrome, in which mothers who have these antibodies in their serum give birth to babies who are susceptible to transient, photosensitive, lupus-like rashes as neonates and to heart block and cardiomyopathy in utero.

The Ro antigen consists of two forms, with molecular masses of 52 kD and 60 kD. Antibodies against the 52 kD antigen have been associated with a variety of conditions, including myositis with lung disease and others.

Antihistone & Antibodies to DNA-Protein Complexes (Anti-DNP)

Autoantibodies to histone proteins are seen in individuals with some forms of **drug-induced lupus** and drug-induced positive ANAs. An example of a medication associated with the induction of autoimmunity is the cardiac arrhythmia drug, procainamide, which commonly leads to drug-induced ANAs in the sera of patients, some of whom develop clinical manifestations of lupus. Antibodies to histones are not diagnostic of a drug-induced lupus syndrome, however, because antihistone antibodies can also be observed in patients with SLE. Whereas patients with spontaneous SLE produce other autoantibodies such as anti-dsDNA together with the antihistone antibody, the characteristic of drug-induced SLE patients is that antihistone antibodies occur alone, without other positive ANA subset tests. Testing for antihistone antibodies can be helpful in confirming the clinical suspicion of drug-induced lupus, but such testing does not help in the diagnosis of patients already known to produce other lupus-associated ANA subset antibodies.

Antibodies to DNA-histone complexes and to other DNA-protein complexes ("anti-DNP") are produced in patients with SLE, but also in other conditions. Finding anti-DNP antibodies in the serum of a patient therefore has little value in and of itself in clinical diagnosis. These tests are not used widely.

Antibodies Involved in the Coagulation System

Deficient function of ADAMTS13 is known to be responsible for the development of thrombotic thrombocytopenic purpura (TTP). Some patients with SLE acquire TTP because of the development of antibodies to the ADAMTS13 protein. TTP physiology may account for clinical features attributed to SLE flares in a small number of SLE cases, because both conditions can demonstrate prominent thrombocytopenia, renal disease, central nervous system disease, hemolytic anemia, and fever. If such patients develop a prominent microangiopathic hemolytic picture with prominent schistocytes, a test for ADAMTS13 and its inhibitory antibodies may be indicated to lead to appropriate therapy for TTP.

Anti-erythrocyte Antibodies

Patients with lupus develop autoimmune hemolytic anemia, with antibodies directed against red cells detected by the direct antiglobulin test (DAT, also known as the direct Coombs test). DAT tests in SLE patients can detect both IgG and the complement C3 protein on the erythrocyte. These tests can be positive even in some lupus patients without overt hemolytic anemia. Patients with SLE may develop antibodies directed against platelets, neutrophils, and lymphocytes, but assays for antibodies against these cell types are not often performed.

Other Autoantibodies

A variety of other autoantibodies are seen in patients with SLE, though many of these are not widely available for clinical use. Antibodies directed against neuronal cell antigens, particularly the N-methyl-D-aspartate (NMDA) glutamate receptor, are seen in some patients with lupus, particularly the subset of patients with diffuse neurocognitive and psychiatric disease manifestations. Antibodies directed against C1q, the first component of complement, are associated with diffuse forms of lupus nephritis. A variety of other nuclear antigens are known to be recognized by some lupus IgG.

ANTIPHOSPHOLIPID SYNDROME & ANTIPHOSPHOLIPID ANTIBODIES

Antiphospholipid syndrome (APS) may be secondary to lupus or other autoimmune connective tissue diseases but may also be primary, without another cause. Antibodies (both IgG and IgM) directed against the phospholipid cardiolipin and to the phospholipid-binding protein beta-2-glycoprotein I are commonly seen in patients with SLE, especially in association with APS (see later). These antibodies are a common cause of biologic false-positive tests for syphilis (BFPTS), that is, false-positive nontreponemal tests such as the rapid plasma reagin (RPR) and Venereal Disease Research Laboratory (VDRL) tests. Presence of the lupus inhibitor/lupus anticoagulant is also part of the antiphospholipid set of antibody tests.

The international consensus criteria for APS designate that the diagnosis of APS requires at least two positive tests performed at least 12 weeks apart for either IgG or IgM anticardiolipin antibodies; antibodies to the phospholipid binding protein beta-2-glycoprotein I; or detection of the lupus inhibitor/lupus anticoagulant through an accepted functional test.

Tests for lupus anticoagulant can be performed by screening with a dilute Russell viper venom time and a similar phospholipid-limited coagulation test. Such tests include a lupus inhibitor-sensitive partial thromboplastin time. Demonstration of an abnormally prolonged test is then repeated with a mixing study using normal plasma to prove the presence of an inhibitor. The addition of an excess phospholipid source such as hexagonal phase phospholipids can demonstrate correction of the prolonged time by phospholipids as additional confirmation. The presence of a lupus anticoagulant is the best predictor of the occurrence of a clinical event secondary to APS. Anticoagulants and acute thrombosis can affect lupus anticoagulant tests because they are functional assays. In contrast, tests for antibodies to cardiolipin and to beta-2-glycoprotein I can be performed even when patients are anticoagulated.

An increased number of antiphospholipid antibodies are associated with higher risk of adverse associations. For example, women positive for anticardiolipin and anti-beta2-glycorotein I and lupus anticoagulant are more likely to have adverse pregnancy outcomes than those positive for only one of the antibodies. However, low-titer positive tests for individual antiphospholipid antibodies are relatively common and very nonspecific. Such findings are usually transient, particularly among inpatient populations, and caution must be used in ascribing importance to such findings for the purpose of clinical decision-making.

Some laboratories offer assays for antibodies to phospholipids that are not part of the classification criteria. These include IgA antibodies to cardiolipin and to beta-2-glycoprotein I, and antibodies to other phospholipids such as phosphatidyl serine and phosphatidyl ethanolamine. The role of these noncriteria autoantibodies in diagnosis and management is controversial.

Chan EKL, Damoiseaux J, Carballo OG, et al. Report of the First International Consensus on Standardized Nomenclature of Antinuclear Antibody HEp-2 Cell Patterns (ICAP) 2014-2015. *Front Immunol*. 2015, Aug 20;6:412. International Consensus on ANA Patterns (ICAP). https://www.anapatterns.org/index.php.

Ippolito A, Wallace DJ, Gladman D, et al. Autoantibodies in systemic lupus erythematosus: comparison of historical and current assessment of seropositivity. *Lupus*. 2011;20:250-255. [PMID: 21362750]

Leuchten N, Annika Hoyer A, Brinks R, et al. Performance of Antinuclear Antibodies for Classifying Systemic Lupus Erythematosus: A Systematic Literature Review and Meta-Regression of Diagnostic Data. Arthritis Care Res 2018;70: 428-438. PMID: 28544593

Pengo V, Tripodi A, Reber G, et al. Update of the guidelines for lupus anticoagulant testing. *J Thomb Haemost*. 2009;7: 1737-1740. [PMID: 19624461]

Pisetsky DS. Antinuclear antibody testing—misunderstood or misbegotten? Perspective. *Nature Rev Rheum*. 2017;13:495-502. [PMID: 28541299]

Saccone G, Berghella V, Maruotti GM, et al. PREGNANTS (PREGNancy in women with ANTiphospholipid Syndrome) working group. Antiphospholipid antibody profile-based obstetric outcomes of primary antiphospholipid syndrome: the PREGNANTS study. *Am J Obstet Gynecol*. 2017;216:525.e1-525. e12. [PMID: 28153662]

Sebastiani GD, Galeazzi M, Tincani A, et al. Anticardiolipin and anti-beta2GPI antibodies in a large series of European patients with systemic lupus erythematosus. Prevalence and clinical associations. European Concerted Action on the Immunogenetics of SLE. *Scand J Rheumatol*. 1999;28:344-351. [PMID: 10665739]

COMPLEMENT TESTING

The complement system is a complex network of at least 20 proteins that function as enzymes, and regulatory proteins; pathogen-related pattern recognition and binding proteins; and cell binding and activation peptides. The main functions of the complement system are to protect against pathogens by amplification of inflammatory pathways and to promote clearance of pathogenic factors from the circulation. Complement proteins are positive acute phase reactants whose serum concentrations tend to increase during most forms of inflammation. In contrast, during flares of some autoimmune rheumatic diseases, complement activation leads to consumption of complement proteins and subnormal serum concentrations. As examples, patients with diseases associated with immune-complex deposition as a major tissue injury mechanism are often found to be hypocomplementemic. Such diseases include SLE and mixed cryoglobulinemia, among others.

There are three pathways of complement activation: the classic pathway, alternative pathway, and lectin pathway. The **classic pathway** is initiated by the binding of immune complexes (ie, antigen-antibody complexes) to C1q, an immunoglobulin Fc-binding protein. The **alternative pathway** is initiated by the binding of complement factor B to either pathogens or exposed negative charges. Finally, the **lectin pathway** is initiated by binding pathogen-associated sugars and glycopeptides to the complement protein mannan-binding protein (also known as mannan-binding lectin).

All these three activation pathways have a terminal pathway common to all, which promotes the clearance of immune complexes (opsonin function) and activation of leukocytes through C3 activation. The terminal pathway of complement activation also leads to the recruitment of neutrophils via the activation of C5 and the production of C5 protein fragments, and to the assembly of the C5-9 complement components into the membrane attack complex (MAC). The MAC results in target cell killing through the creation of holes in the cell membrane, leading to the death of target cells (Figure 3–6).

The main clinical utility of complement testing in rheumatology is to assist in the diagnosis and monitoring of diseases such as SLE, mixed cryoglobulinemia, and certain other conditions associated with immune complex deposition in tissues. Immune complexes activate complement via the classic pathway. As a result, all of the proteins involved in the classic pathway tend to have decreased concentrations during SLE flares, for example. Clinical laboratories typically measure and report the concentrations of complement proteins C3 and C4.

Laboratories may also measure complement by assaying total hemolytic complement, a functional assay requiring the entire complement cascade from C1q to the MAC. The usual method for reporting hemolytic complement activity utilizes RBCs as reagents in the assay. The assay quantifies the amount of complement present required to lyse 50% of the RBCs. This assay is therefore known as the CH50 (CH for "complement hemolysis") test. During active lupus, the expected finding is that C3, C4, and total hemolytic complement all are present at subnormal concentrations. These typically return toward normal as the disease is controlled, provided the patient does not have a heritable deficiency of one or more complement proteins.

One of the genetic contributions to the risk of lupus is inherited partial or complete deficiency of complement C4

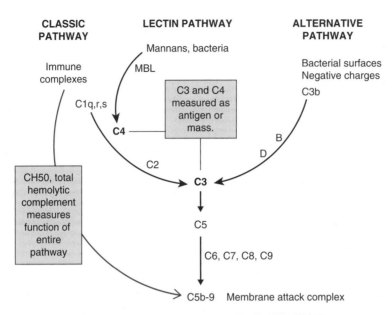

CLASSIC PATHWAY — Immune complexes — C1q,r,s

LECTIN PATHWAY — Mannans, bacteria — MBL

ALTERNATIVE PATHWAY — Bacterial surfaces / Negative charges — C3b

C3 and C4 measured as antigen or mass.

C4

C2

CH50, total hemolytic complement measures function of entire pathway

B

D

C3

C5

C6, C7, C8, C9

C5b-9   Membrane attack complex

▲ **Figure 3–6. Complement cascade.** Complement cascade schematic, showing the three activation pathways (classic, alternative, and lectin) leading to a common terminal pathway. The routine clinical assays for complement measure the concentrations of C4 and C3 as proteins, and the function of the entire classic pathway in the test for hemolytic complement activity, the CH50 test.

due to a null gene at one or more of the four C4 gene loci. Partial C4 deficiency is relatively common in northern Europeans, and individuals with partial C4 deficiency usually have lower serum concentrations of C4 than subjects with all four active genes. In patients with lupus and partial C4 deficiency, the C4 may remain low even when clinically stable. Direct measurement of the serum concentration of complement activation products (the enzymatically produced complement protein fragments) either in plasma or bound to cells may help clarify whether low concentrations of complement are due to increased activation as opposed to low production. Complement fragment concentrations increase only when consumption is increased. Assays to measure complement fragment concentrations, however, are not routine.

The total hemolytic complement concentrations generally correlate with C3 and C4 concentrations, so routine measurement of total complement is not usually necessary. Very low or absent hemolytic complement activity may result not only from in vivo consumption of complement due to active disease but also as an artifact of in vitro specimen handling. If a serum specimen remains at room temperature or above, the function of complement proteins may be lost, because they are heat-labile. Very low hemolytic complement activity with normal or minimally depressed C3 or C4 in a specimen that has been handled and processed correctly suggests the possibility of congenital deficiency of one of the complement components other than (or in addition to) C3 or C4. Deficiency of the classic activation phase proteins C1q and C2, for example, is associated with lupus. C2 deficiencies predispose

patients to potentially life-threatening pneumococcal infections. Deficiencies of other complement proteins can also be associated with other types of recurrent infections. Deficiency of the C5-C9 proteins is especially associated with risk of disseminated gonococcemia and meningococcemia.

Activation and dysregulation of the alternative pathway of complement activation are associated with hemolytic-uremic syndrome and thrombotic microangiopathic disease. Measurement of alternative pathway complement protein concentrations and function and identification of the DNA sequence of complement-related genes may be indicated in rare cases but are not part of the routine evaluation of patients with SLE or other autoimmune rheumatic diseases.

Gandino IJ, Scolnik M, Bertiller E, Scaglioni V, Catoggio LJ, Soriano ER. Complement levels and risk of organ involvement in patients with systemic lupus erythematosus. *Lupus Sci Med.* 2017;4(1):e000209. [PMID: 29259790]

Ramsey-Goldman R, Li J, Dervieux T, Alexander RV. Cell-bound complement activation products in SLE. *Lupus Sci Med.* 2017;4:e000236. [PMID: 29214038]

VASCULITIS-ASSOCIATED TESTS

▶ Anti-neutrophil Cytoplasmic Antibodies

Patients with certain forms of vasculitis make autoantibodies to antigens in the cytoplasmic granules of neutrophilic polymorphonuclear leukocytes (PMNs) and monocytes. These antibodies are detectable in clinical labs using immunofluorescence assays and by solid phase immunoassays such as ELISA tests for antibodies to specific proteins. The autoantigens most tightly linked with vasculitis are proteinase-3 (PR3) and myeloperoxidase (MPO). Antibodies against both are routinely assayed in clinical laboratories. These antibodies, termed collectively "antineutrophil cytoplasmic antibodies" (ANCA), play an important role in the diagnosis of ANCA-associated vasculitides such as granulomatosis with polyangiitis (formerly known as Wegener granulomatosis), microscopic polyangiitis, and eosinophilic granulomatosis with polyangiitis (previously known as Churg-Strauss syndrome).

The substrate used for immunofluorescence is usually PMNs derived from peripheral blood, applied to a glass slide, and fixed on the slide with laboratory fixatives. When a strong fixative such as formaldehyde is used, both the MPO and PR3 antigens remain within the cytoplasmic granules. Antibodies to either antigen stain with a granular cytoplasmic pattern. However, when a relatively weak fixative such as ethanol is used, the myeloperoxidase protein (which carries a strong electrostatic charge) leaves the granules and is attracted toward the nucleus, resulting in a perinuclear location. Anti-MPO applied to these cells stain the cells with a perinuclear pattern (P-ANCA staining). In contrast, even with ethanol fixation, the PR3 antigen remains within the neutrophil granules, and anti-PR3 antibodies stain the neutrophils with a cytoplasmic granular pattern (C-ANCA staining). Clinical laboratories use weak ethanol-fixed cells to distinguish the P-ANCA staining pattern associated with anti-MPO antibodies from the C-ANCA staining pattern associated with anti-PR3 antibodies (Figure 3–7). Antimyeloperoxidase antibodies are often referred to as MPO-ANCA, and antiproteinase 3 antibodies are often termed PR3-ANCA.

The combination of a P-ANCA immunofluorescence staining pattern and MPO-ANCA is most likely to be associated with microscopic polyangiitis. In contrast, the combination of C-ANCA immunofluorescence and PR3-ANCA has a high specificity for granulomatosis with polyangiitis. Overlap situations occasionally occur, however. For example, approximately 10% of granulomatosis cases with polyangiitis have MPO-ANCA rather than PR3-ANCA. The utility of ANCA

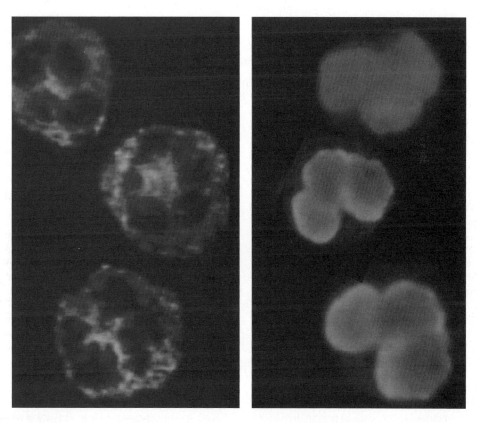

▲ **Figure 3–7. Antibodies to neutrophil cytoplasmic antigens (ANCA) detected by immunofluorescence assay microscopy.** ANCA tests performed on ethanol fixed neutrophils. The cytoplasmic cANCA pattern on the left shows granular staining throughout the cytoplasm, sparing the nucleus. The perinuclear pANCA pattern on the right demonstrates staining that covers the nucleus. In clinical laboratories, this test would also be confirmed using formalin fixed cells, which demonstrates a diffuse cytoplasmic staining pattern for both cANCA and pANCA antibodies. (See color insert.)

testing in the diagnosis of ANCA-associated vasculitides is discussed in greater detail in the chapters on the individual diseases and in the chapter on miscellaneous vasculitides (drug-induced ANCA-associated vasculitis).

Chehroudi C, Booth RA, Milman N. Diagnostic outcome and indications for testing in patients with positive ANCA at a Canadian tertiary care centre. *Rheumatol Int.* 2018;38(4):641-647. [PMID: 29243051]

Radice A, Bianchi L, Sinico RA. Anti-neutrophil cytoplasmic autoantibodies: methodological aspects and clinical significance in systemic vasculitis. *Autoimmunity Rev.* 2013;13:487-495. [PMID: 22921790]

Rao JK, Weinberger M, Oddone EZ, Allen NB, Landsman P, Feussner JR. The role of antineutrophil cytoplasmic antibody (c-ANCA) testing in the diagnosis of Wegener granulomatosis. A literature review and meta-analysis. *Ann Intern Med.* 1995;123:925-932. [PMID: 7486487]

▶ A. Cryoglobulins

Cryoglobulins are immunoglobulins that reversibly precipitate in the cold ("cryo" from the Greek "kruos" for frost). It should be noted that "cold" refers to the temperatures to which the proteins are to in the laboratory—for example, 4°C—temperatures far lower than patients achieve in clinical settings or even in the coldest winter. Although cryoglobulins are often pathogenic proteins in humans, behaving aberrantly and resulting in tissue injury, their pathogenicity is not linked directly to the properties demonstrated in laboratory settings.

The test for cryoglobulins involves placing serum in a refrigerator and assessing the formation of a precipitate. The precipitate may be quantified as a "cryocrit," based on the percent volume occupied by the precipitate after centrifugation. Another approach to quantitation involves redissolving the washed cryoprecipitate and determining the concentration of immunoglobulins in the precipitate. Cryoglobulins should redissolve when heated to 37°C, demonstrating that the precipitation is reversible.

Some cryoglobulins precipitate at room temperature rather quickly, such that the cryoprecipitate would be lost during routine specimen handling. Therefore, specimens to be tested for cryoglobulins should be rapidly placed at 37°C immediately after phlebotomy. The laboratory staff must also keep the specimen warm during centrifugation.

Cryoglobulins are classified immunochemically into three types: Type 1 consists entirely of a monoclonal immunoglobulin that undergoes temperature- and concentration-dependent self-association or self-aggregation. Type 1 cryoglobulins are usually associated with a lymphoma or myeloma producing large amounts of a monoclonal protein. In contrast to the monoclonal nature of type 1 cryoglobulins, types 2 and 3 are known as "mixed" cryoglobulins because they comprise more than one class of immunoglobulin. Type 2 mixed cryoglobulins consist of both a monoclonal component and a polyclonal component in the cryoprecipitate. Typically the monoclonal component is IgM with RF activity, and the polyclonal component is IgG. Type 3 consists of all polyclonal immunoglobulins, usually with polyclonal IgM containing RF activity, and polyclonal IgG. Because of the RF activity of the IgM components of mixed cryoglobulinemias, patients with mixed cryoglobulinemia typically have positive assays for RF. (Remember that RF activity is defined simply as the ability on an immunoglobulin to bind to the Fc portion of IgG.)

Mixed cryoglobulins are commonly associated with chronic hepatitis C virus infection but also may be present in patients with Sjögren syndrome, rheumatoid arthritis, and some other chronic infections. Very low levels of cryoglobulinemia may also be seen in healthy people. The mixed cryoglobulinemia syndrome and cryoglobulinemic vasculitis involves deposition of immune complexes in tissues. The cryoglobulins are part of the pathogenic immune complexes in these syndromes. Because of the high level of immune complexes, virtually all patients with active mixed cryoglobulinemia syndrome and vasculitis also have depressed levels of C4 complement. The C4 hypocomplementemia, typically low out of proportion to C3, can be an important clue to the presence of cryoglobulins.

SYSTEMIC SCLEROSIS/SCLERODERMA

Nearly all patients with systemic sclerosis (scleroderma) are ANA positive when tested by an immunofluorescence assay using HEp2 cells. The pattern of ANA staining can provide a clue as the specific antibody in the patient's serum. An anticentromere pattern is strongly associated with limited cutaneous disease. A nucleolar staining pattern, on the other hand, is characteristic of the autoantibodies associated with diffuse cutaneous systemic sclerosis.

▶ Anticentromere Antibody

The centromere is the area on chromosomes that attaches to the spindle apparatus during mitosis and meiosis. Although there are multiple centromere proteins, patients with systemic sclerosis make autoantibodies to centromere proteins A and B. Assays for antibodies to those specific proteins are available by ELISA or in the multiplex ANA testing platforms, but since the anticentromere immunofluorescence pattern is so characteristic, it usually does not require confirmation by another method. A large majority of anticentromere antibody-positive patients have the CREST (calcinosis, Raynaud phenomenon, esophageal dysmotility, sclerodactyly, telangiectasia) syndrome variant of limited cutaneous systemic sclerosis, but a few develop diffuse cutaneous disease. Anticentromere antibodies are often present early in the course of disease, when the only clinical manifestation of systemic sclerosis may be Raynaud phenomenon. The presence of anticentromere antibodies in serum of a patient with Raynaud phenomenon, together with presence of abnormal periungual nailfold capillaries, is the predictor of systemic sclerosis.

Anti-topoisomerase 1/Scl70

Antibodies to the DNA coiling/uncoiling enzyme topoisomerase I are strongly associated with systemic sclerosis. They predict a worse prognosis in patients with systemic sclerosis, with greater risk for development of interstitial lung disease, more severe cutaneous disease, and higher mortality. A minority of patients with systemic sclerosis develop anti-Scl70 (low sensitivity), but positive results provide strong support for a diagnosis of systemic sclerosis that is likely to be severe.

Antibodies to RNA Polymerase III (Anti-RNAP3)

Anti-RNAP3 antibodies are associated with systemic sclerosis with worse prognosis for ILD and advanced disease. In addition, they are associated with a higher risk for development of scleroderma renal crisis. They are also associated with a higher risk for cancer, particularly breast cancer, diagnosed within a few years before or after the diagnosis of systemic sclerosis. Some authorities recommend an age-appropriate cancer screen in patients with recent onset of systemic sclerosis and the presence of anti-RNAP3.

Other Autoantibodies

A variety of other autoantibodies have been associated with scleroderma, but most of them are present in a small proportion of patients, have been studied in relatively few patients, and are not routinely available in clinical laboratories. Table 3–8 summarizes autoantibodies associated with scleroderma.

Table 3–8. Autoantibodies associated with scleroderma.

Autoantibody	Clinical Features
Topoisomerase (Scl70)	Diffuse cutaneous systemic sclerosis, interstitial lung disease risk
Anticentromere (centromere protein B)	Limited cutaneous systemic sclerosis, CREST syndrome, pulmonary hypertension
RNA polymerase III	Diffuse cutaneous systemic sclerosis, increased risk for renal involvement and scleroderma renal crisis, increased risk for synchronous malignancy, especially breast cancer
Fibrillarin (U3RNP)	Diffuse cutaneous systemic sclerosis, nucleolar ANA
Th/To	Limited cutaneous systemic sclerosis, pulmonary fibrosis
PM/Scl	Overlap of scleroderma and myositis
Ku	Overlap of scleroderma and myositis
SSA/Ro	Overlap of scleroderma and Sjögren syndrome

MYOSITIS & NECROTIZING MYOPATHY

Patients with active inflammatory myopathy, including dermatomyositis, polymyositis, and necrotizing myopathy, usually have elevated concentrations of proteins released from damaged myocytes. Autoantibodies are also found in many patients. Updated classification criteria for inflammatory myopathy include the muscle damage tests creatine kinase (CK), lactate dehydrogenase (LD), aspartate aminotransferase (AST), and alanine aminotransferase (ALT). Despite substantial interest in myositis-specific autoantibodies, the only autoantibody test that is included in the criteria is anti-Jo-1.

Muscle Damage Markers

A. Myocyte-Specific Damage Markers

Elevated serum levels of CK and myoglobin are very specific for muscle cell damage or leakiness. They are elevated in both skeletal and cardiac muscle damage. Since the CK isoform CK-MB is disproportionately present in cardiomyocytes, CK-MB measurement can help differentiate whether an elevated total CK elevation is due to cardiac rather than skeletal muscle injury. The measurement of cardiac troponin has a similar utility. Mild to moderate increases in serum CK and myoglobin may also be associated with increased muscle mass, recent heavy exercise, and genetic factors.

B. Myocyte-Associated Damage Markers

Many proteins that are released from damaged myocytes are also released from other damaged cells. These include aldolase, the aminotransferases (transaminases) ALT and AST, and LD. Aldolase is often tested as a measure of muscle damage since the enzyme has relatively high concentrations in muscle, but it also can be elevated in patients with liver disease in the absence of muscle damage. Conversely, the aminotransferases are often tested as measures of liver disease, but they can be elevated in patients with muscle disease even in the absence of liver disease. LD can be elevated due to damage to many cell types, including RBCs, hepatocytes, myocytes, and others.

C. Autoantibodies in Myositis

Myositis specific autoantibodies are those found only in inflammatory myopathies (polymyositis and dermatomyositis), in necrotizing myopathies, and in the antisynthetase syndrome (Table 3–9). Antibodies that are found not only in patients with inflammatory myopathy but also in other autoimmune rheumatic diseases are termed myositis-associated autoantibodies (MAA).

A. Myositis-Specific Autoantibodies

More than one-half of adult patients with idiopathic inflammatory myopathy have an identifiable myositis-specific autoantibody (MSA), but the only MSA assay that is commonly

Table 3–9. Myositis-specific autoantibodies.

Antibody	Antigen	Clinical	Approximate % of Adult Myositis
Jo-1 PL-7, PL-12, EJ, OJ, KS, Zo, Ha	His-tRNA synthetase Various RNA synthetases	**Synthetase syndrome:** myositis, mechanic's hands, high-frequency ILD, Gottron papules, arthritis, Raynaud phenomenon.	20 1–4 each antibody
Mi-2	Nucleosome deacetylase ATPase	**Skin disease (classic dermatomyositis).** Myositis with good response to treatment.	10
p155/140, TIF1γ	Transcription intermediary factor 1-γ	**Cancer-associated dermatomyositis in adults,** severe skin disease. Juvenile dermatomyositis.	10–15
NXP-2 (MJ)	Nuclear matrix protein-2	**Calcinosis** in dermatomyositis. Associated with malignancy. Juvenile dermatomyositis.	1–5
MDA-5 (CADM-140)	Melanoma differentiation factor 5, an RNA helicase	**Skin disease (dermatomyositis) and rapidly progressive lung disease.** Often without overt muscle disease = **"Amyopathic dermatomyositis"**	15
SAE	Small ubiquitin-like modifier-activating enzyme	**Skin disease, dysphagia.** Possible cancer association.	1
SRP	Signal recognition peptide	**Necrotizing myopathy, often poor treatment response,** cardiac myositis.	5
HMG CoA reductase	3-hydroxy-3-methyl-glutaryl-CoA reductase (target of statin therapy)	**Necrotizing myopathy. Often associated with statin use.** Responds to immunosuppressives.	5–10

available as a standardized clinical test detects antibodies directed against the Jo-1 antigen. Anti-Jo-1 antibodies are found in approximately 20% of patients with inflammatory myopathy. The antigen recognized by anti-Jo-1 antibodies is histidyl transfer RNA synthetase, the enzyme responsible for adding high-energy phosphate to the tRNA that adds the peptide histidine in the ribosome. Multiple other RNA synthetases are also occasionally the targets of autoantibodies, including the PL-7, PL-12, EJ, KS, and OJ antigens. Patients with antisynthetase autoantibodies may have myositis, characteristic rashes, polyarthritis, and interstitial lung disease, collectively considered the "antisynthetase syndrome."

Anti-melanoma differentiation-associated 5 (MDA5) antibodies are notable because they are associated with prominent dermatologic findings of dermatomyositis and the potential for rapid progression of interstitial lung disease or alveolitis, sometimes with little overt muscle inflammation or weakness. Antibodies to HMG CoA reductase (the enzyme inhibited by statin drugs) are associated with the necrotizing myopathy that can follow treatment with statins. Patients with benign myalgias associated with statin use, in contrast, do not develop these autoantibodies. Autoantibodies to TIF1γ and NXP-2 are associated with malignancy. Other MSAs include anti-SRP, which typically is associated with a relatively refractory necrotizing myopathy.

B. Myositis-Associated Autoantibodies

Some autoantibodies present in patients with inflammatory myopathies can also be detected in patients with other autoimmune rheumatic diseases. These include anti-SSA/Ro antibodies (also present in SLE, Sjögren syndrome, systemic sclerosis, and rheumatoid arthritis); anti-U1-RNP antibodies (also found with SLE, mixed connective tissue disease, and systemic sclerosis); anti-PM/Scl antibodies (detected in scleroderma/myositis overlap); and anti-Ku antibodies (seen in systemic sclerosis and SLE). Approximately one-third of patients with inclusion body myositis have antibodies to cytosolic 5'-nucleotidase 1A, but the autoantibody is also seen in a variety of other rheumatologic conditions.

Lundberg IE, Tjärnlund A, Bottai M, et al. 2017 European League Against Rheumatism/American College of Rheumatology Classification Criteria for Adult and Juvenile Idiopathic Inflammatory Myopathies and Their Major Subgroups. Arthritis Rheumatol. 2017;69:2271-2282. [PMID: 29106061]

Nathwani RA, Pais S, Reynolds TB, Kaplowitz N. Serum alanine aminotransferase in skeletal muscle diseases. Hepatology. 2005;41:380-382. [PMID: 15660433]

Pisetsky DS. Antinuclear antibody testing—misunderstood or misbegotten? Perspective. Nature Rev Rheum. 2017;13:495-502. [PMID: 28541299]

Satoh M, Tanaka S, Ceribelli A, et al. A comprehensive overview on myositis-specific antibodies: new and old biomarkers in idiopathic inflammatory myopathy. Clin Rev Allergy Immunol. 2017;52:1-19. [PMID: 26424665]

GENETIC TESTING

▶ HLA Typing

Multiple genetic factors contribute to the pathogenesis and etiology of inflammatory rheumatic diseases. For most inflammatory rheumatic diseases, the dominant genetic risk contributors lie in the major histocompatibility complex (MHC), and within the MHC, the most important genes are in the human leukocyte antigen (HLA) loci. For the rheumatic diseases with prominent autoantibodies, class II HLA loci (HLA-DR, -DQ, and -DP) are responsible for the highest risk. Autoantibody responses and HLA associations are often closely linked. This is because class II HLA molecules govern the ability of antigen-presenting cells to present peptide antigens to T cells, promote a robust immune response with T-cell help, and to produce high levels of high-affinity antibodies. This has an important practical implication in rheumatoid arthritis. Although HLA-DR*0401 and other shared epitope HLA types are closely linked and provide important prognostic information in rheumatoid arthritis, the presence of the shared epitope is closely linked to the development of ACPA/antiCCP antibodies. Autoantibody testing is more convenient, less expensive, and more clinically predictive than testing HLA type in symptomatic patients with inflammatory arthritis. For these reasons, even though the association between the shared epitope within the HLA region and the diagnosis of rheumatoid arthritis is strong and biologically important, HLA typing is not indicated outside of research settings in patients with rheumatoid arthritis.

The seronegative spondyloarthropathies with axial skeleton involvement are strongly linked to HLA-B27, an HLA class I antigen. Up to 90% of patients with ankylosing spondylitis have HLA-B27. Although the relative risk of having a spondyloarthropathy in someone who inherited HLA-B27 is high compared with the general population, only a minority of HLA-B27+ individuals develop a spondyloarthropathy (approximately 8% of Caucasians are HLA-B27+). It is also important to bear in mind that even HLA-B27-negative individuals can develop ankylosing spondylitis.

Although the majority of individuals who are HLA-B27 positive do not develop spondyloarthropathy, testing for HLA-B27 does have a role in clarifying the diagnosis. The ASAS (Assessment of SpondyloArthritis International Society) criteria for spondyloarthropathies include the presence of HLA-B27. Testing for HLA-B27 is most likely to be informative in patients with possible inflammatory back pain in the absence of imaging features that are diagnostic of a spondyloarthritis.

Another rheumatic disease linked to HLA class I genes is Behcet disease, a form of vasculitis linked to HLA-B51.

Depending on what population is studied, about one-third to two-thirds of patients with Behcet disease carry the HLA-B51 allele, but only a small minority of patients with the allele develop the disease. Given this lack of sensitivity and specificity, testing for the presence of the allele has a limited role, but HLA typing for HLA-B51 may be useful in borderline or equivocal cases.

Jutkowitz E, Dubreuil M, Lu N, Kuntz KM, Choi HK. The cost-effectiveness of HLA-B*5801 screening to guide initial urate-lowering therapy for gout in the United States. *Semin Arthritis Rheum.* 2017;46:594-600. [PMID: 27916277]

Lim CSE, Sengupta R, Gaffney K. The clinical utility of human leucocyte antigen B27 in axial spondyloarthritis. *Rheumatology (Oxford).* 2018;57(6):959-968. [PMID: 29029331]

The metabolism and immune and inflammatory responses to medications are under genetic control. HLA typing can help predict toxicity of certain medications, including allopurinol. The risk for cutaneous and systemic reactions to allopurinol, which can be severe and life-threatening, is strongly associated with HLA-B*5801. There is substantial geographic variation in the frequency of that allotype, with higher prevalence in East Asia and in parts of Africa than in Europe. American College of Rheumatology guidelines for treatment of gout indicate that testing for HLA-B*5801 is conditionally recommended in those of Southeast Asian descent (eg, Han Chinese, Korean, or Thai) and African-Americans.

DIAGNOSTIC & CLINICAL UTILITY

To avoid unnecessary health care costs, it is worth considering if laboratory tests are necessary or cost-effective for a given patient. In general, the history, physical examination, and routine laboratory tests including hematology and chemistry studies and urinalysis can guide the diagnostic autoantibody laboratory workup. Laboratory tests generally help to confirm the clinical diagnosis already suspected by prior evaluation, and are particularly useful when the pretest probability (clinical suspicion of disease) is in the 20–90% range. Diagnostic and prognostic laboratory tests should be ordered if they help establish an unknown or uncertain diagnosis, or if the result will lead to a change in treatment or other management.

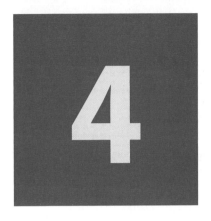

Hand & Wrist Pain:
A Systematic Approach

Janice He, MD

Neal Chen, MD

A large number of diagnoses are possible when a patient presents with pain in the hand, wrist, or elbow. However, a clinician can often reduce the broad differential diagnosis to either one most likely possibility or a small number of potential considerations by taking a systematic approach to history and examination. When etiology, anatomic location, and epidemiology are cross-referenced relative to one another, the number of possible diagnoses narrows substantially.

We begin this chapter with a review of the hand and wrist anatomy.

▶ Hand & Wrist Anatomy

A. Bones and Joints

- Two forearm bones, the radius and ulna, which articulate at the distal radioulnar joint. These bones permit forearm rotation (pronation and supination).
- Eight carpal bones arranged into two rows, referred to as the "proximal row" (scaphoid, lunate, triquetrum, pisiform) and the "distal row" (trapezium, trapezoid, capitate, hamate).
- Five metacarpal bones, one for the thumb and each of the other digits.
- The thumb has two phalanges; each of the remaining digits has three phalanges.
- The joints between the carpal bones and metacarpal bones are known as carpometacarpal (CMC) joints.
- The joints between the metacarpal and the proximal phalanges are known as metacarpophalangeal (MCP) joints.
- The joints between the phalanges make up the proximal and distal interphalangeal (PIP and DIP) joints.

B. Extrinsic Digital Extensors

- Extension of the digits is controlled by muscles in the dorsal forearm, which terminate as tendons that insert terminally on the dorsal aspect of the distal phalanges.

- The extensor digitorum communis (EDC), the main digital extensor, gives off a tendon to each digit except the thumb.
- The index and small fingers each have their own extensor in addition (extensor indicis proprius and extensor digiti quinti, respectively). These muscles provide independent extension of those two digits.
- The thumb has its own extensor, extensor pollicis longus (EPL).
- The sagittal bands, an expansion of connective tissue over the MCP joints, keep the extensor tendon centralized over the MCP joint. Rupture, typically of the radial-sided sagittal band, causes extensor tendon dislocation in an ulnar direction, eventually leading to ulnar drift of the digits.

C. Extrinsic Digital Flexors & Pulley System

- Digital flexion is controlled by muscles in the volar forearm. These muscles terminate as tendons that insert on the middle and distal phalanges.
- Each nonthumb digit has two flexor tendons. The flexor digitorum superficialis (FDS) flexes at the PIP joint and the flexor digitorum profundus (FDP) flexes the digits at the DIP joint. To test tendon integrity, motion across the PIP and DIP joints must be tested separately.
- The thumb has its own flexor, the flexor pollicis longus (FPL).
- The flexor tendons are constrained against the bone by bands of connective tissue called pulleys. These maximize tendon excursion. Rupture of a pulley may result in bowstringing: The tendon moves away from the bone, limiting both excursion and increasing the moment arm of the tendon on the joints, giving a mechanical advantage to the flexors compared to the extensors. This results in a digit that is unable to actively reach full extension or full flexion.

D. Intrinsic Muscles

- The intrinsic muscles are those that arise from the hand, as opposed to extrinsic muscles which arise from the forearm.
- Intrinsic muscles include the thenar muscles (abductor pollicis brevis, opponens pollicis, flexor pollicis brevis); the hypothenar muscles (abductor digiti minimi, opponens digit minimi, flexor digiti minimi brevis); the interossei (4 dorsal and 3 palmar); and the lumbricals (4).
- The thenar muscles are responsible for complex motion of the thumb. The hypothenar muscles are responsible for complex motion of the small finger. Together they allow for opposition of the thumb to small finger.
- The dorsal interossei allow the digits to abduct and the palmar interossei to adduct.
- The lumbricals extend the digits at the PIP and DIP joints, and flex at the MCP joints.

E. Nerves

- The median nerve innervates the thenar muscles, as well as the two more radial lumbricals. The median nerve, along with its branch the anterior interosseus nerve, also innervates the extrinsic flexors of the digits and thumb. It provides sensation to the volar aspect of the hand and the thumb, index, long fingers, and the radial half of the ring finger.
- The ulnar nerve innervates all of the intrinsic muscles not innervated by the median nerve. It provides sensation to the ulnar aspect of the ring finger and the small finger, on both the volar and dorsal sides.
- The radial nerve innervates the extrinsic extensors of the fingers. It provides sensation to the radial half of the dorsal hand, including the thumb and first webspace.
- The median, ulnar, and radial nerves terminate as the digital nerves. Each digit has a radial and ulnar digital nerve that covers half of the digit respectively. These digital nerves can be tested separately.

F. Vessels

- The radial and ulnar arteries supply the hand and wrist.
- These two arteries form the superficial and deep palmar arches, which give off two digital arteries to each finger.
- Patients with complete palmar arches only require either the radial or the ulnar arteries, but not both, to be patent to supply the hand. Those with incomplete palmar arches may have ischemia if either artery is thrombosed or injured.
- Each digit only requires one patent digital artery.

▶ Approaching Hand, Wrist, & Elbow Pain

A useful method of approaching hand, wrist, and elbow pain is to have a framework to organize common diagnoses and to maintain a systematic approach when the diagnosis remains unclear following the initial assessment. Diagnosis groups can be considered by anatomic structure:

Bone and joints: Pain related to bones and joints is commonly the result of fractures, degenerative joint disease, or inflammatory arthritides. Less commonly, the pain may be a result of bony tumors, avascular necrosis following trauma, or idiopathic osteonecrosis. Pathology within a joint may manifest itself as a loss of passive range of motion (PROM).

Soft tissue: Pain within soft tissues is most frequently secondary to tendinopathy, tenosynovitis, or tendon/ligament strain or rupture. In such situations, the pain is usually localized to the structure involved but can also appear to affect the joint above or below the affected tendon if the structure involved traverses multiple joints. Tendon rupture results in loss of specific function, for example, the ability to flex or extend a specific joint. Ligament laxity or rupture, in contrast, leads to a loss of stability. Infection usually manifests with swelling, erythema, and pain.

Vascular: Pain may be associated with ischemia. This may be the result of thromboembolic events, injury, or vasospasm. In these situations, it is important to consider the proximal vascular anatomy. Ischemic pain presents with changes in circulation and color.

Nervous: Compression neuropathies and nerve injury may also be a cause of pain in the hand and wrist. Compression neuropathies are prevalent and usually present with numbness or paresthesias, but can also present as a painful extremity. This is especially true in the cases of acute onset nerve compression, such as in trauma. Patients may have both a sensation deficit in the distribution of the nerve, but also a focal area of pain at the site of nerve laceration.

Referred: Pain in the hand may also be referred from another part of the body. As an example, cervical spine pathology frequently results in symptoms of the hand and forearm.

A. History

History alone can diagnose many conditions affecting the hand, wrist, and elbow. The diagnosis strongly suspected on the strength of the history can then be confirmed by physical examination findings or other studies selected on the basis of the history.

1. History of present illness—Important historical factors include the following:

1. Specific anatomic location.
2. **Time course of onset:** Critical distinctions exist between conditions that are chronic in nature and those that are acute. The time course of symptoms, for example, can

distinguish among a fracture at the base of the first metacarpal, a nonunited fracture at the base of the first metacarpal, and late arthrosis after a malunited fracture at the base of the first metacarpal. It is also useful to characterize the progression of the problem over time. Was there an acute event superimposed upon a chronic process?

3. **Aggravating and alleviating factors:** Pain that is worse with use is a frequent complaint in patients with symptomatic osteoarthritis. Patients with osteoarthritis at the base of the thumb—the first CMC joint—often have greater pain with specific activities such as pinching or repetitive use of the thumb. Symptoms that occur with specific movements focus the diagnosis quickly. For example, patients with subluxation of the extensor carpi ulnaris (ECU) tendon typically have pain with circumduction of the wrist. Compressive neuropathies are often aggravated by specific positions. A prime illustration of this is the patient with cubital tunnel syndrome observes that holding a cell phone to his ear exacerbates the symptoms tingling in the little and ring fingers.

4. **Associated symptoms:** Consideration of constitutional symptoms as well as symptoms at other sites of the musculoskeletal system can be crucial in piecing together complex diagnoses that present with symptoms in the hand and wrist. Axial neck pain with radicular symptoms can help identify foraminal stenosis in the cervical spine.

2. Demographics—Many conditions have predilections for specific age groups or affect the genders in an unequal manner. de Quervain tenosynovitis, for example, commonly causes pain on the radial side of the wrist and is an occupational exposure for women who are either pregnant or postpartum.

3. Past medical and surgical history—Inflammatory arthropathies and systemic illnesses sometimes come to medical attention because of symptoms focusing on hands and wrists. Diabetes mellitus not only predisposes patients to musculoskeletal disorders such a median nerve entrapment (carpal tunnel syndrome) and trigger finger, but it is also a comorbidity that may impact treatment considerations. Poorly controlled diabetics may have problems with blood glucose regulation after a glucocorticoid injection.

4. Social history—The patient's hand dominance, occupation, and preferred recreational activities may contribute to symptoms. Smoking and injection drug history may play a role in vascular problems or infections.

B. Physical Examination

A systematic approach to the hand examination is essential, but the focus will vary according to information obtained in the history.

1. Inspection—Every hand exam begins with inspection for skin quality, deformity, resting position, and contour and bulk of the musculature. Notable findings may be thin skin, ulcerations, changes in pigmentation, or rubor. Plaques or rashes may be the result of a broader systemic illness. In patients with peripheral neuropathy, the skin in the affected distribution may be noticeably drier. Ecchymoses often accompany fractures. Fingernails may demonstrate pitting in psoriatic arthritis. A dark stripe in the fingernail (melanonychia) can be a manifestation of melanoma. Digital clubbing may reflect a pulmonary process.

Bone and soft tissue tumors, fractures, and arthritis may be associated with a noticeable deformity on examination. Ganglia typically occur on the dorsal wrist, on the volar-radial wrist, at the volar MCP joint, and the dorsal DIP joint (mucous cyst). It is worthwhile to be aware of general patterns as this can help predict what type of mass may be present. Arthritis at the base of the thumb may present with deformity at that site, but some patients also develop a compensatory hyperextension of the MCP joint of the thumb.

A patient's resting hand posture may also provide specific clues. A patient with flexor tenosynovitis will hold the affected digit in a semiflexed position. A patient long-standing ulnar neuropathy may demonstrate clawing, with slightly flexed positioning of the ring and small fingers. Patients with rheumatoid arthritis or lupus may present with swan neck or boutonniere deformities of the fingers, ulnar deviation, or subluxation of the MCP joints.

In patients with long-standing peripheral neuropathy or cervical radiculopathy, muscle atrophy and contour changes may be present. Ulnar neuropathy or a C8 radiculopathy can result in atrophy of the interossei, where the muscle between the metacarpals becomes sunken. Severe median neuropathy leads to loss of the thenar musculature on the thumb.

2. Palpation—Palpation can be useful to find areas of tenderness that can help localize the pathology. When a mass is encountered, it is important to consider whether the mass is fixed to other structures, if it is firm or soft, and if there are any areas of proximal lymphadenopathy. Scaphoid fractures are notably tender in the "anatomic snuffbox" or scaphoid tubercle. Important areas of tenderness are demonstrated in Figure 4–1.

3. Range of motion—Loss of range of motion can arise from an intrinsic limitation of a joint or an extrinsic limitation such as a contracture of a muscle or other soft tissue. An assessment of range of motion is performed in two parts. Active range of motion (AROM) is the degree of movement that the patient generates volitionally. In contrast, PROM is the range of motion the examiner can achieve by moving the joint. If AROM is less than PROM, it is likely that the joint is sound but that there is a problem with a muscle or a tendon. A reduction in PROM, however, may result from either an intrinsic or extrinsic limitation.

Many conditions may cause progressive loss of motion, such as with osteoarthritis and Dupuytren's contracture.

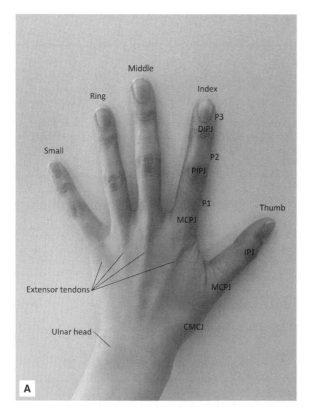

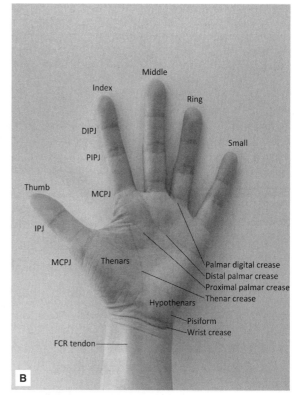

▲ **Figure 4–1. A.** Dorsal hand. **B.** Volar hand.

Masses or traumatic injuries may cause blocks to motion, such as with a malunited fracture that limits flexion or extension of a joint. Important joints to test are as follows:

1. **Wrist:** flexion, extension, pronation, supination, radial deviation, ulnar deviation
2. **Digits:** flexion and extension at MCP, PIP, and DIP joints
3. **Thumb:** flexion and extension at the IP joint, radial abduction, palmar abduction, and composite opposition of the thumb to the little finger

4. Sensation—Sensation is checked in the peripheral nerve distributions of the hand, which include the median, ulnar and radial nerves. Thorough sensation testing includes the evaluation of light touch two-point discrimination, vibration, and pressure testing.

5. Motor—Loss of motor function can result from a central lesion, peripheral nerve dysfunction, muscle disease, and mechanical limitation of a joint.

Patterns of motor loss are important to recognize. Patients with cervical root compression, brachial plexopathy, or peripheral nerve compression will present with specific patterns of weakness. Nerve injury presents with different patterns of motor and sensory deficit. Patients with rheumatoid arthritis and inability to extend the fingers may have either extensor tendon subluxation of the fingers, tendon ruptures, or radial nerve palsy at the elbow. Specific muscle testing is used to distinguish between these different possibilities (Table 4–1).

In compressive neuropathies, sensory deficits typically appear first, with the emergence of motor deficits as the compressive neuropathy progresses. For example, in carpal tunnel syndrome, numbness of the radial three digits is often the presenting complaint. However, as the compressive neuropathy worsens, thenar weakness and muscle atrophy become noticeable.

6. Strength—Strength testing is useful in quantifying hand function and tracking a patient's progress and recovery. Manual muscle strength is tested by direct confrontation of a muscle group by the examiner.

7. Vascular—Large vessels such as the radial and ulnar arteries should be palpable. A pulsatile mass may represent an aneurysm. Thrills may be palpable. An Allen test is performed to evaluate whether the ulnar and radial arteries are connected distally in the hand or if they are separate systems. If the ulnar and radial arteries are separate systems,

Table 4–1. Muscles and nerves of the upper extremity.

Action	Muscle(s)	Peripheral Nerve	Nerve Roots
Shoulder abduction	Deltoid	Axillary	C5
Shoulder internal rotation	Subscapularis	Subscapular	C5
Shoulder external rotation	Infraspinatus	Suprascapular	C5
Elbow flexion with forearm supinated	Biceps and brachialis	Musculocutaneous	C5
Elbow flexion with forearm pronated	Brachioradalis	Radial	C5
Wrist extension	Extensor carpi radialis longus (ECRL)	Radial	C6
Wrist supination	Supinator	Radial	C6
Elbow extension	Triceps	Radial	C7
Wrist flexion	Flexor carpi radialis (FCR)	Median	C7
Wrist pronation	Pronator teres and pronator quadratus	Median	C7
Digit flexion at metacarpophalangeal (MCP) joint and proximal interphalangeal (PIP) joint	Flexor digitorum superficialis (FDS)	Median	C8
Digit flexion at distal interphalangeal (DIP) joint	Flexor digitorum profundus (FDP)	AIN (1st and 2nd), ulnar (3rd and 4th)	C8
Thumb extension	Extensor pollicis longus (EPL)	PIN	C8
Digit abduction	Dorsal interossei	Ulnar	T1

one should take caution in performing any procedure to either vessel.

An Allen test begins by having the examiner exert digital pressure to occlude both the radial and ulnar arteries. The patient then closes the hand repeatedly until the palm and digits blanch. The radial artery is released and the time until capillary refill returns is measured. This maneuver is repeated for the ulnar artery. If the refill takes longer than 7 seconds, then the radial and ulnar systems are likely to be independent.

Capillary refill is another way to assess vascular inflow. This is assessed by putting pressure on a distal finger (eg, the skin of the distal phalanx), compressing briefly so as to make the skin blanch, and assessing the time it takes for the finger to return to a pink color. Normal capillary refill time is less than 2 seconds.

8. Special Tests—There are a multitude of examination maneuvers described to help discriminate one condition from another (Table 4–2). For instance, in patients with base of thumb pain, Finkelstein maneuver and the grind test are helpful to distinguish between de Quervain tenosynovitis and basal joint arthritis.

C. Imaging

1. Radiographs—Many conditions do not require imaging, because the sources of pain caused by soft tissue, nervous or vascular conditions have unambiguous findings on physical

examination. Radiographs are beneficial, however, for cases in which bone involvement is suspected or when the diagnosis is unclear. They are not only useful for fractures but also show tumors, arthritic conditions, osteonecrosis, and soft tissue injuries that have led to disruption of the normal relationship between bones.

2. Ultrasound—Ultrasound facilitates the evaluation of soft tissue masses in the hand and is particularly useful in evaluating masses to determine whether they are solid or cystic, and for the evaluation of suspected aneurysms.

3. Computed tomography (CT) scan—CT is useful to delineate complex bony anatomy. In situations of complex fractures, a CT scan can provide a three-dimensional view to characterize fractures in a comprehensive manner. For example, CT scanning is extremely useful to evaluate displacement in scaphoid fractures and intra-articular interphalangeal joint fractures.

4. Magnetic resonance imaging (MRI)—MRI is useful in evaluating soft tissue within the limits of resolution. Evaluation of small structures, such as intercarpal ligaments and the triangulofibrocartilage complex, depends on the quality of the MRI magnet and coil. The interpretation of these films is highly dependent upon the radiologist.

MRI is valuable for evaluating occult scaphoid and other fractures that are not apparent on radiographs. MRI has some

Table 4–2. Provocative exam maneuvers.

Test	Condition	Maneuver
CMC grind	Basal joint arthritis	Grip first metacarpal and rotate while applying axial load. A positive test elicits pain.
Finkelstein	de Quervain tenosynovitis	The patient closes their fingers over the thumb and ulnarly deviate at the wrist. A positive test elicits pain.
Scaphoid shift (Watson)	SL ligament rupture	Place thumb over volar aspect of distal pole of scaphoid. With constant pressure over the distal pole, move wrist from extension/ulnar deviation into flexion/radial deviation. Positive test when maneuver elicits dorsal wrist pain and a clunk.
Tinel	Nerve compression or injury	Tap over the site of nerve compression or nerve compression. A positive test elicits electric shock sensations in that nerve distribution.
Phalen	Carpal tunnel syndrome	The patient is asked to maximally flex their wrists with the dorsal aspects of their metacarpals touching each other in front of their chest. A positive test reproduces carpal tunnel symptoms when held in this position for 30 seconds.
Durkan	Carpal tunnel syndrome	Place thumb over carpal tunnel on palmar aspect of hand. A positive test reproduces carpal tunnel symptoms when compressed for 30 seconds.
Wartenberg	Ulnar neuropathy	The small finger appears to be abducted due to unopposed action of EDQ and weakness of the intrinsics.
Jeanne	Ulnar neuropathy	The patient is asked to make an "OK" sign by touching their thumb to their index finger. A positive test elicits involuntary thumb IP flexion and CMC hyperextension.
Spurling	Cervical radiculopathy	Turn the patient's head to the affected side and slightly extend the neck. A positive sign reproduces radicular symptoms.
Tenodesis	Tendon rupture	The patient is asked to relax. The examiner holds the forearm and the wrist is passively flexed and extended. When the wrist is extended, the fingers should flex. When the wrist is flexed, the fingers should extend. Abnormal movement or cascade of digits suggests tendon injury.

CMC, carpometacarpal; EDQ, extensor digiti quinti; IP, interphalangeal; SL, scapholunate.

role in evaluating intra-articular injuries. Depending on the institution, an arthrogram may be utilized to study intra-articular pathology such as scapholunate ligament injury and triangular fibrocartilage complex (TFCC) tears.

D. Other Tests

1. Electromyography/nerve conduction velocity (EMG/NCV)—Neurodiagnostic tests are typically used to evaluate compressive neuropathy. EMG/NCV gives information about the speed of conduction, amplitude of the electrical signal, and physiologic changes in the muscle. These variables correspond to demyelination of the nerve, axonal loss, and atrophy or regeneration of the muscle. An EMG may also be useful in differentiating compressive peripheral neuropathy from either a brachial plexopathy or cervical radiculopathy, but the sensitivity of EMG/NCV for these latter two lesions is limited.

▶ Differential Diagnosis

In general, our approach is to constructing a differential diagnosis involves organization by anatomic area.

Elbow

Elbow pain can be due to arthritis but is also commonly caused by tendinopathy of the wrist extensors, wrist flexors,

and distal biceps. Prior elbow injury, participation in sports, occupational risk factors, and history of inflammatory arthritis are important to note. Arthritis of the elbow is most frequently inflammatory or posttraumatic in nature and is characterized by progressive pain and loss of range of motion. Tendonitis is often associated with specific occupations or sports as they are overuse injuries. Tendonitis can be diagnosed on examination by eliciting pain when the patient fires the involved muscle group against resistance. Common musculoskeletal conditions affecting the elbow are shown in Table 4–3.

Base of Thumb/Radial Side of Wrist

Most cases of pain on the radial side of the wrist can be attributed to three major problems: (1) arthritis of the trapeziometacarpal joint (also known as basal joint arthritis or CMC arthritis); (2) de Quervain tenosynovitis; or (3) a scaphoid fracture. Two physical examination maneuvers are useful in the evaluation of pain in the radial wrist area. First, Finkelstein maneuver involves circling the four fingers around the thumb and then deviating the wrist in an ulnar direction (Figure 4–2). This is particularly useful in diagnosing cases of de Quervain tenosynovitis. Second, palpation of the "anatomical snuffbox," that is, the space bounded by the first dorsal extensor compartment, the third dorsal extensor

Table 4–3. Disorders of the elbow.

Degenerative arthritis	**HPI:** Progressive pain worse with use, loss of terminal range of motion, mechanical locking or clicking with use, commonly posttraumatic from prior fracture or from rheumatoid arthritis. Rarely caused by primary osteoarthritis. **Exam:** Diminished range of motion, with loss of terminal flexion and extension first, followed by loss of pronation-supination in later disease. **Studies:** Radiographs show loss of joint space, cystic changes, osteophyte formation, loose bodies. **Non-op Tx:** Activity modification, NSAIDs, glucocorticoid injection. **Surgery:** Elbow arthroscopy and loose body removal. Elbow arthroplasty rarely used.
Lateral epicondylitis	**HPI:** Usually atraumatic, subacute onset. Aggravated by gripping. **Exam:** Pain with resisted wrist and long finger extension. Diminished grip strength. Tenderness over common extensor origin at lateral epicondyle. **Studies:** Radiographs usually negative. May show calcifications. **Non-op Tx:** Activity modification, physical therapy, NSAIDs, glucocorticoid injection. **Surgery:** Rarely indicated.
Medial epicondylitis	**HPI:** Usually atraumatic, with subacute onset, often seen as overuse injury in throwing athletes, associated with cubital tunnel and valgus instability. **Exam:** Pain with resisted pronation and wrist flexion. Tenderness over medial epicondyle. **Studies:** Radiographs usually negative. May show calcifications. **Non-op Tx:** Activity modification, physical therapy, NSAIDs, glucocorticoid injection. **Surgery:** Debridement and reattachment of tendon. Rarely indicated.
Distal biceps tendinopathy	**HPI:** Anterior elbow pain. Subacute in onset. **Exam:** Pain with resisted elbow flexion and supination. **Studies:** Radiographs are normal. **Non-op Tx:** Activity modification, physical therapy, NSAIDs. **Surgery:** Debridement and reattachment of tendon. Rarely indicated.
Distal biceps rupture	**HPI:** Acute anterior elbow pain as the patient moves from flexion to extension while holding a weight in the hand. **Exam:** An examiner is normally able to the hook index finger under patient's distal biceps tendon when the patient's elbow is flexed at 90 degrees and the forearm is fully supinated. Inability to feel the tendon constitutes a positive test. **Studies:** Radiographs are normal. MRI is useful to distinguish between full- and partial-thickness tears, as well as to gauge the amount of retraction. **Non-op Tx:** Physical therapy for those with partial tears or for elderly, low-demand patients. **Surgery:** Surgical repair in those with full-thickness tears or for partial-thickness tears that do not respond to nonoperative treatment.

MRI, magnetic resonance imaging; NSAIDs, nonsteroidal anti-inflammatory drugs.

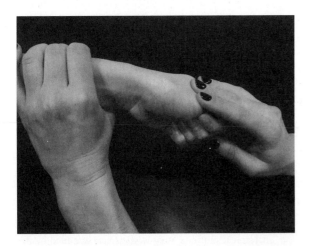

▲ **Figure 4–2.** Finkelstein test.

compartment, and the radial styloid, elicits tenderness in the setting of scaphoid fractures (Table 4–4).

Thumb Metacarpophalangeal Joint

The two most common causes of pain at the thumb MCP joint include trigger thumb and ulnar collateral injury. Trigger thumb is typically an overuse injury leading to thickening and stenosis of the A1 pulley on the palmar side of the joint. Skiier thumb is an acute injury to the ulnar collateral ligament. Gamekeeper' thumb represents a more chronic injury.

Trigger thumb and ulnar collateral injury can usually be distinguished on the basis of history, and the diagnostic suspicion can be confirmed easily on physical examination. Special maneuvers to distinguish between the two include (1) detection of palpable clicking over the A1 pulley when the patient is asked to flex the IP joint of the thumb and (2) instability at the thumb MCP joint with radial stress (Table 4–5).

Table 4–4. Disorders of the radial side of the wrist.

Basal joint arthritis	**HPI:** Atraumatic, subacute onset; worse with use. **Exam:** + CMC grind test (Figure 4–3), diminished pinch strength compared to contralateral hand. **Studies:** XR shows degenerative change of the CMC joint. **Non-op Tx:** Glucocorticoid injection, splinting (particularly at night). **Surgery:** Usually trapziectomy, although technique is highly variable.
STT arthritis	**HPI:** Atraumatic, subacute onset; worse with use. **Exam:** Pain with loading of the thumb metacarpal, diminished pinch strength compared to contralateral side. **Studies:** XR with degenerative change of the STT joint. **Non-op Tx:** Glucocorticoid injection, splinting. **Surgery:** Multiple options including fusion or partial excision.
de Quervain tenosynovitis	**HPI:** Atraumatic, subacute onset; worse with use; more common in younger women. Frequently seen in pregnant/postpartum women and in diabetics. **Exam:** Tenderness over first dorsal extensor compartment, + Finkelstein test. **Studies:** Unnecessary. **Non-op Tx:** Glucocorticoid injection. **Surgery:** Surgical release of first extensor compartment if recurs after injection. **Pathophysiology:** Inflammation and edema of extensor tendons (APL + EPB) in the first extensor compartment.
Scaphoid fracture	**HPI:** Acute onset after fall onto a hyperextended wrist. More common in young men. **Exam:** Tenderness in anatomic snuffbox, possible swelling although not always present. **Studies:** Standard wrist XR may be negative. Scaphoid view has higher sensitivity. CT scan needed to assess displacement (which might be an indication for surgery). **Non-op Tx:** Thumb spica casting for fractures with <1 mm displacement. **Surgery:** ORIF[a] if displacement >1 mm.

[a]ORIF = open reduction, internal fixation.
APL, abductor pollicis longus; CMC, carpometacarpal; CT, computed tomography; EPB, extensor pollicis brevis; STT, scaphotrapezoid trapezial; XR, x-ray.

Dorsal Wrist

Dorsal wrist pain is most frequently attributable to fracture, extensor tendinitis, occult dorsal ganglia, metacarpal boss, or scapholunate ligament injury.

Palpation of specific anatomic structures, such as the radiocarpal joint, radioscaphoid interval, and distal radial-ulnar joint (DRUJ), is also helpful in parsing the variety of pathologies associated with dorsal wrist pain (Table 4–6).

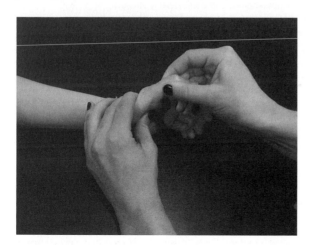

▲ **Figure 4–3.** Grind test.

Table 4–5. Disorders of the first carpometacarpal joint.

Trigger thumb	**HPI:** Atraumatic, subacute onset. Pain over A1 pulley. Clicking or locking with flexion of the IP joint of the thumb. Awakening with locked thumb. **Exam:** Tenderness over A1 pulley. Reproducible, palpable clicking over A1 when the patient flexes or extends the IP joint. **Studies:** Unnecessary. **Non-op Tx:** Glucocorticoid injection, opponens splinting. **Surgery:** Surgical release of A1 pulley if injection and splinting fail to relieve symptoms. **Pathophysiology:** Stenosis of the A1 pulley.
Ulnar collateral Ligament injury (skiier or gamekeeper thumb)	**HPI:** History of thumb injury or sprain. **Exam:** Localized swelling. Instability with radial stress at the MCP joint. **Studies:** Helpful to exclude thumb fractures, particularly avulsion fracture. **Non-op Tx:** Thumb spica casting or splinting. **Surgery:** Ligament repair, especially in high-demand patients. Acute repair is necessary in the presence of a Stener lesion (when the adductor aponeurosis becomes interposed between the ulnar collateral ligament and its attachment site).

IP, interphalangeal; MCP, metacarpophalangeal.

Table 4–6. Disorders of the dorsal wrist.

Distal radius fracture	**HPI:** History of trauma, usually with a fall onto an outstretched hand. **Exam:** Swelling, ecchymoses, sometimes obvious wrist deformity. **Studies:** Plain radiographs for diagnosis. CT scan occasionally required. **Non-op Tx:** Closed reduction and splinting with serial XR to ensure no loss of reduction, nonoperative management typically for elderly and low-demand patients, even if there is some displacement. **Surgery:** ORIF if unacceptable alignment.
Extensor tenosynovitis	**HPI:** Insidious onset of pain with finger extension. Can occur with overuse or in the setting of systemic inflammation. **Exam:** Tenderness over the extensor tendons of the wrist; crepitus with digital motion. **Studies:** MRI (rarely obtained) shows extensor tenosynovitis. **Non-op Tx:** Splinting, medication aimed toward inflammation, injection. **Surgery:** Tenosynovectomy.
Occult dorsal ganglion	**HPI:** Pain with wrist extension, especially with push-ups. **Exam:** Focal dorsal wrist tenderness. **Studies:** XR usually negative, occasionally associated with scapholunate dissociation. **Non-op Tx:** Splinting, observation, ultrasound-guided aspiration. **Surgery:** Excision.
Metacarpal boss	**HPI:** Pain with loading activities. Pain may be inconsistent. **Exam:** Hypertrophic index CMC joint, pain with focal palpation. **Studies:** Narrowing of the index CMC joint. **Non-op Tx:** Splinting, glucocorticoid injection. **Surgery:** Removal of metacarpal boss.
Scapholunate ligament injury	**HPI:** History of wrist sprain (may be remote). Patient may describe "clicking" of the wrist with motion. **Exam:** Tenderness over the scapholunate interval. Positive Watson test. **Studies:** PA or grip view showing widening scapholunate interval. **Non-op Tx:** Splinting, occupational therapy. **Surgery:** Surgical repair or reconstruction in traumatic ruptures without fixed carpal malalignment or arthritis. Arthrodesis in chronic cases with irreducible carpal deformity or arthrosis.

CMC, carpometacarpal; MRI, magnetic resonance imaging; ORIF, open reduction, internal fixation; PA, posteroanterior; XR, x-ray.

Ulnar Wrist

Causes of ulnar-sided wrist pain include pisotriquetral arthritis, hook of hamate fracture, and pathology of either the ECU or TFCC. Wrist MRI is often helpful in cases of ulnar wrist pain to distinguish between pain relating to the ECU and the TFCC, because these pathologies are not visible on plain films. Helpful examination maneuvers include ranging the patient's wrist through pronation, supination, and radial and ulnar deviation. An unstable ECU tendon will subluxate with pronation and supination. Radial and ulnar deviation will exacerbate pain caused by TFCC pathology (Table 4–7).

Global Wrist Pain

Global wrist pain may be caused by osteoarthritis, inflammatory arthritis, or Kienböck disease (osteonecrosis of the lunate). This is usually accompanied by limitations in range of motion (Table 4–8).

Digits

A variety of pathologies can cause pain within the digits. Careful physical examination is crucial in distinguishing these pathologies, because radiologic studies are unremarkable in many of these cases (Table 4–9).

Bony & Soft Tissue Tumors

Tumors can cause symptoms from either a mass effect or rapid growth. The primary decision point is whether a tumor is likely to be benign or malignant. This is usually determined by clinical characteristics such as location, firmness, and mobility. Common benign tumors such as ganglion cysts can be observed, but atypical masses or growths suspicious for malignancy warrant advanced imaging and possible biopsy. The most common benign soft tissue tumors of the hand and upper extremity include ganglion cysts, giant cell tumors of tendon sheath, and epidermal inclusion cysts.

Ganglion cysts are relatively thin, acellular masses. Dorsal ganglions arise predominantly from the scapholunate joint. Volar ganglions, in contrast, commonly arise from radioscaphoid joint. When small, they may not be apparent on physical examination. However, patients complain of pain at terminal flexion or extension due to mass effect of the cyst. Treatment consists of observation if it poses no functional problem. Aspiration and surgical excision are typically performed in cases of symptomatic ganglions.

Giant cell tumors of the tendon sheath are firm, mobile, rubbery masses that grow within the tendon sheath. These benign tumors are histologically similar to pigmented villonodular synovitis (see Chapter 10). They are palpated easily on examination. Treatment is surgical excision, but they can recur.

Epidermal inclusion cysts occur when epidermis is introduced into dermal layers secondary to traumatic event, forming a keratin-filled cyst. This is usually painless, patients do

Table 4–7. Disorders of the ulnar wrist.

ECU tendinosis	**HPI:** Pain with repetitive wrist motions in office workers, golfers, rowers. Atraumatic onset. **Exam:** Pain with resisted wrist extension and ulnar deviation. Decreased grip strength. Must assess for subluxation as this is associated with tendinosis. **Studies:** Plain radiographs are negative. MRI may show fluid around the tendon as well as signal within tendon in cases of tendinosis. MRI also demonstrates tendon rupture. **Non-op Tx:** Glucocorticoid injection, rest, splinting. **Surgery:** Tendon debridement or repair.
Subluxating ECU	**HPI:** Acute onset, snapping of ulnar wrist, common in tennis players and golfers. A substantial portion of the general population has asymptomatic subluxation. **Exam:** ECU subluxates with pronation and supination. **Studies:** Plain radiographs negative but both ultrasound and MRI can reveal subluxation. **Non-op Tx:** Rest, splinting. **Surgery:** ECU subsheath repair or reconstruction.
Pisotriquetral arthritis	**HPI:** Chronic ulnar-sided wrist pain. **Exam:** Tenderness over the pisiform. Ulnar nerve symptoms may be elicited. **Studies:** Plain radiographs show degenerative changes, best appreciated on supinated oblique hand view. **Non-op Tx:** Rest, glucocorticoid injection. **Surgery:** Pisiform excision.
Hook of hamate fracture	**HPI:** May be associated with history of fall or sports (baseball). **Exam:** Tenderness over the hook of hamate. **Studies:** Hook fracture on carpal tunnel view. CT or MRI often necessary for diagnosis. **Non-op Tx:** Splinting or cast reasonable in acute fractures of the base. **Surgery:** Excision of the fractured hook.
TFCC tears	**HPI:** Traumatic onset after fall. Common after distal radius fracture. Ulnar impaction can be associated with a degenerative tear. **Exam:** Tenderness over fovea. Pain with radial and ulnar deviation. **Studies:** Plain radiographs usually negative but may reveal that the ulna is longer than the radius. MRI shows increased signal in the TFCC. **Non-op Tx:** Rest, splinting. **Surgery:** Arthroscopic debridement or repair.
DRUJ instability and arthritis	**HPI:** Acute dislocation instability can occur with trauma, especially in conjunction with forearm fractures. Arthrosis usually long-standing. **Exam:** Tenderness over DRUJ. Pain and limited ROM with pronation/supination. **Studies:** Plain radiographs show degenerative changes to DRUJ. Dynamic CT scan of wrist in pronation and supination can show translation. **Non-op Tx:** Rest, splinting, glucocorticoid injection. **Surgery:** Reconstructions may involve resection of the distal ulna or fusion of the DRUJ.

CT, computed tomography; DRUJ, distal radial-ulnar joint; ECU, extensor carpi ulnaris; MRI, magnetic resonance imaging; ROM, range of motion; TFCC, triangular fibrocartilage complex.

Table 4–8. Causes of the global wrist pain.

Osteoarthritis	**HPI:** Global wrist pain with stiffness and weakness, aggravated by loading across wrist. **Exam:** Limited range of motion. Decreased grip strength. **Studies:** Plain radiographs show narrowing of spaces between carpal bones. In the setting of prior scapholunate ligament injury or scaphoid nonunion, arthrosis progresses in this manner: 1. Radial styloid beaking; degenerative changes of radioscaphoid joint. 2. Degenerative changes of capitolunate joint. The capitate may migrate proximally. 3. Pancarpal arthritis. **Non-op Tx:** Rest, splinting for mild disease. **Surgery:** Proximal row carpectomy, partial carpal fusion, total wrist fusion. **Pathophysiology:** Chronically incompetent scapholunate ligament is speculated to lead to progressive wrist instability, which leads to arthritis.
Kienbock's disease (osteonecrosis of the lunate)	**HPI:** Atraumatic onset of symptoms. Some cases are probably asymptomatic. **Exam:** Tenderness over radiocarpal joint. Decreased flexion-extension range of motion. Decreased grip strength. **Studies:** Plain radiographs showing sclerosis of the lunate. Advanced cases may demonstrate lunate collapse or arthrosis of the wrist. MRI useful for seeing early disease not visible on XR. **Non-op Tx:** Rest, splinting. **Surgery:** Various joint-leveling procedures. In late cases with arthrosis, salvage surgery consisting of removal of the scaphoid, lunate, and triquetrum (proximal row carpectomy) or wrist fusion is an option. **Pathophysiology:** Not entirely clear. May be related to repetitive micro-trauma and biomechanical factors related to ulnar negative variance.
Inflammatory arthritis of the wrist	**HPi:** Joint or hand pain, worse in the morning. **Exam:** Limited range of motion. Decreased grip and pinch strength. Tenderness and synovitis. **Studies:** Plain radiographs may demonstrate erosions and loss of joint space. **Non-op Tx:** Covered in other chapters. **Surgery:** Surgical options include wrist arthroplasty or fusion.

MRI, magnetic resonance imaging; XR, x-ray.

complain of tethering of the mass to skin, which makes the skin immobile.

Benign bony tumors of the hand may present with pain, deformity or pathologic fracture. The most common benign tumor of bone is an enchondroma. These are usually asymptomatic and are an incidental finding but may present with pathologic fracture or night pain. On plain

Table 4–9. Causes of the pain in the digits.

Trigger finger	**HPI:** Atraumatic subacute onset. Pain over the A1 pulley. Clicking or locking with flexion of the IP joint of the digit, waking up with locked digit. **Exam:** Tenderness over A1 pulley, reproducible palpable clicking over A1 when the patient flexes or extends the IP joint of the digit. **Studies:** XR unremarkable. **Non-op Tx:** Glucocorticoid injection. **Surgery:** Surgical release if injection fails.
Sagittal band rupture	**Definition:** The sagittal band refers to connective tissue over the dorsal MCPs that hold the extensor tends in place over those joints. **HPI:** Acute trauma to fingers with forceful flexion or extension or a direct blow to MCP joint. Commonly seen in boxers. Can be atraumatic in those with inflammatory arthritis. **Exam:** Tendon snapping and subluxation. Pain with MCP extension can mimic trigger finger. **Studies:** Plain radiographs to assess other injury and to assess for the presence of erosions in inflammatory arthritis. MRI will confirm diagnosis of rupture. **Non-op Tx:** Extension splinting for acute injuries. **Surgery:** Direct sagittal band repair.
Collateral ligament rupture of the MCP joint	**HPI:** Traumatic event, usually resulting from a "jammed finger." **Exam:** Pain and swelling at involved joint. Instability with ulnar or radial stress at involved joint when maximally flexed. Instability with pinch is observed injuries to the radial side of the index finger. **Studies:** Stress radiographs may aid in diagnosis, sometimes identifying avulsion fractures. **Non-op Tx:** "Buddy taping" to adjacent finger. **Surgery:** Repair indicated for radial-sided injuries to the index finger.
Pulley rupture	**HPI:** Acute onset of pain during forceful digital flexion. Common among rock climbers. **Exam:** Pain and swelling over associated pulley. Bowstringing of the associated tendon is evident in severe cases. **Studies:** XR normal but are needed to rule out other injury. **Non-op Tx:** Taping of the digit at the level of the affected pulley. **Surgery:** Repair, typically requiring use of grafts.
Mallet finger	**HPI:** Sudden onset extensor lag at the DIP joint, usually related to trauma. **Exam:** Pain and swelling over the DIP joint. No active DIP extension. **Studies:** Finger XR needed to assess congruence of DIP joint. May show a bony mallet with avulsed bone fragment. **Non-op Tx:** Extension splinting if less than 50% of the articular surface is affected and there is no DIP subluxation. **Surgery:** Closed reduction and pinning versus ORIF if involves more than 50% of the articular surface is involved or if there is DIP subluxation. Chronic injuries previously unaddressed may also require surgical repair.
Fractures	**HPI:** Trauma with acute swelling and pain +/− ecchymosis at location of fracture. **Exam:** Tenderness and swelling at location of fracture, there may be obvious deformity, need to check for malrotation of digit. **Studies:** XR will show the fracture. CT may define fracture pattern better and estimate fracture displacement in intra-articular fractures. **Non-op Tx:** Varies by fracture pattern/location. **Surgery:** Varies from pinning, plate-and-screw fixation, to bone grafting.

CT, computed tomography; DIP, distal interphalangeal; IP, interphalangeal; MCP, metacarpophalangeal; MRI, magnetic resonance imaging; ORIF, open reduction, internal fixation; XR, x-ray.

radiographs they appear as a lytic lesion, sometimes with stippling calcification.

Giant cell tumors are most frequently seen in the distal radius and arises in the metaphysis and diaphysis of bones. They are benign but locally aggressive and can transform into malignant tumors. They are expansile lesions which can cause significant pain and decreased range of motion secondary to mass effect. Treatment consists of curettage.

Soft tissue and bony sarcomas of the hand and upper extremity are uncommon but warrant consideration. Of the soft tissue sarcomas, undifferentiated pleomorphic sarcoma, epithelioid sarcoma, and synovial cell sarcoma are the most

frequently seen. Of the bony tumors, osteosarcoma is the most frequently seen.

Nerve/Referred Pain

Most patients presenting with nerve symptoms complain of numbness or paresthesias. The majority of cases are either a compressive neuropathy or cervical radiculopathy. However, it is important to consider central causes of weakness such as stroke or multiple sclerosis. Other notable causes of upper limb weakness are tendon rupture (such as a rotator cuff tear) or the Parsonage-Turner syndrome.

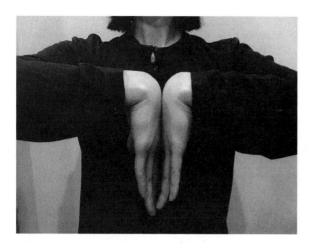

▲ **Figure 4–4.** Phalen test.

When nerve pathology is suspected, examination of the cervical spine and the respective myotomes and dermatomes is important. In addition, provocative maneuvers are useful in distinguishing between different types of compressive neuropathy. Notable tests for carpal tunnel syndrome include Durkan and Phalen tests (Figures 4–4 and 4–5). Elbow flexion testing can help identify cubital tunnel syndrome (Table 4–10).

Vascular

Pain from vascular injury arises from tissue ischemia and is confined to the distribution of the blood supply of the involved vessel. History is important to pinpoint cause of vascular insufficiency that may be from a laceration due to penetrating trauma or prior surgery, vasospasm secondary autoimmune phenomena, or from thromboembolic disease.

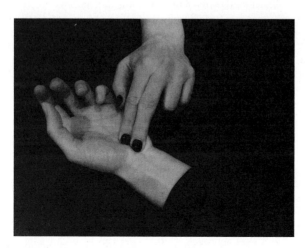

▲ **Figure 4–5.** Durkan test.

Table 4–10. Syndromes of nerve entrapment involving the upper extremity.

Carpal tunnel syndrome	**HPI:** Insidious onset of numbness and paresthesias in the median nerve distribution. The median distribution includes the thumb, index finger, long finger, and the radial half of the ring finger. Symptoms are usually worse at night, when fluid shifts increase pressure within the carpal tunnel. Patients with advanced cases may have atrophy of the thenar muscle, leading to thumb weakness. **Exam:** Sensory deficit in median distribution. Thenar atrophy. Weakness of palmar abduction of the thumb. Positive Durkan, Tinel, and Phalen signs. **Studies:** Nerve conduction studies can confirm the diagnosis if in question. **Non-op Tx:** Nighttime wrist splinting in neutral for mild disease. Carpal tunnel injections are *not* recommended. If splinting does not provide adequate relief, the optimal approach to treatment is surgery. **Surgery:** Carpal tunnel release.
Cubital tunnel syndrome	**HPI:** Insidious onset of numbness and paresthesias in the ulnar nerve distribution, including the ulnar half of the ring finger and small finger. Cubital tunnel syndrome may be exacerbated by cell phone use or other activities involving a flexed elbow. Atrophy of the intrinsic muscles of the hands occurs in severe cases. **Exam:** Sensory deficit in ulnar distribution. Intrinsic muscle atrophy and weakness. Positive Froment (Figure 4–6) sign and positive Jeanne, Wartenberg, and Tinel signs over the cubital tunnel. Ulnar claw hand. Can be associated with and unstable ulnar nerve at the elbow, with subluxation over the medial epicondyle. **Studies:** Nerve conduction studies can confirm the diagnosis. **Non-op Tx:** Extension splinting at elbow. Ergonomic assessment of workspace **Surgery:** Release of the cubital tunnel at the elbow.
Cervical radiculopathy	**HPI:** Usually insidious onset, but can be precipitated by acute trauma. **Exam:** Sensory and/or motor deficits in a peripheral nerve distribution. **Studies:** MRI of cervical spine. **Non-op Tx:** Physical therapy may be beneficial in some cases. **Surgery:** Decompression of nerve root and possible fusion.

MRI, magnetic resonance imaging.

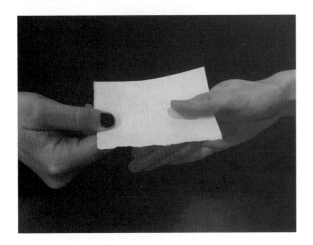

▲ **Figure 4–6.** Froment test.

Doppler ultrasonography is helpful in identifying thrombus in the large vessels of the wrist. CT angiography, MR angiography, and regular angiography may be useful localizing the areas of vascular compromise.

COMMON PATTERNS OF UPPER EXTREMITY FINDINGS IN SYSTEMIC DISEASES

Rheumatoid Arthritis

Rheumatoid arthritis presents in the hands, wrist, and elbow in a variety of ways (see Chapter 13). We describe some general observations and patterns below:

1. **Caput ulnae syndrome:** The caput ulnae syndrome is also known as the "head of the ulna" or "top of ulna" syndrome. Caput ulnae refers to a pattern of wrist involvement in which wrist synovitis has led to a pronatory deformity of the carpus relative to the ulnar head. Synovitis of the MCP joints and radial erosions of the sagittal bands over the joints lead to ulnar deviation of the digits because of the pull of the digital extensors. The extensor tendons become subluxed. Tenosynovitis of the extensor tendons leads to wear and tear at the prominent ulnar head. The ulnar digital extensors may rupture at the site of the ulnar styloid.

2. Mannerfelt syndrome refers to rupture of the FPL secondary to attrition in the carpal tunnel.

3. The DIP joints of the hand are typically spared in RA.

4. Subcutaneous rheumatoid nodules may be observed, which appear over the interphalangeal joints, the olecranon, and the ulnar border of the forearm.

5. A boutonneire deformity of the finger occurs when synovitis in the PIP joint results in volar subluxation of the sagittal bands of the extensor hood. This volar subluxation results in hyperextension of the DIP joint and flexion of the PIP joint.

6. A swan-neck deformity in inflammatory arthritis results when the synovitis of the PIP joint results in laxity of the volar plate. This leads to hyperextension of the PIP joint and reciprocal dorsal subluxation of the lateral bands, resulting in a swan-neck deformity.

Lupus

Lupus (see Chapter 19) may present in the hands with ligamentous laxity that may result in hypermobility of joints, notably the thumb CMC joint and MP joints. The fingers commonly present with swan neck deformities secondary to ligamentous laxity rather than synovitis.

Psoriatic Arthritis

Psoriatic arthritis, a seronegative spondyloarthropathy, commonly presents with rash with plaques over the extensor surfaces. Patients may present with DIP arthritis on x-ray demonstrating a characteristic "pencil-in-cup" deformity. Patients may also present with dactylitis as well as characteristic nail pitting. A small subgroup of patients develops arthritis mutilans, manifesting severe bone destruction and telescoping of the fingers in a manner that has been described as "opera-glass fingers."

APPROACH TO UNCLEAR DIAGNOSIS

History, physical examination, and carefully selected but readily available studies lead to a clear diagnosis in most patients with disorders of the hands, wrists, and elbow. For the unusual cases in which the cause of pain is unclear, several approaches may be considered:

1. If fracture and other acute injury have been excluded, rest and activity modification with or without occupational therapy combined with the judicious of NSAIDs is reasonable. Splinting is another option during this period. It may be useful for patients to try this for a period of time and return to clinic for reexamination after a few weeks.

2. In patients with normal plain radiographs, an unrevealing examination, and pain that is functionally limiting or does not improve with rest, advanced imaging such as MRI, CT, or bone scan may be considered.

3. Diagnostic injection may help distinguish between different pain generators. For example, an injection may be helpful in discriminating between CMC arthritis and de Quervain tenosynovitis.

4. Second opinion: Overall, the approach to the unclear diagnosis can be challenging, and obtaining secondary opinions either within or outside the same specialty is a wise approach if no answer can be found after a few visits.

Approach to the Patient with Foot & Ankle Pain

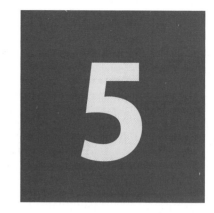

Mark Yakavonis, MD

Craig Lareau, MD

Daniel Guss, MD, MBA

INTRODUCTION

The foot and ankle are the anatomic result of evolution from species that primarily used their feet to grasp objects into a species that relies on their feet principally for bipedal gait. Inherent to this transformation was the ability to transmit the physiologic forces of upright gait through an interconnected network of 26 separate foot bones. These bones are linked through a series of joints, stabilizing ligaments, and tendons. Many conditions can compromise these interconnections, including trauma, which abruptly disrupts normal anatomy, or rheumatologic conditions, which may gradually compromise or erode these links. Persistent application of a substantial physiologic load through such compromised structures can result in the pain and deformity frequently observed among afflicted patients. Understanding and diagnosing such pathology in the foot and ankle requires an intricate knowledge of the underlying anatomy, as well as a recognition of how disruption of one facet of normal anatomy may predicate pathology elsewhere.

ANATOMY

There are 7 tarsal, 5 metatarsal, and 14 phalangeal bones. An additional two sesamoid bones are located within the short flexor tendon of the hallux, and accessory ossicles may also be present in various locations. The bones of the foot are generally divided into the hindfoot (calcaneus and talus), midfoot (navicular, three cuneiforms, and cuboid), and forefoot (metatarsals, phalanges, and sesamoids).

▶ Ankle

The ankle (tibiotalar) joint allows dorsiflexion and plantar flexion range of motion. The mortise, which articulates with the talus, is comprised of the tibial plafond (the horizontal weight-bearing portion of the distal tibia), the medial malleolus, and the lateral malleolus. The deltoid ligament linking the medial malleolus to the talus is the main ligamentous ankle stabilizer during the stance phase and resists an outward valgus and external rotation force on the ankle. Three lateral ankle ligaments of the ankle resist an inward varus force.

The ankle is a mortise joint, a reference to a carpentry term in which a recess is cut into a piece of wood in order to stabilize its linkage to another piece of wood that is inserted into the mortise. The ankle mortise specifically consists of the fibula and tibia, which in turn stabilize the talus between them. To do so, the fibula and tibia are linked together by multiple ligaments which, in concert, span the inferior tibiofibular joint in a complex known as the syndesmosis. The syndesmosis consists of four ligaments, the strongest of which is the posterior inferior tibiofibular ligament.

▶ Hindfoot

Hindfoot joints include the subtalar and transverse tarsal (Chopart) joints (the talonavicular and calcaneocuboid joints). While the ankle joint allows the foot to dorsi- and plantarflex, the subtalar joint is an oblique-axis joint that allows 20 degrees of hindfoot inversion and 10 degrees of hindfoot eversion. The spring (plantar calcaneonavicular) ligament spans the inferior medial calcaneus to the navicular and is critical in maintaining the arch of the foot. Attenuation of this ligament can precipitate a pes planovalgus deformity.

▶ Midfoot

The midfoot joints include the naviculocuneiform, intercuneiform, and tarsometatarsal (Lisfranc) joints. The Lisfranc ligament connects the medial cuneiform to the second metatarsal. There is no ligamentous connection between the bases of the first and second metatarsals, and traumatic tearing of the Lisfranc ligament can allow the lesser metatarsals to sublux laterally off their respective tarsal bones.

Forefoot

The metatarsophalangeal (MTP) joints allow dorsiflexion and plantar flexion of the toes. Lateral collateral ligaments resist varus stress, and medial collateral ligaments resist valgus stress. The plantar plate is the primary stabilizer of the MTP joints, preventing dorsal subluxation or dislocation. Lesser toe plantar plate rupture can lead to dorsal dislocations and crossover toe deformities. Turf toe injuries result from injury to the great toe plantar plate, often due to a forced dorsiflexion injury on artificial turf among athletes. The sesamoids articulate with the plantar aspect of the first metatarsal head. Analogous to the patella, the sesamoids provide a fulcrum that increase first MTP flexion power.

Muscles

Muscles can be categorized as extrinsic and intrinsic. Major tendons that cross the ankle joint into the foot are extrinsic muscles. Anterior intrinsic muscles are the tibialis anterior, extensor hallucis longus, extensor digitorum longus, and peroneus tertius. Lateral extrinsic muscles are the peroneus longus and brevis. The peroneus longus tendon is more likely to dislocate and the peroneus brevis tendon is more likely to tear, possibly because the brevis tendon immediately abuts the posterior fibula. Posterior extrinsic muscles are the Achilles, which is a confluence of the gastrocnemius and soleus muscles. The Achilles is the strongest and largest tendon in the body. The posteromedial extrinsic muscles are the posterior tibialis, flexor digitorum longus, and flexor hallucis longus (FHL), which form the deep flexors of the leg and can plantarflex the foot even in the presence of an Achilles rupture. The posterior tibial tendon also initiates hindfoot inversion during gait, critical to effectively using the foot as a lever arm during gait.

Nerves

Of the five peripheral nerves that innervate the foot, three run superficial to the fascia at the level of the tibiotalar joint (superficial peroneal, sural, and saphenous nerves) and two run deep to the fascia (deep peroneal and tibial nerves). As described above, the superficial peroneal nerve (SPN) supplies sensation to the dorsum of the foot except the dorsal first web space, which is supplied by the deep peroneal nerve. The deep peroneal nerve innervates the muscles in the anterior compartment of the leg (tibialis anterior, extensor digitorum longus, and extensor hallucis longus), and the SPN innervates the muscles in the lateral compartment of the leg (peroneus longus and peroneus brevis). Anterior tarsal tunnel syndrome can occur due to deep peroneal nerve entrapment beneath the inferior extensor retinaculum in the dorsal aspect of the foot, while entrapment of the SPN can occur as it pierces through the peroneal muscles and their fascia as it transitions to becoming a superficial nerve.

The tibial nerve travels in the tarsal tunnel posteromedial to the ankle beneath the flexor retinaculum before splitting into the medial plantar nerve, lateral plantar nerve, and calcaneal sensory nerve. It supplies all the intrinsic muscles of the foot except the extensor digitorum brevis, which is innervated by the deep peroneal nerve. The first branch of the lateral plantar nerve supplies the abductor digiti quinti, and can sometimes be compressed by the fascia of the abductor hallucis as the nerve pierces laterally. The saphenous nerve supplies sensation to the medial foot, and the sural nerve supplies sensation to the lateral aspect of the foot. Morton's neuromas develop in the interdigital nerves, which run plantar to the intermetatarsal ligaments.

PHYSICAL EXAMINATION

Effective evaluation of patients with foot and ankle conditions is largely dependent on the physical examination. The vast majority of foot and ankle anatomy is subcutaneous, permitting the easy visualization and palpation of involved structures. Screening radiographs may supplement the physical examination and are ideally attained as weight-bearing views so that they can reveal anatomy while under physiologic load. Cross-sectional imaging modalities such as computed tomography (CT) and magnetic resonance imaging (MRI) play important roles in selected patients, but generally only when the clinician employs these technologists to answer a specific anatomic question, the results of which may alter the treatment plan. Ultrasound is also becoming increasing relevant given its accessibility at the point of care. Clinicians must bear in mind, however, that many of these imaging modalities often identify abnormalities that may or may not relate directly to the patient's complaints. Therefore, careful correlation between imaging findings and the history and physical examination is critical.

The physical examination of the foot and ankle begins with an observation of the patient's gait before he or she even enters the examining room. The degree of antalgia often underscores the severity of the patient's condition. Assessment of the foot and ankle alignment while the patient is still standing is also critical. Normal alignment of the hindfoot is in approximately 5 degrees of valgus; that is, the ankle equivalent of being slightly knock-kneed. An alignment that is overly valgus, however, will strain medial structures of the ankle such as the deltoid ligament and posterior tibial tendon, potentially causing medial pain (Figure 5–1). If severe enough, as the foot swings outward the lateral fibula may impinge against the calcaneus, generating lateral symptoms. In contrast, when the ankle is in a varus position, the ankle equivalent of being bowlegged, the pathology is likely to be along the lateral aspect of the foot and ankle. Strain to the lateral structures may include a propensity to sprains, peroneal tendon issues, or even lateral foot overload as the fifth metatarsal bears a disproportionate amount of force.

It is useful to have the patient situated such that the feet are dangling above the ground, allowing freedom of motion. If symptoms are unilateral, initial examination of the

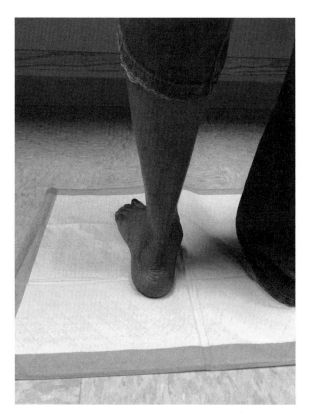

▲ **Figure 5–1.** An alignment that is overly valgus, however, will strain medial structures of the ankle such as the deltoid ligament and posterior tibial tendon, potentially causing medial pain.

contralateral, unaffected limb affords a ready comparison to the involved extremity. Joints in the foot and ankle have traditionally been identified as being either "essential" or "nonessential" joints. Essential joints are those whose motion is important for normal function. These include the tibiotalar joint, subtalar joint, transverse tarsal joints (the talonavicular and calcaneocuboid joint), and the MTP joints. The fourth and fifth tarsometatarsal (TMT) joints are also important in accommodating uneven ground. The other joints, such as the naviculocuneiform and the first through third TMT joints, however, can undergo procedures such as fusions with few functional repercussions. Their principal features are stiffness, which is necessary for bipedal gait.

Active range of motion examination focuses heavily on the ankle and hindfoot regions. The anatomic course of a given tendon predicates its motion. Anterior to the ankle cross the tibialis anterior, the extensor hallucis longus, and the extensor digitorum longus (see Figure 5–1). The tibialis anterior, by virtue of attaching dorsomedially to the midfoot at the medial cuneiform and first metatarsal base, elevates the ankle and inverts the hindfoot. Loss of this tendon results in a foot drop.

Lateral to the ankle lie the peroneus brevis and peroneus longus tendons, which angle around the posterior fibula toward their attachment sites at the base of the fifth metatarsal and the plantar aspect of the first metatarsal, respectively. The peroneus brevis therefore acts to plantarflex and evert the hindfoot, while the peroneus longus everts the foot but also plantarflexes the first ray. Testing of these tendons therefore entails resisted eversion with the ankle held in a dorsiflexed postion.

Posteromedially to the ankle lie the posterior tibial tendon, the flexor digitorum longus, and the flexor halluces longus tendons. The posterior tibial tendon, through its multiple plantar-medial attachment sites at the navicular and midfoot, acts to plantarflex and invert the ankle and hindfoot, as well as plays an important role in maintaining the arch. Testing of this tendon therefore entails resisted inversion with the foot in a full plantarflexed position. The Achilles directly posterior to the ankle draws jointly from the gastrocnemius and soleus muscles and, as the largest tendon in the body, is the strongest plantarflexor of the ankle. Loss of this tendon results in a "positive" Thompson's test, wherein squeezing the calf does not result in associated motion of the foot. Notably, however, patients with an Achilles rupture will still generally be able to plantarflex through the intact deep flexors, such as the posterior tibialis.

Sensory exam to the foot relies on five major nerves: (1) superficial peroneal nerve (SPN), (2) deep peroneal nerve, (3) tibial nerve, (4) sural nerve, and (5) the saphenous nerve. All but the saphenous nerve, which is a sensory continuation of the femoral nerve, are branches off the sciatic nerve. The SPN gives sensation to the dorsum of the foot apart from the first web space, which is the purview of the deep peroneal nerve. The tibial nerve innervates the plantar aspect of the foot, while the sural and saphenous nerves innervate the lateral and medial ankle and hindfoot, respectively. In the setting of neuropathy, loss of monofilament sensation overlying the hallux is an early presentation, but hallux proprioception, the perception of the location of the toe in space, may also be lost as neuropathy progresses.

Vascular exam includes the dorsal pedis pulse, felt dorsally in the midfoot region at the level of the ankle. The posterior tibial pulse, in turn, is felt posteromedially at the ankle behind the medial malleolus.

Direct palpation of anatomy is critical to determining sources of painful pathology, and key knowledge of the involved anatomic structures is critical, as highlighted in the various pathologies discussed later.

▼ FOREFOOT PAIN

METATARSALGIA

ESSENTIALS OF DIAGNOSIS

▶ Pain under the plantar surface of the lesser metatarsal heads.

▶ Clinical Findings

A. Symptoms and Signs

Metatarsalgia is a stress syndrome associated with abnormal loading of the plantar lesser metatarsal heads. An appreciable deformity such as hallux valgus often leads to the abnormal loading. Hallux valgus translates the larger first ray outward leaving the smaller second ray to bear more of the forefoot forces inherent to gait. A second ray that is longer than the first can create a similar situation. Over time, as the metatarsal head becomes progressively loaded, the underlying soft tissues may become painful and are often marked by a plantar callus underlying the involved metatarsal. An associated MTP synovitis may also develop, leading to pain within the joint itself. The principal symptom is pain along the plantar aspect of the foot, most notable during weight bearing, especially when barefoot on hard surfaces. Patients may also have pain in the web space as a result of inflammation about the digital nerve, but most of the tenderness is under the metatarsal head.

B. Imaging Studies and Special Tests

The diagnosis is generally made by direct palpation during the physical examination. Weight-bearing radiographs consisting of AP, oblique, and lateral views of the foot should be obtained.

▶ Treatment

Nonoperative treatment principally involves shoe wear modification, NSAID, and orthotics. Metatarsal pads, a soft felt prominence placed proximal to the metatarsal heads, may be added to the shoes or orthotics to offload the forefoot. A rocker-bottom shoe may also mitigate forefoot pressures during gait. If symptoms persist despite a full course of conservative management and precipitating deformities are present, such as hallux valgus or long second rays, patients may consider operative correction of the underlying deformity. The vast majority of cases of metatarsalgia, however, are managed nonoperatively.

PLANTAR PLATE RUPTURE (TURF TOE & LESSER MTP INSTABILITY)

ESSENTIALS OF DIAGNOSIS

▶ Hyperextension injury to great toe causing pain over plantar first MTP joint; that is, turf toe.

▶ Instability determined with dorsal draw test wherein the proximal phalanx is unstable when shucked on the metatarsal head.

▶ Clinical Findings

A. Symptoms and Signs

Plantar plate injury or instability can occur at the MTP joint in any toe, though at the great toe it is commonly referred to as turf toe. Turf toe in particular is commonly found in contact sports played on rigid surfaces. Its main mechanism of injury is hyperextension with forced axial loading of the first MTP joint, causing plantar plate or phalangeal-sesamoid ligament disruption. Patients will complain of acute pain and stiffness at the first MTP joint with diminished strength and pain with push-off of the toe.

Instability of the lesser MTP joints is less likely to be associated with a particular inciting event. Instead it develops as a result of chronic stress exerted on the plantar plate and collateral ligaments resulting in attenuation or stretching of the stabilizing ligaments.

Visual inspection of the toe will often times reveal plantar swelling and ecchymosis in turf toe, and callosities may be appreciated in cases of lesser toe MTP instability. Pain will be reproduced with both active and passive range of motion of the great toe MTP joint.

B. Imaging Studies and Special Tests

Plantar plate ruptures can initially be evaluated with weight-bearing AP, lateral, and oblique radiographs of the foot. When assessing for turf toe, additional views may be considered, including sesamoid axial and forced dorsiflexion views, the latter to understand whether the sesamoids follow the hallux as it is dorsiflexed or whether they are disrupted. It is important radiographically to assess displacement of the sesamoids relative to the MTP joint. If an injury is suspected but plain radiographs are inadequate, an MRI may be ordered to better assess the plantar plate. Plantar plate attenuation in the lesser toes may demonstrate a subluxation or dislocation of the involved MTP joint.

▶ Treatment

Initial treatment is largely conservative for plantar plate rupture and involves rest and immobilization with stiff-soled shoes or a walking boot, versus casting with the hallux plantarflexed in more severe cases of turf toe. If a turf toe injury is suspected, it is important to immobilize the foot early to allow stabilization and scarring of the involved structures. If a stiff-soled shoe is not tolerated in patients with turf toe, an orthotic with a Morton's extension over the first ray may help splint the great toe. Taping can also be used to restrict movement. In cases that fail conservative treatment or with gross joint instability, the patient should be referred to a foot and ankle specialist for consideration of surgical intervention. Early treatment often entails a plantar plate repair, and surgery may also be indicated for chronic instability.

METATARSAL STRESS FRACTURE

ESSENTIALS OF DIAGNOSIS

▶ Pain with palpation over the metatarsal shaft.

▶ Pain associated with activity.

▶ Clinical Findings

A. Symptoms and Signs

Metatarsal stress fractures have earned the eponym "March Fractures" because of their association with the initiation of rigorous military basic training. They occur as an overuse phenomenon whereby the foot sees stresses and microtrauma repetitively and is unable to adequately repair or regenerate itself before the next trauma ensues. They can happen in each of the metatarsals and typically occur in the distal shaft with the exception of the fifth metatarsal where they occur in the metadiaphyseal junction. Patients with metatarsal stress fractures will present with pain and swelling over the metatarsal shaft, usually associated with activity or weight bearing. They frequently also report a new exercise regimen or recent increase in high-impact exercise.

B. Imaging Studies and Special Tests

Initial radiographic workup consists of plain radiographs of the foot. Characteristic findings of stress fractures will be a periosteal reaction about the metatarsal shaft. It is important to note that this finding takes time to develop, so if patients are imaged in the acute setting the radiographs may be normal. If a high clinical suspicion exists, patient may be brought back for repeat radiographs a few weeks after initial presentation for repeat radiographs. Alternatively, MRI has a high sensitivity in identifying early stress fractures but may not alter early treatment protocols, which generally entail rigid immobilization.

▶ Treatment

Treatment consists of immobilization in either a postoperative shoe or fracture boot for up to 4–6 weeks. Weight bearing should be allowed as tolerated but rest is recommended as long as the patient has pain. Return to activity is predicated by radiographic healing, but absence of symptoms is of equal importance. Avoidance of risk factors, including glucocorticoid use and smoking, is recommended.

HAMMERTOE

ESSENTIALS OF DIAGNOSIS

▶ Pain on the dorsal surface of the toe with shoe wear.

▶ Extension of the distal interphalangeal (DIP) joint and flexion of the proximal interphalangeal (PIP) joint.

▶ Clinical Findings

A. Symptoms and Signs

Hammertoes are the most commonly treated lesser toe deformity, with a higher prevalence in women. The characteristic deformity is PIP flexion with DIP extension; the MTP joint can be either neutral or extended. Pain is associated either with shoes causing pressure on the dorsal surface of the toe or pressure from the ground on the tip of the toe. During visual inspection, it is not unusual to find callous formation in the respective locations of pressure.

It is important to delineate fixed or flexible deformities using a push-up test. When dorsal pressure is exerted under the plantar surface of the metatarsal a flexible deformity with correct to a straight toe while a fixed deformity will not. During this exam, the clinician may also be able to appreciate if the proximal phalanx is dislocated off of the metatarsal head.

B. Imaging Studies and Special Tests

Imaging for the diagnosis of hammertoes consists of weight-bearing AP, lateral, and oblique foot radiographs. It is important to assess the MTP joint to ensure that the proximal phalanx is reduced on the head of the metatarsal and not dislocated dorsally.

▶ Treatment

Treatment is largely symptomatic and directed to decrease the pressure on the dorsum or plantar aspect of the toe. This consists of shoes with deeper toe boxes, toe pads, and foam or silicone gel sleeves for the toes. Flexible deformities can be treated with Budin splints which pull the toe downward, decreasing PIP pressure. In turn, Crest pads underneath the toe can elevate it to offload pressure on the tip of the toe. Conservative measures can frequently alleviate symptoms but refractory pain or recurrent wounds, especially with fixed deformities, may require surgical treatment. If a second hammertoe is associated with a crossover deformity, wherein a hallux valgus places the hallux underneath the second toe, the hallux valgus must be addressed at the same time.

CLAW TOE

ESSENTIALS OF DIAGNOSIS

▶ Pain at the MTP joint.

▶ Flexion of the PIP and DIP joints, extension of the MTP joint.

Clinical Findings

A. Symptoms and Signs

Clawing is attributed to muscular imbalance between the intrinsic and extrinsic musculature in the foot. As it is associated with neuromuscular causes, it can often be found bilaterally. However, other origins exist, including trauma or synovitis. Classically, the proximal phalanx is extended at the MTP joint and the middle and distal phalanges are flexed. This causes the metatarsal head to be driven into the ground leading to pain at the metatarsal head. Often patients will have callosities at both the plantar metatarsal head as well as dorsally over the IP joints. The deformity can be fixed or flexible.

B. Imaging Studies and Special Tests

Weight-bearing radiographs of the foot, including AP, lateral, and oblique, can be useful in assessing the stability of the MTP joint.

Treatment

First-line treatment involves shoe wear modifications, including shoes with deeper toe boxes, as well as orthotics with metatarsal pads or bars to shield the metatarsal head. For flexible deformities, crest pads and Budin splints can be used to correct the deformity. Patients who fail conservative measures are treated similarly to hammertoe deformities with soft-tissue procedures for flexible deformities and interphalageal fusion with possible metatarsal shortening osteotomies for rigid claw toes.

MALLET TOE

ESSENTIALS OF DIAGNOSIS

▶ Pain at the dorsum of the DIP or tip of the toe with ambulation.
▶ Isolated flexed distal phalanx.

Clinical Findings

A. Symptoms and Signs

Mallet toes can result from trauma to the DIP joint or extensor mechanism, or again it can also be degenerative in nature and associated with ill-fitting shoe wear. It is defined as neutral MTP and PIP joints with a flexed DIP joint. On inspection of the foot, patients will have callosities formed at the tip of the toe, which can cause pain with ambulation. The deformity can be flexible or rigid.

B. Imaging Studies and Special Tests

Weight-bearing radiographs of the foot, including AP, lateral, and oblique films, can be useful in assessing for trauma as a cause of mallet toe.

Treatment

Initial treatment is conservative with shoes with deep toe boxes or toe caps and sleeves to prevent callosities. However, patients who have continued pain may be treated surgically. Flexible deformities can be treated with flexor tendon release, while rigid deformities are often treated with either DIP resection arthroplasty or fusion.

MORTON NEUROMA

ESSENTIALS OF DIAGNOSIS

▶ Pain in the interdigital web space.
▶ Worse with weight bearing and constrictive shoe wear.
▶ A positive Mulder's click sign—crepitus in web space elicited by squeezing the metatarsals together—is characteristic.

Clinical Findings

A. Symptoms and Signs

A Morton's neuroma is a compressive neuropathy of an interdigital nerve. The nature of its development is controversial, but the principal etiology is compression on the nerve by the transverse intermetatarsal ligament which spans dorsally to the interdigital nerve between the metatarsal heads. It is most commonly found in the third web space and is more common in females. Pain is typically felt in the involved web space of the forefoot and is exacerbated by constrictive shoe wear. It may also be associated with symptoms of burning distal to the web space. Pain may be elicited on exam by compressing the web spaces. Moreover, a "Mulder's click" may be appreciated as a click in the web space that occurs when the metatarsals are squeezed together, pushing the enlarged nerve in a plantar direction.

B. Imaging Studies and Special Tests

Plain weight-bearing radiographs should be obtained, including AP, oblique, and lateral films. These are typically unremarkable, but may point to a bony structural cause of the pain. MRI and ultrasound have limited utility. Lidocaine and steroid injections to the web space may alleviate pain and help with the diagnosis of a neuroma, though extravasation of the injection elsewhere may also relieve pain from other sources. Electrodiagnostic studies are not useful in the evaluation of symptoms in this region.

Treatment

Initial treatment consists of shoe wear modification, NSAIDs, and activity modification. Wide, soft-laced shoes with a low heel and rubber sole are comfortable. Metatarsal pads or bars will also help relieve pressure from the neuroma. If these measure fail, a glucocorticoid injection may be considered but the patient and clinician must be aware of the risk of ligament and capsular weakening from repeated use. Recalcitrant cases may be considered for nerve release or excision.

HALLUX RIGIDUS

ESSENTIALS OF DIAGNOSIS

▶ Pain with first MTP joint motion, particularly dorsiflexion.
▶ Limited ROM of the first MTP joint.

Clinical Findings

A. Symptoms and Signs

Hallux rigidus is caused by degenerative arthritis at the first MTP joint. Like most degenerative arthritis the cause is often idiopathic though traumatic origins have been implicated. The hallmark of early hallux rigidus is formation of a dorsal osteophyte causing dorsal impingement, and as more of the joint is involved the ROM of the great toe decreases. Patients present with pain over their first MTP joint that is particularly painful with push off during gait. They may also complain of irritation of the dorsal osteophyte with constrictive shoe wear. Patients may also report increased symptoms when walking barefoot due to excessive stress placed on the MTP joint. Examination will reveal limited range of motion, particularly dorsiflexion, and as degenerative changes progress pain elicited with a grind test of the MTP joint.

B. Imaging Studies and Special Tests

Imaging studies for the workup of hallux rigidus consists of plain weight-bearing radiographs of the foot, including AP, oblique, and lateral views. Findings will depend on the grade of disease present. In early cases, the only finding will be a dorsal metatarsal head osteophyte with a preserved joint space, often with subtle squaring of the metatarsal head at its margins, whereas at the end stage of arthritis there will be associated joint space narrowing with subchondral sclerosis and cysts.

Treatment

Initial treatment for hallux rigidus consists of orthotics and NSAIDs. Patients may be instructed to avoid activities that require dorsiflexion of the great toe. The principal orthotic used consists of a Morton's extension with a stiff foot plate that minimizes dorsiflexion forces on the hallux. If patients prefer to avoid orthotics, often shoes with stiff soles will restrict motion at the joint and relieve pain in an analogous fashion. If patients fail conservative management, they may be considered for surgical treatment. For early stage disease, a dorsal cheilectomy may temporarily improve symptoms of dorsal impingement. Definitive surgical treatment has traditionally involved first MTP fusion. Joint arthroplasty is gaining in popularity, especially with more recent implants that require less bony resection, but first MTP fusion remains the gold standard for end-stage first MTP arthritis.

HALLUX VALGUS

ESSENTIALS OF DIAGNOSIS

▶ Pain over the medial eminence of the first MTP joint.

Clinical Findings

A. Symptoms and Signs

Hallux valgus is not simply a medial bone overgrowth, but instead a complex deformity of the first ray involving the relative imbalance of multiple structures. At a basic level, it involves lateral deviation of the great toe on a medially deviated first metatarsal. Over time the sesamoids may erode the cristae that separate them, permitting lateral dislocation and worsening of the deformity. As the flexor and extensor tendons move with the hallux laterally to the mechanical axis, the deformity may further worsen. There is a significant hereditary component, and patients will frequently report relatives with a history of hallux valgus. Other contributors include female gender, ligamentous laxity, and constrictive shoe wear. Primarily patients will present with pain with shoe wear due to medial irritation over the bony prominence. However, some will also describe paresthesias in the great toe secondary to compression of the dorsomedial cutaneous sensory nerve. On examination, there will be a valgus deformity at the first MTP joint that may be passively correctable. It is important to also examine for other deformities, such as hammertoes or metatarsalgia, of the second toe that can develop as a result of altered mechanics in the foot.

B. Imaging Studies and Special Tests

Radiographic evaluation begins with standard weight-bearing AP, oblique, and lateral plain films. Findings will consist of a medial eminence with lateral subluxation of the sesamoids from underneath the MTP joint. There may be an increased angle between the first and second metatarsals and a valgus angle at the MTP joint.

Treatment

Conservative treatment is directed at relieving symptoms. It is important to note that there is no way to ameliorate the progression of a bunion over time with any braces or spacers. The primary initial treatment consists of shoe wear modification with open toe shoes or those with a wide, tall toe box. Toe straps, spacers, and splints may alleviate symptoms. Orthotics may help with symptoms secondary to metatarsalgia but have a limited role in the treatment of hallux valgus as they can crowd shoes and worsen irritation overlying the medial eminence. When conservative measures fail and the patient desires more definitive treatment due to severe pain, surgery may be indicated, often entailing either an osteotomy of the first metatarsal or the proximal phalanx or an arthrodesis procedure of either the first MTP joint or first TMT joint.

BUNIONETTE

ESSENTIALS OF DIAGNOSIS

▶ Lateral prominence and pain over the fifth metatarsal head.

Clinical Findings

A. Symptoms and Signs

A bunionette is a painful lateral bony prominence of the fifth metatarsal head, also known as a "tailor's bunion" due to its historically common occurrence in the profession. The deformity is graded based on the degree of the intermetatarsal and MTP joint angles. Its prevalence is higher in women and is associated with constrictive shoe wear. On examination patients will have a lateral prominence over the fifth metatarsal head, often associated with a medial deviation of the fifth toe with plantar or lateral hyperkeratosis with erythema. Typically, the pain is not associated with range of motion rather direct pressure from shoe wear.

B. Imaging Studies and Special Tests

Weight-bearing radiographs of the foot, including AP, lateral, and oblique images, are useful in determining the width of the fifth metatarsal head as well as intermetatarsal and MTP joint angles.

Treatment

Nonoperative treatment consists of shoe wear modification, keratosis padding, and callous shaving. In patients whom fail conservative measures, treatment is guided by the classification or level of intermetatarsal angle. Patients without an increased intermetatarsal angle may undergo lateral condylectomy of the fifth metatarsal, while patients with an increased angle require a fifth metatarsal osteotomy to correct this angle.

▼ MIDFOOT PAIN

MIDFOOT ARTHRITIS

ESSENTIALS OF DIAGNOSIS

▶ Pain in the midfoot and arch with push off during gait.
▶ Palpable osteophytes on the dorsum of the foot.

Clinical Findings

A. Symptoms and Signs

Many patients with midfoot arthritis indicate a history of trauma or autoimmune conditions, idiopathic osteoarthritis in the absence of a known predisposing condition is also common. When considering arthritis as a diagnosis, the most common complaint is midfoot pain, exacerbated with shoe wear that compresses against prominent dorsal bony osteophytes as well as from any metatarsal alignment deformities resulting from degenerative changes. Physical examination generally demonstrates dorsal tenderness to palpation overlying the TMT joints with varying degrees of osteophyte formation. A weight-bearing examination is also essential to determine the degree and extent of deformity. In this setting, patients will have a flatfoot appearance with pronation, dorsiflexion, and abduction of the medial column.

B. Imaging Studies and Special Tests

Plain weight-bearing radiographs consisting of AP, oblique, and lateral views should be ordered. Typical radiographic findings are narrowing of the involved TMT joints, most commonly the second TMT. With severe cases that have concordant deformity, a collapse of the longitudinal may be visible.

Treatment

Treatment of midfoot arthritis initially involves NSAIDs, stiffer shoes, and orthotics to support the arch. If bony osteophytes are the main complaint, patients may obtain pressure relief with padding and stretching of the overlying shoe or simply wearing a shoe that has a soft, mesh-like upper. Selective glucocorticoid injections can be both therapeutic and diagnostic for midfoot arthritis, and fluoroscopic or ultrasound guidance may be considered to avoid steroids leaching into the surrounding tissue which in rare cases may lead to ulcerations or extensor tendon ruptures. If these modalities are unsuccessful in alleviating pain, patients may be referred to a foot and ankle surgeon for consideration of midfoot arthrodesis of the involved joints.

LISFRANC MIDFOOT DISLOCATION

 ESSENTIALS OF DIAGNOSIS

▶ Tenderness to palpation about the midfoot.
▶ Pain associated with ROM.
▶ Disruption or malalignment of the TMT articulations on weight-bearing radiographs.

▶ Clinical Findings

A. Symptoms and Signs

Lisfranc injuries classically occur secondary to either a high-energy mechanism such as a motor vehicle accident or a fall from height. Lower-energy twisting injuries can also lead to this lesion, however. An estimated 20% of such injuries may be missed on initial examinations, and therefore clinicians must have a high degree of suspicion, especially if the injury is purely ligamentous and not appreciated on non–weight-bearing radiographs. On examination there is a variable degree of swelling and deformity initially, and patients almost universally have pain in the midfoot. A pathognomonic finding is ecchymosis in the plantar midarch region.

B. Imaging Studies and Special Tests

Radiologic evaluation for midfoot instability includes standard AP, oblique, and lateral weight-bearing radiographs of the involved foot with a low threshold for comparison views of the contralateral, unaffected limb. Instability will manifest as often subtle malalignment of the metatarsal with its corresponding midfoot bone. On the AP view, the medial border of the second metatarsal should form a continuous line with the medial border of the middle cuneiform, and the intermetatarsal space between the first and second metatarsals should be roughly equivalent to that on the contralateral side. On the oblique view, the medial border of the fourth metatarsal forms a continuous line with the medial border of the cuboid, and the lateral border of the third metatarsal forms a straight line with the lateral border of the lateral cuneiform. On the lateral radiograph, there may be evidence of dorsal or less commonly plantar displacement of the metatarsals relative to the tarsal bones.

▶ Treatment

All patients with a Lisfranc injury should be referred to an orthopaedic foot and ankle surgeon. There is a very limited role for nonsurgical treatment of midfoot instability. Surgical treatment entails either early fixation of the injury or a midfoot fusion.

DEEP PERONEAL NERVE ENTRAPMENT

 ESSENTIALS OF DIAGNOSIS

▶ Pain and paresthesia in the first web space.
▶ Positive Tinel sign with percussion.

▶ Clinical Findings

A. Symptoms and Signs

A compression neuropathy involving the deep peroneal nerve is called the anterior tarsal tunnel syndrome. Entrapment may occur via intrinsic space occupying lesions such as osteophytes or cysts pushing the nerve against the inferior extensor retinaculum in the foot. Alternatively, pressure external to the foot such as tightly laced shoes may also produce the same symptoms.

Patients with deep peroneal nerve entrapment present with paresthesias or dysesthesias in the dorsal first web space. Pain will be present at rest, but may be aggravated with plantar flexion of the foot which stretches the nerve. Depending on the location of the compression, weakness of the extensor hallucis brevis may result, causing weakness to hallux extension with resistance placed against the proximal phalanx. A Tinel test should be performed by percussing the deep peroneal nerve as it crosses the dorsal foot. A positive test will reproduce the painful symptoms.

B. Imaging Studies and Special Tests

Radiologic evaluation begins with weight-bearing foot plain films, including AP, oblique, and lateral views. They may point to an etiology of compression such as osteophyte formation or other bony deformity. MRI may be a useful adjuvant to assess for ganglion cysts or other masses that may be causing compression.

▶ Treatment

Initial treatment consists of NSAIDs, rest, and shoe wear modification. Well-padded shoe tongues or alternative lacing can help alleviate compression of the DPN. Medications directed at neuropathic pain may be used, but can be associated with systemic side effects such as drowsiness. In severe acute cases, immobilization and injections may be considered. If all conservative measures fail, referral for decompression and neurolysis is warranted.

▼ HINDFOOT PAIN

SUBTALAR ARTHRITIS

ESSENTIALS OF DIAGNOSIS

▶ Pain in the sinus tarsi region and difficulty walking on uneven surfaces.
▶ Subtalar glucocorticoid injection can be therapeutic and diagnostic.

▶ Clinical Findings

A. Symptoms and Signs

Hindfoot degenerative disease is largely the sequel of trauma or inflammatory processes. Subtalar arthritis typically causes pain over the sinus tarsi area, but pain is not the only symptom. Patients will also often complain of swelling, stiffness, and difficulty with walking on uneven surfaces. Occasionally, there will be a progressive hindfoot valgus deformity. Subtalar motion will be restricted and reproduce the symptoms. It is important to remember the complex nature of foot and ankle motion and the different joints which contribute to both axial and sagittal plane motion.

B. Imaging Studies and Special Tests

Radiographic evaluation begins with routine weight-bearing AP, oblique, and lateral radiographs of the foot and ankle. Views that uniquely image the subtalar joint include Broden views that specifically highlight the posterior facet of the subtalar joint by overly internally rotating the ankle during an AP view. Findings on imaging will be joint space narrowing, osteophyte formation, and subchondral sclerosis. CT scans are often helpful to view the subtalar joint as the unique orientation of the articular surfaces often make them difficult to appreciate on plain films. Sometimes, MRI can also be helpful to differentiate between articular or other sinus tarsi soft-tissue pathology.

▶ Treatment

Nonsurgical management of subtalar arthritis begins with NSAIDs, bracing, shoe modifications, and activity restrictions. AFOs such as the Arizona brace can be very helpful with controlling hindfoot deformity. Glucocorticoid injections can also be considered. When nonsurgical management fails to control symptoms, arthrodesis is the gold standard of treatment, with excellent pain relief.

PES PLANOVALGUS WITH SUBFIBULAR IMPINGMENT

ESSENTIALS OF DIAGNOSIS

▶ Flatfoot on weight-bearing examination.
▶ Pain just distal to the tip of the lateral malleolus.

▶ Clinical Findings

A. Symptoms and Signs

Although patients with progressive flatfoot deformities at the level of the ankle often initially complain of medial pain overlying the posterior tibial tendon, with time and worsening deformity the pain may actually localize laterally over the hindfoot. In such a scenario, pain is attributed to extraarticular lateral hindfoot impingement, including talocalcaneal and subfibular impingement. This pain usually begins in older individuals who have been known to have hindfoot valgus deformities for an extended time. Pain is typically worse with weight bearing and focused just distal to the tip of the lateral malleolus. On physical examination, patients will have significant hindfoot valgus which may be fixed or flexible in nature. It is important to evaluate for possible subluxation or dislocation of the peroneal tendons during routine exam given that lateral pressure from the calcaneus may dislodge them from the groove.

B. Imaging Studies and Special Tests

Radiographic evaluation begins with plain weight-bearing AP, oblique, and lateral foot and ankle films showing a pes planovalgus deformity. Cross-sectional imaging, such as MRI, may be ordered and would show subcortical bone marrow edema in the fibula and calcaneus alongside changes to the posterior tibial and peroneal tendons. CT scans often show subcortical sclerosis and cystic changes at the same location.

▶ Treatment

Conservative treatment of subfibular impingement largely depends on whether the deformity remains flexible or has become rigid. In select cases of flexible flat foot deformities, bracing, orthotics, and physical therapy can be considered initially, the idea being to create a medial post to the hindfoot swinging the calcaneus away from the distal fibula. Rigid deformities may benefit from an attempt at bracing. In refractory cases, surgical treatment is necessary. For flexible deformities, joint sparing osteotomies at both the calcaneus and other sites within the foot, depending on the origin of the flatfoot, may be considered to bring the hindfoot out of valgus and to eliminate the source of impingement. For fixed deformities, treatment generally entails either a double (subtalar and talonavicular) or triple (subtalar, talonavicular, and calcaneocuboid) hindfoot arthrodesis.

TARSAL COALITION

 ESSENTIALS OF DIAGNOSIS

▶ Flatfoot that is rigid and an arch that does not reconstitute upon heel rise.
▶ History of recurrent ankle sprains.
▶ Pain that generally presents in late childhood or teenage years, more rarely as a young adult.

▶ Clinical Findings

A. Symptoms and Signs

Tarsal coalitions occur most commonly in two locations, calcaneonavicular and talocalcaneal, but can occur in other joints as well. Their origin is a failure of segmentation of bones during development. This can result in altered hindfoot motion, and the classic deformity found in feet with coalitions includes flattening of the longitundinal arch with abduction of the forefoot and a valgus hindfoot. Most patients are asymptomatic and these coalitions are found incidentally. When painful, however, patients will frequently localize the source to the sinus tarsi in the setting of calcaneonavicular coalitions, and overlying the subtalar joint versus distal to the medial malleolus in the setting of talocalcaneal coalitions which tend to involve the middle facet of the subtalar joint. Pain is often associated activity-dependent. On physical examination, the hindfoot will demonstrate limited motion, and the medial foot longitudinal arch will not reconstitute upon heel-rise. Patients may present with a history of multiple prior ankle sprains.

B. Imaging Studies and Special Tests

Radiographic evaluation initially consists of weight-bearing AP, oblique, and lateral foot plain radiographs. The oblique image is best for evaluating calcaneonavicular coalitions. Lateral radiographs will show either an "anteater sign" (elongated anterior process of the calcaneus) with calcanonavicular coalitions or a "c-sign" (C-shaped arc formed by the medial outline of the talar dome and the posteroinferior aspect of the sustentaculum tali) with talocalcaneal coalitions. CT scans can be used to determine the size, location, and extent of the coalition. Not all coalitions are bony and can also be fibrous or cartilaginous.

▶ Treatment

In most cases, a coalition will be found incidentally and no intervention is needed. In the case of a painful coalition, initial treatment consists of immobilization in a walking cast or boot for 6 weeks followed by progressive return to activity. If patients have persistent symptoms, referral to a foot and ankle surgeon for surgical reconstruction should be considered. Surgical treatment generally entails resection of the coalition, with or without osteotomies to correct associated foot deformity, versus a fusion procedure in cases of more advanced deformity or more extensive coalition joint involvement.

HEEL PAIN

A range of disorders manifest as heel pain (Table 5–1). Accurate diagnosis starts with identifying the location of the pain source. Most heel pain occurs under the plantar, weight-bearing surface, or over the posterior aspect.

PLANTAR FASCIITIS

 ESSENTIALS OF DIAGNOSIS

▶ Pain with the first steps in the morning (start-up pain).
▶ Pain elicited by deep palpation of the plantar fascia origin.

Table 5–1. Causes of heel pain.

Infracalcaneal pain
  Plantar fasciitis
  Infracalcaneal nerve entrapment
  Fat pad atrophy
  Infracalcaneal bursitis
  Calcaneal stress fracture
  Tarsal tunnel syndrome
  Radiculopathy
  Spondyloarthropathy
  Infection
  Tumor
  Fractured heel spur
Retrocalcaneal heel pain
  Achilles tendinitis
  Haglund deformity
  Pre-Achilles bursitis
  Retrocalcaneal bursitis
  Posterior lateral calcaneal exostosis
  Lateral calcaneal adventitious bursitis
Tenderness with lateral compression of the heel
  Stress fracture of the calcaneus
  Osteomyelitis (especially in children)
  Calcaneal apophysitis (ie, Sever disease, especially in boys ages 8–15 years)

▶ Clinical Findings

A. Symptoms and Signs

Plantar fasciitis is a benign, generally self-limited enthesopathy that occurs at the origin of the plantar fascia on the plantar medial tubercle of the calcaneus (Figure 5–2). The plantar fascia is a band of tissue that supports the arch of the foot. Fasciitis is thought to occur as an overuse phenomenon leading to microtrauma to the fascia causing degenerative changes, though the exact etiology is unknown. Risk factors include elevated body mass, gastrocnemius or equinus contracture, employment that requires prolonged standing, and pes planus. Patients will characteristically describe atraumatic onset of pinpoint tenderness at the insertion of the fascia on the calcaneus. Pain may also be located along the medial aspect of the plantar fascia as it courses along the foot. The pain is typically worse after initially getting out of bed or rising after a period of prolonged sitting, and is somewhat relieved after taking the first initial steps. It is important to note ankle ROM as plantar fasciitis often occurs in the setting of a tight Achilles tendon.

B. Imaging Studies and Special Tests

Plantar fasciitis is generally a clinical diagnosis. Radiographs of the affected foot may show a plantar heel enthesophyte or spur. These findings are not causative of the pain and are found in a high proportion of asymptomatic adults, and do not have to be removed accordingly.

▶ Treatment

Most cases of plantar fasciitis resolve with time given that it tends to be a *self-limited condition*. It is important to educate the patient that pain does not disappear quickly with treatment, but typically diminishes slowly over the course of months. Initial treatment focuses on gastrocnemius and plantar fascial stretching, NSAIDs, and use of a heel cushion

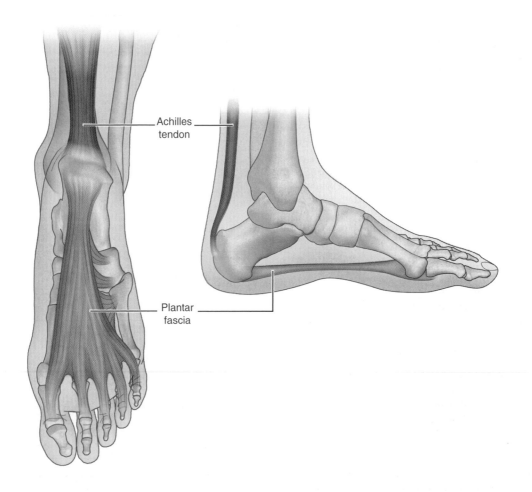

Achilles tendon

Plantar fascia

▲ **Figure 5–2.** Plantar fascia is the thick band of tissue that covers the bones on the bottom of the foot.

to provide symptomatic relief. Regular calf and hamstring stretching should be attempted first as this is noninvasive and often provides significant relief. Night splints are effective in patients for whom pain is particularly bothersome in the morning. Prefabricated shoe inserts are just as effective as custom orthotics in pain relief, though neither has been definitively proven to hasten recovery. Many patients inquire about glucocorticoid injections, but they must be educated that there is an associated risk of fat pad atrophy or atraumatic plantar fascia rupture associated with their use. If patients present with a limp, a period of immobilization in a walking cast or boot may be considered.

In refractory cases, extracorporeal shock wave therapy (ESWT) is a safe and often effective option, but can initially be a painful treatment for patients and generally is not covered by insurance plans.

Surgical release of the plantar fascia is considered only in the most refractory of cases as it can be associated with negative sequela such as loss of the medial longitudinal arch of the foot and a painful scar. It is rarely necessary.

BAXTER NERVE SYNDROME (ENTRAPMENT OF THE FIRST BRANCH OF THE LATERAL PLANTAR NERVE)

 ESSENTIALS OF DIAGNOSIS

▶ Pain to direct palpation over the region of the Baxter nerve.
▶ Burning pain proximally or distally from the point of compression.

▶ Clinical Findings

An uncommon etiology of heel pain entails entrapment of the first branch of the *lateral plantar nerve* (ie, *Baxter nerve*). Compression in this condition occurs as the first branch traverses between the deep fascia of the abductor halluces muscle and the medial margin of the quadratus plantae muscle. The location is somewhat more proximal to the origin of the plantar fascia and overlies the flesh muscle origin of the abductor hallucis. The condition is more common in running athletes in their late thirties, but may occur in nonathletes. Patients will complain of chronic heel pain that can radiate proximally or distally into the foot or ankle. Similar to plantar fasciitis, pain may be worst in the morning, but little relief will be found with stretching, NSAIDs, or orthotics. The pathognomonic physical examination finding is tenderness to palpation over the first branch of the lateral plantar nerve, deep to the abductor hallucis. Continued pressure in the same area causes reproduction of symptoms.

▶ Treatment

Upon arriving at the diagnosis, treatment may begin with a trial of orthotics with a soft arch to decrease pressure. Patients should be warned that orthotics may increase symptoms by crowding the shoe and having the opposite of the desired effect. Neuropathic pain medications can also be helpful. Surgical release of the abductor hallucis fascia is considered when symptoms persist though results may be unpredictable.

FAT PAD ATROPHY

 ESSENTIALS OF DIAGNOSIS

▶ Diffuse, central heel pain aggravated by impact loading activity.
▶ Palpable atrophy of the heel pad.

▶ Clinical Findings

The fat pad of the heel consists of irreplaceable, specialized, separate hydraulic fat chambers designed to absorb shock and transmit mechanical forces to the calcaneus. Fat pad degeneration may occur with increasing age, certain rheumatologic diseases, vascular disease, multiple glucocorticoid injections, and trauma. With atrophy, the resultant heel pain is central and diffuse. In severe cases, the underlying bone may be palpable.

▶ Treatment

There is no surgical solution for this condition. Treatment consists of shoe modification and flexible heel cups that provide external cushion and absorb shock. Glucocorticoid injections are to be avoided because they may exacerbate fat pad atrophy.

TARSAL TUNNEL SYNDROME

 ESSENTIALS OF DIAGNOSIS

▶ Entrapment of the posterior tibial nerve in the tarsal tunnel typically produces unilateral pain, paresthesias, or dysesthesias along the plantar aspect of the foot and toes.
▶ Percussion (Tinel sign) or compression of the posterior tibial nerve along the posteromedial heel elicits symptoms.

Clinical Findings

A. Symptoms and Signs

Tarsal tunnel syndrome is a compression of the tibial nerve as it passes through a fibro-osseous tunnel in the posteromedial heel, posterior and distal to the medial malleolus. The tunnel is created by the flexor retinaculum and the medial talus and calcaneus. Contents of the tunnel include the tibial nerve, along with the posterior tibial artery, flexor hallucis longus tendon, flexor digitorum longus tendon, and the tibialis posterior tendon. Compression of the posterior tibial nerve within the tarsal tunnel may result from a space-occupying lesion, bony deformity, or trauma, or may be idiopathic. Patients present with vague radiating and burning pain in the foot, made worse with activity. Paresthesias may be reported in the plantar foot with a varied distribution based on the location of compression and the level of tibial nerve bifurcation. On examination, patients will have reproducible pain and paresthesias with percussion of the tibial nerve in the tarsal tunnel (Tinel sign). Direct compression of the nerve will recreate symptoms and a dorsiflexion-eversion test can also help make the diagnosis. Neurologic examination is often unremarkable. It is important to perform a standing examination of the foot to evaluate for foot deformity given that tarsal tunnel syndrome can be associated with pes planovalgus.

B. Imaging Studies and Special Tests

Radiographic analysis begins with plain weight-bearing films of the foot to evaluate for obvious bony pathology or deformity leading to nerve compression. MRI may be considered to further evaluate the presence of a space-occupying lesion within the tunnel. Electrodiagnositc studies are equivocally useful in detecting tarsal tunnel syndrome though they may distinguish this diagnosis from lumbar radiculopathy. They should not, however, replace history and physical examination, and even a positive study may not automatically predicate a positive outcome with surgical treatment.

Treatment

First-line treatment consists of activity modification, ice, NSAIDs, and immobilization. In cases secondary to foot deformity, orthotics may be used to correct deformity and eliminate tension on the tibial nerve. Glucocorticoid injections can be helpful, though one must be aware of the risks of tendon rupture secondary to degeneration. Medications for neuropathic pain as well as topical anesthetics may also be effective.

In refractory cases, surgical release of the tibial nerve may be considered. This is generally more successful in eliminating symptoms when there is a documented space-occupying lesion, but less so in cases without obvious causes of compression. Among the latter, some studies suggest that over 40% of patients may do quite poorly after release. Caution should be exercised when considering release in patients without a space-occupying lesion.

NONINSERTIONAL & INSERTIONAL ACHILLES TENDINOSIS

 ESSENTIALS OF DIAGNOSIS

▶ Pain with direct palpation of Achilles tendon.
▶ Fusiform swelling of the tendon.

Clinical Findings

A. Symptoms and Signs

There are a series of conditions related to the Achilles tendon leading to posterior heel pain. Pain may originate from the Achilles itself, a posterior prominence on the posterior calcaneus known as Haglund deformity, a posterior spur formed at the Achilles insertion, or in the bursal space between the Achilles tendon and posterior aspect of the calcaneus.

Achilles tendinopathy may affect the tendon in one of two locations: at the insertion of the tendon on the calcaneus or 2–6 cm proximal to its insertion. Hence, the terms **insertional** and **noninsertional tendinosis.** When the pain originates at the insertion of the Achilles it is often accompanied by retrocalcaneal bursitis and a Haglund deformity of the calcaneus. A prominent bony spur may also form at its insertion. Patients with more proximal tendinosis often present with fusiform swelling of the involved tendon. Achilles tendinosis can be due to overuse, and is often associated with tight heel cords. Disease can occur in both active and sedentary persons, and tendon rupture can occur but is uncommon.

Patients will report a slow onset of pain in the posterior ankle that can be aggravated by shoe wear with a prominent counter. Pain may be particularly bothersome when rising after sitting or resting for prolonged periods.

On examination, pain is reproduced by direct palpation over the diseased portion of the tendon. Often times one will find swelling and bogginess over the area of the affected tendon. Retrocalcaneal bursitis when accompanying Achilles tendinosis may be appreciated as medial and lateral swelling immediately anterior to the tendon. The differential diagnosis of Achilles tendinopathy is shown in Table 5–2.

Table 5–2. Differential diagnosis of Achilles tendinopathy.

Rheumatoid arthritis
Gout
Seronegative arthropathies
Diffuse idiopathic skeletal hyperostosis (DISH)
Fluoroquinolone antibiotic treatment
Systemic glucocorticoids

B. Imaging Studies and Special Tests

Radiographic evaluation begins with weight-bearing plain films of the foot. On the lateral radiograph, one may observe the presence of a large Haglund deformity on the calcaneus or an insertional spur. A thickened soft-tissue shadow depicting the Achilles tendon may be appreciated. MRI is not generally necessary for diagnosis.

▶ Treatment

The mainstay of initial treatment is physical therapy focusing on eccentric exercises and stretching of the gastrocsoleus complex. Heel lifts and activity modification are often recommended. Shoes may be adjusted to avoid direct pressure from the counter of the shoe, and often patients find that they benefit from going up a half or full size in their shoes. NSAIDs may be effective in relieving periods of acute pain. In patients who present with an acute limp and severe pain, a period of immobilization in a walking boot may be considered. Patients may inquire about use of a glucocorticoid injection, but this should be avoided given the significant associated risk of tendon rupture.

When conservative measures fail to provide acceptable relief for insertional Achilles tendinosis and when in the context of significant bony prominences such as an insertional spur or Haglund deformity, surgery may be considered. Surgical intervention involves debridement of diseased tendon and excision of associated spurs and Haglund deformities. The latter requires detachment of the Achilles tendon from its bony insertion with subsequent reattachment, and patients must therefore be aware of the significant associated recovery period. Surgery plays less of a role in the treatment of noninsertional Achilles tendinosis, though more recent studies have suggested that recession of a tight gastrocnemius muscle may play a role.

ACHILLES TENDON RUPTURE

ESSENTIALS OF DIAGNOSIS

▶ Patient reports pop in heel during sporting activity.
▶ Thompson Test—Lack of ankle plantar flexion when calf is squeezed.

▶ Clinical Findings

A. Symptoms and Signs

Achilles tendon ruptures are an important injury to consider among patients with posterior ankle pain. They risk being misdiagnosed as ankle sprains, and studies highlight that patients with elevated BMI, increasing age, and non–sports-related injury mechanisms are at heightened risk of misdiagnosis. The typical presentation involves a perceived pop during forced plantar flexion of the ankle, often while engaged in athletic activities, followed by self-described weakness and

pain in the posterior ankle. Patients will often have a palpable gap at the site of tendon rupture, though this among the least reliable of clinical findings. The Thompson test, the most sensitive physical examination maneuver, entails squeezing the patient's calf with the knee straight and foot hanging over the table edge and assessing the resultant foot motion. If the Achilles tendon is ruptured, patients will lack plantar flexion with this test, especially as compared to the contralateral side. The ability to actively plantarflex the foot, however, may be preserved due to the intact deep flexors of the leg.

B. Imaging Studies and Special Tests

Radiographic workup of this injury consists of AP, oblique, and lateral radiographs of the ankle. It is important to look at the lateral view to ensure that there is no bony avulsion of the tendon off of the calcaneus.

▶ Treatment

After diagnosing an acute Achilles tendon rupture, the patient should immediately be placed in a splint in maximum equinus and referred to a foot or ankle surgeon. Treatment can be either operative or nonoperative depending on a discussion with the patient. Nonoperative treatment consists of a brief period of splinting followed by functional bracing, whereas surgical treatment involves end-to-end suture repair. Traditionally, it was thought that nonoperative treatment led to a relative increase in the risk of rerupture of the tendon, though more modern functional rehabilitation protocols have mitigated some of this risk.

▼ ANKLE PAIN

ANKLE ARTHRITIS

ESSENTIALS OF DIAGNOSIS

▶ Pain and mechanical symptoms at the anterior aspect of the ankle joint.
▶ Decreased range of motion at the ankle that elicits pain.

▶ Clinical Findings

A. Symptoms and Signs

A history and physical examination is the most important diagnostic tool for ankle arthritis. The majority of ankle arthritis is posttraumatic in origin, and patients will present with pain and mechanical symptoms of locking and stiffness at the anterior aspect of the ankle. The pain is increased with weight bearing and relieved with rest. Stiffness will commonly be worse in the morning or after sitting for prolong periods. Physical examination should be complete, including gait analysis, assessment of alignment, inspection, palpation, neurovascular examination, range of motion, strength testing, and stability testing. Gait in the setting of ankle arthritis will often reveal a decreased velocity and stride length. Range of motion will be severely limited with end-stage arthritis.

B. Imaging Studies and Special Tests

Degenerative joint disease of the ankle is best visualized using standard weight-bearing plain ankle radiographs, including AP, mortise, and lateral views. Findings will consist of joint space narrowing, subchondral sclerosis, cystic changes, and osteophyte formation. Sometimes, radiographs may point to inflammatory causes of arthritis. In rheumatoid arthritis, radiographs may show periarticular osteopenia and marginal erosions. Crystalline arthropathies, such as gout, can create punched out erosions beneath the joint surfaces and pseudo-gout will lead to chondrocalcinosis within the joint.

▶ Treatment

There are many options for conservative treatment of ankle arthritis. Similar to arthritis in other regions, NSAIDs, ambulatory aids, and bracing are options for providing pain relief. Local injections of corticosteroids into the ankle combined with a local anesthetic can be diagnostic and therapeutic for these patients. A custom-molded AFO is the gold standard brace for ankle arthritis, but flexible lace-up braces may be tolerated better by some patients. Treatment should be aligned with the patient's preferences and likelihood of compliance. Shoe modifications may also be considered. A rocker bottom shoe has been shown to improve both gait and pain in the setting of ankle arthritis.

If these nonoperative mechanisms fail, surgical management may be considered. The gold standard treatment is tibiotalar arthrodesis, which is often successful at decreasing pain. However, adjacent joint degeneration and altered joint mechanics can be complications associated with this fusion. Ankle arthroplasty is gaining in popularity in the United States and results have improved with modern-generation prostheses, though its indications are more limited in younger and higher-demand patients. Choosing between these tibiotalar arthrodesis and ankle arthroplasty can be a complicated decision, and patients should be educated about the associated risks, with patient selection critical for success.

OSTEOCHONDRAL LESIONS OF THE TALUS (OSTEOCHONDRITIS DISSECANS)

 ESSENTIALS OF DIAGNOSIS

▶ Ankle joint pain exacerbated by weight-bearing activity.

▶ No pathognomonic clinical examination findings.

▶ Advanced imaging (MRI or CT scan) often necessary to make diagnosis.

▶ Clinical Findings

A. Symptoms and Signs

An osteochondral lesion of the talus can be described as a local condition that results in the detachment of a segment of cartilage and its corresponding subchondral bone from an articular surface. The etiology is most commonly traumatic, though many cases are idiopathic. The location of the lesion may provide information as to the nature of the injury. Medial lesions are more common, can be atraumatic or congenital, and tend to be deeper and more posterior than lateral lesions. Lateral lesions are almost always secondary to a known trauma and tend to be more anterior and shallower. Unfortunately, lateral lesions also are more commonly displaced. In acute cases, the signs and symptoms are similar to those found in ankle sprains: ecchymosis, ligament pain, ankle swelling, and limited range of motion. Mechanical locking can occur but is not a common complaint. In chronic cases, stiffness, activity-related pain, and intermittent swelling are typical complaints. There are essentially no pathognomonic clinical signs of osteochondral lesions of the talus.

B. Imaging Studies and Special Tests

Initial radiographic evaluation consists of AP, oblique, and lateral views of the ankle. If these are negative, and one has a high index of suspicion, either MRI or CT scan is indicated, as many lesions are undetectable on plain radiographs. MRI is useful in detecting the presence of a lesion, whereas a CT scan is helpful in determining the extent of bony involvement, including underlying cyst formation.

▶ Treatment

When osteochondral lesions of the talus are asymptomatic and discovered as incidental findings on imaging studies, they require no treatment. For symptomatic lesions, treatment depends on the chronicity, stage, and size of the defect. For nondisplaced lesions, a period of immobilization in a cast or walking boot is recommended along with temporary avoidance of impact-loading activities. Lesions in young patients with open growth plates tend to heal more successfully with this treatment. For unstable lesions, surgery is usually required to alleviate symptoms. Surgical treatment involves arthroscopic evaluation of the lesion followed by either stabilization of the fragment or debridement followed by a mix of cartilage restoration procedures depending on the size and extent of the lesion.

CHRONIC ANKLE IMPINGEMENT

 ESSENTIALS OF DIAGNOSIS

▶ Pain in the anterior ankle.

▶ Limited dorsiflexion of the ankle with pain.

Clinical Findings

A. Symptoms and Signs

Anterior tibiotalar impingement is caused by anterior osteophytes or soft-tissue abnormalities arising from the result of trauma or degeneration. The classic presentation is one of pain in the anterior ankle that is worse with forced dorsiflexion. If there is a mechanical block, the patient may have limited dorsiflexion on exam.

B. Imaging Studies and Special Tests

Radiographic evaluation consists of AP, oblique, and lateral weight-bearing views of the ankle which will display osteophytes in the anterior distal tibial or dorsal aspect of the talus. A CT scan may be performed to better delineate the location of the osteophytes. MRI may be ordered to determine soft-tissue impingement as well as associated intra-articular pathology such as osteochondral defects.

Treatment

Initial treatment involves NSAIDs, physical therapy, and bracing or shoe wear modification. A local glucocorticoid injection in combination with a local anesthetic can be both diagnostic and therapeutic. If pain persists, patients can be referred to a foot and ankle surgeon for consideration of debridement and excision of associated bone spurs or soft-tissue lesions, often arthroscopically.

EXTRA-ARTICULAR CAUSES OF ANKLE PAIN

Extra-articular causes of ankle pain tend to localize to the posterior medial, the posterior lateral, or the anterolateral aspects of the ankle and produce characteristic findings depending on which structures are involved (Table 5–3).

Table 5–3. Extra-articular causes of ankle pain.

Posterior medial ankle pain
Flexor hallucis longus dysfunction
Tibialis posterior tendon dysfunction
Tarsal tunnel syndrome
Posterior lateral ankle pain
Posterior talar impingement syndrome
Peroneal tendinopathy
Tarsal coalition of the subtalar joint posterior facet
Sural nerve neuropathy
Anterior lateral ankle pain
Sinus tarsi syndrome
Superficial peroneal nerve neuropathy
Lateral ankle ligament pathology
Coalition of the talocalcaneal or calcaneal-navicular joints

1. Posterior Tibial Tendinosis

ESSENTIALS OF DIAGNOSIS

▶ Pain over posterior tibial tendon in early stages.

▶ Progressive planovalgus deformity characterized by a valgus heel, collapsed medial arch, and abducted forefoot.

Clinical Findings

A. Symptoms and Signs

Posterior tibial tendon insufficiency or tendonosis is a degenerative process that most commonly presents around the fifth or sixth decade of life, with a higher prevalence in women. The tendon is susceptible to degeneration as it exits the tarsal tunnel and loops around the medial malleolus. Among patients with flat feet, the posterior tibial tendon may be under increased stretch, exacerbating any preexisting wear. While it is not automatically pathological to have flatfeet, it is pathologic to have progressive flattening of the foot, and this results in collapse and worsening flatfoot deformity. As a result of this complex interaction, patients with posterior tibial tendinosis are staged based on the degree of hindfoot deformity. Stage 1 tendinosis is characterized by pain and swelling localized to the posterior tibial tendon with no deformity in the foot. The tendon functions normally and is demonstrated by preforming a single leg heel rise. In stage 2, the tendon becomes elongated reducing its ability to function, and patients will no longer be able to preform a single limb heel rise. The result is progressive deformity of the foot that consists of a flattening arch, a valgus hindfoot posture and an abducted forefoot. Despite worsening deformity, the hindfoot remains flexible and the heel may be passively returned to varus and the forefoot may be easily rotated. With increasing chronicity of symptoms, patients may paradoxically report a relief of their medially based pain as a result of ultimate failure of the tendon but may develop lateral pain as the calcaneus swings outward impinging on the fibula. Stage 3 correlates with a rigid deformity, and stage 4 indicates involvement of the ankle joint with valgus malalignment due to deltoid ligament insufficiency. In all patients, ankle range of motion should be documented as concomitant equinus contractures are frequently present.

B. Imaging Studies and Special Tests

Radiographic evaluation begins with AP, oblique, and lateral weight-bearing plain films of the foot and ankle. These images help to assess the severity of a planovalgus deformity as well as assess for any associated hindfoot arthritis. MRI or ultrasound may be considered if the initial diagnosis of posterior tibial tendonosis is unclear, though this can generally be made clinically.

▶ Treatment

Conservative treatment begins in a stepwise manner. Patients presenting in acute pain with an antalgic gait may undergo a period of immobilization in a walking boot. This is followed by a course of formal physical therapy in conjunction with the use of a medial hindfoot post orthotic to take pressure of the medial tendon. If orthotics alone are insufficient in correcting deformity, bracing may be considered. Surgery is indicated for refractory pain. Surgical treatment depends on the stage of disease. Surgery for flexible deformities seek to address and correct the deforming forces, including debridement or resection of the diseased posterior tibial tendon, flexor digitorum longus tendon transfer to the navicular, medializing calcaneal osteotomy, and selected midfoot fusions, and osteotomies. For rigid deformities, the alignment may only be corrected with hindfoot fusion.

2. Peroneal Tendonitis

ESSENTIALS OF DIAGNOSIS

▶ Pain about the posterolateral hindfoot.
▶ Pain with resisted ankle eversion.

▶ Clinical Findings

A. Symptoms and Signs

Peroneal tendonitis can occur at many levels along the course of the peroneal tendon, and may be secondary to trauma, overuse, or inflammatory disease. Patients will typically complain of vague pain on the posterolateral hindfoot that is worse with activity and better with rest. They will be tender to palpation along the peroneal tendons either immediately posterior to the distal fibula or distal to the lateral malleolus at the site of the peroneal tubercle, and there may be a palpable thickening located in this region. There may also be pain with active eversion of the ankle. It is important to evaluate the alignment of the hindfoot given that patients will often times have hindfoot varus, causing abnormal stress on the peroneal tendons, and predisposing to such conditions.

B. Imaging Studies and Special Tests

Radiographs of the ankle may be useful in ruling out other pathology or diagnosing hindfoot deformity. To most clearly image the peroneal tendons, MRI should be considered. Ultrasound may be useful to not only assess tears but also to evaluated for dynamic issues such as tendon instability.

▶ Treatment

Nonsurgical manamement for peroneal tendonitis includes orthotics, physical therapy, or even a period of supportive immobilization in a CAM boot or a brace. Some advocate for

a local injection of corticosteroid combined with a local anesthetic, though there is an inherent risk of atraumatic rupture of the peroneal tendons. If patients have persistent pain and swelling, referral should be made to a foot and ankle surgeon for consideration of peroneal tenosynovectomy, debridement, and possible repair.

3. Posterior Ankle Impingement (Os Trigonum Syndrome)

ESSENTIALS OF DIAGNOSIS

▶ Posterolateral or direct posterior ankle pain.
▶ Pain is reproducible with forced plantar flexion of the ankle.

▶ Clinical Findings

A. Symptoms and Signs

Posterior ankle impingement occurs as the dorsal aspect of the calcaneal body approaches the posterior aspect of the tibial plafond entrapping the local bony or soft tissues with ankle plantar flexion. This presents as pain over the posterolateral aspect of the ankle or, less often, over the posterior aspect of the ankle deep to the Achilles tendon. Pain is worst when the foot is forced to maximal plantar flexion. The etiology may be repetitive activity in the plantarflexed position or a single traumatic plantar flexion injury. The presence of an os trigonum predisposes to posterior impingement, but is more commonly asymptomatic. Physical examination reveals reproduction of pain with forced plantar flexion of the foot. There may also be slight swelling over the posterior ankle.

When evaluating patients who recall a recent history of trauma, one must be aware that fractures of the posterior process of the talus can mimic posterior impingement, and this must be ruled out when making the diagnosis.

B. Imaging Studies and Special Tests

Radiographic evaluation begins with AP, lateral, and oblique plain films of the ankle. The lateral image allows for identification of an os trigonum. A CT scan may be helpful in ruling out a talus fracture if the radiographs are inconclusive. MRI may be obtained, and will characteristically show bone marrow edema and thickening of the posterior capsule.

▶ Treatment

Conservative treatment begins with NSAIDs, splinting, and activity modification. In acute cases, patients may be immobilized in a walking boot or cast followed by avoidance of offending activities. Steroid injections may provide pain relief in patients with continued symptoms. When nonsurgical measures fail, surgical intervention with posterior ankle and subtalar arthroscopy and excision of offending tissue or os trigonum may be considered.

4. Flexor Hallucis Longus Tendinopathy

ESSENTIALS OF DIAGNOSIS

▶ Pain with palpation of the flexor hallucis longus (FHL) tendon.

▶ Pain with active plantar flexion of the hallux against resistance.

▶ Clinical Findings

A. Symptoms and Signs

FHL tendonosis develops from repetitive use. Risk factors include activities requiring excessive plantar flexion of the great toe, such as in ballet dancers. Tendinosis most commonly occurs posterior to the talus in the fibro-osseus tunnel, but rarely can also occur distally in the foot at the knot of Henry.

Patients with proximal tendinosis will complain of posteromedial ankle pain. On examination, the pain is reproduced with active plantar flexion of the hallux IP joint against resistance. Crepitus may be felt about the posteromedial ankle. In chronic cases, patients may develop a nodule in the tendon, which is appreciated clinically by triggering of the hallux with motion as the nodule is forced to pass through the fibro-osseous tunnel.

B. Imaging Studies and Special Tests

Radiographic evaluation begins with plain weight-bearing radiographs of the ankle to rule out other causes of pain. MRI may be ordered to confirm a suspected diagnosis and will show fluid surrounding the tendon with possible intrasubstance tendon tears. It should be cautioned that fluid around the FHL is commonly seen on MRI in asymptomatic individuals, and should be interpreted only in concert with physical exam findings.

▶ Treatment

Initial treatment consists of rest, NSAIDs, and activity modification. Patients with acute pain may benefit from a period of immobilization in a walking boot or cast, followed by a course of physical therapy. If conservative

measures fail, surgical decompression of the FHL tendon with tenosynovectomy and debridement or repair of the tendon may be warranted.

5. Extensor Tendinopathy

ESSENTIALS OF DIAGNOSIS

▶ Pain over anterior ankle and foot.

▶ Pain with active dorsiflexion of the ankle against resistance.

▶ Clinical Findings

A. Symptoms and Signs

Extensor tendinopathy is typically an overuse phenomenon, most commonly affecting the tibialis anterior tendon. Symptoms consist of pain on the dorsum of the foot and ankle that is worse with activity and better with rest. Patients will sometimes describe having recently started a new repetitive activity. Edema may be found diffusely about the dorsum of the foot. Pain is worst on exam with resisted dorsiflexion of the foot and/or great toe; however, it may also be felt with passive curling of the toes. One of its most distinguishing symptoms is the absence of pain with passive dorsiflexion of the foot, which differentiates extensor tendinopathy from other pathologies.

B. Imaging Studies and Special Tests

Diagnosis is best made by physical examination, but plain radiographs of the foot or ankle may be useful in ruling out other conditions. If there is profound weakness on exam and there is concern for rupture of an extensor tendon, MRI may be useful to evaluate the extent of the injury.

▶ Treatment

Activity modification and rest is the mainstay of treatment for extensor tendinopathy. A period of supportive immobilization in a CAM boot may be useful if pain is severe enough to cause a limp. Patients may also benefit from a course of formal physical therapy. If the patient is found to have sustained a rupture of an extensor tendon, they should be referred to a foot and ankle surgeon for surgical repair.

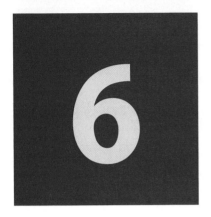

6

Approach to the Patient with Shoulder Pain

John H. Wilckens, MD

Michael T. Freehill, MD

Scott Weiner, DO

Umasuthan Srikumaran, MD

Johnathan A. Bernard, MD

The shoulder complex consists of four joints—the glenohumeral, acromioclavicular (AC), sternoclavicular (SC), and scapulothoracic joints—with encapsulating ligaments and muscles (Figure 6–1). It is the most mobile joint of the body, with the primary role of positioning the hand in space to function. A detailed history and physical examination with appropriate imaging can help narrow the extensive differential diagnosis and guide treatment. Most conditions can be treated initially with medication, glucocorticoid injections, and physical therapy. Resistant shoulder pain should be referred for orthopedic consultation.

► History

Much like pain elsewhere, shoulder pain can be categorized initially by the time of symptom onset, the qualitative character of the pain, and by the activities or strategies that relieve and aggravate it.

The onset of pain may follow a recent injury (≤4 weeks) or remote injury (>4 weeks). Recent injury usually has an acute onset of pain, whereas a remote injury may be episodic or insidious. Because the shoulder is involved in many repetitive functions, pain can result from overuse.

Character, location, timing, and radiation of pain can also be helpful. Sharp or stabbing pain usually suggests a structural cause. Dull and aching pain, especially related to early mornings and weather changes, suggests arthritis. Burning and radiating pain suggests a neurologic cause. Localization to the lateral upper arm is typical of rotator cuff pain. Pain radiating below the elbow or to the medial border of the scapula suggests a cervical spine or neurologic source of the pain. Pain at night is also typical of rotator cuff disease, but it can be noted in metastatic bone disease. Pain with overhead activity is a very common symptom and can be generally categorized as "impingement" pain. It is most commonly caused by rotator cuff dysfunction or disease. Constitutional symptoms, such as fever and weight loss, should alert the clinician that the cause of pain is infectious, metabolic, or neoplastic.

Other symptoms associated with shoulder pain include stiffness, weakness, and instability. A helpful way to frame the magnitude of shoulder pain is to identify the activities that are limited by the pain, such as overhead use, lifting, dressing, combing or shampooing hair, and personal hygiene. Recreational and occupational limitations should also be sought.

► Physical Examination

For an accurate examination, the shoulder needs to be visible; for female patients, privacy can be respected by using special examination gowns or by having the patient wear a sports bra, swimsuit top, or strapless blouse.

Both shoulders should be examined not only from the front but also from the back and side. Particular attention should be paid to shoulder symmetry to allow the clinician to appreciate subtle muscle atrophy. Atrophy suggests neurologic injury or chronicity of the underlying problem.

Palpating the shoulder and assessing its range of motion (ROM) are the next steps in the physical examination.

A. Palpation

Palpation begins at the SC joint and moves laterally over the clavicle to the AC joint. The clinician should be sensitive to deformity, pain, and crepitance. The presence of SC and AC joint pain or deformity can suggest injury, arthritis, or both. A painful acromion may indicate an os acromiale. Next, the greater and lesser tuberosities should be palpated. These are the insertion sites of the supraspinatus and subscapularis, respectively. If tenderness is present at these sites, a rotator cuff abnormality should be suspected. Between the tubercles, the intertubercular groove through which the long head of the biceps courses can be palpated.

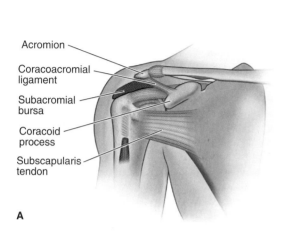

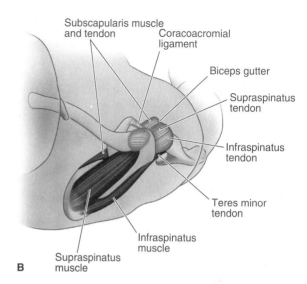

▲ **Figure 6–1.** Shoulder and rotator cuff muscle anatomy, frontal (**A**) and superior (**B**) views.

Tenderness at this location suggests biceps tendinitis, which can occur on its own or with rotator cuff abnormality and superior labral tears.

B. Range of Motion

Because of the shoulder's mobility, its ROM should be checked in several planes, in overhead elevation, and in internal and external rotation. In addition, ROM should be assessed actively and passively. Overhead motion should be observed from the front and back of the patient. From the back, asymmetry of excursion of the scapulae should be assessed. Winging can be observed with serratus anterior, trapezius, and infraspinatus weakness. More subtle medial border elevation is commonly seen with the painful shoulder from weak or misfiring scapular stabilizers, which contribute to the closing of the coracoacromial arch and shoulder impingement.

Internal rotation can be measured by having patients place their thumbs midline on their spines as high as they can. The level of the vertebrae touched should be recorded (Figures 6–2 and 6–3). In addition, internal and external rotation can be measured with the arm abducted 90 degrees and the elbow flexed 90 degrees.

ROM of the affected shoulder should be compared with that of the opposite side. Active ROM that is more painful and restricted than passive ROM suggests a rotator cuff component to the pain. Painful restricted passive ROM, particularly end point pain, is seen in adhesive capsulitis, or "frozen shoulder." The painful arc of motion should also be noted.

Restricted or painful neck motion can refer pain to the shoulder. Therefore, ROM of the cervical spine should also be examined in flexion, extension, lateral bending, and rotation.

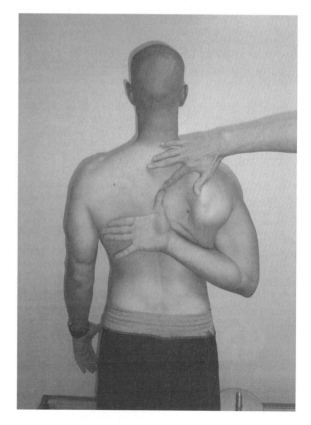

▲ **Figure 6–2.** Measure internal rotation by documenting the vertebral level reached by both the right and left hands.

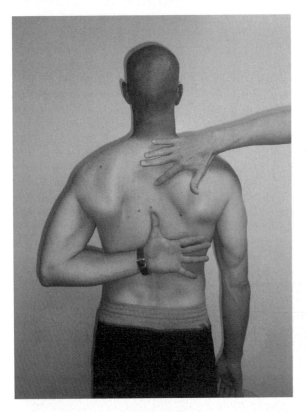

▲ **Figure 6–3.** Measure internal rotation by documenting the vertebral level reached by both the right and left hands.

▶ Neurologic Examination

Muscle testing should be performed next, with special attention to assessment of rotator cuff strength. Abduction against resistance tests the supraspinatus. External rotation versus resistance tests the posterior rotator cuff muscles—the infraspinatus and teres minor. The "belly-press" test and "lift-off" tests assess the anterior rotator cuff muscle, the subscapularis (Figures 6–4 and 6–5).

If cervical neck abnormality is considered, a more formal neurologic examination should be conducted, including an assessment of the patient's sensory modalities, distal motor function, and reflexes.

▶ Special Tests

In addition to the basic examination of the shoulder, numerous abnormality-specific tests or maneuvers can be used to help determine the cause of shoulder pain or dysfunction. Examination of adjacent anatomy (arm, elbow, forearm, hand, and cervical spine) should be performed before these tests. However, many of these tests can elicit pain and apprehension and should therefore be performed after less painful aspects of the

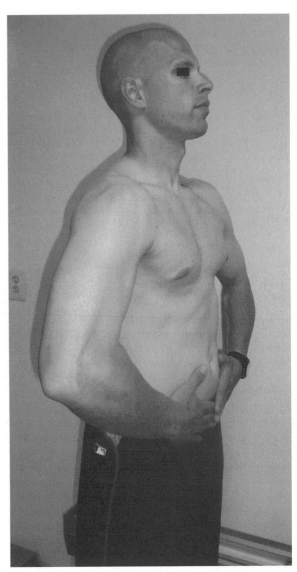

▲ **Figure 6–4.** The belly-press test is used to evaluate the subscapularis.

examination. The findings in the affected shoulder should be compared with those of the normal side. Special tests, including the sulcus sign test, load and shift test, apprehension and relocation test, the Neer test, the Hawkins test, the Yergason test, the Speed test, and the O'Brien test, can be used to assess for abnormalities ranging from instability and rotator cuff impingement, to labral and biceps tendon disease, to disorders of the AC joint.

A. Instability

The shoulder joint is inherently lax, affording it a great degree of mobility. Abnormal laxity represents a spectrum

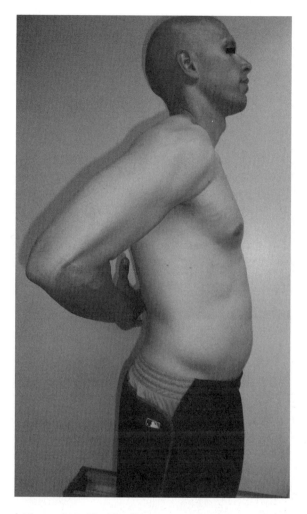

▲ **Figure 6–5.** The lift-off test is used to evaluate the subscapularis.

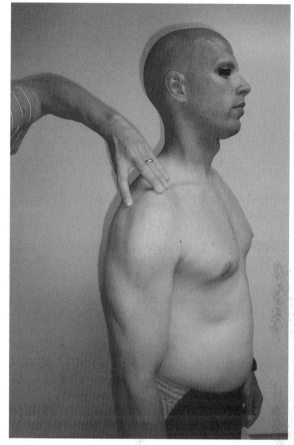

▲ **Figure 6–6.** The sulcus sign test evaluates inferior shoulder laxity.

of disease, ranging from painful subluxation to traumatic dislocation. Because there is a wide range of normal laxity, a determination of abnormal laxity should be made only with consideration of the individual history, baseline examination, or contralateral "normal" examination. Conditions resulting in generalized laxity of several joints should also be considered. These include Marfans Syndrome, Ehlers Danlos Syndrome and other genetic abnormalities. The following are specific tests to evaluate and characterize shoulder instability.

1. Sulcus sign test—The goal of this test is to evaluate for inferior shoulder laxity. With the patient seated, the degree of translation between the lateral border of the acromion and the humeral head is noted as downward force is applied to the distal arm in neutral rotation (Figure 6–6). A "sulcus," or depression in the skin between the acromion and humeral head, is seen. Some practitioners suggest this result should

be graded (grade 0, no translation; grade I [≤1 cm], mild translation; grade II [1–2 cm], moderate translation; grade III [>2 cm], severe translation), whereas others suggest the result should simply be reported as positive or negative. A positive or high-grade sulcus sign in both shoulders may suggest multidirectional instability, whereas a unilateral sulcus sign may suggest inferior instability, particularly if associated with pain or symptoms of instability.

2. Load and shift test—The load and shift test measures humeral translation on the glenoid in the anterior and posterior directions. With the patient seated, the examiner places one hand over the top of the shoulder from the posterior position. The other hand grasps the upper arm, gaining control of the humeral head and controlling rotation (neutral). The first part of this maneuver involves "loading" the joint by applying axial pressure through the arm, centering the humeral head in the glenoid. From this position, anterior or posterior force can be applied (Figures 6–7 and 6–8). The examiner should then note and grade the degree of translation or subluxation

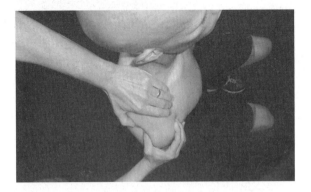

▲ **Figure 6–7.** The load and shift test evaluates the degree of anterior instability.

that is felt as the humeral head slides over the glenoid surface. The modified Hawkins classification assigns three translation grades: I, the humeral head may move up to but not over the glenoid rim; II, the humeral head moves over the rim but returns to a central position; and III, the humeral head moves beyond the rim and requires a reduction maneuver to return to anatomic position. The load and shift test has a high negative predictive value: a negative result excludes anterior or posterior instability.

3. Apprehension and relocation tests—The apprehension test evaluates anterior instability by attempting to reproduce symptoms with the arm in a position of abduction and external rotation. The test can be performed with the patient seated or supine. The examiner positions the patient's arm in increasing amounts of abduction and external rotation while determining whether the patient becomes apprehensive about impending subluxation or dislocation (Figures 6–9 and 6–10). A positive test, indicated by the patient's feeling of apprehension, not simply pain, is suggestive of anterior instability. The positive predictive value of this test approaches 98%.

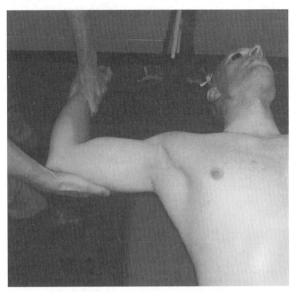

▲ **Figure 6–9.** Anterior instability is evaluated by the apprehension test.

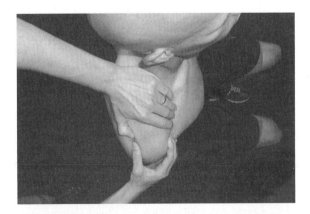

▲ **Figure 6–8.** The load and shift test evaluates the degree of posterior instability.

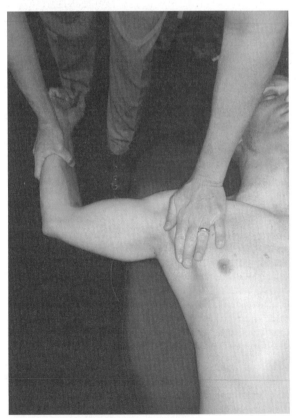

▲ **Figure 6–10.** Anterior instability is evaluated by the Jobe relocation maneuver.

The relocation test is performed in the supine position after the patient's arm is in a position that produces apprehension. The examiner then places one hand anteriorly on the shoulder and applies a posterior force, reducing any humeral head translation. The test is considered positive if this maneuver relieves the sense of apprehension. This test is also very specific and has a 100% positive predictive value for anterior instability.

B. Rotator Cuff Impingement

Patients with rotator cuff pain often note positional pain at night and with overhead activity; however, the pain is usually poorly localized around the anterior or lateral aspect of the shoulder. The Neer and Hawkins tests are frequently used to reproduce this pain and assess for "impingement," which is believed to be a major cause of rotator cuff tendinitis.

1. Neer test—The Neer test is performed by first stabilizing the scapula and then passively raising the patient's arm in forward elevation (Figure 6–11). The patient's report of pain constitutes a positive result and usually occurs at approximately 80 degrees to 120 degrees of elevation (the point at which the anterior rotator cuff impinges on the undersurface of the acromion). This test is nonspecific for rotator cuff abnormality and

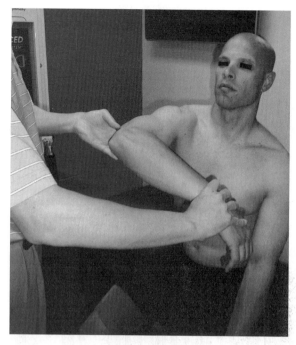

▲ **Figure 6–12.** The Hawkins test evaluates rotator cuff impingement.

may yield a positive result for other conditions, such as adhesive capsulitis, subacromial bursitis, instability, and arthritis.

2. Hawkins test—The Hawkins test is a variation of the Neer test and involves the examiner internally rotating the patient's 90-degree forward-elevated arm with the elbow in flexion (Figure 6–12). The exact anatomic mechanism for pain generation with this maneuver is unclear, but the occurrence of pain implies a rotator cuff abnormality with a high sensitivity and low specificity.

C. Biceps and Labral Abnormality

Abnormality of the biceps tendon is difficult to diagnose because tenderness of the anterior aspect of the shoulder is difficult to isolate anatomically. Likewise, lesions of the labrum (such as superior labrum anterior and posterior [SLAP] lesions) can also be difficult to isolate with the physical examination. Nevertheless, the following tests can help suggest abnormality of these structures.

1. Yergason test—The Yergason test attempts to evaluate for biceps tendon synovitis. With the patient's elbow held at 90 degrees of flexion and the forearm fully pronated, the examiner holds the wrist and resists active supination by the patient (Figure 6–13). Reproduction of pain isolated to the region of the bicipital groove indicates a positive test and likely biceps tendon inflammation. Patients with a rotator cuff tear who also experience anterior shoulder pain should

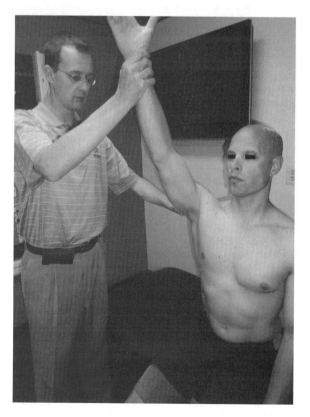

▲ **Figure 6–11.** The Neer test evaluates rotator cuff impingement.

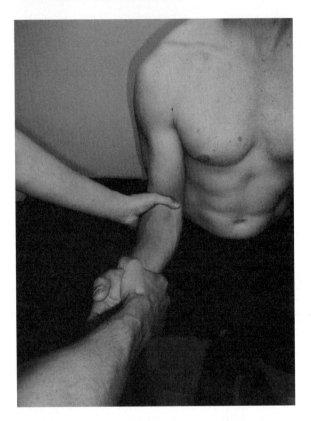

▲ **Figure 6–13.** The Yergason test evaluates biceps tendinitis.

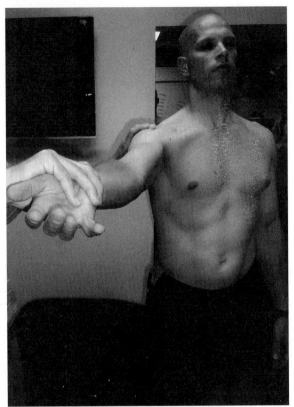

▲ **Figure 6–14.** The Speed test evaluates biceps tendinitis.

have a negative Yergason test. This test has been found to have moderate accuracy with a specificity of 79%.

2. Speed test—The Speed test also attempts to assess for biceps tendon synovitis. The test is performed by having the patient forward-flex the shoulder with the elbow in extension and the forearm in supination against resistance from the examiner at 60 degrees to 90 degrees (Figure 6–14). A positive test causes pain at the bicipital groove. This test has been found to have a specificity of 75% and a sensitivity of 32% in some studies, whereas in others, it has had a sensitivity of 72% and a specificity of 28% for detecting type II SLAP lesions.

3. O'Brien test (active compression sign)—The O'Brien test attempts to discern SLAP lesions. The test is performed by having the patient stand and forward-flex the shoulder to 90 degrees at 10 degrees of adduction, with the elbow extended, the forearm in pronation, and the thumb pointing down. The examiner then applies a downward-directed force on the patient's arm preferably near the wrist. The test is then repeated with the forearm in supination (Figure 6–15). The patient's description of a "click" or pain deep within the shoulder when the arm is pronated, combined with relief or minimal pain with the arm in supination, is considered a positive result and suggestive of a SLAP tear.

D. AC Joint Abnormality

Osteoarthritis, AC separations, and osteolysis are common conditions causing pain around the AC joint. Pain in this anterior region of the shoulder can also be caused by rotator cuff or labral abnormality. In addition to information garnered from the history and physical examination (inspection, palpation), the cross-arm adduction test can help localize pain to the AC joint.

This test is performed by compressing the AC joint by passively adducting the arm at 90 degrees of forward elevation (Figure 6–16). Pain localized to the AC joint is considered a positive test. Sensitivity and specificity are moderately high at 77% and 79%, respectively.

▶ Imaging

A. Radiographs

Radiographs are often used as the initial imaging modality approach to the patient with shoulder pain and can help evaluate the integrity of osseous structures and their anatomic relationship in the shoulder girdle. Radiographs may reveal additional findings that suggest a diagnosis such as the

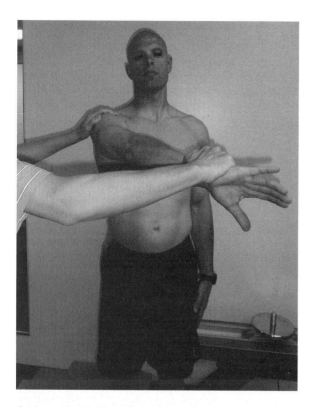

▲ **Figure 6–15.** The O'Brien test evaluates superior labrum anterior and posterior (SLAP) lesions.

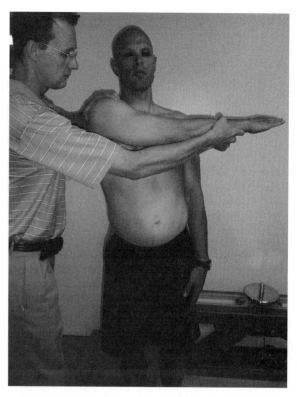

▲ **Figure 6–16.** The cross-arm adduction test evaluates for AC joint abnormality.

so-called "vacuum phenomenon" seen with an intact rotator cuff. In addition, radiographs can document the lack of normal anatomic findings, which may indicate inflammatory conditions. For example, the absence of the peribursal fat plane may indicate rheumatoid arthritis or calcific tendinitis. Signs of rotator cuff impingement, including acromial and supraspinatus outlet morphology, can also be noted on radiographs.

Because there is an association among cuff tears and greater tuberosity sclerosis and hyperostosis, osteophytes, subchondral cysts, and osteolysis in the shoulder, radiography is a reasonable first-line imaging modality for identifying such findings. There are four variations of acromial morphology: flat, curved, convex, and hooked. The hooked type has the highest prevalence for subacromial spurs. Similarly, acromial angle and ossification of the coracoacromial ligament, best seen on outlet view, are also associated with clinical impingement and rotator cuff tears.

There are many radiographic views, all of which yield varying degrees of diagnostic value. A Grashey or true anteroposterior (AP) view with internal or external rotation can be used to assess acute problems. This view is particularly useful in the setting of trauma to identify fractures or dislocations. It can also be useful in chronic conditions, such

as the identification of any narrowing of the glenohumeral space consistent with osteoarthritic changes. However, the true AP view is not useful for the detection of an anterior or posterior dislocation, nor does it help evaluate the lateral shoulder. On the other hand, dislocations can be evaluated on the scapular Y view because this view allows the assessment of the humeral head within the glenoid fossa. The axillary view also allows evaluation of the humeral head and glenoid, making it another study useful for evaluating anterior or posterior subluxation or dislocation. It can also be used to evaluate bony Bankart lesion of the glenoid rim. The West Point view is another option for evaluating the glenoid rim and can be used to identify a bony Bankart lesion. Conversely, the Stryker notch view allows for evaluation of the posterolateral aspect of the humeral head and can document any condition that alters its integrity (eg, a Hill-Sachs or Bennett lesion).

B. Arthrography

Shoulder arthrography can be helpful in diagnosing and treating adhesive capsulitis. Increased resistance on injection of a small amount of the radiopaque contrast agent into the glenohumeral joint and documentation of a small axillary pouch and subscapular recess are diagnostic of adhesive capsulitis.

Shoulder arthrography is also still used on occasion to evaluate full-thickness rotator cuff tears, rupture of the long head of the biceps, and diagnosis and treatment of adhesive capsulitis. This imaging modality, which can be performed as a single-contrast or double-contrast study, involves the fluoroscopic injection of a radiopaque contrast agent into the glenohumeral joint space. Arthrography is effective at defining normal shoulder anatomy and detecting rotator cuff tears. With arthrography, detection of full-thickness rotator cuff tears approaches 98–99%. Leakage of contrast from the glenohumeral joint into the subacromial bursa or the subdeltoid bursa, which represents the rupture of the joint capsule, is indicative of a rotator cuff tear.

Limitations of shoulder arthrography include false-negative results, which can occur when the glenohumeral joint capsule is not ruptured despite the presence of a rotator cuff tear. Shoulder arthrography is also not helpful in identifying partial-thickness tears, and its utility for the assessment of soft-tissue pathology is limited. Moreover, the value of arthrography in evaluating the rotator cuff assessment is inferior to that of magnetic resonance imaging (MRI), and its ability to identify labral injuries is limited. For these reasons, shoulder arthrography has been increasingly replaced by computed tomography (CT) or MRI for the assessment of most types of shoulder abnormalities.

C. Ultrasound

Ultrasound is a dynamic examination that is able to evaluate tendons and bursa of the rotator cuff. It can also be useful in the evaluation of the patient with shoulder instability, and in the postoperative patient with hardware where MRI findings may be obscured by metal artifact. However, it requires the use of an experienced technician and appropriate ultrasound equipment, notably a high-resolution transducer, to generate the most accurate and reliable information.

Ultrasound is useful for rotator cuff disease, including partial-thickness and full-thickness tears. Full-thickness tears have been more completely characterized than partial-thickness tears. Findings of full-thickness tears on ultrasound include nonvisualization, focal thinning, and discontinuity of the rotator cuff. Partial-thickness tears assessed by ultrasound often have increased echogenicity secondary to granulation tissue or hypertrophied synovium and focal thinning around the rotator cuff. The sensitivity of ultrasound drops from 100% for full-thickness tears to 47% for partial-thickness tears, whereas the specificity for both is 98%.

Ultrasound can provide information about the appearance of the biceps tendon and supraspinatus tendon. It can also help evaluate bursal surfaces, including the subacromial bursa and subdeltoid bursa, Hill-Sachs lesions, glenoid rim fractures, and glenohumeral ligaments. In addition, ultrasound can be used to evaluate the labrum under dynamic conditions to assess for degeneration, tears, and inflammatory joint disease.

D. Computed Tomography and Computed Arthrotomography

Computed Tomography (CT) is most useful in evaluating the integrity of bony morphology of the shoulder. Through the delivery of ionizing radiation in the axial plane, multidetector CT can reconstruct sagittal and coronal projections, giving great insight to the complicated three-dimensional anatomy of the shoulder girdle. Although it does not detect soft-tissue abnormalities well, CT is of great use in evaluating shoulder pain in the trauma patient, where assessment of complicated osseous structures, such as the body of the scapula, glenohumeral articular surfaces, and humeral head fractures, is essential.

The combination of CT and arthrography allows for extensive evaluation of the glenoid labrum and may be important for patients with recurrent glenohumeral instability. CT imaging can detect osseous lesions associated with instability, such as Hill-Sachs defects, periosteal reaction, and loose fragments.

E. Magnetic Resonance Imaging

Magnetic resonance imaging (MRI) is an extremely useful imaging modality in the evaluation of the patient with a painful shoulder. MRI is used to assess the rotator cuff, glenoid labrum, articular surfaces, bony anatomy, and surrounding soft tissues. The AC joint can be evaluated for osteoarthritis, capsular hypertrophy, or spurs. Similarly, the morphology of the acromion, whether it is downsloping, lateral, or anterior overhang, can be assessed as the cause of shoulder pain. The subacromial space can be evaluated for bursitis or to find evidence for a clinical diagnosis of subacromial impingement. MRI also provides a detailed look at all of the muscles that comprise the rotator cuff. Information generated from MRI about the rotator cuff muscles includes degree of tendinopathy, partial- or full-thickness tear, atrophy of the muscle, and calcific tendinitis.

In addition to the rotator cuff tendons, the biceps tendon can also be evaluated. Like the rotator cuff, the biceps tendon can be evaluated for a partial- or full-thickness tear and for tendinopathy. The biceps tendon insertion is also evaluated, yielding information about the integrity of the superior labrum of the glenoid. MRI can effectively provide information about the glenohumeral joint and structures, including Hill-Sachs lesions of the humeral head, nondisplaced fractures of the humeral head, and osteonecrosis of the proximal humerus. It can also identify osseous Bankart lesions of the glenoid rim and a glenohumeral joint effusion. Furthermore, it can yield information about the superior, middle, and inferior glenohumeral ligaments, information about the capsule, and the cause of the related abnormality (degeneration or inflammation). MRI also provides information about the rotator interval (disruption of which can be the source of anterior shoulder pain) and about osseous and soft tissue tumors of the shoulder. Such tumors are relatively infrequent, but when they do occur, they can be assessed for various characteristics, such as size, aggressiveness, and metastases.

▶ Diagnosis & Treatment

With a detailed history, physical examination, and indicated imaging, the differential diagnosis for shoulder pain can be narrowed. The differential diagnosis includes the following conditions: rotator cuff disease, instability, adhesive capsulitis, arthritis, cervical abnormality, neurologic disorders, congenital anomalies, and tumors.

A. Rotator Cuff Disease

Rotator cuff abnormality can be secondary to a spectrum of disease processes, including inflammation, partial- or full-thickness tears, and cuff tear arthropathy. Factors underlying rotator cuff disease include intrinsic degeneration because of senescence and tearing because of avascular regions in the tendons, mechanical impingement, or trauma.

Physical examination with observation and maneuvers can lead the physician to a high suspicion for rotator cuff tears. Atrophy in the supraspinatus or infraspinatus fossa compared with the contralateral side, weakness, or pain with the examination all raise suspicion for the diagnosis of rotator cuff abnormality. Weakness or pain against resistance in internal or external rotation with the elbow at the side and bent to 90 degrees is often present with a rotator cuff insult. Likewise, the empty can test against resistance at 45 degrees from the midline and forward flexion to 90 degrees is also a good indication of supraspinatus abnormality. Palpation of the greater tuberosity should be firm, but not hard enough to elicit a painful response from pressing on the periosteum of the bone. The affected shoulder should always be compared to the contralateral one.

Impingement syndrome is one of the most common causes of shoulder pain. A decreased space between the humeral head and the acromion suggests subacromial impingement. A distance of less than 5 mm between these structures as shown on an AP radiograph usually confirms the diagnosis of rotator cuff abnormality. An outlet view can show the presence of subacromial bone spurring and abnormal acromial morphology. A subacromial injection of lidocaine is useful in diagnosing impingement and as an initial treatment modality. Physical therapy for rotator cuff strengthening, stretching, ROM, and modalities for pain relief are other first-line treatments options. If nonoperative management fails, the treatment is acromioplasty. If rotator cuff strength is compromised with the pain secondary to the impingement, suspicion should be high for an associated rotator cuff tear. Along with weakness, rotator cuff tears are often associated with recalcitrant pain and night pain. Rolling over in bed is extremely uncomfortable for these patients, and effective treatment of the problem often constitutes a big boost in quality of life.

Imaging modalities are extremely useful for the diagnosis of rotator cuff tears. Conventional MRIs have been found to have a sensitivity of 100% and specificity of 95% for diagnosing full-thickness rotator cuff tears, and a sensitivity of 82% and specificity of 85% for partial-thickness rotator cuff tears. Partial-thickness tears are best visualized with an MRI arthrogram. Although ultrasound has been found to be a valuable tool for diagnosing full-thickness rotator cuff tears, it is extremely operator-dependent and therefore less practical in many settings.

The treatment of rotator cuff tears varies depending on the size of the tear size and should be individualized to each patient according to his or her overall health profile and goals. Most partial-thickness tears are treated initially without surgery. Arthroscopic evaluation, acromioplasty, rotator cuff debridement, and possible repair are recommended in cases of recurrent symptoms. A full-thickness rotator cuff is not an absolute indication for surgery. Indications for repair of the torn rotator cuff include severity of pain, functional limitations, the demands placed upon the shoulder by the patient's work or recreating, and an unsuccessful trial of nonoperative treatment.

Early surgical intervention is usually recommended for acute traumatic tears or when weakness is prominent or progressive. There is a high rate of cuff tears in the asymptomatic population, however: 51% of patients older than 80 have rotator cuff tears. It is important to understand that patients with rotator cuff tears can exhibit relatively normal shoulder function. A longitudinal analysis of asymptomatic rotator cuff tears detected by ultrasound found that of 58 patients with a symptomatic rotator cuff tear and contralateral asymptomatic rotator cuff tear, only 51% of the asymptomatic cuff tears became symptomatic over a mean of 2.8 years. The natural disease progression of rotator cuff tears remains largely unknown.

B. Instability

Instability includes the spectrum from acute traumatic dislocation to multidirectional instability secondary to generalized ligamentous laxity. The most common sequela of traumatic anterior shoulder dislocation is recurrence. The recurrence rate is documented in the literature as greater than or equal to 90% in patients less than 20 years old.

After a fracture or dislocation, pain and guarding of the arm will be present. ROM is limited and the contour of the shoulder compared with the contralateral side is altered. A thorough neurovascular examination is essential because an associated axillary neuropraxia occurs in 5–35% of first-time dislocators. Comparing the light touch sensation over the lateral deltoid is the best method of evaluating the competency of the axillary nerve.

After a traumatic dislocation, associated rotator cuff tears need to be excluded. As a general rule, young patients suffer ligamentous injuries after dislocation, whereas patients more than 50 years old have a higher incidence of rotator cuff tears.

Axillary neuropraxia can be differentiated from rotator cuff tears by testing the sensation over the lateral deltoid.

Imaging modalities include AP, Grashey (true AP in the plane of the glenoid), and axillary radiographic views for the assessment of the glenohumeral articulation. An axillary view is critical in this setting; an inability to obtain this view makes a CT scan mandatory. The axillary radiographic view and CT are good for the examination of bony abnormality or fracture of the inferior glenoid. MRI is used to diagnose a rotator cuff tear, ligamentous injury or labral pathology.

Closed reduction of the dislocated shoulder can be obtained via one of several reduction maneuvers, usually with conscious sedation. Postreduction attempts should always be evaluated with conventional radiographic imaging, including an axillary view. Immobilization in a sling is warranted after reduction but when a glenoid fracture or gross instability is present, an abduction brace with the shoulder held in internal rotation aids in immobilization.

Treatment is aimed at physical therapy with strengthening of the rotator cuff and scapular stabilizers. In the active population, acute surgical stabilization should be considered. Recurrent episodes of instability with failed nonoperative management may require surgical intervention. Depending on the injury (soft-tissue vs bony involvement), an arthroscopic or open procedure may be used. Repair of the capsulolabral tissue, with possible stabilization of a bony Bankart lesion, of the glenoid is the goal of the procedure. Patients with significant glenoid bone loss may be indicated for larger reconstructive procedures such as coracoid transfers or cadaveric allograft placement.

Overhead athletes, including gymnasts, swimmers, and weight-lifters, are predisposed to multidirectional instability, that is, symptomatic subluxation or dislocation in more than one plane (anterior, posterior, or inferior). The cause of the instability in this setting is a loose shoulder capsule. Physical examination maneuvers show gross ligamentous laxity in both shoulders. Prolonged physical therapy emphasizing strengthening and conditioning of the large and small muscles of the shoulder is instituted. Differentiation from voluntary dislocators must be established because, historically, such patients are poor surgical candidates. If nonoperative management fails after more than or equal to 6 months, surgical stabilization aimed at tightening and decreasing the shoulder capsular volume is recommended.

C. Adhesive Capsulitis

Adhesive capsulitis, or "frozen shoulder," is a common cause of shoulder pain. With this condition, pain is constant, deep, poorly localized, and made worse with any motion. Patients typically have pain at night, generated by rolling over on the shoulder in the course of natural position changes during sleep. Onset can be insidious or acute after incidental trauma. It is seen with endocrine disorders, most commonly diabetes. Many times, the cause is unknown. The hallmark of this condition is a restricted passive ROM, especially internal and external rotation, making activities of daily living difficult. Imaging, particularly MRI, is not helpful with this diagnosis but is used to exclude other causes of shoulder pain.

Although a benign and self-limited condition (1–2 years), most patients seek treatment because the pain and restricted motion have profound effects on their daily activities. Most patients respond to supervised physical therapy that stretches and mobilizes the shoulder joint. Severe and recalcitrant cases can undergo manipulation under anesthesia to restore motion. Arthroscopic capsular release can be conducted to restore motion in the most resistant cases. Because pain occurs at the limits of ROM, pain becomes less problematic as the patient regains ROM.

D. Arthritis

Arthritis can involve the glenohumeral, AC, or SC joints. The cause of the arthritis can be degenerative, infectious, or inflammatory. Physical examination and radiographic appearances are the mainstays of diagnosing the anatomic site and type of arthritis. A long history of repetitive motion (from manual labor or overhead sporting activities) with chronic pain is more suggestive of degenerative arthritis. The insidious onset of pain, with a positive family history and the presence of rashes, fevers, or involvement of multiple joints, may indicate an inflammatory arthritis. An acute onset of fevers, erythema, warmth, or pain with movement makes concern about a possible infectious cause of arthritis higher. Limited, painful passive ROM with fevers and elevated inflammatory markers correlates strongly with an infectious process. Aspiration of the joint and synovial fluid can confirm the diagnosis; white cell counts greater than 50,000 cells/mL strongly suggest infection.

AC arthritis is diagnosed by the finding of local tenderness at the AC joint. This finding is the *sine qua non* of diagnosing AC joint abnormality. The "one-finger" test is useful for determining the precise location of the pain. Generally, the patient will point directly to the AC joint at the top of the shoulder. Local tenderness at the AC joint when compressed by forcible adduction of the arm across the chest is also diagnostic of AC joint arthritis. Although sepsis of the AC joint produces pain and swelling, other symptoms such as fever, redness, and warmth will likely be present. A higher index of suspicion should be present in immunosuppressed individuals or patients with other risk factors for the development of a blood-borne infection.

SC arthritis is the most common diagnosis at the SC joint when there is pain without associated trauma or swelling. Tenderness to palpation is usually present over the joint in the region of the proximal clavicle sternal attachment. In an infectious process of the SC joint, pain, swelling, warmth, and erythema are present. The SC joint can be readily evaluated by comparing both sides of the disrobed patient.

Conventional radiographs of patients with degenerative arthritis usually show sclerosis, asymmetric joint space narrowing, and osteophytes. Infectious arthritis can have normal radiographs in the early stages, and joint destruction and a mixed pattern of sclerosis and osteopenia in later stages. Arthritis secondary to an inflammatory process usually is associated with symmetric joint space narrowing, a lack of osteophytes, and osteopenia.

The initial treatment of degenerative and inflammatory arthritis is composed of nonoperative interventions such as non steroidal anti-inflammatory medication (NSAIDs), oral steroids, and physical therapy, including ROM, strengthening, and local modalities. Intra-articular injection of a glucocorticoid preparation can be administered to the glenohumeral or AC joint to relieve symptoms of pain. If nonoperative treatment fails, degenerative arthritis can be treated with total shoulder arthroplasty or hemiarthroplasty. AC and SC joint arthritis can be treated with distal clavicle excision or medial clavicle excision, respectively. A diagnosis of septic arthritis requires immediate surgical irrigation and debridement of the involved joint with appropriate antibiotics to which the pathogenic organism is extensive.

E. Cervical Abnormality

Cervical disc disease and spondylosis can refer pain to the shoulder. Typically, such patients have restricted cervical ROM and, in the presence of a radicular component, distal neurologic findings. Radiographs, CT scans, and MRI scans are all helpful in making this diagnosis and localizing the level(s) of abnormalities. Early nonoperative treatment includes medication, physical therapy, and a soft cervical collar. More severe and resistant cases should be referred to pain management specialists for more sophisticated treatment modalities and/or a spine surgeon, if a surgical indication exists.

F. Neurologic Disorders

Several neurologic disorders about the shoulder can create pain. Brachial plexopathy can involve a stretch or compression injury, typically from trauma, such as a tackle in football or a fall. Patients complain of "burning" or "stinging" pain. Usually such injuries are self-limited. Persistent symptoms necessitate a workup, including MRI, to rule out cervical root injury. Less common causes of brachial plexopathy include tumor, viral illness, and vaccinations.

Stretch or compression to the long thoracic nerve (that innervates the serratus anterior) or the accessory nerve (that innervates the trapezius) can cause shoulder pain. Because these muscles are scapular stabilizers, these neurologic conditions cause scapular winging. Most of the palsies are self-limited, with recovery over a 12- to 18-month period.

Electromyography or a nerve conduction study can assist in making this diagnosis, and serial studies can monitor recovery. Physical therapy during this period can be helpful in improving function.

The suprascapular nerve innervates the supraspinatus and infraspinatus, and compression of this nerve can cause posterior shoulder pain and muscles weakness and/or atrophy. In addition to compression at the suprascapular notch or spinoglenoid notch, the nerve can be compressed by a perilabral ganglion cyst. Electromyography or a nerve conduction study and MRI can help locate the area of compression. If symptoms persist for more than 6 months, decompression at the site of compression is indicated. Ganglion cyst decompression can be achieved with image-guided aspiration, arthroscopic decompression, or open excision.

G. Congenital Anomalies

Congenital anomalies represent a rare cause of shoulder pain. Such conditions include disorders of the bones, muscles, and neurovascular system. Workup and treatment of these conditions requires the appropriate subspecialist.

H. Tumor

Tumors represent an uncommon cause of shoulder pain. Primary soft-tissue and bony tumors are identified by radiography and MRI. Once suspected, a systematic workup to include biopsy is best conducted by an oncologist. In addition, metastatic disease should be considered for a patient with shoulder pain who has a history of cancer. Referral to an oncologist for workup is recommended.

Karjalainen TV, Jain NB, Page CM, et al. Subacromial decompression surgery for rotator cuff disease. *Cochrane Database Syst Rev.* 2019;1:CD005619. [PMID: 30707445]

Ogbeivor C, Bandaru S, Milton C. A comparison of the effectiveness of lateral versus posterior approach to shoulder injection in patients with subacromial impingement syndrome: a pragmatic randomized controlled trial. *Musculoskeletal Care.* 2019;17(3):257. [PMID: 31373430]

Redler LH, Dennis ER. Treatment of adhesive capsulitis of the shoulder. *J Am Acad Orthop Surg.* 2019;27(12):e544. [PMID: 30632986]

Thangarajah T, Lambert S. Management of the unstable shoulder. *Br J Sports Med.* 2016;50(7):440. [PMID: 26983713]

Wang W, Shi M, Zhou C, et al. Effectiveness of corticosteroid injections in adhesive capsulitis of shoulder: a meta-analysis. *Medicine (Baltimore).* 2017;96(28):e7529. [PMID: 28700506]

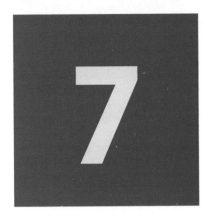

7

Approach to the Patient with Neck Pain

David Borenstein, MD

Neck pain is a common musculoskeletal symptom, accounting for millions of visits to physicians annually in the United States. Of individuals with neck pain, more than 80% are between the ages of 18 and 64 years. Mechanical disorders cause 90% of neck pain episodes. Mechanical neck pain is defined as that which is caused by overuse of a normal anatomic structure, by deformity of an anatomic structure, or by trauma (Figure 7–1). Mechanical disorders are characterized by exacerbation and alleviation of pain in direct correlation with particular physical activities. Neck pain due to mechanical disorders decreases within 2–4 weeks in more than 50% of patients, and symptoms usually resolve entirely within 2–3 months.

INITIAL EVALUATION

The goal of the initial evaluation is to differentiate patients with probable mechanical disorders from those with neck pain that requires more thorough immediate evaluation (Figure 7–2). A history and physical examination should be performed in all patients with new-onset neck pain. The neurologic portion of the examination is designed to determine whether there are any signs of cervical nerve root or cervical cord involvement (ie, spastic weakness, hyperreflexia, clonus, and positive Babinski signs).

Laboratory tests and imaging studies are not necessary during the initial evaluation of patients with probable mechanical neck pain. These tests, however, are indicated for patients whose history and physical findings suggest persistent compression of the spinal cord or nerve roots or raise the possibility of neck pain as a component of an underlying systemic disease.

▶ History

The history should establish the onset, location, and character of the pain, and determine if the pain is associated with radiation to regions beyond the neck, for example, down the arm. The history should also probe any factors that aggravate or alleviate the pain. Mechanical disorders cause pain that increases with activity. The end of the day is associated with more severe distress. In contrast, recumbency and rest are associated with improvement. Tingling pain that radiates down an arm is suggestive of nerve impingement. Aching pain of slow onset that localizes to the base of the cervical spine suggests muscle or joint involvement. The history should determine whether the neck pain has unusual qualities that suggest a focal destructive process (due to tumor or infection), whether it might be referred pain from the heart or other viscera, and whether there might exist an underlying systemic disease presenting with symptoms in the neck (Table 7–1).

The duration of mechanical neck pain is typically a few days to weeks. Disk herniations may require 8–12 weeks to resolve. Medical conditions tend to cause persistent chronic pain.

▶ Physical Examination

Abnormalities of the cervical spine may be observed while the spine is in motion or static. Observation of the spine from 360 degrees identifies any malalignments of the neck or shoulders. Pain in the neck may cause deviation that can be toward or away from the painful side.

Palpation can detect painful structures as well as increased paraspinous muscle tension. Posterior elements of the cervical spine are more easily identified than those located anteriorly. In general, midline tenderness is related to an intrinsic spinal disorder, while sensitivity to pressure in structures of the midline suggests soft-tissue pathology.

Active range of motion in all planes is helpful in documenting the extent but not the cause of cervical spine problems. Active and passive movement of the shoulders can help discriminate abnormalities of the appendicular skeleton from those of the cervical spine.

Neurologic evaluation, including reflex, sensory, and motor function both in the upper and lower extremities,

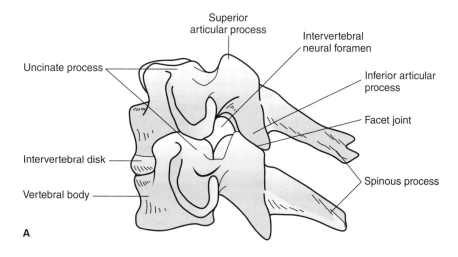

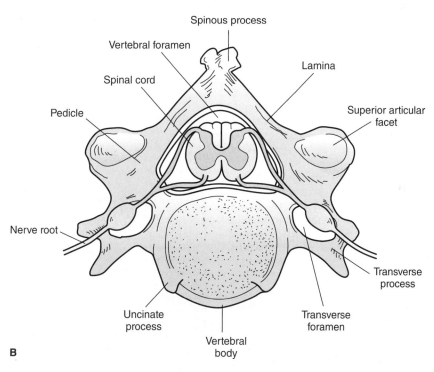

▲ **Figure 7–1.** Schematic representation of a lateral view of the mid-cervical spine (**A**) and the superior aspect of C5 (**B**). The inferior articular processes from synovial-lined **facet joints** (also called **apophyseal joints**) with the superior articular processes of the vertebra below. The uncinate processes or posterolateral lips located on the superior aspect of the vertebral bodies interact with the inferolateral aspects of the vertebral body above, forming the small, nonsynovial-lined **uncovertebral joints** (also referred to as the joints of Luschka). The spinal cord lies within the vertebral foramen formed by the vertebral body anteriorly, the pedicles laterally, and the laminae posteriorly. The cervical nerve roots course along "gutters" formed by the pedicles and exit through an intervertebral foramen. The vertebral artery passes through the transverse foramen. (Reproduced, with permission, from Polley HF, Hunder GS. *Rheumatologic Interviewing and Physical Examination of the Joints,* 2nd ed. WB Saunders; 1978.)

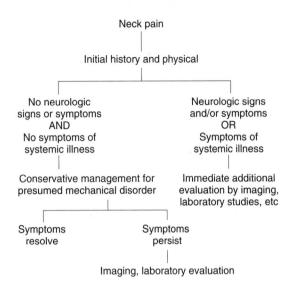

Neck pain
|
Initial history and physical
|
- No neurologic signs or symptoms AND No symptoms of systemic illness
  - Conservative management for presumed mechanical disorder
    - Symptoms resolve
    - Symptoms persist
      - Imaging, laboratory evaluation
- Neurologic signs and/or symptoms OR Symptoms of systemic illness
  - Immediate additional evaluation by imaging, laboratory studies, etc

▲ **Figure 7–2.** The initial evaluation of the patient with neck pain.

is essential to determine the extent of compromise of the central and peripheral nervous systems. The presence of long-tract signs is indicative of more severe spinal cord compression.

The Spurling maneuver is performed by extending and rotating the head to one side and then the other. A positive result is the reproduction of radicular pain. This test is useful in confirming the presence of a cervical radiculopathy.

The Adson test for thoracic outlet obstruction is performed by palpating the pulse at the wrist while abducting, extending, and externally rotating the arm. The patient takes a deep breath and rotates the head to the affected side. If there is compression of the subclavian artery, a marked diminution of the radial pulse is observed, constituting a positive test.

Table 7–1. Symptoms that point to the need for urgent evaluation in a patient with neck pain.

- Constitutional symptoms such as fever, night sweats, weight loss
- Unusual quality of the neck pain
  Greatest at night; exacerbated by recumbency
  Well-localized within the neck
  Occurring in a regular pattern and extending to structures outside the neck
- Neurologic symptoms
  Lower extremity weakness; difficulty walking
  Combination of upper and lower extremity symptoms
  Rectal or urinary incontinence (or both)
- Associated medical conditions
  Cancer, diabetes mellitus, AIDS, and injection drug use, for example

Laboratory Tests

Laboratory tests are not necessary for the diagnosis of mechanical neck pain. Erythrocyte sedimentation rate and C-reactive protein tests are useful in the minority of patients with a systemic disorder causing neck pain.

Imaging Studies

Radiology studies are needed for the small minority of patients who do not respond to a 6–8 week course of medical therapy, who demonstrate severe neurologic compromise, or who have signs or symptoms of a systemic illness. Plain radiographs are easily obtained but offer few specific findings that identify the cause of neck pain. Many anatomic abnormalities are asymptomatic. However, individuals who have dysphagia (Figure 7–3) or new onset of neurologic symptoms (Figure 7–4) may have specific findings that correspond with the clinical complaints. Many anatomic abnormalities are asymptomatic.

MRI is a useful technique for individuals with clinical symptoms and signs of nerve compression who do not respond to medical therapy. MRI is a sensitive means of

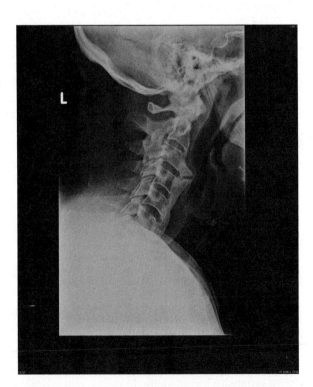

▲ **Figure 7–3.** 56-year-old man with stiff neck and difficulty swallowing caused by diffuse idiopathic skeletal hyperostosis. Lateral view of the cervical spine with flowing osteophytes indenting the esophagus.

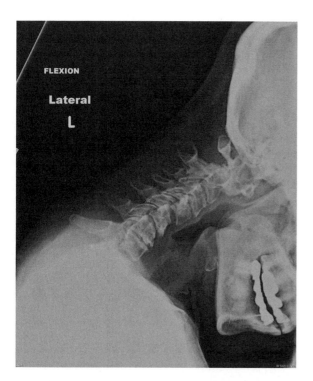

▲ Figure 7–4. 58-year-old woman with long-standing rheumatoid arthritis. Lateral, flexion view of the cervical spine with C1-2 subluxation of 14 mm, indicative of an unstable cervical spine.

identifying disk herniations, narrowing of the spinal canal, and increased inflammation in osseous and soft-tissue structures. CT is a better technique for delineating bony structures. A disadvantage of CT is the exposure to ionizing radiation needed to obtain images of the spine.

▶ Special Tests

Electrodiagnostic tests, electromyography, and nerve conduction tests are useful in the differentiation of central versus peripheral nerve compression (a more difficult distinction with cervical spine disorders compared with lumbar spine problems). For example, electromyography and nerve conduction tests can help distinguish between the individual who has median nerve compression at the wrist and the patient with a C6 or C7 spinal nerve compression from a herniated cervical disk.

DISORDERS REQUIRING URGENT EVALUATION

Suspected cervical myelopathy and neck pain in the setting of systemic disease require urgent evaluation in the form of imaging studies, laboratory investigation, and often, referral to the appropriate specialist.

1. Cervical Myelopathy

ESSENTIALS OF DIAGNOSIS

▶ Symptoms of weakness in upper and lower extremities; urinary or rectal incontinence.

▶ Upper motor neuron signs on examination of the lower extremities.

▶ General Considerations

Cervical myelopathy occurs secondary to compression of the neural elements (spinal cord or nerve roots) in the cervical spinal canal. Cervical spondylitic myelopathy is the most common cause of spinal cord dysfunction in persons older than 55 years. The cause of the compression is usually a combination of osteophytes and degenerative disk disease that leads to a decrease in the volume of the spinal canal. The distribution and severity of symptoms depend on the location, duration, and size of the lesion.

▶ Clinical Findings

A. Symptoms and Signs

The most frequent presentation of myelopathy is a combination of arm and leg dysfunction. Patients with cervical myelopathy may have symptoms in four limbs, difficulty walking, and urinary or rectal incontinence. Only one-third of patients with cervical myelopathy mention neck pain. Older patients may describe leg stiffness, foot shuffling, and a fear of falling. Physical examination reveals weakness of the appendages in association with spasticity. Hyperreflexia, clonus, and a Babinski sign are findings in the lower extremities.

B. Imaging Studies

MRI detects the extent of spinal cord compression and is the imaging test of choice for most cases. CT myelogram helps distinguish between osteophytes and protruding disks. Plain radiographs reveal advanced degenerative disease with narrowed disk spaces, facet joint sclerosis, and osteophytes but do not image neural compression.

▶ Treatment

The natural history of cervical spondylitic myelopathy is gradual progression. Although some patients improve with conservative therapy, progressive myelopathy requires surgery to prevent further cord compression, vascular compromise, and myelomalacia. Outcomes are best when surgery is performed before severe neurologic deficits appear.

2. Neck Pain Associated with Systemic Medical Illness

ESSENTIALS OF DIAGNOSIS

▶ The history and physical examination help identify patients whose neck pain is not due to a mechanical disorder.

▶ The differential diagnosis and clinical context of each case determine the urgency and nature of the evaluation.

▶ Clinical Findings

Patients with neck pain require urgent evaluation if they have constitutional symptoms, symptoms that suggest either a focal process or referred pain, a history of cancer, or a condition that predisposes to infection (see Table 7–1). If present, signs or symptoms of radiculopathy or spinal cord compression add to the urgency of the situation. The differential diagnosis, clinical setting, and findings of the individual case dictate the use of imaging, laboratory investigations, and need for consultations.

▶ Differential Diagnosis

Neck pain in the presence of fever, night sweats, weight loss, or a predisposing condition (such as injection drug use, AIDS, or diabetes) raises the possibility of **infection.** Blood cultures should be performed if serious consideration is given to an infection. MRI and CT are indicated in cases of suspected vertebral osteomyelitis, diskitis, and epidural abscess. In these conditions, radiographs of the cervical spine may demonstrate alterations of bone integrity but are often unrevealing, especially early in the disease course.

Spinal cord infiltrative processes and vertebral column **tumors** tend to produce pain that is greatest at night or with recumbency. Patients with these symptoms and neurologic signs should undergo MRI of the central nervous system. Patients with nocturnal pain and with normal neurologic examinations may have a bone tumor. Benign bone tumors affect the posterior elements of vertebral bodies, while malignant lesions tend to affect the vertebral bodies. If plain radiographs are unable to detect alterations in bone architecture, bone scan is a sensitive means to detect lesions over the entire axial skeleton. CT scan clarifies the nature of abnormalities seen on bone scan.

Pain localized directly over the bony structures of the cervical spine is usually associated with either **fracture** or **expansion of bone.** Any condition that replaces bone with abnormal cells or increases mineral loss from trabeculae causes fractures that occur spontaneously or with minimal trauma. Fractures cause pain in the area of the lesion. Physical examination identifies the maximum point of tenderness. A bone scan may identify the area of fracture if the radiograph is normal. MRI can identify the presence of malignancies, such as **myeloma**, that do not stimulate osteoblast activity and thus are not detected by bone scan.

The **spondyloarthropathies** and **rheumatoid arthritis** can cause early morning stiffness of the cervical spine lasting for hours. Patients with neck symptoms due to these diseases usually have extensive disease of other joints, but women with ankylosing spondylitis may have neck disease without low back pain. Flexion-extension views of the cervical spine can reveal the presence of C1–C2 subluxation in either the spondyloarthropathies or rheumatoid arthritis. MRI is an important technique to identify synovitis affecting the C1–C2 articulation in rheumatoid arthritis. MRI can also visualize the presence of bone marrow inflammation and edema in vertebral structures affected by ankylosing spondylitis.

Patients with **viscerogenic pain** (ie, neck pain secondary to cardiovascular, gastrointestinal, or neurologic disorders) have symptoms that recur in a regular pattern in structures that extend beyond the cervical spine. Pain with exertion raises the possibility of myocardial ischemia. Carotidynia is pain and tenderness over the carotid arteries. Esophageal disorders should be considered if neck pain occurs in association with eating. Posterior esophageal lesions, in particular, may affect the prevertebral space, causing neck pain. Disorders of the cranial nerves can cause cervical spine and facial pain.

Patients with **polymyalgia rheumatica** are over 50 years of age and have severe early morning muscle stiffness. Pain is localized to the proximal muscles of the shoulders and thighs. The erythrocyte sedimentation rate is elevated in most cases but the most useful test is a careful history. Patients with polymyalgia rheumatica often have pain at night in the shoulders and neck when rolling over in bed.

ACUTE NECK PAIN DUE TO A PROBABLE MECHANICAL DISORDER

ESSENTIALS OF DIAGNOSIS

▶ There are no signs or symptoms of systemic disease, and the neurologic examination is normal.

▶ A trial of nonsurgical therapy is indicated.

▶ General Considerations

Patients with neck pain but without symptoms or signs of myelopathy or an associated systemic disorder should receive nonsurgical therapy for 3–6 weeks. In general, imaging studies and laboratory investigations are not necessary unless the neck pain persists.

APPROACH TO THE PATIENT WITH NECK PAIN   89

Treatment

Nonselective nonsteroidal anti-inflammatory drugs (NSAIDs) help decrease pain and localized inflammation that is associated with acute neck pain. Nonsurgical management also includes muscle relaxants, nonopioid analgesics, temperature modalities, local injections, and range of motion and strengthening exercises.

Medications that have rapid onset of action and are effective analgesics are preferred. In addition, drugs with sustained relief properties may offer more constant pain relief with fewer tablets each day. Muscle relaxants do not produce peripheral muscle relaxation but do offer additional pain relief for persons with increased paracervical muscle contractions. Patients must be informed of the potential sedative effects of these medications. Patients may use ice massage on painful areas for 10 minutes for additional analgesia. Some patients may find the application of heat to the neck improves range of motion by decreasing muscle tightness. A local injection with 10 mg of triamcinolone and 2–4 mL of lidocaine into the area of maximum tenderness in the paravertebral musculature or trapezii may decrease pain.

Because of the pain, patients often have difficulty complying with the recommendation of returning to normal motion of the cervical spine. Patients will limit motion and prefer to wear a cervical collar. Short-term immobilization is useful, particularly at night when motion during sleep increases neck pain. A soft collar that does not extend the neck is appropriate in most cases. Patients should understand that the eventual goal of therapy is a return to normal neck motion. Therefore, the collar should be used less frequently as neck pain improves.

PERSISTENT NECK PAIN

Most patients, including those with cervical radiculopathy, improve within 2 months. If initial nonsurgical treatment fails after 6 weeks, symptomatic patients are separated into two groups: patients with neck pain alone and patients with arm pain as the predominant complaint.

1. Neck Pain Predominant

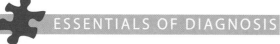

ESSENTIALS OF DIAGNOSIS

▶ Osteoarthritis is a frequent cause of local neck pain.
▶ Muscle tightness is a common exacerbating factor.

Differential Diagnosis & Treatment

Cervical strain causes pain in the middle or lower portion of the posterior aspect of the neck. The pain may cover a diffuse area or both sides of the spine. Physical examination reveals local tenderness in the paracervical muscles, decreased range of motion, and loss of cervical lordosis. No abnormalities are found on neurologic or shoulder examination. Laboratory tests are normal. Cervical spine radiographs of patients with cervical strain may be normal or demonstrate a loss of cervical lordosis. Management of chronic cervical strain includes pharmacotherapy with NSAID, muscle relaxant, and local injections as well as nonpharmacotherapy with neck exercises, including strengthening and range of motion.

Cervical spondylosis is associated with disk degeneration and the approximation of articular structures. This instability results in osteoarthritis with osteophyte formation in the uncovertebral and apophyseal joints. Neck pain is diffuse and may radiate to the shoulders, occipital area, or the interscapular muscles. Physical examination may reveal midline tenderness and pain at the limit of motion with extension and lateral flexion. Factors that exacerbate and alleviate neck pain help differentiate among the various causes of mechanical neck pain. Plain radiographs of the cervical spine demonstrate intervertebral narrowing and facet joint sclerosis. MRI of the neck reveals degenerative disk disease in over 50% of persons 40 years of age or older, many of whom are asymptomatic. The radiographic findings are significant only if they correlate with the clinical symptoms of the patient. Therapy for osteoarthritis of the cervical spine requires a balance between stability and maintenance of motion. Patient education is essential to maximize neck flexibility with range of motion exercises while decreasing pain by restricting neck movement with a cervical collar. NSAIDs and local injections may also diminish neck and referred pain. Most patients with cervical spondylosis have a relapsing course with recurrent exacerbations of acute neck pain.

Cervical hyperextension injuries (whiplash) of the neck are most often associated with rear-impact motor vehicle accidents, but diving, falls, and other sports injuries also cause whiplash. Whiplash is an acceleration-deceleration injury to the soft-tissue structures in the neck. Paracervical muscles are stretched or torn, and with severe injury, cervical intervertebral disk injuries occur. Severe whiplash also can damage the sympathetic ganglia, resulting in Horner syndrome, nausea, hoarseness, or dizziness. Symptoms of stiffness and pain on motion generally develop 12–24 hours after the accident. Patients may have difficulty swallowing or chewing. Physical examination reveals soreness of the neck with palpation, paracervical muscle contraction, and decreased range of motion. Neurologic examination is unrevealing, and radiographs demonstrate loss of cervical lordosis. Structural damage identified on radiographs occurs in patients with severe injuries that require immediate stabilizing therapy. Treatment of most whiplash injuries includes the use of a cervical collar for a minimal period of time. Longer use of collars may result in greater pain and decreased motion. Nonopioid analgesics, NSAIDs, and muscle relaxants decrease pain and facilitate motion of the neck. Patients with persistent symptoms have pain secondary to apophyseal joint injury. Patients with persistent symptoms for greater than 6 months rarely experience significant improvement.

If a patient with persistent neck pain does not have muscle tenderness and if the neurologic examination and imaging studies are unrevealing, the patient should have a complete psychosocial evaluation. Patients with neck pain who have psychiatric conditions may have conversion reactions or substance dependence as the cause of their symptoms.

2. Arm Pain Predominant

ESSENTIALS OF DIAGNOSIS

▶ Herniated intervertebral disks are a frequent cause of radicular pain.

▶ Cervical spinal stenosis is a cause of radicular pain in older persons.

▶ Differential Diagnosis & Treatment

Patients with arm pain refractory to nonsurgical management frequently have symptoms and signs owing to mechanical pressure from a herniated disk or hypertrophic bone and secondary inflammation of the involved nerve roots. Cervical disk herniation occurs with the sudden exertion of heavy lifting. A **herniated cervical disk** causes radicular pain that radiates from the shoulder to the forearm and hand. The pain may be so severe that the use of the arm is limited. Neck pain is minimal or absent. Physical examination reveals increased radicular pain with any maneuver that narrows the intervertebral foramen and places tension on the affected nerve. Compression, extension, and lateral flexion of the cervical spine (Spurling sign) cause radicular pain. Neurologic examination reveals sensory abnormalities, reflex asymmetry, or motor weakness corresponding to the damaged spinal nerve root and degree of impingement (Table 7–2). MRI is the best technique to identify the location of disk herniation and nerve root impingement. Electromyography and nerve conduction tests document nerve dysfunction and are able to differentiate nerve root impingement from peripheral entrapment syndromes (eg, carpal tunnel syndrome).

If arm pain occurs during exertion, vascular evaluation is indicated. Patients who complain of neck and arm pain that occurs with exertion should be evaluated for coronary artery disease, particularly if chest pain occurs in conjunction with arm pain. If the exertional pain is limited to the arm alone, an evaluation for thoracic outlet syndrome, using the Adson test, is also appropriate. Patients with thoracic outlet syndrome should be evaluated by appropriate imaging to rule out a Pancoast tumor (apical lung tumor). Patients with idiopathic thoracic outlet obstruction may benefit from isometric shoulder girdle exercises, improved posture, and limiting movements of the arm above the head. Surgery is helpful in a minority of patients.

Nonsurgical treatment for radiculopathy secondary to an acute herniated cervical disk is successful in 80% of patients. Nonsurgical therapy includes patient education of natural history of improvement, limited use of cervical collars, therapeutic exercises, cervical traction, and NSAIDs. Low-dose glucocorticoids, administered orally or epidurally, may have additional benefit in relieving radicular pain. However, the benefit compared to placebo has not been demonstrated consistently in clinical trials. For patients in whom nonsurgical therapy fails, anterior diskectomy with fusion relieves arm pain in over 90% of patients. Cervical disk arthroplasty has been offered as an alternate surgical approach as a means of maintaining spinal motion while relieving nerve root compression. Selecting appropriate patients is essential for a good outcome with disk replacement. Contraindications to cervical disk replacement include facet joint arthritis, vertebral body deformity, spinal instability, predominant neck pain, poor bone quality, or severe spondylosis.

Cohen SP. Epidemiology, diagnosis, and treatment of neck pain. *Mayo Clin Proc.* 2015;90(2):284-299. [PMID: 25659245]

Enquist M, Lofgren H, Oberg B, et al. Surgery versus nonsurgical treatment of cervical radiculopathy: a prospective, randomized study comparing surgery plus physiotherapy with physiotherapy alone with a 2 year follow-up. *Spine.* 2013;38:1715. [PMID: 23778373]

Enquist M, Lofgren H, Oberg B, et al. Factors affecting the outcome of surgical radiculopathy: a randomized, controlled study. *Spine* 2015;40:1553. [PMID: 26192721]

Vijiaratnam N, Williams DR, Bertram KL. Neck pain: what if it is not musculoskeletal? *Aust J Gen Pract.* 2018;47(5):279-282. [PMID: 29779295]

Table 7–2. Characteristics of radicular pain caused by cervical nerve root compression.

Nerve Root	Area of Pain	Sensory Loss	Motor Loss	Reflex loss
C5	Neck to outer shoulder, arm	Shoulder	Deltoid	Biceps, supinator
C6	Outer arm to thumb, index finger	Index finger, thumb	Biceps	Biceps, supinator
C7	Outer arm to middle finger	Index, middle fingers	Triceps	Triceps
C8	Inner arm to ring and little fingers	Ring, little fingers	Hand muscles	None

Approach to the Patient with Low Back Pain

8

Rajiv K. Dixit, MD

ESSENTIALS OF DIAGNOSIS

▶ Low back pain (LBP) affects as many as 80% of individuals. Degenerative changes of the lumbar spine are the most common cause.

▶ More than 90% of these patients are substantially better within 8 weeks, although recurrences are common.

▶ The initial evaluation should focus on identification of the few patients with neurologic involvement, fracture, or possible systemic disease (infection, malignancy, or spondyloarthritis), the management of whom may require an urgent or specific intervention.

▶ Early imaging is rarely indicated in the absence of significant neurologic involvement, trauma, or suspicion of systemic disease.

▶ Imaging abnormalities, often the result of age-related degenerative changes, should be carefully interpreted because they are frequently present in asymptomatic individuals and may not be the cause of the patient's pain.

▶ Persistent LBP should be treated with an individually tailored program that includes analgesia, core strengthening, stretching, aerobic conditioning, loss of excess weight, and patient education.

▶ There is no evidence for the effectiveness of epidural corticosteroid injections in patients without radiculopathy secondary to disk herniation.

▶ A large number of injection techniques, physical therapy modalities, and nonsurgical interventional therapies lack evidence of efficacy.

▶ The major indication for back surgery is presence of a serious or progressive neurologic deficit.

▶ A pathoanatomic diagnosis and precise identification of the pain generator cannot be made in up to 85% of patients. Thus, the results of back surgery (especially spinal fusion) are disappointing when the goal is relief of LBP rather than relief of radicular symptoms or treatment for the relief of neurogenic signs.

General Considerations

Low back pain (LBP) affects the area between the lower rib cage and gluteal folds. It is the most common musculoskeletal complaint, the number one cause of disability globally, the most prevalent chronic pain syndrome, and the leading cause of limitation of activity in patients younger than 45 years. An estimated 65–85% of the population will experience LBP during their lifetime. LBP is uncommon in the first decade of life, but prevalence increases steeply during the teenage years. Approximately 40% of children between the ages of 9 and 18 years report having LBP. The prevalence increases with age until around 70 years, then gradually declines. LBP is more common in women.

The natural history of LBP, especially the duration and chronicity, is somewhat controversial. Back pain is increasingly understood as a long-lasting condition with a variable course rather than episodes of unrelated occurrences. Acute LBP improves substantially in most patients within days to weeks, and more than 90% are better at 8 weeks. However, two-thirds of these patients still report low-grade discomfort at 3 and 12 months. Recurrences of acute LBP are common and also tend to be brief. Approximately 10% of patients develop chronic persistent, and at times disabling, LBP that is affected by a range of biophysical, psychological, and social factors. These individuals with chronic pain are largely responsible for the associated high costs, currently estimated to be well over $100 billion annually in the United States.

A number of risk factors have been associated with LBP, including heredity, psychosocial factors, heavy lifting, obesity, pregnancy, weaker trunk strength, cigarette smoking, and low income and educational status. Persistence of disabling LBP has been associated with the presence of maladaptive pain coping behavior, functional impairment, poor general health status, and psychiatric comorbidities.

▶ Anatomy

The lumbar spine is composed of five vertebrae. It has a slight lordotic (convex) curvature. Each vertebra (Figure 8–1) consists of a body anteriorly and a neural arch that encloses the spinal canal posteriorly. Cartilaginous end plates cover the superior and inferior surfaces of the vertebral body.

Adjacent vertebrae are united by an intervertebral disk forming the diskovertebral joint. The outer circumference of the disk is made up of concentric layers of dense tough fibrous tissue, the annulus fibrosus. The annulus encloses a shock-absorbing gelatinous nucleus pulposus. In addition to the anteriorly placed diskovertebral joint, at each level of the lumbar spine there are two posterolaterally placed synovial facet (apophyseal) joints. These are formed by articulation of the superior and inferior articular processes of adjacent vertebrae. The vertebral column is stabilized by ligaments and paraspinal muscles (erector spinae, trunk, and abdominal muscles).

The sacroiliac joints join the spinal column to the pelvis. The anterior and inferior part of the joint is lined with synovium, whereas the posterior and superior part is fibrous. There is little or no movement at the sacroiliac joint.

The spinal cord ends as the conus medullaris at the L1 vertebral level (hence cord compression is generally not a feature of lumbar pathology). Lumbar and sacral nerve roots then course down the spinal canal, forming the cauda equina, until they exit at their respective intervertebral neural foramina.

▶ Clinical Findings

LBP is a symptom, not a disease, and can result from several different abnormalities or conditions. The spectrum of clinical presentation is broad. Many individuals have self-limited episodes of acute LBP that resolve without specific treatment, but a minority develop chronic LBP often characterized by periods of acute exacerbation. A thorough history is the most important part of the clinical evaluation. Imaging is often expensive, wasteful, and unnecessary.

A. History

The major focus in the initial evaluation of a patient with LBP is to identify the small fraction (<5%) of patients who may have neural compression, fracture, or underlying systemic disease as the cause of LBP. Infections, malignancies, and spondyloarthritis are the biggest concerns. Patients with these conditions require early imaging and may require specific treatment (eg, antibiotics for vertebral osteomyelitis) or urgent surgical treatment (eg, decompression in a patient with major or progressive neural compression). Thus, clues to the presence of these conditions—"red flags" in the evaluation of a patient with LBP—should be carefully sought (Table 8–1). The prevalence of serious spine disorders is low,

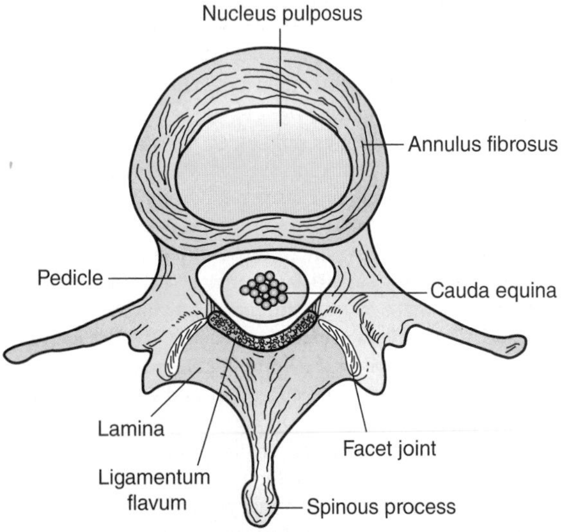

▲ **Figure 8–1.** Schematic drawing showing a cross-sectional view through a normal lumbar vertebra. The facet joints are formed by the articulation between the superior facet of the vertebra below and the inferior facet of the vertebra above.

Table 8–1. "Red flags" for potentially serious causes of low back pain (LBP) that indicate need for early diagnostic testing.

Spinal fracture
Significant trauma
Prolonged glucocorticoid use
Age >50 years
Infection or cancer
History of cancer
Unexplained weight loss
Immunosuppression
Injection drug use
Nocturnal pain
Age >50 years
Cauda equina syndrome
Urinary retention
Overflow incontinence
Fecal incontinence
Bilateral or progressive motor deficit
Saddle anesthesia
Spondyloarthritis
Marked morning stiffness in the back that lasts >30 min
Low back pain that improves with activity but not rest
Alternating buttock pain
Age <40 years

and the sensitivity and specificity of individual red flags to detect these is also low. Imaging should therefore be guided by the full clinical picture rather than by the uncritical emphasis on individual red flags.

Mechanical LBP is due to an anatomic or functional abnormality in the spine that is not associated with inflammatory, infectious, or neoplastic disease. It typically increases with physical activity and upright posture and tends to be relieved by rest and recumbency. More than 95% of LBP is mechanical, with degenerative change in the lumbar spine being the most common cause. Severe, acute mechanical LBP in a postmenopausal woman suggests the possibility of a vertebral compression fracture secondary to osteoporosis. Nocturnal pain, especially when persistent and progressive, suggests the possibility of underlying infection or neoplasm.

Inflammatory LBP as occurs in the spondyloarthropathies usually has an insidious onset and is more common in patients younger than 40 years. It is associated with marked morning stiffness that usually lasts more than half an hour and often awakens patient from sleep in the early morning hours. The pain frequently improves with exercise but not with rest. Even so, only a minority of patients whose symptoms have some features of inflammatory back pain turn out to have spondyloarthritis, and the association between a history of inflammatory back pain and the finding of axial inflammation on magnetic resonance imaging (MRI) is weak.

An important question for the patient is whether or not the back pain radiates into the lower extremities. Radiation of pain into the lower extremities suggests neurogenic claudication caused by spinal stenosis. Neurogenic claudication is often termed "pseudoclaudication" because the symptoms of pain in the lower extremities are caused not by vascular insufficiency as in cases of peripheral vascular disease but rather by compression of nerves as they exit the spinal cord or spinal canal.

Sciatica results from nerve root compression and causes radicular pain. Because the term sciatica has been used inconsistently, "radicular pain" is now the preferred term. **Radicular pain** has a dermatomal distribution. The pain, often accompanied by paresthesias, usually radiates to a level below the knee, and often to the foot or ankle. It frequently worsens during coughing, sneezing, and with the straight leg raise test on physical examination. Radicular pain may be accompanied by **radiculopathy** characterized by a variable combination of muscle weakness, loss of sensation, or loss of a particular reflex associated with a specific nerve root.

Radicular pain must be differentiated from nonneurogenic **sclerotomal pain**. This pain can arise from pathology within the disk, facet joint, or lumbar paraspinal muscles and ligaments. Sclerotomal pain is often referred into the lower extremities, but unlike radicular pain, it is nondermatomal in distribution and usually does not radiate below the knee or have associated paresthesias. Most radiant pain is sclerotomal. Bowel or bladder dysfunction should suggest the possibility of the cauda equina syndrome.

B. Physical Examination

A physical examination usually does not lead to a specific diagnosis. A general physical examination guided closely by the history and including a directed neurologic examination may help identify the few but critically important patients with LBP whose symptoms are related to a systemic disease or who have clinically significant neurologic involvement (see Table 8–1).

Inspection may reveal the presence of scoliosis. This can either be structural or functional. In adults, **structural scoliosis** is usually secondary to degenerative changes and is associated with structural changes of the vertebral column and sometimes the rib cage as well. With forward flexion, structural scoliosis persists. In contrast, **functional scoliosis**, which usually results from paravertebral muscle spasm or leg length discrepancy, usually disappears with forward flexion.

Palpation can detect paravertebral muscle spasm. This often leads to loss of the normal lumbar lordosis. A palpable step-off between adjacent spinous processes indicates spondylolisthesis. Point tenderness on percussion over the spine is reasonably sensitive for vertebral osteomyelitis but not particularly specific in the absence of other suggestive historical features (fevers, risk factors for blood-borne infection, etc).

Limited spinal motion (flexion, extension, lateral bending, and rotation) is not associated with any specific diagnosis because LBP from any cause may limit motion. Range-of-motion measurements, however, can help in monitoring treatment. Chest expansion of less than 2.5 cm has specificity but not sensitivity for ankylosing spondylitis.

The hip joints should be examined because hip arthritis, which normally causes groin pain, may occasionally refer pain to the back. Trochanteric bursitis, with tenderness over the greater trochanter of the femur, can be confused with LBP. The presence of more widespread tender points suggests the possibility that LBP may be secondary to fibromyalgia.

In patients with a history of LBP that radiates into the lower extremities (radicular pain, neurogenic claudication, or referred sclerotomal pain), a **straight leg raising test** should be performed. With the patient lying supine, the examiner places the heel in the palm and raises the patient's leg, keeping the knee fully extended. This movement places tension on the sciatic nerve (that originates from L4, L5, S1, S2, and S3), thereby stretching the nerve roots (especially L5, S1, and S2). If any of these nerve roots is already irritated, such as by impingement from a herniated disk, further tension on the nerve root by straight leg raising will result in radicular pain that extends below the knee. The test is positive if radicular pain is produced when the leg is raised between 30 and 70 degrees. Dorsiflexion of the ankle further stretches the sciatic nerve and increases the sensitivity of the test. Pain experienced in the posterior thigh or knee during straight leg raising is generally from hamstring tightness and does not represent a positive test. The straight leg raising test is sensitive (91%) but not specific (26%) for clinically significant disk herniation at the L4–5 or L5–S1 levels. These are the sites of

Table 8–2. Neurologic features of lumbosacral radiculopathy.

Disk Herniation	Nerve Root	Motor	Sensory (Light Touch)	Reflex
L3–4	L4	Dorsiflexion of foot	Medial foot	Knee
L4–5	L5	Dorsiflexion of great toe	Dorsal foot	None
L5–S1	S1	Plantar flexion of foot	Lateral foot	Ankle

95% of the clinically meaningful disk herniations). False-negative tests are more frequently seen with herniation above the L4–5 level. The straight leg raising test is usually negative in patients with spinal stenosis. The crossed straight leg raising test (with radicular pain reproduced in one leg when the opposite leg is raised) is highly specific but insensitive for a clinically significant disk herniation.

The neurologic evaluation (Table 8–2) of the lower extremities in a patient with radicular pain can often identify the specific nerve root involved. As a general rule of thumb, if a disk herniation results in nerve root compression, the more caudal nerve root is usually impinged. Therefore, for example, L4–5 disk herniation will likely result in L5 nerve root impingement rather than L4 nerve root impingement. The evaluation should include motor testing with focus on dorsiflexion of the foot (L4), great toe dorsiflexion (L5) and foot plantar flexion (S1); determination of knee (L4) and ankle (S1) deep tendon reflexes; and tests for dermatomal sensory loss (Figure 8–2; see Table 8–2). The inability to toe walk (mostly S1) and heel walk (mostly L5) indicate muscle weakness. Muscle atrophy can be detected by circumferential measurements of the calf and thigh at the same level bilaterally.

C. Laboratory Findings

These are used mostly in identifying patients with systemic causes of LBP and play a minor role in the investigation of LBP. A patient with normal blood cell counts, a normal erythrocyte sedimentation rate, and normal radiographs of the lumbar spine is unlikely to have underlying infection or malignancy as the cause of LBP.

D. Imaging Studies

There is concern about overuse of lumbar spine imaging, especially in the United States where imaging capacity is high. Indiscriminate spine imaging leads to a low yield of clinically useful findings, a high yield of misleading findings, substantial radiation exposure, and significant medical expense. The major function of diagnostic testing, especially imaging, is the early identification of pathology in those few patients who have evidence of a major or progressive neurologic deficit and those in whom an underlying systemic disease or vertebral fracture is suspected (see Table 8–1). Otherwise, imaging is not required unless significant symptoms persist beyond 6–8 weeks. More than 90% of the patients will have largely recovered by 8 weeks, with or without imaging.

A significant problem with all imaging studies is that many of the anatomic abnormalities identified in patients with LBP are also commonly present in asymptomatic individuals. These abnormalities, which often result from age-related degenerative changes, frequently have no relationship whatsoever to patients' LBP symptoms. Such age-related abnormalities begin to appear even in early adulthood and are among the earliest degenerative changes in the body. Abnormalities on radiography, such as single-disk degeneration, facet joint degeneration, Schmorl nodes (protrusion of the nucleus pulposus into the spongiosa of a vertebra), spondylolysis, mild spondylolisthesis, transitional vertebrae (the "lumbarization" of S1 or "sacralization" of L5), spina bifida occulta, and mild scoliosis, are equally prevalent in individuals with and without LBP. Given the weak association

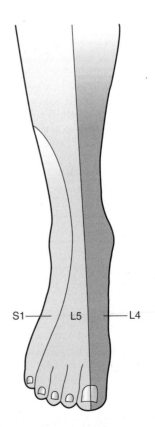

S1 —   L5   — L4

▲ **Figure 8–2.** Lower extremity dermatomes.

between imaging abnormalities and symptoms, it is not surprising that in as many as 85% of patients, a precise patho-anatomic diagnosis with identification of the pain generator cannot be made.

Plain radiographs and MRI are the major modalities used in the evaluation of patients with LBP. In patients with persistent LBP of greater than 6–8 weeks' duration despite standard therapies, radiography may be a reasonable first option if there are no symptoms suggesting radiculopathy or spinal stenosis. Standing anteroposterior and lateral views are usually adequate. Oblique views substantially increase radiation exposure and add little new diagnostic information.

MRI without contrast is generally the best initial test for patients with LBP who require advanced imaging. It is the preferred modality for the detection of spinal infection and cancers, herniated disks, and spinal stenosis. MRI testing for LBP should largely be limited to patients in whom there is a suspicion of systemic disease (such as infection or malignancy), or for the preoperative evaluation of patients who are surgical candidates on clinical grounds (eg, the presence of a significant or progressive neurologic deficit). Disk abnormalities are commonly noted on MRI studies but often have little or no relationship with the patient's symptoms.

A disk bulge is a symmetric circumferential extension of disk material beyond the interspace. A disk herniation is a focal or asymmetric extension. Herniations are subdivided into protrusions and extrusions. Protrusions are broad-based, whereas extrusions have a "neck" so that the base is narrower than the extruded material. Bulges (52%) and protrusions (27%) are common in asymptomatic adults but extrusions are rare.

MRI is generally preferred over computed tomography (CT) scanning in the evaluation of patients with LBP. However, when bone anatomy is critical, CT is superior. This is particularly true when spondylolysis is suspected as this may not be well seen with MRI.

E. Electrodiagnostic Studies

Electrodiagnostic studies can be helpful in the evaluation of some patients with lumbosacral radiculopathy. The main procedures are electromyography and nerve conduction studies. When used in combination, these studies provide information regarding the integrity of spinal nerve roots and their connection with the muscles they innervate. These studies can confirm nerve root compression and define the distribution and severity of involvement. Whereas studies such as MRI can only provide anatomic information, electrodiagnostic studies provide physiologic information that may support or refute the findings on imaging. Electrodiagnostic testing is therefore mostly considered in patients with persistent disabling symptoms of radiculopathy in which there is discordance between the clinical presentation and findings on imaging. Electrodiagnosis is unnecessary in a patient with an obvious radiculopathy. It should be noted that electromyographic changes depend on the development of muscle denervation following nerve injury and may not

be detected for 2–3 weeks after the injury. (In contrast, nerve conduction tests become abnormal immediately after nerve damage.) Another limitation is that electromyographic abnormalities may persist for more than 1 year following decompressive surgery.

▶ Differential Diagnosis

LBP usually originates from pathology within the lumbar spine (Table 8–3). Rarely pain is referred to the back from visceral disease. Most LBP is mechanical, and most mechanical pain is due to degenerative change in the lumbar spine.

A. Lumbar Spondylosis

The current common usage of the term "lumbar spondylosis" includes degenerative changes in both the anteriorly placed diskovertebral joints and the posterolaterally placed facet joints. These degenerative (osteoarthritic) changes are seen radiographically as disk space (or joint space) narrowing, subchondral sclerosis, and osteophytosis (Figure 8–3).

Imaging evidence of lumbar spondylosis is common in the general population, increases with age, and may be unrelated to back symptoms. Complicating matters further, patients with severe mechanical LBP may have minimal radiographic changes, but patients with advanced changes may be asymptomatic.

The clinical spectrum is broad. Patients may present with acute mechanical LBP, often with paravertebral spasm and loss

Table 8–3. Causes of low back pain.

Mechanical
Lumbar spondylosis[a]
Disk herniation[a]
Spondylolisthesis[a]
Spinal stenosis[a]
Fracture (mostly osteoporotic)
Nonspecific (idiopathic)
Neoplastic
Primary
Metastatic
Inflammatory
Spondyloarthritis
Infectious
Vertebral osteomyelitis
Epidural abscess
Septic diskitis
Herpes zoster
Metabolic
Osteoporotic compression fractures
Paget disease
Referred pain to spine
From major viscera, retroperitoneal structures, urogenital system, aorta, or hip

[a]Related to degenerative changes.

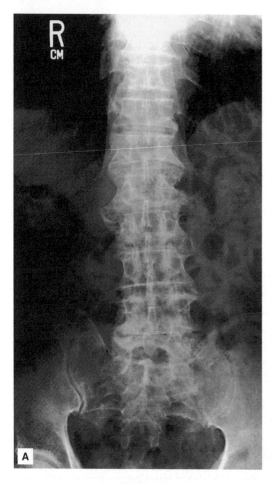

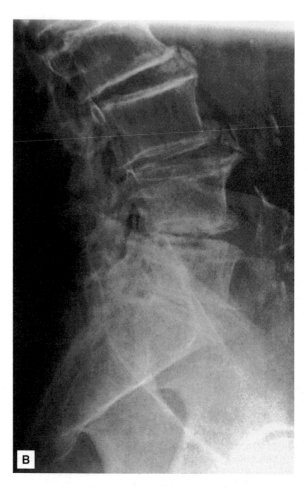

▲ **Figure 8–3.** Lumbar spondylosis. Anteroposterior (**A**) and lateral (**B**) radiographs of the lumbar spine show the cardinal features of disk-space narrowing, marginal osteophytes, and endplate sclerosis. (Used with permission from John Crues, MD, University of California, San Diego.)

of lumbar lordosis. Some patients have chronic mechanical LBP often with periods of acute exacerbation. Somatic referral may lead to sclerotomal pain that radiates into the buttocks and thighs. The diffuse degenerative changes that involve not only the joints but also the para-articular structures such as ligaments and joint capsules predispose these patients to intervertebral disk herniation, spondylolisthesis, and spinal stenosis.

Some patients with facet joint osteoarthritis have sclerotomal pain that radiates into the buttock or posterior thigh. This is alleviated by forward flexion and exacerbated by lumbar hyperextension or by bending to the side ipsilateral to the involved joint (**facet syndrome**). In clinical practice, however, it is difficult to isolate symptoms specifically to the facet joints, and the true prevalence of the facet syndrome as a cause of back pain remains controversial.

Modic changes are signal changes related to spinal degeneration in the vertebral endplate and adjacent bone marrow

that are commonly reported on lumbar MRI. Modic type I changes are secondary to marrow edema and inflammation. Modic type II changes represent fatty replacement of marrow. Modic type III changes reflect subchondral bone sclerosis. The prevalence of these changes increases with age and appears to be associated with degenerative disk changes but sometimes regress over time, as well. Modic changes are present in 20–40% of LBP patients but may be seen in as many as 10% of asymptomatic adults. The clinical usefulness with regard to selecting treatment options of these signal changes is unclear.

Focal high signal in the posterior annulus fibrosus as seen on T2-weighted MRI images, sometimes referred to as a **high-intensity zone**, is believed to represent tears in the annulus fibrosus and to correlate with positive findings on provocative diskography. The high prevalence of high-intensity zones in asymptomatic individuals limits its clinical value.

Spinal instability is seen in some patients with lumbar spondylosis. It is identified by demonstrating abnormal vertebral motion (anteroposterior displacement or excessive angular change of adjacent vertebrae) on lateral radiographs in flexion and extension. However, such spinal motion may be seen in asymptomatic persons and its natural history and relationship to LBP is unclear. Thus, in the absence of fractures, infection, neoplastic disease, or spondylolisthesis, the diagnosis of spinal instability as a cause of LBP and its treatment by spinal fusion remain controversial.

B. Disk Herniation

Intervertebral disk herniation occurs when the nucleus pulposus in a degenerated disk prolapses and pushes out the weakened annulus. These events usually occur in the posterolateral region, where the annulus fibrosus is thinner. Imaging evidence of disk abnormalities has a high prevalence in the general population, and disk bulges and herniations are common in asymptomatic adults. Occasionally, however, the herniated disk can cause nerve root impingement that leads to lumbosacral radiculopathy (Figures 8–4 and 8–5).

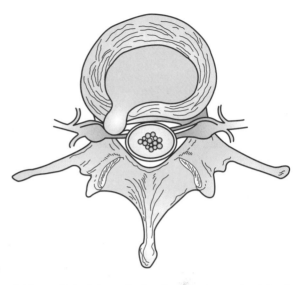

▲ **Figure 8–4.** Schematic drawing showing posterolateral disk herniation resulting in nerve root impingement.

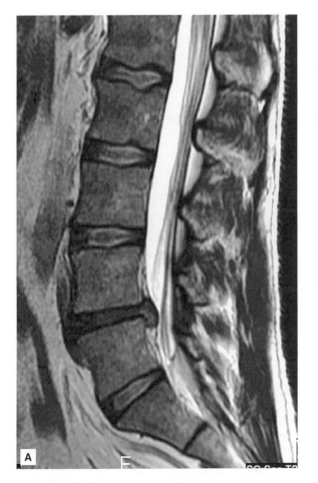

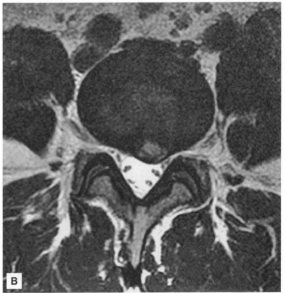

▲ **Figure 8–5.** Lumbar disk extrusion. **A:** The sagittal T2-weighted MRI shows an extruded disk at the L4–5 level. **B:** The axial image through the L4–5 level shows disk extrusion to the left side of the neural canal and compressing the traversing L5 nerve root in the left lateral recess. (Used with permission from John Crues, MD, University of California, San Diego.)

A herniated intervertebral disk is the most common cause of radicular pain in young adults. Up to 95% of clinically significant nerve compression radiculopathies occur at L4–L5 or L5–S1.

The frequency of disk herniation increases with age. The peak frequency of herniations at the L5–S1 and L4–L5 levels is between the ages of 44 and 50 years, with a progressive decline in frequency thereafter.

The genesis of sciatica is felt to have both mechanical and biologic components. The impingement of extruded disk material on a nerve root comprises the mechanical component, but inflammation, vascular invasion, immune responses, and an array of cytokines have also been implicated.

The clinical features of disk herniation resulting in lumbosacral radiculopathy have already been discussed (see sections on history, physical examination, and Table 8–2). Immediate imaging is unnecessary in patients who do not have a clinically significant neurologic deficit or red flags that suggest an underlying systemic pathology (see Table 8–1). Patients with L1 radiculopathy—a rare occurrence—present with pain, paresthesias, and sensory loss in the inguinal region.

L2, L3, and L4 radiculopathies are uncommon and more likely to be seen in older patients with lumbar spinal stenosis.

The natural history of disk herniation is favorable, with progressive improvement expected in most patients. The condition of patients who have motor deficits secondary to herniated disks also improves over time. Only approximately 10% of patients have persistent pain after 6 weeks that is severe enough to justify decompressive surgery.

Large midline disk herniations, usually occurring at L4–5, can compress the cauda equina and lead to the **cauda equina syndrome** (Figure 8–6). These patients present with LBP, bilateral radicular pain, and bilateral motor deficits with leg weakness. Physical examination findings are often asymmetric. Sensory loss in the perineum (saddle anesthesia) is common. The cardinal clinical feature is urinary retention with overflow incontinence (sensitivity 90%, specificity 95%). Fecal incontinence may also occur. Other causes of cauda equina syndrome include neoplasia, epidural abscess, hematoma, and, rarely, lumbar spinal stenosis. Cauda equina syndrome is a surgical emergency because neurologic results are affected by the time

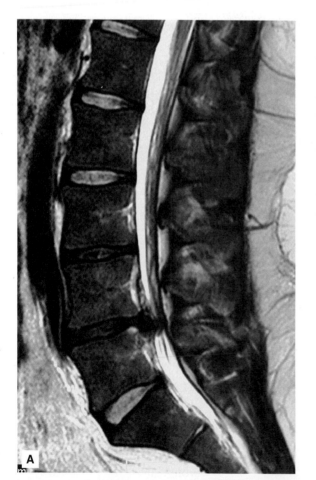

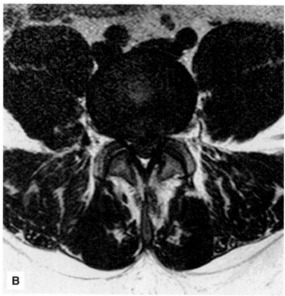

▲ **Figure 8–6.** Cauda equina syndrome. **A:** The sagittal T2-weighted MRI shows an extruded disk at the L4–5 level. **B:** The axial image through this level reveals a large central disk extrusion causing severe loss of cross-sectional area of the thecal sac. (Used with permission from John Crues, MD, University of California, San Diego.)

to decompression. Whenever possible, the cauda equina syndrome should be recognized before established incontinence because once urinary retention has occurred the prognosis is worse.

C. Spondylolisthesis

Spondylolisthesis is the anterior displacement of a vertebra on the one beneath it. There are two major types: isthmic and degenerative. Traumatic spondylolisthesis (following high impact trauma) and pathologic spondylolisthesis (such as secondary to a lytic tumor) occur infrequently.

Isthmic spondylolisthesis (Figure 8–7), most commonly seen at the L5–S1 level, is caused by bilateral spondylolysis. **Spondylolysis** is a unilateral or bilateral defect in the pars interarticularis that is most commonly seen at L5. It is typically a fatigue fracture acquired early in life that is more commonly seen in boys. These abnormalities are surprisingly common. Based on CT imaging, the prevalence of spondylolysis in adults is around 10%. Spondylolysis progresses to spondylolisthesis in approximately 15% of patients. Spondylolisthesis may be missed if standing radiographs are not obtained.

Degenerative spondylolisthesis (Figure 8–8) develops in some patients with severe degenerative changes. Subluxation at the facet joints allows anterior or posterior movement of one vertebra over another. It is usually seen in an older age group (typically age >60 years), is more common in women,

most frequently involves the L4–5 level, and rarely exceeds 30% of vertebral width.

Most patients, especially those with a minor degree of spondylolisthesis, are asymptomatic. Some may complain of an aching mechanical LBP. Neurologic complications may occur in some with greater degrees of spondylolisthesis. Nerve root impingement is more likely to be seen in patients with isthmic spondylolisthesis (especially L5 nerve root). In contrast, with degenerative spondylolisthesis, the more likely clinical presentation is that of spinal stenosis (Figure 8–9). Rarely, extreme slippage results in cauda equina syndrome.

D. Spinal Stenosis

The diagnosis of lumbar spinal stenosis requires both the presence of characteristic symptoms and signs as well as imaging confirmation of narrowing of the lumbar spinal canal or foramina. Radiologic lumbar spinal stenosis, defined as a narrowing of the central spinal canal, its lateral recesses, and neural foramina, diminishes the space available for neural and vascular elements and may result in compression of lumbosacral nerve roots. Spinal stenosis can occur at one or multiple levels, and the narrowing may be asymmetric. It is important to recognize that 20–30% of asymptomatic adults older than 60 years have imaging evidence of spinal stenosis, but radiologic findings often correlate poorly with patients' symptoms. The prevalence of symptomatic lumbar spinal stenosis is not established.

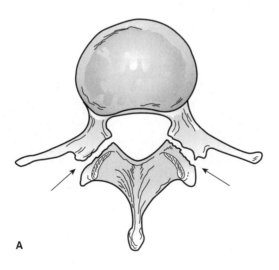

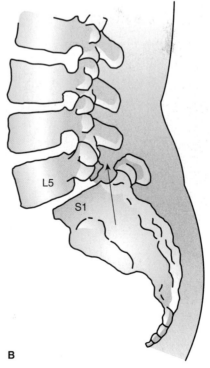

▲ **Figure 8–7. A:** Spondylolysis with bilateral defects in the pars interarticularis (*arrows*). **B:** Spondylolysis of the L5 vertebra (*arrow*) resulting in isthmic spondylolisthesis at L5–S1.

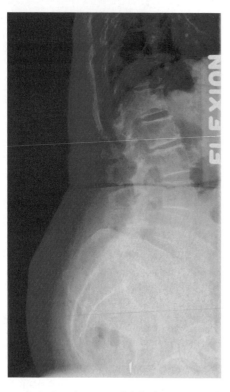

▲ **Figure 8–8.** Lumbar spondylolisthesis. Lateral radiograph of the lumbar spine showing grade 1 anterolisthesis at the levels of L4–5 and L5–S1 related to severe degenerative changes of the facet joints.

Table 8–4. Causes of lumbar spinal stenosis.

Congenital
    Idiopathic
    Achondroplastic
Acquired
    Degenerative
        Hypertrophy of facet joints
        Hypertrophy of ligamentum flavum
        Disc herniation
        Spondylolisthesis
        Scoliosis
    Iatrogenic
        Postlaminectomy
        Postsurgical fusion
    Miscellaneous
        Paget disease
        Fluorosis
        Diffuse idiopathic skeletal hyperostosis

Congenital idiopathic spinal stenosis (Table 8–4) is not uncommon and results from congenitally short pedicles. These patients tend to become symptomatic early (in the third to fifth decade of life) when superimposed mild degenerative changes that would normally be tolerated without symptoms result in narrowing of the spinal canal sufficient to cause symptoms.

Degenerative changes are the cause of spinal stenosis in the vast majority of cases. The intervertebral disk loses height as it degenerates. This results in a bulging or buckling of the

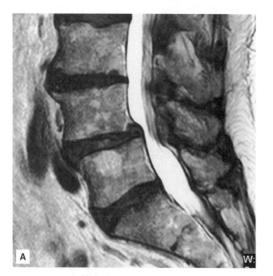

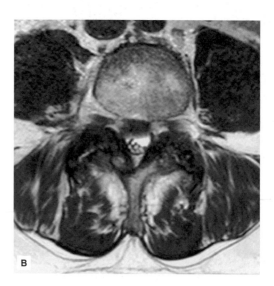

▲ **Figure 8–9.** Degenerative spondylolisthesis. **A:** The sagittal T2-weighted MRI shows an anterior slippage of the L4 vertebral body with respect to the L5 vertebral body compromising the thecal sac at this level. **B:** The axial image through the L4–5 disk space confirms the loss of cross-sectional area of the thecal sac leading to spinal stenosis. (Used with permission from John Crues, MD, University of California, San Diego.)

now redundant and often hypertrophied ligamentum flavum into the posterior part of the canal. Any herniation of the degenerated disk narrows the anterior part of the canal, whereas hypertrophied facets and osteophytes may compress nerve roots in the lateral recess or intervertebral foramen (Figures 8–10 and 8–11). Any degree of spondylolisthesis will further exacerbate spinal canal narrowing.

The hallmark of spinal stenosis is **neurogenic claudication** (pseudoclaudication). The symptoms of neurogenic claudication are usually bilateral but often asymmetric. The patient's primary complaint is of pain in the buttocks, thighs, and legs. The pain may be accompanied by paresthesias. The history is the key to the diagnosis of neurogenic claudication. Neurogenic claudication is induced by standing erect or walking and relieved by sitting or flexing forward. A useful question to ask patients is if their symptoms are improved by leaning forward, as when pushing a grocery cart (the "shopping cart sign"). Forward flexion increases the spinal canal dimensions and alleviates pressure on nerves. Relief through this maneuver may lead the patient to adopt a simian stance. Many patients with lumbar spinal stenosis cannot walk far with becoming symptomatic yet exhibit surprising endurance while pedaling a stationary bicycle.

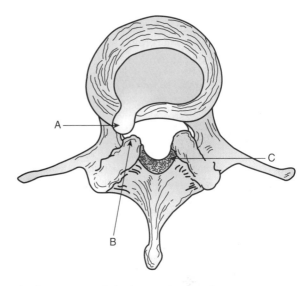

▲ **Figure 8–10.** Spinal stenosis secondary to a combination of disk herniation (**A**), facet joint hypertrophy (**B**), and hypertrophy of the ligamentum flavum (**C**).

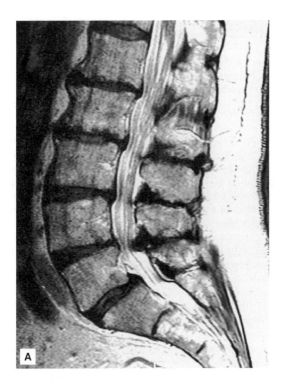

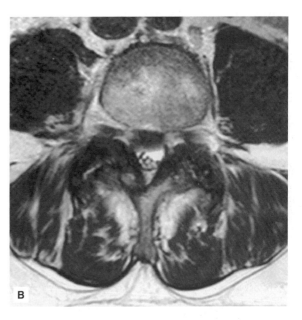

▲ **Figure 8–11.** Degenerative spinal stenosis. **A:** The sagittal T2-weighted MRI shows decreased anteroposterior diameter of the neural canal at the L4–5 level due to redundancy of the ligamentum flavum. **B:** The axial image through the L4–5 disk shows decreased cross-sectional area of the thecal sac from hypertrophic changes of the facet joints posterolateral to the thecal sac. (Used with permission from John Crues, MD, University of California, San Diego.)

The symptoms of neurogenic claudication probably represent intermittent disruption of lumbosacral nerve root function by both mechanical and ischemic mechanisms. Patients often have a sense of weakness in the lower extremities. Unsteadiness of gait, related to compression of proprioceptive fibers, is a frequent complaint. The finding of a wide-based gait in a patient with LBP has more than 90% specificity for lumbar spinal stenosis. Factors that favor a diagnosis of neurogenic claudication as opposed to vascular claudication include preservation of pedal pulses, provocation of symptoms by standing erect just as readily as by walking, relief of symptoms with flexion of the spine, and location of maximal discomfort in the thighs rather than the calves. Central canal stenosis predominantly results in neurogenic claudication, and lateral canal stenosis may result in a radiculopathy.

The physical examination of a patient with lumbar spinal stenosis is often unimpressive. Severe neurogenic deficits are uncommon. Lumbar range of motion may be normal or reduced, and the result of straight leg raising is usually negative. An abnormal Romberg test is seen in some patients. Deep tendon reflexes and vibration sense may be reduced. Mild diffuse weakness in the lower extremities may be present in others, but the significance of these findings is often difficult to determine in elderly patients. However, in a few patients with spinal stenosis, a fixed nerve root injury may occur resulting in a lumbosacral radiculopathy or, rarely, a cauda equina syndrome.

The diagnosis of lumbar spinal stenosis is most often suspected when a history of neurogenic claudication is elicited. The diagnosis is best confirmed by MRI.

Spinal stenosis is generally an indolent condition in which the symptoms evolve gradually and the natural history is benign. As such, prophylactic surgical intervention is not warranted.

E. Diffuse Idiopathic Skeletal Hyperostosis

Diffuse idiopathic skeletal hyperostosis (DISH) is characterized by calcification and ossification of the paraspinous ligaments and the entheses. It is a noninflammatory condition of unknown etiology that is not associated with human leukocyte antigen (HLA)-B27 positivity.

DISH has been associated with obesity, diabetes mellitus, and acromegaly. It is rarely diagnosed before 30 years, is more commonly seen in men, and its prevalence rises with age.

The thoracic spine is involved most commonly, but the cervical and lumbar regions may also be affected. Ossification of the anterior longitudinal ligament is best seen on a lateral radiograph of the thoracic spine. The ossification, together with bridging enthesophytes in the spine, gives the appearance of flowing wax (Figure 8–12) on the anterior and right lateral aspects of the spine. Involvement of the left lateral aspect in patients with situs inversus has led to speculation that the descending aorta plays a role in the location of the calcification.

Intervertebral disk spaces and facet joints are preserved unless there is coexisting lumbar spondylosis. The sacroiliac

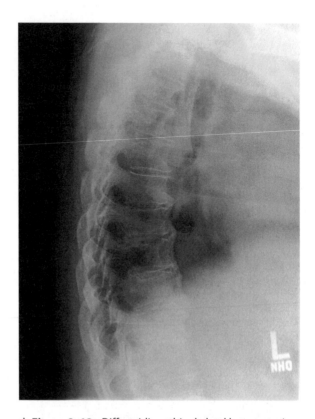

▲ **Figure 8–12.** Diffuse idiopathic skeletal hyperostosis. Lateral radiograph of the thoracic spine demonstrating bridging syndesmophytes, maintained disk spaces, and no fusion of the facet joints.

joints appear normal. This helps to differentiate DISH from spondylosis and the spondylarthritides. Almost any extra spinal osseous or articular site may be affected. Irregular new bone formation ("whiskering") is often best seen at the iliac crests, ischial tuberosities, and femoral trochanters. Ossification of tendons and ligaments at sites of attachment (such as the patella, olecranon process, and calcaneus) and periarticular osteophytes (such as the lateral acetabulum and inferior portion of the sacroiliac joint on pelvic radiographs) may also be seen. Severe ligamentous calcification may be seen in the sacrotuberous and iliolumbar ligaments. Heterotopic bone formation following hip replacement in patients with DISH has been described, but the frequency of that complication in this patient population is not known.

Patients with DISH may be entirely asymptomatic. The most common complaint encountered is of pain and stiffness involving the spine, often the thoracic region. Usually there is only a moderate limitation of spinal motion. The loss of lateral spinal flexion is particularly notable in some patients. Extensive ossification of the anterior longitudinal ligament together with large anterior enthesophytes occasionally compresses the esophagus and causes dysphagia. Ossification of the posterior longitudinal ligament is seen primarily in the cervical spine and may occur either as a discrete disorder or as part of DISH. This can rarely lead to cervical myelopathy. Pain and tenderness may be present at the entheses, and these patients may have findings of lateral or medial humeral epicondylitis, Achilles tendonitis, or plantar fasciitis.

If treatment of DISH is necessary at all, it is directed toward symptom reduction. There is no approach to treating the underlying pathophysiology (still poorly understood) that is known to be effective. Most patients respond to acetaminophen, nonsteroidal anti-inflammatory drugs (NSAIDs), and judicious use of glucocorticoid injections for painful enthesopathy. Knowledge of the indolent nature of the problem and reassurance that they do not have an inflammatory disorder such as ankylosing spondylitis is reassuring to most patients.

F. Nonspecific Low Back Pain

This is defined as pain in the low back that has no identifiable cause (identification of the pain generator) and no clear association with a specific serious underlying anatomical impairment or disease process. This condition is also referred to as idiopathic LBP. A precise pathoanatomic diagnosis with identification of the pain generator cannot be established in as many as 85% of patients with LBP. This is largely because of the nonspecific nature of the symptoms in patients with LBP and the weak association of these symptoms with findings on imaging. Thus, terms such as lumbago, back strain, and back sprain have come into use. These terms have no clinical-radiologic definition and should be avoided. Nonspecific LBP is a more accurate label for these patients, most of whom have a syndrome of acute mechanical LBP that is self-limited. Sometimes the back pain develops immediately after a traumatic event such as lifting a heavy object or a twisting injury, but other patients may simply wake up with LBP. The severity of pain can vary from mild to severe. Most patients are better within 1–4 weeks but remain susceptible to similar future episodes. Chronic nonspecific LBP develops in less than 10% of patients.

Patients with nonspecific LBP are managed conservatively with a goal to relieve pain and restore function.

G. Neoplasm

Neoplasms are an uncommon but nevertheless important cause of LBP. In a primary care setting, neoplasia accounts for less than 1% of cases of LBP. By far the most important predictor for likelihood of underlying cancer as the cause of LBP is a prior history of cancer.

The typical patient with LBP secondary to spinal malignancy presents with persistent, progressive pain that is not alleviated by rest and is often worse at night. In some patients a spinal mass can result in a lumbosacral radiculopathy or cauda equina syndrome. Acute LBP may be the presentation in a patient with a pathologic compression fracture.

Most cases result from involvement of the spine by multiple myeloma or a metastatic carcinoma. The carcinomas most likely to metastasize to the spine are those arising in the prostate, lung, breast, thyroid gland, gastrointestinal tract, or kidney. Vertebral metastases occur in 3–5% of people with cancer, and 97% of spinal tumors are metastatic disease. Metastatic vertebral lesions, detected most often in the thoracic spine, account for 39% of bony metastases in patients with primary neoplasms. Spinal cord tumors, primary vertebral tumors, and retroperitoneal tumors may, in rare cases, be the cause of LBP.

Osteoid osteoma, a benign tumor of bone, typically presents with LBP in the second or third decade of life. The pain is often accompanied by a functional scoliosis secondary to paravertebral spasm. Patients may be seen with pain even before the osteoid osteoma is visible radiographically. Osteoid osteomas predominantly involve the posterior elements of the spine, usually the neural arch. A sclerotic lesion measuring less than 1.5 cm with a lucent nidus is pathognomonic. A bone scan, CT scan, or MRI should be ordered if an osteoid osteoma is suspected but not detected on radiography. Symptoms can often be controlled by NSAIDs, presumably because the nidus produces high levels of prostaglandins. Surgical resection is an option for intolerable pain. Osteoid osteomas spontaneously resolve during the course of several years.

Plain radiographs are less sensitive than other imaging tests in detecting neoplastic lesions. Approximately 50% of trabecular bone must be lost before a lytic lesion is visible. Metastatic lesions may be lytic (radiolucent), blastic (radiodense), or mixed. The majority of metastases are osteolytic. Vertebral bodies are primarily involved (Figure 8–13) because of their rich blood supply associated with red marrow. In contrast to the case with infections of the spine, the disk space is usually spared by metastases. MRI offers the greatest sensitivity and specificity in the evaluation of spinal tumors and is generally the modality of choice. A purely lytic lesion such as multiple myeloma will not be detected by a bone scan.

Radiation therapy is usually helpful in controlling the pain related to skeletal metastases. Decompressive surgery is often required if the spinal mass results in a nerve root compression syndrome.

H. Infection

Vertebral osteomyelitis may be acute (usually pyogenic) or chronic (pyogenic, fungal, or granulomatous). Acute vertebral osteomyelitis evolves during a period of a few days or weeks.

Vertebral osteomyelitis usually results from hematogenous seeding, direct inoculation at the time of spinal surgery, or contiguous spread from an infection in the adjacent soft tissue. The lumbar spine is the most common site of vertebral osteomyelitis. *Staphylococcus aureus* is the most common microorganism (accounting for >50% of cases) followed by

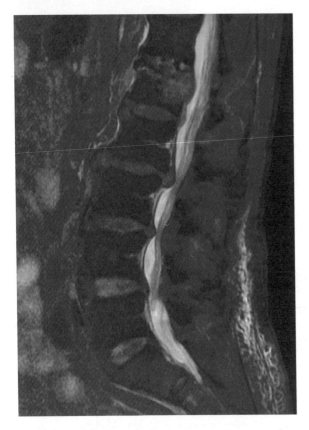

▲ **Figure 8–13.** Vertebral metastasis. Sagittal T2-weighted fat-saturated fast spin echo sequence image of the lumbar spine demonstrating a L1 vertebral bone metastasis typically located in the posterior aspect of the vertebral body with a convex posterior border.

Escherichia coli. Coagulase-negative staphylococci and *Propionibacterium acnes* are almost always the cause of exogenous osteomyelitis after spinal surgery, particularly if internal fixation devices are used.

A source of infection is detected in approximately one-half of the cases, with endocarditis diagnosed in as many as one-third of cases of vertebral osteomyelitis. Other common sites for the primary focus of infection are the urinary tract, skin, soft tissue, a site of vascular access, bursitis, or septic arthritis. Most patients with hematogenous pyogenic vertebral osteomyelitis have underlying medical disorders such as diabetes, coronary artery disease, immunosuppressive disorders, malignancy, and renal failure. Injection drug use is a major risk factor for vertebral osteomyelitis.

Vertebral osteomyelitis may be complicated by an epidural or paravertebral abscess. This may result in neurologic complication such as radiculopathy or cauda equina syndrome. Back pain is the initial symptom in most patients with vertebral osteomyelitis. The back pain usually starts insidiously and progressively worsens over several weeks. The pain tends to be persistent, is present at rest, exacerbated by activity, and, at times, well localized. Point tenderness on percussion over the spine has sensitivity but not specificity for vertebral osteomyelitis. Fever is present in only approximately one-half of the patients. Because most cases of vertebral osteomyelitis result from hematogenous seeding, the dominant manifestations initially may be of the primary infection.

Leukocytosis is seen in only approximately two-thirds of the patients. However, almost all patients have increases in the erythrocyte sedimentation rate and C-reactive protein, with the latter best correlating with clinical response to therapy. Blood cultures are positive in up to 50–70% of patients. If blood cultures are negative in a patient suspected of having vertebral osteomyelitis, a bone biopsy with appropriate culture studies and histopathologic analysis is indicated.

Plain radiography is usually the initial imaging study. Radiographic changes, however, occur relatively late and are nonspecific. Typically there is loss of disk height and loss of cortical definition followed by bony lysis of adjacent vertebral bodies. MRI is the most sensitive and specific imaging technique to detect spinal infections. The classic finding of pyogenic osteomyelitis is involvement of two vertebral bodies with their intervening disk (Figure 8–14). In a patient with neurologic impairment, MRI should be done early to rule out an epidural abscess. Whenever possible, antimicrobial therapy should be directed against an identified susceptible pathogen. Empiric antimicrobial therapy, pending culture results, is warranted in cases of neurologic compromise and sepsis. Empiric treatment, based on the most likely organism to cause infection, is also warranted when cultures are negative, but there is a high index of suspicion. Intravenous therapy of at least 4–6 weeks, and possibly additional oral antibiotic therapy, is usually recommended. Surgery may be necessary to drain an abscess. Surgical debridement is always required when infection is associated with a spinal implant with removal of the implant whenever possible.

Tuberculosis and nontubercular granulomatous infections (blastomycosis, cryptococcosis, actinomycosis, coccidioidomycosis, and brucellosis) of the spine should be considered in the appropriate clinical and geographic setting.

Lumbar nerve roots are commonly involved in patients with herpes zoster. In most cases a single unilateral dermatome is involved. Pain is often severe and may precede the appearance of a maculopapular rash that evolves into vesicles and pustules.

I. Inflammation

Spondylarthritides cause inflammatory LBP (see Table 8–1) and are discussed in detail elsewhere (see Chapter 14).

J. Metabolic Disease

The major consideration in this category is the occurrence of acute mechanical LBP secondary to a vertebral compression

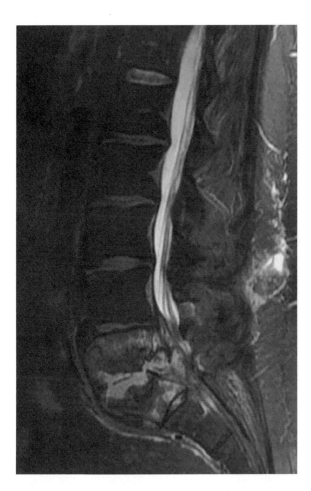

▲ **Figure 8–14.** Lumbar vertebral osteomyelitis. Sagittal T2-weighted fat-saturated fast spin echo sequence image demonstrating severe L5–S1 osteomyelitis with diskitis with destruction of the endplates, fluid in the disk space, and epidural extension of the infection. Also note bone marrow edema pattern in the entire L5 and S1 vertebral bodies.

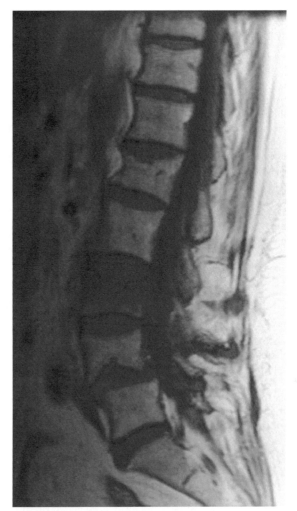

▲ **Figure 8–15.** Osteoporotic fractures. Sagittal T1-weighted fast spin echo image demonstrating chronic fractures at L1 and L4 and more acute fracture at L3 with bone marrow edema pattern.

fracture (Figure 8–15) in a patient with osteoporosis (see Chapter 47). Most patients are postmenopausal women.

Paget disease of bone (see Chapter 48) is most often detected in an asymptomatic patient by the incidental finding of either an elevated alkaline phosphatase or characteristic radiographic abnormality. The spine is the second most commonly affected site after the pelvis. Within the spine, the L4 and L5 vertebrae are most commonly involved. Paget disease of the spine may involve single or multiple levels. The vertebral body is almost always involved together with a variable portion of the neural arch. Radiographically, Paget disease is seen as areas of enlargement of the bone with thickened, coarsened trabeculae. Usually a mixed picture of sclerotic and lytic Paget disease is encountered. The vertebrae may enlarge, weaken, and fracture. LBP may

occur because of the pagetic process itself (with periosteal stretching and vascular engorgement), microfractures, overt fractures, secondary osteoarthritis of the facet joints, spondylolysis with or without spondylolisthesis, or sarcomatous transformation (rare). Neurologic complications secondary to Paget disease of the lumbar spine include radicular pain secondary to nerve root impingement, spinal stenosis, and, rarely, cauda equina syndrome.

K. Visceral Pathology

Disease in organs that share segmental innervation with the spine can cause pain to be referred to the spine. In general, pelvic diseases refer pain to the sacral area, lower abdominal diseases to the lumbar area, and upper abdominal diseases to the lower thoracic spine area. Local signs of disease, such as tenderness to palpation, paravertebral muscle spasm, and increased pain on spinal motion, are absent.

Vascular, gastrointestinal, urogenital, or retroperitoneal pathology may on occasion cause LBP. A partial list of causes includes an expanding aortic aneurysm, pyelonephritis, ureteral obstruction due to renal stones, chronic prostatitis, endometriosis, ovarian cysts, inflammatory bowel disorders, colonic neoplasms, and retroperitoneal hemorrhage (usually in a patient taking anticoagulants).

Most abdominal aortic aneurysms are asymptomatic but may become painful as they expand. Aneurysmal pain is usually a harbinger of rupture. Rarely, the aneurysm may develop leakage. This produces severe pain with abdominal tenderness. Most patients with aortic dissection present with a sudden onset of severe "tearing" pain in the chest or upper back. Pain originating from a hollow viscus such as the ureter or colon is often colicky.

L. Miscellaneous

LBP may be part of the clinical spectrum in innumerable conditions. It would not be practical or useful to discuss all of these entities here. Considered next are some of the more important or controversial causes of LBP.

The **piriformis syndrome** is thought to be an entrapment neuropathy of the sciatic nerve related to anatomic variations in the muscle-nerve relationship or to overuse. The piriformis is a narrow muscle that originates from the anterior part of the sacrum and inserts into the greater trochanter. It is an external rotator of the hip. The sciatic nerve underlies the piriformis muscle. There is, however, debate about the existence of the piriformis syndrome as a discrete entity because of the lack of objective, validated, and standardized tests. The diagnosis is clinical. Patients complain of pain and paresthesias in the gluteal region that may radiate down the leg to the foot. Some patients describe aggravation of pain after sitting. Unlike sciatica from lumbosacral nerve root compression, pain is not restricted to a specific dermatome. The straight leg raising test is usually negative. There may be tenderness over the sciatic notch. Physical examination maneuvers for the diagnosis of piriformis syndrome are based on the notion that stretching the irritated piriformis muscle may provoke sciatic nerve compression. This can be done by internally rotating the hip (Freiburg sign) or by flexion, adduction, and internal rotation (FAIR maneuver) of the hip. Physical therapy that focuses on stretching the piriformis muscle and NSAIDs are generally the treatments offered.

The diagnosis of sacroiliac joints as the source of LBP, in patients without spondyloarthritis, remains controversial. **Sacroiliac joint dysfunction** is a term used to describe pain in the sacroiliac region related to abnormal sacroiliac joint movement or alignment. However, tests of pelvic symmetry or sacroiliac joint movement have low intertester reliability, and fluoroscopically guided sacroiliac joint injections have been unreliable in diagnosis and treatment. Radiographic degenerative changes of the sacroiliac joint are often noted in the evaluation of patients with LBP. Whether these changes are the primary cause of the back pain remains unresolved.

Lumbosacral transitional vertebrae include sacralization of the lowest lumbar vertebral body (assimilation of L5 to the sacrum resulting in four lumbar vertebrae and an enlarged sacral segment) and lumbarization of the uppermost sacral segment (assimilation of S1 to lumbar spine resulting in six lumbar vertebrae and a shortened sacral segment). These common variants can be seen in 15–35% of the general population. The association of these variants with LBP remains controversial.

Epidural lipomatosis may be seen in obese patients, but it is more commonly seen as a rare side effect of long-term use of corticosteroids. There is an increase in epidural adipose tissue that causes a narrowing of the spinal canal. This is usually an incidental finding, although it may lead to compression of neural structures.

LBP during pregnancy is common. The pain usually starts between the fifth and seventh months of pregnancy. The etiology of LBP in pregnancy is unclear. Biomechanical, hormonal, and vascular factors have been implicated. Most women have resolution of their pain postpartum.

Fibromyalgia (see Chapter 11) and polymyalgia rheumatica (see Chapter 26) are two frequently encountered rheumatologic conditions in which LBP may be a prominent part of the clinical syndrome.

▶ Treatment

Specific treatment is available only for the small fraction of patients with LBP who have either evidence of clinically significant neural compression or an underlying systemic disease (cancer, infection, visceral disease, and spondyloarthritis). In the vast majority of patients with LBP, either the precise pathoanatomic cause (ie, the pain generator) cannot be determined or, when the cause is determined, no specific treatment is available. These patients are managed with a conservative program centered on analgesia, education, and physical therapy. Currently a greater emphasis is placed on education, self-management, physical and psychological therapies, and less emphasis on pharmacological, invasive interventional, and surgical procedures. The goal of treatment is relief of pain and restoration of function. Surgery is rarely necessary.

One should be wary of the proliferation of unproven medical, surgical, and alternative therapies. Most have not been rigorously tested in well-designed randomized controlled trials. Uncontrolled studies can produce a misleading impression of efficacy because of fluctuating symptoms and the largely favorable natural history of LBP in most patients.

For management purposes, patients with LBP are considered to have either acute LBP (duration <3 months), chronic LBP (duration >3 months), or a nerve root compression syndrome.

A. Acute Low Back Pain

The typical patient seeks medical attention for sudden onset of severe mechanical LBP. The prognosis for acute LBP is excellent. Indeed, only approximately one-third of these patients seek medical care, and more than 90% recover substantially or completely within 8 weeks or less.

Patients with acute LBP are advised to stay active and continue ordinary daily activities within the limits permitted by pain. This leads to more rapid recovery than bed rest. Bed rest of more than 1 or 2 days is discouraged.

Pharmacologic therapy is used for symptomatic relief and does not affect recovery time. Unfortunately, no medication has consistently been shown to result in large average benefits on pain, and evidence of beneficial effects on function is even more limited. In spite of limited efficacy, it is reasonable to use NSAIDs as first-line analgesics taking into account the patient's age and risk for gastrointestinal, liver, and cardiorenal toxicity. Acetaminophen is an ineffective analgesic in patients with LBP. Short-term use of short-acting opioids is reasonable in patients with severe disabling LBP or in those at high risk of complications because of NSAIDs. Muscle relaxants such as cyclobenzaprine and tizanidine may be tried as second-line pharmacologic therapy for short-term symptomatic relief but have a high prevalence of adverse effects, including drowsiness and dizziness. It is unclear whether these medications truly relax muscles or if their effects are related to sedation or other nonspecific effects. Benzodiazepines have similar efficacy to muscle relaxants for short-term pain relief but are associated with risks for abuse, addiction, and tolerance. There is no convincing evidence for the efficacy of systemic corticosteroids in patients with acute LBP with or without radicular symptoms.

Back exercises are not helpful in the acute phase, and a physical therapy referral is usually unnecessary in the first month. Later, an individually tailored program that focuses on core strengthening, stretching exercises, aerobic conditioning, functional restoration, loss of excess weight, and education is recommended to prevent recurrences. The purpose of back exercises is to stabilize the spine by strengthening trunk muscles. Flexion exercises strengthen the abdominal muscles and extension exercises strengthen the paraspinal muscles. Numerous exercise programs have been developed and appear to be equally effective.

Patient education, including the use of education booklets, is recommended. The information provided should include causes of LBP, basic anatomy, favorable natural history, minimal value of diagnostic testing, importance of remaining active, effective self-care options, and coping techniques.

Spinal manipulation is provided mainly by chiropractors and osteopaths. It may involve low-velocity mobilization or manipulation with a high-velocity thrust that stretches spinal structures beyond the normal range and is frequently accompanied by a cracking or popping sound. For acute LBP, current evidence suggests that manipulative therapy is no more effective than conventional medical therapy. There is no evidence that ongoing manipulation reduces the risk of recurrence of LBP.

Given that most patients with acute LBP improve over time regardless of treatment, it is reasonable to select nonpharmacologic treatment with superficial heat (moderate-quality evidence), massage, acupuncture or spinal manipulation (low-quality evidence).

There is insufficient evidence to recommend the use of corsets and braces. Traction provides no significant benefit for LBP patients with or without radicular pain.

Epidural corticosteroid injections have gained remarkable, but unjustified, popularity. The rationale for their use is that the genesis of radicular pain, when a herniated disk impinges on a nerve root, is at least partly related to locally induced inflammation. There is evidence of a small treatment benefit compared with placebo injection for short-term relief of leg pain in patients with radiculopathy resulting from a herniated nucleus pulposus. However, epidural corticosteroid injections offer no significant functional benefit, nor do they reduce the need for surgery. It is important to note that there is no convincing evidence for the effectiveness of epidural corticosteroid injections in LBP patients without radiculopathy, in patients with spinal stenosis and neurogenic claudication, or for failed back surgery syndrome. Nonetheless, most of the use of epidural steroid injections occurs in these situations of questionable benefit.

A variety of other injection therapies with glucocorticoids or anesthetic agents, often in combination, are used in individuals with LBP with or without radicular pain and other symptoms in the leg. These include injection of trigger points, ligaments, sacroiliac joints, facet joints, and intradiskal steroid injections. There is no convincing evidence of the efficacy of these interventions. Medial branch block for presumed facet joint pain and nerve root blocks for therapeutic or diagnostic purposes are also not recommended.

A number of physical therapy modalities are currently used in the treatment of patients with subacute and chronic LBP. These include transcutaneous electrical nerve stimulation (TENS), percutaneous electrical nerve stimulation, interferential therapy, low-level laser therapy, shortwave diathermy, and ultrasound. There is insufficient evidence of efficacy to recommend their use.

Vertebral compression fractures secondary to osteoporosis are common. There is resolution of pain with fracture healing within a few weeks in most patients. **Vertebroplasty** and balloon **kyphoplasty** are invasive and expensive procedures that are used to treat persistent pain associated with these fractures. Both procedures involve the percutaneous placement of needles into the vertebral body through or lateral to the pedicles, as well as the injection of bone cement to stabilize the fracture. Kyphoplasty differs from vertebroplasty in that the cement is injected into a void in the vertebral body created by inflation of a balloon. Several early studies had suggested a positive treatment effect for vertebroplasty. However, two blinded, randomized, placebo-controlled trials of vertebroplasty for painful osteoporotic spinal fractures found no beneficial effect of vertebroplasty compared with a sham procedure. Therefore, on the basis of current evidence, the routine use of vertebroplasty or indeed kyphoplasty for relief of pain from osteoporotic compression fractures cannot be justified.

B. Chronic Low Back Pain

The clinical spectrum in patients with chronic LBP is wide. Some complain of severe, unrelenting pain, but most have a nagging mechanical LBP that may radiate into the buttocks and upper thighs. Patients with chronic LBP may experience periods of acute exacerbation. These exacerbations are managed according to the principles discussed earlier. A significant number of patients with chronic LBP remain functional and continue working, but overall the results of treatment are unsatisfactory and complete relief of pain is unrealistic for most. There is evidence that in a subset of patients with chronic LBP a pattern of augmented central nervous system pain processing (similar to fibromyalgia) is present, suggesting a component of "centralized pain." Patients with chronic LBP are largely responsible for the high costs associated with LBP. It is, therefore, incumbent on physicians who treat these patients to judiciously use proven therapies.

For patients with chronic LBP clinicians should initially select nonpharmacologic treatment including education, exercise (with a focus on core strengthening and flexibility), aerobic conditioning, and loss of excess weight. Multidisciplinary rehabilitation including cognitive behavioral therapy should be considered if the more conservative measures mentioned fail.

For most patients the initiation of pharmacologic therapy is with NSAIDs. They may provide some degree of analgesia, but the evidence for their long-term efficacy is not compelling. Acetaminophen is ineffective. Randomized clinical trial results do not support initiation of opioid therapy for moderate to severe chronic LBP. Opioid analgesics are an option when used judiciously in a minority of patients with severe disabling pain. Because of substantial risks, including aberrant drug-related behaviors with long-term use in patients vulnerable to abuse or addiction, potential benefits and harms of opioid analgesics should be carefully weighed before starting therapy. The co-prescribing of opioids and benzodiazepines should be avoided. There is no evidence that long-acting, around-the-clock dosing is more effective than short-acting or as-needed dosing, and continuous exposure to opioids could induce tolerance and lead to dose escalations. Tramadol (a weak opioid) and duloxetine (a serotonin-norepinephrine reuptake inhibitor) may be considered for second-line therapy. Muscle relaxants are not recommended for long-term use in patients with chronic

stable LBP. Low-dose tricyclic antidepressants have inconsistent benefits in patients with chronic LBP and adverse side effects are common. There is no evidence of efficacy of selective serotonin reuptake inhibitors for LBP. Depression is, however, common in patients with chronic LBP and should be treated appropriately. There is insufficient evidence to recommend antiepileptic medications, such as gabapentinoids (gabapentin and pregabalin) and topiramate, for pain relief in patients with LBP with or without radiculopathy.

An individually tailored physical therapy program and patient education, as discussed in the earlier section on the treatment of acute LBP, are particularly important aspects in the management of a patient with chronic LBP. The use of physical therapy modalities (as discussed earlier) is also not recommended for patients with chronic LBP. Lumbar supports and traction are ineffective. For most patients with LBP a medium-firm mattress or a back-conforming mattress (waterbed or foam) may be superior to a firm mattress.

A large number of other nonpharmacologic treatments have been evaluated for chronic LBP. The studies reveal that for acupuncture and mindfulness-based stress reduction (moderate-quality evidence), tai chi, yoga, motor control exercise, progressive relaxation, electromyography, biofeedback, low-level laser therapy, operant therapy, and spinal manipulation (low-quality evidence), there is a small to moderate effect on pain and function.

There has been a proliferation of nonsurgical interventional therapies for back pain. Various injection therapies (such as injections of trigger points, facet joints, and nerve root blocks) as discussed under the treatment of acute LBP, lack convincing evidence of efficacy and as such are also not recommended in the treatment of patients with chronic LBP.

Radiofrequency denervation aims to prevent the conduction of nociceptive impulses through the use of an electric current that damages the pain-conducting nerve. It has been used most frequently for treatment of presumed facet joint pain after a positive response to a diagnostic medial branch block. There is a lack of convincing evidence about the long-term effectiveness of this invasive procedure. Intradiskal electrothermal therapy (IDET) and percutaneous intradiskal radiofrequency thermocoagulation (PIRFT) involve placement of an electrode into the intervertebral disk of patients with presumed diskogenic pain and using electric or radiofrequency current to provide heat to thermocoagulate and shrink intradiskal tissue and destroy nerves. Current evidence does not support the use of IDET or PIRFT.

Spinal cord stimulation is a procedure involving the placement of electrodes, percutaneously or by laminotomy, in the epidural space adjacent to the area of the spine presumed to be the source of pain and applying an electric current in order to achieve neuromodulatory effects. Power for the spinal cord stimulator is supplied by an implanted battery or transcutaneously through an external radiofrequency transmitter. Spinal cord stimulation is associated with a greater likelihood for pain relief compared with reoperation or conventional medical management in patients with failed back surgery syndrome with persistent radiculopathy. At present there is no good evidence for the use of spinal cord stimulation for chronic LBP not related to the failed back surgery syndrome with radiculopathy.

Intraspinal drug infusion systems, with use of a subcutaneously implanted pump with attached catheter, have been used in some patients with chronic intractable LBP for the intrathecal delivery of analgesics, usually morphine. Adequate evidence to support this intervention is not available.

Chronic LBP is a complex condition that involves biologic, psychological, and environmental factors. For patients with persistent and disabling nonradicular LBP despite recommended non-multidisciplinary therapies, the clinician should strongly consider intensive multidisciplinary rehabilitation with an emphasis on cognitive-behavioral therapy. Multidisciplinary rehabilitation (also called interdisciplinary therapy) is an intervention that combines and coordinates physical, vocational, and behavioral components, and is provided by multiple health professionals with different clinical backgrounds. Cognitive-behavioral therapy is a psychotherapeutic intervention that involves working with cognitions to change emotions, thoughts, and behaviors. There is strong evidence of improved function and moderate evidence of pain improvement with intensive multidisciplinary rehabilitation programs. The problem lies in the limited availability and affordability of multidisciplinary rehabilitation programs. Functional restoration (also call work hardening) is an intervention that involves simulated or actual work in a supervised environment to enhance job performance skills and improve strength, endurance, flexibility, and cardiovascular fitness in injured workers. When combined with a cognitive-behavioral component, functional restoration is more effective than standard care alone to reduce time lost from work.

As discussed previously, the precise identification of the pain generator in a LBP patient with degenerative changes involving the lumbar spine and no radicular pain is usually not possible in contradistinction to the patient with radicular symptoms. It is, therefore, not surprising that, as a general rule, the results of back surgery are disappointing when the goal is relief of back pain rather than relief of radicular symptoms resulting from neurologic compression. As such, the role of surgical treatment for chronic disabling LBP without neurologic involvement in patients with degenerative disease remains controversial. The most common surgery performed is spinal fusion. In spite of the unclear efficacy, rates of spinal fusion surgery for this indication are rapidly increasing. Interbody fusion is achieved from either a posterior or an anterior approach or both combined for a circumferential fusion. All fusion techniques involve placement of a bone graft between the vertebrae. Instrumentation refers to the use of hardware, such as screws, plates, or cages that serve as an internal splint while the bone graft heals. The rationale for fusion is based on its successful use at painful peripheral joints.

The current evidence is that for nonradicular back pain with degenerative changes fusion is no more effective than intensive interdisciplinary rehabilitation but is associated with small to moderate benefits compared with standard nonsurgical care. Furthermore, the majority of patients who undergo surgery do not experience an optimal outcome defined as no pain, discontinuation or occasional pain medication use, and return to high-level function.

Lumbar disk replacement with a prosthetic disk is a newer alternative to fusion. Disk replacement is approved in the United States for patients with disease limited to one disk between L3–S1 and no spondylolisthesis or neurologic deficit. Approval was based on data showing efficacy equal to that of spinal fusion. This may be faint praise given the controversy regarding the efficacy of spinal fusion for lumbar disk disease. No data support the hypothetical advantage that, unlike spinal fusion, prosthetic disks will protect adjacent levels from further degeneration by preserving motion. At present there is insufficient evidence regarding the long-term benefits and risks of disk replacement to support its recommendation.

Most patients with LBP, including those with neurogenic signs and symptoms, do not require surgical treatment.

C. Nerve Root Compression Syndromes

The precise role of surgery in the care of patients with LBP and neurogenic signs and symptoms is often unclear and controversial. This prompted the National Institute of Arthritis and Musculoskeletal and Skin Diseases (NIAMS) to fund three large parallel randomized Spine Patient Outcomes Research Trial (SPORT) studies in an effort to assess the role of surgery in patients with lumbar disk herniation, lumbar degenerative spondylolisthesis with spinal stenosis or lumbar spinal stenosis. Of note, in each of these milestone studies, all of the patients had radicular leg pain with associated neurologic signs or neurogenic claudication. Patients with serious or progressive neurologic deficits require urgent surgical decompression and, as such, were excluded from all the SPORT studies. Each study included a randomly assigned cohort and an observational cohort. Patients in the observational cohort declined to be randomly assigned in favor of designating their own treatment but agreed to undergo follow-up according to the same protocol. The primary study outcomes were measures of pain, physical function, and disability during a 2-year period. All three studies were compromised by high rates of crossover (as much as 50%) between the assigned treatment, surgical or nonsurgical, in both cohorts. This has caused concern over the validity of the conclusions.

The first study in patients with lumbar disk herniation looked at surgical (diskectomy) versus nonoperative treatment (physical therapy, education, NSAIDs if tolerated) in patients with persistent radicular symptoms despite nonoperative treatment for at least 6 weeks. Both treatment groups improved substantially; the intent-to-treat analysis showed no significant difference in the randomly assigned cohort. Greater improvement with surgery was reported in the observational cohort. However, nonrandomly assigned comparisons of self-reported outcomes are subject to potential confounding and must be interpreted cautiously,

In the second study in patients with lumbar degenerative spondylolisthesis and spinal stenosis, with persistent neurologic symptoms for at least 12 weeks, the intent-to-treat analyses for the randomly assigned cohort showed no significant differences between the surgical (decompressive laminectomy with or without fusion) and usual nonsurgical treatment. The nonrandomly assigned "as treated" comparison that combined both cohorts showed greater improvement in the surgical group. "As treated" analyses are significantly confounded and should be interpreted with caution.

In the final study for patient with lumbar spinal stenosis without spondylolisthesis with persistent neurologic symptoms for at least 12 weeks, both the intent-to-treat and "as treated" analyses showed a significant advantage favoring surgery (posterior decompressive laminectomy).

SPORT data also revealed that in general spinal surgery improved leg pain more than LBP and benefits of surgery diminish with time.

1. Disk herniation—Patients with a herniated disk with radicular pain secondary to nerve root compression should be treated nonsurgically as described in the section on acute LBP unless they have a serious or progressive neurologic deficit (Table 8–5). Only approximately 10% of patients have sufficient pain after 6 weeks of conservative care that surgery is considered. A decision to continue with nonsurgical therapy beyond 6 weeks in these patients does not increase the risk for paralysis or cauda equina syndrome. Surgery in these patients is associated with moderate short-term benefits compared with nonsurgical therapy, although differences in outcome diminish with time and are generally no longer present after 1–2 years. The usual surgery performed is a diskectomy to remove the disk fragment compressing the nerve root.

Epidural corticosteroid injections may offer a small treatment benefit for short-term relief of radicular pain but do not offer significant functional benefit and do not reduce the need for surgery.

There is no convincing evidence of efficacy for the use of systemic corticosteroids or gabapentinoids (gabapentin and pregabalin) in patients with radiculopathy.

2. Spinal stenosis—It is critical to understand the natural history of degenerative lumbar spinal stenosis before making treatment decisions. The symptoms of spinal stenosis remain stable for years in most patients and may improve in some. Dramatic improvement is uncommon. Even when symptoms progress, there is little likelihood of rapid deterioration of neurologic function. Therefore, conservative nonoperative treatment is a rational choice for most patients.

There is a paucity of good data to guide the conservative management of lumbar spinal stenosis. Physical therapy is the mainstay of management, but evidence for the efficacy of specific standardized regimens is not available. Most regimens include core strengthening, stretching, aerobic conditioning, loss of excess weight, and patient education. Exercises that involve lumbar flexion such as bicycling are better tolerated. Strengthening of abdominal muscles may be helpful by promoting lumbar flexion and reducing lumbar lordosis. Lumbar corsets that maintain slight flexion may provide symptomatic relief. They should only be used for a limited number of hours a day to avoid atrophy of paraspinal muscles.

NSAIDs and tramadol are often used for symptomatic relief of pain. Lumbar epidural corticosteroid injections are ineffective in the treatment of patients with neurogenic signs and symptoms of lumbar spinal stenosis.

Surgery is indicated for the few patients with lumbar spinal stenosis who have a serious or progressive neurologic deficit. However, most surgery for lumbar spinal stenosis is elective. The indication for elective surgery is to relieve persistent and disabling symptoms of neurogenic claudication that have not responded to conservative care. In patients without fixed neurologic deficits, delayed surgery produces similar benefits to surgery selected as the initial treatment. The surgical goal is to decompress the central spinal canal and the neural foramina to eliminate pressure on the nerve roots. This is accomplished by laminectomy, partial facetectomy of hypertrophied facet joints, and excision of the hypertrophied ligamentum flavum and any protruding disk material. For most patients with lumbar spinal stenosis, with or without degenerative spondylolisthesis, surgery should be limited to decompression. The addition of instrumented fusion for the treatment of spinal stenosis is no longer the best practice. Its use should be restricted to patients who have proven spinal instability as confirmed on flexion-extension radiographs. Unfortunately there is an alarming increase in spinal fusion surgery with routine use of complex fusion techniques in the absence of evidence of greater efficacy.

Overall, for patients with spinal stenosis, with or without spondylolisthesis, who have disabling symptoms of neurogenic claudication despite conservative care, there is evidence to support the effectiveness of decompressive laminectomy

Table 8–5. Indications for surgical referral.

Disk herniation
Cauda equina syndrome (emergency)
Serious neurologic deficit
Progressive neurologic deficit
Longer than 6 weeks of disabling radicular pain (elective)
Spinal stenosis
Serious neurologic deficit
Progressive neurologic deficit
Persistent and disabling pseudoclaudication (elective)
Spondylolisthesis
Serious or progressive neurologic deficit

in reducing pain and improving function through 1–2 years. Beyond this time frame, the benefits appear to diminish and reoperations are frequently necessary. Given all this, patient preferences should weigh heavily in the decision of whether to have surgery for lumbar spinal stenosis.

A less invasive alternative to decompressive laminectomy is the implantation of a titanium interspinous spacer at one or two vertebral levels. This spacer distracts adjacent spinous processes and thereby imposes lumbar flexion which in turn potentially increases the spinal canal dimensions. There is preliminary evidence of efficacy in patients with one- or two-level spinal stenosis, without spondylolisthesis, and with a history of relief of neurogenic claudication with flexion. It is at present unclear how this newer procedure compares with the standard surgical approach.

3. Spondylolisthesis—The vast majority of patients with spondylolisthesis and chronic LBP are treated conservatively. Rarely a patient may need decompression surgery if a serious or progressive neurologic deficit develops from nerve root impingement or disabling pseudoclaudication secondary to spinal stenosis develops in the patient. A randomized trial involving patients with isthmic spondylolisthesis and disabling isolated LBP or sciatica for at least 1 year suggested fusion surgery produced better results than nonsurgical care although the differences in outcome narrowed during a 5-year follow-up period. As discussed earlier, in most patients with degenerative lumbar spondylolisthesis and spinal stenosis decompressive surgery alone without instrumented fusion is the recommended surgical treatment.

Chou R, Deyo R, Friedly J, et al. Systemic pharmacologic therapies for low back pain: a systematic review for an American College of Physicians Clinical Practice Guideline. *Ann Intern Med.* 2017;166(7):480-492. [PMID: 28192790]

Deyo RA, Mirza SK. Herniated lumbar intervertebral disk. *N Engl J Med.* 2016;374:1732-1772. [PMID: 27144851]

Dixit R. Low back pain. In: Firestein GS, Budd RC, Gabriel SE, et al, eds. *Kelley & Firestein's Textbook of Rheumatology.* 11th ed. Elsevier, Philadelphia, PA, 2020, Chapter 50. In print.

Peul WC, Moojen WA. Fusion for lumbar spinal stenosis—safeguard or superfluous surgical implant? *N Engl J Med.* 2016;374(15):1478-1479. [PMID: 27074071]

Qaseem A, Wilt TJ, McLean RM, et al. Noninvasive treatments for acute, subacute, and chronic low back pain: a clinical practice guideline from the American College of Physicians. *Ann Intern Med.* 2017;166(7):514-530. [PMID: 28192789]

Ropper AH, Zafonte RD. Sciatica. *N Engl J Med.* 2015;372:1240-1248. [PMID: 25806916]

Weinstein J, Lurie J, Tosteson T, et al. Surgical vs nonoperative treatment for lumbar disk herniation. The Spine Patient Outcomes Research Trial (SPORT): observational cohort. *JAMA.* 2006;296:2451-2459. [PMID:17119141]

Weinstein J, Lurie J, Tosteson T, et al. Surgical versus nonsurgical treatment for lumbar degenerative spondylolisthesis. *N Engl J Med.* 2007;356(22):2257-2270. [PMID: 17538085]

Weinstein J, Tosteson T, Lurie J, et al. Surgical vs nonoperative treatment for lumbar disk herniation. The Spine Patient Outcomes Research Trial (SPORT): a randomized trial. *JAMA.* 2006;296:2441-2450. [PMID: 17119140]

Weinstein J, Tosteson T, Lurie J, et al. Surgical versus nonsurgical treatment for lumbar spinal stenosis. *N Engl J Med.* 2008;358(8):794-810. [PMID: 18287602]

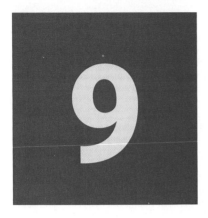

Approach to the Patient with Hip Pain

Lawrence K. O'Malley, MD

Simon C. Mears, MD, PhD

Hip pain is a common complaint that may be referred to the thigh, back, or groin areas. The anatomic location of the true hip joint is unclear to many patients, who confuse pain generated from this area with symptoms arising from the lumbar spine or soft tissues around the hip. The hip joint and its periarticular structures are relatively inaccessible to evaluation by palpation. Accurate assessment of patients with "hip pain" depends on the identification of specific historical features, appropriate physical examination maneuvers, basic insights into common radiographic findings, and a thorough understanding of the differential diagnosis. The likely cause of hip pain in a given patient often has a high correlation with the patient's age.

▶ Clinical Findings

A. History

Taking a careful and astute history is the first essential step in identifying the cause of a patient's hip pain. The history should determine the location of the pain and establish whether the onset of pain was abrupt or gradual. Further, the process of obtaining the history must delineate the circumstances associated with the onset of pain and identify activities that improve or worsen the patient's symptoms.

Pain located primarily in the groin and associated with weight bearing or range of motion is most typical of intra-articular hip abnormalities. Pain beginning in the low back and radiating down the buttock and back of the leg to the side of the calf and lateral side of the foot is more likely caused by a lumbar radiculopathy than an intra-articular hip abnormality. Pain localized to the side of the hip and exacerbated by lying on the affected side is most likely greater trochanteric bursitis. Hip pain due to infections or malignancy is severe, generalized, constant, and often worse at night.

A traumatic event associated with the acute onset of pain strongly suggests fracture or injury to the soft tissues about the hip. In cases of acute onset pain, the history also

should include questions regarding changes in activity, such as new exercise programs or injuries. For example, abnormal mechanics during walking or running, such as injury to the opposite leg or running on oval tracks that lack banks can predispose to trochanteric bursitis. Repetitive loading activities or a sudden increase in the amount of running can result in a femoral stress fracture.

Pain that has been slow and progressive over time is common in arthritic conditions. A person with osteoarthritis of the hip experiences a gradual onset of worsening hip pain and decreasing range of motion. It becomes progressively harder to walk normally, especially going up and down stairs. Hip flexion becomes painful and patients should be asked if they are having trouble tying their shoes.

The age of the patient influences the differential diagnosis of hip pain. Children are susceptible to particular hip problems, such as slipped capital femoral epiphysis and Legg-Calvé-Perthes disease. Adolescents and young adults commonly have avascular necrosis, hip dysplasia, labral tears, or femoroacetabular impingement. Middle-aged and older patients often have osteoarthritis of the hip, low back pain, or trochanteric bursitis.

Snapping in and around the hip suggests one of the "snapping hip syndromes," which are divided into internal and external causes. Internal snapping can be caused by the iliopsoas tendon slipping over the osseous ridge of the lesser trochanter or the anterior acetabulum, or by the iliofemoral ligament riding over the femoral head. Acetabular labral tears or loose bodies can cause intra-articular snapping associated with sharp pain in the groin and anterior thigh. External snapping results from a tight iliotibial band or gluteus maximus tendon riding over the greater tuberosity of the femur. These types of snapping occur during hip flexion and extension, especially during internal rotation.

In rare instances, an intrapelvic, intra-abdominal, or retroperitoneal abnormality may be the cause of hip symptoms. Such causes include uterine fibroids, hernias, and retroperitoneal hematomas or infections.

Another presentation of hip pathology is pain felt in the knee alone. Branches of the obturator nerve innervate both the knee and the hip joint and may cause hip pathology to refer pain to the knee. All patients with knee pain should have an examination of the hip.

B. Physical Examination

A basic understanding of the hip anatomy and biomechanics is the cornerstone of an accurate physical examination of the patient with hip pain. The hip consists of a ball-in-socket joint formed by the proximal femur and its articulation with the pelvis. The bony anatomy of the proximal femur includes the femoral head, the femoral neck, and the greater and lesser trochanters. The acetabulum, the mating socket for the femoral head, is coated with articular cartilage. A rim of fibrocartilage known as the "labrum" lends stability to the hip and circumscribes the outer edge of the acetabulum. The iliotibial band originates along the brim of the iliac wing (along the anterior and posterior margins), consolidates over the greater trochanter, travels laterally along the thigh, and inserts in the proximal leg. These tendinous insertions have associated bursae that decrease friction where the tendon crosses bony protuberances. The trochanteric bursa is located between the gluteus maximus and the greater trochanter; the gluteofemoral bursa between the gluteus maximus and the vastus lateralis origin; and the ischial bursa between the ischial tuberosity and the gluteus maximus. The muscles around the hip can be summarized into four main groups (Figure 9–1).

1. Inspection of gait—Examination of the hip begins with the careful observation of the patient's gait. Two phases of gait need to be observed: stance phase (when the foot is on the ground and bears weight) and swing phase (when the foot moves forward and does not bear weight). Most problems appear during the weight-bearing stance phase. The width of the gait, the shift of pelvis, and flexion of the knee should be observed.

The lumbar spine normally has a slight lordosis. Loss of lordosis may reflect spasm of the paravertebral muscles. Excess lordosis may suggest a flexion deformity of the hip. This observation should always be followed with the assessment of leg-length symmetry. Leg shortening and external rotation with pain suggest hip fracture. The anterior and posterior surfaces of the hip should be inspected for areas of muscle atrophy or bruising related to a traumatic event or neuromuscular disease.

Pain is a common cause of a limp. The characteristic of an **antalgic limp** involves shortened standing time on the affected side. When pain arises in the hip joint, the trunk shifts toward the painful side. Moving the body's center of gravity toward the painful hip decreases the moment arm of body weight to the hip joint, thereby reducing total force on the hip.

An antalgic gait should not be confused with a **Trendelenburg gait**, which is secondary to a weakened gluteus medius muscle. In the Trendelenburg gait pattern, the opposite side of the pelvis tilts downward during the stance phase on the weakened side and, in an effort to compensate for the weakness, the trunk lurches toward the weakened side during the same walking cycle phase (Figures 9–2 and 9–3). This action moves the center of gravity nearer the fulcrum on the weak side and shortens the moment arm from the center of gravity to the hip joint. The result is a characteristic waddle.

A limp is common in patients with substantial hip arthritis or disease in other joints of the lower extremity. The limp may be caused by pain, shortening of the leg, flexion contracture, or weakness of the pelvic girdle muscles or other parts of the lower limb. Thus, a thorough evaluation of the lower extremity muscle strength is essential for diagnosing the cause of a limp. Manual muscle testing is useful for evaluating flexors (iliopsoas and rectus femoris), extensors (gluteus maximus and hamstrings), abductors (gluteus medius and minimus), and adductors (adductor longus, magnus and brevis, pectineus and gracilis). Muscle testing should be performed on the lower leg muscles (ankle and toe dorsiflexors and plantarflexors) to evaluate for weakness as a result of a radiculopathy.

2. Palpation—With the patient supine, the clinician should ask the patient to place the heel of the leg being examined on the opposite knee. This position facilitates palpation along the inguinal ligament. Bulges along the ligament can be inguinal hernias or aneurysms, important secondary causes of hip symptomatology beyond the true hip joint. From lateral to medial, a sequence of nerve, artery, vein, and lymph nodes can be palpated. Enlarged nodes can be present in the setting of a local infection or reflective of systemic inflammation or a hematopoietic malignancy (in which case other lymph node chains are also typically enlarged). Tenderness laterally over the femoral greater trochanter indicates local bursitis rather than arthritis. With the patient lying on the unaffected side and the hip flexed and internally rotated, the trochanteric bursa over the greater trochanter and the bursa over the posterosuperior iliac spine (PSIS) can be palpated (Figure 9–4). The ischiogluteal bursa cannot be palpated unless it is inflamed. When it is inflamed, this bursitis can mimic sciatica. Bursitis is one of the major causes of tenderness around hip joint, but other causes of such tenderness include synovitis of the hip joint or psoas abscess. Tenderness without swelling on the posterolateral surface of the greater trochanter suggests localized tendinitis or muscle spasm from referred hip pain. Crepitus, or a grating sensation in the joint that is either felt by the patient, detected by the examiner, or both is a late manifestation of an arthritic condition but is not a sensitive or specific indicator. Sensory examination of the skin around the hip may reveal a condition called meralgia paresthetica, or compression of the lateral femoral cutaneous nerve. This nerve innervates the lateral aspect of the thigh and may be compressed at the waist by tight belts or clothing, leading to the sensation numbness or pain but not associated with motor weakness.

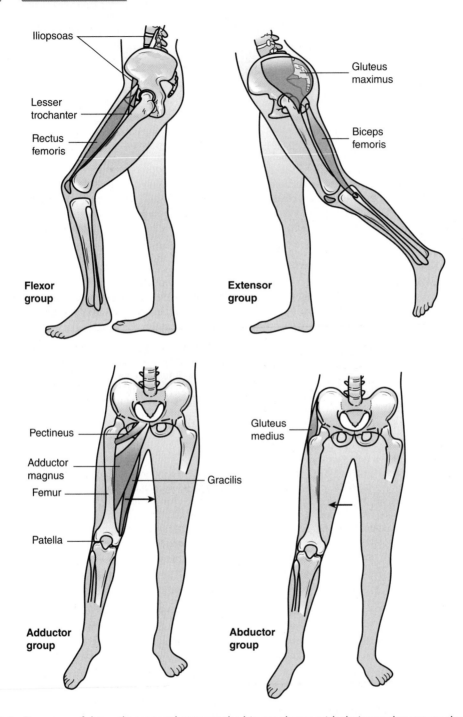

▲ **Figure 9–1.** Four powerful muscle groups that move the hip are shown with their attachments to the femur and pelvis. The primary hip flexor is the iliopsoas tendon, which inserts on the lesser trochanter. The main hip extensor muscle is the gluteus maximus. The hip adductors include the pectineus, adductor brevis, magnus, and longus, and the gracilis. The main abductors of the hip are the gluteus medius and minimus. Abductor function is critical to the hip and weakness leads to a Trendelenburg gait. (Reproduced, with permission, from Bickley LS. The musculoskeletal system. In: *Bates' Guide to Physical Examination and History Taking.* 12th ed. Philadelphia: Lippincott Williams & Wilkins; 2016.)

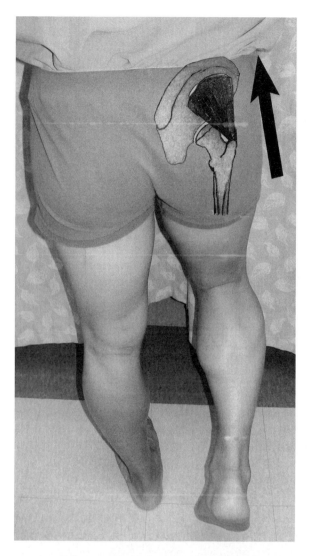

▲ **Figure 9–2.** A Trendelenburg gait results from a weakened gluteus medius muscle (a hip abductor). An intact gluteus medius keeps the pelvis level during a normal single-leg stance.

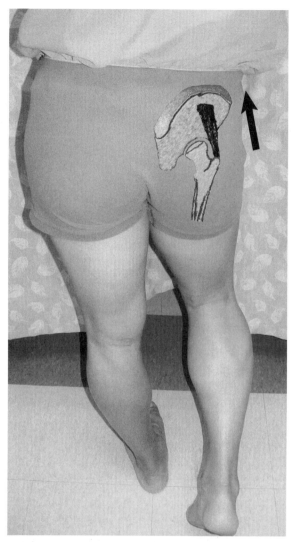

▲ **Figure 9–3.** A Trendelenburg gait results from a weakened gluteus medius muscle (a hip abductor). With a weak gluteus medius, the pelvis droops, and the body then swings laterally over the affected side.

3. Range of motion—Motions of the hip include flexion, extension, abduction, adduction, and rotation (Table 9–1). The hip can flex further when the knee is also flexed. In the case of a hip with a flexion deformity, flexion of the unaffected hip prevents full leg extension of the affected hip, which appears flexed (Figure 9–5). With the patient supine, the examiner places one hand on the patient's iliac crest. As the patient attempts to extend the hip to neutral, the clinician can detect pelvic movement that might be mistaken for hip movement. Flexion deformity may be masked by an increase

in lumbar lordosis and an anterior pelvic tilt. Assessment of the extension can be aided by positioning the patient face down and extending the thigh toward the clinician in a posterior direction.

Restricted abduction is common in hip osteoarthritis. Adduction can be assessed by stabilizing the pelvis and pressing down on the opposite anterosuperior iliac spine with one hand, grasping the ankle with the other, and abducting the extended leg. The normal extent of hip adduction is 45–50 degrees (Figure 9–6). In the same manner, moving the

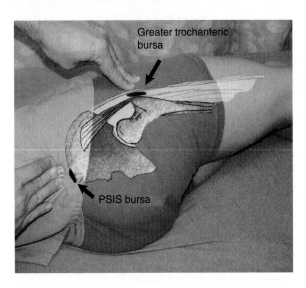

▲ **Figure 9–4.** The bursae around the hip are examined with the patient lying in a lateral position on the unaffected side. The two most common areas of tenderness are over the greater trochanter and over the insertion of the iliacus onto the posterosuperior iliac spine (PSIS). Many patients have tenderness at both of these sites. The ischiogluteal bursa may also be tender over the top of the ischium.

leg medially across the body and over the opposite extremity marks the adduction limit. Flexing the leg to 90 degrees at hip and knee, stabilizing the thigh with one hand, grasping the ankle with the other, and rotating the lower extremity externally (normal, 45 degrees) and internally (normal, 35 degrees) identifies the hip's rotation limits (Figure 9–7). Loss of internal rotation is an especially sensitive indicator of hip disease and is often the earliest change in range of motion. As the disease progresses, prolonged joint stiffness and other limitations of movements become more evident. Limitation of joint movement may be secondary to flexion contractures or mechanical obstructions.

Table 9–1. Normal range of motion of the adult hip.

Motion	Normal Range (degrees)
Flexion	0–135
Extension	0–15
Abduction	0–45
Adduction	0–25
Internal rotation	0–35
External rotation	0–45

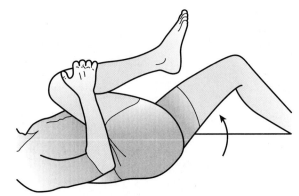

▲ **Figure 9–5.** In flexion deformity of the hip (in this case, the left), the affected hip does not allow full leg extension when the opposite hip is flexed. Therefore, the affected hip appears flexed. (Reproduced, with permission from Bickley LS. The musculoskeletal system. In: *Bates' Guide to Physical Examination and History Taking.* 12th ed. Philadelphia: Lippincott Williams & Wilkins; 2016.)

4. Eliciting hip pain—There are two tests for evaluating elicited hip pain. The Stinchfield resisted hip flexion test evaluates the pain response caused by an increase in hip joint reactive force and is a valuable tool for distinguishing intra-articular and extra-articular hip abnormalities causing groin, thigh, buttock, and even pretibial leg pain. While the

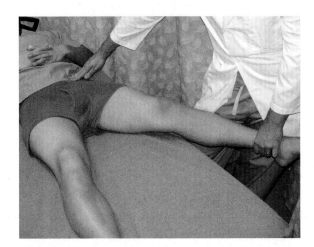

▲ **Figure 9–6.** The limit of hip abduction is determined by stabilizing the pelvis with one hand pressing down on the opposite anterosuperior iliac spine and with the other hand grasping the ankle and abducting the extended leg. The normal abduction of the hip is 45–50 degrees. Limited hip abduction is common in patients with hip arthritis.

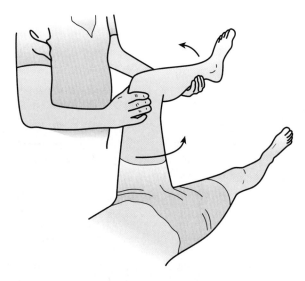

▲ **Figure 9–7.** Establishing the rotation limits of the hip is done by flexing the leg to 90 degrees at the hip and knee, stabilizing the thigh with one hand, and with the other hand grasping the ankle and rotating the lower extremity externally (normal, 45 degrees) and internally (normal, 35 degrees). (Reproduced, with permission, from Bickley LS. The musculoskeletal system. In: *Bates' Guide to Physical Examination and History Taking.* 12th ed. Philadelphia: Lippincott Williams & Wilkins; 2016.)

patient is in a supine position, he or she is asked to elevate the leg while the examiner applies gentle manual resistance to the ankle with the knee extended. Reproduction of pain in a typical pattern related to the sensory innervation of the hip (groin, thigh, buttock, or knee) makes the test positive for a hip abnormality. In the Patrick test, the patient lies supine, and the clinician holds the affected leg and rotates it externally. Pain elicited suggests sacroiliitis, hip abnormality, or an L4 nerve root lesion.

C. Laboratory Findings

Examination and culture of synovial fluid (see Chapter 2) is essential whenever infection of the hip is suspected. Intensely inflammatory effusions suggest pyogenic infection, requiring immediate antibiotic therapy and aspiration or other drainage to establish the diagnosis and prevent joint destruction. Hemorrhagic joint fluid suggests fracture, bleeding diathesis, or malignancy.

Once involvement of the hip joint has been established through the history and physical examination, imaging studies usually take precedence over laboratory tests. Laboratory tests have a more limited role, designed to identify specific systemic causes of hip pain and to exonerate or implicate infection.

D. Imaging Studies

1. Conventional radiography—Conventional radiographs of the hip and pelvis are the first diagnostic tests for patients with symptoms and signs localizing to the hip. Conventional radiographs can delineate the alignment, bone mineralization, articular cartilage, and soft tissue. Alignment abnormality may indicate a fracture, a dislocation, or secondary causes of osteoarthritis, such as congenital dislocation of the hip or slipped capital femoral epiphysis. Bone mineralization may implicate osteoporosis or osteopenia as a risk factor for fracture.

An anteroposterior pelvic radiograph and a "frog-leg" lateral hip radiograph may reveal fractures, provide a better view of the anterolateral femoral head, and help evaluate for osteonecrosis. For patients in the later stages of osteonecrosis, radiographs show a break in the cortex and a rim sign (a linear, black subcortical lucency) characteristic of femoral head collapse. A 40-degree cephalad anteroposterior view is useful for elucidating subtle femoral neck and pubic fractures.

Radiographs may reveal evidence of hip dysplasia shown by the lack of femoral head coverage. Femoroacetabular impingement may be indicated by a "pistol grip" deformity of the femur (such as an osteophyte on the femoral neck causing impingement), or by a deformity on the acetabulum (such as coxa profunda, protrusio, or acetabular retroversion leading to pincer impingement). Impingement may best be seen on the cross-table lateral, Dunn view, or false profile view of the hip.

On conventional radiographs, joint-space narrowing is indicative of articular cartilage loss, spurs or osteophytes are indicative of arthritic change. Segmental radiolucency or sclerotic changes of the femoral head are indicative of avascular necrosis, calcifications are indicative of synovial chondromatosis, and soft-tissue calcification is indicative of calcific tendinitis (Figure 9–8).

2. Arthrography—Arthrography is a useful tool for showing labral abnormalities, especially when it is performed in conjunction with MRI. Magnetic resonance arthrography is the most sensitive and specific test for labral tear of the hip. Injection with local anesthetic agents during the arthrogram can be a powerful tool for the diagnosis of hip abnormalities. If the injection does not help the pain, other diagnoses must be excluded as causes of the pain. Arthrography continues to have a role in the diagnosis of infection and loosening of the prosthesis in the patient with a painful total joint arthroplasty.

3. CT scanning—CT of the hip and pelvis is most useful in the assessment of fractures, particularly complex fractures. Pelvic and acetabular fractures, osseous sequelae of hip dislocation, and intra-articular osseous fragments are visualized more effectively by CT than by conventional radiographs. CT is also useful in characterizing

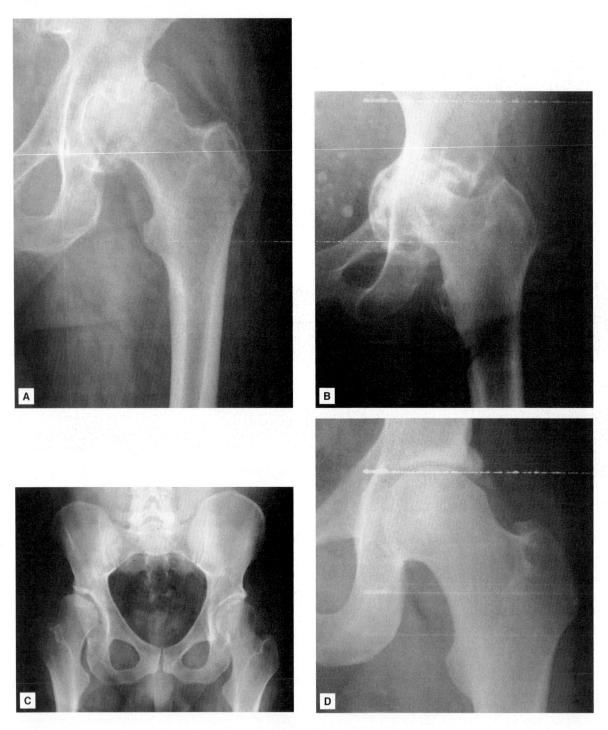

▲ **Figure 9–8.** Common radiographic findings. **A:** Osteoarthritis: asymmetric joint space narrowing, joint sclerosis, osteophytes, subchondral cysts. **B:** Rheumatoid arthritis: symmetric joint space narrowing, protrusio acetabuli. **C:** Dysplasia: acetabular uncovering, increased acetabular slope. **D:** Femoroacetabular impingement: peripheral osteophytes.

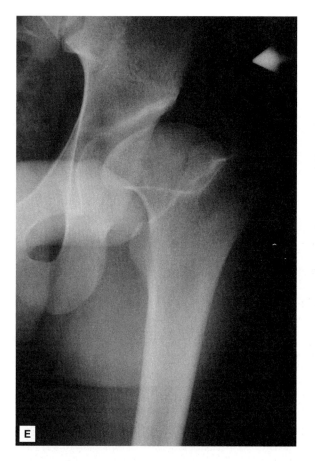

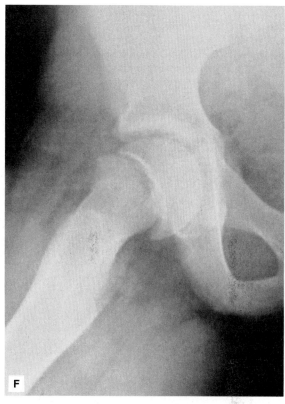

▲ **Figure 9–8.** (*Continued*) **E:** Legg-Calvé-Perthes disease: incongruent joint, misshapen femoral head. **F:** Slipped capital femoral epiphysis: fracture through epiphyseal growth plate.

calcifications secondary to tumor matrix within bone or soft tissue or to ossification, and is the best modality for imaging cortical bone.

4. MRI—MRI provides excellent visualization of medullary bone and soft tissues. The diagnosis of osteonecrosis of the femoral head is made earlier by MRI than by any other technique, including bone scintigraphy, CT, and conventional radiographs. MRI is also the method of choice for the diagnosis of occult hip fracture in the elderly and, despite its expense, can be cost-effective for this purpose. MRI is the most accurate method for the diagnosis of stress fractures around the hip and pelvis, and it is the best test for the diagnosis of transient osteoporosis of the hip. It is also the most valuable test for the staging of bony and soft-tissue tumors around the hip. MRI is frequently helpful in documenting synovitis of the hip joint by revealing effusion (eg, in pigmented villonodular synovitis). Magnetic resonance arthrography is useful in defining labral abnormalities and in examining for evidence of

impingement, such as a high angle or herniation pits in the lateral femur.

5. Bone scans—Bone scans are useful for detecting metastatic disease (when suspected), osteonecrosis, arthritis, and Paget disease of bone. Scintigraphy delineates the regions of increased metabolic activity ("hot spots") by increased uptake of a radioactive tracer.

E. Special Tests

1. Electromyography and nerve conduction velocity studies—Electromyography and nerve conduction velocity studies are used in the differential diagnosis of hip pain to evaluate referred lumbosacral plexopathies and to assess local nerve entrapment or nerve damage from trauma such as meralgia paresthetica, surgery, or other disease states.

2. Injections—Differential block of the hip joint can be a valuable adjunct in differentiating the source of intra-articular hip joint pain. This procedure is best undertaken in the fluoroscopy suite, with arthrography used to confirm the location of the injection. The technique may be particularly useful in distinguishing intra-articular hip abnormalities from referred lumbosacral radiculopathy and possible soft-tissue conditions. Dye injection along the iliopsoas tendon sheath under fluoroscopy sometimes reveals the snapping of the iliopsoas tendon over the pelvic brim and, when accompanied by lidocaine or glucocorticoid injection, may help prove that the tendon condition is the pain generator.

▶ Differential Diagnosis & Treatment

The age of the patient is critical in diagnosing the cause of hip pain (Figure 9–9).

A. Children

Neonates are susceptible to hematogenous infection and can present with an acute septic joint. Children 3- to 10-years-old who have hip pain most commonly have an infection, Legg-Calvé-Perthes disease, or acute transient synovitis. If the child has a fever or sign of infection, hip aspiration should be performed to rule out an acute septic joint. Legg-Calvé-Perthes disease is a condition that causes a portion of the femoral head to develop ischemic necrosis and collapse. Radiographs reveal evidence of Legg-Calvé-Perthes disease (see Figure 9–8E). The hip then gradually remodels; however, later in life, early hip arthritis develops in up to 50% of patients. Children are treated symptomatically and may require realignment surgery if substantial collapse occurs. A normal radiograph and hip pain is most commonly associated with a self-limited condition termed "acute transient synovitis of the hip." This is a diagnosis of exclusion.

The most common diagnosis in children 11- to 16-years-old who have hip pain is slipped capital femoral epiphysis. This condition represents a fracture through the growth plate or epiphysis of the femoral neck (see Figure 9–8F). In 50% of the cases, slipped capital femoral epiphysis occurs bilaterally and is treated surgically to prevent additional slippage, osteonecrosis, and chondrolysis. Fractures occur in different patterns in adolescent patients than in adults. Sudden muscular exertion can cause avulsion injuries and injury at the bony insertion of the tendons around the hip.

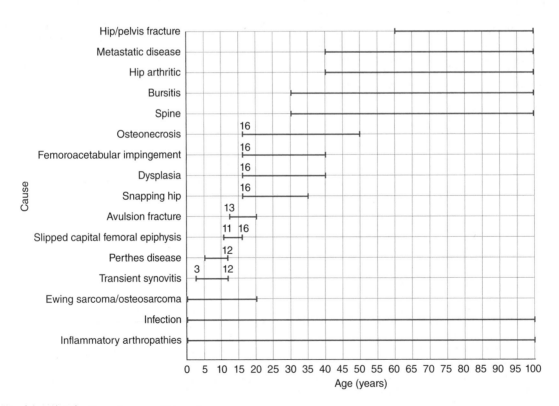

▲ **Figure 9–9.** Timeline of causes of hip pain.

In addition, oncologic problems are different in children compared with adults. In children, primary osteosarcoma and Ewing sarcoma are typical, whereas in adult and elderly patients, metastatic disease is most common. Potential tumors detected by plain radiographs should be further evaluated with MRI scanning.

B. Adults

Stress fractures of the femoral neck may develop in young adults in response to an increase in exercise. Hip pain from several patterns of disease may develop in adults aged 40 years or older, gradually leading to early hip arthritis. The first pattern of disease is hip dysplasia, which occurs when the acetabulum does not develop correctly over the femoral head (see Figure 9–8C). The severity of this process ranges from mild changes to full dislocation. In mild forms, hip dysplasia causes excessive anteversion of the acetabular cup, which leads to gradual wear on the labrum with labral tearing. Wear then begins to occur at the edge of the joint, causing early arthritis. It is possible to reorient the acetabulum surgically with a periacetabular osteotomy to prevent later hip arthritis.

The second condition that can lead to early arthritis and hip pain in the young adult is femoroacetabular impingement. There are two types of femoroacetabular impingement: cam impingement and pincer impingement. These types can occur concurrently. In **cam impingement,** the deformity is on the femoral side of the joint. The upper lateral portion of the femoral neck gradually impinges on the acetabulum, leading to labral tearing, osteophyte formation around the hip (see Figure 9–8D), and ultimately hip stiffness and arthritis. In **pincer impingement,** the deformity is on the acetabular side of the joint. The acetabulum is deeper than normal because of coxa profunda, protrusio acetabuli, or retroversion of the acetabulum. In such settings, the normal femur hits against the enlarged anterior rim of the acetabulum, also culminating in labral damage and arthritis (Figure 9–10A–C).

Impingement can be treated surgically by removing the impinging osteophytes and "reshaping" the femoral head (see Figure 9–10D), or by removing the acetabular osteophytes and reattaching the torn labrum (see Figure 9–10E). There are currently no long-term outcomes to indicate whether these procedures ultimately prevent total hip arthroplasty.

Osteonecrosis of the femoral head may develop in young adults. This condition can be associated with prednisone use, heavy alcohol use, deep sea diving, or coagulopathies. Osteonecrosis, which can develop in multiple joints (but especially the hips and knees), leads to death of subchondral bone in the femoral head. The cartilage above the necrotic bone collapses, and arthritis ensues (Figure 9–11). MRI scans, the most sensitive test for osteonecrosis, are abnormal before the appearance of radiographic changes. In mild cases, decompression or bone grafting procedures may be successful, but in advanced cases, hip replacement surgery is required.

Transient osteoporosis of the hip is a rare condition most often seen in young women during pregnancy. The diagnosis, characterized by the development of acute hip pain, is confirmed by MRI scan. Treatment involves restricted weight bearing and repeated MRI scans to make sure the bone density improves; otherwise, the patient may be at risk for fracture.

Middle-aged patients commonly have hip pain from osteoarthritis of the hip, trochanteric bursitis, or spinal causes. Osteoarthritis of the hip is generally unilateral, and the pain is worse with weight bearing and twisting motions of the hip (see Figure 9–8A). Typically, the pain is in the groin and leads to gradual hip stiffness and limp. Trochanteric bursitis presents with lateral pain that is often worse at night when the patient lies on the affected side. Several other areas around the hip may develop soft-tissue pain (Table 9–2). Spinal problems present with radiculopathy or pain that starts in the lower back and radiates down the leg to the foot. Weakness or numbness may occur with nerve compression in the back.

Hip pain in elderly patients (>60 years old) typically comes from osteoarthritis, metastatic disease, trochanteric bursitis, spinal stenosis, or fracture. Radiographs that reveal lytic lesions of the femoral neck or hip in these patients typically are the result of metastatic disease. Surgery is often needed in such cases to strengthen or replace the bone. Elderly patients with osteoporosis are also at high risk for fracture of the femoral neck or the pelvis. Fracture should be excluded in all elderly patients with acute hip pain. Fractures in this population may occur with even mild trauma as may occur in a seemingly inconsequential fall. Fractures may also occur in the absence of any clear precipitating event and have an insidious onset (insufficiency fractures). Fractures causing hip pain may be located in the proximal femur, the acetabulum, or the pelvis. If radiographs are normal, an MRI scan should be obtained.

C. All Ages

Infections in the hip joint may develop in patients of all ages. Immunosuppressed patients and those who use injection drugs are particularly vulnerable and often do not show systemic signs of infection. Hip joint infections cause unrelenting pain and fevers and should be diagnosed by joint aspiration. Treatment should be intravenous antibiotics and surgical debridement of the hip (Table 9–3). Patients of all ages also are susceptible to a range of inflammatory arthritides, from juvenile idiopathic arthritis in the young patient to rheumatoid arthritis, ankylosing spondylitis, or psoriatic arthritis in the adult patient. Inflammatory

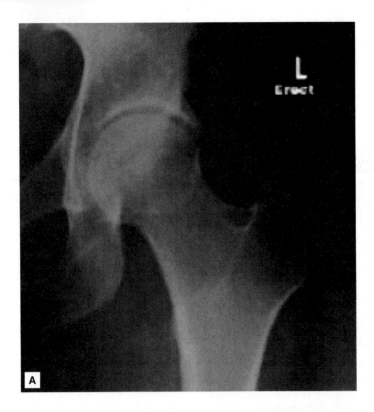

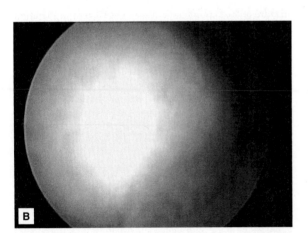

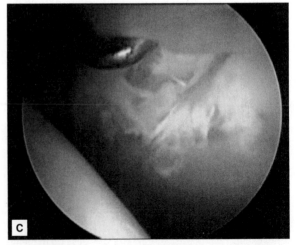

▲ **Figure 9–10.** Pincer impingement. **A:** Radiograph showing a large lateral acetabular osteophyte and corresponding femoral cam lesion causing pincer impingement. **B:** Arthroscopic view of the femoral head showing the cam lesion. **C:** Arthroscopic view of the hip. The hook shows the torn hip labrum.

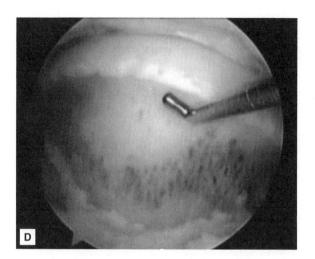

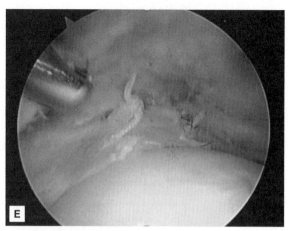

▲ **Figure 9–10.** (*Continued*) **D:** The femoral head cam lesion has been reshaped with a burr. **E:** The labral tear is repaired with suture arthroscopically.

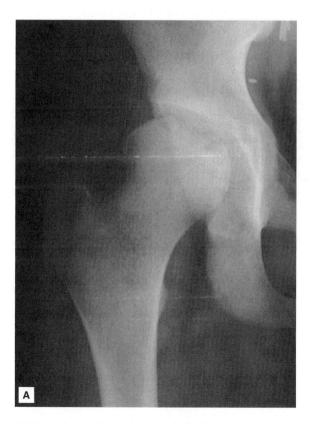

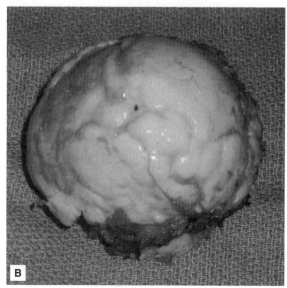

▲ **Figure 9–11.** Osteonecrosis. **A:** Radiographs reveal subchondral lucency and collapse of a segment of femoral head. **B:** At the time of hip arthroplasty, the collapsed bone has delaminated from the cartilage.

Table 9–2. Symptoms of common soft-tissue pains around the hip.

Diagnosis	Symptoms
Iliopsoas bursitis	Deep anterior hip, groin pain with active flexion of the hip, possible audible or palpable snapping of the tendon
Ischial bursitis	Deep pain posteriorly over the ischial tuberosity; pain with sitting
Piriformis syndrome	Deep pain in the buttock region posteriorly
Posterosuperior iliac spine bursitis	Pain in the lateral lower back over the lateral aspect of the pelvic brim, often combined with trochanteric bursitis
Trochanteric bursitis	Lateral pain over the greater trochanter, often with sitting or laying on the side

Table 9–3. Interventions for common hip conditions.

Condition	Intervention
Avulsion fracture	Ice, NSAIDs, activity modification, surgery (rarely)
Dysplasia	NSAIDs, activity modification, surgery for realignment or hip arthroplasty
Femoroacetabular impingement	NSAIDs, activity modification, hip arthroscopy, surgery for hip reshaping or hip arthroplasty, activity modification
Hip fracture	Surgical fixation
Infection	Surgical drainage, intravenous antibiotic
Labral tear	NSAIDs, activity modification, intra-articular steroid injection, hip arthroscopy
Meralgia paresthetica	Relieve pressure on the lateral femoral cutaneous nerve, NSAIDs, surgical decompression
Pelvic fracture	Pain medications, ambulatory aid
Legg-Calvé-Perthes disease	Activity modification, possible surgery
Piriformis syndrome	NSAIDs, activity modification, muscle stretching
Slipped capital femoral epiphysis	Surgical fixation
Snapping syndromes	Muscle stretching, ice, NSAIDs, physiotherapy
Soft-tissue injuries (eg, iliopsoas bursitis)	Muscle stretching, glucocorticoid injection, physiotherapy
Stress fracture	Activity modification, careful observation for the need for surgical stabilization
Transient osteoporosis of the hip	Activity modification, careful observation for the need for surgical stabilization
Trochanteric bursitis	Ice, NSAIDs, muscle stretching, glucocorticoid injection, physiotherapy

NSAIDs, nonsteroidal anti-inflammatory drugs.

arthritis often is bilateral and generally affects both hips as well as other joints throughout the body (see Figure 9–8B).

Buckland AJ, Miyamoto R, Patel RD, Slover J, Razi AE. Differentiating hip pathology from lumbar spine pathology: key points of evaluation and management. *J Am Acad Orthop Surg.* 2017;25(2):e23-e34. [PMID: 28045713]

Gala L, Clohisy JC, Beaulé PE. Hip dysplasia in the young adult. *J Bone Joint Surg Am.* 2016;98(1):63-73. [PMID:26738905]

Redmond JM, Chen AW, Domb BG. Greater trochanteric pain syndrome. *J Am Acad Orthop Surg.* 2016;24(4):231-240. [PMID:26990713]

Approach to the Patient with Knee Pain

10

Andrew Gross, MD

C. Benjamin Ma, MD

Knee pain is a common problem, accounting for several million visits per year to primary care practitioners and emergency departments. By following a systematic approach in evaluating knee pain, physicians can establish the correct diagnosis in an efficient manner and formulate an appropriate therapeutic strategy.

OVERVIEW OF THE CLINICAL ASSESSMENT

The first step in the evaluation of knee pain is a thorough history that includes the core elements outlined in Table 10–1. While obtaining a history, the following key questions should be addressed:

- How long has the pain been present?
- Was there an acute injury?
- Does the pain localize to a specific part of the knee?
- Are there mechanical symptoms?
- Is a joint effusion present?
- Is there evidence of systemic disease?

The answers to these questions help the clinician narrow the differential diagnosis and develop a strategy for additional evaluations of the knee pain.

The examiner should take into account the age and sex of the patient, both of which can influence the differential diagnosis. Finally, the clinician should bear in mind that pain can be referred to the knee from other sites, most notably the ipsilateral hip. Every patient with knee pain should have a careful examination of the hip.

▶ Approach to the Physical Examination of the Knee

Examination of the knee has five major components: observation of stance and gait, range of motion, palpation,

examination for a knee effusion, and stability tests. The clinician can generate a differential diagnosis and then focus the workup accordingly after taking a careful history and then performing a history-guided examination. Examination of the knee is guided by an understanding of the knee's anatomy (Figure 10–1).

A. Observation of Stance and Gait

Physical examination should start with observation of stance and gait. Can the patient bear weight on the affected leg? Is there a limp? Attention should be paid to medial or lateral translation of the knee upon heel strike. Angular deformities (varus = bow-legged; valgus = knock-kneed) can identify bone and cartilage erosion with secondary stretching of the opposite collateral ligament. Varus alignment predisposes medial compartment arthritis. Following gait analysis, patients should be asked to perform a deep squat. Limitations in squatting may be related to patellofemoral or meniscal pathology.

B. Range of Motion

Active and passive range of motion of the knee should be recorded. Normal knee extension is 0 degrees; normal knee flexion ranges from 115 to 160 degrees. It is helpful to compare with the contralateral side.

C. Palpation

The skin overlying the anterior surface of the knee is typically cooler than the skin proximal and distal to the joint. The examiner can discern the likelihood of inflammation within a knee most effectively by using the dorsum of his or her hand to compare the temperature of the skin overlying the patella to the temperature of the skin above and below the knee, and also to the skin overlying the contralateral patella.

Palpation should be gentle but thorough to help localize the knee pain. Palpation around the patella can identify facet tenderness or insertional tenderness of the patella tendon

Table 10–1. Knee pain: core elements of the history.

Age and sex of the patient
Circumstances of the onset of pain
Exacerbating and alleviating factors
Presence of swelling and warmth
Loss of range of motion
Loss of function—inability to bear weight
Presence of mechanical symptoms (locking/catching, instability)
Duration of stiffness when arising in the morning or after inactivity
Localization of symptoms to specific regions of the knee (ie, anterior, posterior, medial, or lateral)
Involvement of other joints
Presence of systemic symptoms

and quadriceps tendon. Palpable defects along the quadriceps or patella tendon can indicate tendon ruptures. Injury along the collateral ligaments can best be identified with pain elicited along their course and at their attachments. Palpation of the joint line is done both medially and laterally to elicit pain that can be caused by meniscal injury. Tenderness at the tibial tubercle can indicate Osgood-Schlatter disease or patella tendon tears.

D. Examination for a Knee Effusion

With the patient supine, an effusion is often visible as fullness in the suprapatellar bursa and loss of the concavity that is usually present on the medial aspect of the knee. The effusion is confirmed by balloting the patella onto the femoral groove while compressing the suprapatellar and infrapatellar bursae. In the absence of fluid, the patella moves directly into the femoral condyles. With large effusions, the patella floats above the condyles, so that when the examiner ballots the patella, a tap is felt as the patella bumps into the condyles.

Smaller effusions can be detected by compressing fluid from the medial compartment of the knee by applying a

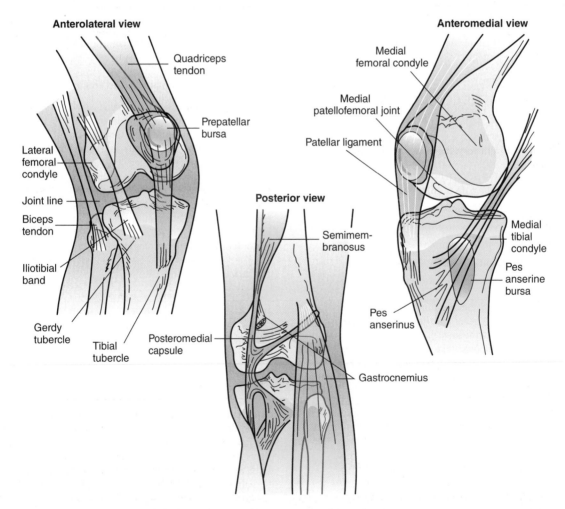

▲ **Figure 10–1.** Functional anatomy of the knee.

sweeping compression motion to the medial and superior aspects of the knee. Compression of the lateral aspect of the knee will generate a fluid wave that can be seen as a small bulge on the medial side. This is known as a "bulge sign."

E. Stability Tests

Stability or provocative tests should be performed when the patient is relaxed. These tests can reproduce symptoms and thus can be uncomfortable. The examiner should determine the direction of instability of the knee: Anterior cruciate ligament (ACL)/posterior cruciate ligament (PCL) tears produce anterior/posterior instability; collateral ligament injuries lead to varus/valgus instability as well as internal/external rotational instability. These tests are described in detail under specific disease entities.

PROBLEMS BY LOCATION OF PAIN WITHIN THE KNEE

Patients often describe pain localized to specific regions of the knee. Although this is not always specific to a particular etiology of the pain, the patient's description of the pain's location can be essential to focusing the examination and narrowing the differential diagnosis.

1. Anterior Knee Pain

ESSENTIALS OF DIAGNOSIS

▶ Pain underneath the patella.
▶ Pain across the patella tendon or quadriceps insertion.
▶ Sensation of swelling in the anterior aspect of the knee.
▶ Patella feels unstable.

▶ General Considerations

Anterior knee pain is a common complaint with a variety of causes (Table 10–2). Several factors are responsible for normal patellofemoral mechanics. The quadriceps tendon guides tracking of the patella. Of the four muscles, the vastus medialis obliquus is the primary stabilizer of the patella against the lateral pull of the vastus lateralis. Other factors that can affect normal patellofemoral mechanics include the shape of the patella, the shape of the trochlea groove, the shape of the femoral condyles, the length of the patella tendon, the patellofemoral articulating cartilage, and tension of the extensor mechanism. Disruption or abnormality in any facet of this complex joint can lead to dysfunction and subsequent pain.

Table 10–2. Causes of anterior knee pain.

Problem	Location
Patellofemoral pain syndrome	Pain underneath patella and along extensor mechanism Usually related to change in activity level; ie, going from a sitting position to initiating walking
Patella instability	Pain over the medial facet of patella Apprehension on examination
Quadriceps tendinitis	Pain at the proximal pole of the patella
Patella tendinitis	Pain at the distal pole of the patella
Osgood-Schlatter disease	Pain and swelling over tibial tubercle Observed generally only in adolescent patients
Anterior horn meniscus tear	Pain along the anterior joint line Can be present in runners or gymnasts Uncommon injury
Patellofemoral osteoarthritis	Pain underneath patella Difficulty with stairs, more with descents Patellofemoral crepitus

▶ Clinical Findings

A. History

When eliciting a history from a patient with anterior knee pain, it is important to attempt to distinguish whether the pain is derived from the anterior structures of the knee, or whether it is referred from the tibial-femoral compartments. The patellofemoral pain syndrome is one of the most common causes of anterior knee pain in the younger patient, especially in women. In contrast, osteoarthritis of the patellofemoral compartment is the most common cause in the older patient. In either case, pain is typically worsened by activity that puts increase load and pressure on the patella, such as ascending and descending stairs, squatting, or even rising from a sitting position.

The history is the key to establishing the diagnosis of the patellofemoral syndrome. Patients typically note pain in the front of the knee after rising from a position of prolonged sitting, such as following a car ride or a movie. The pain subsides as the patients continue to walk. Patients with the patellofemoral syndrome also frequently note the occurrence of symptoms when descending stairs. With knee extension, patients sometimes describe a grinding sensation. Pain typically localizes around or under the patella. Patients may note a sensation of knee buckling or giving way, but this is a nonspecific finding that seems to be largely related to pain rather than pathologic process.

Table 10–3. Prevalent causes of anterior knee pain by age.

Age	Diagnosis	Clinical Characteristics
Skeletal immature	Osgood-Schlatter disease	Pain over tibial tubercle
16–40	Patellofemoral syndrome	Pain underneath patella
20–40	Patella tendinitis/ ruptures	Pain over distal pole For rupture, difficulty with active leg extension, palpable defect between patella and tibial tubercle
50–70	Quadriceps tendinitis and ruptures	Pain over proximal pole For ruptures, difficulty with active leg extension, palpable defect between patella and quadriceps tendon
50–80	Osteoarthritis	Start-up pain Pain under patella

Acute onset of anterior knee pain, with or without trauma, can signify quadriceps tendon rupture (see acute injury section) and prepatellar bursitis. Mild trauma may also result in patellar dislocation in individuals with anatomic malalignment causing excess lateral traction on the patella. It is important to distinguish a true dislocation that required reduction by trained personnel from a sensation of "dislocation" experienced by the patient, because this represents a difference in instability and severity. The cause of subacute or chronic anterior knee pain can often be narrowed based on the age of the patient (Table 10–3).

B. Physical Examination

The examination starts with the evaluation of gait and the evaluation of limb alignment. Any valgus or varus deformity of the limb, internal or external rotation of the leg should be noted. Patients, especially young females, with valgus alignment of their lower limb, commonly complain of anterior knee pain due to a weak quadriceps muscle, lateral pull of the patella, and lateral facet tenderness. The presence or absence of flexion contractures, recurvatum, or abnormal position of the feet should also be noted. Significant recurvatum can reflect generalized ligament laxity that is prone to patella instability. Pronated feet also can lead to valgus alignment, which can lead to lateral subluxation of the patella and anterior knee pain. The examiner should note the position of the patella, whether it is in alta (patella sits high in the patellar grove relative to the femur) or baja (sits low). Patella alta usually leads to increased patella instability as the patella engages

into the trochlea groove at a higher knee flexion angle. Patella baja usually presents after tendon injury or knee surgery and can present with increased anterior knee pain due to increased stress of the patellofemoral joint.

The examination should also include slow, active, unassisted range of motion of the knee to assess patella tracking. The "J" sign can be appreciated when the patella slides laterally at terminal extension of the knee. This can indicate excessive pull of the vastus lateralis muscle, an increased Q angle, patella alta, a shallow trochlea groove, a deficient vastus medialis obliquus, or all of the above.

Through careful palpation, the examiner can identify the source of anterior knee pain (see Table 10–2). Focal tenderness at the superior or inferior pole of the patella represents quadriceps and patella tendinitis. Patients who have acute patella dislocation have tenderness over the medial facet with associated bruising. The patella should then be compressed against the femoral groove to elicit patellar pain. Crepitus during range of motion or pain with "grinding" of the patella on the trochlea groove indicates patellofemoral arthritis. Patellar mobility or glide should also be evaluated. Medial and lateral glide of the patella is performed at full extension and at 30 degrees of flexion. The amount of glide is being quantified using a quadrant system with respect to the widest portion of the patella. The first quadrant means that the patella can be subluxed over the femoral condyle by less than 25% of the widest width of the patella, second quadrant is when the patella can be subluxed between 25% and 50% of the patella width and so forth. It is important to repeat the test at 30 degrees of flexion because most patella dislocations do not occur at full extension. They usually occur at gentle flexion, around 20–30 degrees. The lateral displacement of the patella is also known as the "apprehension test." An increase in pain or apprehension on the part of the patient for fear of the patella dislocating is a positive finding. The apprehension test is the most specific test for patella dislocation or instability. A normal patella should not be displaced beyond the second quadrant in either direction.

The quadriceps, or Q, angle is also an important physical examination. The Q angle is formed by the line of pull of the quadriceps and the patella tendon as they intersect at the patella. The angle is measured for clinical purposes between a line drawn from the anterior-superior iliac spine to the patella and a line drawn from the patella and the tibial tubercle. Normal Q angle should be 8–10 degrees for males and less than 15 degrees for females. The Q angle should be measured at full extension and at 90 degrees of flexion. Any value greater than 10 degrees for males is considered abnormal. Increased Q angle is one of the risk factors for patellofemoral syndrome.

▶ Treatment

Most patellofemoral injuries are treated nonsurgically. Most of these ailments can be treated with physical therapy focusing on quadriceps strengthening, core stability, and hip strengthening exercises. Patients occasionally undergo patellofemoral realignment for chronic problems that do not respond to nonsurgical measures.

Lack S, Neal B, De Oliveira Silva D, Barton C. How to manage patellofemoral pain—understanding the multifactorial nature and treatment options. *Phys Ther Sport*. 2018;32:155-166. [PMID: 29793124]

Vora M, Curry E, Chipman A, Matzkin E, Li X. Patellofemoral pain syndrome in female athletes: a review of diagnoses, etiology and treatment options. *Orthop Rev (Pavia)*. 2018;9(4):7281. [PMID: 29564075]

2. Medial Knee Pain

ESSENTIALS OF DIAGNOSIS

▶ Pain over medial joint line.

▶ Difficulty squatting or twisting.

▶ Pain over anteromedial portion of the proximal tibia.

Several structures on the medial aspect of the knee can cause pain. Careful palpation allows the examiner to localize the source of the discomfort (Table 10–4). Medial meniscus tears have characteristic joint line pain. Patients with medial collateral ligament (MCL) tears have pain along the ligament itself, which extends from the medial epicondyle and the pes anserine area. Pes anserine bursitis causes pain over the pes insertion, which is distal to the joint line over the anteromedial tibia. Bursitis of the pes anserine bursa is very common, particularly in patients with knee osteoarthritis. Localized tenderness of the bursa can be located between the anteromedial tibial metaphysis and the insertion of the sartorius, gracilis, and semitendinosus tendons at the pes anserine. MCL ligament sprain is common following trauma to the lateral aspect of the knee and is associated with valgus laxity. Medial compartment osteoarthritis, as well as tears in the medial horn of the meniscus can also cause medial knee pain.

Table 10–4. Causes of medial knee pain.

Problem	Location
Medial meniscus	Medial joint line, often posterior
Medial collateral ligament	Pain along the course of the ligament from medial epicondyle to pes anserine
Medial compartment osteoarthritis	Medial joint line, but more specifically along the bony edges Varus alignment of the patient's limb ("bow-legged")
Pes anserine	Pain along the anteromedial tibia where the hamstring and sartorius muscles insert

3. Lateral Knee Pain

ESSENTIALS OF DIAGNOSIS

▶ Pain over the lateral joint line.

▶ Difficulty squatting or twisting.

▶ Pain over fibula head.

Lateral knee pain can be caused by damage to several local structures (Table 10–5). In athletes, particularly runners and cyclists, tendinitis of the iliotibial band can develop from friction to the tendon as it passes over the lateral femoral condyle. Compression of the tendon typically causes pain. Lateral compartment osteoarthritis is unusual but can cause lateral joint line tenderness, particularly in patients with valgus deformity. Lateral meniscus tears, which are less common than tears medial meniscus, cause pain along the lateral joint line.

4. Posterior Knee Pain

ESSENTIALS OF DIAGNOSIS

▶ Fullness over the back of the knee.

▶ Difficulty achieving full flexion.

Table 10–5. Causes of lateral knee pain.

Problem	Location
Lateral meniscus	Lateral joint line, often posterior
Lateral collateral ligament sprain	Pain along the course of the ligament from lateral epicondyle to fibular head
Lateral compartment arthritis	Lateral joint line, but more specifically along the bony edges Valgus alignment of the patient's limb
Iliotibial band syndrome	Pain along the Gerdy tubercle or along the iliotibial band near the lateral epicondyle Common with runners or patients who have recent changes in activity level
Biceps femoris tendinitis	Tenderness along the posterior portion of the fibular head and the insertion of the biceps femoris tendon
Peroneal nerve entrapment	Tinel sign along the fibular neck, usually 2 cm distal to the proximal tip of the fibular head

Table 10–6. Causes of posterior knee pain.

Problem	Location
Popliteal cyst	Posterior joint level, can sometimes feel a mass
Gastrocnemius tightness	Tenderness along the heads of the gastrocnemius muscle insertion into the distal portion of the femur, above the joint line
Generalized osteoarthritis	Diffuse pain
Deep venous thrombosis	Common with pain and positive Homan sign (50% of the cases). Distal limb swelling. Occasional with palpable cords

While there are few weight-bearing structures in the posterior knee, there are a few causes of posterior knee pain (Table 10–6). The neurovascular bundle of the leg travels through the popliteal fossa, so vascular events can be manifested by posterior knee pain, including acute arterial thrombosis as well as deep venous thrombosis. Large synovial effusions can cause a Baker cyst to develop in the popliteal fossa. Patients typically complain of symptoms of a synovial effusion, including pain with range of motion and on ambulation, but they may also complain of posterior knee pain or fullness. Occasionally, Baker cysts rupture, resulting in extravasation of synovial fluid into the calf and mimicking a deep venous thrombosis. Finally, tendonitis of the hamstrings or referred pain from lumbar spine osteoarthritis can cause posterior knee pain.

MECHANICAL KNEE SYMPTOMS & NO HISTORY OF ACUTE INJURY

 ESSENTIALS OF DIAGNOSIS

▶ Locking or catching symptoms suggest meniscal tear.

▶ Instability symptoms suggest ligamentous laxity or tear.

▶ Knee buckling is a nonspecific symptom that is associated with knee pain and quadriceps weakness.

▶ Asymptomatic meniscal tears are common findings on MRI in middle-aged and elderly patients.

▶ General Considerations

The middle-aged patient with chronic knee pain in the absence of any recalled trauma is a common and vexing problem. The challenge for the practitioner is to determine whether the source of the pain is from internal derangement (particularly a large meniscal tear that is best managed surgically) or whether the problem is more degenerative in nature and better managed with conservative therapy.

▶ Clinical Findings

A. History

"Mechanical" symptoms can signify the presence of meniscal tears or ligamentous sprain. A locking or catching sensation with knee extension and flexion raises the possibility of a meniscal tear but is a somewhat nonspecific symptom because it can also be caused by loose bodies in the knee. Instability is usually episodic and unpredictable. When given the history of instability, the practitioner should note the severity of these episodes and the presence of swelling after an episode, which can point to the presence of a ligamentous tear.

A third mechanical symptom is that of buckling or "giving way." This is a less specific but extremely common complaint that typically occurs during weight bearing, especially when weight loading is increased such as climbing stairs. The "giving way" is likely to occur as a reflex to pain (from osteoarthritis or meniscus injuries) or from insufficient quadriceps muscle strength to support the knee. Buckling can also be caused by ligamentous tears, but this is relatively uncommon in the absence of trauma. Complaints of buckling should be addressed by the practitioner, since buckling is associated with falls, potentially causing fracture.

B. Physical Examination

Special attention should be focused to specific structures based on the nature of the patient's complaint. When meniscal tear is suspected, patients can be asked to perform deep knee bends to elicit pain. Tenderness elicited by joint line palpation can also suggest meniscal pathology, but both of these tests are nonspecific in the chronic setting (see acute injuries section). The McMurray test and eliciting pain with passive hyperextension have reasonable specificity for meniscal tears but limited sensitivity. Tests for ligamentous instability should be carefully performed for patients with episodes of instability (see acute injuries section). Finally, patients should be assessed for signs of osteoarthritis, including crepitus and bony enlargement, because degenerative disease increases the likelihood of meniscal tears as well as buckling symptoms secondary to pain.

C. Imaging Studies

The plain radiograph can be useful to confirm the presence osteoarthritis but is less helpful to identify the cause of locking symptoms or instability. Patients with abnormal physical examination findings, or complaints highly suggestive of meniscal or ligamentous pathology in the absence of arthritis, should be referred for an MRI.

▶ Treatment

Treatment is typically guided by findings on the MRI study. Careful clinicoradiological correlations is required, however, because the MRI may detect findings that are unrelated to the patient's symptoms.

KNEE EFFUSION

ESSENTIALS OF DIAGNOSIS

▸ Restricted range of motion and pain with ambulation.

▸ An acutely swollen knee with a history of acute injury suggests mechanical derangement, particularly ACL tear.

▸ An acutely swollen knee in the absence of acute injury raises the concern of septic arthritis and demands immediate evaluation.

▸ The presence of an underlying systemic condition must be excluded.

▸ Joint aspiration with synovial fluid analysis is the most helpful test.

▸ General Considerations

Small, asymptomatic effusions commonly occur in healthy individuals. Larger joint effusions, however, signal the presence of intra-articular pathology, the most serious of which is septic arthritis. A variety of pathologic processes cause knee effusions (Table 10–7), and these are typically grouped by fluid characteristics (see Chapter 2).

▸ Clinical Findings

A. History

Patients with joint effusions often complain of swelling and stiffness, as well as loss of knee range of motion. Particularly large effusions can manifest as a Baker cyst in the popliteal fossa and cause posterior knee pain. Occasionally, as noted, very large effusions rupture the synovial capsule, resulting in dependent collection of fluid in the lower leg. Knee involvement is common in systemic causes of inflammation, usually in association with inflammation in multiple joints but

Table 10–7. Differential diagnosis for an acutely swollen knee.

Infection
Bacterial
Mycobacterial
Spirochete (Lyme, syphilis)
Viral
Crystal (gout and pseudogout)
Spondyloarthritis
Reactive arthritis
Inflammatory bowel disease
Hemarthrosis
Acute injury
Osteoarthritis
Osteonecrosis

occasionally confined to a single knee. An early seronegative spondyloarthropathy is a good example of this. Other examples are Lyme disease (characterized by large joint effusions with relatively few inflammatory cells in the synovial fluid), osteoarthritis, and occasionally rheumatoid arthritis. Microcrystalline arthropathies, both gout and pseudogout, can cause repeated episodes of acute knee swelling. Septic arthritis of the knee usually results from hematogenous spread of a pathogen, often associated with endocarditis. Patients with septic arthritis of the knee are often, but not always, febrile.

B. Analysis of Synovial Fluid

Arthrocentesis and subsequent synovial fluid analysis are indicated for all cases of unexplained knee effusion. The aspirated fluid should be sent for cell counts, Gram stain, cultures, and crystal analysis. Hemarthrosis is commonly caused by joint trauma, as described above. Fat droplets (detected by polarized microscopy) also indicate articular fracture. Hemophilia and other clotting disorders can cause hemarthrosis in the absence of trauma. The most common cause of noninflammatory effusions of the knee (synovial fluid white blood cell count <2000 cells/mcL) is osteoarthritis. Other causes include osteonecrosis, Charcot arthropathy, amyloidosis, hypothyroidism, and acromegaly. Inflammatory arthritis (synovial fluid white blood cell >2000 cells/mcL) can be caused by infection, autoimmune disease, and crystal-induced arthritis. Aspiration of dark brown serosanguinous fluid should raise the possibility of pigmented villonodular synovitis.

C. Imaging Studies

Moderate to large knee effusions are apparent on radiographs. Acute nontraumatic arthritis rarely causes additional radiographic abnormalities. In chronic conditions, radiographs can provide valuable information regarding the etiology and severity of the arthritis. Persistent inflammatory arthritis leads to symmetric joint space narrowing as well as marginal erosions and periarticular osteopenia, whereas osteoarthritis (Chapter 39) causes asymmetric joint space narrowing, typically of the medial compartment. Patients with pseudogout of the knee frequently have radiographic evidence of chondrocalcinosis. Osteonecrosis causes a radiolucent lesion and flattening of the femoral condyle.

KNEE PAIN THAT FOLLOWS ACUTE INJURY

ESSENTIALS OF DIAGNOSIS

▸ Mechanism of injury often points to the diagnosis.

▸ "Popping sound" at the time of injury suggests an ACL injury.

▸ Plain radiographs may be indicated to rule out fracture.

▸ Instability suggests ligament injuries.

▸ Locking or catching suggests a meniscal tear.

Table 10–8. Essential features of acute knee injuries.

	Injury Mechanism	Joint Swelling	Characteristics
ACL/PCL tears	Acute injury/trauma	Immediate	Instability
Meniscus	Deep squat or twisting	Delay (first 24 hour)	Pain with twisting
Patella dislocation	Trauma or twisting	Immediate	Pain with palpation of medial facet, lateral femoral condyle
Fractures	Trauma	Immediate	Unable to bear weight

ACL, anterior cruciate ligament; PCL, posterior cruciate ligament.

General Considerations

Acute injuries can lead to fractures, patella dislocation, and internal derangements of the knee, including tears of the ligaments and meniscal cartilage (Table 10–8). Injuries also can cause acute traumatic bursitis as well as tendon strains and tears.

Clinical Findings

A. History

The mechanism of injury is extremely important in the diagnosis of knee injuries (Table 10–9). The injury can be acute or chronic. Most patients can recall the specific knee position during injury and the stresses incurred. Knee injuries can occur from contact forces as well as from falls and twisting injuries not involving contact. An audible "pop" at the time of injury is characteristic of injury to the ACL. It is important to know whether the patient is able to walk following the injury, and whether the injury affects the range of motion of the knee. This information enables the clinician to determine the severity of the injury and the likelihood of intra-articular fractures. Injuries that prevent weight-bearing typically signify a fracture or other severe knee injury.

B. Physical Examination

The patient should be in the supine position on a comfortable examination table. Since the injured knee may be swollen or locked and cannot be fully extended, a pillow can be placed behind the knee to relax it; another pillow can be placed behind the uninjured knee so that both knees can be inspected at the same angle. The uninjured limb should be examined first. Because there is little variation between right and left knees, the uninjured knee can serve as a good indicator for joint motion and laxity prior to injury.

After examining the uninjured knee, the injured knee should first be inspected for its skin integrity and any areas of ecchymosis. Loss of both active and passive range of motion can signify a chronic problem with contractures or a mechanical block, whereas loss of only active motion can signify pain or weakness. Location of pain should be noted during range of motion. For example, displaced meniscus tears can be painful during range of motion and can clue clinicians to the presence of medial or lateral injuries.

The presence and location of swelling is helpful in the evaluation of the acutely injured knee. The majority of acute knee swelling is secondary to hemarthrosis following intra-articular ligament tears, such as ACL tear and patella dislocation. An osteochondral fracture or peripheral tear of the meniscus can also produce a hemarthrosis. The swelling may take longer to occur if ice is applied to the knee immediately following injury. Immediate, brisk swelling should make the examiner suspicious of osteochondral fractures or ACL tears. When the effusion is drained, the presence of fat droplets signifies osteochondral fractures or nondisplaced intra-articular fractures. Swelling that occurs more slowly—over the 24 hours following the injury—likely represents either a meniscus tear or an unstable cartilage injury.

Table 10–9. Mechanisms of injuries.

Scenario	Concern
Fall from a height	Fracture
Twisting injury with foot planted	ACL with or without meniscal tear
Acute pain with deep flexion or twisting	Meniscal tear
Lateral (valgus) blow to the knee	MCL injury
Medial blow (varus) blow	LCL injury
Anterior blow to the knee (dashboard injury)	PCL tear
Misstep with inability to straighten knee	Patella or quadriceps tendon rupture
Acute anterior pain and swelling with twisting motion	Patella dislocation
Gradual onset of discomfort and startup pain	Osteoarthritis or degenerative condition

ACL, anterior cruciate ligament; LCL, lateral collateral ligament; MCL, medial collateral ligament; PCL, posterior cruciate ligament.

C. Imaging Studies

Patients who have difficulty with immediate weight bearing should have anteroposterior and lateral radiographs to exclude

Table 10–10. Ottawa knee rules: indications for obtaining radiographs.

Patient is 55 years or older
Isolated tenderness of the patella
Tenderness of the head of fibula
Inability to flex the knee to 90 degrees
Unable to weight bear for four steps both immediately and at the emergency department
Patients with at least one positive criterion are considered to be at risk for knee fracture and should have a radiograph. Studies indicate the positive predictive value of these criteria for a radiographically confirmed fracture is 85–100%. Patients with normal radiographs but persistent symptoms should undergo follow-up imaging 1–2 weeks later.

fractures. The Ottawa Knee Rules outline indications for obtaining radiographs for this purpose (Table 10–10). The Ottawa Knee Rules consist of five criteria; the absence of all five criteria has a negative predictive value for fracture approaches 100%.

MRI can be helpful in the evaluation of soft-tissue injuries, such as ligament or meniscus injuries. MRI is 75–85% sensitive for detecting meniscal, ligamentous, or cartilage damage. The specificity, however, is lower because of frequent false-positives, particularly in older individuals. Abnormal MRI findings are common, even in asymptomatic knees. Therefore, MRI should be used to confirm a diagnosis rather than as the sole basis for a diagnosis. Careful clinic-radiologic correlation is essential.

▶ Treatment

Protected weight bearing and brace for stabilization can be helpful following acute knee injuries and prior to definitive diagnosis and treatment. Fractures or severe ligament injuries require orthopedic referrals.

Bachmann LM, Haberzeth S, Steurer J, ter Riet G. The accuracy of the Ottawa knee rule to rule out knee fractures: a systematic review. *Ann Intern Med.* 2004;140:121. [PMID: 14734335]

Englund M, Guermazi A, Gale D, et al. Incidental meniscal findings on knee MRI in middle-aged and elderly persons. *N Engl J Med.* 2008;359(11):1108-1115. [PMID: 18784100]

1. Injuries to Collateral Ligaments

▶ Clinical Findings

A. History

Most patients with injuries to collateral ligaments describe injuries on the side of the knee. A lateral blow to the knee leads to injury of the MCL, whereas a medial blow leads to injury of the lateral collateral ligament (LCL).

B. Physical Examination

When testing the MCL, the patient is asked to lie in a supine position with the hip abducted and the knee gently hanging off the edge of the examination table and flexed at 30 degrees. A valgus stress is applied through the examiner's left hand, which supports the ankle. The examination is repeated at full extension. When examining the LCL, an adduction or varus stress is applied. The test is performed similar to the valgus stress test, only with a varus directed force and medial placement of the hand to counteract the stress. The test is performed at full extension and at 30 degrees of flexion.

C. Imaging Studies

MRI is rarely indicated for isolated MCL tears. It is uncommon to have meniscus injuries with MCL tears. However, the ACL can be injured with MCL tears, and these complex injuries should be evaluated by MRI. LCL injuries should necessitate MRI evaluation to determine the significance of injuries. MRI has 80% sensitivity and 90% specificity in the evaluation of acute collateral ligament injuries.

▶ Treatment

MCL injuries are commonly treated with immobilization and bracing. The majority of these injuries heal without the need for surgical stabilization. Grade III (>1-cm opening) injuries are treated with protected weight bearing. LCL or lateral ligament complex injuries do not respond well to nonsurgical treatment and, when recognized, should be urgently referred to an orthopedic surgeon.

Elkin JL, Zamora E, Gallo RA. Combined anterior cruciate ligament and medial collateral ligament knee injuries: anatomy, diagnosis, management recommendations, and return to sport. *Curr Rev Musculoskelet Med.* 2019;12(2):239-244. [PMID: 30929138]

Grawe B, Schroeder AJ, Kakazu R, Messer MS. Lateral collateral ligament injury about the knee: anatomy, evaluation, and management. *J Am Acad Orthop Surg.* 2018;26(6):e120-e127. [PMID: 29443704]

2. Injuries to the Anterior Cruciate Ligament

▶ Clinical Findings

A. History

Typically, the history reveals a twisting injury while the foot is planted. A tear of the ACL can occur with either contact or noncontact mechanisms of injury. Patients commonly describe a "pop" sound.

B. Physical Examination

The **Lachman** or **Ritchey test** is a highly sensitive and specific method for assessing an ACL sprain or tear in the acute setting (Figure 10–2). It consists of an anteriorly directed force with the knee at 30 degrees of flexion; an increase in anterior translation of the tibia compared with the contralateral side constitutes a positive test and signifies injury to the ACL. The anterior drawer test is performed with the knee flexed at

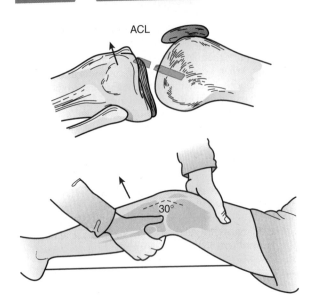

▲ **Figure 10–2.** The Lachman test for tear of the anterior cruciate ligament (ACL). The test is performed at 30 degrees of flexion; the extremity does not have to be lifted or the foot stabilized.

90 degrees and the hip at 45 degrees (Figure 10–3). Difficulty with having the patient relax during the anteriorly directed force can limit the usefulness of this test. The pivot shift test is the most specific test for ACL tear but has low sensitivity for the awake patient. The sensitivity of the test is highly dependent on the examiner's skill and the patient's relaxation.

C. Imaging Studies

MRI is commonly needed to confirm the diagnosis. MRI of the ACL is 93% sensitive and nearly 100% specific. MRI can also identify associated injuries, such as meniscus tear and cartilage injuries, which can affect management.

▶ **Treatment**

The treatment of ACL tears varies on the basis of the needs and activity level of the patient. These injuries are best managed by consultation of an orthopedic surgeon or sports medicine clinician. The patient should be evaluated within 2–3 weeks following the acute injury.

Filbay SR, Grindem H. Evidence-based recommendations for the management of anterior cruciate ligament (ACL) rupture. *Best Pract Res Clin Rheumatol.* 2019;33(1):33-47. [PMID: 31431274]

Puzzitiello RN, Agarwalla A, Zuke WA, Garcia GH, Forsythe B. Imaging diagnosis of injury to the anterolateral ligament in patients with anterior cruciate ligaments: association of anterolateral ligament injury with other types of knee pathology and grade of pivot-shift examination: a systematic review. *Arthroscopy.* 2018;34(9):2728-2738. [PMID: 30037574]

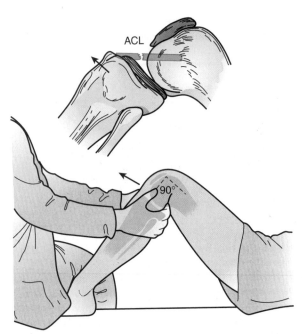

▲ **Figure 10–3.** The anterior drawer test for instability of anterior cruciate ligament (ACL). Flex the knee to 90 degrees and stabilize the foot. Note the forward shift of the tibia.

3. Injuries to the Posterior Cruciate Ligament

▶ **Clinical Findings**

A. History

Injuries to the PCL usually signify significant knee trauma; typically, a significant blow to the anterior portion of the tibia pushes the tibia posteriorly, thereby rupturing the large ligament. A dashboard injury or an injury that occurs when the knee is flexed and the foot is plantarflexed is typical. Associated neurovascular injuries are common and must be ruled out. PCL injuries often occur in combination with other injuries to the knee, such as ACL tears or posterolateral corner injuries.

B. Physical Examination

The most accurate test to identify a PCL injury is the posterior drawer test. This is done in the exact opposite manner as the anterior drawer test: The examiner determines the amount of excess posterior translation when a force is applied to the tibia in a posterior direction with the knee at 90 degrees of flexion. Sometimes, the posterior drawer test is difficult to perform in the acute setting because the patient is unable to flex the swollen knee to 90 degrees.

C. Imaging Studies

Plain radiographs should be obtained to rule out any fractures that may occur with this significant injury. The sensitivity and specificity for MRI for the diagnosis of acute PCL tears approach 90%; MRI also is needed to evaluate possible associated injuries.

Treatment

An urgent referral to an orthopaedic surgeon is needed to rule out other associated injuries. A significant percentage of patients with PCL injuries have injuries to vascular structures, peripheral nerves, other ligaments, and soft tissues.

Bedi A, Musahl V, Cowan JB. Management of posterior cruciate ligament injuries: an evidence-based review. *J Am Acad Orthop Surg.* 2016;24(5):277-289. [PMID: 27097125]

4. Meniscal Injuries

Clinical Findings

A. History

Traumatic lesions of the menisci occur most commonly when there is rotation on the flexed knee as it is moving toward a more extended position. Tears in the medial meniscus usually occur in its posterior horn, possibly because the posterior horn is less mobile and is directly loaded when the knee is flexed. In contrast, tears in the lateral meniscus, which is more mobile and is C-shaped, are usually radial. Meniscal injuries are commonly associated with ACL injuries. In an acute ACL injury, the lateral meniscus is most commonly torn because the lateral tibial plateau subluxes anteriorly on the lateral femoral condyle.

Patients with meniscal tears often complain of a locking and clicking sensation. With larger tears, the knee may lock during range of motion, requiring the patient to stop and twist the knee in order to unlock the displaced meniscus and regain full motion. Small tears of the meniscus produce clicking or catching sensation but not true locking. Meniscal injuries are usually associated with pain and swelling of the knee. Swelling develops over the course of the first day of the injury in contrast to the first 1–2 hours following an ACL tear. Patients may complain of recurrent or chronic swelling in the knee following a twisting injury.

B. Physical Examination

The most important physical finding in patients is localized tenderness along the joint line, with sensitivity and specificity for meniscal tear of 63% and 77%, respectively. The McMurray and the squat tests for meniscal injuries are provocative maneuvers that "trap" the meniscus and generate symptoms. The **McMurray test** is performed with the patient lying supine with the hip and knee flexed to about 90 degrees. With one hand on the knee to apply compression, the examiner uses the other hand to hold the foot and then to maneuver it from external rotation to internal rotation. If positive, this maneuver entraps the torn meniscus, producing a "pop" or "click" that can be felt by the fingers. The McMurray test is 70% sensitive and 71% specific for meniscal tear.

In the **squat test,** the examiner asks the patient to perform a series of full squats, first with legs neutral, then with legs internally rotated, and finally with legs externally rotated. Pain with deep squat indicates the presence of a meniscal tear. If there is more pain with the leg externally rotated, the medial meniscus is most likely injured; conversely, an injured lateral meniscus produces more discomfort when the leg is internally rotated.

C. Imaging Studies

MRI is a very sensitive tool to diagnose meniscal tears. Its specificity is limited due to the occurrence of meniscal tears in asymptomatic individuals. The prevalence of meniscus tears ranges from 19% among women aged 50–59 years to 56% among men aged 70–90 years. Practitioners should use MRI to confirm, not to establish, the diagnosis of meniscal tear.

Treatment

Acute symptomatic meniscal injuries are commonly treated surgically to repair or remove the torn meniscus but more recently a growing emphasis has been placed on preserving the meniscus whenever possible. Chronic or degenerative conditions are usually managed with activity modification and nonsurgical treatment. Surgical debridement can be performed for chronic symptomatic meniscus injuries that did not respond well to nonsurgical treatments.

Beaufils P, Pujol N. Management of traumatic meniscal tear and degenerative meniscal lesions. Save the meniscus. *Orthop Traumatol Surg Res.* 2017;103(8S):S237-S244. [PMID: 28873348]

5. Injuries to the Quadriceps Tendon

Clinical Findings

A. History

Ruptures of the quadriceps tendon are more common at the latter part of life, with a peak incidence from the fifth to seventh decades of life. In addition to age, predisposing factors include systemic conditions, such as diabetes and systemic lupus erythematosus. The rupture typically occurs during eccentric contraction of the knee during a fall, missed step, or twisting injury. The patient usually experiences intense pain over the anterior part of the knee and often is unable to walk. Even when able to ambulate, the patient tends to hold the affected leg straight and to widely circumduct the leg during the swing phase of gait. There is a sensation of instability due to the lack of quadriceps pull.

B. Physical Examination

Common findings are a palpable defect above the patella and a hemarthrosis of the knee. With a complete rupture, the patient is usually unable to extend the knee from a supine position. With varying degrees of rupture, the patients may be able to extend their knee while lying supine but have difficulty when their knee is held in flexion. Quadriceps tendon rupture in the elderly can be subtle; one series reported that up to 30% of the cases were missed initially.

C. Imaging Studies

Radiographs (bilateral flexion weight-bearing standing views and lateral view of the knee) can help evaluate the location of the patella. Quadriceps tendon tear usually leads to patella baja (patella sitting abnormally low). MRI is rarely needed to establish the diagnosis but can be helpful to evaluate partial quadriceps ruptures.

▶ Treatment

Almost all complete quadriceps tendon rupture necessitate surgical repair. Nonsurgical management of quadriceps tendon injuries is reserved only for partial injuries or sedentary individuals.

6. Ruptures of the Patella Tendon

▶ Clinical Findings

A. History

Ruptures of the patella tendon usually occur during violent jumping activities or eccentric contraction. They are less common than ruptures of the quadriceps tendon and usually occur in patients under the age of 40, most often in the setting of preexisting patella tendinitis. Local glucocorticoid injections for patella tendonitis, systemic glucocorticoid use, endocrine abnormalities, and systemic lupus erythematosus predispose to rupture of the patella tendon. Patients usually complain of severe pain and are unable to ambulate.

B. Physical Examination

There is a palpable defect inferior to the patella, which usually has migrated superiorly. Virtually all patients are unable to extend the affected knee.

C. Imaging Studies

Radiographs reveal patella alta (patella sitting abnormally high). MRI is rarely needed to establish the diagnosis but can be helpful to evaluate partial quadriceps ruptures.

▶ Treatment

Ruptures of the patella tendon require urgent repair.

Fibromyalgia

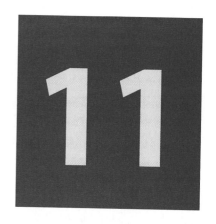

Erin G. Floyd, MD
Andrew Gross, MD

ESSENTIALS OF DIAGNOSIS

▶ Multisite chronic pain: Individuals with fibromyalgia describe widespread pain that waxes and wanes and is experienced for more than 3 months.

▶ Fatigue: Patients report persistent, moderate to severe mental or physical fatigue that is exacerbated by mild exertion.

▶ Nonrestful sleep: Research has shown that patients with fibromyalgia have reduced short-wave sleep (SWS) of non–rapid-eye movement (NREM) sleep during which alpha-rhythm intrudes the normal delta rhythm.

▶ Cognitive symptoms: Patients describe difficulties with executive function, such as working memory and attention. These disease features may be explained by depression and pain.

▶ Exercise and other therapies that address both body and mind issues are essential to successful treatment strategies.

INTRODUCTION

Fibromyalgia is a common condition estimated to affect between 2% and 8% of the population. It is the leading cause of musculoskeletal pain among women aged 20–55 years. Fibromyalgia is more prevalent in patients with autoimmune disease: approximately 16% of patients with rheumatoid arthritis (RA), as well as 22% of those with systemic lupus erythematosus (SLE) and 15% of those with axial spondyloarthritis, meet criteria for fibromyalgia. Patients with fibromyalgia and RA or spondyloarthritis have also been shown to frequently have higher disease activity scores than in patients without fibromyalgia. The co-occurrence of fibromyalgia and inflammatory rheumatologic disorders can therefore confuse management and prevent achievement of "treat-to-target" goals. Thus, effective treatment of symptoms makes it

paramount that rheumatologists consider fibromyalgia when evaluating patients with widespread pain.

Not only is fibromyalgia common, it is also costly to patients and society. The Centers for Disease Control and Prevention has estimated that the total cost of civilian care for fibromyalgia increases at an average of $30 million per year and in 2010 amounted to $232.1 million. Health care costs might be further increased by underdiagnosis of this condition, leading patients to accumulate costs from medical testing and imaging as well as pharmacotherapy and referrals in order to understand and manage their pain levels.

PATHOPHYSIOLOGY OF FIBROMYALGIA: ABNORMAL OBJECTIVE FINDINGS

Patients with fibromyalgia have altered pain processing compared to normal individuals. Not only do patients with fibromyalgia have increased subjective sensitivity to pain, but a body of literature has also provided objective evidence that there is amplified or enhanced pain processing at the level of the central nervous system (CNS) as demonstrated by electromyography (EMG), cerebrospinal fluid (CSF), functional magnetic resonance imaging (fMRI), and positron emission tomography (PET) studies. This is described as central sensitization syndrome. Evidence shows elevations in neurotransmitters associated with potentiation of pain in the CSF, such as substance P, glutamate, excitatory amino acids, and nerve growth factor, as well as reductions in levels of neurotransmitters associated with inhibition of pain, such as norepinephrine. Concentration of natural opioids have also been found to be elevated in patients with fibromyalgia. EMG studies have also demonstrated that patients with fibromyalgia have measurable differences in pain sensitivity compared to patients without fibromyalgia. Specifically, patients with fibromyalgia have been shown to respond to significantly less electrical stimulation in order to elicit a biceps femoris flexion reflex compared to controls, demonstrating a CNS sensitivity to pain stimulation. Finally, neural imaging with fMRI and PET demonstrate that people with fibromyalgia can be distinguished from those with normal pain processing by a set of brain activation patterns during stimulation of pain. In sum, these biochemical, electromyographic, and imaging differences suggest that fibromyalgia results from physiologic changes within the CNS that lead to chronic sensitization to pain.

The mechanism by which these physiologic changes develop is not entirely clear, but genetic predisposition and exposure to trauma seem to be important contributing factors. Genetic studies demonstrate fibromyalgia is associated with allelic variation in pain-related gene products. In fact, it is not uncommon for patients with fibromyalgia to have a family history of chronic pain syndromes.

A body of literature has demonstrated associations between fibromyalgia and exposure to physical trauma/ illness (infections, injuries) or emotional trauma (violence, stress, and loss). Examples of illness resulting in fibromyalgia include Lyme disease, Epstein-Barr virus infections, and parvovirus infections, diseases in which 5–10% of individuals develop chronic widespread pain. Psychological stress or trauma seems to increase the risk of developing fibromyalgia also. For example, experiencing a psychologically stressful event in early life (eg, death of a parent, prolonged hospitalization, severe motor vehicle accident) increases the risk of developing chronic widespread pain by 50–100% later in life. Posttraumatic stress disorder (PTSD) is associated with an even higher risk of developing fibromyalgia.

EXAMPLE CASE

A 48-year-old woman has a history of seropositive RA for 10 years, treated with both methotrexate and etanercept. She now presents to her rheumatologist with ongoing joint pain in her upper and lower extremities as well as pain in her neck and lower back. Her pain worsens with activity. She also reports moderate fatigue and waking up unrefreshed. Her Widespread Pain Index (WPI) score is 11 and her Symptom Severity Scale (SSS) is 7. Physical examination demonstrates joint deformities of the proximal interphalangeal and metacarpophalangeal joints, wrists, and metatarsophalangeal (MTP) joints, consistent with RA. She also has tenderness of many joints in her hands, wrists, elbows, shoulders, knees, ankles, and MTP joints, but no joint swelling is appreciated. Laboratory tests show normal acute phase reactants.

Although the patient has clear signs of RA, her current pain symptoms are out of proportion to the objective findings of arthritis on physical examination. With the combination of widespread pain, fatigue, and nonrestorative sleep as well as her elevated WPI and SSS, the patient meets criteria for fibromyalgia. Ideal symptom management will now address symptoms of fibromyalgia in addition to the longitudinal treatment of RA.

DIAGNOSIS

There is no "gold standard" or objective testing to establish the diagnosis of fibromyalgia. However, the American College of Rheumatology (ACR) 2016 diagnostic criteria provide a useful framework for considering the diagnosis.

▶ ACR 2016 Fibromyalgia Diagnostic Criteria

1. WPI ≥7 and SSS ≥5 *or* WPI 4–6 and SSS score ≥9.
2. Generalized pain, defined as pain in at least four of five regions, is present (left upper, right upper, left lower, right lower, axial).
3. Symptoms have been present at a similar level for at least 3 months.
4. A diagnosis of fibromyalgia is valid regardless of other diagnoses that the patient may have. A diagnosis of fibromyalgia does not exclude the presence of other clinically important illnesses.

One can accurately and efficiently diagnose fibromyalgia by simply asking patients to complete the fibromyalgia symptom questionnaire (Figure 11–1). Such a method can be done in the waiting room or in the exam room before the clinician enters and can be a reliable way to gain insight into the nature of the patient's symptoms, helping to optimize patient counseling time and discussion of the approach to management.

▶ Other Somatic Symptoms of Fibromyalgia

The majority of patients with fibromyalgia have one or more other severe somatic symptoms and many have two or more such symptoms. Such somatic symptoms include those listed in Table 11–1. Many of these are included on the Patient Health Questionnaire Somatic Symptom Short Form (PHQ-SSS). Several of these different symptoms may clue clinicians into the fact that a patient has a diagnosis of fibromyalgia.

A. Physical Examination

A complete physical examination is important to evaluate for other potential causes of pain and fatigue listed in Table 11–2. The presence of multiple allodynic tender points is a typical finding in fibromyalgia. Although a tenderpoint exam was part of the ACR 1990 classification criteria, we do not recommend tenderpoint testing because this test has limited sensitivity and causes unnecessary discomfort to the patient.

B. Laboratory Tests

There are no specific diagnostic tests for fibromyalgia. The sole purpose of laboratory tests when evaluating patients with this possible diagnosis is to exclude alternative diagnoses.

1. Please indicate below if you have had pain or tenderness over the <u>past 7 days</u> in each of the areas listed below. Check the boxes in the diagram below for each area in which you have had pain or tenderness. Be sure to mark right and left sides separately.

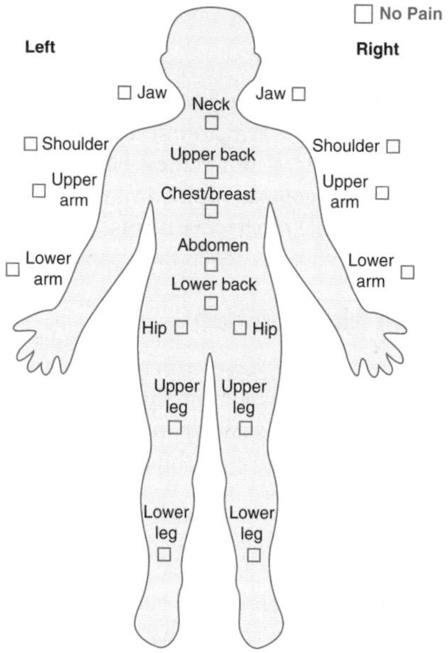

2. Using the following scale, indicate for each item your severity over the past week by checking the appropriate box.

No problem
Slight or mild problems: generally mild or intermittent
Moderate: considerable problems; often present and/or at a moderate level
Severe: continuous, life-disturbing problems

	No problem	Slight or mild	Moderate	Severe
a. Fatigue	☐	☐	☐	☐
b. Trouble thinking or remembering	☐	☐	☐	☐
c. Waking up tired (unrefreshed)	☐	☐	☐	☐

3. During the past 6 months have you had any of the following symptoms?

	No	Yes
a. Pain or cramps in lower abdomen	☐	☐
b. Depression	☐	☐
c. Headache	☐	☐

4. Have the symptoms in questions 2–3 and pain been present at a similar level for <u>at least 3 months</u>? No ☐ Yes ☐

5. Do you have a disorder that would otherwise explain the pain? Yes ☐ No ☐

▲ **Figure 11–1.** Fibromyalgia symptom questionnaire (WPI and SSS). (Reproduced with permission from Clauw DJ. Fibromyalgia and Related Conditions. Mayo Clin Proc. 2015;90(5):680-92.)

Many patients with fibromyalgia undergo a large number of blood tests and imaging studies. Extensive testing often merely begets further testing, as the likelihood of false-positive findings and "red herrings" rises in proportion to the extent of the evaluation. In the absence of relevant clinical symptoms or signs, only a thoughtful and circumscribed laboratory evaluation is justified. In general, the laboratory tests recommended for patients with a diagnosis of fibromyalgia are listed in Table 11–3. Any other tests should be guided by findings from a careful history and physical examination or abnormalities identified in routine testing.

Table 11–1. Somatic symptoms common in fibromyalgia.

Atypical chest pain
Dyspnea
Temporomandibular joint (TMJ) syndrome symptoms
Abdominal pain with bloating and changes in bowel habits (eg, diarrhea/constipation fluctuations)
Headaches
Polyuria/frequency
Dyspareunia/vulvodynia
Dizziness
Pan-positive review of systems (ROS)
Unrevealing evaluation despite extensive testing

Table 11–2. Differential diagnosis for fibromyalgia.

Medications (statins, aromatase inhibitors, fluoroquinolones, vitamin B$_6$ overdose)
Benign joint hypermobility syndrome
Endocrine (thyroid, adrenals)
Polymyalgia rheumatica (PMR)
Systemic lupus erythematosus (SLE)
Primary generalized osteoarthritis
Diffuse idiopathic skeletal hyperostosis (DISH)
Myopathies
Celiac sprue, inflammatory bowel disease (IBD)
Sleep apnea
Ankylosing spondylitis
Parkinson disease
Periostitis (secondary to cancer or drug-induced [eg, voriconazole])
Hypercalcemia (multiple causes including granulomatous inflammation)

Table 11–3. Laboratory tests for patients with fibromyalgia.

Complete blood count (CBC)
Comprehensive metabolic panel (CMP)
Erythrocyte sedimentation rate (ESR)
C-reactive protein (CRP)
Thyroid function tests (eg, thyroid-stimulating hormone [TSH], free T_4 or free T_4 index [FTI])

C. Imaging

Single photon emission computer tomography (SPECT) and functional magnetic resonance imaging (fMRI) have been used experimentally to diagnosis fibromyalgia but are not routinely used by practitioners. We recommend musculoskeletal imaging when there is a concern on the physical exam for joint damage, generally beginning with plain radiographs.

MANAGEMENT OF FIBROMYALGIA SYMPTOMS

A multidisciplinary management approach for fibromyalgia has the highest likelihood of success. Effective management strategies address issues of both the body and mind. Some of these are discussed here.

Exercise

Exercise is the only management modality for fibromyalgia that 100% of the European League Against Rheumatism (EULAR) strongly supported in 2017. Both land-based and aquatic aerobic exercises improve pain and physical function in patients with fibromyalgia. Resistance training also results in significant pain improvement for patients when compared to control. Both aerobic exercise and strength training are effective. It is important to acknowledge to patients that exercise will be painful in the short-term but will improve pain symptoms in the long term. Patients should be encouraged to make any exercise regimen changes slowly and in small increments to decrease chances of extreme pain exacerbation.

Cognitive-Based Therapy

Cognitive-based therapy (CBT) provides some immediate relief in fibromyalgia symptoms, including decreased pain and improved physical functioning, especially in juvenile fibromyalgia. CBT and aerobic exercise have similar effects on key fibromyalgia symptoms (pain, fatigue, and negative mood) immediately following intervention and in long-term follow-up. A 2013 Cochrane Review endorsed exercise (eg, walking) more strongly than CBT as it can be done at no cost, with little to no guidance, and at any time. Multidisciplinary treatment programs that included CBT are more successful than CBT therapy alone, which emphasizes the importance of a multimodality approach for symptom management rather than monotherapy.

Diet & Obesity Management

Fibromyalgia is associated with higher body mass index (BMI). Weight loss in obese patients with fibromyalgia is associated with improved quality of life and function.

Mind-Body Modalities & Hydrotherapy/Spa Therapy

Recent research has shown that some integrative modalities are successful at reducing fibromyalgia symptom severity, including mind-body therapies, such as mindfulness-based stress reduction, qigong, tai chi, and acupuncture. Hydrotherapy and spa therapy may also have a role in effective disease management. In general, more research is needed in these areas.

Sleep Dysfunction Management

Improving sleep hygiene can decrease pain and improve mental well-being. Additionally, symptoms similar to fibromyalgia were observed when healthy people were deprived of stage IV sleep, including musculoskeletal aching and stiffness as well as somatic fatigue.

Patient Education

It is essential to inform patients about the nature of fibromyalgia and also to educate them about what fibromyalgia is not. (eg, it is not an infection, cancer, or an inflammatory immune-mediated condition.) Patient education improves long-term adherence of symptom management. One potential website for patients could be the following: https://www.neurosymptoms.org/welcome/4594357992.

Pharmaceutical Products

Norepinephrine-reuptake inhibitors as well as some antiseizure medication have provided some transient relief for patients with fibromyalgia. However, while duloxetine and milnacipran were shown to reduce pain by 50%, only 28% of the treatment group experienced this reduction compared to 19% of those who received placebo.

Treatment using glucocorticoids and growth hormones should be avoided. Glucocorticoids or growth hormone may lead to transient pain relief in the short term, and any benefit will be overshadowed by the negative side effects associated with long-term use.

Finally, a common occurrence in clinical practice is that each drug approved for fibromyalgia by the Food and Drug Administration (FDA)—milnacipran, duloxetine, and pregabalin—leads to a decrease in some fibromyalgia symptoms; however, this effect usually is transient, lasting on the order of 6 months before subsiding. While patients can be switched to another medication that may provide mild relief, this effect is transient as well. The EULAR 2016 recommendations now only weakly recommend the use of medications for fibromyalgia symptom management. The above modalities are encouraged over drugs.

Arnold LM, Bennett RM, Crofford LJ, Dean LE, Clauw DJ, Goldenberg DL, Fitzcharles MA, Paiva ES, Staud R, Sarzi-Puttini P, Buskila D, Macfarlane GJ. Critical Reviews: AAPT Diagnostic Criteria for Fibromyalgia. *The Journal of Pain.* 2019;20(6):611-628. [PMID: 30453109]

Banic B, Petersen-Felix S, Andersen OK, Radanov BP, Villiger PM, Arendt-Nielsen L, Curatolo M. Evidence for spinal cord hypersensitivity in chronic pain after whiplash injury and in fibromyalgia. *Pain.* 2004;107(1-2):7-15. [PMID: 14715383]

Bennett RM, Burckhardt CS, Clark SR, O'Reilly CA, Wiens AN, Campbell SM. Group treatment of fibromyalgia: a 6 month outpatient program. *J Rheumatol.* 1996;23:521-528. [PMID: 8832996]

Bennett R, Nelson D. Cognitive behavioral therapy for fibromyalgia. *Nature Clinical Practice: Rheumatology.* 2008;2(8):416-424. [PMID: 16932733]

Bernardy K, Klose P, Busch AJ, Choy EHS, Häuser W. Cognitive behavioural therapies for fibromyalgia. *Cochrane Database of Systematic Reviews.* 2013;9:CD009796. DOI: 10.1002/14651858.CD009796.pub2. [PMID: 24018611]

Bidonde J, Busch AJ, Webber SC, et al. Aquatic exercise training for fibromyalgia. *Cochrane Database Syst Rev.* 2014;10:CD011336. [PMID: 25350761]

Brikman S, Furer V, Wollman J, Borok S, Matz H, Polachek A, Elalouf O, Sharabi A, Kaufman I, Paran D, Elkayam O. The Effect of the Presence of Fibromyalgia on Common Clinical Disease Activity Indices in Patients with Psoriatic Arthritis: A Cross-sectional Study. *The Journal of Rheumatology.* 2016;43(9):1749-1754. [PMID: 27252430]

Busch AJ, Webber SC, Richards RS. Resistance exercise training for fibromyalgia. *Cochrane Database Syst Rev.* 2013; 12:CD010884. [PMID: 24362925]

Chinn S, Caldwell W, Gritsenko K. Fibromyalgia Pathogenesis and Treatment Options Update. *Curr Pain Headache Rep.* 2016;20:25. [PMID: 26922414]

Cheng CA, Chiu YW, Wu D, Kuan YC, Chen SN, Tam KW. Effectiveness of Tai Chi on fibromyalgia patients: A meta-analysis of randomized controlled trials. *Complement Ther Med.* 2019;46:1-8. [PMID: 31519264]

Choy EH. The role of sleep in pain and fibromyalgia. *Nat Rev Rheumatol.* 2015;11(9):513-20. [PMID: 25907704]

Clauw DJ. Fibromyalgia: A Clinical Review. *JAMA.* 2014;311(15):1547-1555. [PMID: 24737367]

Clauw DJ. Fibromyalgia and Related Conditions. *Mayo Clin Proc.* 2015;90(5):680-92. [PMID: 25939940]

Clauw DJ, Chrousos GP. Chronic pain and fatigue syndromes: overlapping clinical and neuroendocrine features and potential pathogenic mechanisms. *Neuroimmunomodulation.* 1997;4(3):134-53. [PMID: 9500148]

Deare JC, Zheng Z, Xue CCL, Liu JP, Shang J, Scott SW, Littlejohn G. Acupuncture for treating fibromyalgia. *Cochrane Database of Systematic Reviews.* 2013;5:CD007070. [PMID: 23728665]

Desmeules JA, Cedraschi C, Rapiti E, Baumgartner E, Finckh A, Cohen P, Dayer P, Vischer TL. Neurophysiologic evidence for a central sensitization in patients with fibromyalgia. *Arthritis Rheum.* 2003;48(5):1420-9. [PMID: 12746916]

Diatchenko L, Fillingim RB, Smith SB, Maixner W. The phenotypic and genetic signatures of common musculoskeletal pain conditions. *Nat Rev Rheumatol.* 2013;9(6):340-50. [PMID: 23545734]

Dobkin PL, Abrahamowicz M, Fitzcharles MA, Dritsa M, da Costa D. Maintenance of exercise in women with fibromyalgia. *Arthritis Rheum.* 2005;53:724-731. [PMID: 16208640]

Fietta P, Fietta P, Manganelli P. Fibromyalgia and psychiatric disorders. *Acta Biomed.* 2007;78(2):88-95. [PMID: 17933276]

Goldenberg DL, Burckhardt C, Crofford L. Management of fibromyalgia syndrome. *JAMA.* 2004;292:2388-2395. [PMID: 15547167]

Häuser W, Galek A, Erbslöh-Möller B, et al. Posttraumatic stress disorder in fibromyalgia syndrome: prevalence, temporal relationship between posttraumatic stress and fibromyalgia symptoms, and impact on clinical outcome. *Pain.* 2013;154(8):1216-23. [PMID: 23685006]

Häuser W, Kosseva M, Üceyler N, Klose P, Sommer C. Emotional, physical, and sexual abuse in fibromyalgia syndrome: a systematic review with meta-analysis. *Arthritis Care Res.* 2011;63(6):808-20. [PMID: 20722042]

Häuser W, Urrútia G, Tort S, Uçeyler N, Walitt B. Serotonin and noradrenaline reuptake inhibitors (SNRIs) for fibromyalgia syndrome. *Cochrane Database Syst Rev.* 2013;1:CD010292. [PMID: 23440848]

Jeffery DD, Bulathsinhala L, Kroc M, Dorris J. Prevalence, Health Care Utilization, and Costs of Fibromyalgia, Irritable Bowel, and Chronic Fatigue Syndromes in the Military Health System, 2006-2010. *Military Medicine.* 2014;179(9):1021. [PMID: 25181721]

Jones KD, Liptan GL. Exercise interventions in fibromyalgia: clinical applications from the evidence. *Rheum Dis Clin North Am.* 2009;35:373-91. [PMID: 19647149]

Jorge LL, Amaro E Jr. Brain imaging in fibromyalgia. *Current Pain and Headache Reports.* 2012;16(5):388-398. [PMID: 22717698]

Lauche R, Cramer H, Dobos G, et al. A systematic review and meta-analysis of mindfulness-based stress reduction for the fibromyalgia syndrome. *J Psychosom Res.* 2013;75:500-10. [PMID: 24290038]

Leeb BF, Andel I, Leder S, Leeb BA, Rintelen B. The patient's perspective and rheumatoid arthritis disease activity indexes. *Rheumatology.* 2005;44(3):360-365. [PMID: 15572395]

Macfarlane GJ, Kronisch C, Dean LE, Atzeni F, Häuser W, Fluß E, Choy E, Kosek E, Amris K, Branco J, Dincer F, Leino-Arjas P, Longley K, McCarthy GM, Makri S, Perrot S, Sarzi-Puttini P, Taylor A, Jones GT. EULAR revised recommendations for the management of fibromyalgia. *Ann Rheum Dis.* 2017; 76(2):318-328. [PMID: 27377815]

Nielson WR, Walker C, McCain GA. Cognitive behavioral treatment of fibromyalgia syndrome: preliminary findings. *J Rheumatol.* 1992;19:98-103. [PMID: 1556709]

Okifuji A, Donaldson GW, Barck L, Fine PG. Relationship between fibromyalgia and obesity in pain, function, mood, and sleep. *J Pain.* 2010;11(12):1329-37. [PMID: 20542742]

Perez-Aranda A, Feliu-Soler A, Montero-Marin J, Garcia-Campayo J, Andres-Rodriguez L, et. al. A randomized controlled efficacy trial of Mindfulness-Based Stress Reduction compared with an active control group and usual care for fibromyalgia: the EUDAIMON study. *Pain.* 2019;160(11):2508-2523. [PMID: 31356450]

Ranzolin A, Brenol JC, Bredemeier M, Guarienti J, Rizzatti M, Feldman D, Xavier RM. Association of concomitant fibromyalgia with worse disease activity score in 28 joints, health assessment questionnaire, and short form 36 scores in patients with rheumatoid arthritis. *Arthritis Rheum.* 2009;61(6):794-800. [PMID: 19479706]

Sawynok J. Lynch M. Quigong and fibromyalgia: randomized controlled trials and beyond. *Evid Based Complement Alternat Med.* 2014;379715. [PMID: 25477991]

Schmidt-Wilcke T, Clauw DJ. Fibromyalgia: from pathophysiology to therapy. *Nat Rev Rheumatol.* 2011;7(9):518-27. [PMID: 21769128]

Senna MK, Sallam RA, Ashour HS, et al. Effect of weight reduction on the quality of life in obese patients with fibromyalgia syndrome: a randomized controlled trial. *Clin Rheumatol.* 2012;31(11):1591-7. [PMID: 22948223]

Shapiro JR, Anderson DA, Danoff-Burg S. A pilot study of the effects of behavioral weight loss treatment on fibromyalgia symptoms. *J Psychosom Res.* 2005;59(5):275-82. [PMID: 16253617]

Wach J, Letroublon MC, Coury F, Tebib JG. Fibromyalgia in Spondyloarthritis: Effect on Disease Activity Assessment in Clinical Practice. *The Journal of Rheumatology.* 2016;43(11):2056-2063. [PMID: 27633820]

Welsch P, Üçeyler N, Klose P, Walitt B, Häuser W. Serotonin and noradrenaline reuptake inhibitors (SNRIs) for fibromyalgia. *Cochrane Database Syst Rev.* 2018;2:CD010292. [PMID: 29489029]

Wolfe F, Brähler E, Hinz A, Häuser W. Fibromyalgia prevalence, somatic symptom reporting, and the dimensionality of polysymptomatic distress: results from a survey of the general population. *Arthritis Care Res (Hoboken).* 2013;65(5):777-785. [PMID: 23424058]

Wolfe F, Clauw DJ, Fitzcharles MA, Goldenberg DL, Häuser W, Katz RS, Mease P, Russell AS, Russell IJ, Walitt B. 2016 Revisions to the 2010/2011 fibromyalgia diagnostic criteria. *Seminars in Arthritis and Rheumatism.* 2016;46:319-329. [PMID: 27916278]

Wu YL, Huang CJ, Fang SC, Ko LH, Tsai PS. Cognitive Impairment in Fibromyalgia: A Meta-Analysis of Case-Control Studies. *Psychosom Med.* 2018;80(5):432. [PMID: 29528888]

Yunus MB, Arslan S, Aldag JC. Relationship between body mass index and fibromyalgia features. *Scand J Rheumatol.* 2002;31(1):27-31. [PMID 11922197]

Complex Regional Pain Syndrome (Reflex Sympathetic Dystrophy) & Posttraumatic Neuralgia

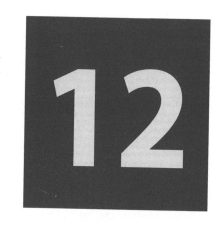

Anne Louise Oaklander, MD, PhD

ESSENTIALS OF DIAGNOSIS

▶ Consider posttraumatic neuralgia (PTN) when an injury causes unexpectedly severe or prolonged distal pain.

▶ Injuries that appear minor, eg, phlebotomy, sometimes injure nerves disproportionately.

▶ Symptoms can be mild and transient, moderate, or severe and prolonged. Children almost always recover.

▶ The complex regional pain syndrome (CRPS) diagnosis requires additional symptoms: eg, asymmetric edema, alterations of cutaneous blood flow or sweating patterns, or movement difficulties.

▶ Full CRPS develops only in the limbs.

▶ Rare cases that are prolonged, bilateral, or not associated with trauma may be related to internal structural causes, underlying systemic inflammation, immune dysregulation, or to small-fiber polyneuropathy. These cases require additional diagnostic approaches and often have specific treatments.

General Considerations

Neuralgia refers to pain caused by injury to nerves rather than other tissues. Complex regional pain syndrome (CRPS) is consensus nomenclature that describes a collection of symptoms in a body region influenced by one or more damaged nerves. Chronic excess pain, often burning, is the cardinal symptom. Symptom onset usually occurs within days of injury. CRPS is likely amplified form of posttraumatic neuralgia (PTN) that includes nonpain symptoms (Table 12–1). Full CRPS develops only in limbs, for reasons that are not entirely clear. In contrast, PTN can develop at any site in the body. By definition, PTN and CRPS are incited by trauma, usually external, but in rare cases the causes are internal. For example, a nerve entrapment or infarction can lead to CRPS. The epicenter of symptoms is usually distal to the injury, reflecting involvement of nerves, blood vessels, and sometimes bone. Symptoms are disproportionate to the external signs of injury which can occur, for example, in venipuncture, when nerve twigs encircling blood vessels might be transected by the needle. Three-fourths of CRPS patients are female, and the median age at onset is in the 40s. CRPS is rare in young children and the elderly. Most patients and virtually all children recover spontaneously. Prolonged or severe CRPS is uncommon but profoundly disabling when it occurs. It should provoke search for complicating endogenous factors that impede healing and require additional treatment for resolution.

Different names have been used for CRPS depending on whether or not nerve injury was evident. **Causalgia,** later **CRPS type II,** was the term used for patients with diagnosed injuries to major nerves, as first described in wounded Civil War soldiers. **Reflex sympathetic dystrophy (RSD),** later known as **CRPS type I,** described patients with seemingly trivial injuries and no overt nerve damage. European names include **algodystrophy** and **Sudeck atrophy.** The divided nomenclature is fading as improved technologies identify subtle nerve injuries in what was formerly called **reflex sympathetic dystrophy (CRPS I).** The incidence overall has been reported as 5.5/100,000 in the United States (Rochester, MN) and 26.2/100,000 in the Netherlands (Marinus et al, 2011). Wrist fractures and those that cause severe pain carry high risk of leading to CRPS.

Pathogenesis

Because CRPS is a very rare complications of common injuries, endogenous biology influences pathogenesis and the persistence of pathology more than the causal injury (Marinus et al, 2011). CRPS primarily involves the unmyelinated C-fibers that have very large receptive fields and innervate bone and blood vessels outside of traditional nerve-map areas (Oaklander and Fields, 2009). From their distal ends, C-fibers release neuropeptides that kindle inflammation (neuroinflammation). Even tiny nerve injuries can further

Table 12–1. The 2012 IASP criteria for complex regional pain syndrome (CRPS).

To make the *clinical* diagnosis, the following criteria must be met:

1. Continuing pain, which is disproportionate to any inciting event
2. Must report at least 1 symptom in *3 of the 4* following categories:
   - Sensory: reports of hyperesthesia and/or allodynia
   - Vasomotor: reports of temperature asymmetry and/asymmetry
   - Sudomotor/edema: reports of edema and/or sweating
   - Motor/trophic: reports of decreased range of motion tremor, dystonia, and/or trophic changes (hair, nails)
3. Must display at least 1 sign *at time of evaluation* in *2 or more* of the following:
   - Sensory: evidence of hyperalgesia (to pinprick) and/or temperature sensation and/or deep somatic pressure
   - Vasomotor: evidence of temperature asymmetry (>asymmetry)
   - Sudomotor/edema: evidence of edema and/or sweating asymmetry
   - Motor/trophic: evidence of decreased range of motion (weakness, tremor, dystonia) and/or trophic changes
4. There is no other diagnosis that better explains the signs and symptoms

For research purposes: Must report at least 1 symptom in *all 4* symptom categories and at least 1 sign (observed categories).
Data from International Association for the Study of Pain (IASP)

trigger extradermatomal symptoms if inflammation spreads to uninjured neighbor axons within nerve trunks, roots, and the spinal cord. Like all chronic pain, CRPS can cause secondary postsynaptic and tertiary network abnormalities in the spinal cord and brain, including changes in neuronal activity, mood, and higher cortical functions. The imaging abnormalities that may be the correlate of central sensitization usually reverse during recovery.

Loss of local microvascular control—required to diagnose CRPS—can cause tissue hypoxia, ischemia, and inflammation that augment and prolong neurogenic inflammation from release of neuropeptides from dysfunctional C-fibers (Figure 12–1). CRPS is linked epidemiologically with asthma and other hypersensitivity syndromes. Some injuries (including rare internal ones) may breach the blood-nerve barrier and initiate chronic neuroinflammation in susceptible individuals.

▶ Prevention

Accidental injuries are the most common cause of CRPS. Fractures cause about 40% of well-characterized cases. About half of causal injuries occur on the job, and some trigger lawsuits. Iatrogenic injuries from medical procedures, including castings and venipuncture, are equally common. Surgeries precede

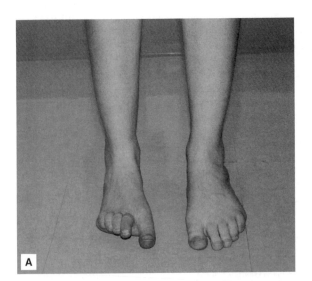 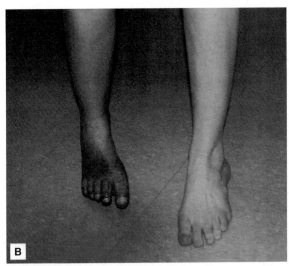

▲ **Figure 12–1.** Progressive right foot and leg CRPS-I beginning at age 13 after soft-tissue trauma with possible occult fracture. She noted dramatic foot edema and reddening within a few hours. She later had two milder CRPS episodes of in her arms caused by venipuncture. Over time her CRPS progressed rather than resolved. Panel A at age 26, shows mild color changes and dystonia accompanying moderate pain. Panel B at age 29, shows microvascular insufficiency causing edema and critical tissue ischemia that worsen pain and prognosis. In addition she developed "total body CRPS" and dysautonomia (tachycardia, hypotension, gastrointestinal dysmotility, and cachexia) that required gastrojejunal and then parental nutrition. Neurological evaluation led to additional diagnoses of Ehlers-Danlos syndrome and small-fiber polyneuropathy, confirmed by left-leg skin biopsy. Multiple treatments, including polypharmacy, spinal cord stimulator, and intrathecal pump, were ineffective or poorly tolerated and IVIg was recommended. (See color insert.)

30% of well-characterized cases (Table 12–2). In addition to avoiding unnecessary procedures, evidence supports avoiding immobilization and supplementing vitamin C. Limb edema, whether from the injury or early CRPS, can create a compartment syndrome under a cast requiring urgent cast removal. Immobilization is a further preventable risk factor. Early CRPS responds better to treatment than established cases, so prompt evaluation and treatment of any suggestion of early CRPS may prevent more serious cases. Smoking cessation, aerobic exercise, and mitigating other contributors to poor tissue perfusion and healing are presumed to be beneficial, also.

▶ Clinical Findings

A. Symptoms and Signs

In 2012, the International Association for the Study of Pain (IASP) approved the "Budapest" consensus diagnostic

Table 12–2. Iatrogenic nerve injuries associated with posttraumatic neuralgia (PTN) and complex regional pain syndrome (CRPS).

Medical Procedure	Location of Worst Pain	Nerve Damaged
Third molar extraction	Mandible	Alveolar nerves of mandible
Lymph-node surgery in neck	Behind ear	Greater auricular nerve
Breast surgery (mastectomy, lumpectomy, axillary node dissection)	Upper inner arm	Intercostobrachial nerve
Thoracotomy or chest tube	Unilateral thoracic dermatome	Intercostal nerve below rib
Carpal tunnel release	Thenar eminence (base of thumb)	Palmar cutaneous branch of median
Venipuncture at antecubital fossa or cephalic or basilic vein	Medial or lateral inner forearm	Medial or lateral antebrachial cutaneous nerves
Venipuncture on back of hand	Back of hand	Radial nerve
Herniorrhaphy	Genitals, inguinal crease	Ilioinguinal or genitofemoral nerve
Endovascular catheterization via femoral artery	Anterior thigh	Femoral nerve
Arthroscopic or open surgery of knee	Lower anterior knee, knee joint, medial lower leg	Infrapatellar branch of saphenous nerve
Below knee casting or compression	Outer lower leg, dorsum of foot	Peroneal nerve against fibula
Saphenous vein stripping	Medial calf, arch of foot (variable)	Descending branch of saphenous nerve

criteria for CRPS that were validated in 2010 (see Table 12–1) (Harden et al, 2010). These include a more rigorous definition for research use with higher specificity.

1. Pain—Pain is required for diagnosis of CRPS. Patients typically report varying neuropathic symptoms that gradually improve. Allodynia, defined as the perception of pain in response to innocuous stimuli such as light touch, is reported in 70–90% of patients. Hyperalgesia, the occurrence of excessive pain in response to a stimulus such as a pinprick that is normally only mildly painful, is also observed. Spontaneous, stimulus-independent pain can be burning, deep and aching, or sharp and shooting. Pain characteristics can guide treatment. Other contributors to CRPS pain include tissue ischemia and inflammation and disuse (eg, contractures, muscle deconditioning). Many patients report worsening in cold weather.

2. Limb edema and skin color and temperature changes—Visible signs of microvascular dysregulation (see Figure 12–1) help distinguish CRPS from PTN. Vasospasm causes pale or blue skin, and hyperperfusion causes redness and warmth. Sometimes, these alternate, perhaps reflecting microvessel hypersensitivity to circulating catecholamines. Denervated arteriovenous shunts lack tone and consequently dump arteriolar blood directly into the venules. Blood then bypasses the capillary beds and produces paradoxical cutaneous flushing and edema, masking deeper tissue hypoxemia. Two-thirds of patients report asymmetric limb edema (Harden et al, 2010). Central sensitization sometimes causes delusions of edema, as a lip numbed by dental anesthesia can falsely feel swollen.

3. Sensory loss—This can be the primary result of underlying nerve injury, the secondary result of tissue ischemia, or the tertiary result of central network changes. CRPS usually arises after subtle, partial nerve injuries and sensation is often relatively preserved as long as tissue perfusion is maintained.

4. Movement disorders—Decreased range of motion and strength, slowed, clumsy movements, and intermittent muscle cramps are common in CRPS. Injury to motor axons rarely causes muscle atrophy and fasciculations. Fewer than 10% of patients develop tremors or dystonia, sustained abnormal postures that can cause contractures that require casting or tendon release.

5. Disorders of sweating, skin, and hair growth (trophic changes)—Half of CRPS patients report reduced regional sweating caused by disordered innervation of sweat glands. The normal surrounding compensatory hyperhidrosis is usually noticed more by patients than is the pathological hypohidrosis. Skin that has lost normal innervation can become thin, shiny, devoid of hair follicles, and vulnerable to injury. Chronic inflammation can cause skin thickening. If allodynia prevents contact and washing, epidermis that does not slough through normal mechanisms can cause a scaly appearance.

6. Bone and joint resorption—Bone metabolism is regulated by C-fibers, the injury to which may increase osteoclast-induced bone absorption and remodeling. These mechanisms contribute to pain and osteopenia and rarely cause pathologic fractures. Joint contractures, common in the most severe cases, can sometimes be prevented with patient education and referrals for physiotherapy and splinting. Established cases may require tendon release. Bone marrow edema is a common MRI finding.

7. Spread of symptoms—CRPS begins in the area of and distal to the site of the inciting injury, but almost half of patients report "mirror" spread to the uninjured limb. Some of this reflects spread through transmidline spinal-cord circuits, but symmetric limb symptoms, or "total body CRPS" associated C-fiber polyneuropathy require neurological evaluation.

B. Laboratory Findings, Imaging Studies, and Special Tests

No diagnostic blood or imaging tests are specific for CRPS. CT or MRI sometimes reveals corroborating edema of bone marrow, joints, or soft tissues, and three-phase bone scan can show the bony hypermetabolism discussed above. However, normal studies do not exclude the diagnosis, which is a clinical one (see Table 12–1). Abnormal results of electrodiagnostic testing (electromyography and nerve conduction study) can help localize a culprit nerve injury, but normal results do not exclude a tiny, distal, small-fiber predominant nerve injury. Ultrasound or MR neurography can help evaluate the health and continuity of larger nerves. Localizing nerve injuries becomes important if surgical exploration or nerve stimulation is considered. Verification of a nerve injury can improve insurance coverage for patients lacking a firm explanation for their symptoms.

▶ Differential Diagnosis

CRPS symptoms are excessive and prolonged versions of normal injury responses. Other causes of chronic limb injury and inflammation, including osteomyelitis and focal causes of arthritis such as gout, should be considered. Arterial or venous occlusion (eg, deep venous thrombosis) can produce limb pain and swelling, and vascular ultrasound is often appropriate at onset. Patients without known trauma may harbor internal causes of nerve damage or irritation (eg, nerve entrapment, infection, infarction, tumor, vasculitis, or vascular malformation). As these may require specific medical or surgical treatment, neuromedical or surgical consultation may be indicated.

The diagnosis of CRPS is too often invoked casually and inappropriately. It is unlikely when there is gradual onset or worsening, when the pain is bilateral or widespread, and when there is no antecedent injury. These suggest generalized nerve damage (polyneuropathy), which most often presents with bilateral foot pain or 4-limb "stocking and glove" sensory complaints. Subclinical systemic inflammation, dysregulated immunity, and polyneuropathy can predispose, potentiate, or prolong CRPS. These must be considered in patients with CRPS that does not resolve. Established causes of poor C-fiber health, such as diabetes, Sjögren syndrome, or neurotoxic medications, should be addressed in order to speed the resolution of CRPS.

▶ Complications

By definition, CRPS is a complication of injury. In severe cases, affected limbs can become immobile, ischemic, infected, and ulcerated. Very rarely, amputation is considered. Although usually ineffective for relief of neuropathic pain since stump pain can persist and phantom pain often develops, rare patients report benefit from removing immobile or ischemic limbs to permit use of limb prostheses. Desperate patients with unremitting severe pain may seek unproven and potentially harmful treatments and rarely commit suicide, so good communication and identifying evidence-supported treatment options is important. CRPS should always inspire compassion and prompt medical attention. Long-lasting severe pain and limb ischemia remain medical emergencies even when prolonged.

▶ Treatment

A. Early CRPS/PTN

Most early cases improve spontaneously or respond well to treatment. Early remobilization and rehabilitation are important as they can head off a downward spiral of pain, disuse, edema, and disability. Patients may require physical and occupational therapy, short-term pain management, and treatment of comorbidities such as depression or smoking. Improved perfusion of affected limbs will speed axonal regeneration, reduce ischemia and inflammation, and reduce maladaptive brain plasticity triggered by chronic pain and disuse. Several trials show efficacy of glucocorticoids and some support the use of free radical scavengers, including vitamin C. Given their safety and low cost, nonsteroidal anti-inflammatory drugs are worth considering even though they have not been studied formally in CRPS with clinical trials. Although sympathetic or somatic nerve blocks—historically a traditional CRPS treatment—may temporarily improve limb perfusion, their cost and potential adverse effects (including nerve damage) argue against routine use. Meta-analyses, in fact, show no long-term benefits.

B. Treatment of Pain

Much of the pain is neuropathic—caused by injury to nociceptive C-fibers—with tissue hypoxia, edema, and inflammation contributing in CRPS. Most trials of pharmacotherapies for CRPS were conducted long ago and do not conform to current standards (Tran et al, 2010). More were conducted in acute than chronic CRPS, where the strongest support is for bisphosphonates and nasal calcitonin, which can reduce painful bone hypermetabolism. Physical therapy and graded motor imagery may provide clinically meaningful improvements in pain and function in CRPS. A recent large trial of lenalidomide, a thalidomide analogue, reported a lack of efficacy, but methodological difficulties may have contributed to this conclusion (Manning et al, 2014). Neridronate, a bisphosphonate approved in Europe for CRPS, is being studied now in the United States.

Evidence-based guidelines for treating neuropathic pain identify the best initial options as the secondary tricyclic amines (nortriptyline, desipramine), serotonin/norepinephrine reuptake inhibitors (venlafaxine, duloxetine), calcium channel $\alpha_2\delta$ ligands (gabapentin, pregabalin), and topical lidocaine. Tramadol and opioid analgesics as well as sodium-channel blockers such as carbamazepine and mexiletine are potential tertiary options for severe, uncontrolled pain.

C. Treatment of Vascular Dysregulation

Nonpharmacologic management is critical to minimize tissue ischemia, for example, avoiding smoking, limb dependency, potentiating or neurotoxic drugs, adding daily aerobic exercise, and wearing compression garments if needed. If these are insufficient, calcium-channel blockers are commonly prescribed. Less often, topical nitroglycerin, phosphodiesterase inhibitors such as sildenafil or surgical sympathectomy are considered.

D. Treatment of Dystonia

These continuous muscle contractions (Figure 12–1A) are painful, disabling, and can lead to contractures. The most effective oral agent is baclofen, which augments GABA-B transmission; muscle relaxants such as cyclobenzaprine or diazepam have little long-term benefit. Intrathecal administration of baclofen through an implanted pump can be considered to reduce systemic adverse effects. Local injection of botulinum toxin type A, which inhibits release of glutamate and substance P from nociceptive nerve endings, as well as inhibit cholinergic activation of muscles is effective for neuropathic pain as well as dystonia. Because benefit lasts only about 3 months it is only practical for small regions. Anticholinergic drugs such as trihexyphenidyl, benztropine, or ethopropazine usually have limited side effects.

E. Surgical Treatment

The possibility of internal structural contributors (eg, nerve entrapment, infection, tumor, or vascular malformation) should be considered for patients with onset in the absence of identifiable trauma and for those with severe nonresolving symptoms. Precise localization is required before recommending surgery. If medical management has been ineffective and surgical exploration not indicated, evidence supports consideration of implanted bipolar neural stimulators, whether on the proximal portion of an injured nerve, spinal cord, motor cortex, or deep within the brain. Stimulating the sensory dorsal columns of the spinal cord is most common because a temporary lead can be placed through a spinal needle to allow a trial before implantation.

F. Tertiary and Emerging Medical Treatments

Completely external (transcranial) magnetic or direct-current stimulation of the motor cortex is effective for neuropathic pain, particularly affecting the hand, but treatments need to be repeated to maintain benefit so long-term utility is unclear. There is emerging evidence of autoimmune contribution to CRPS and C-fiber polyneuropathy. A large trial did not find benefit for low-dose intravenous immunoglobulin (IVIG) (Goebel et al, 2017), but clinical experience shows benefit of higher doses (2 g/kg/4 wk) for select patients with contributing C-fiber inflammation. Preliminary evidence supports tertiary use of lidocaine and ketamine infusions, although ketamine can cause hallucinations and addiction. Ziconotide, a conotoxin administered intrathecally for refractory neuropathic pain, has preliminary case support. There is emerging support for cannabinoids in neuropathic pain, whereas the NMDA (N-methyl-D-aspartate) antagonists, dextromethorphan, memantine, and riluzole, have generally been ineffective (Tran et al, 2010).

▶ Prognosis

Epidemiologic study shows that most patients recover spontaneously and that the prognosis is particularly good in children, presumably due to their great neuroregenerative and other healing capacities. Early diagnosis, remobilization, and pain relief are essential to improve prognosis. In a study of CRPS lasting more than a year, 30% ultimately recovered, 54% were unchanged, and 16% worsened (see Figure 12–1) (Marinus et al, 2011). Barriers to the healing of nerves and blood vessels, including tobacco use, the metabolic syndrome or diabetes, malnutrition, and subclinical polyneuropathy, may require treatment to achieve recovery.

ACKNOWLEDGMENTS

Supported in part by the Public Health Service (NINDS K24NS59892). No commercial funding sources or conflicts of interest.

Goebel A, Bisla J, Carganillo R, et al. Low-dose intravenous immunoglobulin treatment for long-standing complex regional pain syndrome: a randomized trial. *Ann Intern Med.* 2017;167(7):476. [PMID: 28973211]

Harden RN, Bruehl S, Perez RSGM, et al. Validation of proposed diagnostic criteria (the Budapest Criteria) for complex regional pain syndrome. *Pain.* 2010;150(2):268. [PMID: 20493633]

Manning DC, Alexander G, Arezzo JC, et al. Lenalidomide for complex regional pain syndrome type 1: lack of efficacy in a phase II randomized study. *J Pain.* 2014;15(12):1366. [PMID: 25283471]

Marinus J, Moseley GL, Birklein F, et al. Clinical features and pathophysiology of complex regional pain syndrome. *Lancet Neurol.* 2011;10(7):637. [PMID: 21683929]

Oaklander AL, Fields HL. Is reflex sympathetic dystrophy/complex regional pain syndrome type I a small-fiber neuropathy? *Ann Neurol.* 2009;65(6):629. [PMID: 19557864]

Tran DQ, Duong S, Bertini P, Finlayson RJ. Treatment of complex regional pain syndrome: a review of the evidence. *Can J Anaesth.* 2010;57(2):149. [PMID: 20054678]

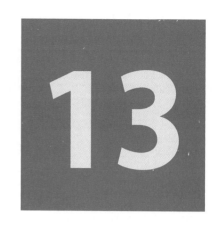

Rheumatoid Arthritis

13

Douglas J. Veale, MD

Ursula Fearon, PhD

Candice Low, MD

Lester D. Miller, MD

Rheumatoid arthritis (RA) is a chronic, systemic autoimmune disease affecting approximately 1% of the adult population worldwide. It may present at any age, but typically affects women in their late childbearing years. In men, RA is more prone to develop in the sixth to eighth decade. The disease occurs more commonly in women (female:male, 3:1) (Table 13–1). The primary pathology is inflammation of the synovial membrane, leading to synovitis and proliferation, which often results in loss of articular cartilage and erosion of juxtarticular bone. The natural history of the disease is one of progressive joint damage and deformity. Moreover, extra-articular manifestations, which occur in a significant minority of patients, are associated with a poor outcome. Recent advances in therapeutic strategies have dramatically altered the prognosis, particularly if RA is diagnosed and treated early. Unfortunately, many patients have suboptimal responses to treatment or tolerate therapies poorly.

The causes of RA remain elusive. The **genetic contribution** to RA is substantial, and more than 100 loci conferring risk for RA have been identified thus far. Most genes linked to RA influence immune responses (eg, T-cell activation, cytokine signaling). The strongest known association is with alleles of *HLADRB1*, which encodes the β chain of HLA-DR, a major histocompatiblity class II molecule directly involved in the presentation of antigen to T cells. Allelic variants of *HLADRB1* associated with risk for RA encode a similar sequence known as the "shared epitope," comprising amino acids 70–74. Although genetics play a significant role in determining risk of RA, most patients have no family history.

Studies of genetic risk reinforce the concept that clinical RA is not a single entity. Most notably, shared-epitope-encoding *HLADRB1* alleles confer risk only for RA associated with **antibodies to citrullinated protein epitopes**. These anticyclic citrullinated peptide antibodies (ACPAs) are present in approximately 70% of all patients with RA. Citrullination—a posttranslational modification of proteins in which arginine residues are converted to citrulline—occurs at sites of inflammation. How patients with RA lose tolerance to citrullinated protein epitopes is uncertain. It is noteworthy that **epidemiologic data** link both smoking (which induces inflammation and citrullinated proteins in the lung) and periodontitis (which is associated with the citrullination of proteins in the oral cavity) to the risk of developing ACPA-positive RA. The combination of shared epitope, ACPA, and smoking increased the risk of RA 40-fold.

ARTICULAR MANIFESTATIONS & TREATMENT

ARTICULAR MANIFESTATIONS OF RA

ESSENTIALS OF DIAGNOSIS

Typical pattern of arthritis is a chronic, symmetric polyarthritis with a tendency to affect the small joints of the hands and feet; for example, the wrists, metacarpophalangeal (MCP), or the metatarsophalangeal (MTP) joints and their corresponding joints in the lower extremities.

▶ Circulating autoantibodies, either rheumatoid factor (RF), ACPAs, or both, occur in approximately in 70% of patients.

▶ Radiographic changes include joint-space narrowing and juxtarticular erosions.

▶ Clinical Findings

A. Symptoms and Signs

1. Onset—In most patients, RA presents with the insidious onset of pain, stiffness, and swelling in multiple joints over the course of weeks to months. The patient may hardly notice the disease onset. Some patients, however, have a fulminant presentation with an abrupt onset of pain and stiffness.

Table 13–1. Classic manifestations.

- Gender: Female (3:1 ratio)
- Age: Women 30–40 years; Men 50–60 years
- Onset: Usually Insidious
- Distribution: Symmetric small joints—wrists, MCP, PIP, and MTP (spares DIP) joints
- Systemic: Fatigue, weight loss, low-grade fevers
- Symptoms: Joint stiffness (worse in morning), pain, swelling
- Laboratory: Anemia, elevated ESR or CRP or both, thrombocytosis, positive rheumatoid factor in 60–80%

CRP, C-reactive protein; DIP, distal interphalangeal; ESR, erythrocyte sedimentation rate; MCP, metacarpophalangeal; MTP, metatarsophalangeal; PIP, proximal interphalangeal.

Alternatively, patients may have persistent monoarthritis or oligoarthritis for prolonged periods before manifesting the more typical pattern of polyarticular involvement. Palindromic rheumatism (episodic, self-limited attacks of polyarthritis) may also evolve into RA. Rarely, extra-articular features of RA (eg, scleritis) may present before the joint problems manifest.

2. Systemic symptoms—Fatigue is a common and prominent symptom and many have low-grade fevers (≤38°C). Significant weight loss can occur but is uncommon in early onset disease.

3. Distribution of involved joints—Figure 13–1 illustrates the different joint distribution in RA and osteoarthritis (OA). RA always spares the distal interphalangeal (DIP) joints (in contrast, these joints are often involved in OA and in patients with psoriatic arthritis). Most patients with RA report involvement of small joints first, classically the wrists, metacarpophalangeal (MCP), metatarsophalangeal (MTP), and proximal interphalangeal (PIP) joints, with involvement of large joints occurring later. In advanced cases, RA may involve the temporomandibular, cricoarytenoid, and sternoclavicular joints. RA may also involve the upper part of the cervical spine, particularly the C1–2 articulation, but unlike the spondyloarthropathies, rarely involves the thoracic or lumbar spine.

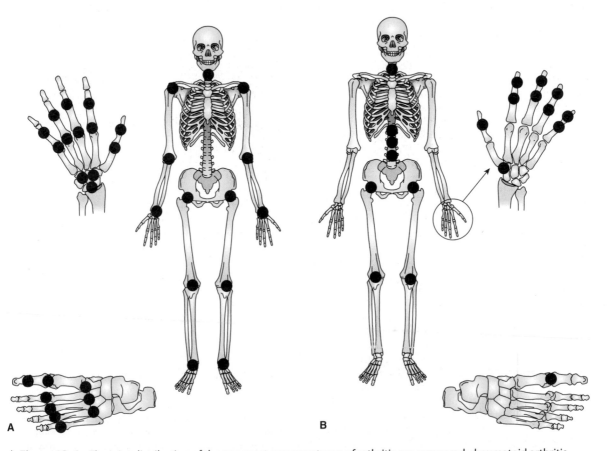

A   **B**

▲ **Figure 13–1.** The joint distribution of the two most common types of arthritis are compared: rheumatoid arthritis (RA) (**A**) and osteoarthritis (OA) (**B**). RA involves almost all synovial joints in the body. OA has a much more limited distribution. Importantly, RA rarely, if ever, involves the distal interphalangeal joints, but OA commonly does.

4. Morning stiffness—Morning stiffness, a hallmark of inflammatory arthritis, is a prominent feature of RA. Patients with RA are characteristically at their worst upon arising in the morning or after prolonged periods of rest. The stiffness often lasts for hours but tends to improve with physical activity. Routine activities like brushing teeth and combing hair may be very difficult early in the morning, and patients sometimes report running warm water over their hands to "get them working."

5. Articular manifestations—Symptoms of the inflammatory arthritis associated with OA include pain, swelling, and stiffness. Joint stiffness often dominates the early morning. Patients with early disease often complain that rings no longer fit on their fingers or pain in their feet, which they liken to walking on a stony beach.

The hands are involved in almost all patients with RA, and hand involvement is responsible for a significant proportion of the disabilities caused by RA. Typical early disease is shown in Figure 13–2A with swelling of the PIP joints. The DIP joints are normal unless the patient has coexistent OA; both diseases are common and occur together, particularly in elderly patients. Radiographs will often detect evidence of articular damage or erosions after 2 years of disease and long before the appearance of joint deformities (Figure 13–3). Late, established disease is often associated with joint damage and deformities such as **ulnar deviation** of the fingers at the MCPs, **swan neck deformities** (hyperextension of the PIP joints and flexion at the DIP joints; Figure 13–2B), and **boutonnière (or buttonhole) deformities** (flexion of the PIP joints and hyperextension of the DIP joints). If the clinical disease remains active, hand function slowly deteriorates.

Wrists are involved in most patients with RA. Early in the course of the disease, synovial proliferation in and around the wrists can compress the median nerve, causing carpal tunnel syndrome. Chronic synovitis can lead to radial deviation of the wrist and, in severe cases, to volar subluxation. Synovial proliferation of the wrist can invade extensor tendons, leading to rupture and the abrupt loss of function of individual fingers.

The feet, particularly the MTP joints, are involved early in many cases of RA and are second only to hand involvement in terms of the problems they cause. Radiographic erosions often occur at an early stage in the feet also. Subluxation of the toes at the MTP joints is common and leads to the dual problem of skin ulceration on the top of the toes and painful ambulation because of loss of the cushioning pads that protect the heads of the metatarsals. Symptoms from MTP subluxation can respond to orthotics but may require surgery later.

Involvement of **large joints** (knees, ankles, elbows, hips, and shoulders) is common but generally occurs at a later stage than small joint involvement. RA characteristically involves the entire joint surface in a symmetric fashion. Therefore, RA is not only symmetric from one side of the body to the other but is also symmetric within an

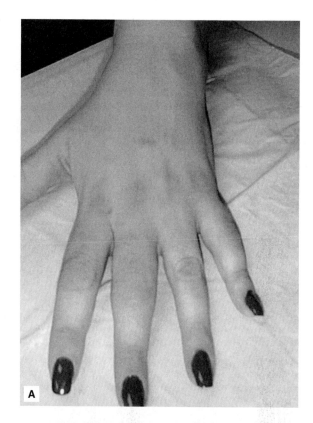

A

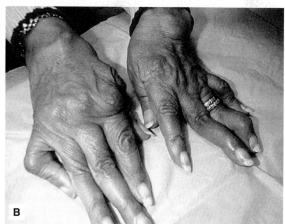

B

▲ **Figure 13–2. A:** A patient with early rheumatoid arthritis (RA). There are no joint deformities, but the soft-tissue synovial swelling around the third and fifth proximal interphalangeal (PIP) joints is easily seen. **B:** A patient with advanced RA with severe joint deformities including subluxation at the metacarpophalangeal joints and swan-neck deformities (hyperextension at the PIP joints).

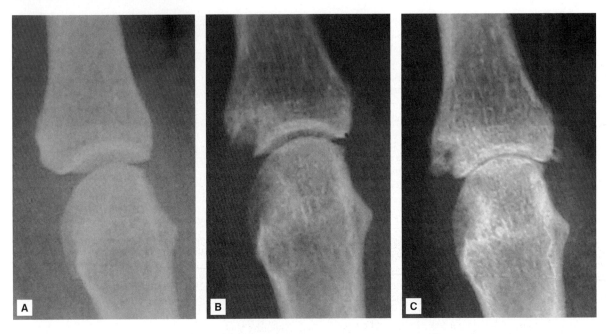

▲ **Figure 13–3.** Progressive destruction of a metacarpophalangeal joint by rheumatoid arthritis (RA). Shown are sequential radiographs of the same second metacarpophalangeal joint. **A:** The joint is normal 1 year prior to the development of RA. **B:** Six months following the onset of RA, there is a bony erosion adjacent to the joint and joint-space narrowing. **C:** After 3 years of disease, diffuse loss of articular cartilage has led to marked joint-space narrowing.

individual joint. In the case of the knee (Figure 13–4A), the medial and lateral compartments are both severely narrowed in RA, whereas OA usually involves only one compartment (Figure 13–4B). Total joint replacements of hips and knees can dramatically improve function and quality of life and should be considered in patients with severe mechanical damage.

Synovial cysts present as fluctuant masses around involved joints (large or small). Synovial cysts from the knee are perhaps the best examples of this phenomenon. The inflamed knee produces excess synovial fluid that can accumulate posteriorly because of a one-way valve effect between the knee joint and the popliteal space (popliteal or **Baker cyst**). Baker cysts cause problems by compressing the popliteal nerve, artery, or veins; by dissecting into the tissues of the calf (usually posteriorly); and by rupturing into calf. Dissection usually produces only minor symptoms such as a feeling of fullness. Rupture of a Baker cyst, however, leads to extravasation of the inflammatory fluid into the calf, producing significant pain and swelling that may be confused with thrombophlebitis (pseudothrombophlebitis syndrome). Ultrasonography of the popliteal fossa and calf is useful to confirm the diagnosis and to rule out thrombophlebitis, which may be precipitated by popliteal cysts. Short-term treatment of popliteal cysts usually involves injecting the knee anteriorly with glucocorticoids to interrupt the inflammatory process.

RA commonly affects **the cervical spine** (especially the C1–C2 articulation) but spares the thoracic, lumbar, and sacral components of the spine. Similar to other synovial joints, bony erosions and ligament damage can affect the odontoid process and disrupt the articulation with C2, leading to subluxation. Most often, subluxation is minor, and patients and caregivers need only be cautious and avoid forcing the neck into positions of flexion. Occasionally, C1–C2 subluxation is severe and requires complex surgical intervention to prevent cervical cord compression.

Wherever synovial tissue exists, RA can cause problems; the temporomandibular, cricoarytenoid, and sternoclavicular joints are examples. The cricoarytenoid joint is responsible for abduction and adduction of the vocal cords. Involvement of this joint may lead to a feeling of fullness in the throat, to hoarseness, or rarely to a syndrome of acute respiratory distress with or without stridor when the cords are essentially frozen in a closed position. Cricoarytenoid joint involvement occasionally precipitates a surgical emergency and the requirement for tracheostomy.

B. Laboratory Findings

Anemia of chronic disease is seen in most patients with RA, and the degree of anemia is proportional to the activity of the disease. Therapy that controls the disease results in a rise of the hemoglobin. White blood cell counts may be elevated, normal,

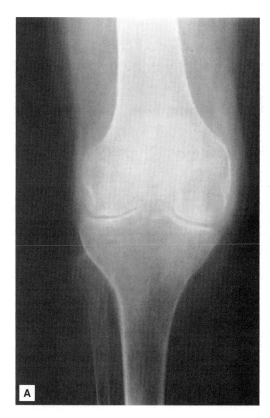
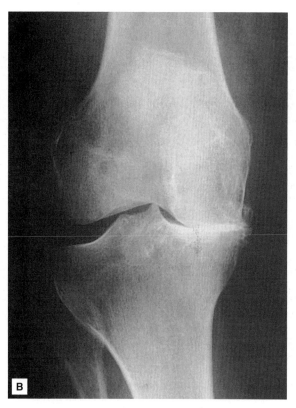

▲ **Figure 13–4.** The radiographic features of rheumatoid arthritis (RA) and osteoarthritis (OA) are compared with regard to large joint involvement. **A:** Symmetric loss of cartilage space that is typical of inflammatory arthritis such as RA. Note that both the medial and lateral compartments are severely narrowed. Despite this severe narrowing, there is very little in the way of subchondral sclerosis or osteophyte formation since these repair mechanisms are generally shut off in active RA. **B:** Complete loss of the cartilage in the medial joint compartment with significant subchondral sclerosis and osteophyte formation. The lateral compartment in this patient is not involved. These features are typical of OA.

or, in the case of Felty syndrome, profoundly depressed. **Thrombocytosis** is common when RA is active, with platelet counts returning to normal as the inflammation is controlled.

An acute phase response, reflected in elevated **erythrocyte sedimentation rates** (ESR) and serum levels of **C-reactive protein** (CRP), often, but not always, parallels the activity of the disease. Persistent elevation of ESR and CRP portends a poor prognosis, both in terms of joint destruction and mortality.

Autoantibodies occur in most patients. The autoantibodies most specific for RA are directed against citrullinated protein epitopes and are detected by use of synthetic cyclic citrullinated peptides (CCP). These **ACPAs** are present in approximately 70% of patients with RA at diagnosis (and often years before diagnosis). ACPAs are 90–98% specific for RA and correlate strongly with erosive disease.

The first autoantibody to be associated with RA was **rheumatoid factor (RF)**, an autoantibody directed against

the constant (Fc) region of IgG. RF is positive in about 50% of cases at presentation and an additional 20–35% of cases become positive in the first 6 months after diagnosis. RF has an unfortunate name because it is not unique to RA and occurs in many other diseases, particularly those characterized by chronic stimulation of the immune system (Table 13–2). In RA, the presence of RF is associated with more severe articular disease, and essentially all patients with the extra-articular features are seropositive for RF. RA is associated with multiple other autoantibodies, including **antinuclear antibodies** (ANA; ~30% of patients) and antineutrophil cytoplasmic antibodies (ANCA), particularly of the perinuclear type (~30% of patients).

Synovial fluid in RA is inflammatory. The white blood cell counts typically range from 5000/mcL to 50,000/mcL with approximately two-thirds of the cells being neutrophils. No synovial fluid findings are pathognomonic of RA.

Table 13–2. Differential of a positive rheumatoid factor.

Rheumatic diseases
Rheumatoid arthritis
Sjögren syndrome
Systemic lupus erythematosus
Others
Infections
Viral: Hepatitis C, EBV, erythrovirus (parvovirus), influenza, others
Bacterial: Endocarditis, osteomyelitis, others
Chronic inflammatory conditions
Liver disease, inflammatory bowel disease, others
Aging

EBV, Epstein-Barr virus.

C. Imaging Studies

Radiographs of rheumatoid joints may demonstrate **juxta-articular demineralization** and **bony erosions**. Early erosions typically occur at the margins of the joint ("marginal erosions"), where synovium directly contacts bone and there is no articular cartilage (see Figure 13–3). Cartilage loss leads to **joint-space narrowing** which, in RA, is uniform (in contrast to OA, which cause irregular narrowing) (see Figures 13–3 and 13–4). Radiographs of the hands and feet are an important component of the evaluation of the patient with RA and should be obtained at the outset and then assessed thereafter at intervals of a year or more. Radiographs are often normal early in the course of RA; the presence of erosions at presentation is associated with a more aggressive course. Erosions of MTPs may be detected prior to radiographic changes in the hands. Progression of erosions and joint-space narrowing is an indication of ongoing joint damage. Radiographs are not sensitive for early changes in hips, knees, elbows, and other large joints but can be very helpful in the assessment of damage in these joints in chronic disease. Radiographs of the cervical spine in flexion and extension can demonstrate C1–C2 subluxation; MRI is the preferred imaging technique to evaluate possible impingement on the spinal cord.

▶ Making the Diagnosis

No single finding on physical examination or laboratory testing is diagnostic of RA. Instead, the diagnosis of RA is a clinical one, requiring a collection of historical and physical features, identified by an astute clinician. The diagnosis of RA requires the objective evidence of joint inflammation (swelling or warmth or both) on examination.

In 1987 the American College of Rheumatology provided classification criteria that, although not designed specifically for the purpose, were widely used as an aid to diagnosis of RA (Table 13–3). The first five criteria—morning stiffness, arthritis of three joint areas, arthritis of the hands, symmetrical arthritis, and rheumatoid nodules—are clinical. The first four of these criteria must be present for at least 6 weeks

Table 13–3. 1987 the American College of Rheumatology classification criteria for rheumatoid arthritis.

• Morning stiffness[a]
• Arthritis of three joint areas[a]
• Arthritis of the hands[a]
• Symmetric arthritis[a]
• Rheumatoid nodules
• Serum rheumatoid factor
• Radiographic changes

[a]These criteria must be present for more than 6 weeks.

before a patient can be classified as having RA. This time requirement was imposed because a number of conditions, most notably viral-related syndromes, can cause self-limited polyarthritis that is indistinguishable from RA (Table 13–4). Such viral syndromes, for example, that caused by parvovirus, generally have a duration of 2–4 weeks.

The 1987 classification criteria perform well for the diagnosis of established RA but are of limited utility for the diagnosis of early disease and do not incorporate testing for anti-CCP antibodies, which are highly specific for RA. In 2010 the American College of Rheumatology and the European League Against Rheumatism collaborated to develop new classification criteria with the explicit goal of improved sensitivity and specificity for early RA. The 2010 classification criteria, which require synovitis in at least one joint and the absence of a more plausible alternative diagnosis, use a composite scoring system based on four domains: (1) the number and site of affected joints; (2) the presence and level of anti-CCP antibodies and RF; (3) acute phase reactants (ESR and CRP); (4) duration of symptoms for more than 6 weeks (see Table 13–4).

▶ Differential Diagnosis

Many diseases can mimic RA (Table 13–5), and the accurate diagnosis of early RA can be particularly challenging. Acute viral syndromes, especially acute hepatitis B, erythrovirus (parvovirus B19), rubella (infection or vaccination), and Epstein-Barr virus can produce a polyarthritis that mimics early RA but is self-limited, usually resolving over 2–4 weeks. Atypical early presentations of RA can be difficult to distinguish from the initial stages of undifferentiated spondyloarthropathy, psoriatic arthritis, and reactive arthritis. A careful history and physical examination, however, may elucidate distinctive clinical features associated with these diseases, such as rash, oral ulcers, nail changes, dactylitis, and urethritis. There can be considerable clinical and serologic overlap between RA and systemic lupus erythematosus. Anti-Jo-1-positive polymyositis can present with an erosive polyarthritis, a positive test for serum RF, and minimal muscle symptoms. Chronic infection with hepatitis C commonly causes polyarthralgias (less often, polyarthritis)

Table 13–4. The 2010 classification criteria for rheumatoid arthritis.

Criteria[a,b]	Score
A. Joint involvement	0
1 large joint	1
2–10 large joints	3
1–3 small joints	4
>10 joints (at least 1 small joint)	
B. Serology	0
Negative RF and anti-CCP	2
Low-positive RF or anti-CCP	3
High-positive RF or anti-CCP	
C. Acute phase reactants	0
Normal CRP and ESR	1
Abnormal CRP or ESR	
D. Duration of symptoms	0
<6 weeks	1
≥6 weeks	

[a]Criteria apply only to patients who have objective signs of synovitis in at least 1 joint and who do not have a better alternative explanation for synovitis.
[b]A patient is classified as having rheumatoid arthritis if the sum of A–D is >6.
CCP, citrullinated peptides; CRP, C-reactive protein; ESR, erythrocyte sedimentation rate; RF, rheumatoid factor.
Adapted from Aletaha D, Neogi T, Silman AJ, et al. 2010 Rheumatoid arthritis classification criteria: an American College of Rheumatology/European League Against Rheumatism collaborative initiative. *Arthritis Rheum.* 2010;62:2569.

in a joint distribution similar to that of RA. Moreover, patients with chronic hepatitis C infections are often RF positive—particularly if they also have circulating cryoglobulins. Hepatitis C patients are not, however, generally ACPA positive, nor do they have radiographic erosions. In some patients, of course, RA and hepatitis C viral infections can both be present, by virtue of their relatively high prevalence.

In an elderly patient with the abrupt onset of polyarthritis, remitting seronegative symmetric synovitis with pitting edema (RS3PE), paraneoplastic syndromes, and drug-induced

Table 13–5. Differential diagnosis.

Viral syndromes, especially hepatitis B and C, Epstein-Barr virus, erythrovirus (parvovirus), rubella
Psoriatic arthritis, reactive arthritis
Tophaceous gout
Systemic lupus erythematosus
Calcium pyrophosphate disease
Polymyalgia rheumatica
Paraneoplastic syndromes
Osteoarthritis, especially hereditary osteoarthritis of the hand
Sarcoidosis, Lyme disease, rheumatic fever, etc

lupus should be considered. Chronic tophaceous gout can also mimic severe nodular RA, and chondrocalcinosis can cause a destructive "pseudorheumatoid" arthropathy of the wrists and MCPs. Finally, OA with severe deformities of the hands from bony proliferation of the DIP and PIP joints (Heberden and Bouchard nodes) may confuse inexperienced clinicians; the keys here are DIP joint involvement and the bony, instead of soft tissue, joint abnormalities.

Complications

RA is a lifelong, progressive disease that can produce significant morbidity and premature mortality. Long-term studies have found that 50% or more RA patients have to stop working after 5–10 years (approximately 10 times the average rate). Patients who have anti-CCP antibodies, who are RF positive, or who have *HLADRB1* alleles expressing the shared epitope have a worse prognosis with more erosions and more extra-articular disease. Once deformities are found on examination or erosions on radiography, the damage is largely irreversible. Erosions develop in the majority of patients in the first 1 or 2 years of disease, but early effective therapy clearly slows the rate of radiographic damage.

TREATMENT

RA is a chronic disease requiring lifelong treatment for most patients. Fortunately, many new highly effective therapies are now available. Their efficacy is greatest if these treatments are started early in the course of the disease.

Early RA appears to represent a "window of opportunity" in which aggressive treatment with disease-modifying antirheumatic drugs (DMARDs) can lead to better long-term outcomes. Therapy may be escalated, or introduced in combination and subsequently reduced, to ensure maximal suppression of disease while making efforts to minimize toxicity and expense.

Therapeutic approaches should be more aggressive for patients with early RA and features of poor prognosis (eg, seropositivity for RF or ACPA, erosive disease on radiographs, the presence of extra-articular disease manifestations, or major functional limitation at diagnosis). In such cases, aggressive therapy is important because once deformities are present the mechanical component is refractory to medical therapy.

Because RA is a dynamic disease and because its therapeutic regimens are complex, it is essential that rheumatologists monitor patients regularly. Treat-to-target approaches that involve frequent evaluations and medication adjustments aimed to achieve optimal suppression of inflammation and disease control are associated with more successful outcomes.

Pharmacotherapy

There are many more medications that are effective in managing RA compared to the mid-1990s, before the development of biologic therapies. Conventional synthetic DMARDs

Table 13–6. Conventional synthetic disease-modifying antirheumatic drugs.

Methotrexate
Hydroxychloroquine
Sulfasalazine
Leflunomide

(Table 13–6), biologic DMARDs, and newer small-molecule inhibitors (Table 13–7) all have roles in the treatment of RA. Glucocorticoids and nonsteroidal anti-inflammatory drugs (NSAIDs) also continue to play a role in the treatment of many patients, though the goal increasingly is to obviate the need for their use entirely. Almost all patients require more than one type of medication.

A. Glucocorticoids

Low-dose glucocorticoids (eg, prednisone 5–10 mg daily) can provide rapid symptomatic improvement of articular disease and significantly slow the radiographic progression of RA. Glucocorticoids are not appropriate as monotherapy for RA but can help control synovial inflammation before the effects of slow-acting csDMARDs have become apparent or if the response to csDMARDs is suboptimal. The toxicities of long-term glucocorticoid therapy are considerable and are mostly dose-dependent. Therefore, prednisone, the most commonly used glucocorticoid, generally should not be used in doses higher than 10 mg daily to treat articular disease and, after initiation of DMARD therapy, should be slowly tapered off or to the lowest effective dose. Long-term therapy with prednisone in doses of greater than or equal to 7.5 mg/day orally

is associated with an increased risk of vertebral and hip fractures and other glucocorticoid toxicities, and some patients have important toxicities at lower doses than 5 mg/day.

Intra-articular injections of glucocorticoids (see Chapter 2) can suppress joint inflammation for several months and can be a useful addition to DMARD therapy, especially when there is residual activity in large joints (eg, wrists, knees). In many cases, patients benefit from consultation with physical and occupational therapists regarding range of motion exercises, joint protection, and assistive devices.

B. Nonsteroidal Anti-Inflammatory Drugs

Nonsteroidal anti-inflammatory drugs (NSAIDs) play only a minor role, if any, in slowing progression of RA. These medications should not be used as the sole therapy for RA but they still provide an important measure of symptomatic relief in some patients. The gastrointestinal toxicity of NSAIDs is a major issue for RA patients, who often have multiple risk factors for gastrointestinal toxicity. The use of protein pump inhibitors reduces the incidence of clinically significant gastrointestinal side effects.

C. Disease-Modifying Antirheumatic Drugs

With rare exceptions, all patients should receive DMARD therapy. Optimal control of disease activity often requires combinations of different synthetic DMARDs or combinations of synthetic DMARDs and a biologic DMARD. Prior to starting DMARD therapy, patients should receive vaccinations (see recommendations of the American College of Rheumatology). Live attenuated vaccines are contraindicated once individuals have started biologic DMARDs, so careful planning is required when initiating therapy.

Table 13–7. Biologic disease-modifying antirheumatic drugs and small-molecule inhibitors.

Agent	Structure	Target	Route of Administration
Infliximab	Chimeric mouse/human IgG1 mAb	TNF-α	Intravenous infusion
Etanercept	Fusion of human p75 TNF receptor and human IgG1 Fc	TNF-α Lymphotoxin	Subcutaneous injection
Adalimumab	Human IgG1 mAb	TNF-α	Subcutaneous injection
Golimumab	Human IgG1 mAb	TNF-α	Subcutaneous injection
Certolizumab pegol[a]	Humanized Fab' linked to PEG	TNF-α	Subcutaneous injection
Abatacept	Fusion protein of human CTLA4 and Fc of human IgG1	CD80, CD86	Intravenous infusion or subcutaneous injection
Rituximab	Chimeric mouse/human IgG1 mAb	CD20	Intravenous infusion
Tocilizumab	Chimeric mouse/human IgG1 mAb	Interleukin-6 receptor	Intravenous infusion or subcutaneous injection
Sarilumab	Human IgG mAb	Interleukin-6 receptor	Subcutaneous injection
Baricitinib	Small-molecule inhibitor	Jak1 and Jak2	Oral
Tofacitinib	Small-molecule inhibitor	Jak1 and Jak3	Oral
Upadacitinib	Small-molecule inhibitor	Jak1	Oral

[a]PEG, polyethylene glycol.

D. Conventional Synthetic Disease-Modifying Antirheumatic Drugs

Conventional synthetic (cs) DMARDs are a group of medications that modify or change the disease course of RA. Drugs included in this class have met the "gold standard" of halting or slowing the radiographic progression of disease. The synthetic DMARDs in current use are methotrexate, sulfasalazine, hydroxychloroquine, leflunomide, and minocycline. These medications take at least 12 weeks to reach maximal effect. Therefore, other measures, such as low-dose glucocorticoid therapy, may provide control of the disease while these medications are starting to work. The choice of csDMARD depends on the activity of the disease, comorbid conditions, concerns about toxicity, and monitoring issues. They are often used in combination with one another (most often, various combinations of methotrexate, sulfasalazine, and hydroxychloroquine) or with a biologic DMARD.

Methotrexate is the csDMARD prescribed most frequently by most rheumatologists. Many patients with RA have a durable, clinically meaningful response to methotrexate, which also slows radiographic progression of the disease. Although often effective as monotherapy, methotrexate is also the anchor drug in most successful combinations of csDMARDs. Combination use of methotrexate with most types of biologic DMARDs has shown synergy with regard to disease control and improved clinical outcomes compared with either methotrexate or the biological DMARD alone.

Methotrexate is administered as a **single dose once a week**—never on a daily basis—because toxicity is substantially greater when the same amount of drug is administered on a daily basis rather than as a weekly pulse. The typical starting dose is 7.5–10 mg orally once a week. This dose then is increased by 2.5–5 mg increments as needed to a maximum of 25 mg. Because oral absorption of methotrexate is variable, subcutaneous methotrexate may be effective if the response to oral methotrexate is suboptimal. Parenteral administration of methotrexate is now more and more common. Oral folate (1–4 mg daily) reduces side effects and should be administered concomitantly. Monitoring of blood cell counts, liver transaminase levels, and serum creatinine should be performed every 2–4 weeks during initiation or after dose adjustments, and then every 3 months thereafter for the duration of methotrexate therapy. Serious toxicities are rare with careful monitoring.

Contraindications to methotrexate include preexisting liver disease, infection with hepatitis B or C, ongoing excess alcohol use, and renal impairment (creatinine clearance <30 mL/min). Oral ulcers, nausea, hepatotoxicity, bone marrow suppression, and pneumonitis are the most commonly encountered toxicities. With the exception of pneumonitis (which may result as a hypersensitivity reaction), these toxicities respond to dose adjustments and are reduced by the concomitant use of folic acid. Renal function is critical for clearance of methotrexate and its active metabolites; previously stable patients may experience severe toxicities when renal function deteriorates. Pneumonitis, while rare, is unpredictable and may be fatal, particularly if the methotrexate is not stopped or is restarted.

Hydroxychloroquine is frequently used for the initial treatment of mild RA, often in combination with other csDMARDs, particularly methotrexate. It has the least toxicity of all the csDMARDs but also is the least effective as monotherapy. Hydroxychloroquine is administered orally at a dose of 200–400 mg daily. An uncommon but serious complication is retinal toxicity, which correlates with cumulative dose and is more likely to occur in patients of small stature are treated at full doses. The incidence of hydroxychloroquine, which may be irreversible, can be reduced by regular screening by an ophthalmologist. The risk of retinal toxicity increases substantially after 5–7 years of use or a cumulative dose of 1000 g. At a minimum, patients should have a baseline ophthalmologic examination and annual screening examinations thereafter. Particular vigilance for hydroxychloroquine retinotoxicity is indicated for patients whose daily dose is greater than 400 mg or greater than 6.5 mg/kg of ideal body weight for patients of short stature, those with kidney or liver dysfunction, those with other forms of retinal disease, and those greater than 60 years of age.

Sulfasalazine is an effective treatment when given in doses of 1–3 g daily, often in combination with methotrexate, hydroxychloroquine, or both. Recommendations for laboratory monitoring are the same as for methotrexate. Sulfasalazine should not be given to patients with a history of sulfa sensitivity.

Leflunomide, a pyrimidine antagonist, appears comparable in effectiveness to methotrexate. It is given daily in an oral dose of 10–20 mg. The most common toxicity is diarrhea, which may respond to dose reduction. Leflunomide can also be associated with hepatotoxicity, and the recommendations for laboratory monitoring with this drug are the same as for methotrexate. Because leflunomide is teratogenic and has an exceptionally long half-life, women who have previously received leflunomide (even if therapy was years ago) should have blood levels drawn if they wish to become pregnant. Oral cholestyramine can rapidly eliminate leflunomide if toxicity occurs or if pregnancy is being considered.

E. Biologic Disease-Modifying Antirheumatic Drugs

Biologic DMARDs, which generally consist of either bioengineered protein monoclonal antibodies or fusion proteins, must be administered by subcutaneous injection or intravenous infusion (see Table 13–7). Biologic DMARDs now target an ever-expanding array of points within the immune system, including the inhibition of tumor necrosis factor-α (anti-TNF agents), the depletion of CD20+ B cells (rituximab), interference with T-cell costimulation (abatacept), and blockade of the receptor for interleukin-6 (tocilizumab). The efficacy of biologic DMARDs is well established, and these medications are among the most carefully studied drugs in the history of pharmacology. All reduce the signs and symptoms of synovitis—even in patients who have active disease despite treatment with methotrexate—and substantially diminish radiographic progression of RA. Moreover, the onset of action of biologic DMARDs is rapid: days to weeks. All have greater efficacy when used in combination with methotrexate. The major disadvantages are cost and concerns about toxicities.

An increased risk of infection is a concern with all biologic DMARDs—as is true for glucocorticoids and many csDMARDs (including methotrexate), as well. All patients under consideration for a biologic agent should be screened for latent tuberculosis with a chest radiograph and either a tuberculin skin test or an interferon-γ-release assay. TNF inhibitors in particular are known to increase the risk of latent tuberculosis reactivation. Active tuberculosis and untreated latent tuberculosis both constitute absolute contraindications to the use of biologic DMARDs. Reactivation of latent tuberculosis has occurred within weeks of starting anti-TNF agents, particularly infliximab, but TNF inhibitors also confer a greatly increased risk of infection with other intracellular pathogens (eg, *Histoplasma capsulatum, Coccidioides immitis,* and *Listeria monocytogenes*).

No biologic DMARDs of any type should be administered to patients with untreated hepatitis B infection or latent hepatitis B infection. Rituximab or other B cell-depleting agents are of particular concern with regard to their propensity to trigger the reactivation of latent hepatitis B. Latent hepatitis B infection, particularly prevalent in a high percentage of patients from Asia and South Asia (who usually acquired the infection at birth), can be detected by antibodies against the hepatitis B core antigen. Patients who are hepatitis B core antibody positive should be considered for prophylaxis against hepatitis B reactivation, regardless of their status with regard to the presence of antibodies to hepatitis B surface antigen. Consultation with an infectious disease expert can be helpful in the interpretation of hepatitis B serologies and decisions around the use of hepatitis B treatment or prophylaxis, which is highly effective and well tolerated. Once patients' hepatitis B status has been addressed adequately, most patients can be treated with appropriate biologic agents for their RA.

There is a paucity of data regarding the use of biologic DMARDs in patients with a history of malignancy. Currently, biologic agents (except rituximab) are not recommended for patients with a solid malignancy or nonmelanoma skin cancer treated within 5 years, a history of treated skin melanoma, or a history of treated lymphoproliferative malignancy.

Anti-TNF agents should not be administered to patients with New York Heart Association class III or IV congestive heart failure or with ejection fractions less than 50%, as this may cause increased heart failure.

F. Janus Kinase (JAK) Inhibitors

Small-molecule inhibitors of the JAK-STAT pathway are the newest class of agents to enter the therapeutic arena for RA. Three agents—tofacitinib, baricitinib, and upadacitinib—are now in widespread use, and more such agents are under development. These agents are slightly lower in price than originator biologic agents but more expensive than biosimilars. They

have the advantage of the oral route of administration. There does appear to be an increased risk of herpes zoster reactivation compared to other available biologic agents.

▶ Assessment of Disease Activity

Accurate assessment of disease activity by objective measures is recommended to judge the effectiveness of treatment but this is often a difficult task. In practice, rheumatologists often gauge activity by their "clinical gestalt" which, in most cases, is heavily influenced by the results of the joint examination. However, the American College of Rheumatology recommends the use of standardized clinical assessments of disease activity to judge the effectiveness of treatment (Table 13–8). Several of these assessments are based solely on self-report (the patient activity scale [PAS], and routine assessment of patient index [RAPID]) or on joint counts and visual analogue scales (the clinical disease activity index [CDAI]). Assessments such as the disease activity scale 28 joints (DAS28) and the simplified disease activity index (SDAI) use joint counts and visual analogue scales but also incorporate a marker of inflammation (the ESR or CRP). Each assessment yields a numeric score and has cut points corresponding to remission and to low, moderate, and high disease activity (see Table 13–8).

▼ EXTRA-ARTICULAR MANIFESTATIONS

Extra-articular disease develops in approximately one-third of patients with RA at some point in the course of their illness. The extra-articular manifestations of RA are diverse (Table 13–9) and range in clinical impact from the minor nuisance of a few isolated subcutaneous nodules to the life-threatening consequences of progressive interstitial pulmonary fibrosis and rheumatoid vasculitis. Extra-articular manifestations occur almost exclusively in patients who are seropositive for RF or ACPA. Moreover, these frequently severe manifestations of RA often cluster together (eg, the co-occurrence of subcutaneous nodules and interstitial fibrosis). The incidence of extra-articular disease appears to be decreasing, probably as a result of the widespread use of aggressive therapy earlier in the course of RA disease (eg, combination csDMARDs plus bDMARDs). Nonetheless, familiarity with the broad spectrum of extra-articular rheumatoid disease is critical for the appropriate management of RA patients.

RHEUMATOID NODULES

ESSENTIALS OF DIAGNOSIS

▶ Usually manifest as subcutaneous nodules over pressure points, such as the extensor surfaces of the elbows and the knuckles.

▶ Strongly associated with RF.

Table 13–8. Standardized assessments disease activity for rheumatoid arthritis.

Assessment	Components	Disease Activity by Numerical Score			
		Remission	Low	Moderate	High
PAS	Questionnaire Pain scale Patient global	≤0.25	0.26 – 3.7	3.71 – <8.0	≥8.0
RAPID3	Questionnaire Pain scale Patient global	≤1.0	>1.0 – 2.0	>2.0 – 4.0	>4.0
CDAI	Patient global Physician global Swollen joints Tender joints	≤2.8	>2.8 – 10.0	>10.0 – 22.0	>22.0
SDAI	Patient global Physician global Swollen joints Tender joints CRP	≤3.3	>3.3 – <11	11.0 – ≤26.0	>26.0
DAS28	Patient global Swollen joints Tender joints ESR or CRP	<2.6	>2.6 – <3.2	≥3.2 – ≤5.1	>5.1

Joints examined: proximal phalangeal joints, interphalangeal joints of thumbs, metacarpophalangeal joints, wrists, elbows, shoulders, knees.

CDAI, clinical disease activity index; CRP, C-reactive protein; DAS28, disease activity score 28 joints; ESR, erythrocyte sedimentation rate; PAS, patient activity scale; RAPID, routine assessment of patient index data; SDAI, simplified disease activity index.

▶ Clinical Findings & Treatment

Subcutaneous nodules occur in 20–35% of patients with RA and are usually nontender, firm, and 1 cm or less in diameter. Subcutaneous nodules can be fixed or mobile and occur most frequently over pressure point areas such as the extensor aspect of the elbows, within the olecranon bursa, and over the Achilles tendon but also can overlie joints (Figures 13–5 and 13-6). Nodulosis over the sacrum, ischial tuberosities, occipital region of the scalp, or borders of the scapulae may develop in bedridden patients. Rarely, nodules develop within organ systems, including the scleral layer of the eye, heart valves, lung, on the dural surface of the brain, or in the larynx.

Rheumatoid nodules are strongly associated with RF, which is positive in more than 95% of cases. Patients with RA who smoke have a higher risk of developing nodules. Strongly seropositive individuals with nodulosis tend to carry a worse prognosis, with a higher propensity toward erosive and destructive rheumatoid disease.

The mimics of subcutaneous rheumatoid nodules include tophi, xanthomas, calcinosis, Garrod knuckle pads (fibrous nodules on the dorsal surfaces of the PIP joints of patients with Dupuytren contractures), the nodules of multicentric reticulohistiocytosis, and, in children, the nodules of acute rheumatic fever. On clinical grounds alone, even experienced rheumatologists may be unable to distinguish RA with olecranon nodulosis from polyarticular gout with olecranon tophi. Excisional biopsy is sometimes necessary to establish the correct diagnosis. Rheumatoid nodules have characteristic—but not specific—histologic findings of central fibrinoid necrosis with a rim of palisading fibroblasts. Histologically, rheumatoid nodules are indistinguishable from granuloma annulare (dermal or subcutaneous nodules not associated with arthritis) or from "benign nodules" that occur exclusively in children less than 18 years of age and are not associated with arthritis or with RF.

Subcutaneous rheumatoid nodules may resolve with effective therapy of the associated articular disease. A subset of rheumatoid patients, however, experiences a paradoxical acceleration of nodulosis with methotrexate therapy. Nodules in these patients are often found over the extensor aspect of the MCP and PIP joints of the fingers. Methotrexate should be discontinued when there is extensive proliferation of nodules, particularly with ulceration of overlying skin. Unfortunately, there is no effective therapy for this situation. Most alternative DMARDs have been tried in these cases but with only occasional success.

Symptomatic subcutaneous nodules located over pressure points can be surgically removed. The effectiveness of this surgical approach, however, is limited by high rates of recurrence of nodules, poor wound healing, and secondary infection at the operative site, often with *S aureus*.

Table 13–9. Extra-articular manifestations.

Dermatologic	Rheumatoid nodules with and without ulceration Vasculitis nailfold infarcts; leg ulcers Pyoderma gangrenosa (rare)
Mucosal	Sicca symptoms Ocular, oral, vaginal mucosa Sjögren syndrome
Ocular	Keratoconjunctivitis sicca Episcleritis Scleritis Scleromalacia perforans Peripheral ulcerative keratitis
Pulmonary	Nonspecific interstitial pneumonitis Usual interstitial pneumonitis Cryptogenic organizing pneumonitis Bronchiectasis Bronchiolitis obliterans Pleuritis and pleural effusion Rheumatoid nodulosis in the lungs Caplan syndrome
Cardiac	Pericarditis and pericardial effusion Constrictive pericarditis Valvular thickening and nodulosis Conduction abnormalities Coronary vasculitis Myocarditis
Hematologic and lymphatic system	Anemia of chronic disease Felty syndrome Large granular lymphocyte leukemia Extremity lymphedema—unilateral or bilateral
Neurologic	Compression neuropathies Atlantoaxial subluxation Peripheral neuropathy Mononeuritis multiplex Rheumatoid pachymeningitis
Renal	AA amyloidosis Necrotizing crescentic glomerulonephritis (rare)

Rheumatoid nodules in the lung may be solitary or multiple, and some are necrotic. Isolated reports suggest a possible link between leflunomide therapy and necrotic pulmonary nodules. Distinguishing rheumatoid pulmonary nodules from carcinoma can be a particularly difficult problem, even after extensive imaging evaluation with computed tomography (CT) and positron emission tomographic scans. CT-guided biopsy is usually the only certain means of differentiating between these possibilities. Rheumatoid nodules in the lung can also be difficult to distinguish from the pulmonary nodules associated with granulomatosis with polyangiitis.

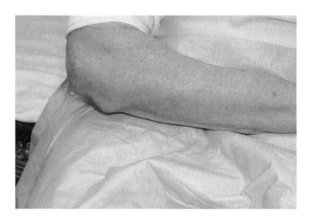

▲ **Figure 13–5.** A rheumatoid nodule in a typical location on the extensor surface of the forearm is apparent in this patient with seropositive, erosive rheumatoid arthritis.

A variant of rheumatoid pulmonary nodulosis is Caplan syndrome. In 1953, Caplan described multiple rheumatoid nodules, some with cavitation, in the lungs of Welsh coal miners with RA. This pattern has also been reported in RA patients exposed to silica dust and asbestos, raising the question of whether Caplan syndrome is a combined "pneumoconiosis—RA" entity.

SJÖGREN SYNDROME

 ESSENTIALS OF DIAGNOSIS

▶ Dryness of eyes and mouth.
▶ The most common ocular manifestation of RA.

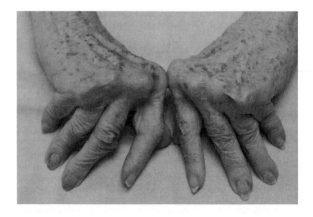

▲ **Figure 13–6.** Prominent rheumatoid nodules over the metacarpophalangeal joints.

Clinical Findings

Approximately 30% of patients with RA have sicca symptoms due to secondary Sjögren syndrome. Mucosal dryness most commonly affects the mouth, the conjunctival surfaces of the eyes, and vagina. Dental caries, gingivitis, and accelerated tooth loss may occur due to the lack of adequate salivary lubrication. Patients frequently experience a chronic "foreign body" sensation in their eyes. Women often develop recurrent monilial infections of the vaginal mucosa.

Care must be exercised in distinguishing typical Sjögren syndrome symptoms from xerostomia due to medications, particularly antidepressants. Chronic hepatitis C infection, which can cause polyarthritis, sicca symptoms, and RF, also can mimic RA with secondary Sjögren syndrome. Finally, it is occasionally difficult to distinguish RA with secondary Sjögren syndrome from primary Sjögren syndrome with polyarthritis.

The diagnostic evaluations to establish xerophthalmia and xerostomia are those used for primary Sjögren syndrome (see Chapter 24). In contrast to primary Sjögren syndrome, antibodies to SS-A/Ro and to SS-B/La are not prevalent in the secondary Sjögren syndrome associated with RA.

Compared to patients with primary Sjögren syndrome, hypergammaglobulinemia, interstitial nephritis, and distal renal tubular acidosis are not typical of patients with RA and secondary Sjögren syndrome. Additional rare complications include the development of non-Hodgkin large B cell lymphomas or mucosa-associated lymphoid tissue (MALT).

Treatment

Treatment of secondary Sjögren syndrome is symptomatic. Artificial tears or cyclosporine 0.05% emulsion drops twice daily can ease ocular symptoms. Pilocarpine hydrochloride 5 mg orally three to four times daily or cevimeline 30 mg three times daily may be effective in promoting increased salivary production but can cause hyperhidrosis.

OCULAR INFLAMMATION

ESSENTIALS OF DIAGNOSIS

▶ RA can cause episcleritis, scleritis, and peripheral ulcerative keratitis.

▶ Nodular scleritis and peripheral ulcerative keratitis threaten vision and require aggressive immunosuppressive therapy.

Clinical Findings & Treatment

Keratoconjunctivitis sicca due to secondary Sjögren syndrome is the most common ocular manifestation of RA.

However, RA can also cause ocular inflammation, leading to episcleritis, scleritis, and peripheral ulcerative keratitis.

Episcleritis, or inflammation of the episclera, manifests as a red eye due to hyperemia of this superficial ocular layer. Episcleritis produces irritation more than pain and does not constitute a vision-threatening condition. Episcleritis occurs occasionally in individuals who do not have RA or any other immune-mediated condition. Episcleritis is often self-limited but can be treated with topical glucocorticoid drops.

Of greater concern is inflammation of the sclera, the deeper, poorly vascularized layer of the eye. **Scleritis** is most commonly seen in patients who have had RA for 10 years or longer. Patients who are both RF and ACPA positive tend to have more intense ocular disease. Scleritis is a painful, persistent, and potentially vision-threatening condition. The eye typically is deep red. With time, thinning of the sclera can occur, imparting a bluish hue from the underlying choroid. Scleritis can be complicated by rheumatoid nodules that form and enlarge within the scleral layer. Unchecked, scleritis can produce scleromalacia perforans and can threaten the structural integrity of the globe. Inadequate or unsuccessful treatment can lead to irreversible blindness. Nodular scleritis is an urgent ophthalmologic problem that requires initiation of intensive immunosuppressive therapy. Cyclophosphamide in combination with high-dose oral prednisone (eg, 1 mg/kg/day) has been the traditional approach. Rituximab is now often considered instead of cyclophosphamide.

An additional serious ocular complication of RA is peripheral ulcerative keratitis, which can be associated with a "melting" of the corneal epithelial layers. Again, this is seen in long-standing RA, often accompanied by rheumatoid vasculitis or other serious extra-articular manifestations. Peripheral ulcerative keratitis must be aggressively as it poses an even more immediate threat to vision than scleritis. In patients who have suffered a corneal melt, a corneal transplant can be performed to salvage vision if the inflammation is successfully ameliorated.

INTERSTITIAL LUNG DISEASE

ESSENTIALS OF DIAGNOSIS

▶ Risk factors include RF, male sex, and smoking.

▶ High-resolution CT is the imaging modality of choice.

▶ Nonspecific interstitial pneumonitis is glucocorticoid-responsive but usual interstitial pneumonitis is often refractory to therapy.

General Considerations

Interstitial fibrosis of the lungs is one of the most dreaded complications of RA and often carries a guarded prognosis.

The prevalence of clinically evident pulmonary fibrosis among RA patients is approximately 2–3%, and the prevalence of asymptomatic pulmonary fibrosis detected by high-resolution CT (HRCT) is substantially higher. The cumulative incidence of clinical pulmonary fibrosis approaches 10%.

▶ Clinical Findings & Treatment

Virtually all patients with interstitial fibrosis are seropositive for RF and have ACPA. Risk factors include male sex and smoking. Patients with interstitial lung disease often have subcutaneous nodules.

Dyspnea on exertion and nonproductive cough are the most common symptoms of interstitial fibrosis. On examination, there may be fine crackles at the bases. The chest radiograph may show an interstitial pattern but is inadequate for assessing the extent of pulmonary fibrosis. HRCT scanning is the current imaging gold standard. Pulmonary function tests reveal a restrictive defect and decreased diffusing capacity.

Nonspecific interstitial pneumonitis (NSIP) and usual interstitial pneumonitis (UIP) are the most common pathologic types of fibrosis encountered. NSIP has a more uniform distribution on plain radiographs and a "ground glass" appearance on HRCT. UIP has a more basilar distribution of fibrosis. HRCT scanning in UIP demonstrates honeycomb patterns and, frequently, traction bronchiectasis (Figure 13–7). If a biopsy is being considered, it is best to obtain a more robust specimen by video-assisted thoracoscopy because transbronchial biopsies through a flexible bronchoscope yield inadequate

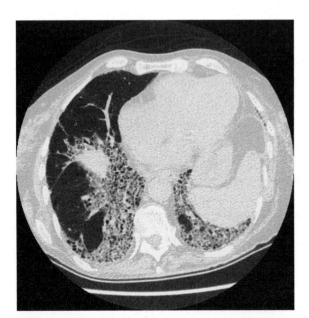

▲ **Figure 13–7.** Rheumatoid interstitial lung disease: usual interstitial pneumonitis.

pathologic material. It is not uncommon to have equivocal or inconsistent interpretations of pulmonary biopsies as specimens may contain pathologic features of both NSIP and UIP.

NSIP is often responsive to glucocorticoids, but there are no current treatments capable of halting the progression of UIP. Nonetheless, most rheumatologists and pulmonologists will initiate a trial of oral prednisone (1 mg/kg/day) regardless of the whether the pathology indicates UIP or NSIP. Prednisone is then tapered in accordance with the clinical picture and the results of serial pulmonary function tests, especially the diffusing capacity. There is little evidence for an ameliorative effect of anti-TNF agents on interstitial fibrosis. Other therapies such as B cell depletion have not been studied adequately but should be considered. There is little evidence that csDMARDs such as azathioprine are useful in this setting. More recently, however, nintedanib has been proven to be effective in interstitial lung disease. This drug appears to have synergy with mycophenolate mofetil, which should also be considered in combination with nintedanib in patients with substantial rheumatoid lung disease.

Patients with preexisting interstitial lung disease may be at increased risk for methotrexate-induced pneumonitis—a hypersensitivity reaction to the drug. Because of this concern, many clinicians obtain a pretreatment chest radiograph and do not use methotrexate if there are radiographic signs of early interstitial lung disease.

OTHER PULMONARY MANIFESTATIONS OF RA

Cryptogenic organizing pneumonia produces a characteristic pattern on HRCT (multiple patches of consolidation in the subpleural areas) and is often responsive to glucocorticoids. Additional pulmonary complications of RA include bronchiectasis, which is present in approximately 3% of patients, and bronchiolitis obliterans, which is rare, poorly responsive to therapy, and frequently leads to severe pulmonary compromise with hypoxia.

PLEURAL INVOLVEMENT

 ESSENTIALS OF DIAGNOSIS

▶ Rheumatoid pleurisy and pleural effusions can precede the articular manifestations of RA.

▶ Very low levels of pleural-fluid glucose are characteristic.

▶ Clinical Findings

Pleurisy or pleural effusion or both can be the initial manifestation of RA, preceding the onset of articular disease. This infrequent event occurs in approximately 1–3% of patients, most of whom are male. Analysis of pleural fluid is necessary to exclude malignancy, bacterial empyema, and infections with *Mycobacterium tuberculosis* and other granulomatous organisms; in some cases, a pleural biopsy is indicated as well. Rheumatoid pleural fluid is exudative and characterized by an extremely low level of pleural-fluid glucose, with the result frequently approaching zero. Some believe that a pleural fluid glucose in this range is diagnostic of a rheumatoid effusion. The low glucose is thought to be secondary to a defect in glucose transport across the pleural membrane.

▶ Treatment

Treatment of rheumatoid pleuritis consists of moderate- to high-dose prednisone tapered in accordance with the clinical response. Pleurodesis or decortication may be required in unresponsive cases.

PERICARDIAL & CARDIAC INVOLVEMENT

Clinically evident **pericarditis** is uncommon in RA, but postmortem and echocardiographic examination reveal evidence of pericardial involvement in 30–50% of patients. Pericardial fluid shows findings similar to those of pleural fluid, notably a very low glucose. Rarely, pericardial involvement leads to **constrictive pericarditis**. This complication requires pericardiectomy with removal of the fibrotic and adherent pericardium. Additional cardiac involvement includes valvular thickening with nodules, valvular insufficiency, conduction abnormalities secondary to localized granulomatous inflammation, coronary vasculitis, and myocarditis. Advances in ultrasonography, particularly transesophageal echocardiography, have uncovered a higher prevalence of these cardiac abnormalities than previously recognized.

FELTY SYNDROME

ESSENTIALS OF DIAGNOSIS

▶ Development of neutropenia and splenomegaly in long-standing seropositive RA.

▶ Increased risk of serious infection and of lower extremity ulcers due to rheumatoid vasculitis.

▶ Large granular lymphocytic leukemia present in 30% of patients.

▶ General Considerations

In 1924, Augustus Felty, then a medical resident, described the co-occurrence of RA, splenomegaly, and neutropenia. Now uncommon, Felty syndrome develops in patients with long-standing, erosive RA who are seropositive for RF and ACPA.

▶ Clinical Findings

The hallmarks of the syndrome are leukopenia (<4000 white blood cells/mcL), neutropenia (<1500 neutrophils/mcL), and splenomegaly. The hematologic components of the syndrome, however, can be present without frank splenomegaly. Approximately 30% of patients with Felty syndrome have large granular lymphocytic leukemia (see next). Chronic neutropenia puts patients with Felty syndrome at risk for serious infections, but many patients remain asymptomatic.

Patients with Felty syndrome often have synovitis that appears bland and "burnt out," but these patients are far from inactive. About one-third have evidence of rheumatoid vasculitis with necrotic leg ulcers. Some are positive for perinuclear antineutrophil cytoplasmic antibodies (P-ANCA), antimyeloperoxidase antibodies, and cryoglobulins.

Rarely, fibrosis develops in the hepatic portal system, which leads to portal hypertension, esophageal varices, congestive splenomegaly, and ascites. Ultrasound or CT imaging of the liver reveals "pseudotumors," which represent the pathologic lesion of nodular regenerative hyperplasia.

▶ Treatment

Treatment of Felty syndrome is directed at the underlying RA. In neutropenic patients considering surgery, such as a total joint arthroplasty, it may be necessary to enhance the neutrophil count by preoperative treatment with granulocyte colony-stimulating factor. Splenectomy can be performed in patients who have complications of neutropenia and who do not respond to DMARD therapy, but the results are not always long-lasting, with late recurrence of neutropenia.

LARGE GRANULAR LYMPHOCYTIC LEUKEMIA

A chronic, indolent form of leukemia due to clonal expansion of T lymphocytes that have the appearance of large granular lymphocytes (T-LGL leukemia) develops in approximately 1% of patients with long-standing RA. The complete blood count, which often is the initial clue to the presence of T-LGL leukemia, reveals neutropenia and a higher than expected percentage of lymphocytes relative to neutrophils (eg, a differential count showing 60% lymphocytes and 35% neutrophils). Approximately 30% of patients with Felty syndrome have T-LGL leukemia. The leukemic cells typically have the cell-surface phenotype CD3$^+$CD8$^+$CD16$^+$CD57$^+$, and Southern blot analysis of T-cell receptor gene rearrangement confirms clonality. T-LGL leukemia patients may respond to low-dose oral methotrexate at standard doses (10–20 mg weekly) for the treatment of RA. Systemic infections remain the major potential danger to these patients.

LYMPHOMA

Non-Hodgkin lymphoma occurs two to three times more frequently in patients with RA than in the general population. RA itself is a risk factor for lymphoma, and the incidence of lymphoma increases in those with very active rheumatoid disease. The most frequently reported form is diffuse large B-cell lymphoma. Development of B-cell lymphomas, particularly those linked to Epstein-Barr virus, is a rare complication of methotrexate therapy for RA. The use of anti-TNF agents is associated with slightly increased risk of lymphoma, but a cause and effect relationship has not been established.

RHEUMATOID VASCULITIS

 ESSENTIALS OF DIAGNOSIS

▶ A complication of long-standing seropositive RA.

▶ Most common form is a smoldering small-vessel vasculitis leading to nailbed infarctions.

▶ Less common is a medium-vessel vasculitis that can cause digital ischemia and mononeuritis multiplex.

▶ Rarely, rheumatoid vasculitis can have a course similar to polyarteritis nodosa.

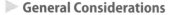

▷ General Considerations

Rheumatoid vasculitis, like other serious extra-articular manifestations of RA, typically develops after 10–15 years of disease and occurs almost exclusively in patients who are seropositive for RF and ACPA. It affects approximately 1–3% of patients.

▷ Clinical Findings

The most common form of rheumatoid vasculitis is a smoldering small-vessel vasculitis that produces painless nailbed infarctions (Figure 13–8), usually in patients with nodular disease. This form of rheumatoid vasculitis usually does not reflect life-threatening systemic vasculitis and can be managed by more aggressive treatment with DMARDs.

Less often, RA causes a medium-vessel vasculitis whose clinical manifestations include necrotic leg ulcers (Figure 13–9), digital gangrene, and mononeuritis multiplex. This form of vasculitis, largely indistinguishable from polyarteritis nodosa, and can lead to infarction of small or large bowel. The ESR and levels of serum CRP are almost always elevated. Cryoglobulinemia and hypocomplementemia are sometimes present. Initial treatment consists of high doses of glucocorticoids and, often, cyclophosphamide. There are reports of successful treatment of refractory cases with rituximab, but more data are required.

NEUROLOGIC MANIFESTATIONS

The most common neurologic complications of RA are compression neuropathies, particularly compression of the median nerve at the wrist (carpal tunnel syndrome) and compression

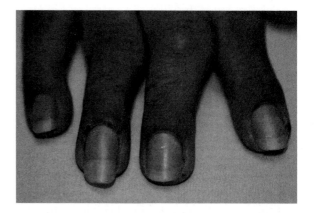

▲ **Figure 13–8.** Rheumatoid vasculitis: periungual and dermal infarcts.

of the ulnar nerve at the elbow or wrist. Rheumatoid vasculitis can cause mononeuritis multiplex and a mixed motor-sensory peripheral neuropathy. Atlanto-axial subluxation and basilar invagination, resulting from rheumatoid synovitis at C1–C2, can produce cervical myelopathy and brainstem compression. An unusual complication of RA is pachymeningitis—inflammation and thickening of dura mater—which presents as a headache, cranial nerve abnormalities, clouded sensorium, and retardation of motor activity (Figure 13–10). Once an infectious etiology has been excluded, pachymeningitis is treated vigorously with glucocorticoids and appropriate DMARDs.

RENAL MANIFESTATIONS

In general, the kidney is spared in RA. Renal impairment in RA patients is most often due to drug toxicity (especially NSAIDs) or to comorbidities such as hypertension or diabetes mellitus. There are, however, rare cases of pauci-immune, necrotizing crescentic glomerulonephritis complicating RA, usually in patients who have antimyeloperoxidase ANCA

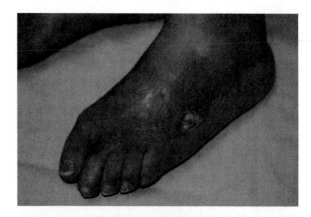

▲ **Figure 13–9.** Rheumatoid vasculitic leg ulcer.

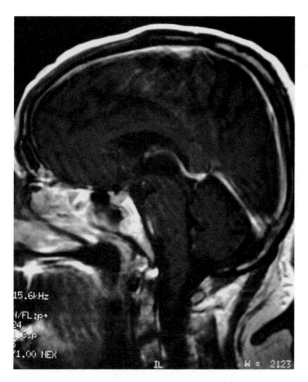

▲ **Figure 13–10.** Magnetic resonance imaging with gadolinium revealing prominent meningeal enhancement of rheumatoid pachymeningitis.

(ie, MPO-ANCA) and evidence of extrarenal vasculitis. Renal amyloidosis is a rare complication of long-standing RA.

AMYLOIDOSIS

Secondary amyloidosis, considered common before effective therapies for RA were available, is now seldom diagnosed in patients with RA.

PYODERMA GANGRENOSUM

Pyoderma gangrenosum is an ulcerative neutrophilic dermatitis of unknown cause. It occurs in less than 1% of patients with RA and usually manifests a lower-extremity, deep ulcer with purplish, overhanging borders. Initial therapy usually involves glucocorticoids, but TNF inhibitors and cyclosporine also have efficacy in this setting.

▶ Managing Comorbidities

Optimal care of patients with RA requires recognition of the comorbid conditions that are associated with RA. These include increased risk of cardiovascular disease, death, osteoporosis, infections, and certain cancers.

The well-documented excess mortality (median life years lost: 8 years for males and 10 years for females) associated with RA is due largely to **cardiovascular disease** that is not explained by the traditional risk factors of family history, smoking, hypertension, diabetes mellitus, and serum cholesterol levels. RA is a systemic inflammatory disease, and chronic systemic inflammation has complex, deleterious effects on lipoproteins and the vascular system. Effective treatment of RA appears to have a beneficial effect on the excess cardiovascular risk. Observational studies suggest that methotrexate and use of anti-TNF agents reduce cardiovascular events and mortality. In addition to RA-directed therapies, clinicians should aggressively address other cardiovascular risk factors (eg, hypertension, serum cholesterol) in these patients.

Osteoporosis is ubiquitous in patients with RA, and early therapy directed at this problem will result in long-term benefits. Patients with RA are at an increased risk for infections, including **septic arthritis** (often due to *Staphylococcus aureus or Streptococcus* species). The risk of infection is further increased by some therapies, especially concomitant glucocorticoids. Patients should be cautioned to seek medical attention early for even minor symptoms suggestive of infection, especially if receiving anti-TNF therapy. All patients with RA should receive pneumococcal and yearly influenza vaccinations (live-attenuated viruses should not be administered to patients receiving biologic therapies).

Finally, patients with RA have an increased risk of **lymphomas**. Occasionally, B-cell lymphomas are associated with immunosuppression and regress after immunosuppression is discontinued. RA patients have significantly decreased risk (odds ratio = 0.2) of developing colon cancer, the explanation for which may be the chronic inhibition of cyclooxygenase by the NSAIDs commonly used in this group of patients.

Coutant F, Miossec P. Evolving concepts of the pathogenesis of rheumatoid arthritis with focus on the early and late stages. *Curr Opin Rheumatol.* 2020 Jan;32(1):57-63. [PMID: 31644463]

De Cock D, Hyrich K. Malignancy and rheumatoid arthritis: epidemiology, risk factors and management. *Best Prac Res Clin Rheumatol.* 2018;32(6):869. [PMID: 31427060]

Deane KD, Holers VM. The natural history of rheumatoid arthritis. *Clin Ther.* 2019 Jul;41(7):1256-1269. [PMID: 31196652]

Favalli EG, Matucci-Cerinic M, Szekanecz Z. The Giants (biologicals) against the Pigmies (small molecules), pros and cons of two different approaches to the disease modifying treatment in rheumatoid arthritis. *Autoimmun Rev.* 2019 Nov 14;19(1):102421. [PMID: 31733368]

Salomon-Escoto K, Kay J. The "treat to target" approach to rheumatoid arthritis. *Rheum Dis Clin North Am.* 2019;45(4):487-504. [PMID: 31564292]

Sparks JA, He X, Huang J, et al. Rheumatoid arthritis disease activity predicting incident clinically-apparent RA-associated interstitial lung disease: a prospective cohort study. *Arthritis Rheumatol.* 2019;71(9):1472. [PMID: 30951251]

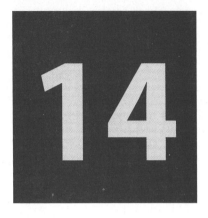

Adult-Onset Still Disease

14

Philippe Guilpain, MD, PhD

Alexandre Maria, MD, PhD

 ESSENTIALS OF DIAGNOSIS

▶ Quotidian fever, frequently greater than 39°C.

▶ Evanescent, salmon-colored macular rash on the trunk and extremities, often coincident with fever spikes, typically in the late afternoon or evening.

▶ Other main clinical features are pharyngitis, polyarthralgia, lymphadenopathy, splenomegaly, and serositis.

▶ Common laboratory abnormalities include a leukocytosis, elevations of the acute phase reactants (erythrocyte sedimentation rate and C-reactive protein), and dramatic increases in the serum ferritin level.

▶ The most striking complication of adult-onset Still disease (AOSD) is reactive hemophagocytic lymphohistiocytosis (RHL), formerly named macrophage activation syndrome.

▶ General Considerations

Adult-onset Still disease (AOSD) is a rare systemic inflammatory disease of unknown etiology. Its reported incidence varies between 0.16 and 0.4 cases per 100,000. The sex ratio varies between 0.5 and 0.7, slightly in favor of women. By definition, AOSD begins after the age of 16 years and tends to affect young adults. The condition occurs after the age of 35 years in only one-quarter of patients and rarely in the elderly.

Patients with AOSD share many clinical similarities with patients who have systemic-onset juvenile idiopathic arthritis (SoJIA), and it is likely that there exists a continuum between these two entities. Common autoinflammatory mechanisms involving inflammatory cytokines such as interleukin (IL)-1-β, tumor necrosis factor-alpha (TNF-α), IL-6, IL-8, IL-18 are operative in both. AOSD has two main clinical presentations (articular form with arthritis at disease onset, and systemic form), and several potential evolutions, including monocyclic, polycyclic, and chronic forms. Its diagnosis is one of exclusion.

▶ Clinical Findings

The classic patient with AOSD has a presentation with four cardinal features: spiking fever, arthralgias, a salmon-pink evanescent maculopapular rash, and peripheral blood leukocytosis.

A. Symptoms and Signs

1. Fever and general signs—The fever of AOSD typically occurs daily, with temperature elevations to greater than or equal to 39°C (sometimes up to 41°C), in the late afternoon or evening. The fever recurs each day with profound sweating and shaking chills that disappear hours later when the temperature returns to normal, even in the absence of antipyretic medications. In some cases, two spikes can be observed daily with a return to normal temperatures in between. In others, however, a low-grade baseline fever persists between spikes. It may therefore present as a prolonged fever of unknown origin and is resistant to antibiotics. General symptoms of fatigue, weight loss, and anorexia accompany the fevers. Patients inevitably endure detailed evaluations for possible infections and malignancies, with multiple cultures, imaging studies, and biopsies (eg, of lymph nodes, liver, and bone marrow) before diagnostic considerations turn to AOSD.

2. Rash—The rash, typically salmon-colored and macular or maculopapular, usually affects the trunk and extremities, sparing the face, palms, and soles (Figure 14–1). The rash is usually asymptomatic and may not be mentioned by the patient, who must therefore be questioned and examined thoroughly. The rash is typically evanescent and transient, occurring during fever spikes and disappearing with return to normal temperature. The Koebner phenomenon may occur following the scratching of uninvolved skin. Atypical distributions and other presentations of skin lesions may occur. For example, urticaria and mild pruritus occur in some cases. Skin biopsy reveals a dermal edema with a polymorphous and/or neutrophilic infiltration of diffuse or perivascular topography. These nonspecific histologic features are found

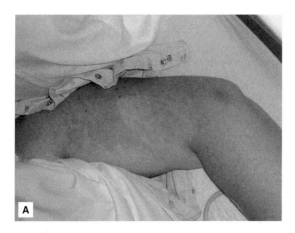
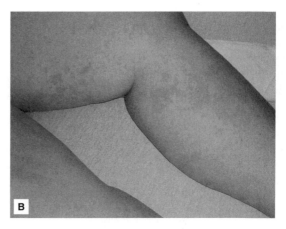

▲ **Figure 14–1.** A 34 year-old woman with adult-onset Still disease who presented with daily fevers, with temperatures as high as 39.7°C daily. She was observed to have this transient but recurring salmon-colored rash on her extremities.

in many dermatologic diseases, including urticaria and cellulitis. Skin biopsies are therefore of little utility in AOSD. The key to the diagnosis is identification of the key clinical features of the rash and appreciating the symptom complex in which the rash has occurred.

3. Pharyngitis—A sore throat due to nonsuppurative aseptic pharyngitis is often the earliest symptom of AOSD. It may antedate the other cardinal symptoms and occur at the time of diseases flares. The presence of a sore throat at the onset of symptoms is an important point about which to ask the patient, since the pharyngitis has often resolved by some days or weeks into the illness.

4. Polyarthralgia and arthritis—Polyarthralgia is common at disease onset and may be associated with synovitis, mainly affecting the large joints (hips, knees, ankles, shoulders, and wrists). The small joints of the hands and feet can be affected to a lesser degree. Joint involvement can persist after resolution of fever and lead to a chronic, destructive arthritis in approximately 20% of patients.

5. Lymphadenopathy—Lymphadenopathy (particularly of cervical nodes) and splenomegaly are frequent, affecting approximately 50% of patients. The distribution of lymphadenopathy within a specific anatomic area suggests the possibility of a malignant process, but lymph node biopsy reveals only reactive hyperplasia.

6. Miscellaneous—Most patients have diffuse myalgias, with sometimes intense pain, particularly during fever spikes. Weakness is uncommon, and creatine phosphokinase levels are usually normal. Symptomatic serositis (pleuritis or pericarditis) is often found. Hepatomegaly is observed in about one-third of patients and increased serum hepatic transaminases 60%.

B. Biological Features

In active AOSD, laboratory findings are highly unspecific but striking. The C-reactive protein and erythrocyte sedimentation rate elevations confirm the presence of systemic inflammation. The leukocytosis (>80% of patients) often exceeds 15,000 cells/µL, primarily comprising neutrophil and is usually associated with a normochromic normocytic anemia or thrombocytosis. The serum albumin is low in the setting of elevated hepatic transaminase concentrations, but the serum creatinine is unperturbed and the urinalysis is normal. Testing for rheumatic disease serologies is usually extensive but unrevealing: assays for antinuclear antibodies, rheumatoid factor, and anticyclic citrullinated peptide antibodies are negative. Serum complement levels are characteristically either normal or increased, as part of the acute phase response.

Increased ferritin levels are observed in most patients, and approximately 30% of patients have extremely high levels (>10,000 ng/mL). Although extremely high ferritin levels are suggestive of AOSD, therefore, even ferritin elevations to levels exceeding 10,000 ng/mL are only about 40% specific. Such levels may also be observed in sepsis or reactive hemophagocytic lymphohistiocytosis (RHL), underscoring the importance of clinic-laboratory correlation in this regard.

A combined examination of the glycosylated ferritin fraction along with the serum ferritin concentration adds greater value as a biomarker in AOSD. The glycosylated ferritin fraction is typically low in active AOSD. A fivefold increase in serum ferritin level combined with a low glycosylated fraction (<20%) has a specificity for AOSD that exceeds 90%. Its sensitivity, on the other hand, is substantially lower—only about 40%. These biomarkers may be most useful in identifying the subgroup of AOSD patients who have RHL, formerly known as the macrophage activation syndrome. These entities are discussed as follows.

▶ Differential Diagnosis

Establishing the diagnosis of AOSD is often complex, because the clinical and biological signs are nonspecific. Physicians must exclude autoinflammatory, autoimmune, infectious, or

Table 14–1. Differential diagnosis of adult-onset Still disease.

Category	Examples
Malignancy	Hodgkin disease Non-Hodgkin lymphoma Renal cell carcinoma Other solid cancers (lung, colic) Myeloproliferative/myelodysplastic syndromes Paraneoplastic syndromes
Acute viral infections	Adenovirus Parvovirus B19 Rubella Epstein-Barr virus Cytomegalovirus Hepatitis B HIV
Other infections	Whipple disease Acute Lyme disease Secondary syphilis Brucellosis Relapsing fever Chronic meningococcemia Subacute bacterial endocarditis Miliary tuberculosis Acute fungal infections (histoplasmosis, coccidioidomycosis, blastomycosis) Parasitic abscess
Postinfectious disorders	Acute rheumatic fever Poststreptococcal arthritis Reactive arthritis
Autoimmune diseases	Systemic lupus erythematosus Seronegative rheumatoid arthritis Inflammatory myopathies Systemic vasculitides (ANCA-associated vasculitis or others) Sarcoidosis
Hereditary periodic fever syndromes	Familial Mediterranean Fever Mevalonate kinase partial deficiency TRAPS
Miscellaneous	Sweet Syndrome Schnitzler syndrome Other reactive hemophagocytic syndromes Drug hypersensitivity

ANCA, antineutrophil cytoplasmic antibody.

malignant conditions that may mimic AOSD (Table 14–1). The complexity of the diagnostic algorithm heightened further by the fact that malignancies or infections may also trigger AOSD flares. The exclusion criteria in the two most commonly used sets of classification criteria for AOSD (Table 14–2, Yamaguchi criteria; Table 14–3, Fautrel criteria) are therefore crucial in the evaluation of a patient with possible AOSD. Lymph node biopsy is often a vital part of

Table 14–2. Yamaguchi classification criteria for adult-onset Still disease.

Major criteria	Fever ≥39°C, intermittent, lasting 1 week or more Arthralgias or arthritis lasting 2 weeks or more Characteristic rash WBC ≥10,000/mcL with neutrophils ≥80%
Minor criteria	Pharyngitis or sore throat Lymphadenopathy Hepatomegaly or splenomegaly Liver enzyme abnormalities Negative tests for rheumatoid factor and antinuclear antibodies
Exclusion criteria	Absence of infection Absence of malignant diseases Absence of inflammatory disease

Classification as adult-onset Still disease requires the presence of five or more criteria, of which at least two must be major criteria.

WBC, white blood cell count.
Data from Yamaguchi M, Ohta A, Tsunematsu T, et al. Preliminary criteria for classification of adult Still's disease. *J Rheumatol.* 1992;19:424-430.

the evaluation for the purpose of excluding Hodgkin disease and non-Hodgkin lymphomas. Other diagnostic tests should be guided by findings on the patient's history and physical examination.

▶ **Complications**

RHL (10–15% of patients), a life-threatening complication, may be the event that brings a patient with AOSD to medical attention or occur later in the disease course, perhaps triggered

Table 14–3. Fautrel classification criteria for adult-onset Still disease.

Major criteria	Spiking fever >39°C Arthralgia Transient erythema Pharyngitis Neutrophil polymorphonuclear count >80% Glycosylated ferritin fraction <20%
Minor criteria	Typical rash Leukocytosis >10,000/mm³

Classification as adult-onset Still disease requires the presence of four major criteria or three major and two minor criteria

Data from Fautrel B, Zing E, Golmard JL, et al. Proposal for a new set of classification criteria for adult-onset still disease. *Medicine (Baltimore).* 2002;81(3):194-200.

by medications or intercurrent infections. RHL is mainly associated with persistent or refractory cases of AOSD and shares a number of features with AOSD that remain uncomplicated, making it difficult to recognize when RHL is emerging. These shared features include fever above 39°C, the classic AOSD rash, lymphadenopathy, hepatosplenomegaly, and markedly increased levels of liver enzymes and serum ferritin. A worsening of the features in a patient with AOSD may indicate the development of RHL as a disease complication. Cytopenia (leukopenia, thrombocytopenia, or both) is a hallmark of RHL, as a consequence of hemophagocytosis. In the context of AOSD, which usually presents with leukocytosis and normal or elevated platelet counts, the finding of cytopenias suggests RHL. Similarly, hypotension, neurologic abnormalities, acute renal failure, acute liver injury, or coagulopathy should prompt the physician to consider the possibility of RHL. Treatments of RHL include glucocorticoids, biologic agents, and etoposide.

Other life-threatening complications include disseminated cytolytic hepatitis, intravascular coagulation (which may occur in the context of RHL or cytolytic hepatitis), and myocarditis.

▶ Treatment

During the initial diagnostic stage, nonsteroidal anti-inflammatory drugs (NSAIDs) can be used, but few patients have an adequate and sustained response. In addition, NSAIDs should be used with caution, because they can cause an increase in serum transaminase levels. Systemic glucocorticoids are required in most cases. Prednisone is given in doses up to 1–2 mg/kg/day, sometimes administered in two divided doses at first to ensure coverage throughout a 24-hour period.

Biologic therapies targeting inflammatory cytokines, particularly IL-1 and IL-6, are the most potent drugs for AOSD and should be employed early if the condition does not come under control quickly with glucocorticoids. The efficacy of TNF-α blockers is limited in AOSD and should be reserved for the treatment of patients with difficult joint symptoms. TNF inhibition is not appropriate for the treatment of RHL. In contrast, IL-1 or IL-6 antagonists can be used in all forms of AOSD. Recent data also suggest the efficacy of IL-18 antagonists. Intravenous immunoglobulins no longer have a role in the treatment

of AOSD or RHL in the era of biologics. Treatment should be escalated quickly to biologics if signs of RHL become apparent.

▶ Prognosis

Cases of life-threatening disease are rare, and the overall prognosis for patients with AOSD is good. Medication should be tapered slowly when remission is obtained. The necessity of maintenance therapy is guided by the evolution of the disease with treatment. AOSD may be divided into three different subtypes, each of which affects approximately one-third of patients. The monocyclic form is characterized by a self-limited course lasting a few months. The polycyclic form is associated with multiple recurrent flares of systemic or articular symptoms that alternate with disease-free intervals. Finally, chronic AOSD is defined by persistently active disease, usually polyarthritis, requiring ongoing therapy.

Gabay C, Fautrel B, Rech J, et al. Open-label, multicentre, dose-escalating phase II clinical trial on the safety and efficacy of tadekinig-alfa (IL-18BP) in adult-onset Still's disease. *Ann Rheum Dis.* 2018;77(6):840-847. [PMID: 29472362]

Kaneko Y, Kameda H, Ikeda K, et al. Tocilizumab in patients with adult-onset Still's disease refractory to glucocorticoid treatment: a randomised, double-blind, placebo-controlled phase III trial. *Ann Rheum Dis.* 2018;77(12):1720-1729. [PMID: 30279267]

Maria AT, Le Quellec A, Jorgensen C, Touitou I, Riviere S, Guilpain P. Adult onset Still's disease (AOSD) in the era of biologic therapies: dichotomous view for cytokine and clinical expressions. *Autoimmun Rev.* 2014;13(11):1149-1159. [PMID: 25183244]

Néel A, Wahbi A, Tessoulin B, et al. Diagnostic and management of life-threatening adult-onset Still disease: a French nationwide multicenter study and systematic literature review. *Crit Care.* 2018;22(1):88. [PMID: 29642928]

Ortiz-Sanjuan F, Blanco R, Riancho-Zarrabeitia L, et al. Efficacy of anakinra in refractory adult-onset Still's disease: multicenter study of 41 patients and literature review. *Medicine (Baltimore).* 2015;94(39):e1554. [PMID: 26426623]

Ruscitti P, Cipriani P, Masedu F, et al. Adult-onset Still's disease: evaluation of prognostic tools and validation of the systemic score by analysis of 100 cases from three centers. *BMC Med.* 2016;14(1):194. [PMID: 27903264]

15

Axial Spondyloarthritis & Arthritis Associated with Inflammatory Bowel Disease

Jean W. Liew, MD

Lianne S. Gensler, MD

▶ The hallmark feature of axial spondyloarthritis (axSpA) is inflammatory back pain (IBP), especially with onset younger than 45 years of age. IBP features include worsening with rest, improvement with activity or exercise, nighttime awakening due to pain and/or stiffness (especially in the second part of the night), and response to nonsteroidal anti-inflammatory drugs (NSAIDs).

▶ Other SpA features include enthesitis, peripheral arthritis, dactylitis, acute anterior uveitis (AAU), psoriasis, and inflammatory bowel disease (IBD).

▶ Among Caucasian individuals with ankylosing spondylitis (AS) (radiographic axSpA), 85–95% are positive for HLA-B27. However, among those who are Black, HLA-B27 is only present in 50%.

▶ Damage to the bilateral sacroiliac (SI) joints is seen on conventional radiographs, although this finding may only develop years after initial symptom onset. Acute inflammation (bone marrow edema) and structural lesions (erosions, ankylosis, and subchondral fat [fat metaplasia]) may be seen earlier on magnetic resonance imaging (MRI) of the SI joints.

▶ General Considerations

Spondyloarthritis (SpA) encompasses a spectrum of diseases characterized by inflammation affecting the sacroiliac (SI) joints, spine, or peripheral joints (Figure 15–1). It is further subdivided into axial and peripheral predominant disease. Ankylosing spondylitis (AS) refers to axial spondyloarthritis (axSpA) with radiographic damage of the SI joints evident on conventional radiography, while nonradiographic axial spondyloarthritis (nr-axSpA) refers to disease in the absence of radiographic damage. The broader category of SpA also includes peripheral involvement,

including psoriatic arthritis (PsA), reactive arthritis, and arthritis associated with inflammatory bowel disease (IBD). The terminology "seronegative spondyloarthropathy" should not be used as it refers to the absence of rheumatoid factor, which is not used in the diagnosis of SpA. Additionally, SpA is preferred over spondyloarthropathy to reflect the inflammatory process.

The prevalence of axSpA in the United States is about 0.9–1.4% of the adult population. Inflammatory back pain (IBP), which has a prevalence of 5–6% among US adults (2009–2010 National Health and Nutrition Examination Survey [NHANES]), is the hallmark feature of axSpA. Symptom onset occurs in the third decade, and the typical male to female distribution is 1:1, though closer to 2–3:1 in the setting of radiographic axSpA (also known as AS). Hereditary factors account for most of the susceptibility of AS. In chronic low back pain, a family history of SpA adds predictive value for a diagnosis of SpA. HLA-B27 is the strongest known risk factor associated with AS, though it only accounts for 20% of the risk. The prevalence of HLA-B27 positivity among the general adult population in NHANES was 6.1%, with a prevalence of 7.5% in non-Hispanic whites and 3.5% in all other racial/ethnic backgrounds. Approximately 80–90% of individuals with AS are positive for HLA-B27, but among those in the general population who are positive for this allele, less than 5% will develop AS. This is because AS is a polygenic disease, requiring multiple alleles and potentially gene-gene interaction (epistasis) to occur.

In addition to inflammation, the pathogenesis of SpA includes inflammation at the sites of ligament or tendon attachment to bone (enthesitis and osteitis), periosteal new bone formation (osteoproliferation), and ankylosis. This is different from rheumatoid arthritis (RA), whose hallmark inflammatory lesion is synovitis and erosion. Although tumor necrosis factor (TNF) is also implicated in SpA, the IL-23/IL-17 axis plays a major role in axSpA pathogenesis and serves as an important therapeutic target.

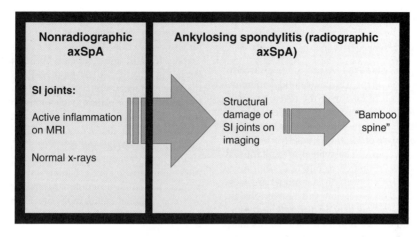

▲ **Figure 15–1.** Spectrum of axSpA. Not all patients progression from nonradiographic axSpA to have structural damage. Per data from cohort studies, about 10% progressed at 2 years and 50% at 10 years.

▶ **Clinical Findings**

A. Signs and Symptoms

1. Axial involvement—The hallmark feature is IBP, which improves with activity or exercise, worsens with rest, may awaken patients at night, and usually has an age of onset younger than 45 years (Table 15–1). Nocturnal back pain and improvement with exercise are the features with the highest positive predictive value to differentiate IBP from mechanical back pain. Mechanical back pain usually worsens with activity and is greatest at the end of the day. Axial involvement may also manifest as buttock pain with an alternating quality, or chest pain due to involvement of the costochondral and costomanubrial joints and the entheses associated with the ribcage.

2. Peripheral arthritis—The prevalence of peripheral arthritis in axSpA ranges from 20% to 52% and does not differ in frequency between AS and nr-axSpA. Large lower extremity joints are more commonly affected than small upper extremity joints. The hip, which is considered an axial or root joint, is affected in about a third of AS patients. Risk factors for hip involvement include juvenile onset of disease (before 16 years old), more severe spinal damage, and the presence of peripheral joint arthritis. Hip disease can result in progressive flexion deformity, contracture, and fusion and is associated with more functional impairment than spinal ankylosis. The shoulder may also be affected, causing joint space narrowing of the glenohumeral joint, erosion, and occasionally ankylosis of the superolateral humeral head.

3. Enthesitis—This occurs in up to 40% at diagnosis and up to 70% over the disease course, with similar frequency in AS and nr-axSpA. Common sites include the Achilles tendon insertion at the calcaneus, the plantar fascia attachment at the calcaneus, the greater trochanter, the epicondyles, and the costochondral joints. Enthesitis may be assessed by putting pressure at entheseal insertion site. However, these sites have low sensitivity to differentiate enthesitis from other causes of pain, such as fibromyalgia, when widespread. Tenderness and swelling at the insertion of the Achilles tendon on the calcaneus or the patellar tendon on the tibial tuberosity may be more discriminatory.

Table 15-1. Inflammatory back pain: classification criteria.

Calin (1977)	Berlin (2006)	ASAS (2009)
Age of onset <40 y	Morning stiffness >30 min	Age of onset <40 y
Duration of back pain >3 mo	Improvement with exercise, not rest	Insidious onset
Insidious onset	Awakening in the second part of the night due to pain	Improvement with exercise
Morning stiffness	Alternating buttock pain	No improvement with rest
Improvement with exercise		Nocturnal pain
Meet criteria: 4/5	Meet criteria: 2/4	Meet criteria: 4/5

Sources: Rudwaleit M, et al. Inflammatory back pain in ankylosing spondylitis: a reassessment of the clinical history for application as classification and diagnostic criteria. *Arthritis Rheum.* 2006;54(2):569–578; Calin A, et al. Clinical history as a screening test for ankylosing spondylitis. *JAMA.* 1977;237(24):2613–2614; and Sieper J, et al. New criteria for inflammatory back pain in patients with chronic back pain: a real patient exercise by experts from the Assessment of SpondyloArthritis international Society (ASAS). *Ann Rheum Dis.* 2009;68(6):784–788.

4. Dactylitis—This refers to the swelling of an entire digit (sausage digit) due to flexor (typically) tenosynovitis. The prevalence in axSpA is 2–6%.

5. Inflammatory eye disease—Acute anterior uveitis (AAU), or inflammation of the iris, ciliary body, and choroid, has a prevalence up to 50% over the disease course. It is the most common extra-articular manifestation in axSpA. About 50% of patients with AAU will be HLA-B27 positive; the majority of HLA-B27 positive individuals with AAU will have SpA. The typical presentation is acute and unilateral, as compared to bilateral, seen more commonly in PsA or IBD. Common symptoms are photophobia, pain with accommodation and blurred vision. On gross examination, the eye may be diffusely red, especially at the edge of the cornea (ciliary flush). On slit-lamp examination, white blood cells will be seen in the anterior chamber. Complications, particularly if untreated, include the formation of synechiae, macular edema leading to blindness, increased intraocular pressure, and cataracts (from topical steroids).

6. Psoriasis—Skin psoriasis occurs in about 10% of patients with axSpA. Common sites of involvement include extensor surfaces (knees and elbows), the umbilicus, gluteal folds, and behind the ears. The nails may also be involved with pitting and onycholysis.

7. Inflammatory bowel disease (IBD)—Clinical IBD has a prevalence of about 5–8% in patients diagnosed with axSpA. However, ileocolonoscopic studies suggest that the prevalence of subclinical IBD may be as high as 50%, with histologic features consistent with both acute and chronic inflammation.

B. Laboratory Findings

The CRP can be in 30–50% of patients with axSpA, typically higher in those with radiographic disease (AS). An elevated CRP is predictive of a response to biologic treatment. The erythrocyte sedimentation rate (ESR) can also be elevated in axSpA, but has less sensitivity and specificity.

HLA-B27 testing can be helpful for diagnostic purposes. However, it cannot rule in or rule out axSpA.

Other laboratory findings may include a mild, normocytic anemia of chronic disease (or anemia of inflammation) and elevated levels of fecal calprotectin, though this can occur from anti-inflammatory drug (NSAID) use too. Occasionally an elevated alkaline phosphatase is found, which more specifically reflects bone-specific alkaline phosphatase.

C. Imaging Studies

Imaging is important in the diagnosis of axSpA and magnetic resonance imaging (MRI) in particular can be considered similar to the information one might obtain from biopsy, which is not performed for axSpA.

1. Conventional radiography—Current guidelines support starting with conventional radiographs of the SI joints (anterior-posterior [AP] view of the pelvis, not SI joint radiographs) in most adult patients. A study has shown no difference in sensitivity between the AP view of the pelvis with the Ferguson view, which is obtained at a 20-degree angle to the head with the patient lying supine. Sacroiliitis is graded from 0 to 4, with 0 being normal and 4 being complete ankylosis (Figure 15–2). Grade 2 is the cutoff for significant radiographic damage and refers to the presence of sclerosis and/or small erosions of the SI joints. However, there is poor inter- and intra-reader reliability even among expert radiologists pertaining to grade 2 sacroiliitis. This, and the fact that conventional radiographs are insensitive to early disease or changes over shorter periods of time, has led to MRI for diagnosis.

2. Computed tomography—CT can capture sclerosis, erosions, and ankylosis of the SI joints. There is a concern for radiation exposure with this modality, though occasionally these images were captured for another clinical indication and can be reviewed for incidental SI joint changes. Low-dose CT protocols are currently being assessed. This modality is not routinely used for diagnosis.

3. Magnetic resonance imaging—MRI without contrast of sacrum or pelvis should be used if conventional radiographs do not demonstrate sacroiliitis and there is still suspicion for axSpA. MRI can confirm the presence of sacroiliitis, as well as define the extent of inflammation and structural changes.

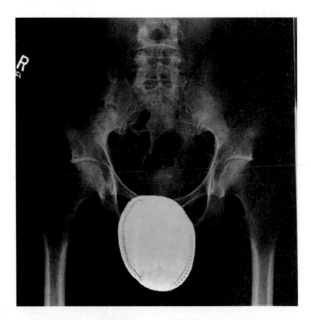

▲ **Figure 15–2. Grade 3 sacroiliitis on x-ray.** X-ray of the pelvis with bilateral grade 3 sacroiliitis. Partial ankylosis is seen of both sacroiliitis joints.

Table 15-2. Inflammatory lesions on MRI characteristic of axSpA.

Lesion	STIR	T1
	Fluid sensitive	*Fat sensitive*
Active inflammation	Hyperintense (bright)	Hypointense (dark)
Fat metaplasia	Hypointense (dark)	Hyperintense (bright)
Sclerosis	Hypointense (dark)	Hypointense (dark)
Erosions	–	Hypointense (dark)

Semicoronal or coronal-oblique views should be obtained with a fluid-sensitive short-tau inversion recovery (STIR) sequence and a fat-sensitive T1 sequence (Table 15–2). Gadolinum is not necessary. On STIR, fluid, including hydrated intervertebral discs and blood vessels are bright (hyperintense); active inflammatory lesions of bone marrow edema (osteitis) around the SI joints representing sacroiliitis are also bright (Figure 15–3). Other inflammatory lesions like enthesitis, capusulitis, and synovitis can occasionally be seen. Structural changes indicative of past inflammation include sclerosis, subchondral fat metaplasia, erosions, and even ankylosis can be seen on the T1 sequence. On T1, bone marrow edema and sclerosis are both dark (hypointense), while fat metaplasia (subchondral fat), which can represent past inflammation, is bright (hyperintense).

Although initially negative MRIs may become positive on follow-up, current guidelines do not recommend routine follow-up MRI examinations. In RCTs, MRIs have been shown to be sensitive to decrease in active inflammatory lesions in response to biologic therapy. There is insufficient data to guide the use of MRI for the monitoring of therapy response.

4. Spine imaging—Conventional radiographs, CT, and MRI can reveal erosions. Repair may lead to the appearance of sclerosis, which is seen as shiny corners (Romanus lesions) on vertebral bodies and/or squaring (Figure 15–4). More advanced changes represent bone formation: the presence of syndesmophytes, bony bridging, and finally, the appearance of a "bamboo spine." The addition of lumbar spine (or other region) MRI does not increase diagnostic yield if both plain film and MRI of the SI joints are unrevealing.

D. Special Examinations

Physical examination should include measures of spinal mobility impairment (metrology). The most sensitive exam maneuver for screening is lateral lumbar flexion, followed by the anterior lumbar flexion (modified Schober test). If considering the diagnosis, this is the only required measure of metrology. There is a hierarchy for the loss of spinal mobility, and it typically proceeds in a cranial fashion with the lumbar spine affected first. A normal lateral lumbar flexion exam is the best predictor for the absence of radiographic structural damage of the spine.

Lateral lumbar flexion is performed with the patient standing upright with their hands at their sides. The examiner measures the difference between the fingertips with the patient in this position as compared to when the patient is asked to bend to one side as far as they can, maintaining the back against the wall and without lifting the contralateral heel off the floor. A normal measurement derived from population-level studies is a difference from neutral to the flexion position greater than 10 cm.

For the modified Schober test, the examiner locates and marks the posterior superior margin of the iliac spines (dimples of Venus) and a site 10 cm above (Figure 15–5). The patient is asked to bend forward at the waist with the knees kept straight, and the distance between the marks is measured. A normal measurement is greater than or equal to 2 cm.

Other measures of spinal mobility include chest expansion and occiput-to-wall. Chest expansion is measured at the level of T4 or the xiphoid notch, for the difference between maximum inhalation and exhalation. A normal

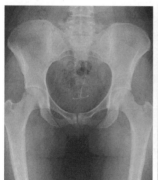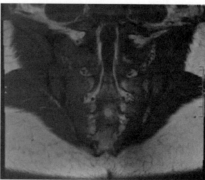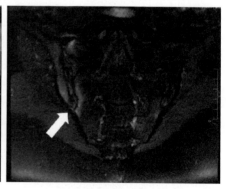

▲ **Figure 15–3.** Comparison of the SI joints on x-ray and MRI. The x-ray does not demonstrate sacroiliitis. The MRI (with T1 and STIR sequences) demonstrates active inflammatory lesions (bone marrow edema) as hyperintense lesions on STIR (*arrow*).

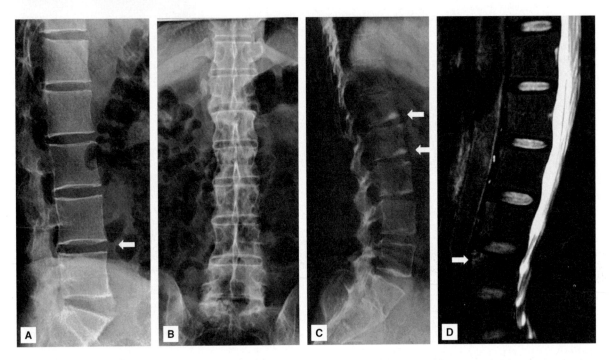

▲ **Figure 15–4.** Structural changes of the lumbar spine. **A:** X-ray of the lumbar spine, lateral view, demonstrating nonbridging syndesmophytes (*arrow*). **B:** AP view of the same study demonstrates lateral bridging syndesmophytes that were not seen on the lateral view. **C:** X-ray of the lumbar spine of a different patient, demonstrating shiny corners (Romanus lesions) (*arrows*). **D:** MRI of the lumbar spine, STIR sequence, with hyperintense, active inflammation of the vertebral corners (*arrow*).

measurement is greater than or equal to 1.9 cm, although this maneuver has poorer performance in obese patients. Occiput-to-wall is measured with the patient standing with their back and heels against the wall and their head in a neutral position. A normal measurement is greater than 0 cm, although abnormal values may be seen in older men in the general population.

Patrick's maneuver, or FABER, is done to elicit pain in the SI joints. With the patient lying supine, their leg is flexed, and hip abducted and externally rotated. This test is neither sensitive nor specific for sacroiliitis and is generally not recommended. Range of motion of the hips should be tested for evidence of hip involvement.

▶ **Classification Criteria**

There are currently no diagnostic criteria for axSpA or AS. There are two main classification criteria in use: the modified New York criteria (1984) for AS, and the Assessment of Spondyloarthritis international Society (ASAS) criteria for axSpA (2009) (Table 15–3). Classification criteria are intended for use in research, where homogeneous populations of patients are desired to be studies. The use of classification criteria for the purpose of diagnosis may result in misdiagnosing people

with axSpA who do not have the disease. In order to apply classification criteria, patients should have received a clinical diagnosis first.

In the older modified New York criteria, the diagnosis of AS is based upon one of three possible clinical criteria and one imaging criterion. For the clinical criteria, the patient should have at least one of the following: chronic IBP, limitation in lumbar flexion, or limitation in chest expansion. The imaging criterion is radiographic damage of the SI joints (grade 2 bilateral or unilateral grade 3 or 4) by conventional radiography. MRI is not included in these criteria.

The newer ASAS criteria are used for axSpA and include AS (also known as radiographic axSpA) and nr-axSpA. The stem requirement for all patients is age of onset before 45 years and at least 3 months of chronic back pain. The criteria are then divided into imaging and clinical arms. In the imaging arm, the presence of sacroiliitis by MRI or at least bilateral grade 2 or unilateral grade 3 or 4 by conventional radiographs and the addition of one or more SpA features are sufficient for the classification of axSpA. In the clinical arm, a positive HLA-B27 and two or more SpA features will fulfill classification criteria for axSpA. A patient is considered as nr-axSpA if they fulfill criteria without having sacroiliitis on a conventional radiograph.

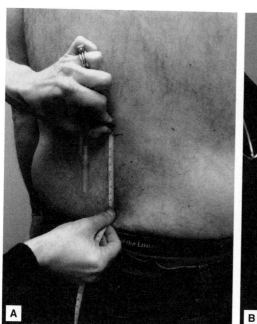
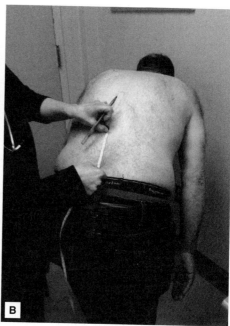

▲ **Figure 15–5. Modified Schober test.** A mark is made at the level of the posterior superior iliac spines, and another mark is made 10 cm above (**A**). The patient is asked to bend forward and the distance between the two lines is measured (**B**).

Table 15-3. Classification criteria.

Modified New York Criteria (1984)	ASAS Criteria (2009)
Definite AS: Fulfilment of radiologic criterion with ≥1 clinical criterion	**AxSpA:** In patients with ≥3 mo of low back pain with onset <45 y, fulfilment of either 1 or 2
1. Clinical criteria	1. Clinical arm
Low back pain >3 mo that improves with exercise but not with rest	HLA-B27 positivity and ≥2 SpA features
Limited mobility of the lumbar spine	2. Imaging arm
Limited chest expansion	Sacroiliitis on imaging[a] and ≥1 SpA feature
2. Radiological criterion	
Sacroiliitis grade 2 bilaterally or grade 3–4 unilaterally	SpA features:
	Inflammatory back pain
	Arthritis
	Enthesitis
	Uveitis
	Dactylitis
	Psoriasis
	Crohn disease or ulcerative colitis
	Good response to NSAIDs
	Family history of SpA
	HLA-B27 positivity
	Elevated CRP

[a]Sacroiliitis on imaging refers to either active inflammation suggestive of SpA seen on MRI or radiographic sacroiliitis according to the Modified New York Criteria.
Sources: van der Linden S, et al. Evaluation of diagnostic criteria for ankylosing spondylitis. *Arthritis Rheum.* 1984;27(4):361-368; and Rudwaleit M, et al. The development of Assessment of SpondyloArthritis international Society classification criteria for axial spondyloarthritis (part II): validation and final selection. *Ann Rheum Dis.* 2009;68(6):777-783.

The definition of AS by the modified New York criteria is interchangeable with AS (radiographic axSpA) defined by the ASAS criteria.

▶ Differential Diagnosis

The differential for sacroiliitis should include infection (unilateral septic sacroiliitis from typical bacteria, tuberculosis, and brucellosis, or osteomyeltis); degenerative changes, which are common in older patients; fracture; and osteitis condenscans ilii (OCI). OCI is a noninflammatory, mechanical condition associated with obesity, the postpartum state, and multiparity. The classic finding is of triangular sclerotic lesions on the iliac side of the SI joint (Figure 15–6). Malignancy is a less common cause of sacroiliitis, and includes solid tumors metastatic to bone and hematologic malignancies. Bone tumors, both malignant and nonmalignant, may also cause sacroiliitis.

Bone marrow edema alone around the SI joints is not specific for axSpA and has been found on MRI studies of other populations, including general population controls, postpartum women, military recruits, runners, and other athletes. In these individuals, the most commonly affected site is the posterior lower ilium.

The main differential diagnoses for spine findings are degenerative disease and diffuse idiopathic skeletal hyperostosis (DISH). DISH has findings of at least three consecutive bridging bulky osteophytes, often sparing the left side of the spine. Patients with DISH can have IBP in up to 80%. Discriminating features include the absence of facet joint ankylosis and association with older age and the metabolic syndrome in DISH.

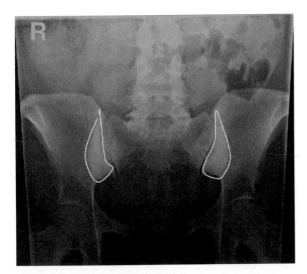

▲ **Figure 15–6. Osteitis condescens ilii.** The classic finding is of triangular sclerotic lesions on the iliac side of the SI joint (outlined). (See color insert.)

▶ Comorbidities & Complications

1. Cardiovascular disease (CVD)—Patients with AS have an increased risk of CVD, including myocardial infarction, stroke, and CVD-related mortality compared to general population comparators of the same age and sex. The prevalence of risk factors for CVD, such as hypertension and diabetes, is also increased. The increased CVD burden is in line with our current understanding in other rheumatic diseases such as lupus and RA. Beyond the contribution of established risk factors, chronic systemic inflammation may also be contributing to heighten this risk.

2. Osteoporosis and fractures—The prevalence of osteoporosis or low bone mass in axSpA is about Abnormal ossification of the spine can falsely elevate bone mineral density scores on routine DXA, though a standard lumbar and hip DXA are still recommended per guidelines. The previously reported prevalence of vertebral fractures in axSpA ranged from 11% to 25%; however, newer studies find that the prevalence ranges from 3% to 20%, with an incidence of 1–6%. The presence of vertebral fracture has been associated with older age, higher body mass index, longer smoking duration, and more spinal mobility impairment at baseline in cohort studies. Cervical spine fracture is an independent predictor of inpatient mortality among hospitalized patients with AS.

3. Fibromyalgia and depression—The prevalence of fibromyalgia in axSpA is about 20%. The diagnosis is associated with higher disease activity scores and a poorer response to therapy. Sleep disturbances and depression are also common comorbidities, and correlated with higher disease activity scores.

4. Other cardiac—Nonischemic cardiac manifestations include aortic root dilatation with 25–50% fibrotic thickening and downward displacement of the aortic valve cusps and resultant aortic regurgitation, and arrhythmias such as atrioventricular block.

5. Pulmonary—Involvement of the thoracic spine and costochondral joints may result in restrictive pulmonary defects. Apical pulmonary fibrosis is a rare entity that is typically asymptomatic. Sleep apnea is more common in AS compared to the gender-matched normal population.

6. Renal—Secondary renal amyloidosis from chronic systemic inflammation, once the most common renal complication of AS, is now rare. Renal impairment can be seen as a result of chronic NSAID use.

7. Neurological—Caution must be taken with AS patients undergoing anesthesia in order to avoid atlantoaxial injury or spinal fracture in those with significant cervical spine disease; for similar reasons, high-velocity chiropractic manipulation should also be avoided. Cauda equina syndrome is a rare complication resulting from arachnoiditis. It can present with pain, sensory loss, and incontinence.

▶ Treatment

A. General Treatment Considerations

1. Physical therapy (PT) and exercise—All patients should be educated about the value of exercise and the types of exercise that are beneficial. Adherence is key. Active PT is recommended over passive PT. Home-based and supervised programs are both beneficial. Land-based exercises are recommended over aquatic exercises due to limitations of access to pools for some patients.

2. Nonsteroidal anti-inflammatory drugs—NSAIDs are the first-line pharmacologic therapy. A good response is seen in 70–80% with optimal effect by 2 weeks. There is no preferred formulation, although long-acting medications like meloxicam may extend symptom relief, especially through the night. With active disease, patients should take NSAIDs continuously, that is, on a daily basis at the full dose for treatment of inflammatory disease. In inactive disease, or once patients have initiated a biologic, NSAIDs may be taken as needed. NSAIDs, in conjunction with biologics, may have a potential disease-modifying effect on radiographic progression. The long-term complications of NSAIDs must also be weighed against their benefits: hypertension, renal dysfunction, and gastrointestinal complications such as gastroesophageal reflux disease or peptic ulcer disease. Selective COX-2 inhibitors such as celecoxib may be provided to avoid gastrointestinal side effects. Proton pump inhibitors may be provided for gastroprotection alongside NSAIDs, especially in older patients.

3. Glucocorticoids—Current axSpA guidelines recommend avoiding the use of systemic glucocorticoids. Directed SI joint glucocorticoid injections can be effective for pain reduction, though are typically temporizing only and address only one side of a typically systemic process.

4. Conventional disease-modifying antirheumatic drugs (cDMARDs)—Sulfasalazine may have modest benefit for peripheral disease, although not for axial disease, as shown in a meta-analysis of multiple older clinical trials. On the other hand, a meta-analysis of methotrexate did not show benefit in either peripheral or axial disease in AS, and its use is not recommended for axSpA symptoms alone.

5. Biologics—TNF inhibitors are recommended as second-line therapy after NSAID inefficacy or intolerance. These include infliximab, adalimumab, etanercept, certolizumab pegol, and golimumab. All are approved in the United States for the treatment of AS. Certolizumab pegol was approved in 2019 for nr-axSpA. While efficacious for the management of disease activity including axial and peripheral disease, less radiographic progression was not seen compared to a historic comparator cohort at 2 years after open-label extension. However, in AS cohort studies, TNF-inhibitor use is associated with slower radiographic progression over longer-term follow-up of 4 years or more, especially if started early. Discontinuation in patients with symptom remission has been associated with high (>50%) rates of relapse, so this is not currently recommended. Retention on TNF inhibitors in axSpA is low; by 5 years, about 50% will no longer be taking the TNF inhibitor that they started on. Primary nonresponse (those who never responded) to the first TNF inhibitor predicts lack of response after switching to a second TNF inhibitor, compared to those who had a secondary loss of response (those who responded initially, but had a loss of efficacy).

After TNF inhibitor loss of response or intolerance, IL-17 inhibitors are recommended. These target the IL-23/IL-17 axis that underlies the pathogenesis of axSpA. Currently, secukinumab, an inhibitor of IL-17A, is approved for the management of AS (but not nr-axSpA).

Other biologics have been studied in AS and have not been found effective. These include the agents used for RA (abatacept, anakinra, sarilumab, rituximab), as well as agents that are effective for PsA or skin psoriasis (apremilast, ustekinumab, risankizumab). Small molecules, including Janus kinuse (JAK) inhibitors, are currently being studied in axSpA (Figure 15–7).

6. Surgery—Total hip arthroplasty (THA) can be helpful for pain and function in those with advanced hip disease. About 5% of axSpA patients with hip disease will need THA. The survival of the prosthetic implant is comparable to those without AS: 99% at 5 years, 97% at 10 years, and 66% at 15 years. The development of ectopic periarticular bone (heterotopic ossification) can complicate this surgery, but preventative strategies such as early mobilization and perioperative NSAID administration can mitigate it. Current guidelines conditionally recommend against elective spinal osteotomy to improve horizontal gaze in those with advanced AS and severe kyphosis (Figure 15–8), unless at a specialized center. This recommendation is based upon the high perioperative mortality of 5% and severe neurological complication rate of 4%.

B. Management of Extra-Articular Manifestations

1. Uveitis—Patients with uveitis should be comanaged with ophthalmology. Glucocorticoid eye drops constitute first-line therapy, and patients with established recurrent uveitis can be advised to take drops at the onset of symptom occurrence, with presentation to ophthalmology as soon as possible. Prednisolone acetate is the recommended formulation, while fluorinated eye drops such as difluprednate should be avoided due to the risk of increasing the intraocular pressure. Refractory inflammatory eye disease may require systemic glucocorticoids or the addition of methotrexate or sulfasalazine. In patients requiring biologic therapy for their axSpA and frequently recurrent uveitis, the monoclonal TNF inhibitors, especially infliximab and adalimumab, though also certolizumab pegol, and golimumab are recommended over etanercept or non-TNF biologics for the evidence supporting prevention of uveitis recurrence. Three phase 3 trials of secukinumab for the treatment of noninfectious uveitis were negative for the primary outcome of uveitis recurrence reduction.

	AS	PsA	PsO	UC	CD
TNF inhibitors					
Etanercept	+++	+++	+++		
Monoclonal antibodies *	+++	+++	+++	+++	+++
IL-17 inhibitors					
Secukinumab (IL-17A)	+++	+++	+++		
Ixekizumab (IL-17A)	+++	+++	+++		
Brodalumab (receptor)		++	+++		
Bimekizumab (IL-17A & F)	++	++	++		
IL12/23 inhibitor					
Ustekinumab		+++	+++		+++
IL23 inhibitors					
Risankizumab		++	+++		
Guselkumab		++	+++		
Tildrakizumab		++	+++		
CTLA-4 fusion protein					
Abatacept		+++			
Integrin $\alpha_4\beta_7$ inhibitor					
Vedolizumab				+++	+++
PDE4 inhibitor					
Apremilast		+++	+++		
JAK inhibitors					
Tofacitinib (JAK1 & 3)	++	+++	+++	+++	+++
Baricitinib (JAK1 & 2)		++	++		
Filgotinib (JAK1)	++	++			++
Upadacitinib (JAK1)				++	

Legend:

+++ Phase 3 efficacy (bold = approved)   ++ Phase 2 efficacy   ▨ Under investigation   ⧄ Trials without benefit   ▦ No RCTs

▲ Figure 15–7. **Biologic and small-molecule therapeutic options for ankylosing spondylitis (AS), psoriatic arthritis (PsA), psoriasis (PsO), ulcerative colitis (UC), and Crohn disease (CD).** *Monoclonal TNF inhibitors: infliximab, adalimumab, certolizumab pegol, golimumab. Only certolizumab pegol is approved for nonradiographic axSpA in the United States. Certolizumab pegol is approved for CD but not UC. Golimumab (subcutaneous) is approved for UC but not CD.

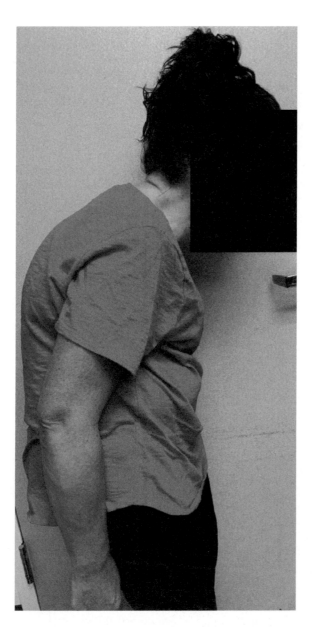

▲ **Figure 15–8. Severe kyphosis.** In advanced AS, involvement of the thoracic spine leads to kyphosis.

2. IBD—Comanagement with gastroenterology is advised, particular to differentiate IBS from IBD initially. Similar to the treatment of uveitis, the preferred biologics are the TNF inhibitors (infliximab, adalimumab, certolizumab pegol, and golimumab). The IL-17A inhibitor secukinumab may worsen or unmask underlying IBD. On the other hand, vedolizumab, an integrin inhibitor targeted to gut mucosa, is effective for the management of IBD but may worsen or unmask arthritis.

3. Psoriasis—In patients with axial disease controlled by NSAIDs, topical therapy can be used for skin disease. For patients on biologics, psoriasis may be better controlled. Ustekinumab was found to be efficacious for psoriasis, but not for axSpA in a phase 3 clinical trial. Combination biologic therapy is not recommended at this time.

C. Monitoring

Borrowing from other diseases such as hypertension, diabetes, and RA, current axSpA guidelines recommend a treat to target strategy. Disease activity should be regularly measured. With active disease and following medication changes, patients should be reevaluated more frequently. The two main measures of disease activity in use are the ASDAS (Ankylosing Spondylitis Disease Activity Score) and the BASDAI (Bath Ankylosing Spondylitis Disease Activity Index) (Table 15–4). The ASDAS is recommended over the BASDAI as the latter only includes subjective, patient-reported measures, while the former incorporates laboratory markers of the inflammation (CRP recommended), is weighted, and reduces redundancy. Other factors associated with radiographic progression include high CRP, presence of syndesmophytes on baseline imaging, and smoking. However, the definition of remission or minimal disease activity is not clear and further work needs to be done in this area (Figure 15–9).

▶ Prognosis

Prognosis is highly variable. Despite natural history studies, the progression of axial disease is poorly understood. A quarter of patients with nr-axSpA progressed to AS over a 15-year follow-up in one US cohort. However, others with nr-axSpA may never develop radiographic sacroiliitis.

AxSpA is associated with poorer health-related quality of life as well as work disability, absenteeism, and presenteeism, compared to the general population. Withdrawal from work is three times more common among individuals with AS than in the general population. This is particularly true of those who perform manual work that involves repetitive bending and twisting.

The major medical comorbidities, especially CVD and osteoporosis, associated axSpA also deserve particular attention, especially as increased mortality compared to the general population is increased in AS and driven by CVD. Preventative and treatment strategies for CVD and osteoporosis should be undertaken per major society guidelines.

▶ When to Refer

IBP alone is not sufficient to make a diagnosis of axSpA; the specificity for this symptom is only 72%. On the other hand, the average delay in diagnosis from the time of symptom onset can be greater than 10 years. In AS, women have

Table 15–4. Measures of disease activity.

ASDAS-CRP	BASDAI
On a numeric rating scale of 0–10, with 0 being not active and 10 being severe, in the past week.	
1. How would you describe the overall level of AS neck, back, or hip pain you have had?	1. How would you describe the overall level of fatigue/tiredness you have experienced?
2. How active was your spondylitis on average?	2. How would you describe the overall level of AS neck, back, or hip pain you have had?
3. How would you describe the overall level of pain/swelling in joints other than neck, back, or hips you have had?	3. How would you describe the overall level of pain/swelling in joints other than neck, back, or hips you have had?
4. How long does your morning stiffness last from the time you wake up? (0: 0 h; 5: 1 h; 10: 2 h or more)	4. How would you describe the overall level of discomfort you have had from any areas tender to touch or pressure?
5. CRP measured in mg/L	5. How would you describe the overall level of morning stiffness you have had from the time you wake up?
Calculation of ASDAS-CRP: 0.1216*Q1+0.1106*Q2+0.0736 *Q3+0.0586*Q4+0.5796Ln (CRP+1).	6. How long does your morning stiffness last from the time you wake up? (0: 0 h; 5: 1 h; 10: 2 h or more)
	Calculation of BASDAI: Compute the mean of questions 5 and 6. Calculate the sum of the values of questions 1–4 and add the result to the mean of questions 5 and 6. Divide the result by 5.

Sources: van der Heijde D, et al. ASDAS, a highly discriminatory ASAS-endorsed disease activity score in patients with ankylosing spondylitis. *Ann Rheum Dis.* 2009;68(12):1811-1818; and Garrett S, et al. A new approach to defining disease status in ankylosing spondylitis: the Bath Ankylosing Spondylitis Disease Activity Index. *J Rheumatol.* 1994;21(12):2286-2291.

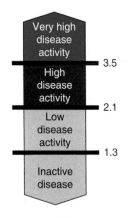

▲ **Figure 15–9. Disease state cut-offs for ASDAS.**

a longer delay to diagnosis than men, with higher patient-reported disease activity and more widespread pain symptoms, but less serologic inflammation and damage. Patients with chronic back pain starting before the age of 45 and other features concerning for SpA should be referred to rheumatology. Other features concerning for SpA include IBP, a positive family history, HLA-B27, anterior uveitis, IBD, psoriasis, enthesitis, dactylitis, and peripheral arthritis.

ARTHRITIS ASSOCIATED WITH INFLAMMATORY BOWEL DISEASE

▶ General Considerations

IBD includes ulcerative colitis and Crohn disease, though one can also consider lymphocytic colitis. Extraintestinal manifestations (overall prevalence of 35%) include arthralgias, arthritis, uveitis, and skin conditions such as psoriasis, erythema nodosum, and pyoderma gangrenosum. The prevalence of enteropathic arthritis among those with IBD is about 20% though some of these patients may be asymptomatic with sacroiliitis incidentally noted on imaging.

Gut dysbiosis and increased gut permeability are implicated in the pathogenesis of IBD. The strongest genetic association is with NOD2 alleles. The prevalence of HLA-B27 among those with IBD and axial arthritis is 70%, lower than in AS without IBD.

▶ Clinical Findings

Arthritis can be axial or peripheral and should be initially be elicited with a careful history.

IBP has a prevalence in IBD ranging from 5% to 30%. AS has a prevalence of 2–10%. In a questionnaire study of patients seen in a specialized IBD clinic, 27% reported a concomitant axSpA diagnosis, and about half had a prior rheumatologic evaluation.

Peripheral arthritis, typically nondestructive, occurs in 5–30% of individuals with IBD. Based on a natural history study, this arthritis is divided into two types. Type 1 (pauciarticular) involves fewer than five joints and is acute in onset and self-limited. It coincides with IBD symptoms and is associated with extraintestinal manifestations. Type 2 (polyarticular) involves five or more joints and is persistent and chronic. The course is independent of IBD manifestations. It is associated with uveitis but less so other extraintestinal manifestations (Table 15–5).

▶ Treatment

In general, NSAIDs should be avoided in patients with IBD, although short courses of COX-2 inhibitors may be considered. Any decision to initiate an NSAID in a patient with IBD should be discussed with the patient's gastroenterologist.

Table 15-5. Arthritis associated with IBD.

	Type I Peripheral	Type II Peripheral	Axial
Prevalence	3–6%	2–4%	~20%
Arthritis type	Oligoarticular	Polyarticular	Sacroiliitis
Joints often affected	Knee	MCPs	SI joint, spine
Timing in disease duration	Early	Later	Chronic
Course	Acute and remitting	Chronic and relapsing	Onset in younger patients
Association with GI activity	Yes	No	No

GI, gastrointestinal; MCP, metacarpophalangeal joints.

Monoclonal TNF inhibitors are recommended for active axSpA with concomitant IBD. If IBD is active, doses should be given per gastroenterology recommendations.

Vedolizumab, is a gut-selective biologic that inhibits $\alpha_4\beta_7$ integrin in the gut mucosa and is approved for use in IBD, may increase the risk of arthritis onset or recurrence.

▶ **When to Refer**

IBD patients should be referred to rheumatology if they have joint pain with inflammatory features. Patients with IBD and concomitant SpA should be comanaged by rheumatology and gastroenterology.

Sieper J, Poddubnyy D. New evidence on the management of spondyloarthritis. *Nat Rev Rheumatol.* 2016;12:282-295. [PMID: 27052489]

Smolen JS, Schöls M, Braun J, et al. Treating axial spondyloarthritis and peripheral spondyloarthritis, especially psoriatic arthritis, to target: 2017 update of recommendations by an international task force. *Ann Rheum Dis.* 2018;77(1): 3-17. [PMID: 28684559]

Spondylitis Association of America (SAA). http://www.spondylitis.org

van der Heijde D, Ramiro S, Landewé R, et al. 2016 update of the ASAS-EULAR management recommendations for axial spondyloarthritis. *Ann Rheum Dis.* 2017;76(6):978-991. [PMID: 28087505]

Ward MM, Deodhar A, Akl EA, et al. American College of Rheumatology/Spondylitis Association of America/Spondyloarthritis Research and Treatment Network 2015 recommendations for the treatment of ankylosing spondylitis and nonradiographic axial spondyloarthritis. *Arthritis Rheumatol.* 2016;68(2):282-298. [PMID: 26401991]

Weber U, Baraliakos X. Imaging in axial spondyloarthritis: changing concepts and thresholds. *Best Pract Res Clin Rheumatol.* 2018;32(3):342-356. [PMID: 31171307]

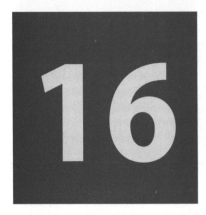

Reactive Arthritis

Sheila L. Arvikar, MD

ESSENTIALS OF DIAGNOSIS

▶ Inflammatory arthritis, developing within days to weeks of gastrointestinal or genitourinary infection, considered to be a form of spondyloarthritis.

▶ Pattern of arthritis is an asymmetric mono- or oligoarthritis tending to affect the lower extremities, associated with enthesitis and dactylitis.

▶ May have extra-articular findings, including ocular inflammation and skin manifestations, particularly keratoderma blennorrhagicum and circinate balanitis.

▶ Many patients have resolution by 6 months, but can result in a chronic arthritis.

▶ First-line treatment is nonsteroidal anti-inflammatory drugs (NSAIDs), followed by glucocorticoids and nonbiologic disease-modifying antirheumatic drugs (DMARDs).

▶ Antibiotic therapy is not of clear benefit once infection has resolved, but antibiotics may have a role in Chlamydia-induced arthritis.

General Considerations

Reactive arthritis (ReA) is a form of inflammatory arthritis that develops days to weeks following an infection, typically involving the gastrointestinal or genitourinary sites. The etiologic agent is most often a bacterial infection, but other types of pathogens can also lead to ReA. Although infection is thought to trigger the disease, organisms are generally not recovered from affected joints, and identification of the specific antecedent infection is not always possible. There are no widely accepted classification or diagnostic criteria for ReA, but proposed criteria require a clinical diagnosis of either a mono- or oligoarthritis following a microbiologically confirmed enteric or genitourinary infection (Kingsley and Sieper, 1996). ReA is generally considered to be a form of

spondyloarthritis, a group of disorders that tend to affect the axial skeleton and periarticular structures as well as peripheral joints. Other spondyloarthritides include ankylosing spondylitis, psoriatic arthritis, inflammatory bowel disease-associated arthritis, and undifferentiated spondyloarthritis.

The term "reactive arthritis," once known as Reiter syndrome, was used in the past to refer to the classic constellation of peripheral arthritis, conjunctivitis, and urethritis or cervicitis. However, it is now recognized that only a subset of patients with ReA present with the full triad of symptoms. ReA is generally characterized by a mono- to oligoarticular arthritis, often of the lower extremities. ReA can also be associated with axial skeleton involvement (particularly the lumbar spine and sacroiliac joints), enthesitis, dactylitis, and extra-articular manifestations that are typical of other forms of spondyloarthritis. The symptoms are often acute and self-limited, resolving within weeks to months, but some patients develop a chronic inflammatory arthritis (symptoms lasting longer than 6 months).

ReA predominantly affects young adults (usual range 20–40 years old) more frequently than children. Both men and women are affected, but ReA resulting from genitourinary infections occurs more commonly in men. Most cases are sporadic, but clusters of ReA cases following outbreaks of foodborne illness have been reported. ReA is the least common of the spondyloarthritis variants, particularly in the United States. Reported incidence and prevalence is variable (reported global incidence between 0.6 and 27 per 100,000), depending on geographic location, methodology for identifying preceding infection, and definition of ReA used (Courcoul et al, 2018). The incidence of ReA after *Chlamydia* infection, the most common cause of ReA, is estimated to be 4–8% (Schmitt, 2017). Enteric infections with *Campylobacter*, *Salmonella*, and *Shigella* are estimated to trigger ReA in approximately 9–12 cases per 1000 infections (Ajene et al, 2013). Some recent studies have indicated that ReA due to *Chlamydia* infection has decreased in recent years, perhaps as a result of earlier recognition and treatment of genitourinary infections. The incidence of ReA induced by enteric pathogens has been stable over time (Mason et al, 2016; Courcoul et al, 2018).

Pathogenesis

Although ReA develops after exposure to an infectious agent, the primary infection site is outside of the joint. Generally speaking, therefore, ReA is not a true septic arthritis in which a pathogen can be cultured from joints. Some studies, however, have demonstrated evidence of pathogens such as *Chlamydia trachomatis* within joints (Taylor-Robinson et al, 1992). Bacterial antigens or debris, perhaps contained within cells, may traffic to joints and trigger inflammation.

The pathogens that have been associated with ReA are shown in Table 16–1. The major enteric pathogens implicated include *Salmonella, Shigella, Campylobacter, and Yersinia.* Cases of ReA triggered by *Escherichia coli* and *Clostridium difficile* are also confirmed. Genitourinary agents include *Chlamydia, Mycoplasma, Ureaplasma,* and HIV. Current diagnostic criteria require microbiologic confirmation of either an enteric or genitourinary pathogen (Kingsley and Sieper, 1996), but respiratory pathogens such as *Chlamydia pneumoniae* and *Mycoplasma pneumoniae* have also been implicated, albeit less frequently. Mycobacterial organisms, such as Bacillus Calmette-Guérin (in the setting of intravesicular cancer treatment) and *Mycobacterium tuberculosis* (Poncet disease), have been linked to ReA. There are also emerging reports of associations with other agents, including *Strongyloides* and *Giardia.* Finally, in 10–25% of cases, there are no symptoms of an infection (Courcoul et al, 2018), which suggests that the list of triggering pathogens is not fully known. Future definitions of ReA may thus need address a broader range of organisms.

It is also not well understood why patients develop ReA following an infection. Host genetic factors may play a role. HLA-B27 is of great interest given its association with spondyloarthritis. Misfolding of HLA-B27 or presentation of arthritogenic peptides, such as microbial peptides mimicking self proteins, may lead to inflammation and autoimmunity. HLA-B27 is also associated with increased disease severity, longer disease duration, and extra-articular manifestations (Leirisalo et al, 1982). However, the presence of HLA-B27 presence is variable across studies. It is found most commonly in Caucasian patients and rarely found in patients from other ethnic groups that develop ReA. In some estimates, HLA-B27 is found in less than or equal to 50% of cases of ReA. Other mechanisms involved in pathogenesis may include induction of IL-17/IL-23 responses by microbes, as shown in *Salmonella* models of ReA (Chaurasia et al, 2016; Noto Llana et al, 2012), or the migration of mucosal T cells that produce IL-17 to the joint. Active infection within synovial tissue has been difficult to demonstrate and reports of this have been controversial, but some investigators have provided evidence that persistence of *Chlamydia* infections within joints could contribute to chronic arthritis (Gerard et al, 2013). Finally, there are ongoing investigations into whether alterations in the gut

Table 16–1. Infectious agents associated with reactive arthritis.

Gastrointestinal
- *Salmonella* (several)[a]
- *Shigella (S flexneri)*[a]
- *Campylobacter jejuni*[a]
- *Yersinia (Y enterocolitica, Y pseudotuberculosis)*[a]
- *Clostridium difficile*

Genitourinary
- *Chlamydia trachomatis*[a,b]
- HIV
- *Neisseria gonorrhoeae* (nondisseminated infection)
- *Mycoplasma genitalium*
- *Ureaplasma urealyticum*

Respiratory
- *Chlamydia pneumoniae*
- *Mycoplasma pneumoniae*

[a]Common; [b]most common.

microbiome, which is also affected by host genetics, can lead to spondyloarthropathies, including ReA.

Clinical Findings

A. Symptoms and Signs

1. Articular manifestations—Patients with ReA present with the acute onset of an asymmetric monoarthritis or oligoarticular arthritis, usually 1–4 weeks following an infection. The latency period may be longer for genitourinary infections. The most commonly affected joints are the medium to large joints of the lower extremities (hips, knees, ankles) (Figure 16–1). Upper extremity involvement, small

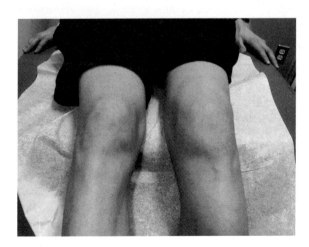

▲ **Figure 16–1.** Monoarthritis of the knee in a patient with *Chlamydia*-associated reactive arthritis. (See color insert.)

joint arthritis, and even a polyarthritis can also be seen, however, and the arthritic findings may be migratory. Inflammatory features such as warmth and swelling of involved joints are present. Axial joint involvement, particularly of the lumbar spine, is also common, and symptoms of inflammatory back pain are present in up to half of patients. The presence of HLA-B27 is associated with axial involvement in ReA.

2. Enthesitis—Enthesitis—inflammation at sites where tendons attach to bone—is a hallmark feature of ReA. Involved sites may be swollen, warm, and tender. The most typical locations for enthesitis at the Achilles tendon and the plantar fascia attachments.

3. Dactylitis—Dactylitis, or swelling of an entire toe or finger, not limited to the joint, also termed "sausage digit," is a common characteristic feature of spondyloarthritides, including ReA, occurring in up to 40% of patients (Schmitt, 2017).

4. Extra-articular involvement—Extra-articular features, particularly mucocutaneous findings, can also be observed in ReA (Table 16–2). Circinate balanitis, an inflammatory penile lesion, presents as hyperkeratotic plaques on the glans penis in circumcised males. In uncircumcised males, vesicles or pustules on the glans penis develop into painless erosions that coalesce into a serpiginous pattern. Another characteristic lesion is keratoderma blennorrhagicum (Figure 16–2), a rash on the palms and soles that begins as erythematous macules and vesicles, progressing to papules, hyperkeratotic plaques, and pustules, resembling pustular psoriasis. Finally, patients may develop oral and genital ulcers, and psoriatic type nail changes such as onychodystrophy.

In terms of other organ involvement, genitourinary tract inflammation (cervicitis, urethritis, prostatitis) may occur, particularly if the inciting infection was genitourinary in

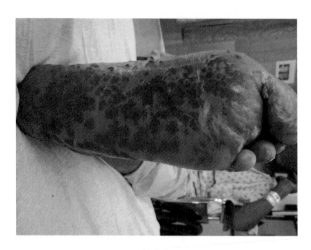

▲ **Figure 16–2.** Keratoderma blennorhagicum. (See color insert.) (Used with permission from Dr. Maureen Dubreuil, MD, MSc, Boston University School of Medicine.)

nature. Ocular involvement, particularly conjunctivitis, but also anterior uveitis, episcleritis, and keratitis may complicate ReA. Cardiac manifestations such as aortic valve regurgitation from inflammation of the aortic root, conduction disturbances, pericarditis, and aortitis all occur rarely.

B. Laboratory Findings

The diagnosis of ReA is based on the finding of an inflammatory arthritis occurring with a compatible pattern of joint involvement and developing after a convincing episode of enteric or genitourinary infection. There are no specific laboratory tests to confirm the diagnosis of ReA. ReA patients are usually seronegative for rheumatoid factor, antibodies to cyclic citrullinated peptides (anti-CCP antibodies, ACPA), and antinuclear antibodies. The erythrocyte sedimentation rate (ESR) and C-reactive protein (CRP) may be elevated, but this is not always the case. Arthrocentesis should usually be performed to exclude a septic arthritis and microcrystalline disease, but the findings on synovial fluid analysis are not diagnostic of ReA. The synovial fluid in ReA is typically inflammatory, with white blood cell counts of 5000–50,000 per microliter, predominantly composed of polymorphonuclear cells. Although the triggering event is infection, synovial fluid is sterile with negative Gram stain and cultures. PCR testing for genitourinary or enteric pathogens in synovial fluid or tissue is not practical in routine clinical practice. Testing for HLA-B27 may provide important prognostic information, portending increased risk for a more severe or chronic course.

It is important to try to identify the triggering pathogen but the pathophysiology of this condition sometimes renders this impossible. Stool cultures should be performed in the setting of gastrointestinal infections, by the diarrhea may have resolved and the inciting pathogen may

Table 16–2. Extra-articular manifestations of reactive arthritis.

Genitourinary
• Urethritis
• Cervicitis
• Prostatitis
Mucocutaneous
• Oral ulcers
• Circinate balanitis
• Keratoderma blennorrhagicum
• Onycholysis
Ocular
• Conjunctivitis
• Uveitis
• Keratitis
Cardiovascular
• Aortic insufficiency
• Aortitis
• Pericarditis

no longer be present by the time the arthritis develops. Serologic tests for enteric pathogens such as *Salmonella, Shigella, Yersinia,* and *Campylobacter* can be performed, but antibody responses may take time to develop and may be falsely negative in the acute setting. Moreover, in areas where these infections are endemic (developing nations), a positive test may not distinguish between past and recent infection. For suspected genitourinary infections, testing for *C trachomatis* or *Neisseria gonorrhoeae* by urine or genital swab nucleic acid amplification should be performed. HIV testing and evaluation for other sexually transmitted disease should also be performed.

C. Imaging Studies

Imaging findings in ReA are nonspecific. In acute disease, plain radiographs may demonstrate only joint effusions. However, periostitis (proliferative changes along shaft of bones), bony erosions, osteolysis, syndesmophytes (ossified spinal ligaments), and ankyloses may develop over time. Radiographic sacroiliitis is usually unilateral, in contrast to the bilateral sacroiliitis seen in ankylosing spondylitis. MRI and ultrasonography may be more revealing than radiographs in early disease. MRI may demonstrate SI joint inflammation and bone marrow edema (Figure 16–3). Ultrasonography may be useful for the detection of enthesitis.

▶ Differential Diagnosis

The differential diagnosis of ReA includes septic arthritis. This is particularly true in the setting of a monoarthritis. Both ReA and septic arthritis can be accompanied by fever and leukocytosis. Although synovial fluid white blood cells counts are generally higher (50,000–150,000 cells/mcL) in a septic joint than in ReA and although synovial fluid Gram stain and cultures are sometimes positive, these distinguishing features are not always present.

The types of pathogens often associated with septic arthritis, for example, *S aureus* and *Streptococci,* are rarely

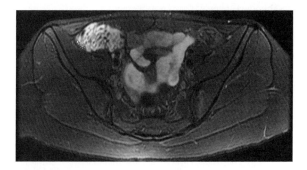

▲ **Figure 16–3.** Asymmetric sacroiliitis (bone marrow edema) of left sacroiliac (SI) joint in a patient with *Campylobacter*-induced reactive arthritis.

associated with ReA. However, a variety of clinical scenarios pose challenges with regard to determining if a syndrome is associated with an active infection as opposed to resulting from an ReA syndrome. Streptococcal infections occasionally trigger a postinfectious arthritis, but this does not include spondyloarthritis features typical of ReA. The migratory arthritis following streptococcal pharyngitis is a well-known albeit now infrequently observed feature of rheumatic fever. Moreover, overlap in the pathogens leading to infectious as opposed to strictly inflammatory arthritides does occur. As an example, *Salmonella* can cause a true septic arthritis and osteomyelitis. *N gonorrhoeae* may disseminate to joints and present with an acute oligoarticular arthritis, usually accompanied by pustular rash and tenosynovitis. In geographic areas endemic for Lyme disease, patients may present with a monoarticular inflammatory arthritis of a knee that resembles ReA. Positive serologic testing for Lyme IgG antibodies by the two-tiered approach of ELISA and Western blot helps to distinguish Lyme arthritis, which requires antibiotic treatment, from ReA. Bacterial endocarditis and viral infections (ie, parvovirus B19, HIV, and Chikungunya) and Whipple disease can also cause oligo or polyarthritis.

In terms of noninfectious causes, microcrystalline disease caused by gout or pseudogout can also mimic ReA in presenting with a monoarthritis or oligoarthritis affecting the lower extremities. Arthrocentesis and synovial fluid analysis is essential to distinguishing these conditions from ReA. Rheumatoid arthritis, most likely to be associated with a symmetrical polyarthritis of the small joints of the hands and feet, can sometimes be confused with ReA by presentations that are less classic, for example, beginning with a monoarthritis. Serologic tests for rheumatoid factor and ACPA are helpful in this setting. Behcet disease shares a number of features with ReA including extra-articular manifestations of uveitis and oral and genital ulcers, as well as sacroiliitis in a minority of cases.

Finally, ReA is sometimes difficult to distinguish from other spondyloarthritides because of their numerous overlapping features. Enthesitis, axial arthritis, HLA-B27 positivity, and extra-articular manifestations are all findings compatible with psoriatic arthritis, ankylosing spondylitis, and inflammatory bowel disease-associated arthritis as well as ReA. Longitudinal follow-up may be required to distinguish these entities. Some patients with features of ReA without evidence of an antecedent infection are categorized as having "undifferentiated spondyloarthritis." Some investigators have found salmonella-specific T-cell responses in patients with undifferentiated spondyloarthritis (Chaurasia et al, 2016), raising the possibility that undifferentiated spondyloarthritis is a "forme fruste" of ReA.

▶ Treatment

Aggressive treatments are usually not warranted at the outset of treatment for ReA, because the duration of the arthritis may be short. First-line therapy for ReA generally consists of anti-inflammatory doses of nonsteroidal anti-inflammatory drugs (NSAIDs), such as naproxen 500 mg orally two times a day or ibuprofen 800 mg four times daily. Patients should be monitored for renal and gastrointestinal side effects and GI prophylaxis should be considered. Patients typically report substantial but often incomplete relief of their symptoms with NSAIDs. In patients who do not respond to NSAIDs, intra-articular steroids can be considered if only one or two joints are involved. For more extensive joint involvement, oral glucocorticoids may be helpful for peripheral arthritis but are usually not effective for axial symptoms. Topical steroid preparations may be useful for ocular and skin manifestations.

Patients who are resistant to NSAIDs and glucocorticoids or who require large doses of glucocorticoids should begin a disease-modifying antirheumatic drug (DMARD). Methotrexate and sulfasalazine are both commonly used options, but unfortunately there are limited data regarding the use of DMARDs in ReA. Sulfasalazine alone has been formally studied and was shown to have a trend toward efficacy at a dose of 2000 mg/day compared to placebo in ReA patients (Clegg et al, 1996). Sulfasalazine is not always well tolerated due to GI side effects, rashes, and cytopenias. Screening for glucose-6-phosphate dehydrogenase deficiency should be performed prior to initiation given risk of hemolytic anemia.

Neither sulfasalazine nor methotrexate is likely to work quickly, so depending on the patient's level of disability from the inflammatory arthritis a biologic DMARD might be a better option. The treatment decision should also take into consideration the fact that certain manifestations of ReA, particularly enthesitis and axial arthritis, respond poorly to nonbiologic DMARDs. Under these circumstances, a tumor necrosis factor (TNF) inhibitor should be utilized. Extrapolation from the efficacy of TNF inhibitors in other forms of seronegative spondyloarthropathies suggests that these agents should be highly effective in ReA, and this is confirmed by the limited clinical experience to date. Early treatment with TNF inhibitors in peripheral spondyloarthritis may result in greater rates of remission (Carron et al, 2017), but whether early biologic treatment in ReA could abort the development of chronic arthritis is not yet known. Finally, given the involvement of IL-17/IL-23 in the pathogenesis of ReA and other spondyloarthritides, therapies directed against these pathways (eg, secukinumab, an IL-17 inhibitors and ustekinumab, an IL12/23 inhibitor) are intuitively appealing. To date, however, they have not yet been formally studied.

In terms of antibiotic treatment in ReA, there is little support for treatment of gastrointestinal infection (Barber et al, 2013), which has usually resolved by the time of arthritis onset. However, if gastrointestinal bacterial infection remains active and the symptoms are severe, treatment directed at the underlying pathogen can be considered.

Patients with C trachomatis or N gonorrhoeae infections should be treated, as should their partners. However, there is less evidence that antibiotic therapy is helpful in the treatment of arthritis once the active infection has resolved

(Barber et al, 2013). Given that there has been more evidence of Chlamydia persistence in joint tissue than for other organisms, there has been greater focus on antibiotic treatment for Chlamydia- induced arthritis. One randomized, double-blind placebo-controlled study found that combination antibiotics (rifampin combined with either doxycycline or azithromycin) were superior to placebo for the treatment of ReA of at least 6 months' duration. All of the patients in that trial had ReA triggered by either C trachomatis or C pneumoniae, as demonstrated by polymerase chain reaction studies of synovial tissue or peripheral blood mononuclear cells (Carter et al, 2010). These findings have not been confirmed by other studies; however, substantial skepticism about the value of antibiotics in this setting persists.

▶ Complications

Although many patients have resolution of arthritis within 6 months, some may develop chronic inflammatory arthritis. Patients with chronic inflammatory arthritis may develop erosions, joint damage, leading to chronic pain, and functional disability.

▶ Prognosis

The course of ReA is variable and may depend on genetic factors as well as the nature of the triggering infection. In many patients, the disease may resolve within weeks to months. However, some patients (~20%) develop chronic or recurrent symptoms (Carron et al, 2017). Some recent studies have reported even higher frequencies of chronic arthritis. One study comparing ReA cases in different decades (1986–1996 vs 2002–2012) found an increased chronicity of ReA in the more recent cohort (55% vs 16%) (Courcoul et al, 2018). Another recent study of Guatemalan patients indicated that half of 32 patients had persistent symptoms at 2 years (Garcia Ferrer et al, 2018). Patients with HLA-B27 positivity or the triad of arthritis, conjunctivitis and urethritis may have more likelihood of developing a chronic spondyloarthritis.

Ajene AN, Fischer Walker CL, Black RE. Enteric pathogens and reactive arthritis: a systematic review of Campylobacter, Salmonella and Shigella-associated reactive arthritis. J Health Popul Nutr. 2013;31:299-307. [PMID: 24288942]

Barber CE, Kim J, Inman RD, et al. Antibiotics for treatment of reactive arthritis: a systemic review and metaanalysis. J Rheumatol. 2013;40:916-28. [PMID: 23588936]

Carron P, Varkas G, Cypers H, et al. Anti-TNF-induced remission in very early peripheral spondyloarthritis: the CRESPA study. Ann Rheum Dis. 76:1389-1395, 2017. [PMID: 28213565]

Carter JD, Espinoza LR, Inman RD, et al. Combination antibiotics as a treatment for chronic chlamydia-induced reactive arthritis: a double-blind, placebo controlled, prospective trial. Arthritis Rheum. 2010;62:1298-307. [PMID: 20155838]

Chaurasia S, Shasany AK, Aggarwal A, et al. Recombinant salmonella typhimurium outer membrane protein A is recognized by synovial CD8 cells and stimulates synovial fluid mononuclear cells to produce interleukin (IL-17)/IL-23 in patients with reactive arthritis and undifferentiated spondyloarthropathy. *Clin Exp Immunol.* 2016;185:210-218. [PMID: 27060348]

Clegg DO, Reda DJ, Weisman MH, et al. Comparison of sulfasalazine and placebo in the treatment of reactive arthritis (Reiter's syndrome): a Department of Veterans Affairs cooperative study. *Arthritis Rheum.* 1996;39:2021-2027. [PMID: 10555027]

Courcoul A, Brinster A, Decullier E, et al. A bicentre retrospective study of features and outcomes of patients with reactive arthritis. *Joint Bone Spine.* 2018;85(2):201-205. [PMID: 28238883]

Garcia Ferrer HR, Azan A, Iraheta I, et al. Potential risk factors for reactive arthritis and persistence of symptoms at 2 years: a case-control study with longitudinal follow-up. *Clin Rheumatol.* 2018;37(2):415-422. [PMID: 29139030]

Gerard HC, Carter JD, Hudson AP. *Chlamydia trachomatis* is present and metabolically active during the remitting phase in synovial tissues from patients with chronic chlamydia-induced reactive arthritis. *Am J Med Sci.* 2013;346:22-25. [PMID: 23792903]

Kingsley G, Sieper J. Third International Workshop on Reactive Arthritis. Report and abstracts. *Ann Rheum Dis.* 1996; 55:564-584. [PMID: 8815821]

Leirisalo M, Skylv G, Kousa M, et al. Follow-up study on patients with Reiter's disease and reactive arthritis, with special reference to HLA-B27. *Arthritis Rheum.* 1982;25:249-259. [PMID: 6978139]

Mason, E. et al. Reactive arthritis at the Sydney Sexual Health Centre 1992–2012: declining despite increasing chlamydia diagnoses. *Int. J. STD AIDS.* 2016;27:882-889. [PMID: 26378192]

Noto Llana M, Sarnacki SH, Vázquez MV, et al. *Salmonella enterica* induces joint inflammation and expression of interleukin-17 in draining lymph nodes early after onset of enterocolitis in mice. *Infect Immun.* 2012;80:2231-2239. [PMID: 22493084]

Schmitt SK. Reactive arthritis. *Infect Dis Clin North Am.* 2017; 31:265-277. [PMID: 28292540]

Taylor-Robinson D, Gilroy CB, Thomas BJ, et al. Detection of *Chlamydia trachomatis* DNA in joints of reactive arthritis patients by polymerase chain reaction. *Lancet.* 1992;340:81-82. [PMID: 24828551]

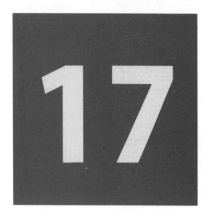

Psoriatic Arthritis

M. Elaine Husni, MD, MPH

▶ Psoriatic arthritis (PsA) is a chronic, immune-mediated disease that affects both the skin and joints.

▶ Clinical manifestations are diverse; however, hallmark features include asymmetric inflammatory arthritis, skin and nail psoriasis, enthesitis, and dactylitis.

▶ About one-third of patients with psoriasis will develop PsA.

▶ Patients with PsA are seronegative, lacking both rheumatoid factor and anti-CCP antibody.

▶ Radiographic findings of erosions, periosteal reaction, ankyloses, and juxta-articular new bone formation can occur.

▶ General Considerations

Psoriatic arthritis (PsA) is a chronic, immune-mediated disease associated with both inflammatory arthritis and skin psoriasis. The prevalence of PsA varies in the United States from 6 to 25 cases per 10,000 people (Ogdie and Weiss, 2015). This wide range in prevalence is attributed to the lack of consensus on the case definition of PsA. The mean age of disease onset ranges from 30 to 55 years, with men and women equally affected. Up to 30% of patients with psoriasis can develop PsA. Patients with PsA often suffer from impaired function and reduced quality of life. PsA is also associated with a higher risk of certain comorbidities, including the increased risk of cardiovascular disease associated with hypertension, hyperlipidemia, diabetes, obesity, and metabolic syndrome, as well as ophthalmologic disease, osteoporosis, and inflammatory bowel disease.

PsA patients present in a heterogeneous manner, the diverse clinical features of which often lead to a delay in diagnosis. Patients can present with either an asymmetric oligoarthritis, an symmetric polyarthritis, or an arthritis of the axial skeleton (ie, the sacroiliac joints and spine). Any of these presentations may be accompanied by periarticular involvement with dactylitis (a "sausage digit") or enthesitis, defined as inflammation at a point at which a tendon inserts into a bone. Skin psoriasis can accompany the joint symptoms, including manifestations such as plaque psoriasis over extensor surfaces, psoriasis predominantly affecting the scalp or nails, or pustular psoriasis on the palms and soles. Despite tremendous growth in the number of approved therapies for patients with PsA, the effects of approved medications are variable with regard to their joint and skin outcomes. The disease heterogeneity of PsA heightens the challenges of selecting the best therapeutic options and improving overall health outcomes.

▶ Pathogenesis

The etiology of PsA is not completely understood, but our understanding of its pathogenesis is evolving. It is hypothesized that both genetic and environmental factors can trigger an aberrant inflammatory response in various organ systems beyond the skin and joint manifestations of PsA. In contrast to rheumatoid arthritis, a disorder in which the synovial is recognized as the primary articular site of inflammation, in PsA the primary site of inflammation is the enthesis. Enthesitis is a distinguishing feature in the pathogenesis of PsA but can also occur more broadly in patients with any of the seronegative spondyloarthropathies (Ferguson et al, 2019).

T cells are important in the pathophysiologies of both psoriasis and PsA. CD8+ T cells in particular play central roles. In addition to Type-17 cells, which include CD4+ and Th17 cells, IL-17A/IL-22-producing cells are increased in psoriatic synovial fluid compared to rheumatoid synovial fluid. Immune cells, including T cells, dendritic cells, macrophages, innate lymphoid cells, MAIT cells, natural killer cells, mast cells, and others, have the ability to synthesize proinflammatory mediators in this process. Tumor necrosis factor (TNF) and interleukin-23/interleukin-17 pathways also contribute to the pathogenesis of PsA and offer compelling treatment targets for both established and emerging therapies.

Preclinical models have provided evidence that further elucidates the physiological response to PsA. In particular, IL-23 overexpression in murine models leads to enthesitis, synovitis, and osteolytic activity (Sherlock et al, 2012), symptoms of features related to both TNF and IL-17. Therapies that do not target cytokines directly, such as Janus kinase (JAK) inhibitors (eg, tofacitinib) and T-cell activation inhibitors (eg, CTLA4-Ig or abatacept), have also been evaluated (Bravo and Kavanaugh, 2019). T-helper 17 (TH17) cells produce IL-17A and are regulated by IL-23. Targeted IL-17 inhibition dramatically ameliorates skin psoriasis, shows moderate efficacy in joint manifestations, reduces progression of radiographic peripheral joint damage, and improves enthesitis and dactylitis (Bravo and Kavanaugh, 2019). Although IL12/23 inhibition has demonstrated efficacy in PsA, it is now recognized that IL-23 may be more relevant to the overall efficacy, especially for cutaneous psoriasis. IL-23 inhibition leads to substantial improvements in both skin and joint outcomes (Bravo and Kavanaugh, 2019).

PsA has a high rate of heritability. The frequencies of HLAB*08, HLAB*27, HLAB*38, and HLAB*39 are all higher in PsA patients compared to the general population (Ritchlin et al, 2017). Environmental exposures to microbes affect the nature of the immune response. With the progression of precision medicine, "multiomics" is becoming a central focus for researchers in the development of advanced therapies. The gut-joint axis is of increasing interest as microbial infections are known triggers of specific types of spondyloarthritis. In addition, PsA patients are more likely than are health controls to experience gut dysbiosis. Genetic and environmental factors are important triggers of disease activity, but the IL-23/IL-17 and TNF pathways remain essential to the propagation joint inflammation (Bravo and Kavanaugh, 2019; Ritchlin et al, 2017).

▶ Clinical Findings

A. Symptoms and Signs (Figure 17–1)

The clinical assessment of PsA can be complicated due to the multiple domains that can be involved. There is no specific diagnostic test for PsA. As a consequence of this, the diagnosis is usually based on recognizing the clinical and imaging features. The presence of inflammatory arthritis, enthesitis, dactylitis, and joint pattern distribution in the setting of psoriasis can provide important clues related to psoriatic disease.

1. Articular involvement—The original description by Moll and Wright described PsA as five different subtypes. These included an asymmetric oligoarthritis of the hands and feet, a symmetric polyarthritis, a distal interphalangeal (DIP) joint predominant pattern, an axial involvement form, and the rarest and most destructive articular manifestation of PsA, arthritis mutilans. These patterns can vary over time, complicating diagnosis.

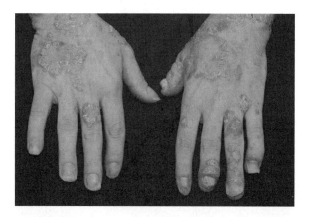

▲ **Figure 17–1.** Patient with psoriatic arthritis affecting the hands showing psoriatic nail changes with onycholysis and typical plaque psoriasis. Telescoping of the L thumb finger and L 3rd DIP joint.

Regardless of the number of symptomatic joints at disease onset, in the absence of effective treatment most patients will progress to additional joint involvement. Ongoing destruction of joints is evidenced clinically by the appearance of joint deformities and radiographically by the development of juxta-articular erosions, joint-space narrowing, and, in some cases, bony ankylosis. The subtype of PsA associated with axial involvement or spondylitis is part of the spondyloarthropathy family of diseases, sharing many features with ankylosing spondylitis, reactive arthritis, and the spondyloarthropathy associated with inflammatory bowel disease. Arthritis mutilans describes the end stage of the destructive process, where loss of bony architecture allows complete subluxation and "telescoping" of the involved digit ("opera-glass finger" or *doigt en lorgnette* in French). Arthritis mutilans, associated with long-standing, poorly controlled disease, is fortunately uncommon.

2. Dactylitis (Figure 17–2)—Dactylitisis, the uniform swelling of a single digit of the fingers or toes, is a distinctive feature of the spondyloarthropathies. Dactylitis affects up to one-third to one-half of PsA patients at some point during the course of the disease. It is often asymmetric and has a predilection for the lower extremities, involving the toes more frequently than the fingers (Brockbank et al, 2005). Advanced imaging modalities such as magnetic resonance imaging (MRI) have allowed better visualization of the joint pathology and demonstrated a close link between dactylitis and enthesitis (Tan et al, 2015).

3. Enthesitis—Enthesitis, an inflammatory process occurring at the site of insertion of tendons into bone, is observed in up to 30–50% of patients. Common sites for enthesitis are the Achilles tendon, the plantar fascia, and the pelvic bones. Entheseal inflammation may evolve to destruction of the adjacent bone and joints. The identification of enthesitis

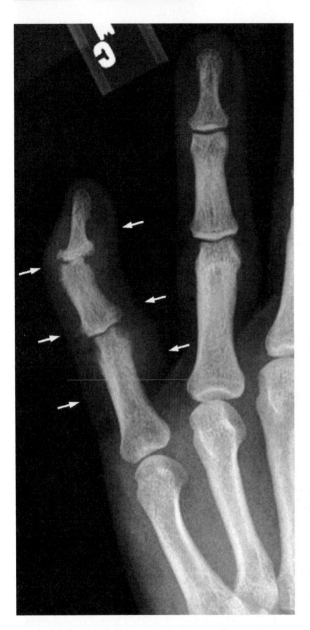

▲ **Figure 17–2.** PA radiograph demonstrates diffuse soft-tissue swelling, or "sausage digit," of the small finger (*arrows*). Note the marginal erosions at the PIP and DIP joints. (Used with permission from Carl S. Winalski, MD, Cleveland Clinic.)

places a patient's diagnosis squarely within the realm of a seronegative spondyloarthropathy. If cutaneous psoriasis is also present, then PsA is the most likely diagnosis.

4. Skin and nail changes (see Figure 17–1)—All forms of psoriasis are associated with arthritis, but classic psoriasis vulgaris is seen most frequently. Typical psoriatic lesions

are erythematous plaques that produce itchy scaling. Many patients with PsA have only mild to moderate skin disease; however, there is no consistent correlation between the degree of psoriasis and the extent of joint involvement. The psoriasis may be subtle. Therefore, careful examination of the entire skin surface must be performed when PsA is suspected, with particular attention to the hairline, scalp, external auditory canal, periumbilical area, and gluteal cleft (Merola et al, 2018).

Nail involvement is common in PsA and can cause changes, including ridging, pitting, onycholysis, and hyperkeratosis. Nails may represent as a sign of psoriasis even in the absence of more characteristic psoriasis skin lesions. Nail changes on the affected finger often correlate with damage to the adjacent DIP joint.

5. Extra-articular manifestations—The most commonly associated conditions are the increased risk of cardiovascular disease and related medical issues, such as hypertension, metabolic syndrome, type 2 diabetes, and fatty liver (Husni et al, 2018; Lucke et al, 2016; Puig et al, 2015). Ocular inflammation (eg, uveitis, iritis, scleritis, and episcleritis), inflammatory bowel disease, subclinical colitis, and osteoporosis can occur in PsA (Husni, 2015).

B. Laboratory Findings

There are no laboratory tests diagnostic for PsA. Because of the systemic, inflammatory nature of the disease, acute phase reactants such as the C-reactive protein and the erythrocyte sedimentation rate may be elevated but are rarely dramatically high. In some patients, elevations of acute phase reactants correlate with disease activity—usually those with a higher number of affected joints. Approximately 25% of patients with PsA are HLA-B27 positive.

Patients with PsA usually do not have rheumatoid factor or anti-CCP antibodies. The reported frequency of anti-CCP antibodies was reported to be approximately 10%, but ranged as low as less than 1% and as high as 20% in some studies. The presence of this antibody has been reported to be associated with a more severe disease phenotype, correlating with polyarthritis, erosive disease, and dactylitis (Kim and Lee, 2019). A positive rheumatoid factor is not an exclusion criterion for the diagnosis of PsA. Antinuclear antibodies are detected in 10–20% of patients, which is comparable to the prevalence of antinuclear antibody positivity in healthy control populations. Hyperuricemia, perhaps a consequence of increased cell turnover associated with psoriasis, is present in 20–30% of patients with PsA (AlJohani et al, 2018). Synovial fluid analysis reveals inflammatory fluid, with white blood cell counts usually in the 5000–50,000/mcL range.

C. Imaging Studies

The most common radiographic findings in PsA are joint-space narrowing and erosions. PsA erosions can be distinguished from RA by their absence of juxta-articular osteopenia and the presence of pathologic new bone formation, a distinctive

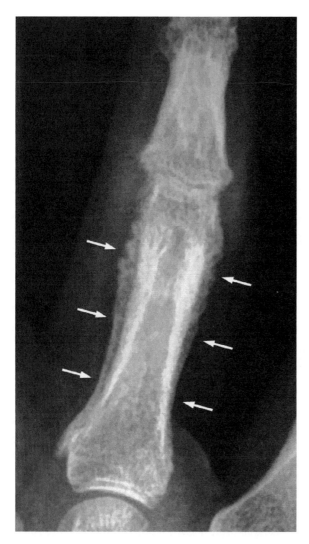

▲ **Figure 17–3.** PA radiograph of the ring finger demonstrates benign appearing periosteal reaction (*arrows*) along the shaft of the proximal phalanx. There is associated soft-tissue swelling of the digit. (Used with permission from Carl S. Winalski, MD, Cleveland Clinic.)

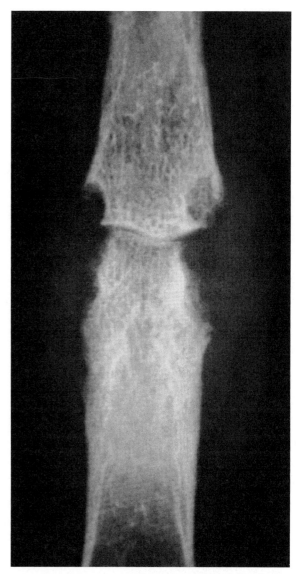

▲ **Figure 17–4.** PA radiograph of the long finger PIP joint demonstrates moderate-sized marginal erosions of the base of the middle phalanx and proximal phalangeal head. There is "fluffy" new bone (periostitis) involved the proximal phalangeal neck (*arrows*). There is also severe joint space narrowing and soft-tissue swelling. (Used with permission from Carl S. Winalski, MD, Cleveland Clinic.)

feature of PsA. This new bone formation often occurs along the shaft of the metacarpal and metatarsal bones and is seen as a fluffy periostitis (Figures 17–3 and 17–4). Rheumatologists and radiologists may use the term "whiskering" to describe these proliferative changes. Typically, these findings are asymmetric, paralleling the pattern of the clinical arthritis.

Severe destructive changes of the joints may occur with longstanding disease but may also develop rapidly in a single joint, resulting in a whittling phenomenon of the bone. When a phalanx is involved, it becomes "penciled," thus giving rise to the classic "pencil-in-cup" deformity when it abuts the

base of an adjacent phalanx (Figure 17–5). For those with axial involvement, unilateral sacroilitis changes can be seen along with syndesmophytes.

Both MRI protocols and power Doppler ultrasound imaging are being performed with increased frequency and can detail synovitis, entheseal inflammation, and erosions earlier

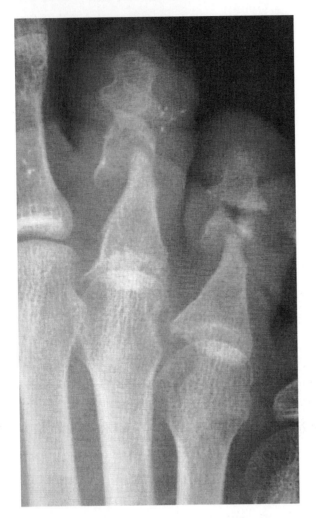

▲ **Figure 17–5.** PA radiograph shows severe osteolysis of the phalanges of the third and fourth toes resulting in "pencil-in-cup" deformities of the PIP joints. (Used with permission from Carl S. Winalski, MD, Cleveland Clinic.)

than plain radiographs. Subchondral bone marrow changes can be detected with MRI.

▶ Differential Diagnosis

The Classification Criteria for Psoriatic Arthritis (CASPAR) criteria are commonly used because of their simplicity and relatively high specificity and sensitivity, but there is not yet consensus on diagnostic criteria. The diagnosis of PsA may be challenging, particularly when skin manifestations are subtle or the arthritis predates skin lesions. The heterogeneity of PsA, the lack of defined diagnostic criteria, and the possibility of overlap syndromes with other rheumatic diseases also add to the complexity of diagnosis.

The differential diagnosis of PsA includes other forms of inflammatory arthritis, particularly rheumatoid arthritis and the other seronegative spondyloarthropathies (ankylosing spondylitis, reactive arthritis, and inflammatory bowel disease–associated arthritis). When acute in onset, the monoarticular and oligoarticular forms of PsA can pose a diagnostic dilemma with the crystal arthropathies (gout and pseudogout) and septic arthritis, necessitating the analysis of synovial fluid to exclude these alternative diagnoses. When performing an arthrocentesis in a patient with psoriasis, it is critical to avoid passing the aspirating needle through psoriatic plaques, which are often heavily contaminated with bacteria.

▶ Treatment

The treatment of PsA is aimed at controlling the inflammatory process. Evidence-based treatment recommendations can be reviewed in publications by several national organizations, including ACR/NPF (American College of Rheumatology/National Psoriasis Foundation) (Singh et al, 2019), EULAR (European Union League AR), and GRAPPA (Group for Research and Assessment of Psoriasis and Psoriatic Arthritis) (Coates et al, 2016). We will briefly review the symptomatic and disease-modifying agents used in PsA.

A. Symptomatic Treatment (Nonsteroidal Anti-Inflammatory Drugs, Glucocorticoids, Local Glucocorticoid Injections)

In patients with PsA, nonsteroidal anti-inflammatory drugs (NSAIDs) may be used to relieve musculoskeletal symptoms of pain and stiffness. NSAIDs are efficacious for joint symptoms and are often used as a first line of treatment in patients with mild, oligoarticular disease. The potential for gastrointestinal and cardiac adverse effects and contraindications need to be considered because high NSAID doses are often required.

Local injections of glucocorticoids provide adjunctive therapy in PsA that can be an important bridge to symptom relief until systemic treatment takes effect. Judicious use of glucocorticoid injections may also be helpful in dactylitis (tendon sheath injections) and in enthesitis, for example, at the elbow or the retrocalcaneal bursae in Achilles enthesitis. Ultrasound guided procedures can help guide these injections if needed. Systemic glucocorticoids may be used with caution at the lowest effective dose in the shortest amount of time. Long-term use of systemic glucocorticoids should be avoided based on the significant risks of adverse events. Systemic glucocorticoids are generally reserved for acute flares and for bridging to other disease-modifying drugs in the short term.

B. Disease-Modifying Antirheumatic Drugs

1. Oral small molecules—For patients with persistent or acute disease activity, disease-modifying antirheumatic drugs (DMARDs) are recommended. Many oral DMARDs have been used in the treatment of PsA, including methotrexate

(MTX), sulfasalazine, leflunomide, and cyclosporine. These have generally demonstrated variable improvement in skin and joint outcomes. Few robust trials have examined specific subsets of psoriatic diseases such as enthesitis-predominant or axial-related PsA.

Methotrexate (MTX) is the most popular oral DMARD used in the peripheral articular manifestations of PsA, and it is often efficacious for skin psoriasis. Careful consideration must be given to identify the efficacious dose in individual patients, because there is much variability. Doses up to 20–25 mg/wk may be required to obtain a clinical response in some patients, but others achieve good effects with lower doses. The subcutaneous route is often recommended in the higher weekly dose range to improve the GI tolerability. The common side effects include nausea, vomiting, abdominal pain, and mouth ulcers. Rare but serious adverse effects include myelosuppression, hepatotoxicity, infection, and pulmonary fibrosis. Daily supplementation with folic or folinic acid (1 mg/day) can alleviate hepatotoxic and gastrointestinal adverse effects.

Sulfasalazine (SSZ) can be effective in improving the symptoms of peripheral synovitis; however, its response is not as robust as newer agents in PsA. SSZ may be utilized in mild PsA, particularly in the absence of more aggressive clinical features. Adverse events such as gastrointestinal intolerance, dizziness, and liver toxicity occur in up to one-third of patients receiving SSZ. Therefore, liver function tests and blood counts should be checked periodically. SSZ may cause allergic reactions, including a rash, and monitoring for these is important. SSZ should be started at a low dose (500 mg twice daily) and slowly increased over weeks to a maximum dose of 2–3 g daily.

Leflunomide inhibits the synthesis of de novo pyrimidine, following which T-cell activation and proliferation is suppressed. Leflunomide (20 mg daily) has a moderate symptom-modifying effect on peripheral synovitis and might improve dactylitis but only a modest effect on the skin psoriasis. There are no data on the effect of leflunomide on enthesitis, spondylitis, or radiographic progression. The more frequent side effects include diarrhea, alopecia, hypertension, and pruritus. Given the drug's prolonged elimination half-life, it is critical to use contraception in women of childbearing age.

Cyclosporine can improve peripheral synovitis and skin psoriasis but has little or no effect on spondylitis and radiographic progression. The medication is limited by adverse events such as hypertension and nephrotoxicity in addition to the numerous drug-drug interactions.

C. PDE4 Inhibitor

Apremilast, an orally administered small molecule that inhibits phosphodiesterase 4 (PDE4), has been effective in reducing the severity of moderate-to-severe plaque psoriasis and difficult-to-treat nail, scalp, and palmoplantar psoriasis. It improves the signs and symptoms of PsA (enthesitis, dactylitis, physical function, and fatigue) in both conventional DMARD-naïve patients and those who have previously received conventional DMARDs. It does not require any specific laboratory monitoring and is generally well-tolerated except for gastrointestinal side effects (diarrhea, nausea), which often improve after the first few weeks of treatment.

D. Biologic Therapies

1. Tumor Necrosis Factor inhibitor (TNFi)—In treatment-naive patients with active PsA, a TNFi can be used. There are numerous randomized clinical trials demonstrating good efficacy for both the skin and joints as well as slowing or halting radiographic progression. There are five available anti-TNF agents (etanercept, infliximab, adalimumab, golimumab, and certolizumab pegol) that inhibit the activity of TNFα. There are also large amounts of data pertaining to the efficacy of these agents for the treatment of enthesitis, dactylitis, and axial disease from trials of these medications in ankylosing spondylitis (Bravo and Kavanaugh, 2019). The common adverse effects include injection site and infusion reactions and issues related to immunosuppression. Reactivation of latent tuberculosis has been seen with all these agents and screening for tuberculosis should be done before initiating an anti-TNF agent. There have been relative contraindications with heart failure or multiple sclerosis patients depending on the severity and risk regarding these concomitant conditions.

2. Ustekinumab—Ustekinumab, an anti-p40 antibody that is directed against the IL-12/23 subunit, inhibits Th17 signaling pathways downstream. Ustekinumab proved to be clinically efficacious in two phase III trials involving PsA patients (PSUMMIT-1 and PSUMMIT-2). It is currently approved for the treatment of PsA following the failure of NSAIDs and conventional DMARDs, and as an alternative to TNFi (25). It has a good safety profile and a convenient Q12 week dosing regimen but appears to be more effective for skin psoriasis than for PsA.

3. Interleukin-17 inhibitors—A newer class of agents include the interleukin-17 (IL-17) inhibitors, secukinumab and ixekizumab, both of which block IL-17; and brodalumab, which binds to and blocks the IL-17 receptor. These IL-17 inhibitors have demonstrated efficacy in both skin and joints (albeit, with better skin psoriasis response compared with joint response) and have demonstrated inhibition of radiographic progression. In addition to their efficacy in treating arthritis, these medications are effective for dactylitis, enthesitis, and skin and nail psoriasis, as well. The reported side effect profiles include an increased risk of candidiasis infection and exacerbation or unmasking of inflammatory bowel disease.

4. CTLA-4IG—**Abatacept**, a cytotoxic-T-lymphocyte-associated antigen 4 (CTLA-4)–Ig human fusion protein, acts to prevent naïve T-cell activation through the inhibition of the CD28 costimulatory pathways. Abatacept is a potential treatment option for a select group of patients with PsA, particularly those with active peripheral arthritis and less skin psoriasis involvement. Although there were trends toward improvement in radiographic progression, enthesitis and dactylitis, abatacept had minimal effects on skin and should not be first line in those with more severe skin involvement or active axial disease. Abatacept has a good safety profile and may be favored in patients with recurrent or serious infection risk.

5. Janus kinase (JAK) inhibitor—Tofacitinib is the first JAK inhibitor approved at a dosage of 5 mg twice daily (BID) or 11 mg extended release dosage for the treatment of active PsA. This can be used in combination with methotrexate for patients who have had an inadequate response or intolerant to a previous other DMARD. Tofacitinib may be used instead of other biologics (TNFi, IL-12/23i, or IL-17i) in patients preferring an oral medication option and may have more mild psoriasis disease. The response in skin psoriasis is not as robust as other available biologics in severe psoriasis.

E. Summary

There are additional biologic agents currently being tested in PsA and this will help patients who do not respond or partially respond to the current treatment options. Most approved drugs for PsA demonstrate greater efficacy for the skin compared to joints, and there is still an unmet need to improve on the joint domain outcome. There should also be an emphasis on wellness strategies to help patients with lifestyle modification (smoking cessation, sleep, stress, exercise, weight management, and controlling stress) to maintain good outcomes and improve quality of life in patients living with PsA.

F. Surgery

As with many inflammatory arthritides, having long-standing erosive, destructive, and uncontrolled disease can lead to extensive joint deformities. If severe destructive disease is present, orthopedic surgery consultation may be considered for joint replacement or stabilization.

▶ Prognosis

Recent research has focused on the early identification of PsA as early therapeutic interventions can lead to better patient outcomes. The strategies used for early recognition include developing patient-oriented questionnaires to identify PsA in a variety of settings, advanced imaging techniques, and the detection of candidate biomarkers to help with both early diagnosis and to follow treatment response. Because the bony destruction associated with PsA is irreversible, prompt diagnosis and early intervention are essential to preserve a patient's functional status and quality of life. If the appropriate diagnosis of a patient is in question, if radiographic damage is detected at presentation, or if a patient does not respond to first-line therapies with NSAIDs, referral to a rheumatologist is appropriate. Furthermore, there is value in greater comanagement with our dermatology colleagues to help improve patient outcomes. There are many unique models of care that involve rheumatologists and dermatologists collaborating in the care of patients with PsA.

The author would like to thank Dr. Xing Qian and MacKenzie Dunlap for their editorial support.

AlJohani R, Polachek A, Ye JY, et al. Characteristic and outcome of psoriatic arthritis patients with hyperuricemia. *J Rheumatol.* 2018;45:(2):213-217. [PMID: 29196385]

Bravo A, Kavanaugh A. Bedside to bench: defining the immunopathogenesis of psoriatic arthritis. *Nat Rev Rheumatol.* 2019;15(11):645-656. [PMID: 31485004]

Brockbank JE, Stein M, Schentag CT, et al. Dactylitis in psoriatic arthritis: a marker for disease severity? *Ann Rheum Dis.* 2005;64:(2):188-190. [PMID: 15271771]

Coates LC, Kavanaugh A, Mease PJ, et al. Group for research and assessment of psoriasis and psoriatic arthritis 2015 treatment recommendations for psoriatic arthritis *Arthritis Rheumatol.* 2016;68:(5):1060-1071. [PMID: 26749174]

Ferguson LD, Siebert S, McInnes IB, et al. Cardiometabolic comorbidities in RA and PsA: lessons learned and future directions. *Nat Rev Rheumatol.* 2019;15:(8):461-474. [PMID: 31292564]

FitzGerald O, Haroon M, Giles JT, et al. Concepts of pathogenesis in psoriatic arthritis: genotype determines clinical phenotype. *Arthritis Res Ther.* 2015;17:115. [PMID: 25948071]

Husni ME. Comorbidities in psoriatic arthritis. *Rheum Dis Clin North Am.* 2015;41:(4):677-698. [PMID: 26476226]

Husni ME, Wilson Tang WH, Lucke M, et al. Correlation of high-density lipoprotein-associated paraoxonase 1 activity with systemic inflammation, disease activity, and cardiovascular risk factors in psoriatic disease. *Arthritis Rheumatol.* 2018;70:(8):1240-1250. [PMID: 29569857]

Kim KY, Lee YH. Anti-cyclic citrullinated peptide antibody in psoriatic arthritis: a meta-analysis of its frequency and association with clinical features. *Z Rheumatol.* 2019. [PMID: 31286191]

Lucke M, Messner W, Kim ES, et al. The impact of identifying carotid plaque on addressing cardiovascular risk in psoriatic arthritis. *Arthritis Res Ther.* 2016;18:178. [PMID: 27485213]

Merola JF, Qureshi A, Husni ME. Underdiagnosed and undertreated psoriasis: nuances of treating psoriasis affecting the scalp, face, intertriginous areas, genitals, hands, feet, and nails. *Dermatol Ther.* 2018;31:(3):e12589. [PMID: 29512290]

Ogdie A, Weiss P. The epidemiology of psoriatic arthritis. *Rheum Dis Clin North Am.* 2015;41:(4):545-568. [PMID: 26476218]

Puig L, Strohal R, Husni ME, et al. Cardiometabolic profile, clinical features, quality of life and treatment outcomes in patients with moderate-to-severe psoriasis and psoriatic arthritis. *J Dermatolog Treat.* 2015;26:(1):7-15. [PMID: 24283931]

Ritchlin CT, Colbert RA, Gladman DD. Psoriatic arthritis. *N Engl J Med.* 2017;376:(10):957-970. [PMID: 28273019]

Sherlock JP, Joyce-Shaikh B, Turner SP, et al. IL-23 induces spondyloarthropathy by acting on ROR-gammat+ CD3+CD4-CD8- entheseal resident T cells. *Nat Med.* 2012;18:(7):1069-1076. [PMID: 22772566]

Singh JA, Guyatt G, Ogdie A, et al. Special Article: 2018 American College of Rheumatology/National Psoriasis Foundation Guideline for the Treatment of Psoriatic Arthritis. *Arthritis Care Res (Hoboken).* 2019;71:(1):2-29. [PMID: 30499259]

Tan AL, Fukuba E, Halliday NA, et al. High-resolution MRI assessment of dactylitis in psoriatic arthritis shows flexor tendon pulley and sheath-related enthesitis. *Ann Rheum Dis.* 2015;74:(1):185-189. [PMID: 25261575]

Juvenile Idiopathic Arthritis

18

Courtney B. Crayne, MD, MSPH

Randy Q. Cron, MD, PhD

ESSENTIALS OF DIAGNOSIS

▶ Juvenile idiopathic arthritis (JIA) is a heterogeneous group of diseases which describe chronic inflammatory arthritis in a child lasting longer than 6 weeks with onset prior to 16 years of age.

▶ Disease subtypes vary with respect to clinical presentation, extra-articular symptoms, and serology.

▶ There is no specific laboratory test or imaging modality that can confirm or exclude a diagnosis of JIA.

▶ Complications of JIA include uveitis, macrophage activation syndrome (MAS), contractures, and growth abnormalities.

▶ Treatment varies with respect to subtype classification.

▶ General Considerations

Juvenile idiopathic arthritis (JIA) refers to a heterogeneous group of diseases, all of which describe chronic inflammatory arthritis lasting longer than 6 weeks with onset prior to 16 years of age. There are three major classification systems: the American College of Rheumatology (ACR), the European League Against Rheumatism (EULAR), and the International League of Associations for Rheumatology (ILAR) (Table 18–1). The ILAR criteria serve to unify the discrepancies between the ACR and EULAR classification criteria and are more widely used in both the clinical setting and research studies. Prior to adaptation of the ILAR criteria, the terms *juvenile rheumatoid arthritis* (JRA) and *juvenile chronic arthritis* (JCA) were used interchangeably per ACR and EULAR criteria, respectively. JRA is a misnomer, as only a small percentage (3–5%) of children predominantly share features of adult rheumatoid arthritis (RA) (Berntson et al, 2001; Brewer et al, 1977; Petty et al, 2001).

In accordance with ILAR classification, JIA is further divided into seven distinct subtypes: oligoarticular, rheumatoid factor (RF)–positive polyarticular, RF-negative polyarticular, systemic, psoriatic, enthesitis-related, and undifferentiated. These subtypes vary with respect to clinical presentation, disease course, and pathophysiology, and subsequently respond differently to treatments currently available. Classification is based on the number of arthritic joints, RF and human leukocyte antigen-B27 (HLA-B27) positivity, medical history, and associated extra-articular manifestations (Table 18–2) (Petty et al, 2001).

Etiology is unknown, hence the term "idiopathic," thereby excluding arthritis associated with other known underlying illnesses, including but not limited to infection-related and connective tissue diseases. JIA occurs in approximately 1 in 1000 children, making it one of the most common chronic diseases of childhood, comparable to childhood diabetes. While the subtypes are phenotypically different, they share many features common to inflammatory arthritis, such as joint stiffness and effusions. If left untreated, JIA can lead to significant disability, including growth disturbances and blindness. This chapter serves as an introduction into the JIA subtypes and their respective therapies.

SUBTYPES

Oligoarticular JIA

Oligoarticular JIA (oligoJIA), historically termed *pauciarticular JRA* per ACR criteria, meets the ILAR criteria for JIA and is further defined as arthritis in four or fewer joints during the first 6 months of disease provided exclusion criteria are met (see Table 18–2). *Persistent* oligoJIA is limited to four or fewer joints during the duration of disease, whereas *extended* oligoJIA involves more than four joints after the first 6 months of disease (Petty et al, 2001). Extended oligoJIA involving a large number of joints mimics polyarticular JIA and can be difficult to treat.

OligoJIA accounts for approximately 30–80% of all JIA diagnoses (depending on geography), occurring most commonly in females and among patients of European descent

Table 18–1. Historical classification of juvenile arthritis.

ACR (JRA)	EULAR (JCA)	ILAR (JIA)
JRA	JCA	JIA
Pauciarticular	Pauciarticular	Oligoarticular Persistent Extended
Polyarticular	Polyarticular JRA	Polyarticular RF-negative RF-positive
	Spondyloarthropathy Juvenile ankylosing spondylitis Juvenile psoriatic	Enthesitis related Psoriatic
Systemic	Systemic IBD-associated arthropathy	Systemic Undifferentiated

ACR, American College of Rheumatology; EULAR, European League Against Rheumatism; IBD, inflammatory bowel disease; ILAR, International League of Associations for Rheumatology; JCA, juvenile chronic arthritis; JIA, juvenile idiopathic arthritis; JRA, juvenile rheumatoid arthritis; RF, rheumatoid factor. Data from Berntson et al, 2001; Brewer et al, 1977; Petty et al, 2001.

compared to other racial populations. Peak age of onset is 1–3 years. Joint distribution tends to be asymmetric, classically affecting large joints, specifically the knees, ankles, and wrists. Involvement of the small joints of the hands foreshadows progression toward a polyarticular course (Al-Matar et al, 2002). Arthritis of the temporomandibular joint (TMJ) is likely underreported and may be evident on imaging studies (Stoll et al, 2012). OligoJIA is often associated with a positive antinuclear antibody (ANA) which increases the risk of asymptomatic uveitis (refer to subheading "Complications" for a more in-depth discussion).

Polyarticular JIA

Polyarticular JIA (polyJIA) is characterized as chronic inflammatory arthritis in five or more joints during the first 6 months of disease. The ILAR classification criteria further divide it into two separate subtypes based on the presence or absence of RF as this seromarker predicts disease prognosis and response to therapies. Seronegative polyJIA refers to a negative RF test, while seropositive polyJIA is used if an RF is positive on two or more occasions separated by at least 3 months. Exclusion criteria are similar to oligoJIA with the exception of the obvious RF status in seropositive polyJIA (see Table 18–2) (Petty et al, 2001).

Polyarthritis occurs in approximately 20% of children with JIA, and of these, about 85% of them are RF negative (Oen and Cheang, 1996). Associated symptoms may include constitutional symptoms, such as weight loss, fatigue, and low-grade fever.

Table 18–2. International League of Associations for Rheumatology (ILAR) classification.

ILAR Category	Definition
Oligoarthritis	Arthritis affecting 1–4 joints during the first 6 months of disease. Persistent: Affecting ≤4 during disease course. Extended: Affecting >4 joints after first 6 months. *Exclusions: a, b, c, d, e*
RF-negative polyarthritis	Arthritis affecting ≥5 joints during the first 6 months of disease plus a negative RF *Exclusions: a, b, c, d, e*
RF-positive polyarthritis	Arthritis affecting ≥5 joints during the first 6 months of disease plus ≥2 positive RF tests at least 3 months apart *Exclusions: a, b, c, e*
Systemic arthritis	Arthritis in ≥1 joints with or preceded by fever of at least 2 weeks' duration documented to be daily quotidian for at least 3 days and accompanied by at least one of the following: evanescent erythematous rash; generalized lymphadenopathy; hepatomegaly and/or splenomegaly; serositis *Exclusions: a, b, c, d*
Psoriatic arthritis	Arthritis and psoriasis OR arthritis and at least two of the following: dactylitis; nail pitting or onycholysis; psoriasis in a first-degree relative *Exclusions: b, c, d, e*
Enthesitis-related arthritis	Arthritis and enthesitis OR arthritis or enthesitis and at least two of the following: sacroiliac joint tenderness (present or historical) and/or inflammatory lumbosacral pain; presence of HLA-B27 antigen; onset of arthritis in a male aged >6 years; acute symptomatic anterior uveitis; history of ankylosing spondylitis, enthesitis-related arthritis, sacroiliitis with inflammatory bowel disease, Reiter syndrome, or acute anterior uveitis in a first-degree relative *Exclusions: a, d, e*
Undifferentiated arthritis	Arthritis that fulfills criteria in no category or in ≥2 of the above categories

Exclusions:
a. Psoriasis or a history of psoriasis in the patient or first-degree relative
b. Arthritis in an HLA-B27–positive male beginning after the 6th birthday
c. History of or a first-degree relative with ankylosing spondylitis, enthesitis-related arthritis, sacroiliitis with inflammatory bowel disease, Reiter syndrome, or acute anterior uveitis in a first-degree relative
d. Presence of IgM RF on at least 2 occasions at least 3 months apart
e. Presence of systemic JIA

HLA-B27, human leukocyte antigen-B27; IgM, immunoglobulin M; RF, rheumatoid factor. Data from Petty RE, Southwood TR, Manners P, et al. International League of Associations for Rheumatology classification of juvenile idiopathic arthritis: second revision, Edmonton, 2001. J Rheumatol. 2004;31(2):390-2.

RF-Negative Polyarticular

Onset of RF-negative polyJIA can occur at any age before 16 years; however, it typically follows a biphasic pattern, peaking between 1 and 3 years and then again in later adolescence. Females are more commonly affected than the male gender. RF-negative polyJIA is similar to oligoJIA in that it classically affects larger joints (eg, knees, ankles, wrists) and may also be associated with a positive ANA, increasing the risk of asymptomatic anterior uveitis. Distribution tends to be more symmetric.

RF-Positive Polyarticular

RF-positive polyJIA parallels adult RA with respect to clinical phenotype, pathology, and serology. Clinically, the main difference between the two diseases is the age of onset. RF-positive polyJIA more frequently affects females with an average age of onset during early adolescence. RF-positive polyarticular JIA is the least common of the subtypes, occurring in only 3–5% of children with JIA.

Unlike oligoJIA, RF-positive JIA is more frequent in non-white children, such as African Americans, Hispanics, and children of Asian descent. Arthritis in RF-positive polyJIA is often erosive, making it one of the most aggressive subtypes of JIA. Joint involvement commonly affects large joints and small joints of the hand and the wrists with symmetric distribution. Subcutaneous nodules and lung disease are rare in children compared to their adult counterparts. Uveitis within this category is rare, even in the presence of ANA.

Systemic JIA

Systemic JIA (sJIA), as the name implies, involves the presence of arthritis in conjunction with systemic features, specifically fever and rash. As defined by the ILAR classification system, sJIA is arthritis in one or more joints with (or preceded by) fever of at least 2 weeks' duration. The fever must be a daily, quotidian (rising once a day and then normalizing or often going lower than normal) pattern for a minimum of 3 days. Additionally, one of the following must be present: evanescent, nonfixed erythematous rash; generalized lymphadenopathy; hepatomegaly and/or splenomegaly; or serositis. The rash, often localized to the trunk and extremities, classically appears in conjunction with the fever and fades as the temperature normalizes (Petty et al, 2004).

Commonly, the systemic features predate the development of arthritis, and while arthritis is required for diagnosis, proper treatment may prevent the onset of clinical arthritis in some patients. Unlike the aforementioned subtypes, sJIA has no gender predominance and occurs throughout childhood with a peak age of onset at 2 years of age. sJIA accounts for roughly 10–15% of children with JIA.

Psoriatic JIA

Strictly defined as arthritis and psoriasis or arthritis plus two of the following: dactylitis, nail pitting or onycholysis, or psoriasis in a first-degree relative. Adolescent psoriatic JIA is considered by some to be a subcategory of spondyloarthropathy as they can develop enthesitis and other related features (Petty et al, 2004; Stoll et al, 2006). Psoriasis in children is uncommon and may be misdiagnosed as atopic dermatitis or eczema. Additionally, onset of arthritis may precede cutaneous manifestations, and without a confirmed diagnosis of psoriasis in either the patient or a first-degree relative, patients may be initially classified within another subtype of JIA. Treatment with disease-modifying agents (discussed in section Treatment) may effectively treat both arthritis and psoriasis, thereby preventing skin findings from ever-manifesting and making the diagnosis of psoriatic JIA tricky without other clinical features.

Psoriatic JIA is thought to have two dichotomous presentations. In younger patients, clinical presentation mimics oligoarthritis and RF-negative polyarticular JIA, whereas older patients follow a disease course comparable to other spondyloarthropathies, such as enthesitis-related arthritis (ERA) and adult psoriatic arthritis (Stoll et al, 2006; Stoll et al, 2013).

Enthesitis-Related Arthritis

Closely related to arthritis is enthesitis, or inflammation at the site where tendons and ligaments insert into the bones. ERA JIA is strongly associated with the presence of HLA-B27 and may progress to ankylosing spondylitis, although axial disease and sacroiliac joint involvement are uncommon at onset in children. Classification is based on the presence of both arthritis and enthesitis or either arthritis or enthesitis, plus two of the following five criteria: (1) sacroiliac joint tenderness or inflammation on imaging, (2) positive HLA-B27, (3) history of acute symptomatic anterior uveitis, (4) a first-degree relative with an HLA-B27–associated disease, or (5) onset of arthritis in a male over 6 years of age (Petty et al, 2004).

ERA JIA occurs more frequently in older males and adolescents. Peripheral arthritis is often localized to the lower extremities and tends to be asymmetric. Like oligoJIA, arthritis in ERA JIA is typically limited to four or fewer joints at onset but can be polyarticular. In the absence of enthesitis, which can be somewhat subjective to elicit on physical exam, age at onset and gender may help distinguish ERA from other JIA subtypes. Additionally, hip involvement should raise suspicion for ERA JIA as this joint is less commonly affected in other subtypes (Weiss, 2016).

Undifferentiated Arthritis

If patients meet criteria for more than one subtype, or no subtype, they are then classified as "undifferentiated." This includes a child with psoriasis and arthritis who has a positive HLA-B27 marker, or children with sJIA who later develop psoriasis (Petty et al, 2004).

Differential Diagnosis

Children who present with monoarthritis of less than 6 weeks' duration by definition do not meet criteria for JIA diagnosis. A broad differential should be considered when

Table 18–3. Differential diagnosis of arthritis and arthropathy in children.

Monoarticular Arthritis	Polyarticular Arthritis	Systemic Arthritis
Oligoarticular JIA	Polyarticular JIA	Systemic JIA
Enthesitis-related JIA	Enthesitis-related JIA	Infection
Psoriatic JIA	Psoriatic JIA	Familial Mediterranean fever syndrome

Infection
  Septic arthritis
  Reactive arthritis
  Osteomyelitis
  Tuberculosis
	Infection
	  Reactive arthritis
	  Lyme disease
	  Acute rheumatic fever
	  Tuberculosis
		Neonatal onset multisystem inflammatory disease
		Other rheumatic disease
		  Systemic lupus erythematosus
		  Sarcoidosis

Malignancy
  Leukemia
  Sarcoma
	Other rheumatic disease
	  Systemic lupus erythematosus
	  Sarcoidosis
	  Sjögren syndrome
	  Mixed connective tissue disease
		Vasculitis
		  Kawasaki disease
		  Henoch-Schönlein purpura
		  Polyarteritis nodosa
		  Granulomatosis with polyangiitis

Sickle cell disease		
Hemophilia		
Trauma		

JIA, juvenile idiopathic arthritis.

assessing these patients (Table 18–3). An acutely warm and exquisitely tender joint or bone pain should raise concern for infection or malignancy. Additionally, nighttime pain that awakens a child from sleep is atypical of arthritis. Malignancy, septic arthritis, and osteomyelitis should always be ruled out prior to initiating systemic therapy for JIA. Until a diagnosis of JIA can be confirmed, initial treatment with nonsteroidal anti-inflammatory drugs (NSAIDs) is appropriate first-line therapy.

▶ Complications

A. Uveitis

One of the most serious complications of JIA is inflammation involving the iris (iritis) and the ciliary body (iridocyclitis), collectively termed "uveitis." Chronic uveitis associated with JIA is one of the most common causes of noninfectious, nongranulomatous uveitis and has been reported in up to 20% of JIA patients (Foeldvari et al, 2015). JIA-associated uveitis tends to be localized to the anterior chamber with clinical presentation dependent on JIA subtype. Oligoarthritis, RF-negative polyJIA, and younger psoriatic JIA patients tend to present with chronic, insidious onset anterior uveitis. Clinically, these patients are asymptomatic (Angeles-Han et al, 2015). Acute, symptomatic uveitis is strongly associated with HLA-B27 positivity and ERA. These patients have a painful, red eye(s), and may be misdiagnosed as having an infection or foreign body.

Eye exams with slit-lamp should be performed at the time of JIA diagnosis and then at regular intervals depending on risk stratification (Table 18–4). A younger age at disease onset, a positive ANA, and a shorter disease duration indicate higher risk for asymptomatic, anterior uveitis in children with oligoJIA and RF-negative polyJIA (Angeles-Han et al, 2015; Angeles-Han and Rabinovich, 2016; Heiligenhaus et al, 2007). Of note, a positive ANA in a child with RF-positive polyarthritis and sJIA does not increase the risk of uveitis, as this complication is rare in those subtypes (Angeles-Han and Rabinovich, 2016; Clarke et al, 2016; Heiligenhaus et al, 2007).

In a small percentage of patients, uveitis may present before the onset of arthritis. In such cases of isolated uveitis in the absence of JIA, physicians should consider rheumatology

Table 18–4. Modified ophthalmologic screening recommendations.

JIA Category	ANA Status	Age of Onset (y)	Disease Duration (y)	Frequency of Eye Exam (mo)
Oligoarthritis/RF-negative Polyarthritis/Psoriatic JIA	+	≤6	≤4	3
			>4	6
			≥7	12
	+	>6	≤2	6
			>2	12
	−	≤6	≤4	6
			>4	12
	−	>6	N/A	12

** For RF+ polyarthritis and enthesitis-related arthritis, systemic JIA annual screening is sufficient regardless of age, disease duration, and ANA status.
ANA, antinuclear antibody; JIA, juvenile idiopathic arthritis; RF, rheumatoid factor.
Data from Heilinghaus et al, 2007.

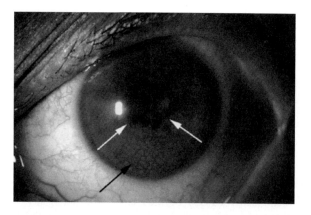

▲ **Figure 18–1.** Acute anterior uveitis with corneal endothelial white cell aggregates (*black arrow*) and posterior synechiae formation (iris adhesions to the lens, *white arrows*). **(See color insert.)** (Reproduced with permission from Chapter 18. Uveitis and Iritis. In: Usatine RP, Smith MA, Chumley HS, Mayeaux EJ, Jr. eds. The Color Atlas of Family Medicine, 2e New York, NY: McGraw-Hill; 2013.)

referrals for disease monitoring. Initial treatment of uveitis typically includes glucocorticoid ophthalmic drops, usually with a mydriatic agent to dilate the pupil aiding in the prevention of synechiae development (Figure 18–1). Chronic use of topical glucocorticoids, however, may lead to cataracts and increased intraocular pressure. Second-line therapy with methotrexate (MTX) and/or anti-TNF (tumor necrosis factor) monoclonal antibodies (eg, adalimumab) can induce remission in children with uveitis refractory to topical steroids (Angeles-Han and Rabinovich, 2016; Cordero-Coma and Sobrin, 2015).

B. Macrophage Activation Syndrome

A potentially life-threatening complication of JIA, almost exclusively within the systemic subtype, is macrophage activation syndrome (MAS). Recognition can be difficult as there is significant clinical overlap with sJIA disease flare, including the presence of fever, markedly elevated serum ferritin, rash, and hepatosplenomegaly. Prevalence of MAS within the sJIA population is reported to be 10%; however, subclinical MAS may be present in as high as 40% of children with sJIA (Behrens et al, 2008; Bleesing et al, 2007). A diagnosis of MAS can be made in any febrile patient with confirmed or suspected sJIA with a serum ferritin level greater than 684 ng/mL plus any two of the following: platelet count less than or equal to 181×109/L, aspartate aminotransferase more than 48 units/L, triglycerides greater than 156 mg/dL, or fibrinogen less than or equal to 360 mg/dL (Ravelli et al, 2016). Treatment of MAS as part of sJIA typically includes high dose corticosteroids, increased doses of interleukin (IL)-1 blockade, and sometimes a calcineurin inhibitor (Stoll ML and Cron, 2013).

C. Joint Destruction

Chronic joint inflammation can lead to joint space narrowing and erosions. Joint destruction is far less common in patients with oligoarthritis compared to the polyarticular subtypes, including sJIA. Bony overgrowth from chronic inflammation can be seen, as in the case of knee involvement with a resulting larger affected knee. Untreated arthritis can progress to leg length discrepancies, contractures, limited range of motion, nearby muscle atrophy, and bony deformities, ultimately causing significant disability, particularly if the wrists, small joints of the hands, and ankles are affected (Cassidy and Petty, 2005; Gowdie and Tse, 2012).

TEMPOROMANDIBULAR JOINT ARTHRITIS

Involvement of the temporomandibular joint (TMJ) is thought to be grossly underreported. Arthritis of this joint tends to be clinically silent, and patients report few, if any, symptoms to suggest inflammation. Suspected prevalence ranges from 63% to 75% based on magnetic resonance imaging (MRI) studies, suggesting TMJ arthritis transcends across several subtypes. Furthermore, JIA may present as isolated TMJ arthritis (Bleesing et al, 2007).

An earlier age of onset is thought to be the most vulnerable time period. Joint damage in TMJ arthritis may manifest as micrognathia, retrognathia, asymmetry, and jaw deviation. Active TMJ arthritis may cause joint destruction and ultimately shorten the affected jaw (Carrasco, 2015; El Assar de la Fuente et al, 2016; Stoll et al, 2012). There is a lot of clinical variability with respect to TMJ arthritis. Additionally, the degree of joint damage does not necessarily correlate with the clinical findings (Carrasco, 2015; El Assar de la Fuente et al, 2016).

CERVICAL SPINE

Like TMJ arthritis, cervical spine involvement is often insidious in onset with subtle clinical findings. Atlantoaxial subluxation, erosions, and spinal fusion may limit range of motion over time. Advanced imaging modalities, specifically MRI, may be required to aid in diagnosis and disease monitoring of these joints (Colebatch-Bourn et al, 2015; Vaid et al, 2014).

GROWTH ABNORMALITIES

Growth disturbances, both generalized and localized, are a well-known complication of JIA. Proinflammatory cytokines (eg, TNF, IL-1, and IL-6) and systemic glucocorticoids interfere with insulin-like growth factor thus resulting in growth restriction. With the advent of more effective immunomodulatory therapies, generalized growth abnormalities, such as short stature, are far less frequent (Bechtold and Simon, 2014; Wong et al, 2016). In recent years, limited disturbances, such as leg length discrepancy, have become more common. These are often localized to one limb and related to one chronically active joint, most commonly the knee. Inflammation at the growth plate can lead to over-stimulation of the ossification center, thus resulting in increased growth of the affected limb. Over time, chronic inflammation can cause premature closure of the epiphyseal plate during puberty and ultimately restrict growth in the affected limb, thereby ultimately resulting in a shorter leg (Fellas et al, 2017).

Pathogenesis & Etiology

As the name implies, the etiology of JIA is unknown and thought to be a complex interaction between genetic and environmental factors. Many studies show an association between JIA and the major histocompatibility complex (MHC, also known as HLA in humans), suggesting the adaptive immune system is responsible for disease pathogenesis. Enteric infections, among other viral illnesses, have been proposed as one immune trigger, particularly in the spondyloarthritis subpopulation; although, no specific organism has been proven to cause JIA (Stoll, 2015). Recently, it has been suggested that the gut microbiome may influence the development of ERA (Stoll and Cron, 2016).

Clinical Findings

A diagnosis of JIA is made in combination with history and physical exam findings. Children with JIA often present with joint stiffness, worse with prolonged inactivity. Joint stiffness is most pronounced in the morning, usually described by parents as an abnormal gait or "walking like an old person." Stiffness usually improves throughout the day with increased activity or with warm showers (Cassidy and Petty, 2005).

Clinical characteristics of active arthritis include joint effusions and limited range of motion. Joints can be warm; however, they are almost never erythematous in JIA. Pain at rest, especially if severe, is rarely associated with arthritis. Pain, however, can be elicited with both passive and active movements. Tenderness to palpation is maximal at the joint line and over inflamed synovium (Cassidy and Petty, 2005).

Joint distribution and pattern vary with respect to subtype (Table 18–5). There is clinical overlap between subtypes, so characteristics should be used as a guide and not as a gold-standard. For example, psoriatic JIA may present with asymmetric polyarticular arthritis or oligoarthritis.

Laboratory Findings

A. Acute Phase Reactants

With the exception of sJIA, which is accompanied by elevated inflammatory markers (eg, white blood cell count, platelets, erythrocyte sedimentation rate, and C-reactive protein), children with JIA often have unremarkable laboratory findings. To further complicate the diagnosis, children with sJIA complicated by MAS may present with normal inflammatory labs due to consumptive coagulopathy. In these cases, ferritin, liver enzymes, fibrinogen, and triglyceride levels can supplement diagnosis. In sJIA, ferritin is often markedly elevated, but not to the degree seen in MAS (Ravelli et al, 2016). JIA remains a clinical diagnosis, and therefore normal labs should not preclude the diagnosis.

B. Autoantibodies

In the setting of confirmed JIA, select serological markers can aid in determination of disease subtype, thereby better guiding treatment. Many of these antibodies are nonspecific and some are frequently present in the general population (eg, ANAs). Additionally, these antibodies can be transiently positive following infections and should not be ordered routinely by general practitioners.

C. Antinuclear Antibody

A positive ANA titer can be present in 20–30% of the healthy population and is subsequently of little diagnostic use. JIA

Table 18–5. Characteristic features based on JIA subtype.

	OligoJIA	PolyJIA	Systemic JIA	Psoriatic JIA	ERA JIA
Gender	F > M	F > M	F = M	F > M	M > F
Age	Toddlers	Bimodal: toddlers and teens	All ages (peak 1–3 years)	Bimodal	Adolescents
Number of joints	<5	≥5	Any	Any	Any
Joint distribution	Large (eg, knees)	Large and small	Any	Any	Lower extremity; hips
Pattern	Asymmetric	Symmetric	—	Asymmetric	Asymmetric
Distinguishing features	ANA+ increases risk of uveitis	Seropositive (RF+) mimics adult RA	Fever, rash	Nail pitting, dactylitis	Enthesitis, HLA-B27+

ANA, antinuclear antibody; ERA, enthesitis-related arthritis; F, female; HLA-B27, human leukocyte antigen-B27; JIA, juvenile idiopathic arthritis; M, male; oligoJIA, oligoarticular JIA; polyJIA, polyarticular JIA; RA, rheumatoid arthritis; RF, rheumatoid factor.

patients with a positive ANA titer are similar with respect to age at disease onset, female gender predominance, and frequency of asymmetric arthritis, thus leading some to hypothesize that ANA positivity represents a homogenous subset within JIA (Ravelli et al, 2011). A low-moderate titer ANA indisputably increases the risk of anterior uveitis and therefore is the most useful in risk stratification for determining the frequency of ophthalmology screening examinations (Angeles-Han et al, 2013).

D. Rheumatoid Factor

Aside from classifying polyJIA as seronegative (RF-negative) versus seropositive (RF-positive), RF titers are seldom diagnostic in juvenile arthritis. Positive IgM RF titers can be seen in a variety of other autoimmune conditions, including Sjogren disease and other connective tissue diseases, as well as in healthy children. In a patient with JIA, presence of RF antibodies may suggest a poorer prognosis (Angeles-Han and Rabinovich, 2016; Brewer et al, 1977). In the absence of clinical findings suggestive of RF+ polyarthritis, an RF is premature and of little diagnostic value.

E. Anticitrullinated Protein Antibodies

Anticitrullinated protein antibodies (ACPA) are a bit more controversial. Studies on the prevalence of ACPA in children with JIA are limited; however, current evidence suggests these autoantibodies may be present in early disease, notably RF-positive polyJIA, and may correlate with higher disease activity (Cassidy and Petty, 2005; Gowdie and Tse, 2012). Preliminary studies also suggest a correlation of ACPA and the presence of IgM RF antibodies. At present time, ACPA do not substantially affect either the diagnosis or management of JIA (El Assar de la Fuente, 2016).

▶ Imaging

Normal images do not exclude a diagnosis of JIA, but they may aid in confirming involvement of questionable joints or exclusion of alternative diagnoses, such as injury. Radiographic changes may show joint space narrowing, bony overgrowth, and erosions depending on the chronicity of inflammation. As one would suspect, the more aggressive the subtype and the longer duration of untreated disease, the more likely changes will be visible on plain radiographs (Giancane at al, 2014).

MRI with contrast can show signs of synovitis, increased intraarticular fluid, and bone marrow edema, thus helping to confirm a suspected diagnosis (Vaid et al, 2014). In cases where joint involvement may be subtle on physical exam, as with TMJ (Figure 18–2), cervical spine arthritis, and with sacroiliitis, MRI may be necessary to monitor disease progression and treatment response (Colebatch-Bourn et al, 2015). The use of MRI should be reserved as a means to help differentiate various causes of joint swelling, as in cases of monoarthritis, and not as a routine diagnostic tool.

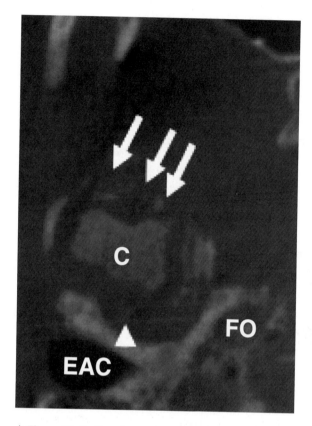

▲ **Figure 18–2.** Cone beam CT image of the right TMJ of an 18-year-old female with polyJIA revealing bony fragments within the anterior (*arrows*) and posterior (*arrowhead*) portion of the TMJ. The condylar head (C), external auditory canal (EAC), and foramen ovale (FO) are indicated.

Ultrasound is a relatively inexpensive and potentially readily accessible mode of imaging that has shown promise in confirming synovitis (Magni-Manzoni et al, 2013). Ultrasound can also be used in guiding arthrocentesis and intraarticular steroid injections. Unlike MRI in the young, ultrasounds can be done without anesthesia; however, results are operator dependent, making them less reliable, particularly with respect to the assessment of TMJ arthritis (Colebatch-Bourn et al, 2015; Muller et al, 2009; Weiss, 2008).

▶ Treatment

Treatment is determined based on subtype classification. Historically, treatment emphasis was placed on NSAIDs. Given the significant disability inflicted if JIA is not properly treated, rheumatologists are shifting toward more aggressive therapy with disease-modifying antirheumatic drugs (DMARDs) as first-line therapy, particularly in polyarthritis (Table 18–6). The 2011 ACR recommendations on the

Table 18–6. Conventional and biologic disease-modifying antirheumatic drugs (DMARDs) with dosing information.

	Dose	Formulation
Conventional DMARDs		
Methotrexate	0.5–1 mg/kg/dose weekly (max 25 mg/week)	Oral or subcutaneous
Leflunomide	<20 kg: Loading dose (100 mg on day 1), then 10 mg every other day	Oral
	20–40 kg: Loading dose (100 mg/ day for 2 days), then 10 mg daily	
	>40 kg: Loading dose (100 mg for 3 days), then 20 mg daily	
Sulfasalazine	30–50 mg/kg/day divided 2–3 times daily	
TNF inhibitors		
Etanercept	<63 kg: 0.8 mg/kg weekly	Subcutaneous injection
	≥63 kg: 25 mg twice a week or 50 mg weekly	Vial, autoinjector, prefilled syringe
	Max: 50 mg weekly	
Adalimumab	10–15 kg: 10 mg every other week	Subcutaneous injection
	15 to <30 kg: 20 mg every other week	Prefilled syringe or pen
	≥30 kg: 40 mg every other week	
Infliximab	3–10 mg/kg/infusion at 0, 2, 4 weeks, then every 4–8 weeks as tolerated	Intravenous infusion
T-cell costimulation inhibitor		
Abatacept	10 mg/kg infusion at 0, 2, 4 weeks, then every 4 weeks	Intravenous infusion
	Max: 1000 mg/dose	Subcutaneous injection
IL-1 inhibition		
Anakinra	1–2 mg/kg/day divided 1–2 times per day	Subcutaneous injection
	Max: 8mg/kg/day	
Canakinumab	≥7.5 kg: 4mg/kg every 4 weeks	Intravenous infusion
Rilonacept	4.4 mg/kg loading followed by 2.2 mg/kg weekly	Subcutaneous injection Subcutaneous injection
IL-6 inhibition		
Tocilizumab	<30 kg: 10 mg/kg every 4 weeks for polyJIA; 12 mg/kg every 2 weeks for sJIA	Intravenous infusion
	≥30 mg: 8 mg/kg every 4 weeks for polyJIA; every 2 weeks for sJIA	Or subcutaneous prefilled syringe

IL, interleukin; PolyJIA, polyarticular juvenile idiopathic arthritis; sJIA, systemic juvenile idiopathic arthritis; TNF, tumor necrosis factor.

treatment of JIA use risk stratification as a guide for the escalation of therapy (Beukelman et al, 2011).

A. Nonsteroidal anti-inflammatory drugs

Once mainstay therapy, NSAIDs are no longer commonly used as monotherapy or for durations longer than 1–2 months (Giancane et al, 2016). As previously stated, NSAIDs are an appropriate first-choice therapy in patients without a confirmed diagnosis of JIA and may be used in oligoarthritis without poor prognostic features and with low disease activity. Chronic NSAID use is not without risk, and periodic lab monitoring is recommended. Serum creatinine, urinalysis, complete blood count (CBC), and liver enzymes should be checked at baseline and then yearly if using three to four times per week or biannually if using daily (Beukelman et al, 2011). Pseudoporphyria is a photodermatitis associated with the use of NSAIDs, particularly naproxen, that resolves with medication discontinuation but can cause permanent scarring (Bryant and Lachman, 2003).

B. Glucocorticoids

Long-term use of systemic glucocorticoids, traditionally administered orally, has a slew of associated adverse consequences, including, but not limited to, infections, osteoporosis, cataracts, hyperglycemia, abnormal weight gain, and adrenal gland suppression. Furthermore, evidence fails to show long-lasting benefits. While systemic glucocorticoids are no longer recommended in treating JIA, they can be used as adjunct therapy in aggressive polyJIA as bridge therapy to temporarily reduce inflammation during DMARD initiation, initially in sJIA, or during flares or MAS to rapidly reduce inflammation (Beukelman et al, 2011; Giancane et al, 2016; Harris et al, 2013; Ringold et al, 2013).

Intra-articular glucocorticoids, on the other hand, are routinely recommended as a treatment for JIA, particularly in patients with four or fewer joints (Beukelman et al, 2011). In patients with active arthritis, intra-articular glucocorticoids may be used as standalone therapy or in conjunction with other medications (Bloom et al, 2011). Moreover, steroid injections may be necessary in order to control local inflammation in spite of systemic therapy, as in the case of refractory TMJ arthritis (Stoll et al, 2012).

Two formulations of intra-articular glucocorticoids are commonly used—triamcinolone hexacetonide and triamcinolone acetonide. In a 2004 double-blind study, the former was found to be superior with regard to rates of remission; however, unfortunately, triamcinolone hexacetonide is currently not available in the United States (Zulian, 2004). Side effects of glucocorticoid injections tend to be localized and may result in skin atrophy and discoloration. Joint infection and systemic side effects are rare (Giancane et al, 2014).

C. Conventional Disease-Modifying Antirheumatic Drugs

DMARDs are a relatively safe and effective alternative to NSAIDs and systemic corticosteroids. Unlike the latter medications, DMARDs aid in the prevention of irreversible joint damage if used early in the disease course.

D. Methotrexate

MTX continues to be the most used DMARD in the management of JIA. MTX is often initiated after failure of an NSAID trial or intra-articular steroid injection. In patients with JIA who have a high disease activity and/or poor prognostic features, it should be used as first-line therapy (Beukelman et al, 2011; Stoll and Cron, 2014). MTX is a folic acid analogue that at high doses competitively inhibits dihydrofolate reductase and subsequently blocks purine synthesis and DNA production. While the exact mechanism of action at lower rheumatic doses remains unknown, it is thought to increase adenosine levels which lead to an anti-inflammatory effect (Harris et al, 2013; Ramanan et al, 2003).

The safety and efficacy were first reported about 25 years ago in a collaborative study between the United States and USSR (Giannini et al, 1992). MTX can be administered either orally or as a subcutaneous (SQ) injection. Differences between the routes remain controversial. Current literature does not strongly support a difference in adverse events, including gastrointestinal (GI) upset; however, recent studies have shown increased bioavailability and improved joint responses with the use of SQ MTX compared to oral MTX (Alsufyani et al, 2004; Falvey et al, 2017; Franova et al, 2016; Stoll and Cron, 2014). These responses were not dose dependent and did not change with dose escalation (Stoll and Cron, 2014).

In general, MTX is well-tolerated. Most commonly, nausea and GI discomfort are reported. Other less common side effects include oral ulcers and alopecia. These side effects likely relate to the folate antagonism, thus adequate folate supplementation may help alleviate negative effects. Likewise, folate antagonism during pregnancy can cause fetal abnormalities. MTX should not be taken during pregnancy, and females should receive appropriate contraceptive counseling (Harris et al, 2013).

Although uncommon, MTX can cause hematologic, liver, and renal toxicity. Because MTX is an immunosuppressive medication, live vaccines are currently contraindicated. Baseline labs should include a CBC, liver enzymes, and creatinine. These labs should be repeated every 12 weeks while on MTX (Beukelman et al, 2011; Harris et al, 2013; Stoll and Cron, 2014; Stoll et al, 2013).

E. Leflunomide

Leflunomide inhibits pyrimidine synthesis and alters cytokine production, ultimately having a similar clinical effect as MTX. In a randomized control trial, MTX was found to be more effective than leflunomide (Silverman et al, 2005). While MTX is the preferred DMARD in patients with JIA, leflunomide is often used as an alternative. Side effects are similar, including GI upset and alopecia. Like MTX, leflunomide is teratogenic and can remain active within the body

for several weeks. Routine lab monitoring of CBC, liver function, and creatinine is indicated as this drug may cause toxicity (Harris et al, 2013; Stoll et al, 2013).

F. Sulfasalazine

Sulfasalazine is more frequently used in enthesitis-related JIA and inflammatory bowel disease (IBD)–associated arthritis; however, studies have shown benefit in both oligoJIA and polyJIA (Chen et al, 2002; van Rossum et al, 1998). Adverse events occur in approximately 30% of children with JIA. Rash and GI upset are more commonly reported. Rare, but serious, side effects include Stevens-Johnson syndrome, drug reaction with eosinophilia and systemic symptoms (DRESS), drug-induced lupus, cytopenia, and hepatotoxicity. Sulfasalazine is contraindicated in any patient with a known hypersensitivity to sulfa drugs, including patients with G6PD deficiency (Harris et al, 2013; Stoll and Cron, 2014; Stoll et al, 2013). It is also contraindicated in sJIA patients because of the potential for severe side effects (Stoll and Cron, 2014). Unlike leflunomide and MTX, sulfasalazine is safe during pregnancy and breast-feeding (Cassidy and Petty, 2005). Routine monitoring should include blood counts and liver function (Harris et al, 2013).

▶ Biologic DMARDs

Biological DMARDs differ from conventional DMARDs in that they target specific biological molecules and are generated with recombinant DNA technology. These drugs are newer with fewer long-term outcome studies available.

A. Tumor Necrosis Factor Inhibitors

The proinflammatory cytokine, TNF, has long since been linked to RA, and as such, it is the main target of the biologic therapies (Stoll and Cron, 2014). Elevated levels of TNF are seen in both the serum and synovial fluid of patients with JIA, suggesting it plays a main role in the pathogenesis of JIA. Three TNF inhibitors have been used extensively in children with JIA: etanercept, adalimumab, and infliximab. The former is a soluble receptor antagonist, and the latter two are monoclonal antibodies directed against TNF. Only adalimumab and etanercept have approval of the Food and Drug Administration (FDA) for use in JIA. While other TNF inhibitors (eg, golimumab and certolizumab) exist, the safety and efficacy in children has not been well studied, and these medications are not currently approved for pediatric use in the United States (Harris et al, 2013; Stoll and Cron, 2014; Sterba and Ilowite, 2016).

At present, TNF inhibitors are recommended by the ACR for use in polyJIA patients with moderate to high disease activity who have not responded to 3 months of MTX. Some pediatric rheumatologists, however, practice a top-down (ie, inverted pyramid) treatment approach, opting to initiate TNF inhibitor therapy early in disease course. Lab monitoring with CBC, liver enzymes, and creatinine should be done prior to initiation and every 3–6 months when receiving anti-TNF biologics. In addition, tuberculosis should be excluded prior to initiation of anti-TNF therapy (Beukelman et al, 2011).

Responses to the different TNF inhibitors may vary. Predictors of successful disease control include shorter disease duration prior to therapy initiation, a younger age at onset, lower baseline disability scores, DMARD use prior to anti-TNF, and a robust response at 4 months (Otten et al, 2011; Wallace et al, 2014); thereby suggesting early aggressive therapy with a TNF inhibitor may maximize treatment outcomes. Results of the TREAT (trial of early aggressive therapy) study showed clinically inactive disease in more than one-third of severe polyJIA patients on early aggressive therapy with etanercept, MTX, and prednisone. The likelihood of disease remission increased with each month earlier that the aggressive treatment was initiated (Wallace et al, 2012).

B. Etanercept

Etanercept, administered as a SQ injection, is a fully humanized soluble TNF receptor linked to the constant portion of immunoglobulin for prolonged stability. Approved by the FDA in 1999 for use in children, it was the first TNF inhibitor studied in JIA (Harris et al, 2013). Lovell et al published the first randomized-control trial comparing etanercept to placebo. Disease flare was seen in 28% of patients treated with etanercept and in 81% of placebo patients. Additionally, they found the time to flare was significantly longer in those who received the TNF inhibitor (116 days compared to 28 days) (Lovell et al, 2000). Disease control was maintained for 8 years in a follow-up report (Lovell et al, 2008). When compared to MTX monotherapy, Giannini et al found no significant difference in treatment response in patients receiving etanercept alone or in combination with MTX; however, it should be noted that patients in the etanercept groups had worse disease activity and many had failed prior MTX treatment (Giannini et al, 2009). Compared to adalimumab and infliximab, etanercept is not as effective in treating JIA-associated uveitis (Cordero-Coma and Sobrin, 2015; Smith et al, 2005).

The safety profile for etanercept is similar to adalimumab with the most frequent adverse event being infections. Of note, there are rare reports of anaphylactic reactions to etanercept (Crayne et al, 2013). Patients treated with etanercept monotherapy have higher incidences of IBD compared to other patients with JIA, including those treated in combination with MTX. The causation remains unclear (Barthel et al, 2015). It is likely that etanercept does not effectively treat IBD like the anti-TNF antibodies (eg, adalimumab and infliximab) rather than etanercept being causative of IBD.

C. Adalimumab

Adalimumab is a fully humanized recombinant IgG monoclonal antibody that directly binds to TNF. It is administered

as a SQ injection at home. In a randomized-control trial, adalimumab was both safe and effective as monotherapy and in combination with MTX in patients with polyJIA. Most frequently reported adverse events were injection site reactions (Lovell et al, 2008). More recently, adalimumab proved to be safe and effective in polyJIA patients aged 2–4 years or weighing less than 15 kg, with infection being the most common reported adverse event in this age range (Kingsbury et al, 2014).

To date, adalimumab is the only noncorticosteroid approved for use in noninfectious intermediate uveitis, posterior uveitis, and panuveitis in adults. While it is not specifically approved for use in children with uveitis, studies show that it is a safe and effective alternative to steroids in children with refractory uveitis, often used in combination with MTX (Hawkins et al, 2016; Ramanan et al, 2003; Ramanan et al, 2014).

D. Infliximab

Infliximab is a chimeric murine-human sequence monoclonal antibody against TNF. Unlike adalimumab and etanercept which are SQ injections, infliximab is administered intravenously. It is not currently approved for use in JIA; however, it is sometimes used off-label (Harris et al, 2013; Stoll and Cron, 2014). Furthermore, studies have shown it to be effective in the treatment of polyJIA after 1 year of treatment; however, the primary efficacy end-point of 14 weeks was not obtained. Transfusion reactions occurred in about one-third of patients receiving infliximab. Presence of anti-infliximab antibodies appeared to increase the risk for a reaction, as did a lower dose (3 mg/kg compared to 6 mg/kg) (Ruperto et al, 2007; Tynjala et al, 2011). Infliximab in combination with MTX reduces the risk of antibody formation and therefore is the preferred regimen (Ruperto et al, 2007).

▶ TNF Inhibitor Safety Profile

As previously mentioned, infections are the most reported side effect associated with anti-TNF therapy. Concomitant use with MTX may increase infection risk. Most often these are mild illnesses, such as upper respiratory infections and skin infections. More serious infections, specifically tuberculosis and fungal infections, can occur. Tuberculosis screening is recommended prior to initiation and then annually (Horneff, 2015a, 2015b).

TNF inhibition has been linked to other autoimmune conditions, notably demyelinating diseases and sarcoidosis; however, it is debatable whether or not the medication is the cause, or if the patient was misdiagnosed at disease onset. Additionally, SLE has been reported in some patients following anti-TNF initiation (Horneff, 2015).

The FDA ordered a black box warning on all TNF inhibitors out of concern for increased rates of malignancy.

Several studies have investigated the relationship between malignancy and JIA, including a notable one published in 2012. Beukelman et al showed no association between the use of medication and occurrence of malignancy. Children with JIA had higher rates of malignancy, irrespective of treatment choice (Beukelman et al, 2012; Mannion et al, 2014).

A. Interleukin-1 Inhibition

IL-1 is a proinflammatory cytokine with a key role in the pathogenesis of inflammation and acute phase response. IL-1 receptor antagonist (IL-1Ra) turns off this inflammatory cascade by acting as a competitive antagonist. Efficacy of IL-1 blockade is limited to systemic disease. Anakinra is structurally identical to IL-1Ra and frequently used as a glucocorticoid steroid sparing therapy in sJIA. Use of anakinra early in disease course when systemic features are most prominent provides the most benefit (Nigrovic, 2014). Additionally, given the clinical overlap, anakinra proves to be efficacious in treating MAS (Nigrovic, 2011). Canakinumab is a monoclonal antibody directed against IL-1, and while mechanistically different, also blocks IL-1 response and is commonly used in the treatment of sJIA (Stoll et al, 2013). Adverse events related to IL-1 inhibition include injection reactions and increased risk of infection. Rilonacept is a dimeric fusion protein that binds and neutralizes IL-1; it consists of the ligand-binding domains of the extracellular portions of the human IL-1 receptor component (IL-1R1) and IL-1 receptor accessory protein (IL-1RAcP) linked in-line to the Fc portion of human IgG1. While not FDA approved for sJIA, rilonacept has been shown to be effective in treating sJIA in a randomized, double-blind, placebo-controlled trial (Ilowite et al, 2014).

B. IL-6 Inhibitor (Tocilizumab)

Tocilizumab is an anti-interleukin-6 (anti-IL-6) receptor monoclonal antibody administered intravenously as an infusion or subcutaneously. Approved for use in sJIA and polyJIA, IL-6 inhibition with tocilizumab shows promise as a therapeutic alternative in the management of polyJIA (Brunner et al, 2015; Sterba and Ilowite, 2016). Horneff et al retrospectively analyzed registry data comparing response rates of tocilizumab to both etanercept and adalimumab in patients with RF-positive and RF-negative polyJIA and extended oligoJIA, finding comparable efficacy among the three treatment groups. Additionally, there were significantly fewer serious adverse events in patients treated with tocilizumab compared to those receiving etanercept (Horneff et al, 2016).

Most recently, tocilizumab has been used to treat severe uveitis refractory to MTX and anti-TNF therapy (Calvo-Rio et al, 2017; Tappeiner et al, 2016). While not approved for use in uveitis, tocilizumab may be an option in patients who fail to respond to conventional therapy.

▶ T-Cell Costimulatory Inhibitor

Abatacept is a soluble CTLA4-IgFcγ fusion protein binding to CD80/CD86 and subsequently inhibiting the T-cell costimulatory pathway. It is FDA approved for use in children 6 years and older with moderate to severe polyJIA. Available as an IV infusion or as an SQ injection, abatacept is recommended as next-line therapy in patients who fail to improve with anti-TNF agents (Harris et al, 2013; Stoll and Cron, 2014). In a randomized, double-blind, placebo-controlled trial, patients received abatacept for the first 4 months before being assigned to the placebo infusion or to continued abatacept for the next 6 months. Compared to the placebo group, patients who received abatacept had significantly fewer disease flares. An open-label extension of the study showed even higher rates of efficacy with long-term abatacept therapy. Even though the mechanisms of action grossly differ, the safety profile for abatacept is similar to the TNF inhibitor agents with nonserious infection comprising a majority of the adverse events. Infusion reactions are uncommon but have been reported (Lovell et al, 2015).

A. Rituximab

Rituximab is a monoclonal antibody targeting the CD20 glycoprotein present on the surface of B cells and is administered as infusions, often every 6 months. It is not routinely used in children; however, case reports suggest it to be efficacious in treating multiple subtypes within JIA (Harris et al, 2013; Stoll et al, 2013; Stoll and Cron, 2014).

THE FUTURE OF JIA TREATMENTS

Treatment advances continue as a better understanding of the pathogenesis of disease unravels. Newer therapies approved for use in adults with RA and psoriatic arthritis are being used off label in children with JIA, particularly those with severe disease refractory to TNF inhibition. Tofacitinib is a Janus kinase (JAK) inhibitor approved for use in adults with RA. Unlike the aforementioned biologics, it is administered orally. There are two ongoing clinical trials studying the safety and efficacy of tofacitinib in children with JIA (Harris et al, 2013). Blockade of other cytokines, such as IL-12 and IL-23, are also being explored in treating JIA (Mannion et al, 2016).

One of the hottest topics lately has been the development of biosimilars, defined as a "biotherapeutic product that is similar in terms of quality, safety, and efficacy to an already licensed reference biotherapeutic product (Isaacs et al, 2016)." They function much like generic medications. Biosimilars, in theory, maintain relative immunogenicity to their reference drug, thereby making the two drugs interchangeable. Economically, biosimilars should theoretically provide a more accessible and relatively cost-effective alternative to biologics (Dorner et al, 2013; Isaacs et al, 2016; Mehr and Brook, 2017).

Originally launched in Europe, biosimilars have been available in other countries since 2006. Only in 2015 was the first biosimilar approved for use by the FDA as per the Biologics Price Competition and Innovation Act within the Patient Protection and Affordable Care Act of 2010. With respect to inflammatory arthritis, the FDA has several approved biosimilars for reference drugs infliximab, etanercept, and adalimumab. To date, only the infliximab biosimilars have been marketed in the United States (Mehr and Brook, 2017). According to the FDA, pharmacists reserve the right to substitute a biosimilar without intervention by the original prescriber. While biosimilars should be clinically comparable to their reference drug, there are few studies evaluating patient outcomes since their introduction.

Prognosis

Disease prognosis varies with respect to JIA subtype; however, the universal treatment goal is clinically inactive disease either on or off medication. About 50% of patients with persistent oligoarthritis go into remission, strictly defined as the absence of active disease while off medication; however, some of these patients will progress to extended oligoarthritis. Extended oligoarthritis is more aggressive with polyarthritis often persisting into adulthood (Shoop-Worrall et al, 2017).

In a Research in Arthritis in Canadian Children emphasizing Outcomes (ReACCh-Out) cohort of 1104 patients with JIA, Guzman et al found the probability of attaining an active joint count of zero within 2 years exceeded 78% on contemporary therapy. Initial treatment included NSAIDs, steroid injections, and conventional DMARDs for polyarthritis. Patients with RF-positive polyarthritis had the worst outcomes; still, the probability of achieving inactive disease at any given point within 5 years was 90%. Within 5 years, 57% of patients with oligoarthritis were in remission off medication, compared to 0% of the RF-positive polyarticular subtype who were unable to discontinue therapy (Guzman et al, 2015).

Many studies report worse outcomes in ERA JIA, with persistent enthesitis and poorer physical function. Axial involvement and progression to ankylosing spondylitis (AS) occurs within 10 years of onset. Risk of AS is higher in patients with a family history of AS and a positive HLA-B27 (Weiss, 2016).

Poor prognostic features include arthritis of the hip, cervical spine, ankles, or wrists, prolonged elevation of inflammatory markers, and radiographic joint damage such as erosions or joint space narrowing (Beukelman et al, 2011). Additionally, a positive RF and/or anti-CCP suggest more aggressive disease and subsequently poorer outcomes. Patients with RF-positive polyarthritis have the lowest rates of remission and often require life-long medication for maintenance (Beukelman et al, 2011; Cassidy and Petty, 2005).

If not adequately treated, inflammation can lead to joint destruction and contractures, causing significant morbidity.

Fortunately, the advent of biologic therapies for treating JIA has markedly improved outcomes (Stoll and Cron, 2014).

Al-Matar MJ, Petty RE, Tucker LB, Malleson PN, Schroeder ML, Cabral DA. The early pattern of joint involvement predicts disease progression in children with oligoarticular (pauciarticular) juvenile rheumatoid arthritis. *Arthritis Rheum.* 2002;46(10):2708-2715. [PMID: 12384930]

Alsufyani K, Ortiz-Alvarez O, Cabral DA, Tucker LB, Petty RE, Malleson PN. The role of subcutaneous administration of methotrexate in children with juvenile idiopathic arthritis who have failed oral methotrexate. *J Rheumatol.* 2004;31(1):179-182. [PMID: 14705239]

Angeles-Han ST, McCracken C, Yeh S, et al. Characteristics of a cohort of children with juvenile idiopathic arthritis and JIA-associated uveitis. *Pediatr Rheumatol Online J.* 2015;13:19. [PMID: 26031738]

Angeles-Han ST, Pelajo CF, Vogler LB, et al. Risk markers of juvenile idiopathic arthritis-associated uveitis in the Childhood Arthritis and Rheumatology Research Alliance (CARRA) Registry. *J Rheumatol.* 2013;40(12):2088-2096. [PMID: 24187099]

Angeles-Han ST, Rabinovich CE. Uveitis in children. *Curr Opin Rheumatol.* 2016;28(5):544-549. [PMID: 27328333]

Barthel D, Ganser G, Kuester RM, et al. Inflammatory bowel disease in juvenile idiopathic arthritis patients treated with biologics. *J Rheumatol.* 2015;42(11):2160-2165. [PMID: 26373564]

Bechtold S, Simon D. Growth abnormalities in children and adolescents with juvenile idiopathic arthritis. *Rheumatol Int.* 2014;34(11):1483-1488. [PMID: 24760485]

Behrens EM, Beukelman T, Gallo L, et al. Evaluation of the presentation of systemic onset juvenile rheumatoid arthritis: data from the Pennsylvania Systemic Onset Juvenile Arthritis Registry (PASOJAR). *J Rheumatol.* 2008;35(2):343-348. [PMID: 18085728]

Berntson L, Fasth A, Andersson-Gare B, et al. Construct validity of ILAR and EULAR criteria in juvenile idiopathic arthritis: a population based incidence study from the Nordic countries. International League of Associations for Rheumatology. European League Against Rheumatism. *J Rheumatol.* 2001;28(12):2737-2743. [PMID: 11764226]

Beukelman T, Haynes K, Curtis JR, et al. Rates of malignancy associated with juvenile idiopathic arthritis and its treatment. *Arthritis Rheum.* 2012;64(4):1263-1271. [PMID: 22328538]

Beukelman T, Patkar NM, Saag KG, et al. 2011 American College of Rheumatology recommendations for the treatment of juvenile idiopathic arthritis: initiation and safety monitoring of therapeutic agents for the treatment of arthritis and systemic features. *Arthritis Care Res (Hoboken).* 2011;63(4):465-482. [PMID: 21452260]

Bleesing J, Prada A, Siegel DM, et al. The diagnostic significance of soluble CD163 and soluble interleukin-2 receptor alpha-chain in macrophage activation syndrome and untreated new-onset systemic juvenile idiopathic arthritis. *Arthritis Rheum.* 2007;56(3):965-971. [PMID: 17328073]

Bloom BJ, Alario AJ, Miller LC. Intra-articular corticosteroid therapy for juvenile idiopathic arthritis: report of an experiential cohort and literature review. *Rheumatol Int.* 2011;31(6):749-756. [PMID: 20155422]

Brewer EJ, Jr., Bass J, Baum J, et al. Current proposed revision of JRA Criteria. JRA Criteria Subcommittee of the Diagnostic and Therapeutic Criteria Committee of the American Rheumatism Section of The Arthritis Foundation. *Arthritis Rheum.* 1977;20(2 Suppl):195-199. [PMID: 318120]

Brunner HI, Ruperto N, Zuber Z, et al. Efficacy and safety of tocilizumab in patients with polyarticular-course juvenile idiopathic arthritis: results from a phase 3, randomised, double-blind withdrawal trial. *Ann Rheum Dis.* 2015;74(6):1110-1117. [PMID: 24834925]

Bryant P, Lachman P. Pseudoporphyria secondary to non-steroidal anti-inflammatory drugs. *Arch Dis Child.* 2003;88(11):961. [PMID: 14612354]

Calvo-Rio V, Santos-Gomez M, Calvo I, et al. Anti-interleukin-6 receptor tocilizumab for severe juvenile idiopathic arthritis-associated uveitis refractory to anti-tumor necrosis factor therapy: a multicenter study of twenty-five patients. *Arthritis Rheum.* 2017;69(3):668-675. [PMID: 27696756]

Carrasco R. Juvenile idiopathic arthritis overview and involvement of the temporomandibular joint: prevalence, systemic therapy. *Oral Maxillofac Surg Clin North Am.* 2015;27(1):1-10. [PMID: 25483440]

Cassidy JT, Petty RE. *Textbook of Pediatric Rheumatology.* 5th ed. Philadelphia, PA: Elsevier Saunders; 2005:xvi, 792.

Chen CC, Lin YT, Yang YH, Chiang BL. Sulfasalazine therapy for juvenile rheumatoid arthritis. *J Formos Med Assoc.* 2002;101(2):110-116. [PMID: 12099201]

Clarke SL, Sen ES, Ramanan AV. Juvenile idiopathic arthritis-associated uveitis. *Pediatr Rheumatol Online J.* 2016;14(1):27. [PMID: 27121190]

Colebatch-Bourn AN, Edwards CJ, et al. EULAR-PReS points to consider for the use of imaging in the diagnosis and management of juvenile idiopathic arthritis in clinical practice. *Ann Rheum Dis.* 2015;74(11):1946-1957. [PMID: 26245755]

Cordero-Coma M, Sobrin L. Anti-tumor necrosis factor-alpha therapy in uveitis. *Surv Ophthalmol.* 2015;60(6):575-589. [PMID: 26164735]

Crayne CB, Gerhold K, Cron RQ. Anaphylaxis to etanercept in two children with juvenile idiopathic arthritis. *J Clin Rheumatol.* 2013;19(3):129-131. [PMID: 23519173]

Dorner T, Strand V, Castaneda-Hernandez G, et al. The role of biosimilars in the treatment of rheumatic diseases. *Ann Rheum Dis.* 2013;72(3):322-328. [PMID: 23253920]

El Assar de la Fuente S, Angenete O, Jellestad S, Tzaribachev N, Koos B, Rosendahl K. Juvenile idiopathic arthritis and the temporomandibular joint: a comprehensive review. *J Craniomaxillofac Surg.* 2016;44(5):597-607. [PMID: 26924432]

Falvey S, Shipman L, Ilowite N, Beukelman T. Methotrexate-induced nausea in the treatment of juvenile idiopathic arthritis. *Pediatr Rheumatol Online J.* 2017;15(1):52. [PMID: 28629458]

Fellas A, Hawke F, Santos D, Coda A. Prevalence, presentation and treatment of lower limb pathologies in juvenile idiopathic arthritis: A narrative review. *J Paediatr Child Health.* 2017;53(9):836-840. [PMID: 28767173]

Foeldvari I, Becker I, Horneff G. Uveitis events during adalimumab, etanercept, and methotrexate therapy in juvenile idiopathic arthritis: data from the biologics in pediatric rheumatology registry. *Arthritis Care Res (Hoboken).* 2015;67(11):1529-1535. [PMID: 25988824]

Franova J, Fingerhutova S, Kobrova K, et al. Methotrexate efficacy, but not its intolerance, is associated with the dose and route of administration. *Pediatr Rheumatol Online J.* 2016;14(1):36. [PMID: 27301536]

Giancane G, Consolaro A, Lanni S, Davi S, Schiappapietra B, Ravelli A. Juvenile idiopathic arthritis: diagnosis and treatment. *Rheumatol Ther.* 2016;3(2):187-207. [PMID: 27747582]

Giancane G, Pederzoli S, Norambuena X, et al. Frequency of radiographic damage and progression in individual joints in children with juvenile idiopathic arthritis. *Arthritis Care Res (Hoboken).* 2014;66(1):27-33. [PMID: 23983211]

Giannini EH, Brewer EJ, Kuzmina N, et al. Methotrexate in resistant juvenile rheumatoid arthritis. Results of the U.S.A.-U.S.S.R. double-blind, placebo-controlled trial. The Pediatric Rheumatology Collaborative Study Group and The Cooperative Children's Study Group. *N Engl J Med.* 1992;326(16):1043-1049. [PMID: 1549149]

Giannini EH, Ilowite NT, Lovell DJ, et al. Long-term safety and effectiveness of etanercept in children with selected categories of juvenile idiopathic arthritis. *Arthritis Rheum.* 2009;60(9):2794-2804. [PMID: 19714630]

Gowdie PJ, Tse SM. Juvenile idiopathic arthritis. *Pediatr Clin North Am.* 2012;59(2):301-327. [PMID: 22560572]

Guzman J, Oen K, Tucker LB, et al. The outcomes of juvenile idiopathic arthritis in children managed with contemporary treatments: results from the ReACCh-Out cohort. *Ann Rheum Dis.* 2015;74(10):1854-1860. [PMID: 24842571]

Harris JG, Kessler EA, Verbsky JW. Update on the treatment of juvenile idiopathic arthritis. *Curr Allergy Asthma Rep.* 2013;13(4):337-346. [PMID: 23605168]

Hawkins MJ, Dick AD, Lee RJ, et al. Managing juvenile idiopathic arthritis-associated uveitis. *Surv Ophthalmol.* 2016;61(2):197-210. [PMID: 26599495]

Heiligenhaus A, Niewerth M, Ganser G, Heinz C, Minden K; German Uveitis in Childhood Study G. Prevalence and complications of uveitis in juvenile idiopathic arthritis in a population-based nation-wide study in Germany: suggested modification of the current screening guidelines. *Rheumatology (Oxford).* 2007;46(6):1015-1019. [PMID: 17403710]

Horneff G. Biologic-associated infections in pediatric rheumatology. *Curr Rheumatol Rep.* 2015a;17(11):66. [PMID: 26385753]

Horneff G. Safety of biologic therapies for the treatment of juvenile idiopathic arthritis. *Expert Opin Drug Saf.* 2015b;14(7):1111-1126. [PMID: 26084637]

Horneff G, Klein A, Klotsche J, et al. Comparison of treatment response, remission rate and drug adherence in polyarticular juvenile idiopathic arthritis patients treated with etanercept, adalimumab or tocilizumab. *Arthritis Res Ther.* 2016;18(1):272. [PMID: 27881144]

Ilowite NT, Prather K, Lokhnygina Y, et al. Randomized, double-blind, placebo-controlled trial of the efficacy and safety of rilonacept in the treatment of systemic juvenile idiopathic arthritis. *Arthritis Rheum.* 2014;66(9):2570-2579. [PMID: 24839206]

Isaacs JD, Cutolo M, Keystone EC, Park W, Braun J. Biosimilars in immune-mediated inflammatory diseases: initial lessons from the first approved biosimilar anti-tumour necrosis factor monoclonal antibody. *J Intern Med.* 2016;279(1):41-59. [PMID: 26403380]

Kingsbury DJ, Bader-Meunier B, Patel G, Arora V, Kalabic J, Kupper H. Safety, effectiveness, and pharmacokinetics of adalimumab in children with polyarticular juvenile idiopathic arthritis aged 2 to 4 years. *Clin Rheumatol.* 2014;33(10):1433-1441. [PMID: 24487484]

Lovell DJ, Giannini EH, Reiff A, et al. Etanercept in children with polyarticular juvenile rheumatoid arthritis. Pediatric Rheumatology Collaborative Study Group. *N Engl J Med.* 2000;342(11):763-769. [PMID: 10717011]

Lovell DJ, Reiff A, Ilowite NT, et al. Safety and efficacy of up to eight years of continuous etanercept therapy in patients with juvenile rheumatoid arthritis. *Arthritis Rheum.* 2008;58(5):1496-1504. [PMID: 18438876]

Lovell DJ, Ruperto N, Mouy R, et al. Long-term safety, efficacy, and quality of life in patients with juvenile idiopathic arthritis treated with intravenous abatacept for up to seven years. *Arthritis Rheum.* 2015;67(10):2759-2770. [PMID: 26097215]

Magni-Manzoni S, Scire CA, Ravelli A, et al. Ultrasound-detected synovial abnormalities are frequent in clinically inactive juvenile idiopathic arthritis, but do not predict a flare of synovitis. *Ann Rheum Dis.* 2013;72(2):223-228. [PMID: 22736098]

Mannion ML, Beukelman T. Risk of malignancy associated with biologic agents in pediatric rheumatic disease. *Curr Opin Rheumatol.* 2014;26(5):538-542. [PMID: 25010437]

Mannion ML, McAllister L, Cron RQ, Stoll ML. Ustekinumab as a therapeutic option for children with refractory enthesitis-related arthritis. *J Clin Rheumatol.* 2016;22(5):282-284. [PMID: 27464779]

Mehr SR, Brook RA. Factors influencing the economics of biosimilars in the US. *J Med Econ.* 2017:1-7. [PMID: 28796564]

Muller L, Kellenberger CJ, Cannizzaro E, et al. Early diagnosis of temporomandibular joint involvement in juvenile idiopathic arthritis: a pilot study comparing clinical examination and ultrasound to magnetic resonance imaging. *Rheumatology (Oxford).* 2009;48(6):680-685. [PMID: 19386819]

Nigrovic PA. Review: is there a window of opportunity for treatment of systemic juvenile idiopathic arthritis? *Arthritis Rheum.* 2014;66(6):1405-1413. [PMID: 24623686]

Nigrovic PA, Mannion M, Prince FH, et al. Anakinra as first-line disease-modifying therapy in systemic juvenile idiopathic arthritis: report of forty-six patients from an international multicenter series. *Arthritis Rheum.* 2011;63(2):545-555. [PMID: 21280009]

Oen KG, Cheang M. Epidemiology of chronic arthritis in childhood. *Semin Arthritis Rheum.* 1996;26(3):575-591. [PMID: 8989803]

Otten MH, Prince FH, Armbrust W, et al. Factors associated with treatment response to etanercept in juvenile idiopathic arthritis. *JAMA.* 2011;306(21):2340-2347. [PMID: 22056397]

Petty RE, Southwood TR, Manners P, et al. International League of Associations for Rheumatology classification of juvenile idiopathic arthritis: second revision, Edmonton, 2001. *J Rheumatol.* 2004;31(2):390-392. [PMID: 14760812]

Ramanan AV, Dick AD, Benton D, et al. A randomised controlled trial of the clinical effectiveness, safety and cost-effectiveness of adalimumab in combination with methotrexate for the treatment of juvenile idiopathic arthritis associated uveitis (SYCAMORE Trial). *Trials.* 2014;15:14. [PMID: 24405833]

Ramanan AV, Whitworth P, Baildam EM. Use of methotrexate in juvenile idiopathic arthritis. *Arch Dis Child.* 2003;88(3):197-200. [PMID: 12598376]

Ravelli A, Minoia F, Davi S, et al. Classification criteria for macrophage activation syndrome complicating systemic juvenile idiopathic arthritis: a European League Against Rheumatism/American College of Rheumatology/Paediatric Rheumatology International Trials Organisation Collaborative Initiative. *Ann Rheum Dis.* 2016;75(3):481-489. [PMID: 26314788]

Ravelli A, Varnier GC, Oliveira S, et al. Antinuclear antibody-positive patients should be grouped as a separate category in the classification of juvenile idiopathic arthritis. *Arthritis Rheum.* 2011;63(1):267-275. [PMID: 20936630]

Ringold S, Weiss PF, Beukelman T, et al. 2013 update of the 2011 American College of Rheumatology recommendations for the treatment of juvenile idiopathic arthritis: recommendations for the medical therapy of children with systemic juvenile idiopathic arthritis and tuberculosis screening among children receiving biologic medications. *Arthritis Rheum.* 2013;65(10):2499-2512. [PMID: 24078300]

Ruperto N, Lovell DJ, Cuttica R, et al. A randomized, placebo-controlled trial of infliximab plus methotrexate for the treatment of polyarticular-course juvenile rheumatoid arthritis. *Arthritis Rheum.* 2007;56(9):3096-3106. [PMID: 17763439]

Shoop-Worrall SJW, Kearsley-Fleet L, Thomson W, Verstappen SMM, Hyrich KL. How common is remission in juvenile idiopathic arthritis: a systematic review. *Semin Arthritis Rheum.* 2017;47(3):331-337. [PMID: 28625712]

Silverman E, Mouy R, Spiegel L, et al. Leflunomide or methotrexate for juvenile rheumatoid arthritis. *N Engl J Med.* 2005;352(16):1655-1666. [PMID: 15843668]

Smith JA, Thompson DJ, Whitcup SM, et al. A randomized, placebo-controlled, double-masked clinical trial of etanercept for the treatment of uveitis associated with juvenile idiopathic arthritis. *Arthritis Rheum.* 2005;53(1):18-23. [PMID: 15696578]

Sterba Y, Ilowite N. Biologics in pediatric rheumatology: quo vadis? *Curr Rheumatol Rep.* 2016;18(7):45. [PMID: 27306623]

Stoll ML. Gut microbes, immunity, and spondyloarthritis. *Clin Immunol.* 2015;159(2):134-142. [PMID: 25967460]

Stoll ML, Cron RQ. Treatment of juvenile idiopathic arthritis in the biologic age. *Rheum Dis Clin North Am.* 2013;39(4):751-766. [PMID: 24182853]

Stoll ML, Cron RQ. Treatment of juvenile idiopathic arthritis: a revolution in care. *Pediatr Rheumatol Online J.* 2014;12:13. [PMID: 24782683]

Stoll ML, Cron RQ. The microbiota in pediatric rheumatic disease: epiphenomenon or therapeutic target? Curr Opin Rheumatol. 2016;28(5):537-543. [PMID: 27286235]

Stoll ML, Good J, Sharpe T, et al. Intra-articular corticosteroid injections to the temporomandibular joints are safe and appear to be effective therapy in children with juvenile idiopathic arthritis. *J Oral Maxillofac Surg.* 2012;70(8):1802-1807. [PMID: 22265164]

Stoll ML, Sharpe T, Beukelman T, Good J, Young D, Cron RQ. Risk factors for temporomandibular joint arthritis in children with juvenile idiopathic arthritis. *J Rheumatol.* 2012;39(9):1880-1887. [PMID: 22589268]

Stoll ML, Zurakowski D, Nigrovic LE, Nichols DP, Sundel RP, Nigrovic PA. Patients with juvenile psoriatic arthritis comprise two distinct populations. *Arthritis Rheum.* 2006;54(11):3564-3572. [PMID: 17075862]

Tappeiner C, Mesquida M, Adan A, et al. Evidence for tocilizumab as a treatment option in refractory uveitis associated with juvenile idiopathic arthritis. *J Rheumatol.* 2016;43(12):2183-2188. [PMID: 27633821]

Tynjala P, Vahasalo P, Tarkiainen M, et al. Aggressive combination drug therapy in very early polyarticular juvenile idiopathic arthritis (ACUTE-JIA): a multicentre randomised open-label clinical trial. *Ann Rheum Dis.* 2011;70(9):1605-1612. [PMID: 21623000]

Vaid YN, Dunnavant FD, Royal SA, Beukelman T, Stoll ML, Cron RQ. Imaging of the temporomandibular joint in juvenile idiopathic arthritis. *Arthritis Care Res (Hoboken).* 2014;66(1):47-54. [PMID: 24106204] van Rossum MA, Fiselier TJ, Franssen MJ, et al. Sulfasalazine in the treatment of juvenile chronic arthritis: a randomized, double-blind, placebo-controlled, multicenter study. Dutch Juvenile Chronic Arthritis Study Group. *Arthritis Rheum.* 1998;41(5):808-816. [PMID: 9588731]

Wallace CA, Giannini EH, Spalding SJ, et al. Trial of early aggressive therapy in polyarticular juvenile idiopathic arthritis. *Arthritis Rheum.* 2012;64(6):2012-2021. [PMID: 22183975]

Wallace CA, Giannini EH, Spalding SJ, et al. Clinically inactive disease in a cohort of children with new-onset polyarticular juvenile idiopathic arthritis treated with early aggressive therapy: time to achievement, total duration, and predictors. *J Rheumatol.* 2014;41(6):1163-1170. [PMID: 24786928]

Weiss PF. Update on enthesitis-related arthritis. *Curr Opin Rheumatol.* 2016;28(5):530-536. [PMID: 27466726]

Weiss PF, Arabshahi B, Johnson A, et al. High prevalence of temporomandibular joint arthritis at disease onset in children with juvenile idiopathic arthritis, as detected by magnetic resonance imaging but not by ultrasound. *Arthritis Rheum.* 2008;58(4):1189-1196. [PMID: 18383394]

Wong SC, Dobie R, Altowati MA, Werther GA, Farquharson C, Ahmed SF. Growth and the Growth hormone-insulin like growth factor 1 axis in children with chronic inflammation: current evidence, gaps in knowledge, and future directions. *Endocr Rev.* 2016;37(1):62-110. [PMID: 26720129]

Zulian F, Martini G, Gobber D, Plebani M, Zacchello F, Manners P. Triamcinolone acetonide and hexacetonide intra-articular treatment of symmetrical joints in juvenile idiopathic arthritis: a double-blind trial. *Rheumatology (Oxford).* 2004;43(10):1288-1291. [PMID: 15252213]

Systemic Lupus Erythematosus

19

Maria Dall'Era, MD

ESSENTIALS OF DIAGNOSIS

▶ Predilection for females of childbearing age.

▶ Multisystem disease that has a tendency to remit and relapse.

▶ Photosensitive rash, polyarthritis, serositis, and fatigue are common flare manifestations.

▶ Renal disease, central nervous system involvement, and complications of antiphospholipid antibodies can cause major morbidity.

▶ Treatment-related morbidity, particularly from glucocorticoids, constitutes a major source of damage associated with having lupus.

▶ Presence of antinuclear antibodies.

▶ Certain autoantibodies (anti-dsDNA and anti-Sm) have great specificity for the diagnosis of systemic lupus erythematosus (SLE) but lack sensitivity.

▶ Hypocomplementemia may occur during flares.

▶ General Considerations

Systemic lupus erythematosus (SLE) is often considered to be the prototype of autoimmune disorders. The disease is characterized by the potential multisystem involvement and the production of an array of autoantibodies. Clinical features in individual patients vary greatly and sometimes change over time, ranging the presence of autoantibodies with relatively few clinical symptoms to skin and joint involvement to organ- and life-threatening disease. Waxing and waning clinical courses are typical, with quiescent periods induced by treatment punctuated by periods of disease flare.

The prevalence of SLE varies across gender, race/ethnicity, and geographic regions. SLE demonstrates a striking female predominance and a peak incidence of disease during patients' reproductive years. In adults, the female-to-male ratio is 10–15:1. This epidemiology often leads to challenging questions surrounding the timing of conception and the maintenance of remission during pregnancy. In the United States, the estimated prevalence is 100 per 100,000 white women and 400 per 100,000 black women. SLE is more common among blacks in the United States but is rare among blacks in Africa. Approximately 160,000–320,000 people in the United States are living with SLE.

Genetic, hormonal, and environmental influences clearly all play role in disease pathogenesis, but the precise ways in which these factors sum to SLE remain uncertain. Genetic studies have revealed strong familial risk for SLE (and other forms of autoimmunity), as evidenced by a disease concordance rate of 24–58% for monozygotic twins compared with only 2–5% for dizygotic twins. Multiple genes have been associated with SLE, including the genes within the major histocompatibility complex and genes that encode components of the complement pathway, Fcγ receptors, protein tyrosine phosphatase nonreceptor type 22 (PTPN22), programmed cell death 1 (PDCD1) gene, and cytotoxic T-lymphocyte–associated antigen 4 (CTLA4).

The reasons for female sex predilection are still unknown. Some observational data suggest that sex hormones might contribute to disease onset. For example, data from the Nurses Health Study suggest that early age at menarche (relative risk 2.1), oral contraceptive use (relative risk 1.5), and use of postmenopausal hormones (relative risk 1.9) all increase the risk of SLE. Moreover, the risk of SLE among men with Klinefelter syndrome (47, XXY) is 14-fold higher compared to male controls. Large controlled trials have confirmed, however, that combined oral contraceptives do not increase the risk of SLE flares in women whose disease is stable. Further, studies examining serum sex hormone levels in patients with lupus compared with patients in a control group have been inconclusive. The overall contribution of hormonal factors to the pathophysiology of SLE, therefore, requires further study.

Various environmental factors have been examined as potential triggers for the development of SLE. Exposure to ultraviolet (UV) light exacerbates both cutaneous and internal organ manifestations of SLE, and the avoidance of UV radiation is an important precept in the disease management of many patients, but there is no clear evidence to suggest that UV light triggers onset of the disease. Smoking is a risk factor for SLE and has been associated with antibodies to double-stranded DNA (anti-dsDNA) production in patients with SLE.

Several viruses have been investigated as possible triggers for SLE, but no conclusive evidence currently links any single pathogen to development of disease. The virus that has received the most attention in this regard is Epstein-Barr virus (EBV). Studies in pediatric and adult patients have demonstrated a higher seroprevalence of antibodies to EBV antigens and a higher EBV viral load in SLE patients versus controls. Molecular mimicry between EBV and self proteins is postulated to play a role in the pathogenesis of SLE, but this long-standing theory still awaits confirmation.

There is increasing evidence that interferon α (IFNα) plays an important role in the pathogenesis of SLE, and this may soon play an important role in the therapy of some patients with the disease (see Chapter 20). Approximately 50% of SLE patients overexpress IFNα-inducible genes, and the degree of overexpression correlates with disease activity and severity. This pattern of gene expression is referred to as the "interferon α signature." One source of IFNα in patients with SLE is plasmacytoid dendritic cells, which have been shown to release IFNα after stimulation with immune complexes containing nucleic acid.

SLE is characterized by the production of a variety of autoantibodies. These autoantibodies are directed against nuclear antigens (antinuclear antibodies [ANA]), cytoplasmic antigens, and cell surface antigens, as well as to soluble antigens in the circulation such as IgG and phospholipids. Subtypes of ANAs are useful for establishing a diagnosis, predicting certain disease manifestations, and (in some patients in the case of some antibodies) monitoring the course of the disease. Antibodies to surface antigens on red blood cells and platelets can lead to autoimmune hemolytic anemia (AIHA) and immune-mediated thrombocytopenia, respectively.

In the majority of SLE patients, the presence of autoantibodies predates the development of symptoms or signs of SLE. Patients accrue different autoantibodies up until the time of diagnosis. One study utilizing the Department of Defense Serum Repository demonstrated that ANA, anti-Ro/SSA antibodies, anti-La/SSB antibodies, and antiphospholipid antibodies were the first to appear and did so at a mean of 3.4 years prior to the diagnosis of SLE. Antibodies to double-stranded DNA (anti-dsDNA) appeared next at a mean of 2.2 years prior to diagnosis, and anti-Smith (anti-Sm) and anti-ribonucleoprotein (anti-RNP) were the last to appear at 1 year before diagnosis. This study also showed that the autoantibody profile at the time of SLE diagnosis remained relatively constant in the years after diagnosis.

▶ Clinical Findings

A. Symptoms and Signs

1. Constitutional—Constitutional symptoms, such as fever, fatigue, and weight changes, are common in SLE. The level of fatigue is often out of proportion to other disease manifestations. In such cases, it is important to consider other factors such as deconditioning, stress, and sleep disturbance. Fever, usually low grade, can occur in active SLE, particularly with serositis. Infection, however, is always a concern when fever develops in a lupus patient, especially in the setting of immunosuppressive therapy.

2. Mucocutaneous—Approximately 80–90% of SLE patients will have mucocutaneous involvement at some point during the course of the disease (Tables 19–1 and 19–2), and 4 of the 11 American College of Rheumatology (ACR) classification criteria describe mucocutaneous manifestations.

Table 19–1. The 1997 update of the 1982 Revised American College of Rheumatology classification criteria for SLE.[a]

Criterion	Definition
Malar rash	Fixed erythema, flat or raised, over the malar eminences, sparing the nasolabial folds
Discoid rash	Erythematous raised patches with adherent keratotic scale and follicular plugging; atrophic scarring may occur in older lesions
Photosensitivity	Skin rash as a result of unusual reaction to sunlight, by patient history or clinician observation
Oral ulcers	Oral or nasopharyngeal ulceration, usually painless, observed by a clinician
Arthritis	Nonerosive arthritis involving two or more peripheral joints, characterized by tenderness, swelling, or effusion
Serositis	a. Pleuritis b. Pericarditis
Renal disorder	a. Persistent proteinuria >0.5 g/day OR b. Cellular casts
Neurologic disorder	a. Seizures OR b. Psychosis
Hematologic disorder	a. Hemolytic anemia OR b. Leukopenia 4000/mcL OR c. Lymphopenia <1500/mcL d. Thrombocytopenia <100,000/mcL
Immunologic disorder	a. Anti-DNA OR b. Anti-Sm OR c. Antiphospholipid antibodies
Positive antinuclear antibody	An abnormal titer of antinuclear antibody by immunofluorescence or an equivalent assay in the absence of a drug

[a]The presence of four or more criteria is required for SLE classification. Exclude all other reasonable diagnoses.
SLE, systemic lupus erythematosus.

Table 19–2. Major clinical manifestations of systemic lupus erythematosus.

Organ	Manifestation
Mouth	Erythema, petechiae, or ulcers occurring most commonly on buccal mucosa, hard palate, or vermillion border
Skin	Malar rash, SCLE, discoid lupus, bullous lesions, panniculitis, palpable purpura, periungual erythema, livedo reticularis, Raynaud phenomenon, chilblain lupus
Lymph nodes	Lymphadenopathy, commonly in cervical and axillary regions
Joints	Symmetric, inflammatory polyarthritis, usually nonerosive; reducible Jaccoud-like arthropathy
Heart	Pericarditis, myocarditis, Libman-Sacks endocarditis, conduction system abnormalities, premature atherosclerosis
Lungs	Pleuritis, pneumonitis, diffuse alveolar hemorrhage, pulmonary hypertension
Gastrointestinal	Peritonitis, hepatitis, pancreatitis, mesenteric vasculitis, intestinal pseudo-obstruction
Kidney	Glomerulonephritis, interstitial nephritis, antiphospholipid nephropathy
Blood	Leukopenia, anemia, thrombocytopenia, arterial/vein thrombosis
Neuropsychiatric	Seizures, headache, acute confusional state, cognitive dysfunction, myelopathy, peripheral neuropathy

SCLE, subacute cutaneous lupus erythematosus.

Photosensitivity, defined by the ACR as "skin rash as a result of unusual reaction to sunlight, by patient history, or physician observation," occurs frequently. Patients may be sensitive to UV-A, UV-B, or visible light. More than 90% of lupus patients have an abnormal skin reaction to UV or visible light. SLE patients also have reported symptoms after exposure to sunlight through car glass windows and to light from fluorescent tubes and photocopiers. The majority of skin reactions occur more than 1 week after sun exposure and last for weeks to months. In addition to skin eruptions, some SLE patients report an exacerbation of systemic symptoms such as fatigue and arthralgias after sun exposure.

Polymorphous light eruption and photosensitizing medications are additional diagnostic considerations when evaluating an SLE patient with a photosensitive rash. In contrast to SLE photosensitivity, polymorphous light eruption is characterized by an intensely pruritic, papular, nonscarring rash that develops hours after sun exposure and resolves after a few days. Polymorphous light eruption may occur in patients with known SLE.

Patchy or diffuse alopecia and thin, friable hair occur during active SLE flares but may also occur as a side effect of certain medications that are commonly used to treat SLE. Hair

regrowth begins 6–8 weeks after disease quiescence or discontinuation of the offending drug. Permanent alopecia can occur following the development of scarring discoid lesions.

Nasal or oral ulcers, which are typically painless, commonly develop in SLE patients. This is in contrast to aphthous stomatitis that is usually painful. Lupus oral ulcers have a gradual onset and can occur anywhere on the oral mucosa. Most lesions present as erythema, petechiae, or ulcerations. They typically occur on the hard palate, buccal mucosa, and vermillion border, and are unilateral or asymmetric. Discoid lupus erythematosus (DLE) can also occur in the oral cavity and are painful. Oral candidiasis and oral lichen planus can resemble the oral ulcers of SLE.

Cutaneous lupus lesions are categorized as "lupus specific" versus "lupus nonspecific" based on the presence or absence of interface dermatitis on histopathology. Acute cutaneous lupus erythematosus (ACLE), subacute cutaneous lupus erythematosus (SCLE), and chronic cutaneous lupus erythematosus (CCLE) are all considered to be lupus specific lesions. ACLE lesions can be localized or generalized. The localized form produces the classic malar or "butterfly" rash, which is characterized by sharply demarcated erythema on the cheeks and bridge of the nose, sparing the nasolabial folds (Figure 19–1). Induration and scaling may occur. The malar rash of SLE is sometimes confused with that of acne rosacea, seborrheic dermatitis, and flushing syndromes. Unlike SLE, rosacea is characterized by the predominance of telangiectasias and pustules that may sting and burn. Heat and alcohol intake worsen the erythema of rosacea.

Seborrheic dermatitis is manifested by scaly erythematous plaques that occur on the eyebrows and the lateral sides of the nose. In contrast to the malar rash of SLE, seborrheic dermatitis is commonly found within the nasolabial folds. If the diagnosis remains unclear after clinical examination,

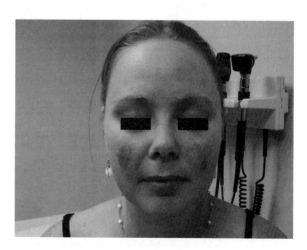

▲ **Figure 19–1.** Malar rash of systemic lupus erythematosus.

biopsy of the rash can be helpful to distinguish SLE from these other dermatologic entities.

Generalized ACLE consists of maculopapular erythematosus lesions involving any area of the body in a photosensitive distribution. The dorsa of the hands and the extensor surfaces of the fingers are commonly involved. The erythema is typically found between the interphalangeal joints, which is to be distinguished from the Gottron papules of dermatomyositis, which occur over the joint. ACLE lesions heal without scarring, although postinflammatory hyperpigmentation can be observed.

The rash of SCLE may be papulosquamous or annular and is believed to be the most photosensitive of all the lupus rashes (Figure 19–2). The scaly, erythematous papules are frequently located on the torso and limbs and spare the face. Neither scarring nor atrophy is present. Patients with such lesions often have anti-SSA/Ro antibody. Compared with other forms of cutaneous lupus, SCLE is more often induced by medications such as hydrochlorothiazide and terbinafine.

Discoid lupus is the most common subtype of CCLE. The term "discoid" refers to the disc shaped appearance of the lesions. Such lesions are raised, erythematous plaques with adherent scale occurring most commonly on the scalp, face, and neck (Figures 19–3 through 19–5; see Figure 19–1). There is usually an erythematous ring around the lesions, which denotes the active component (see Figure 19–3). Over time, discoid lesions can lead to scarring and skin atrophy, resulting in permanent alopecia and disfigurement (see Figures 19–4 and 19–5). DLE can also occur in the oral mucosa. Squamous cell carcinoma has been reported as a late sequela of DLE; thus, surveillance of known lesions and biopsy of changing or suspicions lesions are important.

Other subtypes of CCLE include hypertrophic lupus erythematosus and lupus panniculitis. Lupus panniculitis is a lobular panniculitis that has a predilection for the scalp, face, arms, buttocks, and thighs. When a cutaneous discoid lesion

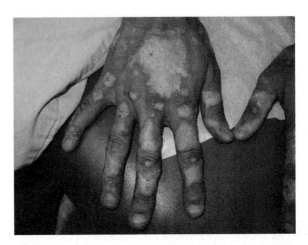

▲ **Figure 19–3.** Discoid lupus with erythematous plaques and scale.

overlies the panniculitis, the entity is referred to as lupus profundus. Lupus panniculitis typically presents as a deep, firm nodule that can lead to cutaneous atrophy and rarely ulceration. Biopsy is often necessary to secure the diagnosis because

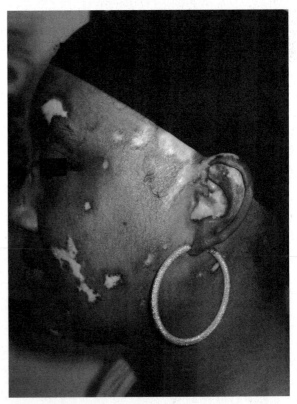

▲ **Figure 19–4.** Discoid lupus with prominent scarring and atrophy.

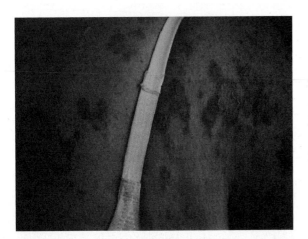

▲ **Figure 19–2.** Annular subtype of subacute cutaneous lupus.

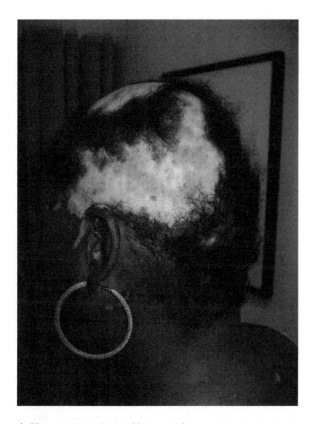

▲ **Figure 19–5.** Discoid lupus with prominent scarring and atrophy and alopecia.

there are reports of T-cell lymphoma mimicking panniculitis. However, biopsy should be performed carefully because lesions have tendency to break down. Lupus panniculitis is one of the few panniculitides that can occur above the waist.

Lupus nonspecific skin findings, such as bullous lesions, periungual erythema, chilblain lupus, and livedo racemosa, can also develop in SLE patients. Bullous lupus erythematosus is a rare cutaneous manifestation that presents as blistering skin lesions. SLE may also be associated with other bullous disorders such as bullous pemphigoid and dermatitis herpetiformis. The physical examination finding of periungual erythema represents dilatation of the capillaries at the base of the nail. These capillaries can be visualized at the bedside with a dermatoscope or ophthalmoscope. Other disorders associated with periungual erythema include scleroderma and mixed connective tissue disease (MCTD). Unlike scleroderma and MCTD, SLE is not associated with capillary dropout. Chilblain lupus is characterized by the presence of erythematous or violaceous macules or plaques (or both) on acral surfaces that worsen after exposure to a cold, humid weather. Livedo racemosa is characterized by an erythematous to violaceous reticular or net-like pattern of the skin. It is also highly associated with the antiphospholipid antibody syndrome.

3. Lymphadenopathy—Lymphadenopathy is a common feature of SLE and can be localized or diffuse. The lymph nodes are soft and nontender, and the cervical and axillary chains are most frequently involved. Biopsy reveals reactive hyperplasia. A change in the pattern of a patient's lymphadenopathy or unusually enlarging or hard lymph nodes should prompt an evaluation for lymphoma, which has an increased incidence in SLE.

4. Musculoskeletal—Arthritis and arthralgias are noted in up to 95% of SLE patients at some time during the course of the illness and frequently involve the wrists and small joints of the hands. Swan-neck deformities and ligamental laxity are often noted (Figure 19–6). Unlike the joint findings in rheumatoid arthritis and MCTD, bony erosions rarely occur in SLE, and the swan-neck deformities are usually reducible (Jaccoud-like arthropathy).

5. Lupus nephritis—Renal involvement is common in SLE and is a significant cause of morbidity and mortality. Although clinically significant nephritis develops in only 50% of people with SLE, up to 90% of SLE patients have pathologic evidence of nephritis on biopsy. Lupus nephritis typically develops in the first 36 months of the disease, but exceptions to this rule occur. Immune complex glomerulonephritis is the most common form of SLE renal involvement, but tubulointerstitial disease and vascular disease may also be present. The clinical presentation of lupus nephritis is highly variable, ranging from asymptomatic hematuria or proteinuria (or both) to frank nephrotic syndrome to rapidly progressive glomerulonephritis with loss of renal function.

Routine screening for the presence of lupus nephritis is a critical component of the ongoing evaluation and management of SLE patients. Screening procedures include asking about new-onset polyuria, nocturia, or foamy urine and looking for the presence of hypertension or lower extremity edema. Performance of a urinalysis with microscopy is

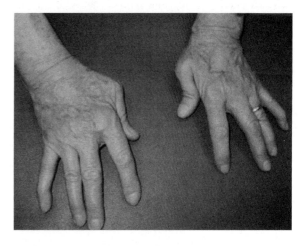

▲ **Figure 19–6.** Jaccoud-like arthropathy.

essential. Hematuria, pyuria, dysmorphic red blood cells, and red blood cell casts may all be present. Accurate measurement of proteinuria is critical because proteinuria is a very sensitive indicator of glomerular damage. Measurements of spot urine protein to creatinine ratios are extremely useful in most cases and far more convenient to check that timed 24-hour urine protein collections. Normal daily protein excretion is less than 150 mg, and rising urine protein:creatinine ratios signal the presence of increasing glomerular proteinuria. It should be borne in mind that the spot ratio often may not be representative of the findings in a timed collection, especially in the range of 0.5–3.0 g/24 h, which is the range of most lupus nephritis flares. In addition, the spot ratio is less accurate in patients who are either extremely muscular or cachectic.

Urine dipsticks should not be used for the quantification of proteinuria because they reflect the concentration of the urine protein, which varies depending on the volume of the sample. Screening SLE patients at regular intervals for the presence of proteinuria and hematuria is recommended. In patients with active SLE, screening at intervals not less than every 3 months is wise. Hematuria in the absence of proteinuria might also be due to urolithiasis, menstrual contamination, or bladder pathology, particularly transitional cell carcinoma in a patient with previous cyclophosphamide exposure.

Renal biopsy is a critical part of the evaluation of a patient with possible lupus nephritis. The International Society of Nephrology/Renal Pathology Society system classifies the glomerular pathology into six categories (Table 19–3) based on light microscopic, immunofluorescent, and electron-micrographic findings. An individual biopsy might exhibit just one of the pathologic classes or a combination of classes. In **class I lupus nephritis**, glomeruli appear normal on light microscopy and immune deposits shown by immunofluorescence are limited to the mesangium. **Class II disease** is characterized by mesangial proliferation on light microscopy and mesangial deposits on immunofluorescence.

Classes III and IV lupus nephritis are highly inflammatory lesions with immune complex deposition in the subendothelial space. These forms of lupus nephritis are described as "proliferative" because of the presence of proliferating endocapillary cells within the glomeruli. Class III denotes that less than 50% of glomeruli are involved and class

IV denotes that more than or equal to 50% of glomeruli are involved. Class IV lesions are subcategorized according to whether the majority of glomeruli show focal involvement (<50% of the glomerular tuft) or global involvement (>50% of the glomerular tuft). Class IV lesions are further described as active (A), chronic (C), or a mixture of both (A/C).

Class V lupus nephritis is characterized by immune complex deposition in the subepithelial space resulting in thickened capillary loops. This lesion commonly manifests clinically as nephrotic range proteinuria. Class V nephritis may occur in a pure histopathologic form or in combination with features of class III or IV nephritis. Finally, **class VI nephritis** is defined by the presence of more than 90% globally sclerotic glomeruli.

In addition to glomerular pathology, renal histopathologic changes may include tubulointerstitial inflammation or fibrosis and a variety of vascular lesions including hyaline thrombi and thrombotic microangiopathy. Thrombotic microangiopathy is highly associated with the presence of antiphospholipid antibodies and should prompt the consideration of antiphospholipid nephropathy.

When an SLE patient has clinical or laboratory features that suggest the presence of nephritis, a renal biopsy should be performed in order to confirm the diagnosis, evaluate the degree of disease activity, and determine an appropriate course of treatment. A biopsy is especially important because urinary parameters, such as hematuria and the degree of proteinuria, imperfectly predict the underlying renal pathology. Hematuria might be absent in patients with severe class IV nephritis, and proteinuria can be modest in patients with class V nephritis.

Each histopathologic class portends a different renal prognosis. Classes I and II nephritis are associated with excellent renal prognoses and do not require any specific therapy. In contrast, the long-term renal prognosis of class III–IV nephritis is extremely poor in the absence of immunosuppression. The long-term prognosis of class V nephritis, more favorable than that of class III–IV lesions, is defined largely by the concurrent finding of associated proliferative lesions, the presence of which portends a worse prognosis.

Follow-up renal biopsies are indicated in certain clinical settings, for example, if a patient is not responding appropriately to therapy or if a patient unexpectedly worsens after having achieved a good response to therapy. Repeat renal biopsies are also the only means of detecting class transformations, which occur in 15–50% of lupus nephritis patients during the course of the disease.

6. Cardiovascular—Cardiovascular disease, a common feature of SLE, may involve the pericardium, valves, myocardium, and coronary arteries. Pericarditis may be asymptomatic. Pericardial effusions in lupus are typically small and usually do not lead to hemodynamic compromise. Occasionally, however, lupus pericarditis leads to life-threatening hemodynamic complications. Valvular heart disease predominantly affects the mitral and aortic valves as

Table 19–3. International Society of Nephrology/Renal Pathology Society classification of lupus nephritis.

Class	Description
I	Minimal mesangial
II	Mesangial proliferative
III	Focal nephritis
IV	Diffuse nephritis
V	Membranous
VI	Advanced sclerosing

valve leaflet thickening, with or without nonbacterial vegetations (Libman-Sacks endocarditis). One echocardiographic study in SLE patients cited a prevalence of valvular abnormalities of 61% compared to 9% of controls. The presence of valvular disease was not associated with other clinical or serologic features of lupus disease activity. Myocarditis and conduction defects are rarer manifestations. SLE is associated with accelerated atherosclerosis, and the diagnosis of SLE itself comprises an important risk factor for cardiovascular disease (see later, Complications). The most common form of peripheral vascular disease in SLE is Raynaud phenomenon (see Chapter 22), which affects approximately 30% of SLE patients. Raynaud phenomenon in SLE is typically less severe than in cases of systemic sclerosis (scleroderma).

7. Pulmonary—Pleuritis is the most common pulmonary manifestation of SLE. Pleural effusions, typically small, develop in up to 50% of patients during the course of the disease. Many patients experience pleuritic chest pain, but some effusions are asymptomatic. When evaluating an SLE patient with a pleural effusion, it is important to exclude other potential etiologies such as infection, malignancy, and heart failure.

Lupus pneumonitis, characterized by an acute respiratory illness with fever, cough, and pulmonary infiltrates, is but associated with a high mortality. Chronic interstitial lung disease, also a rare complication of SLE, develops in an insidious fashion or after one or more episodes of acute lupus pneumonitis. Chest radiographs may be normal early in the disease course, but high-resolution computed tomography (CT) may show characteristic findings of lung fibrosis. Pulmonary function studies reveal a restrictive pattern.

Diffuse alveolar hemorrhage is extremely rare in lupus but associated with a high mortality rate. Dyspnea and cough are among the presenting symptoms, and hemoptysis is not a universal feature at the time the patient is recognized to be ill. Clinicians should suspect diffuse alveolar hemorrhage in the setting of acute pulmonary infiltrates, a falling hematocrit, and a hemorrhagic bronchoalveolar lavage. Lupus nephritis frequently occurs concomitantly with diffuse alveolar hemorrhage as part of a pulmonary-renal syndrome.

Isolated pulmonary arterial hypertension is an uncommon manifestation of SLE but is more likely to be present in patients with features of mixed connective tissue disease MCTD (eg, positive anti-RNP antibodies).

8. Gastrointestinal—SLE may involve any part of the gastrointestinal system. Abdominal pain has been reported in up to 40% of SLE patients and can be due to SLE-related causes, medication side effects, and other non–SLE-related etiologies such as infection. When evaluating an SLE patient with abdominal pain, it is critical to exclude first non-SLE conditions—which are more likely—and to bear in mind that treatment with glucocorticoids or other immunosuppressives can both contribute to abdominal symptomatology and mask the clinical signs of an acute abdomen.

SLE-related causes of abdominal pain include peritonitis, pancreatitis, mesenteric vasculitis, and intestinal pseudo-obstruction. Pancreatitis, an uncommon complication of SLE, is usually associated with active SLE in other organs. When considering the potential diagnosis of pancreatitis, it is important to note that elevated serum amylase concentrations can be misleading because they are often observed in SLE patients in the absence of pancreatitis. Although glucocorticoids and azathioprine have been associated with the development of pancreatitis in patients who do not have SLE, these medications do not seem to play a major role in the development of pancreatitis in patients who do have SLE. Mesenteric vasculitis is a very rare manifestation of SLE, usually occurs in the presence of active SLE elsewhere, and typically involves the small vessels (arterioles and venules) of the small bowel submucosa. Thus, mesenteric angiography is usually nondiagnostic.

Abnormalities of liver tests occur frequently in SLE patients during the course of the illness (see later, Liver Tests). Once medications and infections have been excluded as possible culprits, persistent liver test abnormalities should prompt an investigation with an abdominal ultrasound and possibly a liver biopsy. Lupus hepatitis is an entity distinct from autoimmune hepatitis, although these conditions were often equated in the past; autoimmune hepatitis was once frequently referred to as "lupoid hepatitis." Lupus hepatitis is typically characterized by lobular inflammation with a paucity of lymphoid infiltrates. These findings contrast with those of autoimmune hepatitis in which periportal inflammation and dense plasma cell infiltrates usually dominate. Finally, disorders of the liver such as Budd-Chiari syndrome, hepatic veno-occlusive disease, and hepatic infarction are prone to occur in patients with SLE, particularly those with antiphospholipid antibodies.

9. Neuropsychiatric—Neuropsychiatric manifestations can involve any aspect of the central or peripheral nervous system. Involvement of the nervous system is associated with a poorer prognosis.

The ACR categorized the neuropsychiatric manifestations of SLE into 19 distinct syndromes encompassing both the central and peripheral nervous systems (Table 19–4). Headaches, cerebrovascular disease, seizures, mood changes, and cognitive dysfunction are the most frequent neuropsychiatric manifestations of SLE. The pathogenic mechanisms underlying these manifestations are varied and may involve small vessel vasculopathy in some cases, thromboses of arteries and veins in others, as well as atherosclerotic disease, demyelination, intrathecal production of proinflammatory cytokines, and likely other inflammatory pathways.

Central nervous system (CNS) events occur more frequently than peripheral nervous system events. The histopathologic correlates in CNS lupus are vascular hyalinization, perivascular lymphocytosis, or endothelial proliferation, all representative of a small-vessel vasculopathy; multifocal infarctions; hemorrhage cortical atrophy; and demyelinating

Table 19–4. American College of Rheumatology classification of neuropsychiatric syndromes in SLE.

Central Nervous System	Peripheral Nervous System
Aseptic meningitis	Guillain-Barré syndrome
Cerebrovascular disease	Autonomic disorder
Demyelinating syndrome	Mononeuropathy, single/multiplex
Headache	Myasthenia gravis
Movement disorder	Cranial neuropathy
Myelopathy	Plexopathy
Seizure	Polyneuropathy
Acute confusional state	
Anxiety disorder	
Cognitive dysfunction	
Mood disorder	
Psychosis	

SLE, systemic lupus erythematosus.

lesions resembling those found in multiple sclerosis. True CNS vasculitis is rare. The most common findings on brain MRI include T2 hyperintense focal lesions in the periventricular and subcortical white matter. These are similar to those that occur in multiple sclerosis.

A lumbar puncture should be performed in any patient with suspected CNS involvement, the primary purpose of which is to exclude a CNS infection. Cerebrospinal fluid findings are neither sufficiently sensitive nor specific to confirm a diagnosis of neuropsychiatric SLE. Some SLE patients demonstrate a pleocytosis or elevated protein (or both), but cerebrospinal fluid findings may also be entirely within normal limits.

Cognitive dysfunction, manifested primarily by deficits in thinking, memory, and concentration, is increasingly recognized in SLE patients. Cognitive dysfunction may be associated with antiphospholipid antibodies, but these antibodies are not invariably present in patients with such symptoms. Acute myelopathy or "transverse myelitis," an uncommon but devastating neuropsychiatric manifestation characterized by the onset of bilateral lower extremity paresthesia, numbness, and weakness, can rapidly progress to upper limb and respiratory muscle involvement. A sensory level is usually present. Magnetic resonance imaging (MRI) of the spinal cord is in the confirmation of a myelopathy, which generally demonstrates both T1 and T2 signal abnormalities and widening of the spinal cord as a result of inflammation and edema. Urgent treatment is necessary if permanent neurologic damage is to be avoided. SLE myelopathy should be distinguished from neuromyelitis optica (NMO)—once referred to commonly as "longitudinal myelitis"—which causes both spinal cord inflammation and optic neuritis in the setting of a positive anti-NMO IgG antibody. The myelitis and optic neuritis are not necessarily both obvious at presentation, so a high index of suspicion for the possibility of anti-NMO antibodies must be maintained.

Some of the most dramatic and devastating CNS manifestations of SLE reflect systemic features of the disease rather than processes localized to the brain or spinal cord. As an example, the occurrence of a stroke in a patient with SLE is often linked to the presence of antiphospholipid antibodies and a cerebral thrombosis in the absence of focal inflammatory pathology in the CNS per se.

Peripheral neuropathy in SLE is typically characterized by a symmetric, length-dependent sensory or sensorimotor polyneuropathy. Small nerve fibers are likely the site of pathology in such cases, and therefore both clinical neurological examinations and nerve conduction studies are often unrevealing. Patients typically have fluctuating numbness and tingling of the upper extremities and hands. A large-fiber vasculitic neuropathy can also occur in patients with SLE. This manifestation warrants urgent treatment to prevent ongoing and irreversible nerve damage. Autonomic neuropathies and cranial neuropathies may also develop in patients with SLE.

When evaluating an SLE patient with possible neuropsychiatric manifestations, it is important to distinguish if the neurologic symptoms are due to SLE-mediated damage or to secondary factors (such as metabolic abnormalities; severe hypertension; infection; or adverse effects of medications, such as glucocorticoids). No laboratory or imaging study is sufficiently sensitive or specific to confirm the diagnosis of neuropsychiatric SLE. Instead, the diagnosis is based on a thorough clinical evaluation supported by data from brain imaging, serologic testing, lumbar puncture, and neuropsychiatric assessment.

B. Laboratory Findings

1. Hematology—All three blood cell lines can be affected in SLE. Anemia can be due to anemia of chronic disease (most common cause), AIHA, microangiopathic hemolytic anemia (MAHA), blood loss, renal insufficiency, pure red cell aplasia, and aplastic anemia.

Patients with AIHA demonstrate an increased serum unconjugated bilirubin, increased lactate dehydrogenase, increased reticulocyte count, and reduced serum haptoglobin. The direct Coombs test, usually mediated by warm reacting IgG antierythrocyte antibodies, is typically positive. The peripheral blood smear often shows spherocytosis. There is an association between AIHA and the presence of anticardiolipin antibodies. AIHA may be the presenting manifestation of SLE but also may predate full-blown SLE by many years.

MAHA, characterized by the presence of schistocytes on peripheral blood smear, should prompt the consideration of thrombotic thrombocytopenic purpura—a syndrome that consists of MAHA, thrombocytopenia, fever, neurologic symptoms, and renal involvement and which occurs with increased frequency in SLE. Because MAHA, thrombocytopenia, neurologic symptoms, and renal involvement can also occur in catastrophic antiphospholipid antibody syndrome, antiphospholipid antibodies should always be measured as part of the evaluation.

Leukopenia occurs in approximately 50% of SLE patients and can be secondary to lymphopenia or neutropenia or both. The presence of lymphocytotoxic antibodies in some SLE patients correlates with lymphopenia. Thrombocytopenia is noted in up to 25% of SLE patients and can manifest in a severe fashion similar to immune thrombocytopenia. Chronic, low level thrombocytopenia is also a characteristic feature of the antiphospholipid antibody syndrome. Similar to AIHA, isolated immune thrombocytopenia has been shown to predate the development of complete SLE by several years. When evaluating a patient with the hematologic abnormalities described above, it is always important to consider the potential of bone marrow suppression from such medications as methotrexate, azathioprine, mycophenolate mofetil, and cyclophosphamide. Glucocorticoids are a common cause of lymphopenia.

2. Chemistry—Hyperkalemia can occur as part of renal tubular acidosis in a patient with lupus nephritis. Hyperkalemia may also be encountered in lupus nephritis patients with renal insufficiency, particularly if they are being treated with an angiotensin-converting enzyme inhibitor. Serum creatinine may be elevated in lupus nephritis patients.

3. Liver tests—Liver test abnormalities have been described in up to 60% of SLE patients at some point during the course of the illness, but clinically significant liver disease is rarely a direct manifestation of SLE. For this reason, the presence of liver disease should prompt a search for other causes, including medications such as nonsteroidal anti-inflammatory drugs, methotrexate, and azathioprine, all of which can cause hepatotoxicity. Glucocorticoids can lead to hepatic steatosis. Elevated transaminases also can be seen in the setting of SLE-associated hepatitis and pancreatitis.

4. Muscle enzymes—Creatine kinase can be elevated in the setting of SLE-associated myositis but is more commonly elevated in patients with MCTD.

5. Acute phase reactants—The erythrocyte sedimentation rate (ESR) sometimes correlates with SLE disease activity, but the test is very nonspecific. One of the principal drivers of an elevated ESR is an increase in serum immunoglobulin levels, which most lupus patients have at baseline. Anemia and renal disease, both common in SLE patients, also elevate the ESR. The majority of SLE patients have a mild elevation in the C-reactive protein (CRP) level, but very few have a marked elevation. Notable exceptions are those patients with serositis or concomitant infection in which the CRP level can be quite high (>60 mg/L). In contrast to ESR, CRP levels are not thought to correlate well with SLE disease activity.

C. Special Tests

1. Autoantibodies—The standard method for the detection of ANA is via indirect immunofluorescence using a human tumor cell line substrate (the HEp-2 cell line). When this method is used, ANA are present in virtually all SLE patients (Table 19–5). More recently, enzyme-linked immunosorbent

Table 19–5. Autoantibodies and clinical significance in systemic lupus erythematosus (SLE).

Autoantibody	Prevalence in SLE (%)	Clinical Significance
ANA		
Anti-dsDNA	70	95% specificity for SLE; fluctuates with disease activity; associated with glomerulonephritis
Anti-Sm	20	99% specificity for SLE; associated with anti-U1RNP antibodies
Anti-U1RNP	30	Defining antibody in MCTD; associated with lower frequency of glomerulonephritis
Anti-Ro/SSA	30	Associated with Sjögren syndrome, photosensitivity, SCLE, neonatal lupus, congenital heart block
Anti-La/SSB	20	Associated with Sjögren syndrome, SCLE, neonatal lupus, congenital heart block, anti-Ro/SSA
Anti-histone	70	Associated with drug-induced lupus
Antiphospholipid	30	Associated with arterial and venous thrombosis, pregnancy morbidity

MCTD, mixed connective tissue disease; SCLE, subacute cutaneous lupus erythematosus.

assays (ELISA) containing a mixture of nuclear antigens are being used to detect ANA. These ELISA tests have a lower sensitivity for the detection of ANA than the HEp-2 cell immunofluorescence technique. Thus, if suspicion for SLE remains high following a careful clinical evaluation, a negative ANA by ELISA should be repeated on a HEp-2 cell line.

The ANA is a nonspecific test and may be positive in a variety of other conditions including infection, malignancy, and other autoimmune diseases such as scleroderma and autoimmune thyroid disease. Approximately 30% of healthy people have an ANA titer of 1:40 and 3% have a titer of 1:320. Thus, while a negative ANA typically excludes SLE, a positive ANA does not secure the diagnosis. Once a patient with a positive ANA and characteristic symptoms receives a diagnosis of SLE, there is usually no need to repeat the ANA test.

Anti-dsDNA antibodies are highly specific for SLE and may fluctuate with disease activity. Anti-dsDNA antibodies correlate reasonably well but imperfectly with the presence of lupus nephritis. Anti-Sm and anti-RNP antibodies are antibodies to small ribonucleoprotein particles that are found in some SLE patients. Anti-Sm is highly specific for the diagnosis of SLE. High titers of anti-RNP strongly suggest MCTD. Anti-Ro/SSA and anti-La/SSB antibodies are associated with the development of neonatal lupus and congenital heart block. In SLE patients, it is very rare to detect anti-La/SSB antibodies in the absence of anti-Ro/SSA antibodies. Anti-Ro/SSA antibodies are also associated with SCLE. Both antibodies are also commonly detected in patients with primary Sjögren syndrome.

Antiphospholipid antibodies are antibodies that are directed against phospholipids or to plasma proteins that bind to phospholipids. They are present in up to 50% of SLE patients and are associated with venous and arterial thrombosis and fetal loss. Some reports suggest an association between antiphospholipid antibodies, AIHA, and immune thrombocytopenia. Antiphospholipid antibodies are discussed further in Chapter 21.

2. Complement—Hypocomplementemia may occur during SLE flares as a result of complement activation and consumption, resulting in low C4, C3, and CH50. Because other diseases that cause hypocomplementemia are uncommon, low complement levels can be a useful clinical indicator in SLE. Hereditary deficiencies of the early components of the classic pathway occur with increased frequency in patients with SLE. Thus, complement deficiencies should be considered before attributing hypocomplementemia to active SLE. This distinction is most relevant when evaluating a patient with low C4. C4 is encoded by two genes: C4A and C4B. Partial deficiency of C4 is common. In fact, it is estimated that 1% of whites are homozygous for C4A null alleles and 3% of whites are homozygous for C4B deficiency. Up to 15% of whites with SLE are C4A deficient. Thus, it may be difficult to discern if low C4 in a patient with SLE is due to complement consumption or to an inherited deficiency of C4.

Ongoing complement consumption due to active SLE is more likely to result in reduced levels of multiple complement components (eg, reduction in the levels of C3 as well as C4) and the levels of C4 fluctuate with disease activity. In contrast, an inherited deficiency of C4 results in a fixed low level of C4 that does not vary with disease activity. Although rare, C1q deficiency is the complement deficiency that is most highly associated with SLE. Homozygous deficiency of C2 also confers increased risk for the development of SLE as well as an increased risk of certain types of infections (eg, pneumococcus).

3. Biopsy—A skin biopsy can aid in the diagnosis of cutaneous lupus in the setting of an atypical clinical presentation. Immunofluorescence should always be performed along with conventional histology. Histopathologic findings include vacuolar degeneration of keratinocytes in the basal layer and interface dermatitis. Dermal mucinosis is often observed. Discoid lupus lesions show follicular plugging. Immunofluorescence demonstrates deposition of IgG, IgA, IgM, and complement components along the dermoepidermal junction. IgM is the most frequent, and IgA is the least frequent immunoglobulin class deposited. The skin biopsy in dermatomyositis can appear identical to that of SLE.

D. Imaging Studies

Chest radiography is the appropriate initial study for the detection of pleural effusions or alveolar infiltrates in the evaluation of pleuritic chest pain or dyspnea. However, high-resolution CT has a higher sensitivity for the diagnosis of lupus pneumonitis or diffuse alveolar hemorrhage. Echocardiography is useful for the detection of pericardial effusions, valvular lesions, and as a screening test for pulmonary hypertension. Transesophageal echocardiography provides better resolution in the evaluation of valvular abnormalities. MRI of the brain or spinal cord is often crucial for the evaluation of neuropsychiatric lupus.

▶ Diagnostic Criteria

Establishing the diagnosis of lupus can be quite challenging because of the remarkable heterogeneity in clinical presentation and the lack of a definitive diagnostic test. The ACR has developed classification criteria for SLE (see Table 19–1) that are often cited to support a lupus diagnosis. A person must fulfill 4 of 11 criteria in order to be classified as having SLE, presuming that all other reasonable diagnoses have been excluded. It should be emphasized, however, that these classification criteria were developed in an effort to standardize patients being enrolled into clinical trials, and they should not be relied upon for diagnosis and the basis a treatment decisions. For example, a person with unequivocal biopsy proven lupus nephritis might only meet two of the classification criteria. At the other end of the spectrum, a person with an acute parvovirus B19 infection might fulfill four criteria. Although these criteria cannot always be relied upon for diagnostic purposes, they serve as useful reminders of the myriad of symptoms and signs that can be seen in SLE.

▶ Differential Diagnosis

Because of the involvement of multiple organ systems and the lack of specificity of some of the early symptoms, SLE can be readily mimicked by a variety of systemic diseases. A thorough evaluation for infectious, malignant, and other autoimmune diseases must be undertaken before SLE is diagnosed in a patient.

A number of viral infections can produce a constellation of symptoms and signs similar to SLE. Such viral infections can also trigger the production of autoantibodies. A careful patient history and appropriate serologic testing for the potential offending virus should lead to the correct diagnosis. Parvovirus B19 presents with fever, rash, anemia, and a symmetric inflammatory polyarthritis. A positive ANA assay, anti-dsDNA antibodies, and hypocomplementemia have also been reported in such patients. Cytomegalovirus and EBV can present with constitutional symptoms; cytopenias; and gastrointestinal, hepatic, and lung abnormalities that can mimic an SLE flare. Acute HIV infection typically presents with fever, lymphadenopathy, and mucosal ulcers.

Hepatitis B and C infection can also cause an inflammatory arthritis with positive autoantibodies.

Malignancy, particularly non-Hodgkin lymphoma, can present with constitutional symptoms, arthralgias, cytopenias, rash, and a positive ANA. Clinicians must be especially concerned about the possibility of malignancy in an older patient who has a new lupus-like syndrome. It is critical to ensure that the patient is up-to-date on all of their age appropriate malignancy screening tests.

Other autoimmune diseases, such as rheumatoid arthritis and dermatomyositis, can share similar features with SLE. A symmetric inflammatory arthritis with a predilection for the wrists and small joints of the hands develops in patients with rheumatoid arthritis and SLE. ANA and rheumatoid factor may be elevated in both disorders, although anticyclic citrullinated peptide antibody is usually absent in SLE. The photosensitive, erythematous rashes of dermatomyositis and SLE can appear clinically and histopathologically identical. A careful patient history and supporting serologic tests aid in making the correct diagnosis. MCTD must also be considered when evaluating a patient for possible SLE. MCTD is a syndrome characterized by a high titer anti-RNP antibody in conjunction with clinical features that are often present in SLE, scleroderma, and polymyositis. Patients frequently have puffy, swollen hands and Raynaud phenomenon. In contrast to SLE, an erosive arthritis that resembles rheumatoid arthritis can develop in patients with MCTD. Pulmonary arterial hypertension is a leading cause of morbidity and mortality in MCTD.

Drug-induced lupus usually manifests as polyarthritis, myalgia, fever, and serositis. A wide variety of drugs have been implicated in the development of drug-induced lupus; minocycline, procainamide, hydralazine, isoniazid, INFα, and anti-tumor necrosis factor (TNF) agents are well known culprits. Hydrochlorothiazide is associated with SCLE. All these drugs cause a positive ANA and, with the exception of minocycline, antihistone antibodies. Although characteristic of drug-induced lupus, antihistone antibodies also are present in up to 80% of idiopathic SLE patients and cannot be used to distinguish drug-induced lupus from idiopathic SLE. Minocycline and hydralazine also can trigger production of perinuclear-staining antineutrophil cytoplasmic antibodies (pANCAs), contributing further to diagnostic confusion. Anti-TNF agents often cause anti-dsDNA antibodies and a subset of these patients develop clinical features of SLE that resolve following the discontinuation of TNF inhibition.

▶ Complications

A. Accelerated Atherosclerosis

SLE patients are at increased risk for the development of premature atherosclerotic coronary artery disease, which has an estimated prevalence of 6–10% among all SLE patients. Myocardial infarction in women with SLE is 50-fold more common than in age-matched controls. Traditional cardiovascular risk factors do not explain this increased risk of coronary artery disease. Thus, SLE itself is thought to be an independent risk factor. Evaluation for and treatment of modifiable cardiovascular risk factors such as obesity, smoking, hypertension, and hyperlipidemia are important in mitigating the development of atherosclerotic disease.

B. End-Stage Renal Disease

It is estimated that up to 10% of lupus nephritis patients progress to end-stage renal disease requiring dialysis. Some patients experience a decrease in SLE activity following the onset of end-stage renal disease, while others continue to have active extrarenal manifestations and elevated serologies. SLE patients are typically good candidates for renal transplantation, although it is recommended that patients are given a 3-month dialysis period in order to allow for the possibility of recovery of renal function. The incidence of recurrent lupus nephritis in the allograft is low and does not universally result in allograft loss.

C. Infection

Infections are a major cause of illness and death in patients with SLE. Immunosuppressive medications (especially glucocorticoids and cyclophosphamide) and the immunologic abnormalities associated with SLE itself all contribute to the increased risk of infection. Bacterial, viral, and opportunistic pathogens have all been described.

Progressive multifocal leukoencephalopathy (PML) is a very rare and usually fatal demyelinating disease caused by reactivation of the JC polyomavirus. Although PML has been well recognized in patients with human immunodeficiency virus (HIV) and in patients receiving heavy immunosuppression for treatment of malignancy, it has also been described in patients with rheumatic disease. The majority of reported cases of PML in the setting of rheumatic diseases have occurred in patients with SLE. Although some such patients have a history of treatment with rituximab and many have histories of treatment with multiple other immunosuppressive agents, as well, PML has also been reported in lupus patients whose immunosuppressive therapy was quite mild. Therefore, new, progressive neurologic deficits and white matter lesions on brain imaging should prompt an evaluation for PML in any lupus patient. The diagnosis of PML is confirmed by the detection of JC virus by polymerase chain reaction of the cerebrospinal fluid.

Vaccination with inactivated vaccines such as the Pneumovax and the inactivated influenza vaccine is an important practice to reduce risk of certain infections. Vaccinations against shingles should also be considered in SLE patients because patients are at an increased risk of shingles even before receiving immunosuppression. Prophylaxis against *Pneumocystis jiroveci* should be offered to selected patients, particularly those being treated with cyclophosphamide, high doses of prednisone, or combinations of immunosuppressive therapies.

D. Avascular Necrosis and Osteoporosis

Glucocorticoids are a major risk factor for the development of avascular necrosis and osteoporosis in SLE patients. Avascular necrosis often involves multiple joints in SLE patients with the femoral head being most commonly affected. SLE is an independent risk factor for avascular necrosis, even in the absence of glucocorticoid therapy. Thus, the diagnosis should be considered in any SLE patient with persistent pain in any joint that is not explained by SLE activity. Raynaud phenomenon and hyperlipidemia may be additional risk factors for avascular necrosis in patients with SLE. MRI is the most sensitive imaging modality to detect early avascular necrosis. It is important to use the lowest possible dose of prednisone to control SLE disease activity. Patients should be routinely screened for low bone mineral density, and daily calcium and vitamin D supplementation should be emphasized. The use of bisphosphonates in women of childbearing age remains highly controversial due to the prolonged half-life of those agents.

E. Malignancy

Patients with SLE have an increased risk of malignancy, the most common types being non-Hodgkin lymphoma, Hodgkin lymphoma, lung cancer, and cervical cancer. Interestingly, the increased cancer risk is highest in the early years after SLE diagnosis rather than after many years of disease. SLE patients should undergo age appropriate cancer screening including yearly cervical cancer screening.

▶ Prognosis

The prognosis of SLE patients has improved dramatically over the past 50 years from a 50% survival at 2 years in the 1950s to 90% survival at 10 years in developed countries in the current era. The reasons for this improvement are likely multifactorial and include earlier diagnosis, more effective treatment (glucocorticoids were introduced in the 1950s), and better medical management of such complications as infection and renal disease. However, as SLE patients live longer, complications from long-standing disease and side effects of treatments emerge. The bimodal mortality pattern in SLE was first described over 30 years ago; patient deaths early in the course of the disease are from active disease or infection, while deaths in long-standing disease are due to atherosclerotic coronary disease. Malignancy also is a cause of excess mortality in patients with long-standing disease. The survival curve of patients with mild disease is similar to that of patients with severe disease up until 10–15 years after diagnosis at which time there is a decline in survival in the severe group. Recognition of long-term complications of disease and implementation of appropriate preventive strategies to prevent and screen for atherosclerosis and malignancy are imperative in the ongoing care of SLE patients.

Aringer M, Costenbader K, Daikh D, et al. 2019 European League Against Rheumatism/American College of Rheumatology Classification Criteria for Systemic Lupus Erythematosus. *Arthritis Rheumatol.* 2019;71(9):1400-1412. [PMID: 31385462]

Ayoub I, Cassol C, Almaani S, Rovin B, Parikh SV. The kidney biopsy in systemic lupus erythematosus: a view of the past and a vision of the future. *Adv Chronic Kidney Dis.* 2019;26(5):360-368. Review. [PMID: 31733720]

Hanly JG, Urowitz MB, Gordon C, et al. Neuropsychiatric events in systemic lupus erythematosus: a longitudinal analysis of outcomes in an international inception cohort using a multistate model approach. *Ann Rheum Dis.* 2020;79(3):356-362. [PMID: 31915121]

Pisetsky DS. Evolving story of autoantibodies in systemic lupus erythematosus. *J Autoimmun.* 2019 Dec 3:102356. doi: 10.1016/j.jaut.2019.102356. Review. [Epub ahead of print] [PMID: 31810857]

Ribero S, Sciascia S, Borradori L, Lipsker D. The cutaneous spectrum of lupus erythematosus. *Clin Rev Allergy Immunol.* 2017;53(3):291-305. [PMID: 28752372]

Treatment of Systemic Lupus Erythematosus

20

Arezou Khosroshahi, MD

S. Sam Lim, MD, MPH

Systemic lupus erythematosus (SLE or lupus) is an autoimmune disease associated with autoantibody production and immune complex deposition. The disease is heterogeneous in its clinical presentation, course, and prognosis. Despite many advances in understanding of the human immune system in recent decades, diagnostic and treatment approaches in SLE remain mostly the same. Patients with SLE have significantly increased morbidity and mortality. The risk of death in SLE patients is reported to be two to five times higher than the general population. Although the survival rate of patients with SLE has improved from a 4-year survival rate of 50% in 1950 to a 15-year survival rate of 85% in 2013, the mortality remains high compared to the general population and lupus nephritis (LN) outcomes have not changed in the past 30 years. Successful treatments, as measured by long-term remission, are limited, and at this time only one new medication—belimumab—has been approved for SLE in more than 60 years. Patients with SLE rarely achieve complete disease remissions with the currently available treatments.

Since SLE is a significantly heterogenous condition, the approach to management of patients should be tailored to each individual. In this chapter, we focus on current standard treatment approaches and discuss common associated issues.

GENERAL MEASURES

Taking care of lupus patients is not merely about administering medications to treat their disease activity and manage their lupus-related symptoms but also about improving the quality of their lives through the prudent use of current therapies and preventing the damage that can result from both disease and treatment. Rheumatologists should pay specific attention to their patients' lifestyles and encourage modifications that may be appropriate. Discussions about diet, exercise, smoking cessation, family planning, and sun protection are as important as the disease-specific treatments.

Most lupus patients see their rheumatologists more frequently than their primary care doctors. They have greater risk of cardiovascular disease compared to their age-matched group in general population. It becomes the rheumatologists' responsibility to coordinate efforts to achieve better blood pressure and lipid metabolism in order to improve patients' health and life expectancy.

Another complication of their disease and prolonged glucocorticoid treatment is osteoporosis. Rheumatologists taking care of lupus patients should assess their calcium and vitamin D intake regularly and screen them for osteoporosis. Majority of lupus patients have low serum levels of vitamin D, due at least in part to the avoidance of sun exposure and the use of sunscreens. Vitamin D levels should be monitored and repleted as needed.

Lupus patients are at increased risk of malignancy due to their proinflammatory state and immunosuppressive medication use. Routine screening for malignancy according to the guidelines for general population and preventive measures, such as human papillomavirus (HPV) vaccinations, are recommended.

Infection is still among the leading causes of death in lupus patients. Vaccination following the Centers for Disease Control and Prevention guidelines for immunocompromised patients, specifically vaccination for influenza and pneumonia, is strongly encouraged in SLE.

LUPUS-SPECIFIC TREATMENTS

In many chronic nonrheumatic conditions, including diabetes and hypertension, the therapeutic strategy has evolved to a target-based approach to achieve a better outcome. An international task force recommended a treat-to-target strategy for SLE, suggesting that treatment should target remission in order to prevent damage and improve health-related quality of life in SLE patients.

SLE is a chronic disease requiring long-term or lifelong treatment. In most cases, patients experience a relapsing and remitting course with periods of unpredictable flares and remission. We use multiple treatments to induce and maintain remission, defined by experts as a durable state of no disease activity. In many cases, achieving low disease activity can improve outcome.

The European League Against Rheumatism (EULAR) Task Force on SLE recently updated its recommendations for management of SLE. These recommendations are formed by an approach that combines research-based evidence and expert opinion consensus. Table 20–1 addresses the main statements from the updated EULAR recommendations.

Table 20–1. Recommendations for the management of patients with systemic lupus erythematosus (SLE).

Lupus care is based on shared patient-physician decision making and should consider medical and societal costs and impact.

Treatment goals include long-term patient survival, prevention of organ damage, and improvement of quality of life.

Treatment in SLE should aim at remission or low disease activity and prevention of flares, with the lowest possible dose of glucocorticoids that maximize effect.

Flares of SLE can be treated according to the severity by adjusting ongoing glucocorticoids or immunosuppressive agents or switching/adding new therapies.

Hydroxychloroquine is recommended for all patients with SLE, unless contraindicated, at a dose not exceeding 5 mg/kg/real body weight.

Glucocorticoids can be used at variable doses, depending on the type and severity of organ involvement.

For chronic maintenance treatment, glucocorticoids should be minimized to <7.5 mg/day (prednisone equivalent) and, when possible, stopped after an appropriate tapering schedule, if needed.

Prompt initiation of immunosuppressive agents, such as methotrexate, azathioprine or mycophenolate, can facilitate tapering and discontinuation of glucocorticoids.

Cyclophosphamide can be used for severe organ threatening or life-threatening SLE.

Early recognition of signs of renal involvement, performance of a diagnostic renal biopsy, and prompt treatment are essential for optimal outcomes.

Mycophenolate mofetil or intravenous cyclophosphamide are recommended as induction treatment of lupus nephritis. Mycophenolate mofetil or azathioprine should be used for maintenance therapy.

Comorbidities should be assessed regularly.

Patients with SLE with a high-risk antiphospholipid profile (persistently positive medium/high titers or multiple positivity, especially with a recurrent history of thromboembolic events and/or recurrent miscarriages) may receive primary prophylaxis with antiplatelet agents.

General preventative measures (including immunizations) and early recognition and treatment of infection/sepsis are recommended.

Patients should have regular assessment for risk of cardiovascular disease, including persistently active SLE, increased disease duration, high titers of antiphospholipid antibodies, renal involvement, and chronic use of glucocorticoids. Based on their cardiovascular risk profile, they may be candidates for preventive strategies, including low-dose aspirin and/or lipid-lowering agents along with lifestyle modifications.

Therapeutic approaches in SLE vary widely, often lacking data from controlled trials. However, some general therapeutic recommendations apply to all patients and are in line with the treat-to-target approach:

- Regardless of the organ manifestation or severity of the disease, all lupus patients should be treated with an antimalarial agent, either hydroxychloroquine (HCQ) or chloroquine (CQ).
- Although glucocorticoids remain the mainstay in treatment of moderate to severe manifestations of SLE, providers should limit the cumulative dose and length of glucocorticoid use in these patients.
- Most patients require a glucocorticoid-sparing medication for remission maintenance therapy. Glucocorticoids should be reserved for the treatment of acute flares.
- Patients should be counseled to avoid pregnancy during periods of active SLE. Pregnancy can heighten the severity of SLE flares.
- Use of medications containing sulfonamides should be avoided, because sulfonamides increase the risk of lupus flare in patients with SLE.

We now discuss the treatment of SLE by therapeutic agent. Treatment of cutaneous lupus and the renal and central nervous system (CNS) manifestations of this disease are discussed separately.

Glucocorticoids

Despite the considerable side effects associated with glucocorticoids, they are still the mainstay and first-line therapy for most lupus manifestations. Moreover, most lupus patients require treatment with glucocorticoids for their flares. Rheumatologists decide on dosing based on the perceived severity of flares. Most patients with lupus arthritis and skin lesions respond to low-to-medium doses of glucocorticoids, typically in the range of 5–20 mg/day of prednisone. For more severe manifestations, including myositis, cardiopulmonary involvement (eg, pericarditis, myocarditis, or pleuritis), and hematologic manifestations such as thrombocytopenia, medium-to-high doses on the order of 30–60 mg/day are begun and generally tapered to low doses over a 2- to 3-month period.

Life- or organ-threatening manifestations of SLE such as alveolar hemorrhage, LN, or CNS disease dictates the use of high doses of glucocorticoids. Such treatment is often initiated with "pulse" intravenous (IV) doses of methylprednisolone (125 mg–1 g/day) for 3–5 days, followed by prednisone at 0.5–1 mg/kg/day. The dose of glucocorticoids should be tapered according to clinical response with a goal of reaching less than 5.0–7.5 mg/day within 3 months. In almost all cases, a glucocorticoid-sparing agent (see later) should be added early in the course of treatment to facilitate tapering and the maintenance of response. An apparent inability to taper glucocorticoids should trigger concerns about adherence or the presence of an underlying infection, leading to a reevaluation of the overall situation.

Glucocorticoids are life-saving treatments in lupus and improve functional status of these patients. However, serious adverse effects associated with both the cumulative lifetime doses and the mean daily doses of glucocorticoids demand that practitioners employ these agents cautiously and grudgingly. A multidisciplinary EULAR taskforce showed that the risk of harm is low for the majority of patients with rheumatic diseases at long-term doses of 5 mg/day of prednisone or less. Similarly, other large cohort studies of lupus patients have shown minimal impact on damage accrual with glucocorticoid doses of less than 6 mg/day. Because lupus patients often require multiple courses of glucocorticoids at varying doses for the management of acute flares over their lifetimes, we recommend minimizing or discontinuing glucocorticoids as soon as possible, encouraging rigorous adherence to a steady tapering schedule.

Antimalarial Agents

Antimalarial agents, particularly HCQ and CQ, are first-line systemic therapies for lupus and should be employed liberally. HCQ, the most commonly used antimalarial in Canada and the United States, has a side-effect profile superior to that of CQ. The efficacy of HCQ has been proven in randomized clinical trials for the treatment of both SLE and cutaneous lupus. HCQ not only leads to a reduction in disease activity and lowers the risk of major and minor flares in patients with SLE, but it also has antithrombotic and lipid-lowering effects that are beneficial to this population of patients at high risk of cardiac mortality.

HCQ has an independent protective effect on damage accrual and is associated with a survival benefit in patients with SLE. The drug is usually well tolerated, with rash and gastrointestinal upset being the most commonly reported adverse effects. Both of these complications are unusual. The most feared adverse effect of HCQ is an irreversible retinopathy caused by deposition of drug within the retina. The risk of retinopathy depends on daily dose and duration of treatment. HCQ retinopathy is rare with the drug being dosed appropriately and can be avoided by insisting upon regular retinal screenings. The daily dose of HCQ should not exceed 5 mg/kg of real body weight. At this recommended dose, the risk of HCQ retinopathy is less than 1% at 5 years and less than 2% at 10 years, but it increases to about 20% after 20 years of treatment. Comorbidities such as chronic kidney disease and concomitant use of tamoxifen increase the risk of HCQ toxicity. It is recommended that patients have an ophthalmology examination at the initiation of treatment to exclude any preexisting retinal problems and to include annual screenings by an ophthalmologist starting with the fifth year of HCQ treatment. Automated visual field and spectral domain optical coherence tomography (SD-OCT) are the two recommended tests. Patients of Asian descent can have a pattern of toxicity that extends beyond the macula, requiring a broader examination.

Glucocorticoid-Sparing Agents

▶ Conventional Therapies

Immunosuppressives play important roles in treating lupus patients who have persistently active disease despite antimalarial therapy. The majority of patients with arthritis, myositis, serositis, significant cutaneous disease, hematologic, and CNS manifestations as well as all patients with active renal disease will require a glucocorticoid-sparing agent for maintenance of their remission after the initial glucocorticoid treatment. The decision to select a specific medication is mostly based on the severity of the manifestation, cost and tolerability of medication, and the status of family and contraceptive planning, as many of these agents are contraindicated during pregnancy. Evidence-based data with regard to efficacy of these medications in different manifestations of disease are generally lacking, except in renal disease. Examples of immunosuppressive agents that may be used in lupus patients include azathioprine (AZA), mycophenolate mofetil (MMF), methotrexate (MTX), leflunomide (LEF), cyclosporine, cyclophosphamide (CYC), and tacrolimus.

A. Azathioprine

Azathioprine (AZA) is considered a safe and effective maintenance therapy for lupus and is usually the first immunosuppressive agent added to HCQ for treatment of nonrenal manifestations of the disease due to its relatively favorable side-effect profile and availability. It also has the advantage of safety during pregnancy, as many lupus patients are women of childbearing age.

AZA, a purine antimetabolite, is catalyzed by an enzyme called thiopurine methyltransferase (TPMT). Only 0.3% (1 in 300) of the population is homozygous for mutations of TPMT, a genotype that results in no enzyme activity. The use of AZA in a patient who is homozygous negative for TPMT can lead to catastrophic bone marrow suppression and liver toxicity resulting from the accumulation of abnormally high concentrations of certain AZA metabolites. Either the enzyme levels or the patient's genotype should be measured before AZA is begun.

B. Mycophenolate Mofetil

Mycophenolic acid (MPA) is a relatively selective antimetabolite that inhibits T- and B-lymphocyte activation. MPA has two oral formulations: (1) mycophenolate mofetil (MMF), and (2) enteric-coated mycophenolate sodium (eMPA).

The roles of MMF and eMPA in induction and maintenance therapy for LN is discussed separately. A number of studies, including randomized clinical trials, have shown efficacy of MMF in the treatment of nonrenal lupus manifestations. In a recent randomized, open-label trial in nonrenal SLE, eMPA was superior to AZA in achieving remission and reducing flares. However, its higher cost compared to AZA or MTX and its teratogenicity are the main reasons it is not used as a first-line immunosuppressive in women of childbearing age with nonrenal lupus manifestations. It is usually used in doses of 1–2 g/day for maintenance therapy in nonrenal SLE. Gastrointestinal intolerance is another limiting factor in its universal use.

C. Methotrexate

Methotrexate (MTX) is an efficacious medication in some lupus patients. It is usually selected over AZA and MMF when patients have prominent inflammatory arthritis, similar in approach to rheumatoid arthritis. A systematic review of nine studies, including lupus patients with mostly mucocutaneous or musculoskeletal manifestations, found that MTX treatment led to a significant reduction in disease activity and lowered the average glucocorticoid doses used by lupus patients. MTX should be used cautiously in patients with kidney involvement.

D. Leflunomide

Leflunomide (LEF) has been used in SLE patients with mostly cutaneous and musculoskeletal features refractory to MTX, AZA, or MMF.

E. Cyclophosphamide

Cyclophosphamide (CYC) is an alkylating agent with cytotoxicity to both resting and dividing lymphocytes. IV CYC treatment is a standard approach to remission induction treatment of the most severe manifestations of lupus. Monthly CYC doses of 0.5–1 g/m^2 IV for six cycles followed by AZA or MMF for maintenance therapy are a commonly used regimen. CYC is usually employed to treat lupus cerebritis, vasculitis of the CNS, and other organ- or life-threatening manifestations. Its role in LN is discussed separately.

Treatment with CYC is associated with the potential for considerable toxicity, including increased risk of malignancy and gonadal dysfunction, leading to premature ovarian failure and infertility. These associations are dependent on both the age of the patient and cumulative CYC dose. Many efforts have been made to study the effectiveness of lower doses of CYC for treatment in SLE.

F. Intravenous Immunoglobulin

Intravenous immunoglobulin (IVIG) has been used in the treatment of hematologic manifestations of SLE, including severe thrombocytopenia, hemolytic anemia, and immune-mediated neutropenia. IVIG has established a role in the treatment of other refractory features of SLE, particularly during a systemic infection when immunosuppressive agents are being avoided.

▷ Biologic therapies

A. Belimumab

Belimumab is the only SLE medication approved by the US Food and Drug Administration since 1955, the year that HCQ was approved. Belimumab is a fully human, monoclonal antibody directed against B-lymphocyte stimulator (BLyS), also known as B cell–activating factor (BAFF), which is the costimulator for B-cell survival and function. Belimumab has been successful in clinical trials of extrarenal SLE for patients with inadequate disease activity control on standard of care treatment. Most of these studies have included patients with mucocutaneous and musculoskeletal manifestations of the disease. Although limited by cost and relative lack of real-world outcomes data, belimumab should be considered in combination with HCQ in patients with nonrenal SLE who have ongoing disease activity or frequent flares.

Belimumab is relatively safe compared to many of the other immunosuppressives used in lupus. Further studies of the effectiveness of belimumab in certain SLE manifestations such as pleuropericarditis, hematologic features, CNS involvement, and renal disease are required, as are investigations of the timing of belimumab use relative to other immunosuppressive medications.

B. Rituximab

Rituximab (RTX) has shown promising efficacy in SLE in different cohorts despite disappointingly negative results in clinical trial. Many clinicians taking of SLE patients use RTX for the treatment of refractory disease manifestations, including arthritis, serositis, myositis, and nephritis. RTX has become the next line treatment after glucocorticoids for the majority of hematologic manifestations of SLE, such as thrombocytopenia, hemolytic anemia, and antiphospholipid syndrome. Most rheumatologists use the rheumatic disease dose of 1000 mg for two doses in the treatment of SLE, but the lymphoma dosing (375 mg/m^2 for four doses) can also be used. RTX has also been used in combination with IV CYC in patients with severe, organ- or life-threatening SLE.

The results observed in daily clinical practice in patients with refractory SLE treated with RTX often stand in contrast to the disappointing results of the Exploratory Phase II/III SLE Evaluation of Rituximab (EXPLORER) and Lupus Nephritis Assessment with Rituximab (LUNAR) trials. Explanations offered for these negative clinical trial results include unreliable outcome measures, poor patient selection, and excessive concomitant treatment. The promising results of many open-label studies of RTX and the data from national registries led both the American College of Rheumatology (ACR) and the EULAR to recommend RTX as a treatment for difficult-to-treat lupus.

CUTANEOUS MANIFESTATIONS

The approach to the treatment of cutaneous lupus varies by subtype. Photoprotection, however, is a central tenet to the management of all forms of cutaneous lupus. Subacute cutaneous lupus erythematosus (SCLE), discoid lupus erythematosus (DLE), and malar rash are among the most photosensitive skin lesions. Patients with SLE should be advised to avoid prolonged exposure to sunlight and other sources of ultraviolet (UV) light, including halogen and fluorescent lights. They should also use sunscreens that block both UV-A and UV-B radiation, with a recommended sun protection factor of 50 or greater. Physical protection with hats and clothing is recommended during the outdoor activities, particularly during peak daylight.

Smoking also impacts the severity of the skin lesions in lupus in a negative manner. Patients should be educated about this information and encouraged to quit.

▶ Topical Therapies

Topical glucocorticoids are usually the first line of treatment for cutaneous lupus lesions. Selection of a particular class or agent is mostly based on clinical experience and historical case series. Most practitioners start the treatment by using a nonfluorinated, low-potency topical glucocorticoid and escalate to higher-potency fluorinated glucocorticoids based on response to treatment. The use of high-potency preparations should be limited to 2 weeks, and use on facial lesions should be avoided. Long-term use of topical glucocorticoids is associated with skin atrophy, telangiectasia, dyspigmentation, striae, and acne. It is recommended to apply hydrocortisone cream for cutaneous lesions on the face and to save ointment preparations of medium potency, such as triamcinolone acetonide or betamethasone valerate, for the limbs and trunk. Higher-potency agents such as clobetasol ointment can be used for severe manifestations.

Topical calcineurin inhibitors (pimecrolimus and tacrolimus) are considered second-line treatment for cutaneous lupus lesions and can minimize chronic topical steroid use.

Intralesional glucocorticoid injections are reserved for discoid lesions that have not responded to either topical steroids or calcineurin inhibitors. Skin atrophy and depigmentation are more common with intralesional injections.

▶ Systemic Therapies

When patients fail topical therapies or have widespread lesions, systemic treatment is recommended. Antimalarials, HCQ and CQ, are first-line systemic therapies for cutaneous lupus. Quinacrine, another antimalarial agent that has no or little retinal toxicity, can be added safely to HCQ or CQ for synergy. Quinacrine is available only through compounding pharmacies and can therefore be expensive. Long-term use can lead to yellow discoloration of the skin. Patients who fail to respond to systemic antimalarial treatment may benefit from systemic immunosuppressive medications that were discussed for other lupus manifestations such as MTX, AZA, and MMF.

Dapsone, a synthetic sulfone, has a specific role in the treatment of bullous lupus lesions and also has efficacy for other cutaneous manifestations in refractory cases. Dapsone cannot be used for patients with sulfa allergies and also needs to be employed cautiously in patients with glucose-6-phosphate

dehydrogenase deficiency. Thalidomide can be successful in selected patients with SCLE, but its use is limited due to its well-known teratogenicity and possible neuropathy.

Systemic retinoids, lenalidomide, cyclosporine, CYC, and IVIG have been reported for use in refractory cases of cutaneous lupus. Belimumab has shown efficacy in cutaneous manifestations of SLE. Finally, short-term, low-dose systemic glucocorticoid treatment can be initiated while waiting for the effect of antimalarial or other medications. Systemic glucocorticoids are not recommended for SCLE and DLE, however, because of both poor efficacy and the long-term treatment typically required by those subtypes of cutaneous lupus.

LUPUS NEPHRITIS

Lupus nephritis (LN) is a relatively common manifestation of SLE with a range of severity. The approach to management is similar to extrarenal manifestations in that expert clinical assessment is required, and potential confounding factors such as hypertension must be considered. Evaluations of potentially active LN can exploit serum and urinary biomarkers such as complement levels, anti-dsDNA antibody levels, and urinary protein:creatinine ratios. However, the gold standard for establishing the diagnosis and determining the optimal therapeutic approach is renal histology. The current pathologic classification is known as the International Society of Nephrology/Renal Pathology Society (ISN/RPS) classification.

LN classes I and II involve immune complexes in the glomerular mesangium and do not require significant immunosuppressive therapy. Class VI LN has significant glomerular sclerosis and lacks inflammation. Therefore, this section focuses on pharmaceutical therapies for those with proliferative LN (classes III or IV) and membranous LN (class V). In the case of mixed histologic types, any significant proliferative component leads to consideration of the patient as having a class III/IV LN for the purposes of therapy. Involvement of the interstitium as well as the glomeruli has an additional impact on renal outcomes, but there is currently no standard approach to incorporating the extent of interstitial disease into treatment decisions.

Regardless of the type of LN and immunosuppressive strategy chosen, clinicians should not underestimate the importance of general renal protective measures. Data on blood pressure goals for patients with chronic kidney disease should be considered and applied to patients with LN. Aggressive management with agents that block the renin-angiotensin system is considered first-line therapy, particularly for patients with significant proteinuria. The nondihydropyridine calcium channel blockers such as verapamil and diltiazem also have a beneficial effect in those with proteinuria. Hypercholesterolemia will often require the use of statins. Metabolic acidosis should be corrected. Sodium should be restricted from the diet to no more than 2–2.5 g/day. Nonsteroidal anti-inflammatory drugs and other nephrotoxic medications must be avoided. In order to maximize adherence and avoid malnutrition, reduction of dietary protein should focus on consumption of healthy proteins while maintaining adequate caloric intake. Associated comorbidities, which may include smoking and morbid obesity, should be addressed. Hyperuricemia will often result from renal impairment and the use of diuretics, but correction is not indicated unless recurrent gout attacks are demonstrated. With significant proteinuria, there should be consideration of antiplatelet or even anticoagulation to prevent thrombosis.

Classes III & IV Lupus Nephritis

The treatment of proliferative disease (classes III and IV) is divided into two consecutive phases: induction and maintenance. The induction phase, designed to control inflammation rapidly and limit damage accrual, is generally considered to be 3–6 months long. The dose, duration, and modality (oral vs IV) of glucocorticoids have not been defined, specifically by randomized controlled trials. Most clinicians prescribe 0.5–1 mg/kg/day for the first 4 weeks and then taper over the next 4–6 months to a goal of less than or equal to 7.5 mg/day (or, preferably, off completely). One of the following regimens must be used in conjunction with glucocorticoids:

- The modified National Institutes of Health (NIH) regimen utilizes monthly IV CYC at 0.5–0.75 g/m² for six doses.

- The Aspreva Lupus Management Study (ALMS) regimen uses MMF at 0.5 g twice daily for the first week, then 1 g twice daily to a target of 1.5 g twice daily, as tolerated, by week 3.

- The Euro-Lupus regimen uses IV CYC at 500 mg every 2 weeks for six doses.

The Euro-Lupus regimen was originally shown to be as effective after 5 and 10 years of follow-up in a predominantly European Caucasian cohort as the modified NIH regimen. Although subsequent studies have shown similarly positive outcomes of the Euro-Lupus regimen in other racial/ethnic groups, caution must be taken as long-term data are still lacking. In general, studies show that IV CYC and MMF are generally equally efficacious in induction. When weighing the differences in potential benefits and side effects, consideration should also be given to the modality. MMF has gained popularity given the convenience of oral therapy and lack of certain potential side effects of CYC (malignancy, infertility). IV CYC can be beneficial when poor medication adherence and/or limited oral intake/absorption are concerns.

There are limited data about the utility of other drugs. AZA and LEF have shown some efficacy. Other than glucocorticoids, AZA is the only drug that can be used during pregnancy for LN. Calcineurin inhibitors have been evaluated for induction in LN but mostly in smaller Asian studies and may be more effective when used in combination with MMF.

The maintenance phase aims to maintain the improvement or remission achieved with induction therapy and to decrease the chance of another future renal flare, which is not uncommon and can occur years after the initial LN event. Relative stability of symptoms, insufficient education about the importance of vigilance for recurrence, and decreased frequencies of visits following the induction of remission lead to a high-risk period for LN patients, when decreased adherence and loss to follow-up can contribute to poor outcomes. It is crucial to educate patients about the long-term nature of LN treatment from the beginning therapy and to emphasize the importance of adherence, even after the induction phase is over.

Quarterly dosing of IV CYC has been one primary remission maintenance regimen. This approach is superior to the use of glucocorticoids alone but is associated with significant toxicities characteristic of long-term CYC use (eg, malignancy, infertility, and infection). Subsequent studies established the use of MMF and AZA for remission maintenance, with MMF superior to AZA. AZA remains a good alternative in those who cannot tolerate MMF, who become pregnant or are at high risk for becoming pregnant.

There is no established guideline for the discontinuation of maintenance therapy.

Patients who achieve only partial remission should continue immunosuppression, either prolonging their current induction regimen or switching to another regimen/agent. If possible, strong consideration should be given to repeating a kidney biopsy, which defines the degree of improvement and, more importantly, the degree of activity and chronicity that may define the choice and intensity of future immunosuppression.

Class V Lupus Nephritis

Class V LN can be present with a proliferative component, in which case it should be treated as previously discussed for proliferative LN. Pure class V lesions have not been as comprehensively studied as proliferative LN. If proteinuria is below nephrotic range with normal renal function, treatment should be conservative and focus on reducing proteinuria with diet restriction of salt, tight blood pressure control, and use of agents that block the renin-angiotensin system. Those with nephrotic range proteinuria and worsening renal function, immunosuppressive therapy should be started. Similar to proliferative disease, the use of CYC or cyclosporine with glucocorticoids was superior to glucocorticoids alone, but CYC treatment is associated with a more durable response. A post hoc analysis of the ALMS trial of those with pure class V LN suggested that MMF and IV CYC were no different with regard to efficacy. AZA has been shown to have results comparable to those of MMF. In current practice, MMF and IV CYC are most commonly used in severe class V LN. Calcineurin inhibitors and AZA are alternatives.

Class VI Lupus Nephritis

In most cases, class VI LN will result in eventual kidney failure or end-stage renal disease (ESRD). As ESRDs become inevitable, kidney transplantation should be explored as it improves survival, costs, and quality of life compared to dialysis. Recurrence of LN in a transplanted kidney occurs in less than 4% of cases. Rejection remains the leading cause of transplant failure. Some advocate early education and awareness of renal transplantation to the point that it may lead to more preemptive (before instituting dialysis) transplants, which leads to higher survival but is less common in ESRD secondary to LN versus other causes. There is no evidence to support delaying renal transplantation after the initiation of dialysis to ensure lowering of disease activity in order to optimize outcomes and, in fact, may worsen the risk of eventual transplant failure and death. Although some suggest a reduction in systemic lupus activity near or during ESRD, the risk of lupus flares is clearly not zero and should warrant ongoing surveillance.

NEUROPSYCHIATRIC SLE

The first step in the management of neuropsychiatric (NP) manifestations of lupus is to determine whether the feature is attributed to SLE activity or it is a complication of treatment, infection, or coincidental existence of a non–SLE-related process.

Although many NP symptoms in lupus patients occasionally reflect manifestations of SLE due to organic nervous system involvement, most are functional disorders unrelated to SLE and should be managed as we would have approached them in other patients.

Cognitive dysfunction, headache, and mood disorders are among the most common NP manifestations in SLE patients, but these are usually not directly related to lupus activity and do not respond to immunosuppression. The approaches to these manifestations are similar to any other patient with these symptoms, including the exclusion of other common etiologies.

Treatment of NP manifestations of lupus is based on the underlying etiology. If NP symptoms are due to medications, such as glucocorticoids, appropriate dose reductions are essential. Cerebrovascular disease is common among lupus patients, particularly in the setting of antiphospholipid antibodies, proteinuria, and comorbidities such as hypertension. Antiplatelet or anticoagulation therapy is indicated to prevent further events. Seizures in SLE are usually treated with the same anticonvulsant medications used in individuals without SLE. In a limited number of patients with ongoing inflammatory processes, seizures can represent CNS inflammation from SLE and requires immunosuppressive therapy.

Treatments with glucocorticoids and immunosuppressive agents are indicated when NP symptoms are thought to reflect an inflammatory process, such as optic neuritis, transverse myelitis, refractory seizures, psychosis, acute confusional state with laboratory and imaging findings supportive of CNS inflammation in the presence of generalized lupus activity. No placebo-controlled trials have looked at the different approaches to the treatment of CNS involvement in SLE, but the common approach is usually initiation of high dose IV glucocorticoids followed by IV CYC, similar to the induction regimen for LN. AZA or MMF are typically used for maintenance therapy in these patients. In severe NP SLE refractory to standard immunosuppressive therapy, plasma exchange, IVIG, and RTX have been used.

Alarcon GS, McGwin G, Bertoli AM, et al. Effect of hydroxychloroquine on the survival of patients with systemic lupus erythematosus: data from LUMINA, a multiethnic US cohort (LUMINA L). *Ann Rheum Dis.* 2007;66(9):1168-1172. [PMID: 17389655]

Appel GB, Contreras G, Dooley MA, et al. Mycophenolate mofetil versus cyclophosphamide for induction treatment of lupus nephritis. *J Am Soc Nephrol.* 2009;20(5):1103-1112. [PMID: 19369404]

Fanouriakis A, Kostopoulou M, Alunno A, et al. 2019 update of the EULAR recommendations for the management of systemic lupus erythematosus. *Ann Rheum Dis.* 2019;78(6):736-745. [PMID: 30926722]

Houssiau FA, Vasconcelos C, D'Cruz D, et al. The 10-year follow-up data of the Euro-Lupus Nephritis Trial comparing low-dose and high-dose intravenous cyclophosphamide. *Ann Rheum Dis.* 2010;69(1):61-64. [PMID: 19155235]

van Vollenhoven RF, Mosca M, Bertsias G, et al. Treat-to-target in systemic lupus erythematosus: recommendations from an international task force. *Ann Rheum Dis.* 2014;73(6):958-967. [PMID: 24739325]

Weening JJ, D'Agati VD, Schwartz MM, et al. The classification of glomerulonephritis in systemic lupus erythematosus revisited. *Kidney Int.* 2004;65(2):521-530. [PMID: 14717922]

Yokogawa N, Eto H, Tanikawa A, et al. Effects of hydroxychloroquine in patients with cutaneous lupus erythematosus: a multicenter, double-blind, randomized, parallel-group trial. *Arthritis Rheumatol.* 2017;69(4):791-799. [PMID: 27992698]

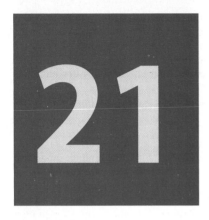

Antiphospholipid Syndrome

Elena Gkrouzman, MD

Doruk Erkan, MD, MPH

ESSENTIALS OF DIAGNOSIS

▶ Persistent antiphospholipid antibodies (lupus anticoagulant test, anticardiolipin [aCL] antibodies, and anti–β_2-glycoprotein-I antibodies [aβ2GPI]) measureable in the peripheral blood.

▶ Arterial and venous thrombosis affecting the micro- and/or macro-vasculature.

▶ Pregnancy morbidity, including pregnancy losses beyond the first trimester.

▶ Nonthrombotic manifestations such as thrombocytopenia or cardiac valve disease.

▶ Wide spectrum of manifestations including multiple organ thromboses (catastrophic antiphospholipid syndrome).

▶ Traditional thrombosis and cardiovascular disease risk factors also contribute to clinical events.

▶ General Considerations

Antiphospholipid syndrome (APS) is defined as thrombosis (venous, arterial, or microvascular) or pregnancy morbidity occurring in individuals with antibodies against phospholipid-binding plasma proteins (antiphospholipid antibodies [aPL]). The most common aPL are anticardiolipin antibodies (aCL), anti–β_2 glycoprotein-I antibodies (aβ_2GPI), and lupus anticoagulants (LA). APS may be seen in patients with other autoimmune diseases, such as systemic lupus erythematosus (SLE), or in otherwise healthy persons (primary APS).

Livedo racemosa, cardiac valve disease, thrombocytopenia, hemolytic anemia, aPL-associated nephropathy, cognitive dysfunction, and subcortical white-matter changes are recognized as clinically relevant manifestations in aPL-positive patients. Because these manifestations are not currently part of the APS classification criteria, however, they are now generally termed as "noncriteria" manifestations.

The clinical manifestations of aPL-positive patients comprise a spectrum of features (Figure 21–1). aPL-related vascular events range from superficial venous thrombosis to multiple simultaneous organ thromboses (catastrophic APS). In addition, patients may present solely with obstetric morbidity or nonthrombotic manifestations, for example, thrombocytopenia. The presence of aPL positivity in the absence of clinical manifestations characteristic of APS does not equate to an APS diagnosis.

Suspicion for APS should be raised when individuals of young age develop thromboses that are recurrent or at unusual sites, especially when unprovoked. Unexplained pregnancy morbidity, such as late pregnancy losses, severe preeclampsia, or the HELLP syndrome (Hemolysis, Elevated Liver enzyme levels and Low Platelet count) may also be indicative of APS. Livedo racemosa (Figure 21–2), particularly in young patients with history of vascular or pregnancy events, should alert physicians to the possibility of aPL positivity. Patients with prolonged activated partial thromboplastin time (aPTT) and false-positive screening tests for syphilis (rapid plasma reagin [RPR]; Venereal Disease Research Laboratory [VDRL]) should be screened for aPL in the appropriate clinical setting.

The prevalence of aPL in the general population is not well known due to lack of large-scale, population-based studies. In healthy blood donors, positive aCL have been noted in 10% of the samples. At 1 year of follow-up, however, less than 1% of these donors remained positive, and LA assays were negative in all tested donors at baseline. This is consistent with the consensus that false-positive aCL tests are common, but patients with positive LA assays typically have a higher risk of developing APS.

Based on a systematic review, the aPL frequency is estimated as 6% for the general population patients with pregnancy morbidity, 10% for deep venous thrombosis (DVT), 11% for myocardial infarction, and 14% for stroke, although limitations of the literature, for example, lack of confirmation of aPL-positivity, were significant. Approximately 30–40%

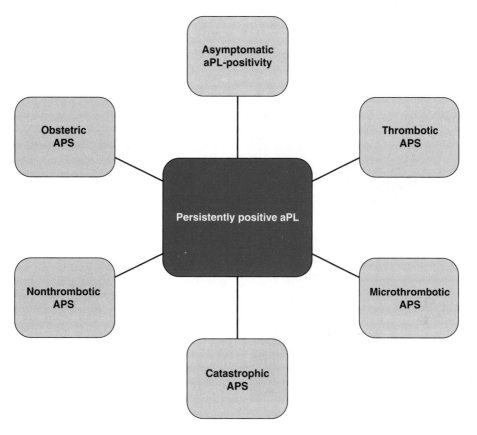

▲ **Figure 21–1.** Spectrum of clinical manifestations in persistently antiphospholipid antibody (aPL)–positive individuals.

of patients with SLE have persistent moderate-to-high-titer aPL.

Andreoli L, Chighizola CB, Banzato A, Pons-Estel GJ, Ramire de Jesus G, Erkan D. Estimated frequency of antiphospholipid antibodies in patients with pregnancy morbidity, stroke, myocardial infarction, and deep vein thrombosis: a critical review of the literature. *Arthritis Care Res (Hoboken)*. 2013;65:1869. [PMID: 23861221]

Miyakis S, Lockshin MD, Atsumi T, et al. International consensus statement on an update of the classification criteria for definite antiphospholipid syndrome (APS). *J Thromb Haemost*. 2006;4:295. [PMID: 16420554]

Vila P, Hernandez MC, Lopez-Fernandez MF, Batlle J. Prevalence, follow-up and clinical significance of the anticardiolipin antibodies in normal subjects. *Thromb Haemost*. 1994;72:209. [PMID: 7831653]

▶ Clinical Findings

A. Signs and Symptoms

1. Thrombotic manifestations—Deep venous thrombosis, often accompanied by pulmonary embolism (PE), is the most common manifestation of APS. Unusual venous distributions may be affected, for example, the arterial or venous circulation of the eye, renal or splenic vein thrombosis, Budd-Chiari syndrome, or portal, sagittal sinus or mesenteric thrombosis. Stroke and transient ischemic attack, which comprise nearly one-quarter of initial APS presentations, are the most common arterial events. However, arterial thrombosis may develop at unusual locations, for example, peripheral and mesenteric thrombosis leading to extremity gangrene and bowel ischemia, respectively. Myocardial infarctions can also occur in aPL-positive patients. Moreover, intracardiac thrombosis may mimic myxoma.

2. Microthrombotic manifestations—Some of the organs that can be affected include the skin, kidney, heart, liver, and lung. Livedo reticularis, generally manifested by symmetrical mottling of the skin, has poor specificity for any disease and is found most commonly, in fact, in healthy individuals, induced by the cold. In contrast, livedo racemosa (broken asymmetrical mottling of the skin) is more specific for APS (see Figure 21–2). Cutaneous necrosis or ulcerations may develop due to underlying livedoid vasculopathy, often leading to the clinical finding of atrophie blanche.

The renal vasculature—arteries, arterioles, and glomerular capillaries—can also be affected in APS, leading to a condition

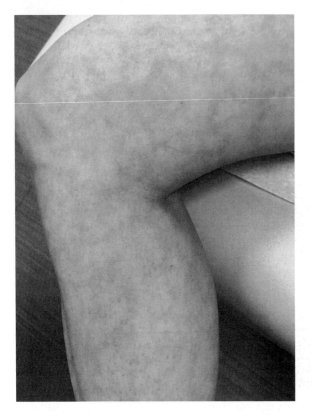

▲ **Figure 21–2.** Livedo racemosa in a patient with persistent antiphospholipid antibodies.

termed aPL-nephropathy. Kidney biopsies in aPL-nephropathy patients can demonstrate acute lesions, for example, thrombotic microangiopathy, or chronic lesions, including focal cortical atrophy, arterial fibrous intimal hyperplasia, and fibrous or fibrocellular occlusions of arteries and arterioles. Cardiac microthrombosis can result in coronary artery disease–related symptoms despite normal coronary angiogram. Patients with microvascular lung involvement commonly present with diffuse alveolar hemorrhage. In such patients, lung biopsy sometimes reveals a leukocytoclastic vasculitis, indistinguishable from pulmonary-renal syndromes such as antineutrophil cytoplasmic antibody (ANCA)–associated vasculitis. The presence of vasculitis, however, is often difficult to demonstrate because the size of the affected blood vessels is small.

Catastrophic APS is a rare, life-threatening complication of aPL that occurs in multiple organs over a period of days. Multiple thromboses of small-, medium-, and even large-sized vessels may develop despite adequate anticoagulation, usually associated with thrombotic microangiopathy.

3. Nonthrombotic manifestations of APS—Thrombocytopenia (usually >100 × 10⁹/L) is common. Despite their low platelet counts, however, APS patients remain at risk for

thrombosis and the foundation of therapy still involves anticoagulation. Both Coombs-positive hemolytic anemia (without schistocytes) and microangiopathic hemolytic anemia (with schistocytes) may occur in APS. Valvular heart disease (vegetations and/or valve thickening) is the most common aPL-related cardiac involvement. Both aortic and mitral insufficiencies are common and lead to valve replacement in severe cases. Neurologic involvement in the form of cognitive dysfunction that is independent of overt cerebrovascular disease, chorea, transverse myelitis, multiple sclerosis-like syndrome, and seizures are reported in aPL-positive patients, but these features are rare and controversial.

4. Obstetric manifestations—Unexplained death of a morphologically normal fetus at or beyond the 10th week of gestation is considered the most specific criterion for obstetric APS. Other manifestations of APS, based on the Updated Sapporo APS Classification Criteria, include premature birth of a morphologically normal neonate before the 34th week of gestation due to severe preeclampsia or eclampsia, and three or more unexplained consecutive spontaneous abortions before the 10th week of gestation, assuming the exclusion of other causes such as chromosomal, maternal anatomic, or hormonal abnormalities.

Asherson RA, Cervera R, de Groot PG, et al. Catastrophic antiphospholipid syndrome: international consensus statement on classification criteria and treatment guidelines. *Lupus.* 2003;12:530. [PMID: 12892393]

Garcia D, Erkan D. Diagnosis and management of the antiphospholipid syndrome. *N Engl J Med.* 2018;378: 2010. [PMID: 29791828]

Miyakis S, Lockshin MD, Atsumi T, et al. International consensus statement on an update of the classification criteria for definite antiphospholipid syndrome. *J Thromb Haemost.* 2006;4:295. [PMID: 16420554]

B. Laboratory Findings

The laboratory diagnosis of APS relies on detection of aPL through a coagulation assay (LA test) and immunoassays (aCL and aβ₂GPI).

The **lupus anticoagulant test** is a three-step functional coagulation assay that measures the ability of aPL to inhibit the conversion of prothrombin to thrombin. Final confirmation of a positive LA test requires the following steps: (a) prolongation of a screening test such as dilute Russell viper venom time (dRVVT) or aPTT (screening phase); (b) failure to correct the prolonged coagulation time by mixing studies where patient plasma is mixed 1:1 with normal pooled plasma (mixing phase; ruling out a clotting factor deficiency); (c) correction of prolonged coagulation by addition of excess phospholipids (proving that the inhibitor is phospholipid dependent) (confirmation phase); and (d) exclusion of other coagulopathies.

Anticardiolipin antibodies are detected by aCL enzyme-linked immunosorbent assay (ELISA). The presence of β₂-glycoprotein I (β₂GPI) is a requirement for binding of autoimmune aCL to cardiolipin-coated plates in the standard ELISA. **aβ_2GPI** directly target β_2GPI and can also be detected by ELISA. aPL assays other than the LA test, aCL, and aβ_2GPI ELISA are currently not well standardized and routinely used in clinical practice.

Pengo V, Tripodi A, Reber G, et al. Update of the guidelines for lupus anticoagulant detection. Subcommittee on Lupus Anticoagulant/Antiphospholipid Antibody of the Scientific and Standardisation Committee of the International Society on Thrombosis and Haemostasis. *J Thromb Haemost.* 2009;7:1737. [PMID: 19624461]

▶ Diagnostic Considerations

There are no diagnostic criteria for APS. The Updated Sapporo APS Classification Criteria, which were published in 2006, require at least one clinical (thrombotic or obstetric) and one laboratory criterion for a patient to be classified as having APS. The purpose of the classification criteria is to facilitate the inclusion of homogeneous patient groups for research; thus, these criteria should not be used as the only diagnostic tool. However, they may serve as a guide during the diagnostic assessment of aPL-positive patients, for which a step-by-step approach is summarized in Table 21–1. Both LA positivity and triple aPL-positivity for LA, aCL, and aβ_2GPI, especially with moderate-to-high aPL ELISA titers, correlate well with the likelihood of clinical events that would confirm an APS diagnosis.

Concomitant thrombosis risk factors may promote aPL-associated events in an additive manner and should be explored in aPL-positive patients, as this may also influence treatment strategies. In aPL-positive patients with pregnancy morbidities, the contribution of concomitant gynecologic, genetic, and hormonal conditions should be considered. Other

thrombotic microangiopathic syndromes such as disseminated intravascular coagulation, heparin-induced thrombocytopenia, thrombotic thrombocytopenic purpura, hemolytic uremic syndrome, or HELLP syndrome may share similar features with catastrophic APS, and sometimes overlap.

Chayoua W, Kelchtermans H, Moore GW, et al. Identification of high thrombotic risk triple-positive antiphospholipid syndrome patients is dependent on anti-cardiolipin and anti-beta2glycoprotein I antibody detection assays. *J Thromb Haemost.* 2018;16:2016. [PMID: 30079628]

Galli M, Luciani D, Bertolini G, Barbui T. Lupus anticoagulants are stronger risk factors for thrombosis than anticardiolipin antibodies in the antiphospholipid syndrome: a systematic review of the literature. *Blood.* 2003;101:1827. [PMID: 12393574]

Kelchtermans H, Pelkmans L, de Laat B, Devreese KM. IgG/IgM antiphospholipid antibodies present in the classification criteria for the antiphospholipid syndrome: a critical review of their association with thrombosis. *J Thromb Haemost.* 2016;14:1530. [PMID: 27279342]

Lockshin MD, Kim M, Laskin CA, et al. Prediction of adverse pregnancy outcome by the presence of lupus anticoagulant, but not anticardiolipin antibody, in patients with antiphospholipid antibodies. *Arthritis Rheum.* 2012;64:2311. [PMID: 22275304]

Miyakis S, Lockshin MD, Atsumi T, et al. International consensus statement on an update of the classification criteria for definite antiphospholipid syndrome (APS). *J Thromb Haemost.* 2006;4:295. [PMID: 16420554]

Ortel TL, Erkan D, Kitchens CS. How I treat catastrophic thrombotic syndromes. *Blood.* 2015;126:1285. [PMID: 26179082]

Pengo V, Ruffatti A, Legnani C, et al. Clinical course of high-risk patients diagnosed with antiphospholipid syndrome. *J Thromb Haemost.* 2010;8:237. [PMID: 19874470]

Pengo V, Ruffatti A, Legnani C, et al. Incidence of a first thromboembolic event in asymptomatic carriers of high-risk antiphospholipid antibody profile: a multicenter prospective study. *Blood.* 2011;118:4714. [PMID: 21765019]

Table 21–1. Diagnostic assessment of antiphospholipid antibody (aPL)–positive patients.

	Assessment of aPL Tests		
	Anticardiolipin (aCL) and Anti-β_2-Glycoprotein-I (aβ_2GPI) Antibodies		
Lupus Anticoagulant (LA) Test	**IgG**	**IgM**	**IgA**
When truly positive, associated with highest risk for clinical events, compared to aCL and aβ_2GPI	Moderate-to-high titers (≥40 GPL or MPL units) have higher association with clinical events compared to lower titers		Isolated positivity, irrespective of titer, is of unknown clinical significance
Caution in anticoagulated patients due to false-positive results	IgG positivity has a stronger association with clinical events compared to IgM		
The above tests must be positive on two separate occasions at least 12 weeks apart; they can be transiently positive during infections.			
Assessment of aPL Profile			
High-risk aPL profile	Positive LA test with or without moderate-to-high titer aCL or aβ_2GPI IgG or IgM (≥40 GPL or MPL units)		
Moderate-risk aPL profile	Negative LA with moderate-to-high titer aCL or aβ_2GPI IgG or IgM (≥40 GPL or MPL units)		
Low-risk aPL profile	Negative LA test with low titer aCL or aβ_2GPI IgG or IgM (20–39 GPL or MPL units)		

Adapted with permission from Garcia D, Erkan D. Diagnosis and management of the antiphospholipid syndrome. *N Engl J Med.* 2018;378:2010.

> ## Prevention & Treatment

Primary Thrombosis Prevention

Modification of reversible thrombotic risk factors (such as smoking or oral contraceptives) and cardiovascular disease risk factors (such as hypertension or hyperlipidemia), prophylaxis during high thrombosis risk periods (such as surgical interventions or prolonged immobilization), and optimal management of other systemic autoimmune diseases (such as lupus) are critical, especially in patients with moderate-to-high risk aPL profiles. Low-dose aspirin was not shown to be beneficial for primary thrombosis prophylaxis neither in a randomized, double-blind, placebo-controlled clinical trial nor in prospective cohort studies. Nevertheless, low-dose aspirin is prescribed by some physicians because of data from retrospective studies implying that it may be protective against first thrombosis. Our approach is low-dose aspirin only if patients have additional cardiovascular disease risk factors. Hydroxychloroquine (HCQ) has antithrombotic effects in mouse models and in SLE patients, but no prospective, controlled studies in aPL-positive patients without systemic autoimmune diseases have been performed.

Secondary Thrombosis Prevention

Warfarin remains the cornerstone for long-term treatment of patients with thromboses with a target international normalized ratio (INR) of 2–3. Despite retrospective cohort studies demonstrating that high-intensity (INR 3–4) anticoagulation is more effective than moderate intensity (INR 2–3), two prospective randomized trials of moderate- versus high-intensity warfarin in APS patients did not show any difference between the treatment groups in the prevention of recurrent thrombosis. However, patients with history of arterial events comprised only one-fifth of the patients in those prospective investigations. Thus, although physicians are generally comfortable with the use of moderate-intensity anticoagulation after the first venous thromboembolism, some centers still prefer high-intensity anticoagulation for arterial thromboses. Our approach is warfarin with a target INR of 2.5–3, adding low-dose aspirin if patients have additional cardiovascular disease risk factors. This approach is similar to the recommendations from a working group of the 15th International Congress on aPL (September 2016).

In patients who experience recurrent arterial or venous thrombosis despite therapeutic range INR, options can include higher intensity warfarin (INR 3–4) or switching to low-molecular-weight heparin. The addition of low-dose aspirin, HCQ, or a statin—or some combination of these therapies—can also be considered.

Lifelong anticoagulation is generally recommended for APS patients with vascular events. The need for lifelong anticoagulation is less clear, however, when patients develop a provoked vascular event and are found to have aPL in the course of evaluation.

Direct oral anticoagulants (DOACs) are currently not recommended for secondary prevention of thrombosis. The effectiveness of rivaroxaban for secondary thrombosis prevention in APS patients and history of venous thromboembolism was evaluated in an open-label, phase 2/3, noninferiority randomized controlled trial (RCT). This study demonstrated that rivaroxaban was inferior to warfarin with respect to the percentage change in endogenous thrombin potential (a quantitative measurement of thrombin generation) on day 42, which was the primary outcome measure of the study. However, no patients in either group developed thrombosis during the 6-month safety period. A subsequent open-label, multicenter, noninferiority RCT (warfarin vs rivaroxaban), investigating triple aPL-positive patients with history of arterial or venous thrombosis, was terminated early due to increased risk of thrombosis and bleeding in the rivaroxaban group. Future studies will help us understand the role of DOACs in APS. Another RCT comparing apixaban to warfarin for secondary prevention of thrombosis in APS patients with history of venous thromboses is ongoing.

Microthrombotic Manifestations

Microthrombotic manifestations of APS pose a treatment challenge because they do not always respond to anticoagulation and may develop while a patient is receiving anticoagulation at therapeutic levels. Evidence-based approaches are limited. Both glucocorticoids and immunosuppressive agents are used based on anecdotal experience.

For aPL-related skin ulcers, antiplatelet agents (low-dose aspirin in combination with dipyridamole or pentoxifylline) and/or anticoagulation have been used with variable results. Rituximab was effective in a small phase II pilot study of non-criteria manifestations of APS, including skin ulcers. Referral to a vascular surgery team should be considered to exclude peripheral arterial disease and venous hypertension, which can interfere with wound healing. Supportive measures such as compression stockings for venous insufficiency are recommended to promote healing.

Plasma exchange is generally used in the acute thrombotic microangiopathy phase of aPL nephropathy. Intravenous immunoglobulin (IVIG), rituximab, or eculizumab also have been used in resistant cases. Chronic aPL-nephropathy patients are usually treated with mycophenolate mofetil and/or rituximab, sometimes with the addition of glucocorticoids. Mechanistic target of rapamycin (mTOR) inhibitor sirolimus improved renal graft survival and decreased renal lesions in aPL-positive patients who had received a renal transplant, but additional studies of this therapeutic approach are needed.

Patients with diffuse alveolar hemorrhage are generally treated with glucocorticoids during the acute phase. Many patients also require a steroid sparing agent to achieve remission; cyclophosphamide, rituximab, mycophenolate mofetil, azathioprine, plasmapheresis, and IVIG have all been used with varying degrees of success.

Catastrophic APS

Early intervention and communication among all specialists are of critical importance in managing patients with catastrophic APS. The highest survival rate is achieved with the combination of anticoagulation (unfractionated intravenous heparin), glucocorticoids, and plasma exchange and/or IVIG. Plasma exchange with fresh frozen plasma should be considered if features of microangiopathic hemolytic anemia—that is, schistocytes—are present. Antiplatelet agents such as aspirin can be used as an additional therapy after weighing risks and benefits of potential bleeding complications when combined with therapeutic dose heparin. Rituximab or eculizumab (in patients with hematological manifestations and/or thrombotic microangiopathy) may be considered in refractory cases, but evidence is based only on case reports or series.

Nonthrombotic Manifestations

Thrombocytopenia usually does not require any treatment in and of itself because the degree of thrombocytopenia is rarely severe ($<50 \times 10^9$ L). Glucocorticoids and/or IVIG are first line treatments for platelet counts less than 50×10^9 L. Besides IVIG, immunomodulatory medications such as HCQ, azathioprine, mycophenolate mofetil, or rituximab may be considered in glucocorticoid-resistant cases. Hemolytic anemia may be treated with corticosteroids, azathioprine, or mycophenolate mofetil. Rituximab has also been used in aPL-positive patients with thrombocytopenia and/or hemolytic anemia. Cardiac valve thickening increases the risk for arterial/embolic events. Corticosteroids and anticoagulation do not lead to regression of such lesions, but antithrombotic treatment is usually administered to decrease risk of embolic events.

Obstetric Manifestations

In women with obstetrical complications of APS who have not experienced thrombosis, low-dose aspirin and prophylactic doses of enoxaparin during pregnancy and 8- to 12-week postpartum are recommended. In women with a history of thrombotic events and APS, low-dose aspirin and therapeutic-dose enoxaparin should be used during pregnancy even in the absence of any history of pregnancy complications. For patients with positive aPL but no obstetric or thrombotic history, a prophylactic dose of enoxaparin is recommended during the 8- to 12-week postpartum period, but not during pregnancy. Low-dose aspirin has been generally used in this setting without supportive prospective data.

Perioperative Management

Patients with APS have a higher risk for thrombosis when they undergo surgery and perioperative complications may occur despite prophylaxis. Perioperative assessment and planning prior to any surgical procedure are of importance to avoid postoperative complications. Periods without anticoagulation should be minimized, and pharmacological and physical antithrombotic interventions should be applied. Any deviation from a normal postoperative course should be assessed in light of underlying APS.

Arnaud L, Mathian A, Ruffatti A, et al. Efficacy of aspirin for the primary prevention of thrombosis in patients with antiphospholipid antibodies: an international and collaborative meta-analysis. *Autoimmun Rev.* 2014;13:281. [PMID: 24189281]

Cohen H, Hunt BJ, Efthymiou M, et al. Rivaroxaban versus warfarin to treat patients with thrombotic antiphospholipid syndrome, with or without systemic lupus erythematosus (RAPS): a randomised, controlled, open-label, phase 2/3, non-inferiority trial. *Lancet Haematol.* 2016;3:e426. [PMID: 27570089]

Crowther MA, Ginsberg JS, Julian J, et al. A comparison of two intensities of warfarin for the prevention of recurrent thrombosis in patients with the antiphospholipid antibody syndrome. *N Engl J Med.* 2003;349:1133. [PMID: 13679527]

Erkan D, Harrison MJ, Levy R, et al. Aspirin for primary thrombosis prevention in the antiphospholipid syndrome: a randomized, double-blind, placebo-controlled trial in asymptomatic antiphospholipid antibody-positive individuals. *Arthritis Rheum.* 2007;56:2382. [PMID: 17599766]

Erkan D, Vega J, Ramon G, Kozora E, Lockshin MD. A pilot open-label phase II trial of rituximab for non-criteria manifestations of antiphospholipid syndrome. *Arthritis Rheum.* 2013;65:464. [PMID 23124321]

Finazzi G, Marchioli R, Brancaccio V, et al. A randomized clinical trial of high-intensity warfarin vs. conventional antithrombotic therapy for the prevention of recurrent thrombosis in patients with the antiphospholipid syndrome (WAPS). *J Thromb Haemost.* 2005;3:848. [PMID: 15869575]

Pengo V, Denas G, Zoppellaro G, et al. Rivaroxaban vs warfarin in high-risk patients with antiphospholipid syndrome. *Blood.* 2018;132:1365. [PMID: 30002145]

Woller SC, Stevens SM, Kaplan DA, et al. Apixaban for the Secondary Prevention of Thrombosis Among Patients With Antiphospholipid Syndrome: Study Rationale and Design (ASTRO-APS). *Clin Appl Thromb Hemost.* 2016;22:239. [PMID 26566669]

▶ Prognosis

Prognosis varies in different aPL-positive individuals according to presentation. The mortality rate from a large European cohort of 1000 APS patients with a 10-year follow up was estimated to be 5%, with most deaths resulting from thromboses, infections, and hemorrhage. In catastrophic APS, the mortality ranges between 33 and 48% and is worse in patients with underlying SLE. Catastrophic APS seldom recurs. Patients who survive the initial episode generally have a stable course with continued anticoagulation.

Cervera R, Serrano R, Pons-Estel GJ, et al. Morbidity and mortality in the antiphospholipid syndrome during a 10-year period: a multicentre prospective study of 1000 patients. *Ann Rheum Dis.* 2015;74:1011. [PMID: 24464962]

Rodriguez-Pinto I, Moitinho M, Santacreu I, et al. Catastrophic antiphospholipid syndrome (CAPS): descriptive analysis of 500 patients from the International CAPS Registry. *Autoimmun Rev.* 2016;15:1120. [PMID: 27639837]

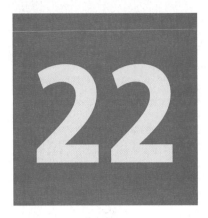

Raynaud Phenomenon

Nadia D. Morgan*, MD, MHS

Fredrick M. Wigley, MD

ESSENTIALS OF DIAGNOSIS

▶ Raynaud phenomenon (RP) is an exaggeration of the normal vasospastic reaction to cold environments or emotional stress.

▶ Characterized by well-demarcated color changes (pallor, cyanosis, hyperemia) involving the peripheral digits (fingers and toes).

▶ Classified clinically into primary or secondary forms.

▶ Primary RP is idiopathic and functional in nature, the integrity of the blood vessel architecture is preserved.

▶ Secondary RP is associated with an underlying structural vasculopathy and may be complicated by digital ischemia, recurrent digital ulcerations, rapid deep tissue necrosis, and amputation.

▶ The principal approach in the management of RP entails preventative measures through the avoidance of cold environments and use of protective clothing to maintain adequately warm core and peripheral body temperatures.

▶ Therapeutic agents are indicated if quality of life is affected adversely or if there are complications of tissue ischemia, including digital ulcers.

▶ General Considerations

Raynaud phenomenon (RP) is classified into two categories: primary and secondary. **Primary RP** accounts for the majority (80–90%) of cases. It occurs in the absence of an identifiable disease and is due to vasospastic events precipitated by exposure to cold environments or emotional stress. Primary RP occurs more commonly in otherwise healthy females, with an onset of symptoms around 15–30 years of age. A positive family history of RP in first-degree relatives is reported

in 30–50% of patients. The RP attacks are typically bilateral and symmetrical, affecting the hands. The thumb is generally spared. It is not complicated by progression to tissue necrosis or gangrene. Nailfold capillaroscopy (see later) and physical examination findings are normal. If a patient meets criteria for primary RP and no new symptoms develop over 2 years of follow-up, the development of secondary disease is unlikely to occur. The presence of abnormal nailfold capillaries on capillaroscopy or specific autoantibodies are strong predictors of secondary RP associated with an underlying autoimmune disease (Overbury et al, 2015).

Secondary RP is seen in a variety of disorders that disturb normal vascular reactivity. It is often observed in patients with autoimmune diseases, particularly systemic sclerosis (SSc), systemic lupus erythematosus (SLE), Sjögren syndrome, and dermatomyositis. In 10–20% of cases, it presents as the initial manifestation of an underlying autoimmune disease but often it goes unrecognized for years and is not appreciated fully until other disease manifestations occur (Goundry et al, 2012). RP is associated with pathology that alters regional blood flow by various mechanisms, including damaging blood vessels, interfering with neural circulatory control, and changes in the physical properties of blood or the levels of circulating mediators that regulate digital and cutaneous circulation (Herrick, 2012). Patients with secondary RP generally have more severe, painful RP that may be associated with digital ulceration and gangrene. In fact, the occurrence of such tissue injury places a patient's case of RP clearly in the secondary RP category.

▶ Pathogenesis

Involvement of the skin of the fingers, toes, and tips of the nose and ears occurs preferentially in RP. These sites have a unique circulatory system with specialized structural and functional thermoregulatory mechanisms. Local blood flow is regulated by a complex interaction of neural signals, cellular mediators, and circulating vasoactive molecules (Flavahan, 2015; Herrick, 2012). Temperature responses are mediated principally via the sympathetic nervous system, which is capable of

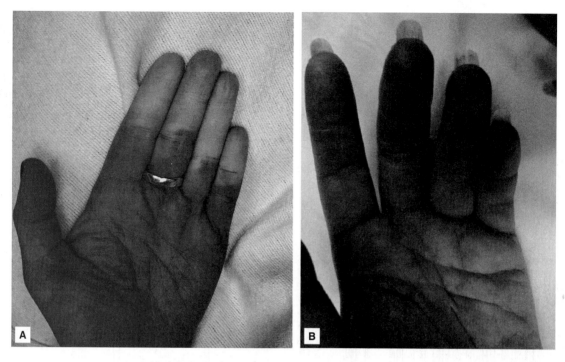

▲ **Figure 22–1. A:** Typical Raynaud phenomenon attack characterized by sharp demarcations of skin pallor. **B:** Cyanosis of the digits.

altering cutaneous blood flow rapidly through arteriovenous shunts. In hot weather, these shunts vasodilate allowing heat to dissipate. In contrast, in cold environments, the shunts constrict, shifting blood centrally, and helping to maintain a stable core body temperature.

RP is transient digital ischemia occurring in the setting of cold temperatures or emotional stress. The vasoconstriction of digital arteries, precapillary arterioles, and cutaneous arteriovenous shunts leads to a sharp demarcation of skin pallor or cyanosis of the digits (Figure 22–1). The ischemic phase is followed by recovery of blood flow that appears as cutaneous erythema, caused by rapid digital reperfusion (Flavahan, 2015).

▶ Clinical Findings

The clinical assessment—the history and physical examination—remains of paramount importance in the evaluation of a patient with suspected RP. All patients with a history of RP should be asked about symptoms suggestive of an autoimmune disease, such as arthritis, rash and tightening or thickening of the skin, dry eyes or dry mouth, myalgia, fevers, or shortness of breath. Careful physical examination should include evaluation of the pulses, auscultation over large arteries (eg, the subclavians), and nailfold capillaroscopy, as well as inspection for the presence of digital ulcers and gangrene. If an underlying autoimmune disease is suspected following a

careful history and examination, then there is a role for autoantibody testing (see section Laboratory Findings).

A. Symptoms and Signs

RP most often affects the fingers, although toes and occasionally areas of the face (tips of the nose and ears) may also be affected (Figure 22–2). A typical RP attack is characterized by

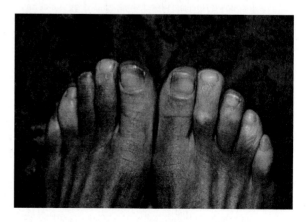

▲ **Figure 22–2.** Raynaud phenomenon attack involving the toes, with evidence of skin pallor.

the sudden onset of cold digits associated with a demarcation of skin pallor (a "white attack") or cyanosis (a "blue attack"). After rewarming, there is vascular reperfusion, resulting in the erythema (a "red attack") secondary to rebound of blood flow. RP attacks typically start in a single digit and then spread to other digits of the same or both hands. The index, middle, and ring fingers are involved most commonly. White attacks may lead to critical digital ischemia due to the intense constriction of arterial inflow. In contrast, blue attacks are mainly the result of sluggish blood flow and venous congestion. Low blood flow to the digits may persist for 15 minutes after rewarming. Physicians should pay careful attention to painful RP attacks: They are a symptom of ischemia and are therefore more likely to be associated with a secondary disease process.

A diagnosis of RP may be made if a patient has a history of both cold sensitivity and associated color changes of the skin (pallor, cyanosis, or both) limited to the digits. The diagnosis of RP can be made by asking the following questions: (1) "Are your fingers unusually sensitive to cold?" ("Compare your fingers to your friends' fingers"); (2) "Do your fingers change color when they are exposed to cold?"; and (3) "Do they turn either white or blue (or both)?" The diagnosis of RP is confirmed if there is a positive response to all three questions but is excluded if responses to the latter two are negative (Maverakis et al, 2014). Color changes, in short, are the *sine qua non* of RP.

B. Laboratory Findings

Patients with clear clinical evidence for primary RP do not need further laboratory testing. This includes patients with symmetric attacks, no evidence of peripheral vascular disease, no digital gangrene or digital pitting (small skin defects secondary to previous injury), and a normal nailfold capillary examination. Appropriate clinical follow-up is important to ensure that no secondary process emerges, but it is important to reassure patients that their prognosis is excellent and that they can make a major impact on their symptoms through behavior modification (warm clothing). If a secondary cause of RP is suspected, specific blood work guided by the clinical findings should include antinuclear antibody (ANA) testing (see later), serum chemistries, a complete blood cell count, thyroid function tests, serum and urine protein electrophoresis, and testing for cryoglobulins and cryofibrinogens. In addition, elevated inflammatory markers, such as the erythrocyte sedimentation rate or C-reactive protein, are associated with some but not all causes of secondary RP.

ANA testing and assays for specific autoantibodies are essential in the evaluation of patients suspected of having secondary RP. A positive ANA assay was one of the strongest predictors of progression to SSc in a study of 586 patients monitored for approximately 3200 person-years. The pattern of ANA can provide clues to the underlying autoimmune disease. An anticentromere pattern detected on ANA testing is associated strongly with limited scleroderma (ie, the CREST [calcinosis, Raynaud phenomenon, esophageal dysmotility, sclerodactyly, telangiectasia] syndrome). Antitopoisomerase antibodies are usually found in patients with diffuse SSc and interstitial lung disease. Anti-dsDNA, anti-Ro/SS-A, anti-La/SS-B, anti-Smith, and anti-RNP antibodies are more commonly encountered in patients with SLE, Sjögren syndrome, or mixed connective tissue disease. Anti-Jo-1 and other antisynthetase antibodies are typically associated with inflammatory myopathies, some of which have RP and other signs of organ dysfunction out of proportion to the degree of muscle weakness, which may or may not be present.

C. Special Tests

Examination of nailfold capillaries is important for the differentiation of primary and secondary RP (Pavlov-Dolijanovic et al, 2013). Nailfold capillaries may be visualized using high magnification videocapillaroscopy, widefield microscopy, a dermatoscope, or the more easily accessible ophthalmoscope. To perform nailfold capillaroscopy, a drop of grade B immersion oil is placed on the patient's skin at the base of the fingernail. This area is then viewed using a dermatoscope or an ophthalmoscope set to 40 diopters or a stereoscopic microscope. Normal capillaries appear as symmetric, nondilated loops. In contrast, distorted, dilated, or absent capillaries suggest a secondary disease process (Figure 22–3).

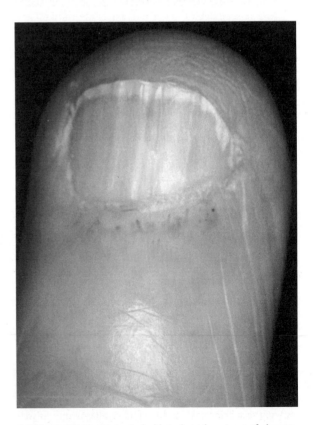

▲ **Figure 22–3.** Distorted, dilated, and regions of absent nailfold capillaries. (See color insert.)

Abnormalities of the nailfold capillaries are strong independent predictors of rheumatic conditions, particularly SSc, SLE, and dermatomyositis.

Evaluation with arterial Doppler studies and large vessel imaging is warranted if an atypical presentation of RP is noted, such as unilateral digital involvement and decreased peripheral pulses.

Differential Diagnosis

RP is a clinical diagnosis, based on a patient's report of sudden, episodic color changes of the digits provoked by cold temperature or emotional stress. However, true RP should be distinguished from the sensitivity to cold or the nondemarcated mottling seen in a normal response to cool temperatures. True RP must also be distinguished from acrocyanosis, a syndrome characterized by persistent discoloration, absence of blanching, and extension beyond the digits to involve the hands and feet. Although acrocyanosis is aggravated by cold temperatures, episodic attacks with sharp demarcations of digital color changes are notably absent.

Mechanical stress on the nerves or vessels in the hand or fingers may also cause sensitivity to cold temperatures. For instance, industrial injuries such as the hand-arm vibration syndrome (HAVS), which can be triggered by the continuous use of vibrating hand-held machinery, may lead to white fingers that resemble RP. Patients with complaints of color changes and concomitant numbness should be evaluated for carpal tunnel syndrome or neuropathy.

Paraproteinemias and hyperviscosity syndromes are also in the differential diagnosis. RP in these patients results from sluggish blood flow through cutaneous and digital vessels. Patients with cryoglobulinemia may also have RP due to the presence of cold-sensitive proteins. In 30% of patients with cryoglobulinemia, RP is the presenting symptom. A high index of suspicion should be maintained for this differential especially in patients with concomitant cutaneous lesions due to leukocytoclastic vasculitis.

The use of certain drugs (eg, sympathomimetic agents) that induce vasoconstriction can aggravate or cause RP. In addition, patients with hypothyroidism often have cold hands, acrocyanosis, or RP.

Distinguishing primary from secondary RP is critical. The connective tissue diseases are the most common secondary disorders that the internist will encounter. Thus, a thorough review of systems focusing on symptoms of connective tissue diseases is essential. Patients should be asked about dry eyes or mouth (Sjögren syndrome); painful joints or morning stiffness (arthritis); rashes, photosensitivity, or cardiopulmonary abnormalities (SLE); and skin tightening, respiratory distress, or gastrointestinal disease (SSc); and muscle weakness (inflammatory myopathy).

Most patients with RP report symmetric involvement of the digits. A vascular occlusion, such as atherosclerosis, emboli, or arterial occlusions, should be considered in patients with asymmetric RP. In particular, RP in the feet associated with lesions of digital ischemia warrants a workup for macrovascular disease. In such cases, vascular imaging such as a magnetic resonance arteriogram is appropriate.

Prevention

Primary and first-line interventions in the management of RP include preventative strategies focusing on cold avoidance and stress management. Emotional stressors and cold environments activate thermoregulatory vessels in the skin which are under sympathetic adrenergic control, resulting in vasoconstriction and reduced blood flow to the peripheries. Emphasis should therefore be placed on keeping the whole body warm by wearing multiple layers of loose-fitting clothing, hats, mittens or warm gloves, and wool socks. Commercially available hand warmers may also be utilized. Even in the summer months, RP attacks may be precipitated by damp, windy weather, or rapid shifts in the ambient temperature. Air-conditioned environments at home, in the work place, and the supermarket often trigger RP attacks. Patients should therefore be encouraged to utilize protective clothing as needed throughout the year.

Emotional stressors may provoke RP attacks by lowering the threshold for temperature-induced attacks. Thus, stress control and relaxation techniques also have an important role in the prevention of RP attacks.

Vasoconstricting agents, such as nonselective beta blockers and other sympathomimetic drugs (decongestants, diet pills, ephedra, amphetamines) and serotonin agonists (sumatriptan), should be avoided because they can cause vasoconstriction of peripheral arteries precipitating RP attacks. In addition, chemotherapeutic agents, including bleomycin, cisplatin, carboplatin, and vinblastine, may cause vascular occlusion and RP attacks. Opioids can also cause cutaneous vessel vasoconstriction and should be used with caution. Smoking cessation is of paramount importance, as nicotine reduces cutaneous and digital blood flow.

Treatment

A. Medications

The preventative strategies outlined above are often sufficient to minimize the frequency and severity of RP attacks. Most patients with primary RP do not require therapeutic intervention. Initiation of therapeutic agents (Table 22–1) is indicated if RP attacks impact quality of life negatively or are complicated by digital ischemia.

1. Calcium channel blockers—Dihydropyridine calcium channel blockers are the first-line agents of choice for both primary and secondary RP in patients exhibiting a suboptimal response to supportive measures (Kowal-Bielecka et al, 2017). In a Cochrane review of randomized controlled trials

Table 22–1. Approach to the management of Raynaud phenomenon.

Preventative strategies and supportive care
• Cold avoidance
• Protective clothing to ensure warmth
• Stress management
• Avoid vasoconstrictive agents
• Smoking cessation
Therapeutic agents
First line therapy
Dihydropyridine calcium channel blocker
Second line therapy
Phosphodiesterase type 5 inhibitors
Topical Nitrates
Prostacyclin
Alternative therapies
Fluoxetine (selective serotonin reuptake inhibitor)
Losartan (angiotensin II receptor antagonist)
Atorvastatin
Botulinum toxin A

evaluating the efficacy of oral calcium channel blockers in the treatment of primary RP, these agents were shown to decrease the frequency of attacks (Ennis et al, 2016). Calcium channel blockers differ in their peripheral vasodilatory properties. Dihydropyridine calcium channel blockers, such as nifedipine, amlodipine, felodipine, and isradipine, have more potent vasodilatory effects compared to nondihydropyridines such as diltiazem and verapamil, which are less selective for vascular smooth muscle. Therapy should be commenced at the lowest dose and titrated to achieve therapeutic efficacy with no or minimal side effects. If one calcium channel blocker is ineffective, patients may be switched to another. Individual responses may vary. Slow-release preparations of calcium channel blockers are preferred due to the safer side-effect profile. Side effects of calcium-channel blocker therapy include headache, hypotension, tachycardia, lower extremity edema, and rarely aggravation of gastroesophageal reflux.

2. Phosphodiesterase inhibitors—These agents are used alone or in combination with calcium channel blockers in instances of suboptimal response to calcium-channel blocker monotherapy (eg, the development of digital ulcers). Phosphodiesterase inhibitors regulate levels of intracellular cyclic nucleotides such as cyclic adenosine monophosphate (cAMP) and cyclic guanosine monophosphate (cGMP), to mediate intracellular responses to prostacyclin and nitrous oxide, inducing vascular smooth muscle relaxation and vasodilation. Selective phosphodiesterase type 5 (PDE5) inhibitors include sildenafil, tadalafil, and vardenafil. These agents have been shown to reduce the frequency, severity, and duration of RP attacks (Roustit et al, 2013). Sildenafil is initially initiated at low doses (20 mg daily) and increased as tolerated to the maximum dose (20 mg three times daily). Phosphodiesterase inhibitors are generally more expensive than calcium

channel blockers and should not be used in combination with topical nitrates because of the risk of hypotension.

3. Topical vasodilators—Topical nitrates are another alternative that may be used in patients with a poor response to calcium-channel blocker monotherapy. Formulations include ointments, gels, creams, tapes, and sustained-release transdermal patches. The use of these agents is generally reserved for management of RP attacks characterized by disproportional involvement of 1 or only a few digits, in order to provide rapid targeted relief and minimize ischemia. Topical nitroglycerin ointment is frequently used alone or in combination with other vasodilator therapy. Improvement in RP may be noted with the daily application of 0.25–0.5 inches of 2% nitroglycerin ointment. The medication is absorbed systemically and patients often experience side effects of headaches or hypotension. Systemic side effects may be minimized by placing very small quantities of the nitroglycerine ointment directly on the fingers of affected hands. Desensitization or tachyphylaxis may occur with prolonged use of topical nitroglycerin resulting in reduced efficacy.

4. Prostaglandins—Prostaglandins are not first-line agents, but prostaglandins may be utilized when symptoms persist and other options have been exhausted. Prostacyclin is a potent vasodilator with inhibitory effects on platelet aggregation and antiproliferative properties on smooth muscle cells. Iloprost, a prostacyclin analogue, is beneficial in the treatment of RP secondary to SSc. Therapy with iloprost (0.5–2 ng/kg/min intravenous infusion for 5 days) can provide relief for several weeks with significant improvement in the number and duration of vasospastic RP attacks. However, in the United States, iloprost is only available as an inhaled medication for the treatment of pulmonary hypertension. Epoprostenol and treprostinil may be beneficial for severe refractory RP and digital ulcerations secondary to scleroderma. Intravenous administration is required and is generally reserved for resistant cases. While oral preparations of prostacyclin analogs have shown potential in the management of pulmonary hypertension, evidence from clinical trials has been mixed. More studies are needed to support the efficacy of prostaglandins in the treatment of RP.

5. Alternative therapies—The following agents have been utilized as adjunctive therapy in special circumstances where comorbid conditions exist, but are often modest in efficacy:

1. **Selective serotonin reuptake inhibitors:** Serotonin is a potent circulating vasoconstrictor. Its role in RP is not clearly defined, but several reports have noted improvement in RP in patients treated with selective serotonin reuptake inhibitors. In a 6-week crossover study with nifedipine, fluoxetine reduced the frequency and severity of RP attacks. The use of selective serotonin reuptake inhibitors can be considered particularly if the patient's baseline blood pressure is low.

2. **Angiotensin II receptor blocker:** Losartan, an angiotensin II receptor blocker, decreased the number and severity of RP attacks in both primary and secondary RP.

3. **Atorvastatin:** This lipid-lowering agent was shown to reduce the number of digital ulcers in SSc patients with secondary RP, when administered in conjunction with vasodilator therapy.

4. **Botulinum toxin type A:** Evidence supporting the use of botulinum toxin injections is primarily derived from uncontrolled case series (Iorio et al, 2012). A recent controlled trial evaluating its use in SSc patients with severe RP revealed administration of botulinum toxin to be no better than placebo (Bello et al, 2017).

5. **Anticoagulation:** Antiplatelet therapy with aspirin (81 mg/day) is recommended in selected patients with severe secondary RP who are at risk for digital ulceration or larger-artery thrombotic events. Heparin may be used during an acute ischemic crisis to prevent further digital vessel thrombosis, but long-term anticoagulation with heparin or warfarin is not recommended unless there is evidence of a hypercoagulable disorder such as antiphospholipid syndrome or thrombosis associated with malignancy.

B. Surgical Interventions

More invasive approaches are required in the management of RP when cases are refractory to medical management and complications of acute ischemic pain or painful digital ulcers ensue. The primary goals of surgical intervention are pain relief, restoration of blood flow to the peripheries, and protection against progressive permanent dysfunction. Surgical sympathectomy may be used to disrupt the sympathetic nerves that cause vasoconstriction. A chemical sympathectomy with a digital or wrist block using lidocaine or bupivacaine without epinephrine can rapidly reverse digital artery vasospasm. The localized peripheral approach (digital, ulnar, and radial sympathectomy) is preferred to more regional approaches (cervical sympathectomy) because of the potential adverse effects of cervical sympathectomy, which include reduction of the inherent risks of cervical sympathectomy. These include neuralgia, decreased localized sweating, and Horner syndrome.

The return of increased sympathetic tone may occur within weeks of cervical or digital sympathectomy, making some of the benefits of this procedure therefore short-lived. However, the RP attacks are usually less severe following digital sympathectomy. Digital sympathectomy can be especially helpful in an acute digital ischemic crisis and it is best reserved for patients who have not responded to medical therapy and continue to have severe RP or ischemia threatening the digits.

▶ Complications

The impact of RP on patients can vary from a mild inconvenience to recurrent ischemia and digital ulceration. Primary RP is not associated with critical ischemia or digital ulcerations, but cold sensitivity, digital numbness, and discomfort can alter hand function, force alterations in planned activities, and affect quality of life. Emotional problems can occur from the social stigma of cold hands with unsightly skin color changes, especially in adolescents.

Digital ischemia may occur in patients with secondary RP, leading to recurrent digital ulcerations, rapid deep tissue necrosis, and amputation. These patients, unlike patients with primary RP, have structurally abnormal digital vessels or disruption of the normal neurologic and/or hormonal regulation of regional blood flow. Pain severe enough to prompt patients to seek medical attention or to place the hand in a dependent position to improve blood flow indicates critical ischemia and impending ulceration. This constitutes a medical emergency, and hospitalization is indicated.

Such patients with critical ischemia should be kept as warm as possible, encouraged to exert emotional regulation over their symptoms, and treated with pain control (often with narcotics) to minimize sympathetic vasoconstriction. Vasodilator therapy with a short-acting calcium channel blocker (eg, nifedipine 10–20 mg orally every 8 hours) should be started in combination with aspirin. If symptoms progress, more aggressive therapy should be utilized, including a combination of vasodilators (eg, a calcium channel blocker and topical nitroglycerin) or an intravenous vasodilator such as prostaglandin infusion (eg, epoprostenol) in the setting of poor response to oral agents. A temporary chemical digital sympathectomy (eg, xylocaine) may rapidly reverse vasospasm if severe structural disease or vascular occlusion has not occurred. Anticoagulation (intravenous heparin or enoxaparin) for 48–72 hours should be considered if acute macrovascular occlusive disease is occurring. Long-term anticoagulation is not recommended unless a hypercoagulable state is discovered. Surgical digital sympathectomy may be considered if ischemia persists despite vasodilator therapy.

Macrovascular disease may complicate the situation and should be considered, because if present macrovascular disease can be amenable to surgical intervention leading to reversal of symptoms. Other complicating factors, such as hypercoagulable disorders, embolic disease, or underlying vasculitis, need to be considered and treated if present. Early intervention with hospitalization and vasodilator therapy is the key to preventing irreversible vessel occlusion and breaking the cycle of vasospasm and digital ischemia.

Digital ulcerations from recurrent tissue ischemia may develop in patients who have secondary RP. These ulcers should be kept as clean as possible with soap and water and appropriate protective dressing in order to avoid infection. Topical or systemic antibiotics are used if an infection develops. Bosentan, a dual endothelin receptor antagonist, has been shown to decrease the frequency of recurrent digital ulcers in patients with SSc. Although bosentan does not decrease the frequency of RP attacks, it may be used in this select group to reduce the occurrence of new digital ulcers. Conversely, treatment with macitentan, another dual endothelin receptor antagonist, did not reduce the frequency of new digital ulcerations in patients with SSc (Khanna et al, 2016).

Prognosis

Nonpharmacological supportive interventions are often sufficient for symptomatic control in many patients with primary and secondary RP. Patients with primary RP may be treated effectively by the primary care provider. Initial care is focused on preventive measures such as warm clothing and minimizing emotional stress in order to avoid RP attacks. Every effort should be made to manage RP with conservative preventative strategies before commencing therapeutic agents. Patients with secondary RP due to a connective tissue disease or RP from an unknown cause should be referred to a specialist for further management. Any patient with critical digital ischemia should be referred for hospitalization and immediate inpatient management. A vascular surgeon should be consulted early in the hospitalization for chemical or surgical digital sympathectomy or vascular repair if the ischemia is unresponsive to oral or intravenous vasodilators.

Bello RJ, Cooney CM, Melamed E, et al. The therapeutic efficacy of botulinum toxin in treating scleroderma-associated Raynaud's phenomenon: a randomized, double-blind, placebo-controlled clinical trial. *Arthritis Rheumatol (Hoboken, NJ).* 2017;69(8):1661-1669. [PMID: 28426903]

Ennis H, Hughes M, Anderson ME, Wilkinson J, Herrick AL. Calcium channel blockers for primary Raynaud's phenomenon. *Cochrane Database Syst Rev.* 2016;2:Cd002069. [PMID: 24482037]

Flavahan NA. A vascular mechanistic approach to understanding Raynaud phenomenon. *Nat Rev Rheumatol.* 2015;11(3):146-158. [PMID: 25536485]

Goundry B, Bell L, Langtree M, Moorthy A. Diagnosis and management of Raynaud's phenomenon. *BMJ.* 2012;344:e289. [PMID: 22315243]

Herrick AL. The pathogenesis, diagnosis and treatment of Raynaud phenomenon. *Nat Rev Rheumatol.* 2012;8(8):469-479. [PMID: 22782008]

Iorio ML, Masden DL, Higgins JP. Botulinum toxin A treatment of Raynaud's phenomenon: a review. *Semin Arthritis Rheum.* 2012;41(4):599-603. [PMID: 21868066]

Khanna D, Denton CP, Merkel PA, et al. Effect of macitentan on the development of new ischemic digital ulcers in patients with systemic sclerosis: DUAL-1 and DUAL-2 randomized clinical trials. *JAMA.* 2016;315(18):1975-1988. [PMID: 27163986]

Kowal-Bielecka O, Fransen J, Avouac J, et al. Update of EULAR recommendations for the treatment of systemic sclerosis. *Ann Rheum Dis.* 2017;76(8):1327-1339. [PMID: 27941129]

Maverakis E, Patel F, Kronenberg DG, et al. International consensus criteria for the diagnosis of Raynaud's phenomenon. *J Autoimmun.* 2014;48-49:60-65. [PMID: 24491823]

Overbury R, Murtaugh MA, Fischer A, Frech TM. Primary care assessment of capillaroscopy abnormalities in patients with Raynaud's phenomenon. *Clin Rheumatol.* 2015;34(12):2135-2140.

Pavlov-Dolijanovic SR, Damjanov NS, Vujasinovic Stupar NZ, Baltic S, Babic DD. The value of pattern capillary changes and antibodies to predict the development of systemic sclerosis in patients with primary Raynaud's phenomenon. *Rheumatol Int.* 2013;33(12):2967-2973. [PMID: 23934522]

Roustit M, Blaise S, Allanore Y, Carpentier PH, Caglayan E, Cracowski JL. Phosphodiesterase-5 inhibitors for the treatment of secondary Raynaud's phenomenon: systematic review and meta-analysis of randomised trials. *Ann Rheum Dis.* 2013;72(10):1696-1699. [PMID: 23426043]

Scleroderma (Systemic Sclerosis)

Jennifer Mandal, MD

Francesco Boin, MD

ESSENTIALS OF DIAGNOSIS

- ▶ Scleroderma (systemic sclerosis) is a systemic autoimmune disease characterized by varying degrees of skin fibrosis, vascular damage, and a wide array of internal organ dysfunction.

- ▶ Most manifestations of scleroderma fall into two main categories: fibrotic disease (such as skin tightening and interstitial lung disease [ILD]) and vascular disease (such as Raynaud phenomenon [RP] and pulmonary arterial hypertension [PAH]).

- ▶ In limited cutaneous scleroderma, skin involvement remains confined to the distal extremities (fingers, toes) and face. In contrast, in the diffuse form of scleroderma, skin tightening extends proximal to the elbows and knees as well as the trunk. Both limited and diffuse scleroderma can have significant internal organ involvement.

- ▶ RP and antinuclear antibodies (ANA) positivity are each present in more than 95% of scleroderma patients. When either of these features is missing, an alternative diagnosis should be strongly considered.

- ▶ Some patients with scleroderma develop clinical features overlapping with other rheumatic disorders such as rheumatoid arthritis, systemic lupus erythematosus, inflammatory myopathy, and Sjögren syndrome.

- ▶ It is helpful to take an organized organ-by-organ approach to assess an individual patient's specific manifestations, disease activity, extent of damage, and treatment options.

- ▶ There is no "universal" pharmacologic intervention for scleroderma that treats the disease as a whole. Combination therapy is most effective to address the heterogeneous nature of this disease manifestation.

General Considerations

Patients with scleroderma differ significantly from one another in regard to the timing of disease onset and progression, the combinations of organ-specific manifestations, the severity of their illness, and the response to therapy. This extreme variability makes it impossible to take a "one size fits all" approach to diagnosis and treatment. Effective care of scleroderma requires individualized attention to each patient's unique characteristics and disease course. This is what makes treating scleroderma patients so challenging but also ultimately so rewarding.

Scleroderma is rare, affecting approximately 20 people per million per year, with an estimated prevalence in the United States of 100–300 cases per million. It affects women more commonly than men (4:1), and the average age at diagnosis is 30–50 years old. African Americans and Native Americans tend to have a more severe disease course and worse outcomes compared to Caucasians.

Survival in patients with scleroderma is often limited directly by the underlying disease manifestations. Prognosis is highly variable, depending on the disease subtype, the type and severity of internal organ involvement, and responsiveness to treatment. In particular, the following characteristics are associated with higher mortality:

- Older age at onset
- Male gender
- African American ethnicity
- Diffuse skin disease
- Interstitial lung disease (ILD)
- Pulmonary arterial hypertension (PAH)
- Myocardial dysfunction
- Scleroderma renal crisis
- Severe gastrointestinal (GI) dysmotility

The 5-year survival rate for patients with limited scleroderma is approximately 90%, compared to 70–80% in diffuse scleroderma. Among patients with scleroderma, the most common cause of death is cardiac involvement (approximately 30%) followed by lung disease (approximately 25%).

Early diagnosis and treatment during the active, inflammatory stage of scleroderma can substantially reduce morbidity and mortality. In patients with established disease, vigilant monitoring for new or worsening disease manifestations and adjustment of medication regimens as disease activity waxes and wanes are crucial to achieving good outcomes.

Primary care physicians are encouraged to connect all their scleroderma patients with a rheumatologist, whenever possible. For patients with severe or complex disease, providers should strongly consider referring them to a specialty center with experience treating a high volume of scleroderma cases. Despite the challenges of managing this complex and often cruel disease, there is great hope on the horizon for a better understanding of the underlying causes of scleroderma and new breakthroughs in therapies.

When to Suspect Scleroderma

Early diagnosis of scleroderma is critical for the reduction of suffering and mortality associated with this condition. While the clinical onset can differ greatly from one patient to another, there are early clinical findings that should alert the provider to the possibility of scleroderma. Most common is Raynaud phenomenon (RP), characterized by episodic vasoconstriction of the arterial circulation to the digits, which occurs in more than 95% of patients. New-onset RP (particularly in subjects over the age of 20, in men, or when associated with complications such as digital ulcerations) should prompt the consideration of an underlying connective tissue disease such as scleroderma (see section Raynaud Phenomenon). Autoantibody positivity can also be a useful hint. Antinuclear antibodies (ANA) assays are positive in more than 95% of scleroderma patients but constitutes a highly nonspecific finding in and of itself. However, there are a number of specific autoantibodies that are strongly associated with scleroderma and its unique manifestations (see section Autoantibodies).

The most readily recognizable feature of scleroderma is skin tightening, which is caused by excessive collagen deposition (fibrosis). This can have a "limited" distribution, affecting only the hands, feet, and/or face, or a "diffuse" distribution, extending in a progressive proximal manner to the elbows and knees and ultimately impacting the trunk, as well. During early phases, skin changes may include edematous swelling of the hands ("puffy fingers"), itching/burning in the distal extremities, and skin hardening with progression from distal to proximal sites. Any of these skin features, particularly in someone with RP and positive ANA, should prompt referral to a rheumatologist to evaluate for the possibility of scleroderma.

Terminology

The terminology used to classify different forms of scleroderma is a common source of confusion. Broadly, scleroderma is divided into two major categories: **localized scleroderma** and **systemic sclerosis (systemic scleroderma)** (Figure 23–1).

Localized scleroderma (which will not be covered in this chapter) is characterized by skin changes presenting in discrete areas without internal organ involvement. It includes several subtypes such as localized morphea, generalized morphea, and linear scleroderma. Localized scleroderma tends to be self-limited and is not life-threatening.

This chapter focuses exclusively on the systemic form of scleroderma (systemic sclerosis). Systemic sclerosis is divided into three main subtypes, based on the extent of skin thickening:

1. **Limited scleroderma (65%):** Skin thickening confined to the extremities, distal to the elbows and knees. The face is also often involved.
2. **Diffuse scleroderma (30%):** Skin thickening extending to the proximal portion of the extremities and/or the trunk.
3. **Scleroderma sine scleroderma (5%):** Rare subtype without obvious skin thickening.

Patients and providers commonly misinterpret the term "limited scleroderma" to mean a lack of internal organ involvement (or only mild or "limited" organ involvement). In fact, patients with the limited form of scleroderma can manifest a wide array of internal organ presentations, ranging from mild to severe.

The term "CREST syndrome" was previously used as a synonym for limited scleroderma. The acronym describes common manifestations of limited scleroderma: **C**alcinosis, **R**aynaud phenomenon, **E**sophageal dysmotility, **S**clerodactyly, and **T**elangiectasias. However, this term has fallen out of favor, as many patients with limited scleroderma do not have all five of these manifestations. More importantly, patients with diffuse scleroderma can have all of these features as well, the "CREST" is no longer considered to denote limited scleroderma and should generally be discarded from the scleroderma lexicon.

Limited and diffuse scleroderma share many clinical manifestations—in fact, nearly any internal organ can be affected in either scleroderma subtype. However, disease features tend to present with different frequency and severity in one form of the disease or the other. These are summarized in Table 23–1.

Classification Criteria

Classification criteria for scleroderma were developed for the purpose of enrolling patients into research studies. Although these criteria are not intended for the purpose of diagnosis, they still serve as a useful guide in the clinical setting.

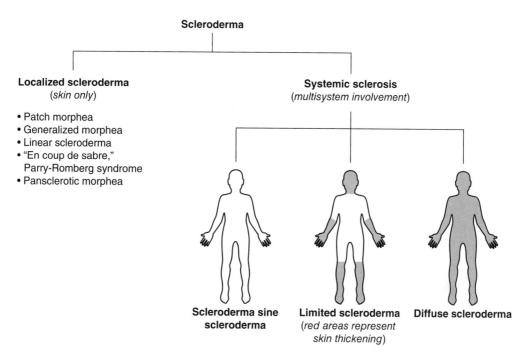

▲ **Figure 23-1.** Classification of scleroderma subsets.

The 2013 European League Against Rheumatism (EULAR)/ American College of Rheumatology (ACR) classification criteria for systemic sclerosis are shown in Table 23-2.

Autoantibodies

There is no specific laboratory test (or set of tests) that can definitively confirm or exclude a diagnosis of scleroderma. While this is true also for autoantibodies, their determination remains very important to help establish the proper diagnosis and to estimate the risk for unique scleroderma disease manifestations.

As noted above, ANA are positive in more than 95% of patients, frequently in association with unique specificities of scleroderma-specific autoantibodies. These can be detected in patient subsets exhibiting distinct disease manifestations (Table 23-3).

Table 23-1. Clinical manifestations associated with limited and diffuse subsets of scleroderma.

	Limited Scleroderma	Diffuse Scleroderma
Skin	Skin tightening of face and extremities (distal to elbows/knees), calcinosis, telangiectasias	Skin tightening of both distal and proximal extremities and/or trunk, prominent flexion contractures.
Raynaud phenomenon	Onset several years before scleroderma diagnosis	Onset close to scleroderma diagnosis
Digital ulcers	Ischemic	Ischemic and traumatic (from subcutaneous atrophy and flexion contractures)
Interstitial lung disease (ILD)	Less frequent (clinically relevant ILD in 20%), can be severe	More frequent (clinically relevant ILD in 70%), can be severe
Pulmonary hypertension	Group 1 (Pulmonary arterial hypertension)	Group 2 (due to left heart disease) and Group 3 (due to lung disease)
Myocardial dysfunction	Rare	More frequent
Scleroderma renal crisis	Rare	More frequent (15%)
Gastrointestinal	Gastroesophageal reflux disease (GERD), dysphagia	More severe dysmotility, even gut failure
Musculoskeletal	Milder, mostly small joints	More severe, small and large joint with contractures
Pain/disability	Mild	Can be severe
Autoantibodies	Anticentromere, anti-Pm-Scl, anti-Th/To	Antitopoisomerase I (Scl-70), anti-RNA polymerase III

Table 23–2. The 2013 European League Against Rheumatism (EULAR)/American College of Rheumatology (ACR) classification criteria for systemic sclerosis (scleroderma).

Item	Score
Skin thickening of both hands extending proximal interphalangeal (PIP) to the metacarpophalangeal (MCP) joints	9
Skin thickening of the fingers: (Only count the higher score)	
• Puffy fingers	2
• Sclerodactyly of fingers (distal to MCPs but proximal to PIPs)	4
Fingertip lesions: (Only count the higher score)	
• Fingertip ulcers	2
• Fingertip pitting	3
Telangiectasias	2
Abnormal nailfold capillaries	2
Pulmonary arterial hypertension or interstitial lung disease	2
Raynaud phenomenon	3
Scleroderma-specific autoantibody (any):	
• Anticentromere	
• Antitopoisomerase I (Scl-70)	
• Anti-RNA polymerase III	3

Patients with a total score ≥9 are classified as having systemic sclerosis.

General Approach to Management

The primary goals of the initial encounter are (1) to confirm the diagnosis of scleroderma; (2) to characterize the patient's clinical phenotype based on a number of key clues, including degree of cutaneous involvement, autoantibody status, and pattern of internal organ dysfunction; and (3) to educate the patient about their diagnosis and expect disease course. There are many prevalent misconceptions about scleroderma (often held by patients and providers alike). Among the most troublesome of these is that scleroderma is an untreatable, universally deforming, and fatal disease. Correcting these misconceptions and establishing a trusting and collaborative relationship with the patient contribute greatly toward improving outcomes.

Given the highly variable nature of scleroderma, it is very helpful to take a systematic organ-by-organ approach when evaluating a patient's specific disease manifestations. At each follow-up visit, the provider should carefully assess the disease activity and severity within each organ system, as well as evaluate possible indications to start, titrate, or stop organ-specific interventions. It is important to recognize that there are no "universal" pharmacologic interventions for the treatment of scleroderma and that all therapeutic decisions must be carefully tailored to the patient's specific symptoms and disease activity. In the following sections, we will break down the clinical manifestations, assessment, and treatment of scleroderma in each organ system.

Table 23–3. Clinical features associated with scleroderma-specific autoantibodies.

Autoantibody	Associated Clinical Features (Common)	Prevalence
Anticentromere	Limited skin involvement, severe Raynaud phenomenon and digital ischemia, pulmonary arterial hypertension, telangiectasias, calcinosis. Overlap with primary biliary cirrhosis, Sjögren syndrome, Hashimoto's thyroiditis. Better overall prognosis	15–40%
Antitopoisomerase I (Anti-Scl-70)	Diffuse skin, pulmonary fibrosis, ischemic and traumatic digital ulcers, cardiac involvement, African American ethnicity. Worse overall prognosis	10–45%
Anti-RNA polymerase III	Rapidly progressive skin tightening (severe), scleroderma renal crisis (±sine scleroderma), myositis, myocarditis. High-risk concurrent malignancy (particularly in older age group)	5–20%
Anti-U3-RNP (Antifibrillarin)	Limited or diffuse skin tightening, pulmonary fibrosis, severe GI dysmotility, cardiac disease, African American ethnicity	5–10%
Anti-U1-RNP	Pulmonary fibrosis, mixed connective tissue disease (overlapping features with SLE, inflammatory arthritis, myositis)	5–7%
Anti-PM-Scl	Limited skin involvement, overlapping features of myositis, pulmonary fibrosis	2–8%
Anti-Th/To	Limited skin involvement, pulmonary fibrosis	1–5%
Anti-Ku	Myositis, arthritis, pulmonary fibrosis, SLE overlap	1–5%

SLE, systemic lupus erythematosus.

Skin

A. Clinical Manifestations

The word scleroderma literally means "hard skin" (from the Greek, *skleros:* hard; *derma:* skin). In fact, skin changes due to excessive collagen deposition (fibrosis) are often the first and most obvious clinical manifestation observed in patients. The extent of skin tightening can be restricted to the face and the extremities distal to the elbows and knees (limited cutaneous scleroderma), or include the proximal portion of the limbs as well as the truncal areas (diffuse cutaneous scleroderma) (Figure 23–2). Patients with an established phenotype of

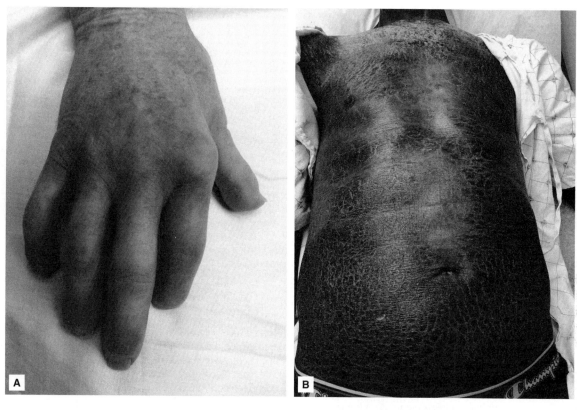

▲ **Figure 23–2.** Skin involvement in scleroderma: (**A**) sclerodactyly; (**B**) diffuse skin disease (trunk).

limited scleroderma do not progress to the diffuse form. Rarely, scleroderma can manifest without any apparent skin thickening. This rare subtype, referred to as "scleroderma sine scleroderma," affects 5% of patients. Some experts prefer the term "undifferentiated connective tissue disease."

Patients with severe and extensive skin thickening are at risk for developing debilitating flexion contractures (particularly of the fingers, wrists, and elbows). They are also prone to developing skin ulcers from mild trauma (such as bumping or scraping a knuckle). Skin involvement on the face is often accompanied by a gradual thinning of the lips, a decrease in oral aperture, vertical perioral furrowing (rhytides), and narrowing of the nose bridge. Hypopigmentation of affected areas (vitiligo-like) and patches with preserved perifollicular pigmentation ("salt-and-pepper" appearance) can develop over face, arms, and trunk. Fibrotic skin changes in diffuse scleroderma begin distally (fingers, toes, and face) and subsequently progress proximally. In a patient presenting with proximal skin thickening but no involvement of hands and feet, an alternative diagnosis such as localized scleroderma or other scleroderma mimics (eg, eosinophilic fasciitis, scleromyxedema, or scleredema) should be strongly considered.

The natural history of skin damage in scleroderma consists of three sequential phases:

1. **Early inflammatory phase:** During this stage, which can last several weeks, the skin may appear erythematous and edematous (ie, nonpitting edema). Patients often complain of pruritus or a burning sensation of the skin surface, or even pain in this phase. Early on, patients with puffy, swollen fingers may be misdiagnosed with rheumatoid arthritis. Wrist and hand discomfort early on may also be mistakenly attributed to carpal tunnel syndrome.

2. **Fibrotic phase:** After the initial inflammatory manifestations, the skin becomes progressively fibrotic, with thickening of the dermis causing typical induration and lack of elasticity. Deeper layers can be affected, including periarticular and even muscle structures, leading to joint contractures and myopathy. Atrophy of subcutaneous adipose tissue and loss of appendages are also typical. During this phase, which can last anywhere from months to years, the pruritus gradually resolves and the skin thickening does not extend to new areas. Patients rarely "relapse" back into skin inflammation after this stage.

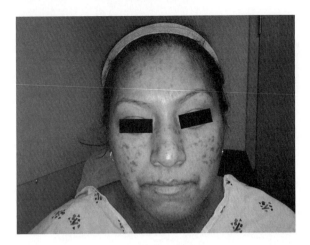

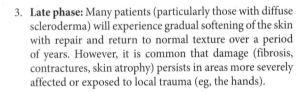

▲ **Figure 23–3.** Facial telangiectasias in patient with limited scleroderma. (See color insert.)

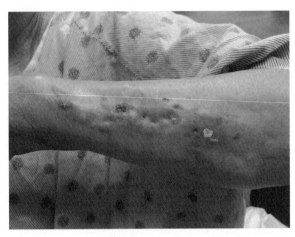

▲ **Figure 23–4.** Extensive forearm calcinosis with skin rapture and calcium extrusion.

3. **Late phase:** Many patients (particularly those with diffuse scleroderma) will experience gradual softening of the skin with repair and return to normal texture over a period of years. However, it is common that damage (fibrosis, contractures, skin atrophy) persists in areas more severely affected or exposed to local trauma (eg, the hands).

Other important skin manifestations in scleroderma include telangiectasias, which are dilated superficial postcapillary venules. These often develop on the hands, face, and chest, presenting with a characteristic "matted" appearance (Figure 23–3).

Telangiectasias tend to become larger and more numerous over time, correlating with the progression of other as other vascular manifestations such as severe RP or pulmonary hypertension. Calcinosis (subcutaneous calcium deposits) can appear in areas of repetitive friction, pressure, or ischemia such as fingertips, extensor surfaces of the forearms, and patellae (Figure 23–4).

The deposits can rupture through the skin causing extrusion of a thick, white material. Calcium accumulation can cluster around joints as well causing bone erosion and inflammation. Telangiectasias and calcinosis are observed both in patients with limited and diffuse scleroderma.

B. Assessment

The degree of skin involvement can be quantified and monitored over time using the modified Rodnan skin score (mRSS), which involves pinching the patient's skin in 17 specified body areas and rating the degree of skin thickening in each area from 0 to 3. While this method is prone to inter-rater variability, it represents a useful tool for assessing the progression (and improvement) of scleroderma skin disease over time, and can be used to guide when to start and/or stop immunosuppressive therapy.

C. Treatment

Treatment of scleroderma skin involvement should be considered during the early active inflammatory phase, particularly in patients with diffuse scleroderma and rapid progression. The main therapeutic approach involves nonselective immunosuppression. Both mycophenolate mofetil (MMF) and cyclophosphamide (CYC) have shown evidence of benefit in the management of active scleroderma skin disease. MMF is typically preferred as first-line therapy due to its milder side-effect profile. Small benefit has also been reported with use of methotrexate (MTX), and this may be a reasonable option to consider in patients with active skin disease and concurrent prominent inflammatory arthritis. Administration of rituximab and intravenous immunoglobulins (IVIGs) have shown promising results in treating skin disease in small open-label studies, and are used alone or in combination with other immunosuppressive drugs (eg, MMF) by some practitioners in patients with inadequate responses to first-line agents. Glucocorticoids (systemic) are generally not recommended to manage skin inflammation. The addition of gabapentin can help with pruritus and burning pain. Once the initial inflammatory phase is controlled and/or the skin exhibits signs of softening, tapering of immunosuppression should be considered. Management of inactive or late skin disease is mostly supportive. Patients should always be counseled to keep their skin very well moisturized, and protected it from excessive sun exposure and trauma.

In a subset of patients with early, severe diffuse scleroderma, more aggressive therapy may be considered. Specifically, a few studies have investigated the use of myeloablative therapy with high-dose CYC followed by autologous hematopoietic stem cell transplantation (HSCT), and found that this approach can be effective in controlling diffuse skin disease, stabilizing lung function (in the setting of ILD), and improving patient-reported measures of quality of life. However, HSCT is associated with significant treatment-related morbidity and mortality (3–10%), and more data are needed to help determine which scleroderma patients are appropriate candidates for this aggressive approach. In addition, long-term data regarding risk for secondary malignancy are still missing.

Patients with only mild skin thickening (as is often the case in limited scleroderma), or patients who are diagnosed at later stages (ie, several years into their disease course), typically do not require any immunosuppression for their skin disease. However, immunosuppression may be considered for other organ-specific manifestations such as ILD or musculoskeletal inflammation.

Telangiectasias can be shrunk with laser therapy (typically performed by a dermatologist) if they are cosmetically bothersome to the patient. However, they tend to redevelop over time at the same sites. There is currently no effective medication to treat calcinosis. Patients should be counseled to avoid repetitive local trauma and friction over affected areas as much as possible (eg, wear soft elbow pads, or silicone cushions on their fingertips), and to optimize tissue blood perfusion. Hypoxia appears to be a significant trigger for calcinosis, particularly in the fingers.

▶ Raynaud Phenomenon

Raynaud phenomenon (RP) is characterized by episodes of exaggerated vasoconstriction of the digital arterial circulation in response to cold temperature or emotional stress. Patients with RP classically experience sharply demarcated blanching and cyanosis of the skin on their fingers and/or toes, followed in some cases by erythema due to reactive hyperemia upon rewarming (Figure 23–5).

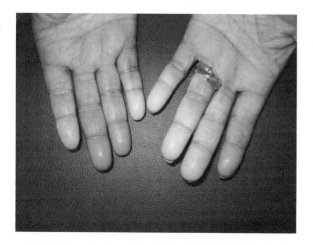

▲ **Figure 23–5.** Raynaud phenomenon presenting with asymmetric digital pallor during vasospastic attack. (See color insert.)

RP is relatively common in the general population, occurring in approximately 5–10% of individuals. It is four times more common in women than men. RP is defined as "primary" when it is not associated with any underlying systemic disease or known trigger. This typically manifests in young women, often in teenagers. Secondary RP occurs in the setting of autoimmune rheumatic disorders (scleroderma, systemic lupus erythematosus, idiopathic inflammatory myopathies, Sjögren syndrome), occupational trauma (vibration-hand syndrome), thoracic outlet syndrome, hematological abnormalities (cryoglobulinemia, cold agglutinins), or in association with use of medications driving peripheral vasoconstriction (see section Treatment). Vessel inflammation (vasculitis) may cause digital ischemia but not RP per se, as the digital ischemia of vasculitis is not preceded by a history of cold-induced, reversible digital color changes.

"Red flags" indicating the possibility of RP secondary to a connective tissue disorder include the following:

- Later age of onset (>20 years old)
- Male
- Asymmetry (manifestations only on one hand or in a dominant digit)
- Severe RP leading to ischemic fingertip ulcerations
- Positivity for ANA or other autoantibodies
- Nailfold capillary abnormalities (see section Assessment)

RP is present in more than 95% of patients with scleroderma and typically represents the first manifestation of the disease. In limited scleroderma, RP can precede onset of other systemic symptoms by years. In contrast, in diffuse scleroderma, RP frequently starts concurrently with other disease features. Symptoms of RP can range from mild and infrequent, to extremely severe. Recurrent attacks can be associated with development of ischemic complications such as exquisitely painful fingertip ulcers or progression to digital gangrene and finger loss (Figure 23–6).

A. Assessment

Careful physical examination of the fingers can provide important information about the severity of RP and guide treatment decisions. Nailfold capillaroscopy is a very helpful tool that can be used at the bedside to help distinguish between primary RP (normal nailfold capillaries) and scleroderma-related RP (abnormal capillary patterns). Capillaroscopy can be conducted under magnification using a variety of tools, including a simple ophthalmoscope with immersion oil, a handheld dermatoscope, or a computerized video system. Normal nailfold capillaries appear like thin, well-organized palisading loops. In scleroderma-related RP, capillaries become dilated (giant loop), tortuous, with areas of microhemorrhages and eventually vessel drop out (avascular) (Figure 23–7).

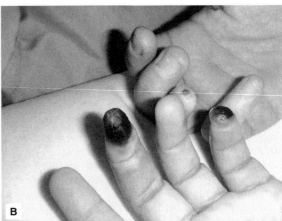

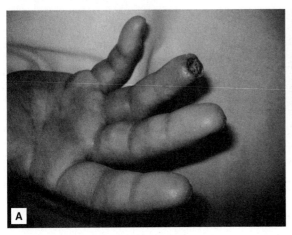

▲ **Figure 23–6.** Ischemic complications from severe Raynaud phenomenon resulting in (**A**) painful fingertip ulceration or (**B**) digital gangrene leading to digital loss. (See color insert.)

Patients with mild RP may have a normal physical examination and only subtle nailfold capillary changes. In contrast, moderate to severe RP can be associated with manifestations suggesting active disease as well as transition to chronic ischemia in affected digits. These can include the following:

- Acute digital vasoconstriction with significant pallor or cyanosis (particularly if the exam room is air conditioned!)
- Digital pitting (small dimples on the tips of the fingers)
- Acro-osteolysis (shortening of the fingers due to reabsorption of the distal bone tufts)
- Active digital ulcers (usually located on the fingertips, these can be exquisitely painful and difficult to heal)
- Digital gangrene (which can lead to partial or complete digit loss)

B. Treatment

The treatment of RP is discussed in detail in Chapter 22.

▶ Interstitial Lung Disease

Interstitial lung disease (ILD) is the most common lung manifestation and one of the most important determinants of morbidity and mortality in scleroderma. Usually, ILD develops early on during the disease course, typically within the first 5 years. The severity of ILD can range from minimal, stable disease (not requiring treatment) to progressive lung involvement necessitating aggressive therapy. In some cases, ILD leads to organ failure and referral to lung transplantation. Clinically relevant ILD can affect up to 60% of patients with diffuse scleroderma and 20% of those with limited disease.

Specific risk factors for more severe ILD include African American or Native American ancestry, the presence of certain specific autoantibodies (namely, antitopoisomerase [Scl-70], anti-U3-RNP, or anti-Th/To), and diffuse skin involvement.

▲ **Figure 23–7.** Abnormal nailfold capillaries with loops dilatation (megacapillaries).

A. Assessment

The possibility of ILD should be evaluated immediately at the time of scleroderma diagnosis and monitored closely thereafter in every patient. Emerging ILD often presents with dyspnea on exertion, fatigue, or dry cough. However, it is important to remember that many patients are asymptomatic early on and that other scleroderma manifestations can be associated with respiratory symptoms (eg, gastroesophageal reflux disease [GERD], anemia, myopathy). The most common finding on physical exam is the presence of fine inspiratory crackles at the lung bases.

Pulmonary function testing is a critical tool for screening and monitoring of ILD. Characteristic PFT findings include a restrictive ventilatory defect, characterized by decreased lung volumes as well as diffusion capacity of carbon monoxide (DLCO). Scleroderma patients without known ILD should have PFTs tested annually or sooner if new pulmonary symptoms manifest. In presence of ILD, monitoring of the lung function (on or off treatment) should be performed more frequently.

High-resolution chest CT (HRCT) is more accurate than chest radiography for assessing ILD. More than two-thirds of patients with scleroderma will show at least some evidence of fibrosis on HRCT. Typical early/mild changes are characterized by increased subpleural lung attenuation in the bibasilar lung fields (some patients will not go beyond this phase). With progression of ILD, more ground glass opacities (suggesting active inflammation) and reticular fibrosis (permanent scarring) develop (Figure 23–8).

The severity of HRCT findings at the time of initial diagnosis is an important prognostic marker. Disease extent of more than 20% on initial HRCT predicts ILD progression and higher mortality. The most common histologic pattern of ILD in scleroderma is nonspecific interstitial pneumonia (NSIP), with a smaller subset demonstrating a usual interstitial pneumonia (UIP) pattern. A diagnosis of scleroderma-related ILD can typically be made on the basis of characteristic PFT and HRCT findings, and lung biopsy is rarely needed. Unlike PFTs, HRCT typically does not need to be repeated on an annual basis. However, repeat HRCT can be useful to investigate sustained decline of lung volumes, unexplained pulmonary symptoms, concern for superimposed infections, and to help guide decisions about therapeutic changes.

B. Treatment of Interstitial Lung Disease

Scleroderma patients with mild fibrosis on HRCT and stable lung volumes often do not require immunosuppressive therapy. In presence of disease progression or when ILD is already advanced at diagnosis, however, treatment should be initiated promptly. The major goal is to prevent further decline of the lung function. Current treatment options are mostly directed to suppress the ongoing immune-driven, inflammatory response. MMF and CYC have both demonstrated modest benefit in stopping or slowing progression of scleroderma-related ILD in randomized clinical trials. The results of the Scleroderma Lung Study II (SLS II) further support the common practice to use MMF as preferred first-line therapy as it provides similar clinical efficacy to CYC but is associated with fewer adverse effects. Oral or IV CYC can be used as a second-line therapy for patients who fail or cannot tolerate MMF.

The use of antifibrotic medications in scleroderma-related ILD has been evaluated in recent clinical trials. Nintedanib, a tyrosine kinase inhibitor, slowed ILD progression in a 52-week randomized placebo-controlled study. This drug appears poised now to play an important role in treating scleroderma ILD, perhaps in combination with MMF.

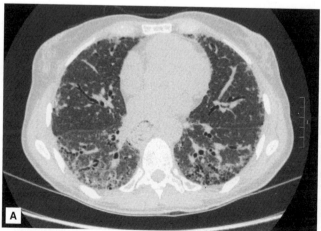
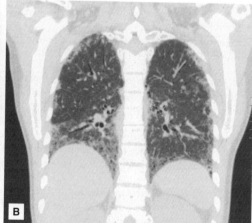

▲ **Figure 23–8.** Scleroderma interstitial lung disease. High-resolution chest CT, (**A**) axial and (**B**) coronal sections showing basilar and peripheral predominant fibrosis, reticulation, bronchiectasis, and diffuse groundglass opacities.

Small observational studies provide some evidence for the use of rituximab (B-cell depletion) as an alternative therapy for refractory ILD. Azathioprine appears to less effective than MMF or CYC, but can be useful in presence of other organ manifestations such as myositis.

Cell-based treatment using myeloablative conditioning regimens followed by autologous HSCT can also be considered in carefully selected patients with ILD, as recently completed studies have confirmed their efficacy in stabilizing lung function.

Lung transplantation is an option and a life-saving intervention in scleroderma patients with very advanced ILD who have failed maximal pharmacologic therapy. Based on data obtained from experienced transplant programs, the morbidity and mortality in scleroderma subjects are similar to those observed in patients undergoing lung transplantation for other fibrotic lung diseases (particularly idiopathic pulmonary fibrosis).

▶ Pulmonary Hypertension

Pulmonary hypertension is another potentially life-threatening manifestation of scleroderma. Pulmonary vascular disease can be a primary process, characterized by luminal narrowing of medium-size, precapillary arteries (pulmonary arterial hypertension, or PAH). Pulmonary hypertension can also present, however, as a complication of other conditions, including those associated with parenchymal lung disease (eg, advanced ILD, emphysema), chronic thromboembolism, or left heart disease.

Risk factors for the development of PAH include the following:

- Older age at diagnosis
- Limited cutaneous involvement
- Numerous and prominent telangiectasias
- Disproportionately low DLCO on PFTs
- Elevated NT-proBNP
- Presence of specific autoantibodies: anticentromere, anti-U1-RNP, anti-U3-RNP

Despite the availability of newer targeted therapies, PAH is still associated with a high mortality in scleroderma. The median survival in patients manifesting PAH is limited to about 4 years. In contrast with ILD, PAH typically manifests later in the course of scleroderma, often more than a decade from disease onset. Despite this, there is evidence indicating that the vascular injury leading to PAH begins much earlier, remaining undetected for many years and in the absence of obvious symptoms. Patients presenting with a progressive drop of the DLCO (disproportioned to the changes of lung volumes) should be considered at high risk for developing PAH. The combination of pulmonary hypertension and ILD carries a worse prognosis compared to either manifestations presenting alone.

A. Assessment

During early stages, PAH is often asymptomatic. As the condition progresses, patients may present with dyspnea on exertion and fatigue. In more advanced cases, hypotension and lower extremity edema may be present. Physical examination may reveal a loud S2 pulmonic component, a systolic murmur (from tricuspid regurgitation), and evidence of right heart failure (elevated jugular venous pressure, hepatomegaly, dependent edema). Severe hypoxia, syncope, or sudden death are complications of severe disease.

All patients with scleroderma should be screened for evidence of PAH with an annual transthoracic echocardiogram (TTE). This is extremely useful to monitor for hemodynamic changes and to exclude dysfunction of the left heart. Detection of elevated right ventricular systolic pressure (RVSP) should prompt further testing for PAH, particularly in presence of progressive respiratory symptoms, dilatation of right cardiac chambers, increased BNP or NT-proBNP levels, or declining of the DLCO disproportionately to the lung volumes. Definitive PAH diagnosis requires a right heart catheterization (RHC) demonstrating a mean pulmonary artery pressure greater than 25 mm Hg with increased peripheral vascular resistances (PVR >3 Woods units) and a normal pulmonary artery wedge pressure (PAWP ≤15 mm Hg).

B. Treatment of Pulmonary Arterial Hypertension

Management of scleroderma-related PAH revolves around the use of vasodilatory drugs, alone or in combination. This is complemented by general adjunctive interventions which include smoking cessation, supplementary oxygen (at rest or with activity), salt restriction, and use of diuretics as needed. Inotropic support (eg, digoxin) can be used in advanced cases. Anticoagulation is not routinely recommended in patients with scleroderma-related PAH as it has been associated with worse outcome. Concurrent manifestations driving or contributing to PH, such as left cardiac disease, parenchymal lung disease, obstructive sleep apnea, and thromboembolic disease, must be identified and managed effectively.

Several classes of agents are currently employed for targeted therapy in scleroderma-PAH. These include the following:

- Endothelin receptor antagonists (ambrisentan, bosentan, macitentan)
- Phosphodiesterase type 5 inhibitors (sildenafil, tadalafil, vardenafil)
- Prostacyclin analogues (epoprostenol, iloprost, treprostinil)
- Selective prostacyclin receptor (IP receptor) agonist (selexipag)
- Soluble guanylate-cyclase stimulator (riociguat)

All these drugs have shown the ability to improve exercise tolerance, quality of life, and some hemodynamic parameters particularly when early treatment is implemented. Clinical trials indicate a survival benefit supporting current guidelines for use of combination therapy early in subjects with new PAH diagnosis, even in presence of milder disease. The combination of ambrisentan and tadalafil has been used for this purpose. Patients with more severe PAH (WHO functional class III or IV) are typically treated with IV prostacyclin analogues in association with one or more oral agents of different classes. Caution is indicated with use of vasodilators in the setting of concurrent severe ILD, as these drugs may acutely worsen alveolocapillary gas exchange due to venous blood shunting through fibrotic lung areas.

High-dose calcium channel blockers do not appear to be effective in scleroderma-related PAH. In severe refractory cases, lung or heart-lung transplantation may be an option for carefully selected patients. A small retrospective study suggests that their survival does not differ from the overall population of lung transplant recipients.

▶ Gastrointestinal

The vast majority of patients with scleroderma experience gastrointestinal symptoms, which can range from mild acid reflux to life-threatening malnourishment and gastrointestinal failure. Scleroderma-related GI dysfunction is mostly driven by failure of visceral smooth muscle contractility resulting in significant hypomotility. While the esophagus is most commonly affected, any portion of the GI tract can be involved.

Perioral skin tightening and facial skin fibrosis can result in decreased oral aperture with difficult intake of larger bites of food. Decreased saliva production further interferes with the ability to chew. Pharyngeal dysfunction can be present due to weakness of the swallowing muscles (myopathy), resulting in increased risk for aspiration of solid food or liquids. GERD affects 75–95% of patients with scleroderma and is usually associated with symptoms of heartburn, hoarseness, regurgitation, and dysphagia. Untreated, reflux and esophageal hypomotility can lead to chronic esophagitis, esophageal strictures/ulcers, and Barrett's esophagus (premalignant mucosal lesions characterized by intestinal metaplasia). It is also important to remember that some pulmonary complaints such as chronic cough, dyspnea, or recurrent "pneumonias" may actually be related to uncontrolled GERD and chronic aspiration.

The stomach involvement ranges from delayed gastric emptying to severe gastroparesis, and can be associated with early satiety, nausea, vomiting, and inability to retain solid food. Gastric ulcers can occur, but upper GI bleeding in scleroderma patients is often the consequence of abnormally dilated mucosal blood vessels and arterial-venous malformations, a condition known as gastric antral vascular ectasia (GAVE) or "watermelon stomach." Patients with other vascular manifestations of scleroderma, such as prominent and numerous cutaneous telangiectasias, severe RP, and PAH are at higher risk for developing GAVE.

Delayed transit in the lower GI tract can result in small intestinal bacterial overgrowth or carbohydrate malabsorption commonly associated with abdominal pain, bloating, and frequent diarrhea. Decreased contractility of the colon and impaired gastrocolic reflex drive constipation. This can be severe, manifesting with colonic dilatation (megacolon), impaction, and even episodes of pseudo-obstruction, which can be mistaken for surgical emergencies due to the intensity of abdominal symptoms, impaired transit and marked dilatation of intestinal segments. Severe and protracted bowel dysfunction leads in some cases to profound malnutrition, weight loss, and global intestinal failure. Anorectal dysfunction can manifest with fecal incontinence and rectal prolapse.

A. Assessment

All scleroderma patients should be asked about upper and lower GI symptoms on a regular basis, including their eating habits, swallowing difficulties, digestion, bowel function, and any unintentional weight loss. Esophagogastroduodenoscopy (EGD) is indicated for patients with symptoms of GI reflux not responding to antacid therapy or worsening dysphagia to assess for complications such as uncontrolled esophagitis, esophageal strictures, superimposed candidiasis, Barrett's esophagus, or malignancy. Barium swallow testing (cine-esophagram) can be helpful to assess pharyngeal and esophageal function as well as the presence of strictures. In some cases, direct measurement of esophageal motility using manometry may be recommended, particularly if the patient presents with atypical pain or concern for recurrent aspiration events. Anorectal manometry and magnetic resonance defecography are useful tools to further evaluate fecal incontinence and presence of pelvic floor dysfunction.

B. Treatment of Gastrointestinal Dysfunction

Careful counseling about behavioral measures, such as avoiding aggravating foods (spicy sauces, alcoholic, caffeinated, and carbonated beverages), eating small frequent meals, dining at least 2–3 hours before bedtime, and sleeping at a 30–35 degree angle with the use of an elevating bed headboard, are critical part of managing scleroderma esophageal dysfunction. Mild GERD symptoms should be treated empirically with agents inhibiting acid secretion such as proton pump inhibitors (PPIs) and histamine H-2 receptor antagonists (H2-blockers). Patients who fail to respond adequately to lifestyle adjustments or background therapy may benefit from higher dose PPIs, combination with H2-blockers and possibly from the addition of promotility agents such as metoclopramide, erythromycin (or other macrolides), or domperidone (not available in the United States). Fundoplication surgeries have often negative outcomes in scleroderma patients due to significant esophageal hypomotility. Thus, they are not recommended. When GERD symptoms are associated with severe dysphagia or swallowing difficulties, endoscopic dilatation of esophageal strictures may be required. EGD can also be useful to explore for presence of

GAVE in the stomach and proximal intestine, and to exert treatment of the bleeding vessels with laser photocoagulation or cryotherapy.

Management of constipation-predominant symptoms revolves around use of stool softeners (such as docusate) and/or intermittent laxatives (such as polyethylene glycol). Bulking agents should be used with caution as they may be poorly tolerated in high quantities. New agents for constipation such as linaclotide, lubiprostone, or prucalopride may be effective in more difficult cases. Persistent diarrheal symptoms may indicate small intestine bacterial overgrowth and can be treated with intermittent courses of rotating antibiotics (such as rifaximin or metronidazole). The addition of a daily probiotic can be appropriate. Other promotility agents, such as octreotide or pyridostigmine, have shown some benefit in severe lower GI dysmotility. In presence of recurrent pseudo-obstruction and progressive gut failure, bowel rest and total parenteral nutrition may be necessary for a prolonged period of time. Placement of gastrostomy tube (PEG, G-tube) or gastrojejunostomy tubes (PEG-J or GJ tubes) is indicated only when decompression of the GI tract may be needed. Management of fecal incontinence includes strategies to increase stool consistency, use of antidiarrheal medications, nerve stimulation, biofeedback techniques, and exercises to improve pelvic floor function. Surgical intervention is rarely used and remains limited to treat complicating factors such as rectal prolapse or severe hemorrhoids.

▶ Renal

Scleroderma renal crisis (SRC) affects approximately 5–10% of patients with scleroderma. It is a medical emergency that requires a rapid diagnosis and prompt treatment in order to prevent irreversible kidney failure and death. Several factors are associated with the development of SRC. These include the following:

- Diffuse cutaneous scleroderma (particularly during phases of progressing involvement progression)
- Early disease (median disease duration at SRC diagnosis is 8 months)
- Ethnicity (more frequent in African Americans)
- Exposure to high-dose corticosteroids (ie, ≥20 mg prednisone daily) or prolonged use
- Anti-RNA polymerase III antibodies (positive in 60% of SRC cases)

Preexisting primary hypertension is not a risk factor for SRC.

SRC classically presents with sudden-onset elevation of the blood pressure (usually higher than 150/90 mm Hg) and typical signs of malignant hypertension such as headache, visual disturbances (hypertensive retinopathy), nosebleeds, signs of heart involvement (pericardial effusion, congestive heart failure or flash pulmonary edema), encephalopathy with altered mental status, or seizures. Concurrent progression to renal failure may occur rapidly. Approximately 10% of patients with SRC present with normal or only mildly elevated blood pressure, making initial recognition and diagnosis more challenging.

A. Assessment

SRC is a medical emergency. Scleroderma patients presenting with new clinical signs indicative of hypertensive urgency should be immediately evaluated and their kidney function assessed. Renal involvement can progress over hours to days and manifest with elevated creatinine, abnormal urinalysis (typically microscopic hematuria or mild proteinuria), evidence of microangiopathic hemolytic anemia (drop in hemoglobin/hematocrit, schistocytes on peripheral blood smear), and/or thrombocytopenia. Assays for ADAMTS-13 can be helpful to distinguish between SRC (normal level) and idiopathic thrombotic thrombocytopenic purpura (low), but the results of these assays are typically not available for days. Therefore, treatment for SRC usually needs to begin without this information.

Early recognition of SRC can be challenging; therefore, it is important to counsel all patients who are at high risk for SRC (patients with early diffuse scleroderma, particularly those with anti-RNA polymerase III) to monitor their blood pressure regularly at home and seek immediate care for any signs of increased blood pressure. SRC patients are commonly admitted to the hospital for prompt management of their hypertensive state. Renal biopsy should be pursued to confirm the diagnosis and clarify prognosis. Measuring the extent of renal damage assists in estimating the possibility of renal recovery. The plan to obtain a renal biopsy should never delay the initiation of ACE inhibitor treatment.

B. Treatment of Scleroderma Renal Crisis

Patients suspected to have SRC should be immediately started on a short-acting ACE inhibitor (ie, captopril) with rapid upward titration to control the hypertensive state. The goal should be to decrease the systolic blood pressure approximately 20 mm Hg every 24 hours. Swifter reductions may lead to renal hypoperfusion. When full-dose ACE inhibitors fail to control blood pressure adequately, additional agents such as calcium channel blockers, angiotensin receptor blockers (less effective than ACE inhibitors when used alone), or other anti-hypertensive drugs should be added. Vasodilators specific to treat scleroderma vascular manifestations should also be considered in refractory cases (eg, endothelin receptor antagonists, prostacyclin).

Prior to the introduction of ACE inhibitors, SRC was the most common cause of death among scleroderma patients. Early diagnosis and rapid initiation of ACE inhibitor therapy have dropped the 1-year mortality rate to less than 15%. Morbidity is still significant as even with aggressive therapy, approximately 50% of SRC patients require dialysis—and only half of these will eventually recover enough to discontinue renal replacement therapy. Approximately 25% of patients eventually have full renal recovery. Renal function can take up to 12 months to improve. Patients with permanent renal failure are considered for renal transplantation. This is associated with an overall survival benefit compared to long-term dialysis. Recurrence of SRC after transplant is uncommon (5%).

Prophylactic use of ACE inhibitors to prevent development of SRC in subjects at risk is not supported. In fact, several studies have demonstrated worse outcomes (including higher mortality) among patients using ACE inhibitors before the onset of SRC.

▶ Musculoskeletal

Musculoskeletal symptoms are extremely common in scleroderma, and can vary from nonspecific stiffness, arthralgias, and myalgias to distinct inflammatory arthritis, myositis, and advanced joint contractures. The type and severity of musculoskeletal pathology depends, in part, on the type of skin involvement (limited vs diffuse), disease duration, and overall disease activity. During early phases of diffuse skin disease, patients may present significant inflammatory manifestations extending from the subcutaneous tissues to the underlying musculoskeletal structures, with presence of joint effusion, tendon friction rubs, and muscle weakness. Late fibrotic stages can be associated with substantial skin atrophy and joint contractures. These can be quite severe and debilitating, especially on the hands, where pain and loss of function can lead to extreme disability. Resorption of the distal finger tufts (acroosteolysis) (Figure 23–9) and deposition of calcium around affected joints can further impair hand function.

A subset of patients can manifest frank synovitis with features of erosive arthritis in apparent overlap condition with rheumatoid arthritis.

Muscle weakness (generalized or focal) is often associated with development of sarcopenia (loss of muscle mass) which can be appreciated in about 20–30% of scleroderma patients. Features of inflammatory polymyositis, typically manifesting with proximal muscle weakness and elevated enzymes, can be present in approximately 5–10% of cases. Patients with positive anti-PM/Scl-100 antibody are at particularly increased risk for this overlapped presentation.

Calcinosis is a typical complication observed in patients with limited or diffuse scleroderma. Calcium deposits usually cluster in areas of limited vascular perfusion and repetitive trauma (digits, extensor surface of forearms, knee caps) or around joints where they can restrict motion. In rare cases, calcium accumulation can become massive and widespread throughout the body surface and soft tissues (tumoral calcinosis).

A. Assessment

Careful physical examination can reveal evidence of synovitis, peritendon inflammation (associated with palpable or even audible tendon friction rubs), muscle atrophy, flexion contractures, or muscle weakness. In patients with prominent

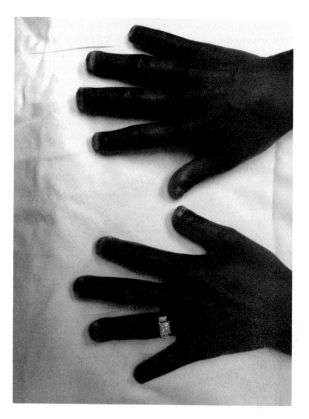

▲ **Figure 23–9.** Acroosteolysis manifesting with resorption of the distal finger tufts.

synovitis, serologic testing to assess positivity for rheumatoid factor and anticitrullinated cyclic protein antibodies and imaging studies to define presence of erosive arthritis are recommended. The nature and severity of muscle involvement should be evaluated with determination of muscle enzymes (creatine phosphokinase, aldolase) levels, electromyography (irritable myopathy), and MRI (inflammation vs atrophy). An excisional muscle biopsy may be considered to confirm the diagnosis and rule out other causes of muscle dysfunction.

B. Treatment of Musculoskeletal Features

Patients who are developing flexion contractures should be encouraged to maintain as much mobility in their joints as possible with daily stretching exercises. Referral to physical therapy and hand therapy can be particularly useful in these cases. Uncontrolled inflammatory joint disease, not responsive to immunomodulation implemented to treat other organ manifestations (eg, skin, lungs), may benefit from the addition to the regimen of MTX and/or TNF-inhibitors. Similarly, patients with overlapping features of inflammatory myopathy may require initiation of myositis-targeted therapy such as MTX, azathioprine, IVIG, or rituximab. In general, the use of glucocorticoids should be minimized in scleroderma patients (particularly in those with diffuse cutaneous disease), due to their association with increased risk of scleroderma renal crisis.

General management of calcinosis revolves around optimizing blood flow to the extremities and avoidance of repeated local trauma, friction, or infection. No pharmacological treatment has shown clear benefit beyond some anecdotal report. Surgical excision of calcinosis or debridement procedures should be limited to cases with significant functional impairment (due to the location and size of calcium deposits), nonhealing superficial ulcerations, or superimposed infections.

Denton CP, Khanna D. Systemic sclerosis. *Lancet.* 2017; 390(10103):1685-1699. [PMID: 28413064]

Distler O, Highland KB, Gahlemann M, et al. Nintedanib for systemic sclerosis-associated interstitial lung disease. *N Engl J Med.* 2019;380(26):2518-2528. [PMID: 31112379]

Kowal-Bielecka O, Fransen J, Avouac J, et al. Update of EULAR recommendations for the treatment of systemic sclerosis. *Ann Rheum Dis.* 2017;76(8):1327-1339. [PMID: 27941129]

Shah RJ, Boin F. Lung transplantation in patients with systemic sclerosis. *Curr Rheumatol Rep.* 2017;19(5):23. [PMID: 28386760]

Sullivan KM, Goldmuntz EA, Keyes-Elstein L, et al. Myeloablative autologous stem-cell transplantation for severe scleroderma. *N Engl J Med.* 2018;378(1):35-47. [PMID: 29298160]

van den Hoogen F, Khanna D, Fransen J, et al. 2013 classification criteria for systemic sclerosis: an American College of Rheumatology/European League against Rheumatism collaborative initiative. *Arthritis Rheum.* 2013;65(11):2737-47. [PMID: 24122180]

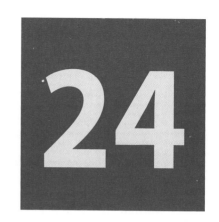

Primary Sjögren Syndrome

Manuel Ramos-Casals, MD, PhD

Pilar Brito-Zerón, MD, PhD

Antoni Sisó-Almirall, MD, PhD

ESSENTIALS OF DIAGNOSIS

- ► Sjögren syndrome (SjS) is a systemic autoimmune disease that presents with sicca symptomatology of mucosal surfaces.

- ► The main sicca features (xerophthalmia and xerostomia) are determined by specific ocular tests (corneal stainings and Schirmer test) and oral investigations (salivary flow measurement and parotid scintigraphy).

- ► The histologic hallmark is a focal lymphocytic infiltration of the exocrine glands, determined by a biopsy of the minor labial salivary glands.

- ► The spectrum of the disease includes systemic features (extraglandular manifestations) in some patients, and is complicated by the development of lymphoma in a small percentage of patients.

- ► Patients with SjS can be characterized by a broad spectrum of laboratory features (cytopenias, hypergammaglobulinemia, and high erythrocyte sedimentation rate) and autoantibodies, of which antinuclear antibodies are the most frequently detected, anti-Ro/SS-A the most specific, and cryoglobulins and hypocomplementemia the main prognostic markers.

► General Considerations

Sjögren syndrome (SjS) is a systemic autoimmune disease that affects the exocrine glands prominently and usually presents as persistent dryness of the mouth and eyes due to functional impairment of the salivary and lacrimal glands. An estimated 2–4 million persons in the United States have SjS, the majority of whom have this condition on a secondary basis—secondary to another underlying rheumatologic disorder. The prevalence of SjS in European countries is estimated to range between 0.05% and 0.72% of the general population, and the annual incidence of primary SjS has been calculated

to be on the order of 3–10 new cases per 100,000/year. SjS primarily affects white perimenopausal women, with a female:male ratio of 14:1 in the largest reported international series. The disease may occur at all ages but typically has its onset in the fourth to sixth decades of life. When sicca symptoms appear in a previously healthy person, the syndrome is classified as primary SjS. When sicca features are found in association with another systemic autoimmune disease, most commonly rheumatoid arthritis, systemic sclerosis, or systemic lupus erythematosus, it is classified as associated SjS.

Major clinical manifestations are summarized in Table 24–1. Although most patients present with sicca symptoms, there are various clinical and laboratory features that may indicate undiagnosed SjS (Table 24–2). The variability in the presentation of SjS may partially explain delays in diagnosis of up to 10 years from the onset of symptoms. SjS is a disease that can be expressed in many guises depending on the specific epidemiologic, clinical, or immunologic features. The management of SjS is centered mainly on the control of sicca features, using substitutive and oral muscarinic agents. Glucocorticoids, immunosuppressive agents, and biologics play a key role in the treatment of systemic disease.

► Clinical Findings

A. Symptoms and Signs

1. Sicca features—Xerostomia, the subjective feeling of oral dryness, is the key feature in the diagnosis of primary SjS, occurring in more than 95% of patients. Other oral symptoms may include soreness, adherence of food to the mucosa, and dysphagia. Reduced salivary volume interferes with basic functions such as speaking or eating. The lack of salivary antimicrobial functions may accelerate local infection, tooth decay, and periodontal disease. Xerostomia can lead to difficulty with dentures and the need for expensive dental restoration, particularly in elderly patients. Various oral signs may be observed in SjS patients. In the early stages, the mouth may appear moist, but as the disease progresses, the usual pooling

Table 24–1. Major clinical manifestations of Sjögren syndrome.

Organ	Manifestations
Mouth	Oral dryness (xerostomia), soreness, caries, periodontal disease, oral candidiasis, parotid swelling
Eyes	Ocular dryness (xerophthalmia), corneal ulcers, conjunctivitis
Nose, ear, and throat	Nasal dryness, chronic cough, sensorineural hearing loss
Skin	Cutaneous dryness, palpable purpura, Ro-associated polycyclic lesions, urticarial lesions
Joints	Arthralgias, nonerosive symmetric arthritis
Lungs	Obstructive chronic pneumopathy, bronchiectasis, interstitial pneumopathy
Cardiovascular	Raynaud phenomenon, pericarditis, autonomic disturbances
Nephro-urologic	Renal tubular acidosis, glomerulonephritis, interstitial cystitis, recurrent renal colic
Peripheral nerve	Mixed polyneuropathy, pure sensitive neuronopathy, mononeuritis multiplex, small-fiber neuropathy
Central nervous system	White matter lesions, cranial nerve involvement (V, VIII, and VII), myelopathy
General symptoms	Low-grade fever, generalized pain, myalgias, fatigue, weakness, polyadenopathies

Table 24–2. Non-sicca manifestations suggestive of Sjögren syndrome.

Clinical features
  Chronic fatigue
  Fever of unknown origin
  Leukocytoclastic vasculitis
  Parotid/submandibular gland swelling (isolated submandibular gland swelling rare)
  Raynaud phenomenon
  Peripheral neuropathy
  Interstitial lung disease
  Renal tubular acidosis
  Annular erythema
  Mother of a baby born with congenital heart block
Laboratory features
  Elevated erythrocyte sedimentation rate (often with normal C-reactive protein)
  Hypergammaglobulinemia
  Leukopenia and thrombocytopenia
  Serum and/or urine monoclonal band
  Positive antinuclear antibodies or rheumatoid factor in an asymptomatic patient

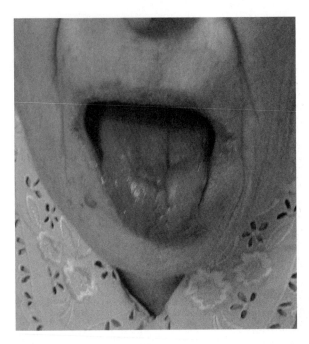

▲ **Figure 24–1.** Dry mouth in a patient with primary SjS: red tongue with depapillation.

of saliva in the floor of the mouth disappears. Typically, the surface of the tongue becomes red and lobulated, with partial or complete depapillation (Figure 24–1). In advanced disease, the oral mucosa appears dry and glazed and tends to form fine wrinkles. Angular cheilitis, erythematous changes of the hard palate, and a red tongue with atrophic papillae strongly suggest *Candida* infection, which occurs frequently in the setting of SjS.

The subjective feeling of ocular dryness is associated with sensations of itching, grittiness, soreness, and dryness, even though the eyes may have a normal appearance. Other ocular complaints include photosensitivity, erythema, eye fatigue, or decreased visual acuity. Environmental irritants, such as smoke, wind, air conditioning, and low humidity, may exacerbate ocular symptoms. Diminished tear secretion may lead to chronic irritation and destruction of corneal and bulbar conjunctival epithelium. This condition is known as *keratoconjunctivitis sicca*. In severe cases, slit-lamp examination may reveal filamentary keratitis, marked by mucus filaments that adhere to damaged areas of the corneal surface (Figure 24–2). Tears also have inherent antimicrobial activity and SjS patients are more susceptible to ocular infections such as blepharitis, bacterial keratitis, and conjunctivitis. Severe ocular complications may include corneal ulceration, vascularization, and opacification.

Reduction or absence of respiratory tract glandular secretions can lead to dryness of the nose, throat, and trachea resulting in persistent hoarseness and chronic, nonproductive

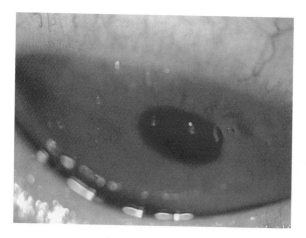

▲ **Figure 24–2.** Dry eye with filamentary keratitis.

cough. Likewise, involvement of the exocrine glands of the skin leads to cutaneous dryness. In female patients with SjS, dryness of the vagina and vulva may result in dyspareunia and pruritus, affecting their quality of life.

Chronic or episodic swelling of the major salivary glands (parotid and submandibular glands) is reported in 10–20% of patients and may commence unilaterally, but often becomes bilateral (Figure 24–3).

2. Systemic manifestations

a. General symptomatology—Patients with primary SjS often have general symptomatology, including generalized pain, fatigue, weakness, sleep disturbances, anxiety, and depression, which may have a much greater impact on the quality of life of patients than sicca features. Fatigue, generalized pain, and weakness are among the most debilitating clinical features of primary SjS. The coexistence of primary SjS with a defined fibromyalgia is reported often. Low-grade fevers may also occur in SjS, usually in young patients with positive immunologic markers.

b. Joint and muscular involvement—Joint involvement, primarily generalized arthralgias, is seen in 50% of patients. Less frequently, joint disease presents as an intermittent symmetric arthritis primarily affecting small joints of the hands (16%). Joint deformity and mild erosions are very rare, except for those cases associated with rheumatoid arthritis. Clinical myopathy is rare but myalgias are frequently observed, often in the setting of concomitant fibromyalgia.

c. Skin—Although the main cutaneous manifestation of patients with primary SjS is skin dryness, a wide spectrum of cutaneous lesions may be observed, the most frequent of which is a small-vessel vasculitis. The skin findings include palpable purpura (Figure 24–4), urticaria, and erythematous macules or papules. The cutaneous vasculitis occurs in the setting of cryoglobulins in 30% of patients. Life-threatening vasculitis is also closely related to cryoglobulinemia.

Primary SjS patients may also have nonvasculitic cutaneous lesions. Some patients with anti-Ro/SS-A antibodies may present with polycyclic, photosensitive cutaneous lesions (Figure 24–5). These lesions are clinically identical to the so-called annular erythema described in Asian SjS patients and subacute cutaneous lupus.

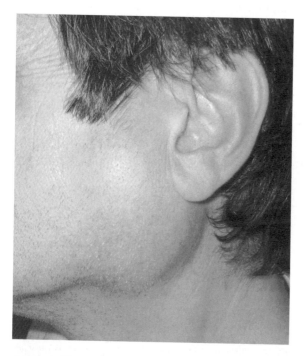

▲ **Figure 24–3.** Parotid enlargement.

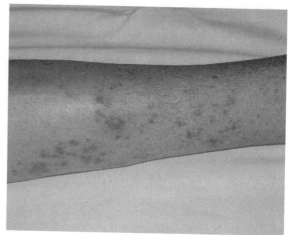

▲ **Figure 24–4.** Cutaneous purpura in the legs in a patient with SjS and cryoglobulinemia.

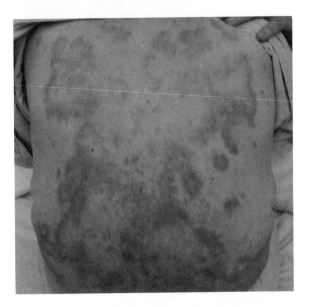

▲ **Figure 24–5.** Polycyclic, photosensitive cutaneous lesions in a 67-year-old woman with primary SjS and anti-Ro/SS-A antibodies.

d. Lungs—Two types of pulmonary involvement, bronchial and interstitial, can complicate primary SjS. Bronchial/bronchiolar involvement is more common than pulmonary fibrosis. The typical symptoms of patients with pulmonary involvement are chronic cough, dyspnea, and recurrent respiratory infections. Studies of respiratory tract involvement in primary SjS have demonstrated that the main underlying pathology in these patients consists of peribronchial infiltrates that lead to small airway disease. CT findings in patients included in large series showed bronchiectasis/bronchiolar abnormalities (50%) and ground glass opacities/interstitial changes (49%) as the most-frequent pulmonary patterns. The most-frequent histopathological diagnoses are nonspecific interstitial pneumonia (45%), bronchiolitis (25%), usual interstitial pneumonia (16%), and lymphocytic interstitial pneumonia (15%). Pleurisy is a rare manifestation of primary SjS and often signals the presence of an additional autoimmune disease, particularly lupus.

e. Cardiovascular features—Raynaud phenomenon, with a prevalence of 10–20%, is probably the most common vascular feature observed in primary SjS. The clinical course of Raynaud phenomenon in primary SjS is mild. The development of vascular complications (eg, digital loss, digital pulp pitting, or fingertip infarctions) suggests the possibility of underlying limited systemic sclerosis. Cardiac involvement is rarely observed, with pericardial effusions (usually mild and asymptomatic) being the most frequent feature. Some studies have described autonomic cardiovascular disturbances.

f. Gut—Gastrointestinal involvement is uncommon in SjS. *Helicobacter pylori* infection should be excluded in patients with gastritis because of the close association with gastric mucosa-associated lymphoid tissue (MALT) lymphoma. Primary biliary cirrhosis and type 1 autoimmune hepatitis also occur with an increased frequency in SjS.

g. Nephro-urologic involvement—Overt renal involvement was found in only 5% of the nearly 10,000 patients included in the largest reported series. The main types of renal involvement described are interstitial renal disease, often associated with renal tubular acidosis, and glomerulonephritis. Renal tubular acidosis is clinically symptomatic in two-thirds of cases but can be lead to a hypokalemic weakness/paralysis that sometimes presents with severe respiratory failure. Renal tubular acidosis can also lead to renal colic induced by nephrocalcinosis, or to osteomalacia and pathological fractures or polyuria/polydipsia (diabetes insipidus). In patients with primary SjS associated with glomerulonephritis, the main results of renal biopsy disclose membranoproliferative (mainly related to cryoglobulinemia), proliferative and membranous GN; a high rate of adverse outcomes has been reported in these patients. Finally, interstitial lymphocytic cystitis, sometimes with severe symptoms, has been reported in some SjS patients.

h. Neurologic involvement—Although earlier studies described central nervous system involvement as a frequent extraglandular manifestation of primary SjS, clinically significant central nervous system involvement is actually very rare. Nevertheless, SjS is occasionally associated with severe, puzzling, and disabling neurological features. A pure sensory neuronopathy (ganglionopathy) is rare but recognized as a characteristic neurologic complication of primary SjS. The ganglionopathy, caused by damage to the sensory neurons of the dorsal root and gasserian ganglia by a process that remains obscure, is associated with striking ataxia and severe deficits in proprioception. As an example, patients are unable to identify objects placed in their hands (eg, keys or coins) if their eyes are closed. Another more common neurologic feature of SjS—but one that still occurs in only a minority of patients—is small-fiber neuropathy. Mononeuritis multiplex develops in some patients with an SjS-associated vasculitis, leading to foot drop and other classic features of that syndrome. A small percentage of patients with SjS develop cranial nerve palsies, usually of the trigeminal (V) or facial (VII) cranial pairs. The pathophysiology of these cranial nerve palsies remains uncertain. Finally, some SjS patients present with transverse myelitis or the combination of a myelopathy and optic neuritis, similar to neuromyelitis optica.

i. Other organs—Nearly one-third of patients with primary SjS have thyroid disease. Subclinical hypothyroidism is the most frequent finding, especially in patients with antithyroid autoantibodies. Although ear, nose, and throat involvement has been little studied in patients with primary SjS, some studies have described sensorineural hearing loss in nearly 25% of

SjS patients. Psychiatric disorders, including depression and anxiety, are frequently described in patients with SjS.

B. Laboratory Findings

The results of routine laboratory tests and immunologic markers in primary SjS are summarized in Table 24–3. The most frequent laboratory findings are cytopenia, elevated erythrocyte sedimentation rate, and hypergammaglobulinemia (20–30%). The differential leukocyte count has been studied in large series of patients with primary SjS and the most commonly reported abnormality was lymphopenia, closely followed by neutropenia. Cytopenias, which are found more commonly in patients with autoantibodies directed against the Ro antigen, are seldom severe enough to cause clinical consequences. Erythrocyte sedimentation rate levels correlate closely with the percentage of circulating gamma globulins (hypergammaglobulinemia), while serum C-reactive protein levels are usually normal. Highly elevated serum C-reactive protein levels in a patient with primary SjS

Table 24–3. The laboratory evaluation in Sjögren syndrome.

Test	Typical Result
Complete blood cell count	• Normochromic, normocytic anemia. Isolated cases of hemolytic anemia • Mild leukopenia (3–4 × 10⁹/L); lymphopenia, neutropenia • Mild thrombocytopenia (80–150 × 10⁹/L)
Erythrocyte sedimentation rate (ESR) and C-reactive protein (CRP)	• Elevated ESR (>50 mm/h) in 20–30% of cases, especially in patients with hypergammaglobulinemia • Normal values of CRP
Serum protein	• Hypergammaglobulinemia • Monoclonal band
Liver function tests	• Raised transaminases (discard hepatitis C virus or autoimmune hepatitis) • Raised alkaline phosphatase and/or bilirubin (discard primary biliary cirrhosis)
Electrolytes and urinalysis	• Proteinuria, hematuria (glomerulonephritis) • Hypokalemia, low plasma bicarbonate, and low blood pH (renal tubular acidosis)
Immunological tests	• Antinuclear antibody: positive in more than 80% • Rheumatoid factor: positive in 40–50% of patients, often leading to diagnostic confusion with rheumatoid arthritis • Positive anti-Ro/SS-A (30–70%) and anti-La/SS-B (25–40%) • Complement levels are decreased in 10–20% of patients • Cryoglobulins present in 10–20% of patients

should raise the suspicion of an infection. Finally, circulating monoclonal immunoglobulins, most commonly monoclonal IgG, are detected in nearly 20% of patients with primary SjS.

C. Special Tests

1. Assessment of oral involvement—Methods used to assess oral involvement include the salivary flow rate, sialochemistry, sialography, or scintigraphy (Table 24–4). These tests are typically cumbersome or expensive, however, and are seldom used in routine clinical practice. Ultrasonography is a noninvasive method that may provide useful information about the etiology of parotid enlargement in undiagnosed patients, but its ability to distinguish SjS reliably from other causes of parotid enlargement remains questionable. The clinical applicability of ultrasonography in SjS remains uncertain at this time.

2. Assessment of ocular involvement—Assessments of ocular dryness are more practical and widely used. The main ocular tests (see Table 24–4) include measurement of lachrymal gland output (Schirmer test) and analysis of the corneal surface by the use of dyes that stain degenerated or dead cells (corneal stainings); several scores are used to categorize the degree of corneal damage (Figure 24–6). The Schirmer test for the eye quantitatively measures tear formation via placement of filter paper in the lower conjunctival sac. The test can be performed with or without the instillation of anesthetic drops to prevent reflex tearing. The test result is positive when less than 5 mm of paper is wetted after 5 minutes. Slit-lamp examination is useful in detecting destroyed conjunctival epithelium caused by desiccation.

3. Immunologic tests—The main immunologic markers found in primary SjS are antinuclear antibodies, anti-Ro/SS-A or anti-La/SS-B antibodies, rheumatoid factor, hypocomplementemia, and cryoglobulins (see Table 24–3). Antinuclear antibodies, detected in more than 80% of cases, are the most frequently detected antibodies in primary SjS. High ANA titers help differentiate SjS from nonautoimmune causes of sicca syndrome and indicate which patients need a more detailed serological evaluation. Anti-Ro/SS-A and La/SS-B antibodies, detected in 30–70% of patients, are highly specific for SjS. Moreover, these autoantibodies are strongly associated with the potential for developing extraglandular features, particularly cutaneous lesions, neurologic features, congenital heart block, and cytopenias. In nearly 50% of cases, patients with primary SjS are rheumatoid factor positive.

Hypocomplementemia and cryoglobulinemia (see Chapter 32) are two closely related immunologic markers that have been linked with more severe SjS. Recent studies have associated low complement levels and cryoglobulins (usually type II, which are found in 10–20% of patients) with an increased risk of lymphoma. Serum monoclonal gammopathy often indicates the presence of an underlying type II mixed cryoglobulinemia.

Table 24–4. Main diagnostic tests for the study of salivary and lachrymal dysfunction in Sjögren syndrome.

Diagnostic Test	Technical Equipment	Abnormal Values	Practical Issues
Unstimulated salivary flow rates (UWF)	Graduated test tube/preweighed tube	<1.5 mL collected over a 15 min (<0.1 mL/min)	Results may be influenced by age, length of disease, comorbidities, temperature, or medications.
Stimulated salivary flow rates (SWF)	Graduated test tube/preweighed tube Chewing gums or lemon juice	<0.2–0.3 mL/min collected over a 15 min	Better correlation with histopathological results or structural glandular damage.
Salivary scintigraphy	Radioactive tracer, technetium 99 Gamma scintillation camera	Schall categorical classification into 4 grades (from normal to very severe involvement)	Severe involvement (grade IV) at diagnosis associated with higher systemic activity and poor outcomes.
Schirmer test I	Filter paper (no. 41 whatman) Anesthesic	≤5 mm of the paper after 5 min	Evaluates baseline secretion
Schirmer test II	Filter paper (no. 41 whatman)	≤10 mm of the paper after 5 min	Measures baseline plus reflex secretion
Corneal stainings	Dyes (fluorescein, rose Bengal, and lissamine green) Slit lamp Blue cobalt filter	van Bijsterveld score ≥4 Oxford scale score ≥III OSS score ≥3	Rose begal (nonvital dye) has been substituted by lissamine green (vital dye) Studies in development are suggesting the increase of abnormal OSS score to 5

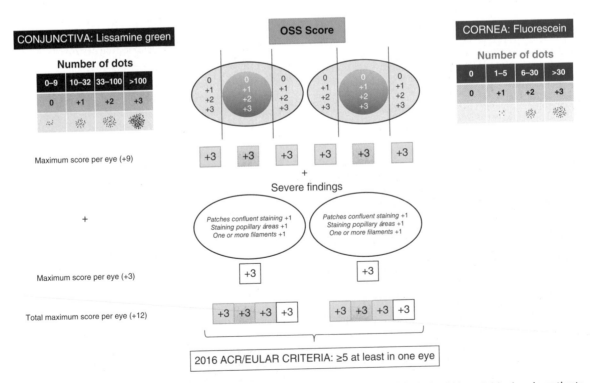

▲ **Figure 24–6.** The Ocular Staining Score (OSS): a quantitative method of grading keratoconjunctivitis sicca in patients with primary SjS.

4. Salivary gland biopsy—Minor salivary gland biopsy, a useful test in the evaluation of patients with possible SjS, is often essential in parsing the differential diagnosis of patients who may present with sicca symptoms (eg, sarcoidosis, amyloidosis, IgG4-RD). Focal lymphocytic sialadenitis, defined as multiple, dense aggregates of 50 or more lymphocytes in perivascular or periductal areas, is the characteristic histopathologic feature of SjS. The key requirements for a correct histologic evaluation are an adequate number of informative lobules (at least four) and the determination of an average "focus score." A focus is defined as a cluster of at least 50 lymphocytes (Figure 24–7). A focus score of 1 is compatible with SjS. Nonspecific inflammatory findings are quite common in biopsy samples of minor salivary glands in healthy control populations, however, so clinicopathological correlation is essential to the correct interpretation of these biopsies.

Differential Diagnosis

Sicca syndrome has many causes. Therefore, the diagnosis of SjS requires not only the presence of sicca symptoms but also objective evidence of dry eyes and mouth and laboratory evidence of autoimmunity. The most frequent cause of the sicca syndrome is the chronic use of medications leading to mucosal dryness. These include antihypertensives, antihistamines, and antidepressants. Assuming that medications are excluded as a cause of sicca syndrome, should be considered (Table 24–5). First, some processes may mimic the clinical picture of SjS through nonlymphocytic infiltration of the exocrine glands by granulomas (sarcoidosis, granulomatosis with polyangiitis, tuberculosis), a lymphoplasmacytic infiltrate (IgG4-related disease), amyloid proteins (amyloidosis), or malignant cells (hematologic neoplasia). Second, extrinsic factors, mainly chronic viral infections such as hepatitis C virus or HIV, may induce a lymphocytic infiltration of exocrine glands. Third, patients may have primary SjS or SjS associated with other autoimmune diseases.

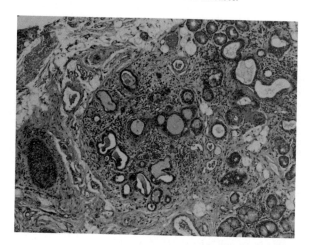

▲ **Figure 24–7.** Focal lymphocytc sialadenitis. (See color insert.)

Table 24–5. Classification of Sjögren syndrome (SjS): primary, associated, and mimicked SjS.

1. **Primary SjS**
2. **Associated SjS**
   Systemic autoimmune diseases
      Systemic lupus erythematosus
      Systemic sclerosis
      Rheumatoid arthritis
      Sarcoidosis
      Inflammatory myopathies
      Mixed connective tissue disease
   Organ-specific autoimmune diseases
      Primary biliary cholangitis
      Autoimmune thyroiditis
      Multiple sclerosis
      Diabetes mellitus
      Celiac disease
   Chronic viral infections
      Chronic HCV infection (Mediterranean countries)
      HTLV-1 infection (Asian countries)
      HIV infection
3. **Mimicked SjS**
   Other diseases infiltrating exocrine glands
      Granulomatous diseases (sarcoidosis and tuberculosis)
      Amyloidosis
      Neoplasias (lymphoma)
      IgG4-related disease
      Type V hyperlipidemia
   Other processes
      Graft-versus-host disease
      Eosinophilia-myalgia syndrome
      Radiation injury
      Medication-related dryness

HCV, hepatitis C virus; HTLV, human T-cell lymphoma virus.

Diagnosis

Sicca symptoms often receive little attention and are often inappropriately considered to be trivial by physicians. These symptoms have a spectrum of severity, however, and are often intensely distressing to patients. Early diagnosis and timely management can relieve symptoms of dry mouth and may prevent or slow the progress of the oral complications of SjS, including dental caries, oral candidiasis, and periodontal disease. Untreated severe dry eye can result in corneal ulcers. Table 24–6 summarizes the current classification criteria, and Figure 24–8 the algorithm diagnostic following these criteria.

Complications

Primary SjS usually progresses slowly, with no rapid deterioration in salivary function or dramatic changes in sicca symptoms. The main exceptions to this benign course are the development of systemic manifestations and the occurrence of lymphoma in a small minority of patients.

Table 24–6. American College of Rheumatology/European League Against Rheumatism classification criteria for primary Sjögren syndrome.

The classification of primary Sjögren syndrome applies to any individual who meets the inclusion criteria, does not have any of the conditions listed as exclusion criteria, and has a score of at least 4 when the weights from the 5 criteria items below are summed.

Inclusion Criteria

1. Patients with ocular and/or oral dryness, defined as a positive response to at least 1 of the following questions:
   - Have you had daily, persistent, troublesome dry eyes for more than 3 months?
   - Do you have a recurrent sensation of sand or gravel in the eyes?
   - Do you use tear substitutes more than three times a day?
   - Have you had a daily feeling of dry mouth for more than 3 months?
   - Do you frequently drink liquids to aid in swallowing dry food?

   or

2. Patients with suspected systemic Sjögren (at least 1 domain with a positive item in the European League Against Rheumatism SS Disease Activity Index questionnaire)

Exclusion Criteria

Prior diagnosis of any of the following conditions, which would exclude diagnosis of SS and participation in SS studies or therapeutic trials because of overlapping clinical features or interference with criteria tests:
   - history of head and neck radiation treatment
   - active hepatitis C infection (with confirmation by polymerase chain reaction)
   - AIDS
   - sarcoidosis
   - amyloidosis
   - graft-versus-host disease
   - IgG4-related disease

Criteria Items (score)

1. Labial salivary gland with focal lymphocytic sialadenitis and focus score of ≥1 foci/4 mm² (*Score = 3*)
   The histopathologic examination should be performed by a pathologist with expertise in the diagnosis of focal lymphocytic sialadenitis and focus score count, using the protocol described by Daniels et al.
2. Anti-SSA/Ro positive (*Score = 3*)
3. Ocular Staining Score (OSS-) ≥5 (or van Bijsterveld score ≥4) in at least one eye (*Score = 1*)
4. Schirmer test ≤5 mm/5 min in at least one eye (*Score = 1*)
5. Unstimulated whole saliva flow rate ≤0.1 mL/min (*Score = 1*)

Primary SjS patients are at higher risk for lymphoma than are healthy individuals and patients with other autoimmune diseases. The long-term risk of lymphoma for patients with primary SjS is often estimated to be 5%, but the risk of this complication is concentrated in a subset of patients with florid clinical and laboratory features of extra-nodal SjS: cryoglobulinemia, hypocomplementemia, CD4-lymphopenia, and palpable purpura. The few studies that have analyzed the causes and rates of mortality in these patients compared to the general population found that the overall mortality of patients with primary SjS increased only in patients with these adverse predictors.

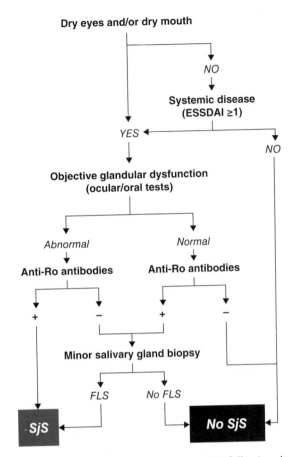

▲ **Figure 24–8.** Diagnostic algorithm of SjS following the 2016 ACR/EULAR classification criteria.

Lymphomas that develop in primary SjS patients are extranodal in 80% of cases. The most common site is the parotid glands. Persistently hard, often asymmetric glandular enlargement should alert the clinician to the possibility of a lymphoma. Ninety percent of primary SjS patients in whom lymphoma develops have histories of major salivary gland enlargement during the disease course. Lymphomas developing in SjS may also occur in the gastrointestinal tract or lungs. They often begin as B cell MALT lymphomas or, in lymph nodes, as marginal zone lymphomas. After years of slow progression, these low-grade tumors may progress to rapidly growing, high-grade lymphomas.

The European League Against Rheumatism (EULAR) has recently promoted an international collaboration between primary SjS experts to develop consensus disease activity indexes. Two indexes have been developed: (1) a patient-administered questionnaire to assess subjective symptoms, called the EULAR Sjögren's Syndrome Patients Reported Index (ESSPRI), and (2) a systemic activity index to assess systemic complications, called the EULAR Sjögren's Syndrome Disease Activity Index (ESSDAI), that includes the main systemic features ordered organ-by-organ (Table 24–7).

Table 24–7. ESSDAI scoring of systemic activity in SjS.

Organ (Weight)	Clinical Features	Low Activity	Moderate Activity	High Activity
Constitutional (3)	Fever/night sweats	37.5°C–38.5°C	>38.5°C	–
	Involuntary weight loss	5–10% of body weight	>10% of body weight	–
Lymphadenopathy (4)	Lymphadenopathy	≥1 cm or ≥2 cm (inguinal region)	≥2 cm or ≥3 cm (inguinal region)	–
	Splenomegaly	–	Clinically palpable or imaging-proven	–
	B-cell neoplasia	–	–	Current
Glandular (2)	Parotid swelling	≤3 cm	>3 cm	–
	Submandibular swelling	Limited	Important	–
	Lachrymal gland swelling	Limited	Important	–
Articular (2)	Arthralgias (hands, wrists, ankles, and feet)	With morning stiffness >30 min	–	–
	Synovitis	–	1–5 joints	≥6 joints
Cutaneous (3)	Erythema multiforma	Clinically proven	–	–
	Cutaneous vasculitis	–	Limited extension	Diffuse extension and/or ulcers
	Urticarial vasculitis	–	Limited extension	Diffuse extension
	Purpura	–	Limited to feet and ankle	Diffuse extension
	Subacute cutaneous lupus	–	Clinically proven	–
Pulmonary (5)	Persistent cough	With normal imaging	–	–
	Bronchial involvement	With normal imaging	–	–
	ILD demonstrated by HRCT with dyspnea grade	NHYA I	NHYA II	NHYA III/IV
	ILD demonstrated by HRCT with DLCO%	>70%	40–70%	<40%
	ILD demonstrated by HRCT with FVC%	>80%	60–80%	<60%
Renal (5)	Tubular acidosis	GFR ≥60 mL/min	GFR <60 mL/min, or biopsy-proven	–
	Proteinuria	0.5–1 g/24 h	1–1.5 g/24 h	>1.5 g/24 h
	Glomerular involvement	–	Extra-membranous (biopsy-proven)	Hematuria, GFR <60 mL/min, proliferative, cryo-related
Muscular (6)	Abnormal EMG or biopsy with	No weakness	Deficit 4/5	Deficit 3 or less/5
	Raised CK values	N <CK ≤ 2N	2N <CK ≤ 4N	CK > 4N
PNS (5)	Pure sensory axonal polyneuropathy	Confirmed by NCS	Cryo-related	–
	Axonal sensory-motor neuropathy or CIPD	–	Motor deficit 4/5	Motor deficit 3 or less/5
	Ganglionopathy or CIPD with ataxia	–	Mild/moderate	Severe
	Mononeuritis multiplex	–	–	Cryo-related
	Peripheral cranial nerve involvement	Trigeminal	Others than V	–
CNS (5)	Central cranial nerve involvement	–	Proven	–
	Multiple sclerosis-like syndrome	–	Pure sensory impairment	Motor deficit
	Cognitive impairment	–	Proven	–
	Cerebral vasculitis presenting with	–	–	Cerebrovascular accident/transient ischemic attack
	Seizures	–	–	Proven
	Transverse myelitis	–	–	Proven
	Lymphocytic meningitis	–	–	Proven
Hematological (2)	Neutrophils	1000–1500/mm^3	500–1000/mm^3	<500/mm^3
	Hemoglobin	10–12 g/dL	8–10 g/dL	<8 g/dL
	Lymphocytes	500–1000/mm^3	≤500/mm^3	–
	Platelets	100,000–150,000/mm^3	50,000–100,000/mm^3	<50,000/mm^3
Biological (1)	Serum immunoelectrophoresis	Clonal component	–	–
	Complement levels	Low C3, C4 and/or CH50	–	–
	Serum igg levels	16–20 g/L	>20 g/L, or <5 g/L	–
	Cryoglobulins	–	Positive	–
	Hypogammaglobulinemia	–	Recent onset	–

Treatment

At present, there is no treatment shown to be consistently capable of modifying the pathophysiology underlying SjS. Limited evidence exists to support the use of most drugs commonly used in primary SjS.

Treatment of sicca manifestations is mainly symptomatic and is typically intended to limit the damage resulting from chronic involvement. For ocular dryness, the frequent use of preservative-free tear substitutes is recommended. Ocular lubricating ointments are usually reserved for nocturnal use. Controlled trials support the use of topical 0.05% cyclosporine twice daily for patients with moderate to severe dry eye disease. Severe cases of ocular dryness should be comanaged with an ophthalmologist.

For oral dryness, sialogogues such as pilocarpine or cevimeline are often highly effective in inducing increases in saliva production. The dose of these medications, which are usually well-tolerated, should be pushed to high levels; for example, 5 mg every 8 hours for pilocarpine and 30 mg every 8 hours for cevimeline. In patients with contraindications or intolerance to muscarinic agonists, N-acetylcysteine may be an alternative. Alcohol and smoking should be avoided and thorough oral hygiene is essential. SjS patients should have dental cleanings every 6 months.

The management of systemic SjS features is generally organ-specific. Glucocorticoids, immunosuppressive agents and biologics are limited to potentially severe scenarios. Nonsteroidal anti-inflammatory drugs usually provide relief from the minor musculoskeletal symptoms of SjS, as well as from painful parotid swelling. Hydroxychloroquine may be used in patients with fatigue, arthralgias, and myalgias. For patients with moderate extraglandular involvement (mainly arthritis, extensive cutaneous purpura, and nonsevere peripheral neuropathy), 0.1–0.3 mg/kg/day of prednisone may suffice. For patients with internal organ involvement (pulmonary alveolitis, glomerulonephritis, or severe neurologic features), a combination of prednisone (using methylprednisolone intravenous pulses in potentially life-threatening involvements) and immunosuppressive agents can be considered. Unfortunately, there is little evidence to support the efficacy of conventional DMARDs such as cyclophosphamide, azathioprine, or mycophenolate mofetil.

Tumor necrosis factor inhibitors have been shown to be ineffective in primary SjS in controlled clinical trials. B-cell targeted agents may be useful in some settings but data supporting their use are inconsistent. Rituximab has been suggested to improve extraglandular features (vasculitis, neuropathy, glomerulonephritis, and arthritis) in uncontrolled studies but does not ameliorate the sicca features of this disease. Rituximab is therefore considered an off-label "rescue" therapy in patients with extraglandular SjS whose disease features are refractory to standard treatment. The medication is generally well tolerated in SjS, however, and if it is to be used some consideration should be given to using it early in patients with extra-grandular disease and findings suggestive of an aggressive course.

Brito-Zerón P, Acar-Denizli N, Zeher M, et al; EULAR-SS Task Force Big Data Consortium. Influence of geolocation and ethnicity on the phenotypic expression of primary Sjögren's syndrome at diagnosis in 8310 patients: a cross-sectional study from the Big Data Sjögren Project Consortium. *Ann Rheum Dis.* 2017;76(6):1042-1050. [PMID: 27899373]

Brito-Zerón P, Baldini C, Bootsma H, et al. Sjögren syndrome. *Nat Rev Dis Primers.* 2016;2:16047. [PMID: 27383445]

Brito-Zerón P, Kostov B, Fraile G, et al; SS Study Group GEAS-SEMI. Characterization and risk estimate of cancer in patients with primary Sjögren syndrome. *J Hematol Oncol.* 2017;10(1):90. [PMID: 28416003]

Brito-Zerón P, Theander E, Baldini C, et al. Early diagnosis of primary Sjögren's syndrome: EULAR-SS task force clinical recommendations. *Expert Rev Clin Immunol.* 2016;12(2):137-56. [PMID: 26691952]

Carsons SE, Vivino FB, Parke A, et al. Treatment guidelines for rheumatologic manifestations of Sjögren's syndrome: use of biologic agents, management of fatigue, and inflammatory musculoskeletal pain. *Arthritis Care Res (Hoboken).* 2017; 69(4):517-527. [PMID: 27390247]

Fisher BA, Jonsson R, Daniels T, et al. Standardisation of labial salivary gland histopathology in clinical trials in primary Sjögren's syndrome. *Ann Rheum Dis.* 2017;76(7):1161-1168. [PMID: 27965259]

Nocturne G, Cornec D, Seror R, Mariette X. Use of biologics in Sjögren's syndrome. *Rheum Dis Clin North Am.* 2016;42(3): 407-17. [PMID: 27431344]

Price EJ, Rauz S, Tappuni AR, et al. The British Society for Rheumatology guideline for the management of adults with primary Sjögren's Syndrome. *Rheumatology (Oxford).* 2017; 56(10):1643-1647. [PMID: 28957572]

Ramos-Casals M, Brito-Zerón P, Seror R, et al. Characterization of systemic disease in primary Sjögren's syndrome: EULAR-SS Task Force recommendations for articular, cutaneous, pulmonary and renal involvements. *Rheumatology (Oxford).* 2015;54(12): 2230-2238. [PMID: 28379527]

Seror R, Theander E, Brun JG, et al. Validation of EULAR primary Sjögren's syndrome disease activity (ESSDAI) and patient indexes (ESSPRI). *Ann Rheum Dis.* 2015;74(5):859-66. [PMID: 24442883]

Shiboski CH, Shiboski SC, Seror R, et al; International Sjögren's Syndrome Criteria Working Group. 2016 American College of Rheumatology/European League Against Rheumatism classification criteria for primary Sjögren's syndrome: A consensus and data-driven methodology involving three international patient cohorts. *Ann Rheum Dis.* 2017;76(1):9-16. [PMID: 27785888]

Zero DT, Brennan MT, Daniels TE, et al; Sjögren's Syndrome Foundation Clinical Practice Guidelines Committee. Clinical practice guidelines for oral management of Sjögren disease: dental caries prevention. *J Am Dent Assoc.* 2016;147(4):295-305. [PMID: 26762707]

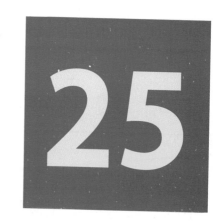

Autoimmune Myopathies, Immune-Mediated Necrotizing Myopathies, & Their Mimickers

25

Brittany Adler, MD

Alex Truong, MD

Andrew L. Mammen, MD, PhD

Lisa Christopher-Stine, MD, MPH

ESSENTIALS OF DIAGNOSIS

- ▶ Symmetric proximal muscle weakness progressing over weeks to months.
- ▶ Elevated muscle enzymes, including creatine kinase (CK), aldolase, aspartate aminotransferase (AST), and alanine aminotransferase (ALT).
- ▶ An "irritable myopathy" shown by electromyography (EMG).
- ▶ Magnetic resonance imaging (MRI) of affected muscles reveals evidence of edema, fasciitis, or both.
- ▶ Heliotrope rash or Gottron sign/papules are pathognomonic of dermatomyositis.
- ▶ Muscle biopsy in dermatomyositis and polymyositis frequently reveals endomysial, perimysial, and perivascular lymphocytic infiltrates. Perifascicular atrophy is pathognomonic of dermatomyositis.
- ▶ Muscle biopsy with necrotizing and regenerating muscle fibers is characteristic of the immune-mediated necrotizing myopathies, including statin-associated autoimmune myopathy.
- ▶ A careful family history, medication list review, physical examination, laboratory evaluation, and muscle biopsy are all critical parts of the evaluation.
- ▶ Exclusion of alternative diagnoses, such as an inherited muscle disease or toxic myopathy, is essential.

General Considerations

Polymyositis, dermatomyositis, and the immune-mediated necrotizing myopathies comprise a group of rare, heterogeneous autoimmune myopathies with an approximate incidence of 1 case per 100,000 per year. Although polymyositis is virtually unheard of in children, juvenile dermatomyositis is well described and occurs most commonly between the ages of 10 and 15 years. Immune-mediated necrotizing myopathy has also been described in children. In adults, the autoimmune myopathies can occur at any age but appear to peak between the ages of 45 and 60 years.

Muscle, skin, and lung are the organs most commonly affected in the autoimmune myopathies. Dermatomyositis is typically distinguished from polymyositis by the presence of a distinct rash, although occasionally a diagnosis of dermatomyositis can be made in the absence of a rash if the classic muscle biopsy features of dermatomyositis are present. These patients are said to have "dermatomyositis sine dermatitis" (Table 25–1). Although most patients with dermatomyositis have both skin and muscle involvement, patients occasionally have only the skin manifestations and are classified as having "dermatomyositis sine myositis" or amyopathic dermatomyositis.

In both polymyositis and dermatomyositis, muscle biopsies are characterized by lymphocytic infiltrates. Perifascicular atrophy is pathognomonic of dermatomyositis. The immune-mediated necrotizing myopathies, which include statin-associated autoimmune myopathy, have a distinct appearance on muscle biopsy: prominent myofiber degeneration, muscle necrosis, and a paucity of inflammatory cells.

Clinical Findings

A. Symptoms and Signs

Symmetric proximal muscle weakness evolving over weeks to months is the presenting symptom in most patients. Typical complaints include difficulty rising from a low chair, walking up steps, and washing one's hair. In more severe cases, weakness of the neck flexors, pharyngeal weakness, and diaphragmatic weakness can cause head drop, dysphagia, and respiratory compromise, respectively. On physical examination, weakness of the proximal arm muscles, especially the deltoids, but often including the biceps and triceps, is expected. Hip flexors are the most commonly affected leg muscles but the hamstrings and quadriceps are also frequently weak. Subtle leg weakness can be detected by having the patient attempt to rise from a 6-inch high stool without using their arms.

Table 25–1. Classification of the autoimmune myopathies.

1. Polymyositis (PM)
2. Immune-mediated necrotizing myopathy (IMNM)
3. Dermatomyositis
   a. Dermatomyositis sine myositis (amyopathic dermatomyositis)
   b. Dermatomyositis sine dermatitis
   c. Juvenile dermatomyositis

As a general rule, distal weakness in the autoimmune myopathies should occur only in the presence of severe proximal muscle weakness. Isolated or even mild distal weakness should always raise doubts about the diagnosis of dermatomyositis, polymyositis, or immune-mediated necrotizing myopathy. The examiner can test whether distal weakness is present by evaluating the strength of wrist flexors, wrist extensors, distal finger flexors, and finger extensors. In the lower extremities, ankle dorsiflexion and ankle plantarflexion strength should be assessed manually and by having the patient attempt to walk on their heels and toes. The presence of facial weakness or scapular winging (Figures 25–1 and 25–2) should

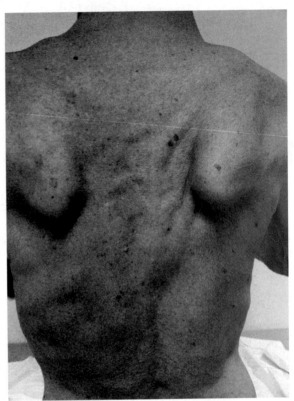

▲ **Figure 25–2.** Scapular winging on attempted forward arm flexion.

be assessed. Both of these findings are extremely atypical in autoimmune myopathy and suggest the possibility of an alternative diagnosis (see section Differential Diagnosis).

Other symptoms in addition to muscle weakness may be present, including arthralgias or frank arthritis, myalgias, severe fatigue, Raynaud phenomenon, or symptoms of another overlapping rheumatologic condition such as systemic lupus erythematosus or systemic sclerosis. Dyspnea may reflect diaphragmatic weakness or, especially in patients with the antisynthetase syndrome (see later), interstitial lung disease. The latter is often associated with a persistent dry cough, velcro-like crackles on chest auscultation, and decreased oxygen saturation with exercise. Serious cardiac manifestations also occur, albeit rarely, in the autoimmune myopathies.

Patients with dermatomyositis may present with cutaneous manifestations either before or after the development of muscle symptoms. **Gottron's papules** are raised, violaceous lesions located at the extensor surfaces of the metacarpophalangeal, proximal interphalangeal, and the distal interphalangeal joints (Figure 25–3). The **Gottron's sign** is an erythematous rash involving these sites that can also be found at the extensor surfaces of the elbows and knees. The heliotrope rash is a red or purplish discoloration of the

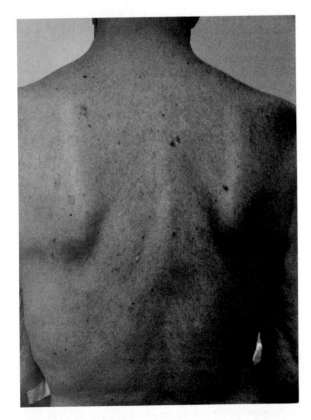

▲ **Figure 25–1.** Evaluation of scapular winging (see Figure 25–2).

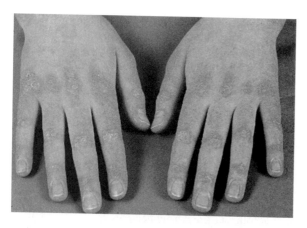

▲ **Figure 25–3.** Dermatomyositis. Gottron papules on the dorsa of the hands and fingers, especially over the metacarpophalangeal and interphalangeal joints. (Reproduced, with permission, from Wolff K, Johnson RA, Suurmond D. *Fitzpatrick's Color Atlas and Synopsis of Clinical Dermatology.* 6th ed. McGraw-Hill, 2009.)

eyelids (Figure 25–4). In patients with dark skin, a heliotrope may appear hyperpigmented.

Both the heliotrope rash and Gottron's papules and sign are pathognomonic for dermatomyositis, but less specific rashes may also be noted. These include an erythematous or poikilodermatous rash across the posterior neck and shoulders (the shawl sign) and a similar rash on the anterior neck and chest (the V-sign). In some patients, dermatomyositis-associated rashes are photosensitive. In others, particularly those with the antisynthetase syndrome (see later), hyperkeratotic skin thickening on the radial surfaces of the fingers or

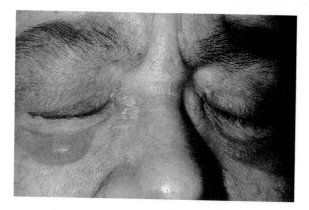

▲ **Figure 25–4.** Dermatomyositis. Heliotrope erythema of upper eyelids and edema of the lower lids. (Reproduced, with permission, from Wolff K, Johnson RA, Suurmond D. *Fitzpatrick's Color Atlas and Synopsis of Clinical Dermatology.* 6th ed. McGraw-Hill, 2009.)

toes (hiker's feet), often with painful cracking, may develop. These findings in the hands and feet are known, respectively, as mechanic's hands or hiker's feet. Periungual telangiectasias and nailfold capillary changes identical to those found in scleroderma may develop.

No definite environmental exposures have been linked with the development of dermatomyositis or polymyositis. Although increased UV light exposure may predispose patients to dermatomyositis, a history of intense sun exposure is elicited only occasionally from patients with this condition. In contrast, a distinct form of immune-mediated necrotizing myopathy is triggered by statin use. Patients with that condition have autoantibodies directed against HMG-CoA reductase, the pharmacologic target of statins (see below).

B. Laboratory Findings

Creatine kinase (CK), aldolase, aspartate aminotransferase (AST), alanine aminotransferase (ALT), and lactate dehydrogenase are released from damaged muscle. Elevated serum concentrations are often but not always found in patients with autoimmune myopathy. In some patients with dermatomyositis and polymyositis, aldolase may be elevated in the presence of a normal CK level. Elevated AST and ALT levels are often misinterpreted as evidence of liver disease in patients with myopathy. To exclude liver disease, a serum gamma-glutamyl transferase (GGT) level can be measured. GGT is usually released along with AST and ALT in liver disease but not from damaged muscle.

As in other systemic autoimmune diseases, there is a strong association of autoantibodies directed against specific autoantigens with distinct clinical phenotypes. The term "myositis-specific autoantibody" has been used to describe these antibodies, which are found in ~60–80% of patients with polymyositis, dermatomyositis, and immune-mediated necrotizing myopathy but usually not other rheumatic diseases or neuromuscular disorders (Table 25–2).

Autoantibodies recognizing one of the aminoacyl tRNA synthetases (eg, anti-Jo-1) are the most common of the myositis-specific autoantibodies and occur in ~30% of patients with polymyositis or dermatomyositis. In addition to an autoimmune myopathy, patients with antisynthetase autoantibodies may have one or more of the following features: interstitial lung disease, arthritis, fevers, Raynaud phenomenon, and mechanic's hands. Patients with one of the antisynthetase autoantibodies and two or more of these features are said to have the antisynthetase syndrome.

The different antisynthetase antibodies appear to be associated with these features at different frequencies. For example, 90% of patients with anti-Jo-1 antibodies have muscle involvement, and 50–75% of patients have interstitial lung disease. In contrast, approximately 50% of patients with anti-PL-12 antibodies have muscle involvement, but interstitial lung disease occurs in 90% of such patients.

A number of different autoantibodies are found exclusively in dermatomyositis. For example, antibodies recognizing the

Table 25–2. Myositis-specific autoantibodies.

Name	Antigen	Clinical Manifestation
Antisynthetase autoantibodies		
Anti-Jo-1	Histidyl t-RNA synthetase	PM or DM with ILD
Anti-PL-7	Threonyl t-RNA synthetase	PM or DM with ILD
Anti-PL-12	Alanyl t-RNA synthetase	ILD more often than Myo
Anti-EJ	Glycyl t-RNA synthetase	PM more often than DM with ILD
Anti-OJ	Isoleucyl t-RNA synthetase	ILD with PM/DM
Anti-KS	Asparaginyl t-RNA synthetase	ILD more often than Myo
Anti-Zo	Phenylalanyl t-RNA synthetase	ILD with Myo
Anti-Ha	Tyrosyl t-RNA synthetase	ILD with Myo
Nonsynthetase autoantibodies		
Dermatomyositis-specific autoantibodies		
Anti-Mi-2	DNA helicase	Dermatomyositis with rash > muscle symptoms, treatment responsive
Anti-MDA5 (anti CADM 140)	Melanoma differentiation-associated gene 5	DM with rapidly progressive lung disease, pneumomediastinum
Anti-TIF1-γ	Transcriptional intermediary factor 1-gamma	CAM, juvenile DM
Anti-NXP-2	Nuclear matrix protein (NXP-2)	Calcinosis, juvenile DM
Anti-SAE	Small ubiquitin-like modifier-activating enzyme	DM: CAM, DM with rapidly progressive lung disease, pneumomediastinum
Immune-mediated necrotizing myopathy–specific autoantibodies		
Anti-SRP	Signal recognition particle	Severe, acute, resistant necrotizing myopathy
Anti-HMGCR (anti 200/100)	HMG CoA Reductase	Necrotizing myopathy, often associated with statin use but not always

CAM, cancer-associated myositis; DM, dermatomyositis; ILD, interstitial lung disease; JDM, juvenile dermatomyositis; myo, myositis (may be either PM or DM); PM, polymyositis; RP, Raynaud phenomenon.

chromatin-remodeling enzyme Mi-2 are found in as many as 20% of patients with dermatomyositis. Despite the fact that these autoantibodies are associated with fulminant cutaneous manifestations, they typically demonstrate excellent responses to treatment and have a lower risk of associated malignancy. In contrast, autoantibodies to TIF1-γ (P155/140) are also found exclusively in patients with dermatomyositis but are associated with an increased malignancy risk, as are patients with anti-NXP-2 autoantibodies. Anti-NXP-2 autoantibodies are also linked to the development of subcutaneous calcium deposits. Anti-MDA5 autoantibodies are associated with amyopathic dermatomyositis, cutaneous ulcerations, and severe interstitial lung disease, especially in Asians. Anti-small ubiquitin-like modifier 1 (SUMO-1) autoantibodies have also been reported in approximately 8% of patients with dermatomyositis.

Anti-TIF1-γ, anti-NXP-2, and anti-MDA5 autoantibodies are also found in children with dermatomyositis. Children with Anti-TIF1-γ have especially severe skin disease and patients with anti-NXP-2 have an increased risk of calcinosis. However, there is no increased risk of malignancy in children with or without these autoantibodies.

Antinuclear antibodies are found in more than half of patients with polymyositis or dermatomyositis and are associated with the presence of antibodies recognizing Mi-2 (a nuclear protein) or an autoantigen associated with one of the other connective tissue diseases. Examples include anti-PM-Scl and anti-Scl-70, autoantibodies found in patients with scleroderma-myositis overlap, and anti-RNP, which is found in patients with mixed connective tissue disease. The erythrocyte sedimentation rate (ESR) and C-reactive protein (CRP) are markedly elevated in only about 20% of myositis patients and are not particularly useful in diagnosis. In fact, an elevated ESR may be indicative of lung disease rather than muscle injury in the inflammatory myopathies.

Two-thirds of patients with immune-mediated necrotizing myopathy have an identifiable myositis-specific antibody, of which anti-SRP and anti-HMGCR are the most common. Anti-SRP autoantibodies, found in approximately 5% of myositis patients, are associated with myofiber degeneration and necrosis, with minimal inflammation on muscle biopsy. These patients tend to have a rapidly progressive myopathy associated with very high CK levels in the thousands or tens of thousands, early muscle atrophy, dysphagia, and, frequently, an incomplete response to immunosuppressive therapy.

Anti-HMGCR antibodies are found in approximately 5% of myositis patients and have a strong association with a necrotizing muscle biopsy and prior statin exposure. The CK is generally elevated in the thousands or tens of thousands. Extra-muscular manifestations, such as ILD, arthritis, and rash, are rare. Among patients with these antibodies over the age of 50, more than 90% report prior statin exposure. Although statins are a significant risk factor, statin exposure is not necessary for the development of anti-HMGCR myopathy, especially in younger patients. Indeed, in younger patients with anti-HMGCR myopathy (less than 50 years of age), the majority of patients have never been exposed to statins. There are reports of anti-HMGCR myopathy in children and even infants, which may mimic a muscular dystrophy. Younger patients with anti-HMGCR myopathy often have more severe disease and a slower recovery compared to their older counterparts.

Statin-associated immune-mediated necrotizing myopathy is a distinct pathologic process that is important to distinguish from the more common self-limited statin myopathy. Although self-limited statin myopathy can present with similar symptoms of fatigue and myalgias, weakness and elevated CK levels are less common. Self-limited statin myopathy also resolves after cessation of the statin. In contrast, statin-associated autoimmune myopathy is a self-perpetuating autoimmune disease in which anti-HMGCR autoantibodies are present; this disease almost always requires immunotherapy. Patients with self-limited statin myopathy do not have myositis-specific autoantibodies, including anti-HMGCR autoantibodies.

C. Imaging Studies

Computer-based image analysis using MRI, CT, and ultrasonography can aid in diagnosis and assessment of disease activity. Of these, MRI with T2-weighted images and fat suppression or short tau inversion recovery (STIR) offers the best imaging of soft tissue and muscle (Figure 25–5). MRI plays an important role in the evaluation and management of autoimmune myopathy because of its ability to evaluate muscle edema (as an indicator of active inflammation) and fatty infiltration (as an indicator of chronic disease).

MRI can detect early or subtle disease changes as well as patchy muscle involvement. Because of these capacities and the fact that it is noninvasive, MRI is superior to EMG in determining the site for muscle biopsy. Use of MRI to guide biopsy may lower the rates of false-negative muscle biopsies, which range from 10% to 25%. Furthermore, MRI can be used to assess degree of fascial involvement as well as to grade muscle involvement in a semiquantitative manner. Thus, MRI is useful in monitoring response to therapy. This point may be particularly useful when trying to differentiate between active myositis and glucocorticoid-induced myopathy. In such situations, the presence of edema in the muscle tissue is indicative of an ongoing inflammatory process. The correlation between changes on MRI and changes in tissue are not perfect, however.

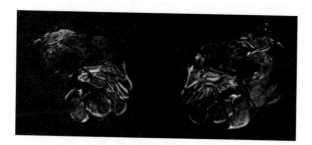

▲ **Figure 25–5.** Axial short tau inversion recovery (STIR) MRI through the midsection of the thighs of a patient with dermatomyositis. There is marked enhancement of the fascia and the quadriceps muscles of both thighs in a symmetric fashion.

Treatment with immunosuppressive medications can result in decreased signal intensity on MRI, but histologically detected inflammation may not change significantly.

Although its clinical use is currently limited, ultrasound provides some potential benefits over CT or MRI in the evaluation of autoimmune myopathies. In particular, in skilled hands, ultrasound provides high spatial resolution and real-time imaging without radiation exposure. Although there are subtle differences among different forms of immune-mediated muscle disease, conventional ultrasound is not yet sensitive enough to differentiate between them. Use of contrast-enhanced ultrasound does not seem to improve sensitivity or positive or negative predictive values.

CT scan with intravenous or radio-opaque contrast is useful in the evaluation of muscle perfusion and mass. However, CT has lower contrast resolution than MRI and is less useful in the evaluation of myositis. However, in the emergency department, it is helpful in the detection of calcification and for the diagnosis of pyomyositis.

D. Special Tests

Nerve conduction tests and EMG may play a critical role in the evaluation of neuromuscular diseases. These tests can aid in determining whether a patient with weakness has a defect of the anterior horn cell, nerve, neuromuscular junction, or muscle. In patients with only autoimmune myopathy, the sensory nerve tests should be normal and the motor nerve tests should be normal or, in very severe cases, notable only for decreased compound muscle action potentials. In patients with myopathy, EMG reveals the early recruitment of small polyphasic motor unit potentials. In those with active disease resulting in myofiber necrosis, abnormal insertional and spontaneous activity (ie, fibrillations and positive sharp waves) are frequently observed. When spontaneous activity occurs in the context of myopathic motor units, a patient is said to have an irritable myopathy. Although classically found in dermatomyositis, polymyositis, and immune-mediated necrotizing myopathy, an irritable myopathy on EMG is not specific for autoimmune muscle disease and can be found in many other myopathic conditions.

Except perhaps in patients with the pathognomonic skin features of dermatomyositis, muscle biopsy is typically recommended in the initial evaluation of patients in whom autoimmune myopathy is suspected. The ideal muscle to biopsy is one that is affected clinically but not one so weak that the study is likely to reveal only end-stage muscle—a sample in which no differentiation can be made between the various etiologies. In general, a deltoid or biceps muscle with 4/5 strength is well-suited to biopsy. One of the quadriceps muscles is also frequently selected for biopsy. Because the muscle pathology may be patchy and all of the quadriceps muscles may not be involved, an MRI study may help guide biopsy to the rectus medialis, rectus femoris, or rectus lateralis muscles.

Perifascicular atrophy is pathognomonic for dermatomyositis, but beyond this finding the autoimmune myopathies do not have specific features on muscle biopsy. Muscle biopsies revealing perivascular inflammation and complement deposition on endomysial capillaries are suggestive of dermatomyositis but not diagnostic of that disease: clinicopathological correlation is required. Similarly, in polymyositis, muscle biopsies typically reveal non-necrotic muscle fibers surrounded and invaded by cytolytic CD8+ T cells, but such findings can also be observed in non–immune-mediated myopathies. The presence of myofibers expressing MHC I on cell surface is more specific for polymyositis, particularly if the fibers are found distant from sites of inflammation.

In some patients with myopathy, the muscle biopsy reveals abundant regenerating, degenerating, and necrotic muscle fibers with scant lymphocytic infiltration (Figure 25–6). These patients may have one of the immune-mediated necrotizing myopathies, but there are also other possible explanations: namely, polymyositis or dermatomyositis in which the inflammation was missed due to sampling error; a toxic myopathy; or a muscular dystrophy. In short, the muscle biopsy findings must be considered carefully and placed into the appropriate clinical context, interpreted in light of physical examination findings, the results of serological investigations, and radiologic studies.

Malignancy screening should be considered for all patients with immune-mediated myopathies—not only dermatomyositis. There is no consensus yet on the optimal cancer screening protocol, but most patients undergo broad conventional cancer screening with thoracoabdominal CT, mammography, gynecologic exam, and tumor marker analysis. Colonoscopy is recommended for patients over the age of 50, and perhaps should be done in all adult patients (regardless of age) in whom immune-mediated myopathy was recently diagnosed. A chest CT has the added benefit of detecting interstitial lung disease. While the utility of "pan-scanning" is currently unknown, most experts recommend imaging of the ovaries by transvaginal ultrasound due to the over-representation of ovarian carcinoma in dermatomyositis and polymyositis, especially when patients have an autoantibody associated with malignancy such as anti-TIF1-γ or anti-NXP-2 antibodies. More research is needed to determine if PET/CT has a role in the detection of malignancy in myositis. For patients who are at high risk for an underlying cancer, age- and gender-specific serial cancer screening should be considered for the first 5 years after presentation, when the risk of presenting with a malignancy is highest.

▶ Differential Diagnosis

Distinguishing patients with an autoimmune myopathy from those with a nonautoimmune process is critical; autoimmune myopathies have muscle weakness that improves significantly with immunosuppression. Absent a classic dermatomyositis rash, the differential diagnosis for a myopathic process is extensive and includes muscular dystrophy, congenital myopathy, metabolic myopathy, mitochondrial myopathy, myotonic dystrophy, inclusion body myositis (IBM), and dermatomyositis without skin involvement (ie, dermatomyositis sine myositis). A diagnosis of polymyositis or immune-mediated necrotizing myopathy can only be established when the possibility of each of these other diseases has been excluded by careful consideration of the history, physical examination findings, laboratory results, EMG, and muscle biopsy findings.

A number of features from the patient's history should suggest the possibility of a diagnosis other than an autoimmune myopathy. First, patients who report a slowly progressive decline over years are unlikely to have immune-mediated disease, which tends to present over weeks to months. However, the converse is not necessarily true; some patients with long-standing muscle disease may not notice weakness until the disease reaches an advanced stage. Second, since autoimmune myopathy is not hereditary, a family history significant for another family member with "polymyositis" strongly suggests both subjects have one of the hereditary myopathies. Third, exercise-induced cramping should suggest the possibility of a metabolic myopathy.

Finally, the lack of markedly improved muscle strength with aggressive immunosuppressive therapy should always raise doubts about a diagnosis of an autoimmune process. Improved CK levels should not be misinterpreted as a positive response, however, because glucocorticoids may dramatically reduce serum CK levels even in patients with non–immune-mediated myopathies. A classic example of this is IBM—although treatment with glucocorticoids may

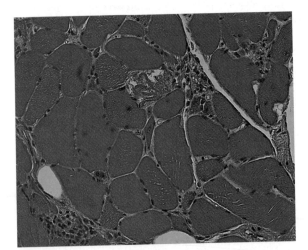

▲ **Figure 25–6.** Muscle biopsy from a patient with immune-mediated necrotizing myopathy. Muscle biopsy is characterized by necrotizing and regenerating muscle fibers with scant lymphocytic infiltration. (See color insert.)

improve or normalize CK concentrations, glucocorticoids do not improve muscle strength in IBM, nor do they impact the long-term prognosis. Glucocorticoids should not be used in the treatment of IBM, regardless of their impact on serum CK levels.

The following describes several pearls that are useful in discriminating patients with autoimmune myopathies from patients with non-immune disorders:

- The presence of proximal muscle weakness supports the diagnosis of an autoimmune myopathy. Patients with autoimmune myopathy generally have distal weakness only in the setting of severe disease. A non–immune-mediated muscle disease should be suspected in patients with wrist and finger weakness. A non–immune-mediated muscle disease should also be considered in patients who cannot walk on their heels or toes (heel-walking requires normal ankle dorsiflexion strength and toe-walking requires normal ankle plantar flexion strength). Rare exceptions to the proximal muscle weakness rule exist. For example, distal weakness has been described in myositis patients with anti-NXP-2 and anti-HMGCR autoantibodies.

- Asymmetry in strength between the same muscle groups on opposite sides of the body should raise doubts about a diagnosis of an autoimmune myopathy.

- The facial muscles are not typically weak in the autoimmune myopathies.

- The presence of scapular winging should initiate a search for one of the genetic muscular dystrophies associated with this feature (Table 25–3).

Myositis-specific autoantibodies are found in ~60% of patients with an autoimmune myopathy and are rarely, if ever, found in patients with other neuromuscular conditions. Consequently, the presence of a myositis-specific antibody is diagnostically very useful. However, not all patients with an autoimmune process have a known myositis-specific antibody. Furthermore, tests for all of the myositis-specific antibodies are not readily commercially available and, even when available, it may take weeks to receive the results.

Electrophysiologic studies often have an important role in distinguishing myopathic processes from neuropathic processes. In patients with active, untreated myositis, EMG usually reveals an irritable myopathy, but this is not specific for immune-mediated myopathies. Furthermore, many patients with partially treated myositis have a non-irritable myopathy on EMG. Certain findings on EMG strongly suggest an alternative diagnosis. For example, the majority of patients with myotonic dystrophy have characteristic myotonic discharges on EMG.

In the absence of definitive skin findings implicating dermatomyositis, muscle biopsy is an essential part of the diagnostic evaluation for any patient in whom an immune-mediated myopathy is suspected. When perifascicular atrophy is observed, a diagnosis of dermatomyositis sine dermatitis can be made even in the absence of rash. However, although inflammatory cell infiltrates are characteristic of polymyositis and dermatomyositis muscle biopsies, their presence is not specific for immune-mediated muscle disease. Rather, abundant inflammatory cells can be found in IBM and even in several of the most common muscular dystrophies (Table 25–4). Certain features of the muscle biopsy (discussed later) should prompt an evaluation for a non–immune-mediated process.

▶ Common Mimickers of Autoimmune Myopathies

A. Inclusion Body Myositis

Inclusion body myositis (IBM) is a slowly progressive myopathic process that generally affects individuals more than 50 years of age and does not respond to immunosuppressive therapy. The typical pattern of muscle involvement includes prominent—and often *asymmetric*—weakness of the triceps, wrist flexors, distal finger flexors, quadriceps, and ankle dorsiflexors. Orbicularis occuli weakness is rarely noticed by the patient but can frequently be detected by the careful examiner when asking the patients to keep eyes tightly shut while

Table 25–3. Myopathies associated with scapular winging.

Dystrophies
  Facioscapulohumeral dystrophy
  Limb-girdle muscular dystrophy (LGMD)
    LGMD 2A (calpain-3)
    LGMD 2E (α-sarcoglycan)
    LGMD 2I (fukutin-related protein gene)
    LGMD 2N (POMT2)
  Emery-Dreifuss muscular dystrophy
Scapulonperoneal syndromes (eg, centronuclear myopathy)
Other neuromuscular conditions
  Hereditary inclusion-body myositis type 2
  Distal spinal muscular atrophy type 4

Table 25–4. Myopathies that may have inflammation on muscle biopsy.

Autoimmune myopathies
  Polymyositis
  Dermatomyositis
Inclusion body myositis
Muscular dystrophies
  Dystrophinopathies (eg, Duchenne and Becker muscular dystrophy)
  Facioscapulohumeral dystrophy
  Limb-girdle muscular dystrophy 2A (calpainopathy)
  Limb-girdle muscular dystrophy 2B (dysferlinopathy)

the clinician attempts to open them. If the clinician attempts to pry open a closed eye but only sees the sclera or the iris and pupil directed superiorly, then the patient is giving a good effort to keep her eyes closed. This is known as Bell's phenomenon.

Dysphagia is another typical feature of IBM. Although hip flexor weakness can occur, knee extensor weakness is generally more significant. Similarly, deltoid weakness can be present but is usually less profound than weakness of the triceps and finger flexors. Both of these points are consistent with the principle that IBM demonstrates a predilection for affecting distal musculature.

Although the underlying pathologic mechanisms remain obscure, it may be that IBM is initiated and/or maintained by both degenerative and immune-mediated processes. For example, the abnormal intracellular accumulation of proteins, such as beta-amyloid, phosphorylated tau, and TDP-43, suggest that IBM is a myodegenerative disease. In contrast, the presence of autoantibodies against cytosolic 5'-nucleotidase 1A (cN1A), found in up to 70% of patients with IBM, suggests that there is also some component of immune dysregulation in this disease. Of note, since anti-cN1A autoantibodies are found in IBM but not in PM, they are useful for distinguishing these two forms of muscle disease. However, anti-cN1A autoantibodies can also be found in other autoimmune disorders, including dermatomyositis, Sjögren syndrome, and systemic lupus erythematosus patients—even those with no clinical evidence of muscle dysfunction.

Routine muscle biopsy classically reveals not only primary inflammation as seen in polymyositis but also red-rimmed vacuoles on the Gömöri trichrome stain, which can be helpful in distinguishing IBM from polymyositis. However, in some patients with clinical features of IBM, no rimmed-vacuoles are found, even on repeat muscle biopsy. Indeed, a recent study showed that more than one-third of patients with primary inflammation and no rimmed vacuoles had the typical clinical features of IBM. Because of the overlapping biopsy features, IBM is very frequently misdiagnosed and treated as polymyositis. Only a very careful physical examination allows the clinician to distinguish between IBM and one of the immune-mediated myopathies for which aggressive immunosuppressive therapy may be warranted.

Patients with IBM do not respond to immunosuppression or IVIG. In fact, some data suggest that the muscle weakness in IBM progresses faster if patients are placed on immunosuppression. A regular exercise program is the one intervention that may improve muscle strength in IBM patients.

B. Facioscapulohumeral Dystrophy

Facioscapulohumeral dystrophy is an autosomal-dominant form of muscular dystrophy. With an incidence of about 4 per million and a prevalence of about 50 per million, facioscapulohumeral dystrophy is the second most common adult-onset muscular dystrophy. In fact, it is approximately as common in the general population as polymyositis or dermatomyositis.

Facial weakness—highly unusual in the autoimmune myopathies—is present in most patients with facioscapulohumeral atrophy by the time they are 30 years old. This facial weakness is usually not appreciated by patients with facioscapulohumeral atrophy. If asked, however, patients may admit to difficulty using straws, blowing up balloons, and whistling. On examination, a transverse smile is characteristic. In many cases, patients do not seek medical attention until they are disabled by weakness of the scapular or humeral muscles, particularly the biceps. The muscle involvement is often asymmetric, and patients may complain that one arm became weak long before the other.

On examination, scapular winging and relative sparing of the deltoids (observed when the scapula is manually fixed to the chest wall by the examiner) are typical. As the disease progresses, proximal and distal muscles (especially the tibialis anterior [used for walking on heels]) may become weak, as well. Laboratory features include a CK in the normal to ~1000 international units/L range and a myopathic EMG. Because genetic testing can usually establish the diagnosis of facioscapulohumeral dystrophy, muscle biopsy is rarely necessary when patients see a clinician who is familiar with this disease. However, ~2–5% of patients with the facioscapulohumeral dystrophy phenotype have an unusual mutation, leading to false-negative genetic testing. When performed, muscle biopsies can sometimes reveal an inflammatory myopathy, occasionally leading to the misdiagnosis of polymyositis, especially when the genetic testing is normal. Unnecessary and potentially harmful treatment can be avoided by recognizing that the patient with a combination of facial weakness and scapular winging is exceedingly unlikely to have an autoimmune myopathy.

C. Limb-Girdle Muscular Dystrophy

The limb-girdle muscular dystrophies (LGMDs), a heterogeneous collection of disorders, can be inherited in either an autosomal-dominant or autosomal-recessive fashion. LGMD 1A through LGMD 1H are inherited in an autosomal dominant manner. In contrast, LGMD 2A through LGMD 2Z are autosomal-recessive diseases. Because they may present in early adulthood without a family history and with symmetric proximal muscle weakness, markedly elevated muscle enzymes, an irritable myopathy on EMG, and an inflammatory muscle biopsy, LGMD 2A (due to mutations in the gene for calpain-3) and LGMD 2B (due to mutations in the dysferlin gene) are frequently misdiagnosed as polymyositis. Indeed, a recent report showed that 25% of genetically confirmed cases of LGMD 2B were initially treated for polymyositis because of the presence of inflammatory infiltrates.

Certain clinical characteristics should raise suspicion and lead to genetic testing for these forms of LGMD. This includes scapular winging, which is found in ~80% of LGMD 2A patients, and ankle plantar flexion weakness (difficulty standing on tiptoe), which is found in many patients with LGMD 2B. Finally, a diagnosis of LGMD should be considered in any patient with "refractory polymyositis."

D. Metabolic Myopathy

The metabolic myopathies are autosomal recessive and X-linked disorders that can be separated into abnormalities of carbohydrate, lipid, and adenine nucleotide metabolism.

1. Disorders of carbohydrate metabolism—There are 14 different enzyme mutations associated with disorders of carbohydrate metabolism (Table 25–5). Six of these present only in infancy or early childhood. Of the remainder, three can present in adulthood with exercise intolerance but are not associated with weakness. Three may present in adulthood with exercise-induced cramping and, rarely, with static weakness. These include patients with defects in (1) amylo-1,4-1,6-transglucosidase (ie, branching enzyme deficiency); (2) myophosphorylase (ie, McCardle disease); and (3) phosphorylase b kinase. Muscle biopsies in these conditions reveal glycogen-containing vacuoles with no inflammation. Each of these enzyme deficiencies can be detected by performing the appropriate commercially available enzyme analysis on frozen muscle specimens.

Because fixed weakness is uncommon in the metabolic myopathies and because muscle biopsies reveal characteristic glycogen accumulation without inflammation, these disorders should not be confused with the autoimmune myopathies if a full evaluation is performed. Patients with debranching enzyme deficiency may have generalized muscle weakness but more often also have significant distal muscle weakness.

Patients with adult-onset acid maltase deficiency (Pompe disease) develop proximal muscle weakness, thereby potentially mimicking one of the immune-mediated myopathies. The diaphragm is often markedly affected and respiratory failure is the presenting feature in some patients with this disease. Although muscle biopsies may reveal glycogen-filled vacuoles, sometimes only nonspecific changes, such as necrotic and regenerating muscle fibers, are found. Therefore, when patients have an autoantibody-negative necrotizing myopathy, it is prudent to perform a dried bloodspot enzyme analysis to rule out the possibility of Pompe disease. This is important not only to avoid unnecessary immunosuppressive treatment, but also because some patients with adult-onset Pompe disease are eligible for enzyme replacement therapy.

2. Disorders of lipid metabolism—Defects affecting both lipid metabolism and the transport of long-chain fatty acids can cause myopathy as well as affect other organ systems. **Carnitine transporter deficiency** can present in early adulthood with progressive proximal muscle weakness and cardiomyopathy. Muscle biopsy reveals abnormal lipid accumulation when the appropriate stain, such as Sudan black or an oil red O stain, is performed. In some patients, oral L-carnitine treatment may be beneficial.

Carnitine palmitoyltransferase 2 deficiency is an autosomal recessive disorder that can present in young adults with myalgias and exercise-induced myoglobinuria. CK levels, muscle strength, and routine muscle biopsies may be normal between episodes of rhabdomyolysis. In suspected cases, carnitine palmitoyltransferase 2 enzyme deficiency can be assessed in frozen muscle tissue and the presence of mutations confirmed by genetic testing.

Very long-chain acyl-CoA dehydrogenase deficiency can also present with exercise-induced myoglobinuria and muscle pain. CK is normal between attacks of rhabdomyolysis, and muscle biopsies may be normal or show abnormal lipid deposits. The diagnosis can be confirmed by genetic testing.

Table 25–5. Disorders of carbohydrate metabolism.

	Enzyme Defect	Adult Presentation?	Fixed Weakness?
Type I	Glucose-6-phosphate	N	N
Type II (Pompe disease)	Acid α-1,4-glucosidase	Y	Y
Type III (Cori-Forbes disease)	Amylo-1,6-glucosidase (debrancher)	Y	Y
Type IV (Anderson disease)	Amylo-1,4-1,6-transglucosidase (brancher)	Y	Y
Type V (McCardle disease)	Myophosphorylase	Y	Y
Type VI	Liver phosphorylase	N	N
Type VII	Phosphofructokinase	N	Y
Type VIII	Phosphorylase b kinase	Y	Y
Type IX	Phosphoglycerate kinase	N	Y
Type X	Phosphoglycerate mutase	Y	N
Type XI	Lactate dehydrogenase	Y	N
Type XII	Aldolase	N	Y
Type XIII	Triosephosphate isomerase	N	Y
Type XIV	β-enolase	Y	N

E. Mitochondrial Myopathy

Defects in mitochondrial oxidative phosphorylation can cause muscle dysfunction, but the clinical picture is frequently dominated by other organ systems, including the central nervous system and heart. Patients with **myoclonic epilepsy and ragged-red fibers** may present in adulthood with myopathy accompanied by myoclonus, seizures, ataxia, dementia, hearing loss, and optic atrophy. **Kearns-Sayre syndrome** occasionally presents in young adults with myopathy associated with progressive external ophthalmoplegia, pigmentary retinopathy, cardiomyopathy, or endocrinopathies. Sometimes, **progressive external ophthalmoplegia** presents with limb weakness. **Mitochondrial neurogastrointestinal encephalopathy** can present with a variety of clinical manifestations, sometimes including distal greater than proximal muscle weakness. Muscle biopsies from each of these entities are characterized by evidence of mitochondrial dysfunction, including the presence of ragged-red fibers on Gömöri trichrome stain or increased staining for succinic dehydrogenase (encoded by nuclear DNA) in the context of reduced staining for cytochrome oxidase (encoded by mitochondrial DNA). Given the other organ system involvement and lack of inflammation on muscle biopsy, mitochondrial myopathies should rarely be misdiagnosed as one of the immune-mediated myopathies.

▶ Treatment of the Autoimmune Inflammatory Myopathies

The autoimmune inflammatory myopathies are a heterogeneous group of diseases that generally respond well to immunomodulating agents. Prompt diagnosis and treatment for these patients is essential. Given that the current understanding of the pathogenesis of the immune-mediated myopathies centers around an overactive immune system leading to inflammation that causes muscle damage, the mainstay of therapy focuses on control of inflammation through immunosuppression. Goals of therapy include increasing muscle strength, controlling pain, enabling patients to manage their activities of daily living, and improving their quality of life. Few randomized clinical trials exist on effective therapies, and current therapeutic regimens, especially in resistant disease, are based on expert opinion and clinical experience. Serum CK concentrations may decrease without parallel improvements in strength, and vice versa. Thus, improvement in strength, function, and skin manifestations (in the case of dermatomyositis) should be the primary goal of therapy. The usefulness of monitoring serum CK levels may be helpful as an indicator of possible flare, but trends in CK levels alone should not be used as the sole measure of the efficacy of therapy, especially in dermatomyositis.

A. Glucocorticoids

Prednisone is generally used as the empiric first-line therapy. In general, prednisone should be started at 1–2 mg/kg/day (or equivalent dose is used) to control acute disease, and then it is tapered after 3–4 weeks, depending on level of clinical improvement. Tapering to the lowest effective dose is preferred in order to reduce comorbidities associated with glucocorticoid therapy. Retrospective studies have demonstrated the effectiveness of glucocorticoids in reducing mortality and improving muscle strength and function. Elevations in serum CK levels in addition to clinical deterioration in strength and function may indicate that glucocorticoids are being tapered too quickly or that additional immunosuppression is necessary. Concomitant glucocorticoid-sparing immunosuppressive therapy is warranted in most adults with immune-mediated myopathy and generally should be started at diagnosis. Indicators that additional immunosuppressants are required include the following: (1) patients are experiencing unacceptable complications from glucocorticoid use, (2) inability to taper glucocorticoid dose without precipitating a myositis flare, (3) ineffectiveness after 2–3 months of therapy (if glucocorticoid-sparing agents were not begun at the outset of treatment), and (4) rapidly progressive disease with respiratory failure.

Patients taking high-dose prednisone (ie, >20 mg/day) are at risk for *Pneumocystis jiroveci* (previously called *Pneumocystis carinii*) infection and should receive prophylaxis. Vitamin D, calcium supplementation, and possibly bisphosphonates should be used in patients who are taking at least 7.5 mg of prednisone or its equivalent for more than 3 months to prevent bone loss, especially in postmenopausal women.

B. Glucocorticoid-Sparing Immunosuppressive Medications

Conventional immunosuppressive medications are usually used in addition to glucocorticoids and have been shown to be effective in some studies, but their use remains largely empiric. In general, methotrexate, azathioprine, and mycophenolate mofetil are all used as first-line glucocorticoid-sparing drugs. There is generally little basis for selecting one of these medications over the others, and the choice is often made in consideration of potential patient comorbidities and clinician experience.

C. Methotrexate

There have not been any randomized, prospective clinical trials of the use of methotrexate that have demonstrated effectiveness in myositis, but several retrospective trials suggest that a majority of patients with dermatomyositis and polymyositis have responded to treatment. One potential side effect of methotrexate therapy is pneumonitis, which may be difficult to differentiate from the interstitial lung disease seen in patients with antisynthetase syndromes; thus, methotrexate should be used with caution in this subset of patients. Either azathioprine or mycophenolate mofetil might be preferred for the antisynthetase syndromes or other patients with disease-related interstitial lung disease.

D. Azathioprine

One clinical trial of azathioprine in addition to prednisone showed no improvements in strength or histologic findings but showed a significant improvement in serum CK levels when compared with patients receiving prednisone alone. (The pitfalls of attaching too much importance to improvements in CK levels have been noted above). Several retrospective studies, however, suggest that azathioprine may be effective, with some beneficial response seen in approximately two-thirds of patients with either polymyositis or dermatomyositis but complete responses (defined as the ability to taper prednisone successfully and the achievement of normal muscle strength) occurring in only about 10%. Patients who were previously responsive to glucocorticoids tend to respond better to the addition of azathioprine than those who have responded poorly to glucocorticoids. The likelihood that azathioprine will salvage a glucocorticoid-refractory patient is low.

E. Mycophenolate Mofetil

Mycophenolate mofetil has shown some benefit in patients with polymyositis and dermatomyositis, and it may be particularly effective for dermatomyositis-related skin disease, even among patients resistant to other therapies.

F. Rituximab

The monoclonal antibody rituximab may be beneficial in some cases of myositis, and is often used as additive therapy when oral immunosuppressants are insufficient. Rituximab appears to be particularly helpful in many cases of dermatomyositis, and in our experience may be particularly effective for SRP-positive myopathy. Though not confirmed by a strong evidence base, a case can be made for using rituximab early in the treatment of autoimmune myopathies in the interest of decreasing glucocorticoid toxicity and effecting good clinical outcomes. Rituximab also appears to be effective for HMGCR-positive myopathy.

G. Intravenous Immunoglobulin

One trial of intravenous immunoglobulin (IVIG) in glucocorticoid-resistant polymyositis and dermatomyositis demonstrated significant improvements in strength, function, and CK levels. However, adverse reactions were seen in 43% of patients, although none required hospitalization. IVIG has been shown to be successful in mitigating the pathologic changes seen on repeated muscle biopsy as well as improving strength in patients with dermatomyositis. IVIG is also effective for HMGCR-positive myopathy, and in some cases can be used as monotherapy in this disease.

H. Cyclophosphamide

Use of cyclophosphamide has shown mixed results, with some case reports indicating positive improvements in patients with severe polymyositis, although this could not be replicated in other studies. It is probably best reserved for severe interstitial lung disease or myopathy nonresponsive to other immunosuppressants. Interstitial cystitis occurs in up to one-third of patients taking the drug orally. This complication can be reduced by administering cyclophosphamide intravenously; however, efficacy of this route of administration is unclear in the immune-mediated myopathies. In severe refractory cases, some patients may benefit from high-dose intravenous cyclophosphamide (50 mg/kg of ideal body weight every day for four consecutive days) without stem cell rescue.

I. Acthar

Acthar Gel is a long-acting analog of adrenocorticotropic hormone (ACTH) that has anti-inflammatory properties through its actions on melanocortin receptors located on immune cells. Acthar Gel has been an FDA-approved treatment for myositis since 1952. Despite FDA approval, use of Acthar in clinical practice has been limited because of a paucity of clinical data. A recent open-label trial of 10 patients with refractory dermatomyositis and polymyositis showed that Acthar Gel led to a clinically significant improvement in 70% of patients. Use of Acthar may become more mainstream in the future, although currently in our practice we reserve it for cases of refractory myositis.

J. Exercise and Supplements

Exercise was once discouraged in patients with inflammatory myopathies but it has become increasingly clear that maintaining daily exercise is beneficial in all stages of the disease. Patients may benefit from formal physical therapy. Isometric exercises are recommended, while heavy weight lifting is discouraged. When supplemented with creatine, exercise may further improve function over exercise alone. Thus, a moderate exercise routine can be beneficial in patients with polymyositis and dermatomyositis without increased rates of myositis flares or injury. In our experience, the same is true for patients with immune-mediated necrotizing myopathy.

▶ Complications

Major complications that develop in patients with inflammatory muscle diseases are most often seen in patients in whom the diagnosis, and thus therapy, was delayed or in patients with refractory disease. Persistent or progressive active muscle disease can result in permanent fatty replacement of skeletal muscle. These patients may become wheelchair-dependent. Patients with dysphagia or dysphonia are at risk for aspiration pneumonia. Those with interstitial lung disease may progress to respiratory failure due to worsening end-stage fibrosis. Cardiomyopathy with congestive heart failure can develop in the few patients with cardiac involvement.

Complications can also result from therapy. Most notable are the side effects and toxicities of glucocorticoid use. Patients treated with these agents can manifest all of the features of iatrogenic Cushing syndrome (including central obesity, hypertension, hyperhidrosis, "moon facies," striae, and hirsutism). Other well-known glucocorticoid-related toxicities include cataracts, acne, emotional lability, hyperlipidemia (especially hypertriglyceridemia), and osteopenia/osteoporosis. Two of the most troubling complications of glucocorticoid treatment are opportunistic infections and glucocorticoid-induced proximal muscle weakness. Opportunistic pulmonary infections such as *P jiroveci* pneumonia can be rapidly fatal. Glucocorticoid-associated myopathy can be particularly frustrating because it complicates the course of a patient who is getting stronger on therapy and confounds the assessment of treatment response. Patients with glucocorticoid-induced myopathy typically show improvement with glucocorticoid therapy and then suddenly plateau or deteriorate. In this setting, it is difficult to determine whether the decrease in muscle strength is due to disease flare or

glucocorticoid toxicity. MRI studies may be useful in making this distinction but differentiation between these diagnoses is often not straightforward.

Allenbach Y, Drouot L, Rigolet A, et al. Anti-HMGCR autoantibodies in European patients with autoimmune necrotizing myopathies: inconstant exposure to statin. *Medicine (Baltimore)*. 2014;93:150-157. [PMID: 247971700]

Benjamin Larman H, Salajegheh M, Nazareno R, et al. Cytosolic 5′-nucleotidase 1A autoimmunity in sporadic inclusion body myositis. *Ann Neurol*. 2013;73:408-418. [PMID: 23596012]

Mammen AL, Tiniakou E. Intravenous immune globulin for statin-triggered autoimmune myopathy. *N Engl J Med*. 2015;373:1680-1682. [PMID: 26488714]

Wolstencroft PW, Chung L, Li S, Casciola-Rosen L, Fiorentino DF. Factors associated with clinical remission of skin disease in dermatomyositis. *JAMA Dermatol*. 2018;154:44-51. [PMID: 29114741]

Giant Cell Arteritis & Polymyalgia Rheumatica

26

Sebastian Unizony, MD

ESSENTIALS OF DIAGNOSIS

Giant Cell Arteritis (GCA)

▶ A granulomatous vasculitis of the aorta and the main aortic branches with tropism for the extracranial tributaries of the carotid arteries.

▶ The most common primary form of vasculitis in adults, with a lifetime risk after the age of 50 of 1% and 0.5% in women and men, respectively.

▶ Presents with cranial signs or symptoms (eg, headaches, scalp tenderness), polymyalgia rheumatica (PMR) symptoms, constitutional symptoms, or clinical manifestations reflecting large artery involvement (eg, extremity claudication).

▶ The most serious complication is blindness, which occurs in up to 20% of patients, usually before the diagnosis is made and prednisone treatment is initiated. Therefore, it is mandatory to start glucocorticoid therapy as soon as GCA is suspected to prevent irreversible vision loss.

▶ Erythrocyte sedimentation rate (ESR) or C-reactive protein (CRP) levels are elevated in more than 95% of patients at disease onset.

▶ Definitive diagnosis requires temporal artery biopsy or vascular imaging.

▶ Most patients respond acutely to prednisone. However, relapse upon prednisone tapering is common and glucocorticoid-sparing immunosuppressive drugs (eg, tocilizumab) are needed for remission maintenance in most cases.

PMR

▶ Is an inflammatory disorder of the shoulder and hip girdles that can occur as part of GCA or, more frequently, as an isolated condition (ie, primary PMR).

▶ The epidemiology of primary PMR overlaps with that of GCA, but PMR is three times more common.

▶ The diagnosis is primarily a clinical one, aided by the fact that most patients have elevated ESR or CRP levels.

▶ The mainstay of treatment is glucocorticoids, but flares upon glucocorticoid dose reduction are common and glucocorticoid-sparing medications are sometimes required.

Giant cell arteritis (GCA) and polymyalgia rheumatica (PMR) are chronic, relapsing inflammatory conditions considered to be part of the same disease spectrum. GCA is the most common form of systemic vasculitis in adults. It is a disorder that affects the aorta and its main branches, demonstrating a predilection for the subdivisions of the extracranial carotid arteries. The most feared complication of GCA is blindness, which can be prevented in the majority of cases by early diagnosis and prompt treatment with glucocorticoids. Other complications may include aortic aneurysm, limb ischemia form arterial stenosis, and treatment-related toxicity from glucocorticoids. PMR is an arthritis and periarthritis of the shoulder and hip girdles that can occur as part of GCA or, more commonly, as an isolated condition (ie, primary PMR).

▶ Etiology & Pathogenesis

The etiology of GCA and primary PMR is unknown, and the understanding of their pathogenesis is only partially understood. It is known, however, that these conditions share risk factors, and probably disease mechanisms as well.

The search for an infectious cause for GCA has been pursued with a number of techniques. Varicella zoster virus has been proposed as a causative agent in studies of temporal artery biopsies, but results have not been replicated. Genome-wide–associated studies (GWAS) and candidate gene studies, however, have identified several human leukocyte antigen (HLA) and non-HLA genetic risk factors in patients with GCA including variants within the loci of

HLA-DRA/HLA-DRB1, HLA-DQA1/HLA-DQA2, HLA-B, PLG, P4HA2, PTPN22, IL-6, IL-17A, IL12B, MMP9, NOS2, VEGFA, REL, and LRRC32.

Granulomatous inflammation with abundant CD4⁺ T cells, macrophages, and giant cells involving large- and medium-sized arteries is the histopathologic hallmark of GCA. The pathogenesis of this vasculitis appears to be initiated by CD4⁺ T cells in the adventitia responding to an unknown antigen presented by dendritic cells. CD4⁺ T cells in GCA lesions mainly demonstrate two effector phenotypes (Deng et al, 2010), T helper (Th)1—producing interferon gamma (IFN-γ) and Th17—producing interleukin (IL)-17. IFN-γ and IL-17 orchestrate downstream events resulting in monocyte recruitment and differentiation of these cells into macrophages (Figure 26–1). Macrophages coalesce in the media, forming multinucleated giant cells secreting metalloproteinases and reactive oxygen species that compromise the vessel's structural integrity.

Through interactions with vascular endothelial growth factor (VEGF)–stimulated endothelial cells of the vasa vasorum that express Jagged 1, NOTCH1⁺ CD4⁺ T cells are instructed to differentiate into Th1 and Th17 cells (Wen et al, 2017). In addition, patients with GCA carry a pathogenic population of regulatory T cells (Tregs) that express a hypofunctional variant of the master regulatory transcription factor Foxp3 (so-called Foxp3Δ2 Tregs) and produce IL-17 (Miyabe et al, 2017). Other mechanisms operating in inflamed GCA arteries include dysfunctional CD8⁺ Tregs, a defective immunoinhibitory PD1/PD1-L1 checkpoint system, and up-regulation of the GM-CSF and JAK-STAT pathways.

IL-6 is a key contributor to the pathogenesis of GCA (see Figure 26–1). This cytokine not only drives the polarization of CD4⁺ T cells toward the Th17 phenotype, but it also suppresses the differentiation and function of Tregs. Moreover, IL-6 participates in the activation of monocytes and macrophages, and induces endothelial cells to acquire the pro-inflammatory phenotype necessary to traffic these and other leukocytes to the sites of inflammation. Confirming the preponderant role of IL-6 in the pathogenesis of GCA is the result of clinical trials of IL-6 blockade demonstrating effective disease control off glucocorticoids (Stone et al, 2017).

The pathogenesis of primary PMR has not been explored as thoroughly, partly because the acquisition of tissue in that disease is more challenging than in GCA. However, both conditions are thought to be part of the same spectrum and to share overlapping molecular and cellular mechanisms.

▶ Epidemiology

More than 95% of cases of primary PMR and GCA occur in Caucasian individuals. The Hispanic population is infrequently affected, and these conditions are exceedingly rare among Asian, Arab, and African American descents (Tuckwell et al, 2017). Age is the strongest risk factor for both, primary PMR and GCA. Both diseases generally develop in persons older

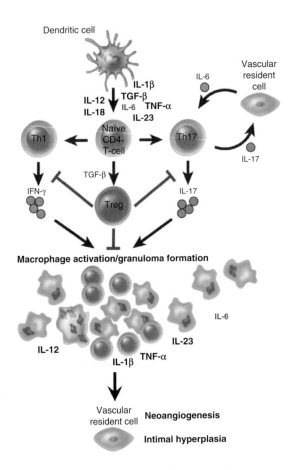

▲ **Figure 26–1.** Pathogenesis of GCA. GCA lesions are mainly composed by CD4⁺ T cells, macrophages, and giant cells. CD4⁺ T cells demonstrate two effector phenotypes, T helper (Th)1—producing interferon gamma (IFN-γ) and Th17—producing interleukin (IL)-17. Patients with GCA also carry a pathogenic population of regulatory T cells (Tregs) in peripheral blood that produce IL-17 and express a hypofunctional variant of the master regulatory transcription factor Foxp3 lacking domain 2 (Foxp3Δ2 Tregs). IL-6, a key pathogenic cytokine in GCA, drives the polarization of CD4⁺ T cells toward the Th17 phenotype, suppresses Treg differentiation and function, participates in the activation of monocytes and macrophages, and induces endothelial cells to acquire a pro-inflammatory phenotype. Vascular resident cells (eg, smooth muscle cells and endothelial cells) respond to the inflammatory insult with different mechanisms including intimal hyperplasia and neoangiogenesis (ie, vascular remodeling). (Reproduced with permission from Unizony S, Kermani TA. IL-6 blockade and its therapeutic success in giant cell arteritis. *J Neuroophthalmol.* 2018;38(4): 551-558.)

than 50 years, with peak incidence in the eighth decade of life. For reasons that are unclear, it is truly exceptional for the diagnosis of GCA to be established before a patient is 50. The diagnosis of PMR is made more frequently among individuals younger than 50, but this, too, is unusual. Females are involved two to three times more often than males.

GCA is the most common form of vasculitis in adults. The incidence and prevalence of this condition has been estimated to vary geographically, ranging from between 10–30 and 25–275 cases per 100,000 persons older than 50 years, respectively. Primary PMR is approximately three times more common than GCA with an incidence and prevalence that range between 41–113 and 600 cases per 100,000 persons older than 50 years, respectively. The Scandinavian Peninsula and other countries of the North of Europe have the highest incidence rates of both disorders. In the United States, more than 228,000 individuals are affected with GCA and more than 711,000 carry the diagnosis of primary PMR (Buttgereit et al, 2016). The lifetime risk for primary PMR and GCA in women is 2.4% and 1%, respectively. The corresponding numbers for men are 1.7% and 0.5%, respectively (Buttgereit et al, 2016).

▶ Clinical Manifestations

The onset of GCA is often subacute, with weeks or months of subclinical symptoms before the diagnosis is established. In contrast, patients are more likely to remember the precise day their PMR symptoms began. Even so, patients with GCA and primary PMR frequently ignore their symptoms for days to weeks, attributing them to "old age" or something else. The most common clinical manifestations of GCA can be divided into four domains, which are not mutually exclusive and often overlap with each other. These domains include cranial manifestations, PMR symptoms, constitutional symptoms, and signs and symptoms of large artery involvement. In addition to PMR symptoms, patients with primary PMR often report constitutional symptoms.

A. Cranial Manifestations

The cranial manifestations of GCA include headache, jaw claudication, scalp tenderness, temporal artery abnormalities, and visual symptoms.

1. Headache—Diffuse or localized headache, the most common symptom in GCA, is seen in about two-thirds of patients. The location of the pain may vary but usually involves the temporal or occipital areas of the head. The headache is frequently described as a dull, aching pain of moderate severity. However, variations in quality and severity occur often. The single most characteristic feature of this symptom is that it is new for the patient. Even if the patient has had migraines or other types of headache in the past, the GCA-related headache is different. Pain tends to be persistent and to respond incompletely to analgesics.

2. Jaw claudication—Jaw claudication, reported as exertional pain localized to the jaw upon mastication, is detected in 30–50% of patients. This symptom develops when the oxygen demand of the masticatory muscles exceeds the supply provided by inflamed narrowed arteries. The onset of jaw claudication is remarkably rapid, occurring after only a short period of chewing. The presence of jaw claudication is a strong predictor of temporal artery biopsy positivity. Many patients do not provide such a classic description of jaw claudication, but instead report a vague sense of discomfort along the jaw or face, with or without protracted chewing.

3. Temporal artery abnormalities and scalp tenderness—Abnormalities involving the superficial temporal artery or its frontal or parietal branches may be detected in 30–70% of the cases. On palpation, these vessels may be enlarged, thickened, nodular, tender, or pulseless. Occasionally, erythema in the topography of these arteries can be seen. In addition, nearly half of patients describe tenderness of the scalp (eg, temporal, parietal or occipital areas), especially when they comb or brush their hair or when they wear eyeglasses or hats. In rare extreme cases, occlusion of the superficial cranial arteries may lead to severe ischemia and scalp necrosis.

4. Ophthalmic complications—About one-third of patients with GCA have visual manifestations. These may include diplopia, blurred vision, amaurosis fugax, and the most serious GCA complication, permanent vision loss or blindness. Blurred vision and amaurosis fugax are episodic and transient and tend to be monocular—at least initially. Blindness, which occurs in 8–20% of patients, is an early event in the course of the disease in the great majority of cases (Vodopivec and Rizzo, 2018). Vision loss typically occurs before the diagnosis of GCA is made. In such cases, it is the event that brings the patient to medical attention, at which time it is too late for glucocorticoids or other treatment to prevent vision loss. This complication can develop abruptly but more often is preceded by episodes of blurred vision or amaurosis fugax. By the time blindness occurs, most patients have increased inflammatory markers in serum and also report other clinical manifestations (eg, headaches, jaw claudication, PMR symptoms). It has been suggested that patients who develop ischemic eye complications tend to have less prominent systemic inflammatory responses in terms of constitutional symptoms and degree of elevation of inflammatory markers, but this observation may be circular: it is because their acute phase reactants are low that their underlying GCA is not recognized until the time of a catastrophic visual event.

In more than 95% of cases, the mechanism of permanent vision loss is the occlusion of the posterior ciliary arteries that perfuse the head of the optic nerve causing anterior ischemic optic neuropathy (AION) (Figure 26–2A). In a minority of cases, vision loss is secondary to the occlusion of the central retinal artery (CRAO) or one of its branches (BRAO). Finally, and very rarely, vision loss in GCA can be

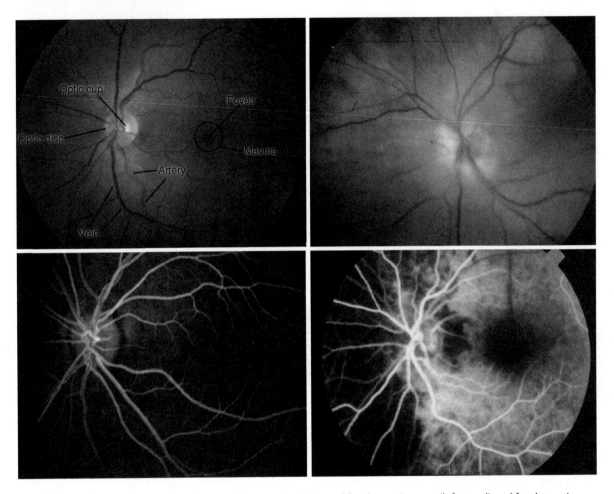

▲ **Figure 26–2.** Acute ischemic optic neuropathy in GCA. **A:** Normal fundoscopic exam (left panel) and fundoscopic exam of a GCA patient with acute ischemic optic neuropathy (AION), which demonstrates a swollen and pale optic disc with diffuse margins (right panel). **B:** Normal fluorescein angiography (left panel) and fluorescein angiography of the GCA patient with AION (right panel) demonstrating patchy choroidal hypoperfusion (dark geographic region) on the nasal side of the fundus. (See color insert.) (Images courtesy of Dr. Joseph Rizzo III, Massachusetts Eye and Ear Infirmary, Boston.)

caused by a stroke involving the occipital cortex in patients with vertebral artery involvement. On examination, patients with AION demonstrate a relative afferent pupillary defect, elicited by moving a shining light from the normal eye to the blind eye and noting that the pupil of the blind eye does not constrict to the light. In the first few hours after optic nerve infarction, the optic disc generally appears normal on funduscopic examination, even in the presence of profound visual loss. Within hours to days, however, disc pallor and swelling, cotton-wool spots, and flame-shaped intraretinal hemorrhages may develop (see Figure 26–2A). Over weeks or months, the disc becomes atrophic. Fluorescein angiography demonstrates a characteristic delay of perfusion and patchy hypoperfusion of either the choroid, retina, or both (Figure 26–2B).

B. Polymyalgia Rheumatica

PMR is a clinical diagnosis defined as inflammatory pain and stiffness in the shoulder and hip girdles. Symptoms may begin unilaterally but quickly become bilateral and symmetric. The shoulders and arms are more commonly involved (70–95%) than the hips and thighs (50–70%). Patients with PMR also often report involvement of the neck and lower back. A characteristic feature of PMR is its worsening after immobilization (eg, morning predominance) and improvement with physical activity. Patients commonly report great difficulty rolling in or getting out of bed, arising from the toilet, or brushing their teeth. Morning stiffness typically lasts from 30 minutes to several hours. Examination of the shoulders and hips is usually unremarkable except for decreased active range of motion early in the morning (passive range of motion is typically much easier for patients). Swelling, erythema, or warmth are usually absent. Patients with PMR occasionally experience arthralgia or even frank arthritis of the sternoclavicular joints, wrists, small joints of the hands, knees, or ankles. Patients with GCA report PMR symptoms in 40–60% of cases, but only 15–20% of patients with primary PMR subsequently develop GCA.

C. Constitutional Manifestations

Most patients with GCA and primary PMR report nonspecific manifestations such as malaise, fatigue, anorexia, or weight loss. A minority of patients present with true fevers, and GCA is a common cause of fever of unknown origin. This is discussed later.

D. Manifestations Associated with Large Vessel Disease

Large vessel involvement, which is seen in nearly 100% of GCA patients according to necropsy studies (Ostberg, 1972), is identified in up to 80% of cases by vascular imaging depending on the imaging modality used. Imaging modalities to look for changes suggesting vasculitis include color duplex ultrasonography (CDS), magnetic resonance imaging (MRI) and magnetic resonance angiography (MRA), computed tomography angiography (CTA), and positron emission tomography (PET).

Despite being virtually universal histologically, large vessel vasculitis in GCA becomes clinically significant in only about 30% of patients (Koster et al, 2018). Vascular inflammation can cause structural damage of the walls of elastic arteries causing dilatation and dissection, and narrowing of the lumens of muscular arteries causing stenosis, occlusion, and distal ischemia. The most frequently affected vessels include the thoracic and abdominal aorta, and the vertebral, carotid, subclavian, axillary, and brachial arteries. GCA of the arteries of the lower extremities is occasionally seen.

Signs and symptoms related to the involvement of the subclavian, brachial, axillary, femoral, and popliteal arteries may include extremity claudication, decreased peripheral pulses, blood pressure asymmetries, and vascular bruits. Involvement of the vertebral, and less often the carotid circulation, may cause transient ischemic attack and stroke. Aortic involvement may lead to aortic aneurysm (mainly in the thoracic aorta) and less frequently aortic dissection. Thoracic aneurysms may present with chest wall pain, aortic regurgitation, myocardial infarction, or dissection. Surgical specimens of the aortic lesions show disarray and loss of elastic fibers with or without inflammatory infiltrates, suggesting a role for both, inflammation and hemodynamic stress in the formation and progression of GCA-related aneurysms. In most patients, however, large artery inflammation and subsequent arterial damage is clinically silent.

Table 26–1. The American College of Rheumatology classification criteria for giant cell arteritis.

Criterion[a]	Definition
Age at disease onset ≥50 years	Development of symptoms or findings beginning at age 50 or older
New headache	New onset or new type of localized pain in the head
Temporal artery abnormality	Temporal artery tenderness to palpation or decreased pulsation, unrelated to arteriosclerosis of cervical arteries
Elevated erythrocyte sedimentation rate (ESR)	ESR ≥50 mm/h by the Westergren method
Abnormal artery biopsy	Biopsy specimen with artery showing vasculitis characterized by a predominance of mononuclear cell infiltration or granulomatous inflammation, usually with multinucleated giant cells

[a]For purposes of classification, a patient is said to have giant cell (temporal) arteritis if at least three of these five criteria are present. Reproduced with permission from Hunder GG, Bloch DA, Michel BA, et al. The American College of Rheumatology 1990 criteria for the classification of giant cell arteritis. *Arthritis Rheum.* 1990;33(8):1122-1128.

GCA patients with large vessel disease tend to be younger, sometimes report only PMR symptoms, and often have negative temporal artery biopsy and lower levels of serum inflammatory markers compared to patients presenting with classic cranial manifestations. Hence, patients with large vessel involvement may not satisfy the 1990 American College of Rheumatology (ACR) classification criteria for GCA (Table 26–1) and experience significant diagnostic delays.

E. Less Common Clinical Manifestations

GCA may present with atypical features. Awareness of these nonclassic presentations maximizes the physician's chance of diagnosing the disease before blindness develops.

Fever is the major clinical manifestation of GCA in about 10% of patients. Moreover, approximately one out of six elderly individuals with fever of unknown origin has GCA. Occasionally, fevers can be high and associated with chills and sweats. Patients with GCA presenting solely with fever tend to be younger and have stronger serologic inflammatory responses (ESR, CRP, IL-6, anemia) compared to patients with classic presentations. Vascular radiology, particularly PET-based imaging, is the diagnostic modality of choice in this scenario because most of these patients have large vessel involvement and because malignancy and infection are in the differential diagnosis.

Respiratory or otolaryngeal symptoms develop in about 10% of GCA patients. The most common symptom is a dry cough, resembling that seen in some patients taking angiotensin-converting enzyme inhibitors. The cause of the cough is obscure because chest imaging studies are normal. The cough may reflect inflammation within the arteries adjacent to cough centers, which are distributed throughout various sites in the respiratory airways, including the larynx, bronchi, and diaphragm. Other respiratory or otolaryngeal manifestations caused by vasculitis of the head and neck arteries include tongue pain, intermittent sore throat, episodic odyno- or dysphagia, transient hoarseness, and anterior cervical tenderness (angiodynia). Tongue ulceration and gangrene occur occasionally, typically on the lateral portion of the tongue on either or both sides.

Central and peripheral nervous system involvement can be seen in GCA. Cerebrovascular accidents (CVAs) are seen in 2–7% of patients. Unlike atherosclerosis-related CVAs, the majority of the vasculitic CVAs occurring in GCA patients involve the posterior circulation by a mechanism of arterioarterial embolization, with origin in the extradural vertebrobasilar system (Samson et al, 2015). True intracranial vasculitis is exceedingly rare. CVAs occurring at the time of GCA diagnosis or within 4 weeks of treatment initiation are generally presumed to be GCA-related. However, it is often difficult to know with certainty whether a brain ischemic event in a GCA patient is related to GCA or other causes (eg, atherosclerosis or thromboembolism unrelated to vascular inflammation). Vestibuloauditory manifestations including sensorineural hearing loss and vertigo have been reported in up to 7% of GCA patients. Peripheral nerve involvement in the form of mononeuritis, mononeuritis multiplex, peripheral neuropathy, and plexopathy (eg, upper brachial plexopathy) complicates the course of GCA in approximately 7% of patients.

Rarely vasculitis in GCA may involve the coronary arteries causing myocardial infarction, the mesenteric arteries causing ischemic colitis or the hepatic arteries causing liver ischemia. Although the renal arteries may be damaged radiologically in up 7% of cases, renal artery stenosis with clinical consequences is virtually never encountered.

In some patients with GCA and primary PMR, diffuse tenosynovitis and inflammatory soft tissue edema of the hands and feet result in marked upper extremity edema that may wax and wane. However, this disorder, termed remitting seronegative symmetrical synovitis with pitting edema (RS3PE), is not specific for GCA or primary PMR and may also occur as an isolated syndrome or in association with other diseases, such as elderlyonset rheumatoid arthritis.

▶ Diagnosis

The diagnosis of GCA is based on a characteristic pattern of symptoms, physical examination findings, elevated serum markers of inflammation, biopsy findings, and vascular imaging. Nevertheless, a group of patients with GCA may have negative biopsy and vascular imaging, receiving the diagnosis on the basis of clinical manifestations, response to glucocorticoids, and characteristic clinical courses (eg, relapse upon prednisone tapering). The diagnosis of primary PMR is based on the presence of classic symptoms, absence of cranial manifestations, elevated serum markers of inflammation, and musculoskeletal imaging. For both GCA and PMR, the most important diagnostic test is a carefully and skillfully taken history.

A. Laboratory Abnormalities

The laboratory hallmark of GCA and primary PMR is the elevation of the inflammatory markers erythrocyte sedimentation rate (ESR) and C-reactive protein (CRP). Increased ESR or CRP is seen in 84% and 86% of GCA patients, respectively (Kermani et al, 2012). Both inflammatory markers are usually concomitantly elevated, but discordant results may be seen in up to 8% of patients. Although ESR and CRP are highly sensitive for the diagnosis of temporal artery biopsy positive GCA, the specificity of these tests is low (~30%). Of note, only approximately 4% of new-onset, untreated GCA patients have both ESR and CRP within normal limits (Kermani et al, 2012). Thus, normal inflammatory markers do not rule out GCA completely. As in GCA, ESR and CRP elevation is seen in more than 90% of patients with primary PMR. Other nonspecific laboratory abnormalities that can be seen in GCA and primary PMR patients include anemia of chronic disease, thrombocytosis, and sometimes leucocytosis and liver alkaline phosphatase elevation.

B. Temporal Artery Biopsy

A characteristic pattern of inflammation in a temporal artery or other arterial biopsy (eg, occipital artery or aorta) is the most specific test for the diagnosis of GCA. However, the estimated sensitivity of temporal artery biopsy varies widely, from approximately 40–85%, and the true sensitivity is likely on the order of 60%.

Typical histologic features include granulomatous infiltrates composed of lymphocytes, macrophages, and giant cells. Mononuclear cell aggregates are most prominent in the adventitia and media. In addition, disruption of the elastic lamina is frequently seen (Figure 26–3). Approximately 50% of biopsies compatible with GCA lack one or more of the above mentioned elements, however, and in some biopsies only an isolated, periadventitial inflammatory infiltrate or vasculitis of small vessels surrounding the temporal artery (vasa vasorum) is present. Fibrinoid necrosis is not a histologic change typical of GCA, and this finding should raise the suspicion for other forms of vasculitis that sometimes mimic GCA, such as polyarteritis nodosa or ANCA associated vasculitis.

Because skip lesions are common in GCA, multiple sections of the artery should be examined to increase the diagnostic yield of a given temporal artery biopsy specimen. Some controversy exists in terms of the ideal biopsy length to maximize the likelihood of making a GCA diagnosis.

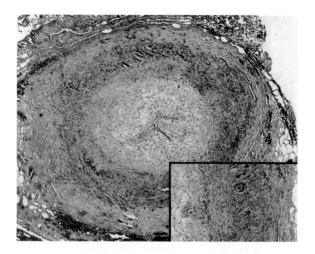

▲ **Figure 26–3.** Giant cell arteritis histopathology. Temporal artery biopsy showing intimal hyperplasia, fragmentation of internal elastic lamina, and infiltration of the adventitia and media by inflammatory cells. Giant cells are especially well seen in the inset. (Reproduced, with permission, from Hellmann DB. Vasculitis. In: Stobo J, et al, eds. *Principles and Practice of Medicine.* Appleton & Lange; 1996.)

However, biopsies with a postfixation length of at least 1–2 cm are generally recommended. In addition, simultaneous or sequential bilateral temporal artery biopsies increase the yield to some degree. Treatment with glucocorticoids initiated within 2–4 weeks before temporal artery sampling does not appear to reduce the likelihood of a positive biopsy significantly. Pathologic changes diagnostic of GCA have been identified in the temporal artery biopsies of patients treated for many months—with apparent clinical success—with glucocorticoids.

C. Vascular Imaging

Vascular imaging plays an increasingly important role in the diagnosis of GCA. Its role in longitudinal management is less clear. Characteristic mural lesions may include circumferential wall thickening or edema, contrast enhancement, and ^{18}fluorine-2-deoxy-D-glucose (18-FDG) uptake. Luminal lesions may include diffuse stenosis, occlusion, and aneurysmal dilatation.

1. Color duplex ultrasound—CDS of the temporal arteries and large vessels is a safe, noninvasive, and cost-effective diagnostic tool in GCA. The most characteristic lesions suggesting vasculitis found with this imaging modality are the halo sign and the compression sign, which are sonographic correlates of arterial wall edema. The halo sign is seen as a rim of hypoechoic thickening surrounding the affected vessels (Figure 26–4). A positive compression sign is defined as the persistence of a visible vessel wall on compression of the lumen with the ultrasound probe.

CDS is operator dependent and requires skilled sonographers. For diagnostic purposes, the recommendation is to scan the complete length of both common superficial temporal arteries with their frontal and parietal branches in transverse and longitudinal views. Several studies and meta-analyses have estimated the sensitivity (55–100%) and specificity (75–100%) of the halo sign following this approach for the diagnosis of GCA compared to clinical diagnosis as the gold standard. Scanning other vascular territories (eg, axillary arteries, subclavian arteries, carotid arteries, facial arteries, occipital arteries, and abdominal aorta) may increase the diagnostic yield. The timing of resolution of CDS findings, once glucocorticoids are initiated, may range from days to months and tends to be longer for larger arteries.

2. Cross-sectional vascular imaging—Radiologic evidence of vasculitis involving the aorta and its primary branches is extremely common in GCA. Cross-sectional imaging has been an important part of classification criteria for inclusion of patients in clinical trials. CTA-defined large vessel arteritis (eg, mural thickening) is seen in up to 70% of GCA patients upon disease diagnosis (Figure 26–5A). Vasculitic involvement is more common in the thoracic and abdominal aorta, brachiocephalic trunk, subclavian arteries and carotid arteries. Arterial wall thickening and contrast uptake usually improve after treatment with glucocorticoids, but residual changes may persist in two-thirds of the patients who have them at diagnosis. Whether persistent mural lesions represent vascular remodeling or smoldering inflammation is unclear. After a mean follow-up time of 10 years, chronic damage in the form of aortic aneurysm or ectasia is seen by CTA in more than 30% of patients. These are frequently detected in patients with disease that is clinically and serologically quiescent.

PET-based imaging demonstrates changes suggestive of arterial inflammation (ie, 18-FDG uptake) in up to 80% of treatment-naïve patients with new-onset disease (Figure 26–5B). The vascular territories commonly affected include subclavian arteries and thoracoabdominal aorta, and less frequently carotid, brachial, and axillary arteries. Shorter disease duration, lower prednisone doses at the time of image acquisition, and clinical disease activity are predictors of a positive PET scan in GCA patients. Studies performing serial PET imaging demonstrate that the intensity of the arterial FDG uptake decreases with treatment but does not resolve entirely in more than half of patients judged to be in remission on the basis of other parameters. This residual abnormality raises speculation about low-grade inflammation as opposed to alterations of the endothelium or smooth muscle caused by vascular remodeling.

Large vessel vasculitis can also be demonstrated using MRI and MRA, which may identify concentric mural thickening with or without edema and/or gadolinium uptake and characteristic luminal changes (Figure 26–5C), respectively. As described with CT- and PET-based imaging, persistent vessel wall MRI signals are often detected during follow-up of treated patients.

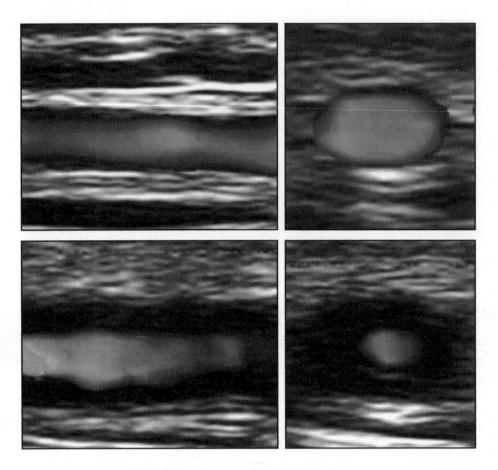

▲ **Figure 26–4.** Duplex ultrasound in GCA. Color duplex ultrasound (CDS) of the temporal arteries in longitudinal and transverse views in a patient without GCA (upper panels) and in a patient with GCA demonstrating the characteristic halo sign (concentric hypoechoic thickening surrounding the affected vessels) (lower panels). (See color insert.)

Besides its frequent use for diagnosis of GCA, vascular imaging has an established role in the assessment of large- and medium-sized arteries when clinical findings suggest the presence of lesions (eg, claudication, pulse deficits, blood pressure asymmetries or vascular bruits), and in the longitudinal monitoring of arterial damage previously identified. Nevertheless, the precise role of vascular imaging with respect to evaluation of response to therapy, monitoring of disease activity, and prediction of disease relapse or long-term arterial damage has not clearly been defined.

D. Musculoskeletal Imaging

Nonspecific bursitis and synovitis of the shoulder, hip, and related structures, including trochanteric bursitis, subacromial bursitis, subdeltoid bursitis, and bicipital tenosynovitis, can be identified by ultrasound, MRI, or PET in patients with PMR (Figure 26–6). In addition, both MRI and PET of the spine may demonstrate interspinous bursitis (see Figure 26–6).

Routine x-ray imaging of shoulders, hips, and spine, however, is not helpful in diagnosing PMR.

▶ Diagnostic Criteria

Five sets of classification criteria have been developed for primary PMR. These criteria summarize the main features of PMR, which include characteristic clinical symptoms (eg, hip/shoulder girdle pain and stiffness), elevation of inflammatory markers, and occurrence in the elderly. Some criteria also include prompt response to low/moderate doses of glucocorticoids. The 2012 provisional PMR criteria (Table 26–2) introduce specific laboratory testing and the optional use of ultrasound of the shoulders and hips into a scoring algorithm. According to these criteria, patients older than 50 years presenting with bilateral shoulder pain without alternative explanations can be classified as having PMR with approximately 70% sensitivity and approximately 80%

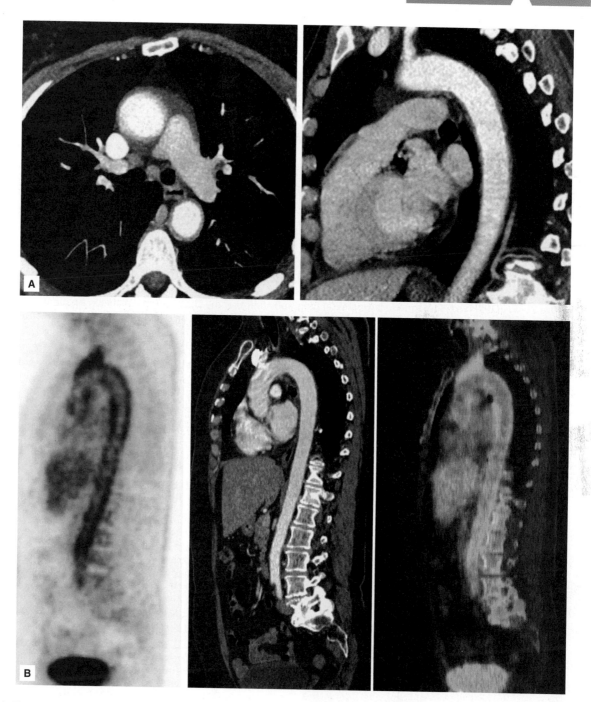

▲ **Figure 26–5.** Noninvasive cross-sectional vascular imaging in GCA. **A:** Computed tomography (CT) angiography of the thorax demonstrating mural thickening of the thoracic aorta in a patient with GCA-related aortitis (transversal and sagittal planes). **B:** Positron emission tomography (PET)/CT scan of the thoracic aorta of a GCA patient demonstrating markedly increased [18]fluorine-2-deoxy-D-glucose (18-FDG) uptake suggesting arterial inflammation (sagittal plane). The panel on the left shows the PET, the middle panel shows the CT, and the third panel shows the overlap of the former two (PET/CT). (See color insert.)

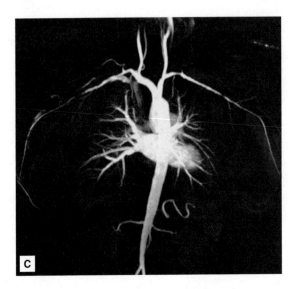

▲ **Figure 26–5.** (*Continued*) **C:** Magnetic resonance angiography (MRA) of the chest (coronal plane) in a patient with GCA showing long segments of diffuse stenosis involving the axillary and brachial arteries in a patient with GCA and arm claudication.

specificity when a combination of the following features are present: morning stiffness more than 45 minutes, elevated CRP and/or ESR, new hip pain/limited range of motion, absence of rheumatoid factor and anticitrullinated protein

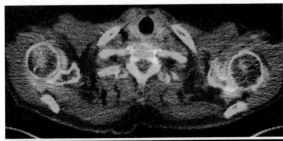

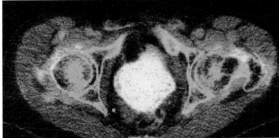

▲ **Figure 26–6.** Imaging in PMR. PET/CT in a patient with PMR demonstrating increased [18]fluorine-2-deoxy-D-glucose (18-FDG) in the structures around the shoulders (upper panel) and hips (lower panel) and in vicinity of the spinous process of the cervical vertebrae (upper panel). (See color insert.)

Table 26–2. 2012 provisional classification criteria for PMR.

Required criteria: age 50 years or older, bilateral shoulder aching, and abnormal CRP and/or ESR		
	Points without US (0–6)	Points with US[a] (0–8)
Morning stiffness lasting >45 minutes	2	2
Hip pain or limited range of motion	1	1
Absence of RF and ACPA	2	2
Absence of other joint involvement	1	1
At least one shoulder with subdeltoid bursitis and/or biceps tenosynovitis and/or glenohumeral synovitis (either posterior or axillary) and at least one hip with synovitis and/or trochanteric bursitis	Not applicable	1
Both shoulders with subdeltoid bursitis, biceps tenosynovitis, or glenohumeral synovitis	Not applicable	1

A score of 4 or more is categorized as PMR in the algorithm without US and a score of 5 or more is categorized as PMR in the algorithm with US.
[a]Optional ultrasound criteria.
ACPA, anticitrullinated protein antibody; CRP, C-reactive protein; ESR, erythrocyte sedimentation rate; PMR, polymyalgia rheumatica; RF, rheumatoid factor; US, ultrasound.
Reproduced with permission from Dasgupta B, Cimmino MA, Maradit-Kremers H, et al. 2012 provisional classification criteria for polymyalgia rheumatica: a European League Against Rheumatism/American College of Rheumatology collaborative initiative. *Ann Rheum Dis.* 2012;71(4):484-492.

antibody, absence of peripheral joint pain and presence of subdeltoid bursitis, biceps tenosynovitis, glenohumeral synovitis, hip synovitis, and/or trochanteric bursitis.

In 1990, the ACR developed classification criteria for GCA (see Table 26–1). These criteria include age more than 50 years, ESR greater than 50 mm/h, the occurrence new-onset headache, temporal artery abnormalities elicited on physical examination (eg, induration), and the presence of mononuclear inflammatory infiltrates in temporal artery biopsy. The sensitivity and specificity of these criteria to differentiate GCA from other vasculitides is approximately 80% and approximately 90%, respectively. The main limitation of the 1990 ACR criteria for GCA is that characteristic clinical manifestations (eg, jaw claudication, PMR symptoms, scalp tenderness, and visual disturbances), CRP elevation, and classic vascular imaging abnormalities are not captured. Modifications of the 1990 ACR classification criteria have been used as part of the inclusion criteria for clinical trials.

Differential Diagnosis

It is important to distinguish patients who have primary PMR from those who have PMR in the setting of GCA. Patients are classified as having primary PMR if they have no "above-the-neck" symptoms, namely, headache, jaw claudication, scalp tenderness, or vision symptoms. Completing a GCA workup in patients presenting with only PMR symptoms is not generally recommended. However, up to 20% of patients with symptoms of PMR alone may have positive temporal artery biopsy or vascular imaging suggesting GCA rather than primary PMR (Tuckwell et al, 2017).

Distinguishing primary PMR from rheumatoid arthritis in an older person can be difficult to impossible, particularly in patients with PMR symptoms who also have a distal polyarthritis. Severe erosive arthritis, rheumatoid nodules, and/or positive rheumatoid factor or anticitrullinated protein antibody make rheumatoid arthritis the more likely diagnosis.

Polymyositis causes objective proximal weakness rather than pain. In contrast, patients with PMR always rate their pain greater than any weakness. The creatine kinase is usually elevated in polymyositis but normal in PMR. Proximal limb pain or stiffness can occur with a variety of endocrine disorders, including hypothyroidism, diabetes, and osteomalacia. PMR is usually easily distinguished from fibromyalgia, which is a condition of diffuse pain—both proximal and distal—typically occurring in young women in the absence of objective findings or abnormal laboratory tests. Other conditions that can mimic PMR include early Parkinson disease, amyloidosis, late-onset systemic lupus erythematosus, endocarditis, myelodysplastic syndrome, and degenerative joint disease. Since absence of shoulder involvement is rare in PMR, patients thought to have "below the waist" PMR are more likely to have lumbar spinal stenosis, which can cause stiffness and pain restricted to the hip-girdle region.

Transient monocular loss of vision (amaurosis fugax) or permanent monocular blindness can also occur from atherosclerotic cerebrovascular or cardiovascular disease. The non-arteritis patients may be distinguished by their lack of other symptoms and normal inflammatory markers (ESR and CRP). Both atherosclerosis and GCA can also cause upper or lower extremity claudication. Angiography can usually differentiate these conditions. GCA produces isolated long segments of smooth narrowing in the midportions of arteries, whereas atherosclerosis tends to be focal and favors branch points.

Some of the clinical features of GCA can be produced by other forms of systemic vasculitis (GCA mimickers). ANCA-associated vasculitis, cryoglobulinemic vasculitis, and polyarteritis nodosa, for example, can cause inflammation of the extracranial arteries and produce headaches, scalp tenderness, and jaw claudication. These disorders can cause biopsy-proven "temporal arteritis" that is not GCA. The distinction is important, because the treatments for these conditions differ from those of GCA. Takayasu arteritis can affect the large vessels as GCA does, but it is usually seen in young women and is more likely than GCA to involve the pulmonary and renal arteries. Multiple myeloma, Waldenström macroglobulinemia, endocarditis, and osteomyelitis can produce systemic features with marked elevations of the ESR. In plasma cell dyscrasias, the ESR is usually disproportionately elevated with respect to the CRP (which is sometimes even normal) because of the excessive quantities of immunoglobulins in the serum. Many patients with diabetes in whom proteinuria has developed feel poorly and can have ESR elevations, as do patients with other forms of renal failure. Other mimickers of GCA may include myelodysplastic syndromes and systemic amyloidosis.

Treatment

Giant Cell Arteritis

There is no curative treatment for GCA. Until recently, prolonged glucocorticoid tapering courses (eg, 12–18 months) were the only option for disease control. Nevertheless, up to 85% of patients treated with 1 full year of glucocorticoids experience disease relapse when this medication is tapered. In addition, almost all GCA patients develop glucocorticoid-related side effects (see Prognosis). Many studies of potential "steroid-sparing" agents have failed or demonstrated only modest efficacy at best—prime examples being methotrexate and tumor necrosis factor inhibitors. Fortunately, the combination of IL-6 receptor (IL-6R) blockade with tocilizumab in combination with shorter glucocorticoid tapers has been shown to be an effective strategy (Stone et al, 2017).

A. Glucocorticoids

Prednisone (40–60 mg/day) should be administered immediately to any patient in whom GCA is strongly suspected while appropriate confirmatory workup is being completed (eg, temporal artery biopsy or large vessel imaging). The initial prednisone dose is typically maintained for about 4 weeks making sure that all symptoms resolve and the inflammatory markers normalize. Intravenous methylprednisolone pulses (eg, 1000 mg/day) for 3–5 days are recommended by some experts in the setting of visual manifestations (eg, amaurosis fugax, vision loss). Once the activity of the disease is controlled, the prednisone taper schedule varies among providers and may also be different depending on whether tocilizumab is being concomitantly used. Before the availability of tocilizumab, classic prednisone tapers for GCA even in the absence of disease flare were typically on the order of a minimum of 12 months and many practitioners never discontinued prednisone entirely. Initial dose reductions of 5–10 mg every 1–2 weeks until the prednisone dose was 20 mg would be followed by tapers of 2.5–5 mg every 1–2 weeks until the patient reached the dose of 10 mg daily. From 10 mg down to zero, the patients would taper 1 mg every 2–4 weeks. Upon disease relapse, the prednisone dose would be increased followed by a new tapering attempt. Not infrequently, many relapsing patients would remain on glucocorticoids for years.

B. Tocilizumab

The pivotal role of IL-6 in the pathogenesis of GCA has been demonstrated in randomized, controlled trials. Tocilizumab therapy leads to a higher rate of sustained remission, less cumulative glucocorticoid exposure, and superior quality of life compared with treatment using glucocorticoids alone. In a phase III GiACTA trial (Stone et al, 2017), 251 patients with active GCA (47% newly diagnosed) were randomized in a 1:1:1:2 ratio to placebo plus 26-week prednisone taper (PBO+26, N = 50), placebo plus 52-week prednisone taper (PBO+52, N = 51), TCZ 162 mg every other week plus 26-week prednisone taper (TCZ Q2W, N = 50) or TCZ 162 mg weekly plus 26-week prednisone taper (TCZ QW, N = 100). The prednisone taper was prespecified and standardized. The primary endpoint was sustained prednisone-free remission at week 52 comparing TCZ QW and TCZ Q2W versus PBO+26.

The primary endpoint of GiACTA was met in 56% of patients in the TCZ QW arm and in 53% of patients in the TCZ Q2W arm, compared to only 14% of patients in the PBO+26 arm ($P < .001$ for both comparisons). A key secondary endpoint was the comparison between the TCZ groups versus the PBO+52 group, which better reflects the previous usual treatment of GCA. Sustained prednisone-free remission was achieved in only 18% of patients in the PBO+52 group, again demonstrating superiority of TCZ QW and TCZ Q2W groups ($P < .01$ for both comparisons). Relapses were observed in 23% of patients in the TCZ QW arm, 26% of patients in the TCZ Q2W arm, 68% of patients in the PBO+26 arm, and 49% of patients in the PBO+52 arm. Furthermore, the cumulative median prednisone dose over 52 weeks was 1.9 mg in each of the TCZ groups compared with 3.3 mg in the PBO+26 group ($P < .01$) and 3.8 mg in the PBO+52 group

($P < .01$). Finally, compared to the PBO+26 and the PBO+52 groups, the TCZ QW group demonstrated better patient reported health-related quality-of-life outcomes.

C. Other Agents

IL-12/23 blockade has a good biologic rationale in GCA, but studies have shown conflicting results. RCTs with the monoclonal antibody against IL-6 sarilumab (ClinicalTrials.gov Identifier: NCT03600805), the JAK/STAT inhibitor upadacitinib (ClinicalTrials.gov Identifier: NCT03725202), and the GM-CSF receptor antagonist mavrilimumab (ClinicalTrials.gov Identifier: NCT03827018) are currently ongoing.

Polymyalgia Rheumatica

A. Glucocorticoids

Primary PMR is treated initially with oral glucocorticoids. Patients with primary PMR require 10–25 mg/day of prednisone or equivalent for induction of remission. After approximately 4 weeks on the initial dose, the prednisone is gradually tapered over 9–12 months. Additional treatment with immunosuppressive agents may be considered on an individual basis, particularly in patients who are unable to taper their prednisone successfully or who are at high risk of glucocorticoid toxicity at baseline. Evidence for a substantial impact of methotrexate is slim, but some experts use methotrexate in patients with risk factors for disease relapse (eg, females), those who have relapsed in the past, those suboptimal disease control with glucocorticoids alone, or those with poor tolerance of glucocorticoids. A more effective strategy is likely to treat such patients with IL-6R blockade (tocilizumab).

▶ Prognosis

GCA is associated with significant morbidity from the disease itself, reduced quality of life, and treatment-related toxicities. The most serious complication of the disease is blindness. Other possible complications include aortic aneurysm, aortic dissection, limb ischemia from large artery stenosis, and stroke. PMR is associated with reduced quality of life and glucocorticoid-related toxicity, although to a lesser extent compared to GCA given the milder nature of the disease and the lower glucocorticoid doses commonly employed.

Blindness

Blindness may occur in up to 20% of GCA patients, typically before the diagnosis is made and treatment with glucocorticoids is initiated. Unfortunately, permanent vision loss is usually severe and irreversible. Bilateral blindness occurs in a minority of patients. Given this risk, prompt initiation of high doses of glucocorticoids is mandatory when GCA is suspected, even before the diagnosis can be confirmed. Vision loss during longitudinal follow-up of patients is rare, but patients must be attuned to the possibility of new or recurrent vision symptoms so that treatment can be escalated appropriately.

Relapse

Depending of the definition used and the duration of follow up, between 34% and 85% of GCA patients treated only with glucocorticoids develop one or more relapses characterized by the recurrence of cranial symptoms, PMR symptoms, or a combination of both. Flares tend to occur within the first 12–24 months, when patients have tapered their prednisone dose below 10–15 mg (Stone et al, 2019). Similarly, relapses are seen in the majority of patients with primary PMR. Of note, up to one-third of relapses in patients with GCA and primary PMR may occur with normal levels of ESR and CRP and require diagnosis solely on the basis of clinical manifestations. In contrast to GCA patients receiving treatment only with glucocorticoids, the relapse rate in GCA patients treated with TCZ in combination with glucocorticoids is approximately 25% (Unizony et al, 2018).

Glucocorticoid-Related Toxicity

The median duration of glucocorticoid use in GCA patients treated with glucocorticoid monotherapy is about 3 years, leading to cumulative doses of approximately 5 g (Broder et al, 2016). Thus, complications from glucocorticoids develop in most patients. Glucocorticoid-related toxicity may include infection, osteoporosis with fragility fractures, avascular necrosis of the bone, diabetes, hypertension, dyslipidemia, psychiatric complications (eg, psychosis, anxiety, mood swings, and insomnia), gastrointestinal bleeding, weight gain, glaucoma, cataracts, myopathy, skin fragility, secondary adrenal insufficiency, and worsening of preexisting cardiovascular and metabolic conditions (eg, hypertension, diabetes, and congestive heart failure). For each 1 g of cumulative glucocorticoid exposure, the risk of toxicity increases by 3–5% (Broder et al, 2016). Glucocorticoid toxicity is also seen in PMR patients, but to a lesser extent.

A key aspect of the care of GCA and PMR patients is to take adequate measures to prevent and manage glucocorticoid-related toxicity. These measures include glucocorticoid-induced osteoporosis prophylaxis and treatment (including the use of bisphosphonates), immunizations (eg, influenza, pneumococcal, and zoster vaccines), and clear communication with the patient's primary care providers to address other glucocorticoid-related side effects that may arise (eg, hypertension, diabetes, psychiatric symptoms). It is important to keep in mind that more than 50% of patients with GCA receiving treatment with glucocorticoids will develop elevated inflammatory markers without clinical signs or symptoms of disease activity at some point of their disease (Unizony et al, 2018) Increasing the prednisone dose to "treat" this laboratory abnormalities is not recommended because it will increase the glucocorticoid exposure and likely lead to further toxicity. Instead, watchful monitoring and treatment modification upon clinical disease relapse are advised.

Large Artery Complications

Large artery complications in GCA include aortic aneurysm, aortic dissection, and large artery stenosis. Compared to the general population, GCA patients have a higher risk of both thoracic and aortic aneurysms. GCA-related aortic aneurysms, which are seen in 10–30% of GCA patients, are usually a late disease manifestation that develops on average 5–7 years after disease diagnosis. The subgroup of GCA patients who develop aortic aneurysms has a more than threefold increased risk of death compared to sex- and age-matched controls. Aortic dissection occurs in about 5% of patients and is an early phenomenon that carries a very high mortality rate. Arterial stenoses (eg, subclavian, axillary or brachial), which develop in 10–15% of patients, are usually diagnosed at the time or within 1 year of diagnosis. Large artery stenosis is not associated with increased mortality and generally improves or stabilizes with treatment. Thus, surgical revascularization is rarely required.

Given the prevalence of large vessel involvement in GCA and the potential clinical consequences of these lesions, early vascular imaging and longitudinal imaging surveillance with technology able to assess for mural and luminal arterial changes (eg, CTA, MRI/MRA, PET/CTA, PET/MRI/MRA) is recommended.

Broder MS, Sarsour K, Chang E, et al. Corticosteroid-related adverse events in patients with giant cell arteritis: a claims-based analysis. *Semin Arthritis Rheum.* 2016;46(2):246-252. [PMID: 27378247]

Buttgereit F, Dejaco C, Matteson EL, Dasgupta B. Polymyalgia rheumatica and giant cell arteritis: a systematic review. *JAMA.* 2016;315(22):2442-2458. [PMID: 27299619]

Deng J, Younge BR, Olshen RA, Goronzy JJ, Weyand CM. Th17 and Th1 T-cell responses in giant cell arteritis. *Circulation.* 2010; 121(7):906-915. [PMID: 20142449]

Kermani TA, Schmidt J, Crowson CS, et al. Utility of erythrocyte sedimentation rate and C-reactive protein for the diagnosis of giant cell arteritis. *Semin Arthritis Rheum.* 2012;41(6):866-871. [PMID: 22119103]

Koster MJ, Matteson EL, Warrington KJ. Large-vessel giant cell arteritis: diagnosis, monitoring and management. *Rheumatology (Oxford).* 2018;57(suppl_2):ii32-ii42. [PMID: 29982778]

Miyabe C, Miyabe Y, Strle K, et al. An expanded population of pathogenic regulatory T cells in giant cell arteritis is abrogated by IL-6 blockade therapy. *Ann Rheum Dis.* 2017;76(5):898-905. [PMID: 27927642]

Ostberg G. Morphological changes in the large arteries in polymyalgia arteritica. *Acta Med Scand Suppl.* 1972;533:135-159. [PMID: 4508179]

Samson M, Jacquin A, Audia S, et al. Stroke associated with giant cell arteritis: a population-based study. *J Neurol Neurosurg Psychiatry.* 2015;86(2):216-221. [PMID: 24780954]

Stone JH, Tuckwell K, Dimonaco S, et al. Glucocorticoid dosages and acute-phase reactant levels at giant cell arteritis flare in a randomized trial of tocilizumab. *Arthritis Rheumatol.* 2019; 71(8):1329-1338. [PMID: 30835950]

Stone JH, Tuckwell K, Dimonaco S, et al. Trial of tocilizumab in giant-cell arteritis. *N Engl J Med.* 2017;377(4):317-328. [PMID: 28745999]

Tuckwell K, Collinson N, Dimonaco S, et al. Newly diagnosed vs. relapsing giant cell arteritis: baseline data from the GiACTA trial. *Semin Arthritis Rheum.* 2017;46(5):657-664. [PMID: 27998620]

Unizony S, Pei J, Sidiropoulos PN, Best JH, Birchwood C, Stone JH. Clinical outcomes of patients with giant cell arteritis treated with tocilizumab in real-world clinical practice. *ACR/ARHP Annual Meeting, Chicago* 2018.

Vodopivec I, Rizzo JF 3rd. Ophthalmic manifestations of giant cell arteritis. *Rheumatology (Oxford).* 2018;57(suppl_2):ii63-ii72. [PMID: 29986083]

Wen Z, Shen Y, Berry G, et al. The microvascular niche instructs T cells in large vessel vasculitis via the VEGF-Jagged1-Notch pathway. *Sci Transl Med.* 2017;9(399). [PMID: 28724574]

Takayasu Arteritis

27

Sebastian Unizony, MD

▶ Takayasu arteritis (TAK) causes granulomatous vasculitis of the aorta, main aortic branches and pulmonary arteries.

▶ Preferentially affects young women.

▶ Often presents with absent pulses, extremity claudication, hypertension, or constitutional symptoms.

▶ Erythrocyte sedimentation rate and C-reactive protein levels are usually elevated.

▶ Definitive diagnosis requires vascular imaging or biopsy.

▶ Patients respond acutely to prednisone. However, relapse upon prednisone tapering is common and glucocorticoid-sparing immunosuppressive drugs are needed for remission maintenance in most cases

▶ Subclinical progression of arterial damage despite treatment can be seen and patients should undergo periodic imaging surveillance.

Takayasu arteritis (TAK), named for the Japanese ophthalmologist who first described the ocular manifestations in 1908, is a granulomatous large-vessel vasculitis that mostly affects women during their reproductive years. The granulomatous arteritis associated with TAK leads both vascular stenoses and ectases, depending on the specifc vessel involved. TAK generally presents two major challenges. First, the diagnosis can be delayed for months or even years due to its rarity and the protean nature of the presenting manifestations. Second, relapse and subclinical disease progression often occur despite treatment. Although TAK is a chronic condition, it usually follows a waxing and waning course that requires careful clinical and imaging monitoring to determine when the disease is active, and immunosuppression is needed. Because of the advances in medical therapy and

surgical treatment of vascular complications such as aortic regurgitation, survival of patients with TAK has increased significantly. Substantial morbidity, however, still occurs in most cases. Morbidity occurs not only as a result of the disease but also from complications of treatment.

▶ Epidemiology

TAK has been reported most extensively in Asia, the Middle East, and Latin America, but cases have been described worldwide and TAK is known to affect patients with diverse ethnic backgrounds (Onen and Akkoc, 2017). The highest prevalence of TAK, 40 cases per million population, was estimated in Japan. The prevalence in the United States has been reported to be 0.9–2.6 cases per million population. The prevalence in European countries varies between 4.7 and 33 per million population. TAK affects women up to eight times more frequently than men (Goel et al, 2018). The average age at diagnosis is in the mid-20s, but the disease may begin as early as age 4 or as late as age 74. Symptoms develop before age 20 in nearly one-third of patients and after age 40 in 10–25% of them. Caucasians tend to be older at the time of diagnosis.

▶ Etiology & Pathogenesis

The cause of TAK remains elusive. However, the geographic clustering of cases suggests genetic or environmental etiologic factors. HLA and non-HLA genetic associations have been identified. These include HLA-Bw52, HLA-B/MICA, HLA-DQB1, HLA-DRB1, FCGR2A, FCGR3A, RPS9/LILRB3, IL6, TNF-α, IL-17F, and IL12B (Carmona et al, 2017; Renauer et al, 2015; Saruhan-Direskeneli et al, 2013). In addition, the predominance of TAK in women of childbearing age suggests that female hormones may play a permissive role, as in other systemic autoimmune conditions.

TAK is characterized by inflammatory injury of the walls of large- and medium-sized arteries. A break in self-immune tolerance, possibly via molecular mimicry between host- and pathogen-derived antigens, is believed to be the initial event. The pathogenic process progresses from a granulomatous inflammatory response early on to a pauci- or noninflammatory remodeling phenomenon characterized by extensive fibrosis, smooth muscle cell proliferation, and intimal hyperplasia in later stages of the disease. The inflammatory infiltrates observed in TAK are more heterogeneous than those of giant cell arteritis. Key cellular players include CD4+ T cells, CD8+ T cells, γδ+ T cells, B cells, natural killer (NK) cells, macrophages, and multinucleated giant cells (Espinoza and Matsumura, 2018). Immunophenotype analysis of the CD4+ T-cell compartment demonstrates phenotypes skewed toward the Th17 and Th1 lineages (eg, IL-17 and IFN-γ production) to the detriment of the regulatory T-cell subset.

One of the putative mechanisms of immune-mediated damage in TAK includes the NK group 2D (NKG2D) receptor expressed on NK cells and various subsets of T cells. NKG2D recognizes the HLA class I molecule MICA that is located on the surface of cells exposed to stress. Certain MICA variants confer risk for TAK, and upregulation of this molecule has been detected in aortic samples derived from affected patients.

Various inflammatory cytokines such as IL-6, IL-12, IL-18, IL-23, IL-17, TNF-α, and IFN-γ, some of which correlate with disease activity (eg, IL-6 and TNF-α), are thought to play roles in the amplification and maintenance of the inflammatory process in TAK (Espinoza and Matsumura, 2018).

▶ Clinical Presentation

TAK can have an acute onset, but the great majority of patients develop subacute or chronic presentations. The severity of the disease at presentation may range from asymptomatic to catastrophic, with stroke caused by uncontrolled (often unrecognized) hypertension or heart failure resulting aortic insufficiency. Unfortunately, the median diagnostic delay is approximately 1 year. Delays are usually longer in patients presenting with normal inflammatory markers.

Although the clinical features of TAK are heterogenous, they can be categorized into two broad domains: those caused by vascular involvement and those caused by systemic inflammation. The separation of these two types of presenting features is not always neatly maintained; many patients have both vascular complications and systemic symptoms, and others have a biphasic presentation, with systemic symptoms dominating early (so-called "acute phase") and vascular features (so-called "chronic phase") becoming more prominent later.

The vessels most commonly involved are the subclavian, carotid, axillary, and renal arteries and the aorta (Table 27–1) (Li et al, 2017). The vertebral, pulmonary, coronary, mesenteric, and iliofemoral arteries are affected less often. Inflammation and intimal proliferation lead to wall thickening and stenotic or occlusive lesions (usually seen in the primary

Table 27–1. Frequency of blood vessel involvement in Takayasu arteritis.

Blood Vessel	% Abnormal
Thoracic aorta	10–60
Abdominal aorta	20–70
Subclavian artery	65–80
Common carotid artery	30–80
Vertebral artery	10–30
Pulmonary artery	5–70
Coronary artery	20–60
Renal artery	20–50
Mesenteric artery	7–30
Iliofemoral artery	10–20

branches of the aorta), while destruction of the elastic and muscularis often leads to aneurysms in the aorta.

Depending on the territory involved, vascular inflammation and subsequent damage may cause a variety of clinical manifestations (Goel et al, 2018). Signs and symptoms of arterial involvement are observed in more than 60% of patients. Bruits can be detected frequently over the carotid arteries, but can also be heard in the supraclavicular or infraclavicular space (reflecting subclavian disease), along the flexor surface of the upper arm (from axillary artery stenosis), in the abdomen (due renal artery involvement), or in the groin (femoral artery disease). Multiple bruits are common. Upper extremity claudication, manifested by exertional arm fatigue and pain, develops more often than lower extremity claudication. Arterial dissection is a possible but uncommon complication of TAK (Sanchez-Alvarez et al, 2019).

Cardiac disease is a major cause of morbidity and mortality in TAK. At some point during the course of the disease, nearly half of patients have cardiac manifestations, which can potentially affect any structure of the heart. Volume overload (ie, aortic insufficiency), pressure overload (ie, hypertension due to aortic narrowing or renal artery stenosis), myocardial ischemia (ie, coronary arteritis), and myocarditis may lead to left ventricular dysfunction. Other cardiac manifestations comprise pericarditis, ischemic heart disease secondary to premature atherosclerosis, arrhythmia, and sudden cardiac death. Symptoms reflecting cardiac involvement may include chest pain, dyspnea, palpitations, and syncope.

Aortic insufficiency is detected in 15–50% of TAK patients depending of the diagnostic methodology used. This complication occurs primarily as a consequence of valvular leaflet separation produced in the context of ascending aortitis and aneurysm formation (Figure 27–1A). The clinical presentation of aortic insufficiency ranges from asymptomatic to rapidly progressive congestive heart failure. Physical examination may elicit a diastolic murmur along the right

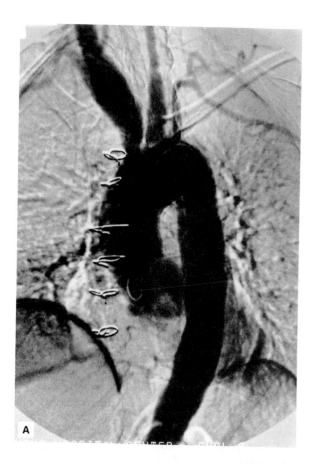

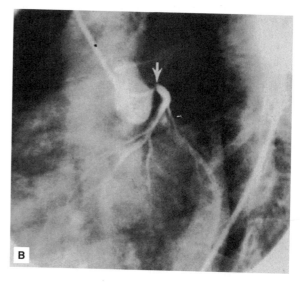

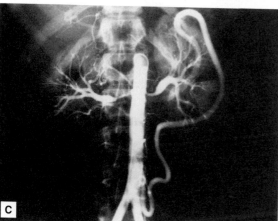

▲ **Figure 27–1.** Conventional angiography in TAK. **A:** Angiogram showing multiple lesions, including dilatations of the ascending aorta (with surgical wires from aortic valve replacement surgery) and the brachiocephalic and proximal right common carotid arteries. The left common carotid artery is occluded distal to its origin **B:** Coronary angiogram showing left coronary ostial stenosis. **C:** Angiogram showing bilateral renal artery stenosis. A large left colic branch of the inferior mesenteric artery provides collateral circulation. (A and B, Reprinted with permission from Hellmann DB, Flynn JA. Clinical presentation and natural history of Takayasu's arteritis and other inflammatory arteritides. In: Perler BA, Becker GJ, eds. *Vascular Intervention: A Clinical Approach.* New York: Thieme Medical; 1998:249-256. **C,** Used with permission from Dr. Michael Jaff, Boston, MA.)

sternal border and widened pulse pressures ("bounding or Corrigan's pulse").

Coronary artery involvement is demonstrated by angiography in up to 60% of patients, but becomes symptomatic in only 5–20% of cases. Clinical presentations may include angina, myocardial infarction, arrhythmia, conduction abnormalities, or congestive failure. Along with aortic valve disease, myocardial ischemia is a leading cause of death in TAK. Stenosis and occlusions tend to occur in the coronary ostia (>70%) and proximal coronary segments (Figure 27–1B). Vascular inflammation is the main mechanism of coronary arteriopathy. In addition, ostial obstructions may also be caused by extension of adjacent aortic remodeling (ie, fibrotic retraction). In many cases, atherosclerosis secondary to hypertension and chronic inflammation is an adjuvant factor for the development of coronary artery disease.

Although up to 50% of the individuals with TAK have some degree of subclinical myocardial inflammation, overt myocarditis is rarely seen. This complication should be suspected in patients presenting with chest pain or heart failure in the absence of pericardial, coronary, or valvular lesions. Secondary cardiomyopathy, on the other hand, can occur in the setting of chronic hypertension, valvulopathy, and ischemic coronary disease.

Neuro-ophthalmologic manifestations are common in TAK. Common symptoms include headaches, dizziness, presyncope and syncope. Stroke and transient ischemic attack develop in 5–15% of patients due to involvement of the carotid or vertebral arteries, and rarely due to inflammation of the intracranial arteries. In contrast, the visual symptoms first described by Takayasu occur rarely today. When present, visual symptoms chiefly result from retinal ischemia produced by narrowing or occlusion of the carotid arteries (ie, Takayasu retinopathy). Fundoscopic examination demonstrates wreath-like anastomosis of the retinal vessels, arteriovenous dilation, microaneurysms, and neovascularization. Fluorescein angiography may reveal delayed choroidal circulation and areas of peripheral ischemia. Occasionally, patients may have such limited blood flow through the supra-aortic arteries that merely turning or tilting the head causes light-headedness or visual loss (ie, visual claudication). In some cases, severe renovascular hypertension is the cause of retinopathy, but in such cases the retina has a different appearance, consistent with that of hypertensive retinopathy.

The pulmonary arteries are affected in up to 50% of patients. Clinically significant pulmonary arterial hypertension is seen in just a quarter of those cases, however. The pulmonary hypertension associated with TAK is generally mild to moderate, and therefore rarely provokes right ventricular dysfunction.

Stenosis of one or both renal arteries, observed in 25–50% of patients, results in significant hypertension in many of those affected (Figure 27–1C). More than half of patients with renal artery involvement develop chronic kidney disease. In a minority of individuals with TAK, hypertension may be due to aortic narrowing from a prior inflammatory insult (ie, aortic coarctation).

About two-thirds of TAK patients experience constitutional or musculoskeletal symptoms, including asthenia, weight loss, fever, night sweats, myalgias, and arthralgias. These features dominate the presentation in nearly one-third of all cases. Prominent back pain, especially in the thoracic region, develops in a few patients. This pain resembles that seen in older patients with thoracic dissection and probably results from stimulation of nociceptive nerve fibers along the inflamed aorta.

Other clinical manifestations may include erythema-nodosum–type lesions, Raynaud phenomenon, livedo reticularis, skin ulcers (sometimes resembling pyoderma gangrenosum), digital gangrene, inflammatory eye disease (eg, uveitis, scleritis, and episcleritis), angiodynia (eg, carotidynia), abdominal angina form mesenteric vasculitis, and rarely, glomerulonephritis. Finally, an association between inflammatory bowel disease and TAK has been reported with approximately 6% of TAK patients carrying the diagnosis of either ulcerative colitis or Crohn disease, usually preceding the onset of vasculitis.

▶ Diagnosis

The diagnosis of TAK requires demonstrating vasculitis in the aorta or its major branches by vascular imaging or biopsy, and excluding the diseases that can produce similar clinical presentations or arterial abnormalities. Two types of presentations should alert the clinician to the possibility of TAK: (1) a systemically ill patient with nonspecific laboratory findings indicative of inflammation; and (2) cardiovascular features, such as limb claudication, hypertension, or inability to palpate a pulse or obtain a blood pressure reading, particularly in a young patient or a patient without risk factors for atherosclerosis. A high index of suspicion, proper evaluation of the patient's history, and meticulous physical examination in search of arterial bruits, pulse deficits, blood pressure asymmetries, and cardiac murmurs all aid in the early diagnosis of TAK.

A. Laboratory Findings

TAK does not cause any specific blood test or urinary abnormalities but is usually associated with elevated acute phase reactants and other indicatiors of inflammation. Nearly 80% of patients have elevated erythrocyte sedimentation rates (ESR) or C-reactive protein (CRP) values, especially during phases of active disease. Unfortunately, no blood test that is a reliable measure of disease activity currently exists. For example, the ESR is normal in 20–30% of patients with active disease and is elevated in 40–50% of patients with inactive disease. Anemia of chronic disease develops in 50% of patients. Thrombocytosis, which occurs in one-third of patients, is often mild but may occasionally exceed 800,000 per microliter. Patients with renal artery involvement may develop elevated serum creatinine and urinalysis abnormalities (eg, mild proteinuria and/or hematuria) from hypertensive nephropathy.

B. Imaging Studies

Vascular imaging is the diagnostic test most frequently used in TAK because abnormalities suggestive of vasculitis

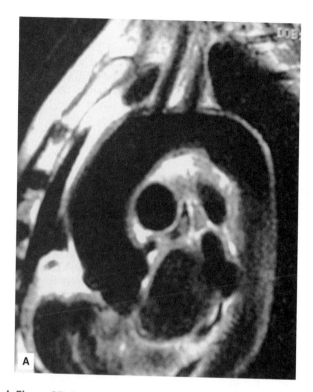 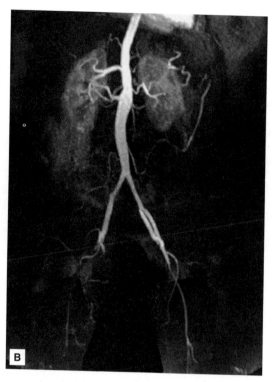

▲ **Figure 27–2.** Magnetic resonance-based imaging in TAK. **A:** Magnetic resonance imaging (MRI) showing thickening of the wall of the ascending and descending thoracic aorta. **B:** Magnetic resonance angiography (MRA) showing a long segment of severe luminal stenosis of the right external iliac artery with reconstitution of the right common femoral artery from collaterals. Suprarenal abdominal aortic narrowing is also observed.

are found in the walls and lumens of large-sized arteries in virtually all cases (Barra et al, 2018) (Figures 27–2 through 27–4; see Figure 27–1). Several imaging modalities are helpful in identifying characteristic vascular lesions, including conventional angiography, magnetic resonance imaging and angiography (MRI/MRA) (see Figure 27–2), computed tomography angiography (CTA) (see Figure 27–3), positron emission tomography (PET) (see Figure 27–4), and vascular ultrasound. Mural findings may include circumferential wall thickening or edema (MRI, CTA, and ultrasound), contrast enhancement (MRI and CTA), and ^{18}fluorine-2-deoxy-D-glucose (FDG) uptake (PET) (Barra et al, 2018; Grayson et al, 2018). Luminal lesions may include stenosis, occlusion, and aneurysmal dilatation (MRA, CTA, angiography, and ultrasound).

Given their ability to detect mural changes, MRI, CTA, PET, and ultrasound may identify arterial lesions before irreversible damage has occurred (eg, stenosis/occlusion and dilatation). Conventional angiography, although unhelpful in determining mural involvement, provides an accurate assessment of the arterial lumens (see Figure 27–1). However, MRA (see Figure 27–2B) and CTA (see Figure 27–3), which delineate vascular lumens noninvasively, have relegated the

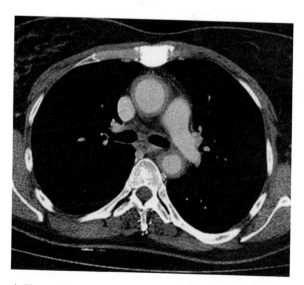

▲ **Figure 27–3.** Computed tomography angiography in TAK. Computed tomography angiography showing thickening of the wall of the ascending and descending thoracic aorta.

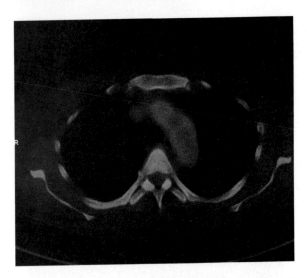

▲ **Figure 27–4.** Positron emission tomography/computed tomography in TAK. Positron emission tomography/computed tomography (PET/CT) showing increased 18-fluorodeoxyglucose uptake in the wall of aortic arch.

use of conventional angiography to selected cases. Because TAK patients often require periodic vascular imaging, MRI/MRA is the technology of choice for longitudinal monitoring of arterial damage to avoid excessive radiation exposure.

C. Biopsy

Tissue from blood vessels is obtained only in the minority of patients requiring surgery, and therefore, is not a widely used diagnostic tool in TAK. Biopsies of involved arteries show granulomatous vasculitis. The initial site of inflammation is the medio-adventitial junction, where the vasa vasora enter the artery wall. Once the disease is well established, all arterial wall layers become affected. Active lesions exhibit diffuse inflammatory infiltrates composed of mononuclear cells, including lymphocytes, macrophages, and giant cells. In addition, medial and adventitial necrosis, as well as intimal fibrocellular hyperplasia and thrombus formation, are often appreciated. In contrast, chronic lesions are characterized by fibrosis involving the media and the adventitia and patchy inflammatory infiltrates.

▶ Diagnostic and Classification Criteria

Several sets of diagnostic and classification criteria have been developed to differentiate TAK from other vasculopathies (Table 27–2). The Ishikawa criteria and the Ishikawa criteria modified by Sharma et al., are based on major and minor criteria including signs, symptoms, inflammatory markers and angiographic lesions. The 1990 American College of Rheumatology (ACR) classification criteria includes age, the presence of extremity claudication, physical findings (eg, decreased pulse, blood pressure discrepancies, and vascular

bruits), and classic angiographic abnormalities. Similarly, the European League Against Rheumatism (EULAR) / Pediatric Rheumatology International Trials Organization (PRINTO) / Pediatric Rheumatology European Society (PRES) classification criteria for childhood TAK requires typical angiographic lesions plus at least one of the following: (1) peripheral pulse deficit or limb claudication; (2) blood pressure asymmetry; (3) bruits; (4) hypertension; and (5) elevated ESR or CRP.

▶ Disease Extension

Hata and Numano et al proposed a radiologic classification of TAK based on the distribution of arterial involvement. According to this classification, type I disease presents involvement of branches of aortic arch; type IIa presents involvement of ascending aorta, aortic arch and its branches; type IIb comprise type IIa plus involvement of thoracic descending aorta; type III presents involvement of thoracic descending aorta, abdominal aorta and/or renal arteries; type IV presents involvement of abdominal aorta and/or renal arteries; and type V represents the combination type IIb plus type IV (ie, entire aorta and its major branches). Whereas type V disease is reported in 50-70% of patients in most cohorts, other vascular distributions demonstrate geographic variation. Indian (30%) and Thai (20%) patients present type III disease more often compared with patients from Japan, Mexico, US, Turkey, Italy, and Korea (1-8%). In contrast, type I and II disease is less frequent in India (15%) and Thailand (10%) compared to the other above mentioned geographic regions (25-45%).

▶ Differential Diagnosis

The biggest impediment to diagnosing TAK is that few physicians are sufficiently familiar with this rare disease to recognize its presenting manifestations. Of the other vasculitides, giant cell arteritis (see Chapter 26) is the form most likely to be confused with TAK. Both diseases cause granulomatous panarteritis and elevation of ESR and CRP. In contrast to TAK, giant cell arteritis exclusively affects patients over the age of 50, typically involves the superficial cranial arteries (eg, temporal arteries), does not involve the pulmonary arteries, and very rarely affects the renal arteries. Cogan syndrome is a rare disease characterized by immune-mediated inner ear disease leading to vestibular-auditory abnormalities (deafness, vertigo) and ocular inflammation (especially inflammation of the cornea) that causes a medium- or large-vessel vasculitis in a minority of patients. Behçet disease (see Chapter 34) is associated with a variable-vessel vasculitis that involves large blood vessels in approximately 10% of cases. The distinctive feature of Behçet disease—recurrent orogenital ulcers—does not occur in TAK. IgG4-related disease can cause aortitis in either the thoracic or abdominal aorta,

Table 27–2. Takayasu arteritis (TAK) diagnostic and classification criteria.

Ishikawa Criteria	Sharma Criteria	ACR Criteria	EULAR/PRINTO/PRES Criteria (Childhood TAK)
Mandatory criterion ≤40 years at onset of characteristic signs or symptoms[a] for >1 month **Major criteria** 1. Left mid-subclavian artery stenosis or occlusion 2. Right mid-subclavian artery stenosis or occlusion **Minor criteria** 1. ESR ≥20 mm/h 2. Carotid artery tenderness 3. Hypertension at age ≤40 4. Aortic regurgitation or annuloaortic ectasia 5. Pulmonary artery stenosis, aneurysm, or luminal irregularity 6. Left common carotid artery stenosis or occlusion 7. Distal brachiocephalic trunk stenosis or occlusion 8. Descending aortic stenosis, aneurysm, or luminal irregularity 9. Abdominal aortic stenosis, aneurysm, or luminal irregularity sparing the aortoiliac region In addition to the mandatory criterion, the presence of 2 major criteria or 1 major plus ≥2 minor criteria, or ≥4 minor criteria provides 84% sensitivity and 100% specificity for the diagnosis of TAK	**Major criteria** 1. Left mid-subclavian artery stenosis or occlusion 2. Right mid-subclavian artery stenosis or occlusion 3. Signs and symptoms[a] for >1 month **Minor criteria** 1. Elevated ESR ≥20 mm/h 2. Carotid artery tenderness 3. Hypertension 4. Aortic regurgitation or annuloaortic ectasia 5. Pulmonary artery stenosis, aneurysm, or luminal irregularity 6. Left common carotid artery stenosis or occlusion 7. Distal brachiocephalic trunk stenosis or occlusion 8. Descending aortic stenosis, aneurysm, or luminal irregularity 9. Abdominal aortic stenosis, aneurysm, or luminal irregularity 10. Coronary artery stenosis, aneurysm, or luminal irregularity below the age of 30 years and in the absence of other risk factors (eg, diabetes) The presence of 2 major or 1 major and ≥2 minor criteria or ≥4 minor criteria provides 92.5% sensitivity and 95% specificity for the diagnosis of TAK	1. Onset at age <40 years 2. Limb claudication 3. Decreased brachial artery pulse 4. Unequal arm blood pressures (>10 mm Hg) 5. Subclavian or aortic bruit 6. Angiographic evidence of narrowing or occlusion of the aorta or its primary branches The presence of ≥3 criteria provides 90.5% sensitivity and 97.8% specificity for the diagnosis of TAK	**Mandatory criterion** Typical angiographic changes detected in the aorta, main aortic branches, and/or pulmonary arteries (eg, dilatation, narrowing, occlusion, or mural thickening) **Nonmandatory criteria** 1. Absence of a peripheral artery pulse or presence of limb claudication 2. >10 mm Hg difference in systolic blood pressure in any extremity 3. Arterial bruits 4. Hypertension 5. ESR ≥20 mm/h and/or CRP above the normal limit In addition to the mandatory criterion, the presence of ≥1 nonmandatory criterion provides 100% sensitivity and 99.9% specificity for the diagnosis of TAK

[a]Characteristic signs and symptoms may include limb claudication, pulselessness or pulse difference, unobtainable or significant blood pressure difference of more than 10 mm Hg in systolic blood pressure, fever, neck pain, transient amaurosis, blurred vision, syncope, dyspnea, or palpitations.

ACR, American College of Rheumatology; CRP, C-reactive protein; ESR, erythrocyte sedimentation rate; EULAR, European League Against Rheumatism; PRES, Pediatric Rheumatology European Society; PRINTO, Pediatric Rheumatology International Trials Organization; TAK, Takayasu arteritis.

occasionally requiring surgery, and is sometimes associated with retroperitoneal fibrosis. Syphilitic aortitis, a prototypical form of large-vessel inflammation, is extremely rare these days but can be excluded by appropriate serologic studies.

A few other inflammatory diseases can affect the aorta or its branches, but almost never do they mimic TAK in a convincing manner (Table 27–3). Relapsing polychrondritis, which results in characteristic changes in cartilage, may also affect the aorta. Rheumatoid vasculitis and ankylosing spondylitis rarely affect the thoracic root. Buerger disease—a form of medium-vessel vasculopathy associated with smoking—may affect the femoral, brachial, and axillary arteries. Noninflammatory conditions should also be considered in the differential diagnosis of TAK. Marfan syndrome and type IV

Ehlers-Danlos syndrome are causes of vascular fragility and aortic aneurysm, but these patients present with other classic phenotypical features (eg, joint hypermobility). Fibromuscular dysplasia may involve the renal, carotid, and vertebral arteries causing characteristic radiologic lesions. Neurofibromatosis and congenital coarctation may affect the abdominal aorta and mesenteric great vessels. Radiation-induced damage can affect any vessel including the aorta. Atherosclerosis of the aorta and major branches rarely develops before age 50 and does not produce the long, smoothly tapered and stenotic segments of arteries that are so characteristic of TAK. In addition, noninflammatory vasculopathies lack radiological (eg, concentric arterial wall thickening) or serological (eg, increased ESR or CPR) evidence of inflammation.

Table 27–3. Differential diagnosis of Takayasu arteritis: other diseases that can affect large and medium-sized arteries.

Inflammatory diseases	Giant cell arteritis, Cogan syndrome, Behçet disease, relapsing polychrondritis, ankylosing spondylitis, rheumatoid arthritis, systemic lupus erythematosus, sarcoidosis, IgG4-related disease (IgG4RD), polyarteritis nodosa (PAN), Kawasaki disease
Infectious diseases	Syphilis, mycotic aneurysm
Noninflammatory vasculopathies	Atherosclerosis, radiation-induced arterial damage, neurofibromatosis, congenital coarctation, Marfan syndrome, EDS type IV, fibromuscular dysplasia (FMD)

▶ Treatment

A. Medical Treatment

1. Glucocorticoids—Glucocorticoids are effective in controlling inflammation and inducing disease remission when used in moderate to high doses in most patients with TAK. Initial therapy consists of prednisone (0.5–1 mg/kg/day) for approximately 1 month, followed by a taper of variable duration (eg, 6–12 months). Often times, TAK patients require low doses of glucocorticoids (eg, prednisone 5–10 mg daily) for maintenance of remission. Unfortunately, relapse is common in patients receiving glucocorticoids alone, and glucocorticoid-induced toxicity is frequently seen (Kerr GS et al. 1994).

2. Conventional immunosuppression—Immunosuppressive medications have been used in TAK to try to prevent disease relapse and spare the use of glucocorticoids. Until recently, however, randomized controlled trials were not available to guide therapy, and most recommendations were based on observational uncontrolled studies. Agents commonly used include methotrexate, azathioprine, mycophenolate, leflunomide, and less frequently, cyclophosphamide. Although better disease outcomes have been reported in patients receiving a combination of oral immunosuppressant and glucocorticoids compared to patients treated only with glucocorticoids, relapse (30–95%) and vascular disease progression (20–50%) still challenge the longitudinal care of patients with TAK (Maksimowicz-McKinnon K et al. 2007).

3. Biologic immunosuppressants—Evidence from uncontrolled studies suggests that TNF-α inhibitors (eg, infliximab, adalimumab, certolizumab, and etanercept) may be effective in maintaining remission and sparing glucocorticoids in TAK patients (Hoffman et al, 2004; Molloy et al, 2008). A review of

20 observational studies, including 120 patients treated with infliximab (N = 109), etanercept (N = 17), or adalimumab (N = 9), showed that remission was achieved in up to 90% of patients and that glucocorticoid discontinuation was possible in 40% of patients (Clifford and Hoffman, 2014). In the majority of cases, however, a nonbiologic immunosuppressive drug was maintained along with the TNF-α blocker. Despite treatment, 37% of patients relapsed and 50% of them required an increase in the dose or a switch to a different TNF-α inhibitor to maintain remission (Clifford and Hoffman, 2014).

Following positive results observed with the IL-6 receptor inhibitor tocilizumab in observational studies, a randomized controlled trial evaluated the efficacy of this agent in 36 patients with relapsing disease (Nakaoka et al, 2018). Patients were randomized in a 1:1 ratio to tocilizumab 162 mg subcutaneously weekly or placebo in combination with a prednisone taper. Relapses were seen in 8 (44%) and 11 (61%) of patients assigned to tocilizumab and placebo, respectively. Analyzed with an intention-to-treat approach, tocilizumab failed to show a significant difference in time to relapse as compared to placebo (hazard ratio [HR] 0.41, 95% confidence interval [CI] 0.15–1.10, $P = 0.06$). However, a significant difference favoring tocilizumab was observed in a per-protocol analysis (HR 0.34, 95% CI 0.11–1.00, $P = 0.03$). As with all other treatment agents, vascular disease progression (often clinically silent) has been reported in TAK patients receiving tocilizumab. Thus, periodic imaging surveillance is recommended even in patients that are judged to be in clinical remission.

Finally, encouraging preliminary results have been reported in patients with refractory TAK using ustekinumab, a monoclonal antibody that inhibits IL-12 and IL-23 signaling (Yachoui et al, 2018).

4. Revascularization—Revascularization of stenotic lesions is frequently unnecessary in TAK, because the slow pace of the disease generally permits the development of abundant collateral blood vessels. Whenever possible, angioplasty or vascular surgery should be deferred until immunomodulatory therapy has suppressed the arterial inflammation.

Surgery can be lifesaving for treating aortic regurgitation, coronary artery lesions, and thoracic aortic aneurysms. Angioplasty with stenting and bypass procedures have been successful in treating cases of refractory hypertension caused by renal artery stenosis and in cases of limb, cerebral, or mesenteric ischemia that is severe and symptomatic despite medial therapy. The rate of restenosis, which seems to be higher after angioplasty compared to bypass surgery, has decreased in the era of drug-eluting stents and with the more frequent use of systemic immunosuppression.

▶ Activity Monitoring, Outcomes, & Prognosis

Most patients with TAK develop relapsing and remitting courses requiring careful monitoring and adjustment of immunosuppressive therapy. Judging disease activity in this

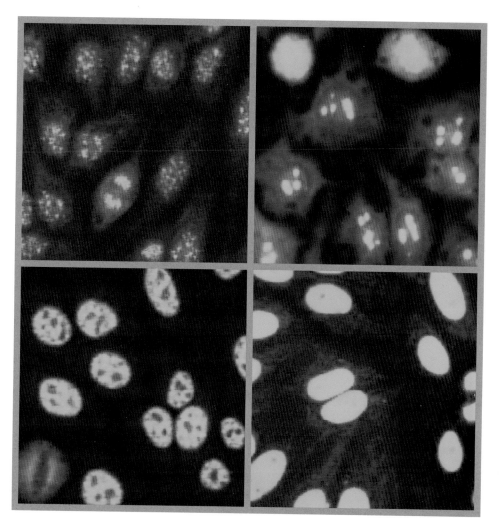

▲ **Figure 3–5. Patterns of antibodies to nuclear antigen (ANA) performed by immunofluorescence microscopy.**
Representative appearance of ANA tests performed by immunofluorescence microscopy on HEp-2 cells. Top left:
anticentromere pattern. Top right: nucleolar pattern. Lower left: speckled pattern. Lower right: diffuse/homogeneous
pattern. (Used with permission from Kathleen Hutchinson.)

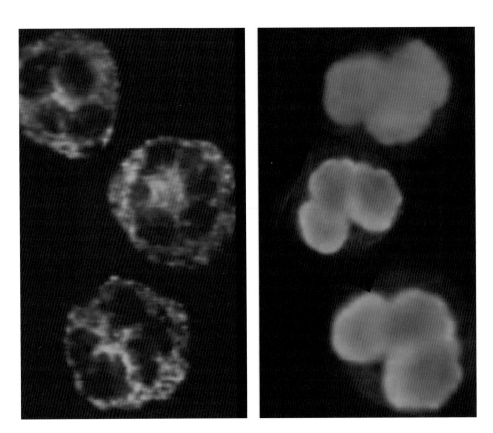

▲ **Figure 3–7. Antibodies to neutrophil cytoplasmic antigens (ANCA) detected by immunofluorescence assay microscopy.** ANCA tests performed on ethanol fixed neutrophils. The cytoplasmic cANCA pattern on the left shows granular staining throughout the cytoplasm, sparing the nucleus. The perinuclear pANCA pattern on the right demonstrates staining that covers the nucleus. In clinical laboratories, this test would also be confirmed using formalin fixed cells, which demonstrates a diffuse cytoplasmic staining pattern for both cANCA and pANCA antibodies.

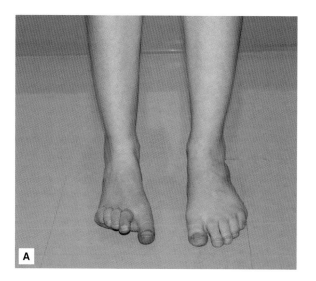

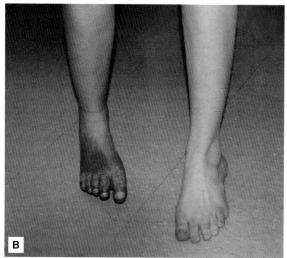

▲ **Figure 12–1.** Progressive right foot and leg CRPS-I beginning at age 13 after soft-tissue trauma with possible occult fracture. She noted dramatic foot edema and reddening within a few hours. She later had two milder CRPS episodes of in her arms caused by venipuncture. Over time her CRPS progressed rather than resolved. Panel A at age 26, shows mild color changes and dystonia accompanying moderate pain. Panel B at age 29, shows microvascular insufficiency causing edema and critical tissue ischemia that worsen pain and prognosis. In addition she developed "total body CRPS" and dysautonomia (tachycardia, hypotension, gastrointestinal dysmotility, and cachexia) that required gastrojejunal and then parental nutrition. Neurological evaluation led to additional diagnoses of Ehlers-Danlos syndrome and small-fiber polyneuropathy, confirmed by left-leg skin biopsy. Multiple treatments, including polypharmacy, spinal cord stimulator, and intrathecal pump, were ineffective or poorly tolerated and IVIg was recommended.

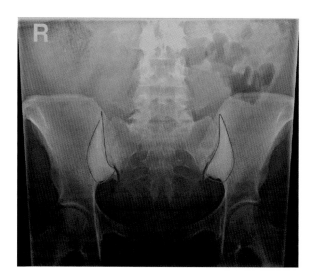

▲ **Figure 15–6. Osteitis condescens ilii.** The classic finding is of triangular sclerotic lesions on the iliac side of the SI joint (outlined).

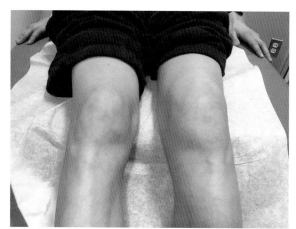

▲ **Figure 16–1.** Monoarthritis of the knee in a patient with *Chlamydia*-associated reactive arthritis.

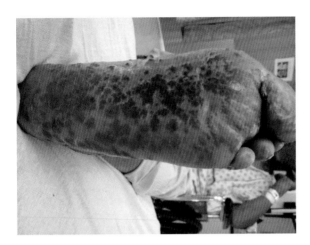

▲ **Figure 16–2.** Keratoderma blennorhagicum. (Used with permission from Dr. Maureen Dubreuil, MD, MSc, Boston University Schoool of Medicine.)

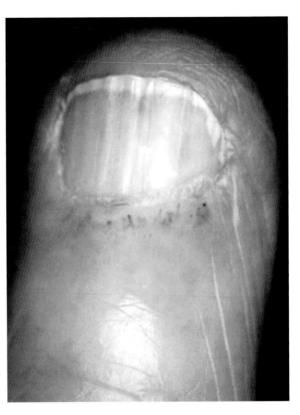

▲ **Figure 22–3.** Distorted, dilated, and regions of absent nailfold capillaries.

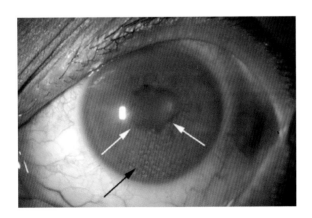

▲ **Figure 18–1.** Acute anterior uveitis with corneal endothelial white cell aggregates (*black arrow*) and posterior synechiae formation (iris adhesions to the lens, *white arrows*). (Reproduced with permission from Chapter 18. Uveitis and Iritis. In: Usatine RP, Smith MA, Chumley HS, Mayeaux EJ, Jr. eds. The Color Atlas of Family Medicine, 2e New York, NY: McGraw-Hill; 2013.)

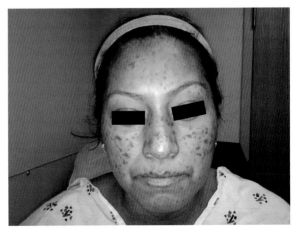

▲ **Figure 23–3.** Facial telangiectasias in patient with limited scleroderma.

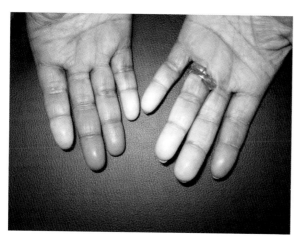

▲ **Figure 23–5.** Raynaud phenomenon presenting with asymmetric digital pallor during vasospastic attack.

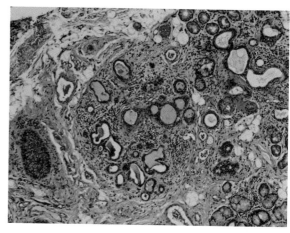

▲ **Figure 24–7.** Focal lymphocytc sialadenitis.

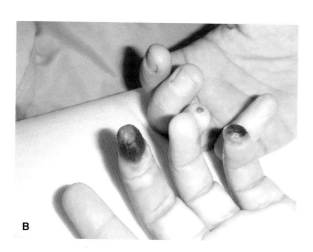

B

▲ **Figure 23–6B.** Ischemic complications from severe Raynaud phenomenon resulting in digital gangrene leading to digital loss.

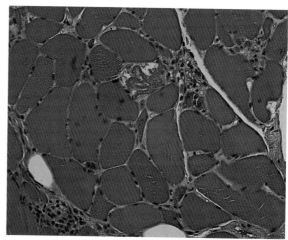

▲ **Figure 25–6.** Muscle biopsy from a patient with immune-mediated necrotizing myopathy. Muscle biopsy is characterized by necrotizing and regenerating muscle fibers with scant lymphocytic infiltration.

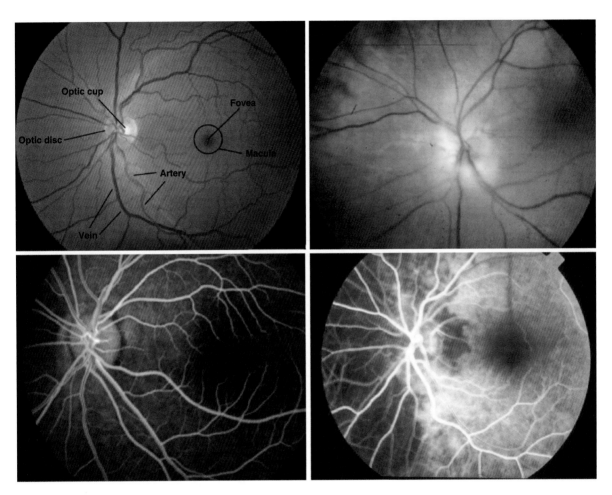

▲ **Figure 26–2.** Acute ischemic optic neuropathy in GCA. **A:** Normal fundoscopic exam (left panel) and fundoscopic exam of a GCA patient with acute ischemic optic neuropathy (AION), which demonstrates a swollen and pale optic disc with diffuse margins (right panel). **B:** Normal fluorescein angiography (left panel) and fluorescein angiography of the GCA patient with AION (right panel) demonstrating patchy choroidal hypoperfusion (dark geographic region) on the nasal side of the fundus. (Images courtesy of Dr. Joseph Rizzo III, Massachusetts Eye and Ear Infirmary, Boston.)

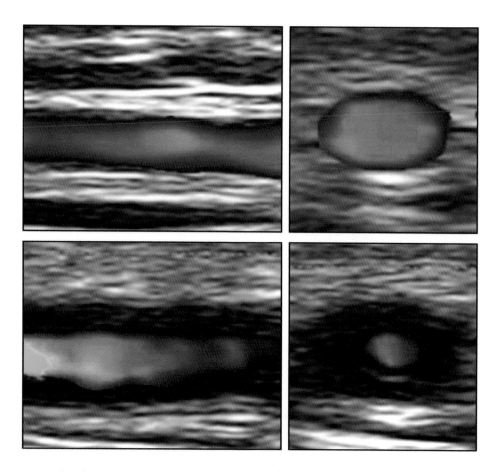

▲ **Figure 26–4.** Duplex ultrasound in GCA. Color duplex ultrasound (CDS) of the temporal arteries in longitudinal and transverse views in a patient without GCA (upper panels) and in a patient with GCA demonstrating the characteristic halo sign (concentric hypoechoic thickening surrounding the affected vessels) (lower panels).

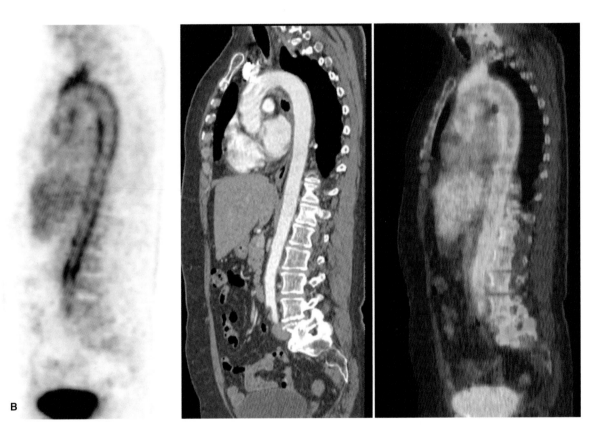

▲ **Figure 26–5B.** Noninvasive cross-sectional vascular imaging in GCA. Positron emission tomography (PET)/CT scan of the thoracic aorta of a GCA patient demonstrating markedly increased [18]fluorine-2-deoxy-D-glucose (18-FDG) uptake suggesting arterial inflammation (sagittal plane). The panel on the left shows the PET, the middle panel shows the CT, and the third panel shows the overlap of the former two (PET/CT).

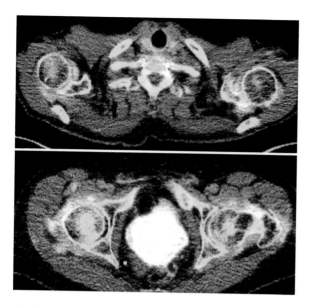

▲ **Figure 26–6.** Imaging in PMR. PET/CT in a patient with PMR demonstrating increased ¹⁸fluorine-2-deoxy-D-glucose (18-FDG) in the structures around the shoulders (upper panel) and hips (lower panel) and in vicinity of the spinous process of the cervical vertebrae (upper panel).

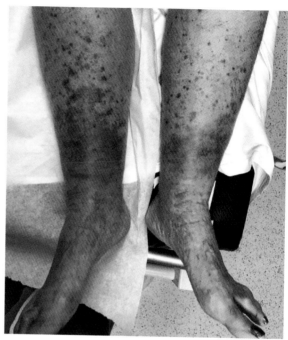

▲ **Figure 32–1.** Small-vessel vasculitis in a patient with mixed cryoglobulinemia. Palpable purpura, a feature of small-vessel vasculitis, is seen predominantly involving the lower extremities.

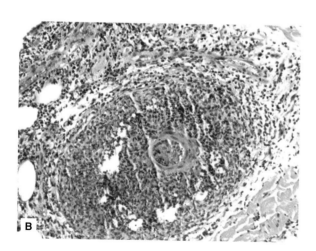

▲ **Figure 31–4B.** The diagnosis of PAN can be made by obtaining biopsy specimens of the skin that capture lobules of subcutaneous fat. Biopsies of nodules, papules, and the edges of ulcers have higher yields than biopsies of livedo racemosa. Deep punch biopsy demonstrating transmural inflammation with an intense mononuclear cell infiltrate in a medium-sized muscular artery.

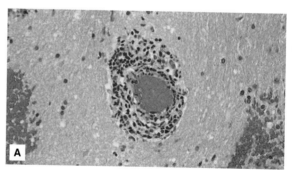

▲ **Figure 36–4A.** Histopathologic findings in CNS vasculitis. Lymphocytic vasculitis with reactive gliosis.

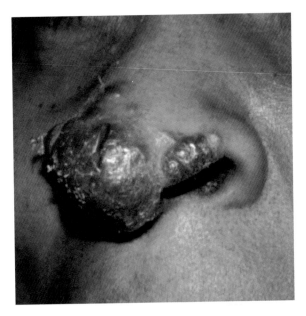

▲ **Figure 46–2.** Lupus pernio. This form of cutaneous eruption in sarcoidosis is typified by violaceous plaques and nodules that involve the nose, nasal alae, malar areas, nasolabial folds, around the eyes, scalp, and along the hairline. (© Bernard Cohen, MD, Dermatlas; http://www.dermatlas.org.)

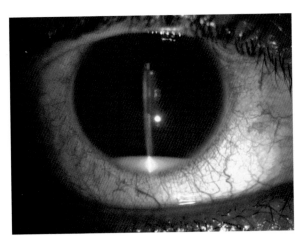

▲ **Figure 49–1.** Patient with HLA-B27–associated uveitis and associated hypopyon (layering of white blood cells within the anterior segment of the eye).

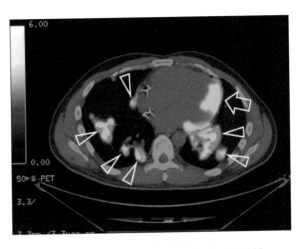

▲ **Figure 46–4.** Cardiac sarcoidosis. Cardiac PET/CT scan demonstrates FDG uptake in the left ventricle lateral wall (*arrow*) of a patient who also has active pulmonary sarcoidosis (*arrowheads*).

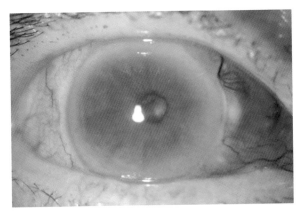

▲ **Figure 49–5.** Patient with rheumatoid arthritis and nasal scleritis with associated scleral melt.

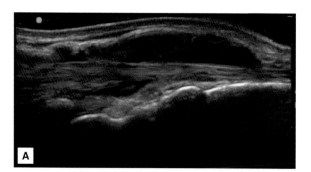

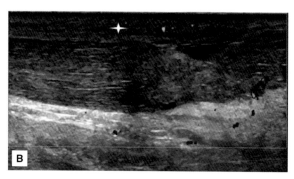

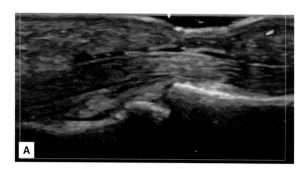

▲ **Figure 54–11B.** Power Doppler signal within tendon and paratenon.

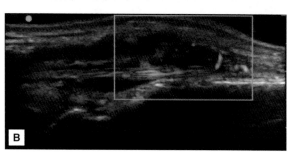

▲ **Figure 54–5.** **A:** Dorsal longitudinal view of wrist tenosynovitis in a rheumatoid arthritis patient. **B:** Dorsal transverse view of wrist tenosynovitis with positive power Doppler signal consistent with active inflammation.

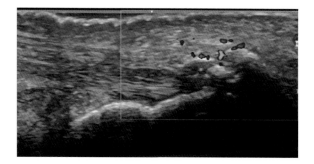

▲ **Figure 54–10.** Posterior longitudinal view: Achilles enthesitis with cortical erosions and positive power Doppler signal.

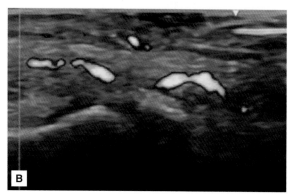

▲ **Figure 54–12.** **A:** Dactylitis. Swelling of tissue, flexor tendon, and PIP synovium. **B:** Dactylitis. Positive power Doppler signal.

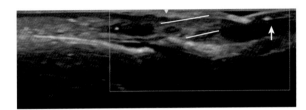

▲ **Figure 54–13.** DIP and nail enthesitis. Swelling around extensor tendon with positive power Doppler signal. Lines outline thickening of extensor tendon as it approaches nail (*arrow*).

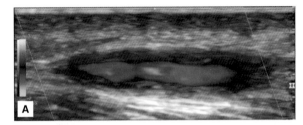

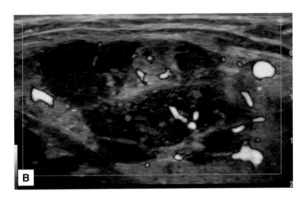

▲ **Figure 54–19B.** Enlarged submandibular gland with hyperemia (increased color power Doppler signal).

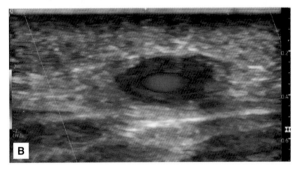

▲ **Figure 54–20.** **A:** Longitudinal view of temporal artery with color flow Doppler and halo sign (thickening of intima medial wall). **B:** Transverse view of temporal artery with color flow Doppler and halo sign (thickening of intima medial wall).

disease is challenging and needs assessment of symptoms, signs, inflammatory markers, and vascular imaging.

One common finding in TAK is the persistence of vascular inflammation in patients who appear to be quiescent. In fact, between 10% and 60% of patients whose disease is clinically silent, develop new arterial lesions during follow-up. Moreover, surgical specimens from patients believed to be in remission have revealed histologic evidence of vasculitis in more than 40% of cases. In one study of patients at routine visits, 46% were noted to have either elevated acute phase reactants but no changes on MRA studies or normal acute phase reactants but the detection of new vessel wall enhancement or edema by MR imaging. The role of vascular imaging as a single instrument to assess disease activity and guide therapy has not been established as several studies have demonstrated residual vascular changes in patients whose disease is otherwise judged to be in clinical remission.

Mortality in patients with TAK has decreased significantly in the recent years so that 10-year survival rates of 80–90% have become common. Mortality causes include congestive heart failure (eg, from severe aortic insufficiency), stroke, myocardial infarction, renal failure, or infectious complications of immunosuppressive treatment. Advances in diagnosis, medical and surgical treatment, and monitoring augur even better prognosis in the future.

Barra L, Kanji T, Malette J, Pagnoux C, CanVasc. Imaging modalities for the diagnosis and disease activity assessment of Takayasu's arteritis: a systematic review and meta-analysis. *Autoimmun Rev.* 2018;17(2):175-187. [PMID: 29313811]

Carmona FD, Coit P, Saruhan-Direskeneli G, et al. Analysis of the common genetic component of large-vessel vasculitides through a meta-Immunochip strategy. *Sci Rep* 2017;7:43953. [PMID: 28277489]

Clifford A, Hoffman GS. Recent advances in the medical management of Takayasu arteritis: an update on use of biologic therapies. *Curr Opin Rheumatol* 2014;26(1):7-15. [PMID: 24225487]

Espinoza JL, Ai S, Matsumura I. New insights on the pathogenesis of Takayasu arteritis: revisiting the microbial theory. *Pathogens.* 2018;7(3):E73. [PMID: 30200570]

Goel R, Danda D, Joseph G, et al. Long-term outcome of 251 patients with Takayasu arteritis on combination immunosuppressant therapy: single centre experience from a large tertiary care teaching hospital in Southern India. *Semin Arthritis Rheum.* 2018;47(5):718-726. [PMID: 29096935]

Grayson PC, Alehashemi S, Bagheri AA, et al. 18F-Fluorodeoxyglucose-Positron Emission Tomography As an Imaging Biomarker in a Prospective, Longitudinal Cohort of Patients With Large Vessel Vasculitis. *Arthritis Rheum.* 2018;70(3):439-449. [PMID: 29145713]

Hoffman GS, Merkel PA, Brasington RD, Lenschow DJ, Liang P. Anti-tumor necrosis factor therapy in patients with difficult to treat Takayasu arteritis. *Arthritis Rheum.* 2004;50(7):2296-2304. [PMID: 15248230]

Kerr GS, Hallahan CW, Giordano J, et al. Takayasu arteritis. *Ann Intern Med.* 1994;120(11):919-929. [PMID: 7909656]

Li J, Sun F, Chen Z, Yang Y, et al. The clinical characteristics of Chinese Takayasu's arteritis patients: a retrospective study of 411 patients over 24 years. *Arthritis Res Ther.* 2017;19(1):107. [PMID: 28545566]

Maksimowicz-McKinnon K, Clark TM, Hoffman GS. Limitations of therapy and a guarded prognosis in an American cohort of Takayasu arteritis patients. *Arthritis Rheum.* 2007;56(3):1000-1009. [PMID: 17328078]

Molloy ES, Langford CA, Clark TM, Gota CE, Hoffman GS. Anti-tumour necrosis factor therapy in patients with refractory Takayasu arteritis: long-term follow-up. *Ann Rheum Dis.* 2008;67(11):1567-1569. [PMID: 18677012]

Nakaoka Y, Isobe M, Takei S, et al. Efficacy and safety of tocilizumab in patients with refractory Takayasu arteritis: results from a randomised, double-blind, placebo-controlled, phase 3 trial in Japan (the TAKT study). *Ann Rheum Dis.* 2018;77(3):348-354. [PMID: 29191819]

Onen F, Akkoc N. Epidemiology of Takayasu arteritis. *Presse Med.* 2017;46(7-8 Pt 2):e197-e203. [PMID: 28756072]

Renauer PA, Saruhan-Direskeneli G, Coit P, et al. Identification of susceptibility loci in IL6, RPS9/LILRB3, and an intergenic locus on chromosome 21q22 in Takayasu arteritis in a genome-wide association study. *Arthritis Rheum.* 2015;67(5):1361-1368. [PMID: 25604533]

Sanchez-Alvarez C, Mertz LE, Thomas CS, Cochuyt JJ, Abril A. Demographic, clinical, and radiologic characteristics of a cohort of patients with Takayasu arteritis. *Am J Med.* 2019;132(5):647-651. [PMID: 30615861]

Saruhan-Direskeneli G, Hughes T, Aksu K, et al. Identification of multiple genetic susceptibility loci in Takayasu arteritis. *Am J Hum Genet.* 2013;93(2):298-305. [PMID: 23830517]

Yachoui R, Kreidy M, Siorek M, Sehgal R. Successful treatment with ustekinumab for corticosteroid- and immunosuppressant-resistant Takayasu's arteritis. *Scand J Rheum.* 2018;47(3):246-247. [PMID: 28276951]

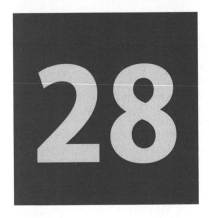

Granulomatosis with Polyangiitis

John H. Stone, MD, MPH

ESSENTIALS OF DIAGNOSIS

▶ Three pathologic hallmarks: granulomatous inflammation, vasculitis, and necrosis.

▶ Classic clinical features are found in multiple organ systems:

- Nonspecific constitutional symptoms, such as fatigue, myalgias, weight loss, and fevers.

- Migratory pauciarticular or polyarticular arthritis.

- Persistent upper respiratory tract and ear "infections" that do not respond to antibiotic therapy.

- Orbital pseudotumor, nearly always associated with chronic nasosinus conditions.

- Nodular or cavitary lung lesions that are misdiagnosed initially as malignancies or infections.

- Rapidly progressive glomerulonephritis.

▶ Antineutrophil cytoplasmic antibody (ANCA) assays are extremely helpful in diagnosis but have significant shortcomings as indicators of disease activity or guides to when to treat. A significant minority of patients with granulomatosis with polyangiitis are ANCA negative, particularly those with "limited" disease.

▶ General Considerations

Granulomatosis with polyangiitis (GPA; formerly called Wegener granulomatosis) is one of the most common forms of systemic vasculitis, with a reported annual incidence of 10 cases per million. The disease involves small- to medium-sized blood vessels (small more often than medium). GPA affects both the arterial and venous circulations, in contrast to polyarteritis nodosa, a disorder in which only arteries and muscular arterioles are affected. The cause of GPA is not known, but the prominence of upper and lower airway involvement suggests a response to an inhaled antigen.

The disease is the prototype of conditions associated with antineutrophil cytoplasmic antibodies (ANCAs), autoantibodies generally believed to amplify rather than to initiate the inflammatory process. GPA occurs in people of all ethnic backgrounds but demonstrates a predilection for whites, particularly those of northern European ancestry. The male:female ratio is approximately 1:1. The mean age at diagnosis is 50 years. The elderly are often affected. The disease is less common but known to occur in children.

GPA typically presents in a subacute fashion. Patients complain of symptoms that appear to be innocuous at first, such as nasal stuffiness, "sinusitis," and decreases in hearing. During this "prodrome," attentive clinicians may suspect and diagnose GPA before the onset of generalized disease. Such early recognition of GPA may prevent the disabling and disfiguring end-organ complications of this disorder such as collapse of the nasal bridge, renal failure, diffuse alveolar hemorrhage, and widespread infarctions of peripheral nerves. Because of the remitting and relapsing nature of many GPA cases and the disease's tendency to recur during or after the stopping of treatment, remission maintenance strategies and early detection of disease flares are important.

Therapies for GPA are associated with substantial treatment-induced morbidity in both the short and long term. The long-term impact of chronic glucocorticoid therapy is frequently underappreciated. Careful follow-up and monitoring of basic laboratory tests (eg, regularly obtaining complete blood cell counts) may prevent some adverse effects of treatment or minimize their impact. More widespread use of rituximab in lieu of cyclophosphamide has also reduced some of the long-term side effects once seen commonly with cyclophosphamide, particularly infertility, malignancy, and opportunistic infection.

▶ Clinical Findings

A. Symptoms and Signs

1. Nose, sinuses, and ears—Approximately 90% of patients with GPA have nasal involvement. This is often the first

Table 28–1. Major clinical manifestations of granulomatosis with polyangiitis (formerly Wegener granulomatosis).

Organ	Manifestation
Nose	Persistent rhinorrhea; bloody, brown nasal crusts; nasal obstruction; nasal septal perforation; saddle-nose deformity
Sinuses	Sinusitis with radiologic evidence of bony erosions
Ears	Conductive hearing loss due to granulomatous inflammation in the middle ear; sensorineural hearing loss; mixed hearing loss common
Mouth	Strawberry gums; tongue or other oral ulcers; occasional purpuric lesions on palate
Eyes	Orbital pseudotumor; scleritis (often necrotizing); episcleritis; conjunctivitis; keratitis (risk of corneal melt); uveitis (anterior)
Trachea	Subglottic stenosis
Lungs	Nodular, cavitary lesions; nonspecific pulmonary infiltrates; alveolar hemorrhage; bronchial lesions
Heart	Occasional valvular lesions, usually not evident during life; pericarditis
Gastrointestinal	Mesenteric vasculitis uncommon; splenic involvement quite common but usually subclinical (detected as splenic infarcts on cross-sectional imaging)

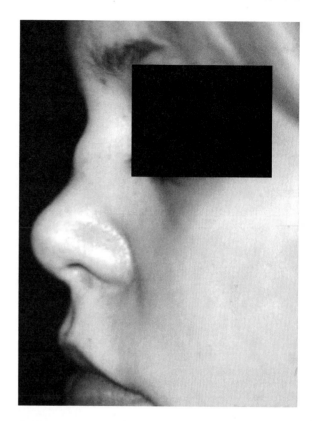

▲ **Figure 28–1.** Cartilaginous inflammation of the nose in granulomatosis with polyangiitis (Wegener granulomatosis) may lead to nasal septal perforation and ultimately to collapse of the nasal bridge ("saddle-nose" deformity).

disease manifestation. The typical symptoms are persistent rhinorrhea, unusually severe nasal obstruction, epistaxis, and bloody or brown nasal crusts (Table 28–1). Cartilaginous inflammation may lead to perforation of the nasal septum and collapse of the nasal bridge (a "saddle-nose" deformity) (Figure 28–1). Bony erosions of the sinus cavities are characteristic of GPA but only develop after long-standing disease (months).

Both conductive and sensorineural forms of hearing loss occur in GPA. The usual pattern of auditory dysfunction is a mixed one, with the simultaneous occurrence of both conductive and sensorineural hearing loss. Conductive hearing loss results from granulomatous inflammation in the middle ear, leading to serous otitis media. Inflammation in the middle ear may also compress the seventh cranial nerve as it courses through the middle ear cavity, leading to a peripheral facial nerve palsy. (This is often misdiagnosed as Bell palsy or Lyme disease.) Sensorineural hearing loss results from inner ear (cochlear) involvement and may also be associated with vestibular dysfunction (eg, nausea, vertigo, tinnitus). However, the sensorineural hearing loss associated with GPA is seldom profound.

2. Eyes—GPA may present with a variety of inflammatory lesions of the eye (Figure 28–2). Orbital pseudotumors in the retrobulbar space may lead to proptosis and vision loss through optic nerve ischemia (compression of the nerve's

blood supply by the space-occupying mass). These lesions can be particularly difficult to differentiate from the orbital lesions of IgG4-related disease. Scleritis causes photophobia and painful, often nodular, scleral erythema. If unchecked, necrotizing scleritis may lead to scleral thinning, scleromalacia perforans, and vision loss. Peripheral ulcerative keratitis (PUK) may cause ulcerations on the margin of the cornea and lead to the syndrome of "corneal melt." This intensely painful complication of eye inflammation associated with GPA can lead to the loss of normal vision in the eye.

Episcleritis and conjunctivitis constitute less serious ocular complications of GPA but are very common. Their occurrence may be the presenting symptom of the disease or the first manifestation of a flare. Nasolacrimal duct obstruction leads to poor outflow of tears such that the eyes in a patient with GPA are characteristically wet. Anterior uveitis is rare in GPA in comparison to other rheumatologic conditions such as ankylosing spondylitis, Behçet disease, and sarcoidosis. Central retinal artery occlusions are a known complication of GPA, but other retinal lesions and posterior uveitis are uncommon.

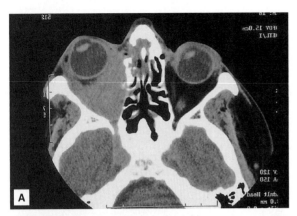

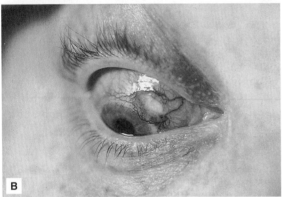

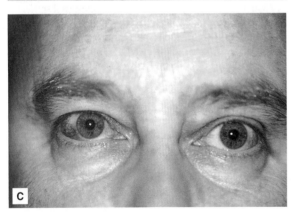

▲ **Figure 28–2. A:** CT scan of the orbit showing an orbital pseudotumor, leading to proptosis and visual loss. **B:** Scleritis with a marginal corneal ulceration. **C:** Painless erythema of the superficial surface of the eye—episcleritis—the most common ocular complication of granulomatosis with polyangiitis (formerly Wegener granulomatosis).

3. Mouth—Two classic mouth lesions of GPA are gum inflammation ("strawberry gums" [Figure 28–3]) and tongue ulcers [Figure 28–4]). The gum inflammation of GPA, which derives its name from the resemblance of the dental papillae

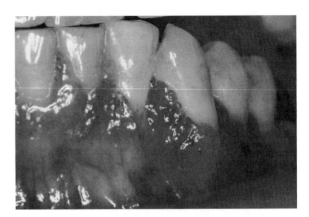

▲ **Figure 28–3.** Granulomatosis with polyangiitis (formerly Wegener granulomatosis) patient with intense inflammation of the gums, a physical finding known as "strawberry gums."

to strawberries, is distinctive among rheumatologic conditions. The oral ulcerations of GPA are not the aphthous ulcers characteristic of Behçet disease or systemic lupus erythematosus, but rather occur typically on the lateral sides of the posterior tongue. These are the result of medium-vessel vasculitis. Strawberry gums and tongue ulcers, both quite painful, respond promptly to glucocorticoids.

4. Trachea—Subglottic stenosis, the result of tracheal inflammation and scarring below the vocal cords, is a potentially disabling manifestation that has a high specificity for GPA. Relapsing polychondritis can also cause lesions at this site. Another diagnosis unrelated to GPA is idiopathic tracheal stenosis. Subglottic involvement is often asymptomatic

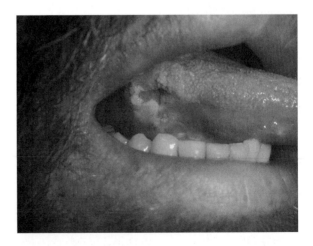

▲ **Figure 28–4.** Tongue ulcer in a patient with granulomatosis with polyangiitis.

and may manifest itself only as a subtle hoarseness. With time, however, airway scarring and profound tracheal narrowing may occur. Pulmonary function tests with flow volume loops can show a fixed extrathoracic obstructive defect, but this may not become apparent until the process is advanced.

5. Lungs—Approximately 80% of patients with GPA have pulmonary lesions during the course of their disease. Pulmonary symptoms include cough, hemoptysis, dyspnea, and sometimes pleuritic chest pain. Lung lesions are often asymptomatic, however, and some are detectable only if chest imaging is performed. The most common radiologic findings are pulmonary infiltrates and nodules (Figure 28–5). The infiltrates, which may wax and wane, are often misdiagnosed initially as pneumonia. Single, large pulmonary nodules are often misdiagnosed as lung cancer. The nodules are usually multiple and bilateral, however, and are often cavitary. Many nodules have peripheral locations and, if wedge-shaped, may be mistaken for pulmonary emboli.

Pulmonary capillaritis can lead to hemoptysis and rapidly changing alveolar infiltrates. Large airway disease leading to significant bronchial stenosis, similar to the findings found in subglottic stenosis, occurs in a minority of GPA patients. Large airway disease may be more common in pediatric than in adult GPA. Bronchial stenosis poses important challenges in diagnosis because in contrast to the situation with advancing subglottic stenosis, patients' status may appear to be well preserved until advances stages on bronchial narrowing. Finally, venous thrombotic events (particularly deep venous thromboses) occur in a substantial proportion of patients, perhaps as a complication of the disease's propensity to involve the venous circulation or the hypercoagulability associated with many inflammatory states. Deep venous thromboses and pulmonary emboli tend to occur in close association with periods of active disease. Pulmonary emboli should be considered in the GPA patient in whom dyspnea, pleuritic chest pain, or other compatible symptoms develop.

6. Kidneys—Renal disease, among the most ominous clinical manifestations of GPA, is often a marker for swift disease progression. Renal involvement, present in approximately 20% of patients with GPA at the time of diagnosis, develops eventually in a substantially higher portion of patients (up to 80%) during the course of the disease. The clinical presentation of renal disease in GPA is rapidly progressive glomerulonephritis: hematuria, red blood cell casts, proteinuria (usually non-nephrotic), and rising serum creatinine. Without appropriate therapy, loss of renal function can ensue within days or weeks. More subacute courses of renal diseases also develop in some patients with GPA, particularly those with antimyeloperoxidase antibodies (MPO-ANCA) as opposed to PR3-ANCA. GPA is also known to present with renal mass lesions that mimic malignancy.

7. Other organs—Nonspecific arthralgias and frank arthritis often occur early in the course of GPA and may assume a variety of patterns. The most common form of arthritis is a pauci- or monoarticular syndrome of lower or upper extremity joints that is often migratory in nature. The return of a migratory oligoarthritis is often a key indicator of a recurrence of disease activity. Polyarthritis of the small joints of the hands can also occur. Digital ischemia and gangrene

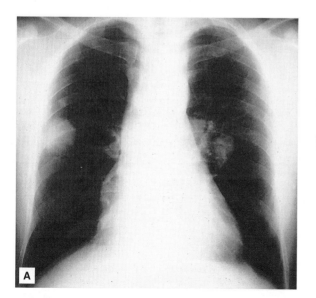

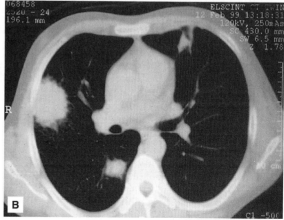

▲ **Figure 28–5.** Chest radiograph and computed tomography scan show multiple bilateral nodules. **A:** Posteroanterior view of the chest shows bilateral lung nodules. **B:** Computed tomography scan of the chest in the same patient shows additional lesions not evident of the radiograph.

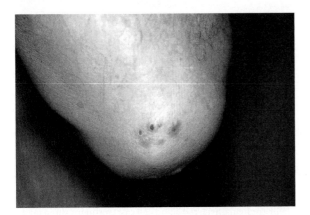

▲ **Figure 28–6.** The patient has granulomatosis with polyangiitis (formerly Wegener granulomatosis) and has a positive test result for rheumatoid factor. The nodule over the extensor surface of the elbow was initially misdiagnosed as a rheumatoid nodule instead of a "Churg-Strauss granuloma" (cutaneous extravascular necrotizing granuloma).

resulting from inflammation in medium-sized digital arteries are occasionally the presenting features of GPA. The skin manifestations of GPA include the full array of findings associated with cutaneous vasculitis: palpable purpura, papules, ulcers, and vesiculobullous lesions. In general, however, the extent of purpura in GPA and in other forms of ANCA-associated vasculitis is less extensive than that observed in patients with forms of small-vessel vasculitis mediated primarily by immune complex deposition, for example, mixed cryoglobulinemia or immunoglobulin A (IgA) vasculitis.

Examination of the skin should include careful inspection for the nodular lesions of "Churg-Strauss granulomas" (cutaneous extravascular necrotizing granulomas). These nodules are located typically on the extensor surfaces of the elbows and other pressure points (Figure 28–6). Splinter hemorrhages may occur in GPA, raising diagnostic confusion with endocarditis. Lesions resembling pyoderma gangrenosum but caused by a medium-vessel vasculitis may also occur. Although involvement of the brain parenchyma with GPA has been reported, meningeal inflammation (presenting as excruciating headaches and cranial neuropathies) is a more typical central nervous system disease manifestation. Mononeuritis multiplex resulting from vasculitic neuropathy can complicate GPA and can be devastating if it occurs, but this feature is less characteristic of this disease than other forms of systemic vasculitis (eg, polyarteritis nodosa, microscopic polyangiitis, and eosinophilic GPA).

B. Laboratory Findings

The results of routine laboratory tests and more specialized assays in GPA are shown in Table 28–2. All of these tests are appropriate at the initial evaluation of a patient with

Table 28–2. The laboratory evaluation in granulomatosis with polyangiitis (formerly Wegener granulomatosis).

Test	Typical Result
Complete blood cell count	• Normochromic, normocytic anemia; acute, severe anemias possible in alveolar hemorrhage • Mild to moderate leukocytosis common, usually not exceeding 18×10^9/L • Moderate to pronounced thrombocytosis typical, ranging from platelet counts of 400×10^9/L to occasionally >1000×10^9/L
Electrolytes	Hyperkalemia in the setting of advanced renal dysfunction
Liver function test	Hepatic involvement is quite unusual in GPA; when present, there can be elevations of transaminases (AST/ALT) in excess of 1000 mg/dL
Urinalysis with microscopy	• Hematuria (ranging from mild to so high that red blood cells are too numerous to count) • Red blood cell casts • Proteinuria (nephritic range proteinuria in a small minority)
Erythrocyte sedimentation rate/C-reactive protein	Dramatic elevations of acute phase reactants are typical, generally with good correlation to disease activity
ANA	Negative
Rheumatoid factor	Positive in 40–50% of patients, often leading to diagnostic confusion with rheumatoid arthritis
C3, C4	Complement levels are normal to elevated in GPA, in contrast to systemic lupus erythematosus, cryoglobulinemia, and other diseases in which immune complexes appear to play major roles
ANCA	Positive in 60–90% of patients with GPA
Anti-GBM	A minority of patients with GPA also have anti-GBM antibodies

ANA, antinuclear antibody; ANCA, antineutrophil cytoplasmic antibody; anti-GBM, antiglomerular basement membrane antibody; AST/ALT, aspartate aminotransferase/alanine aminotransferase; GPA, granulomatosis with polyangiitis.

possible GPA. The exclusion of renal disease through the careful performance of a urinalysis and urine protein:creatinine ratio is essential in the evaluation and follow-up of all patients with GPA. The erythrocyte sedimentation rate and serum C-reactive protein level are useful (albeit imperfect) biomarkers in the longitudinal evaluation of disease activity. The utility of ANCA testing is discussed below.

C. Imaging Studies

Up to one-third of patients with GPA have asymptomatic pulmonary lesions on radiologic imaging. Patients with confirmed or strongly suspected diagnoses of GPA should have CT scans of the chest as baseline studies. Virtually any finding (with the rare exception of hilar and mediastinal adenopathy) may be present on chest imaging in GPA, including pleural effusions and nonspecific infiltrates.

D. Special Tests

1. Biopsy—Because of the numerous potential mimickers of GPA and the frequent shortcomings of ANCA (see next section on ANCA testing), the diagnosis of GPA is most secure when established through biopsy of an involved organ. Among the organs commonly involved in GPA, those most likely to yield tissue that permits a diagnosis are (in descending order): lung, kidney, and upper respiratory tract (nose or sinuses). Alternatively, the finding of vasculitis in a less typical organ (eg, a leukocytoclastic vasculitis in the skin) combined with a strongly positive ANCA with a specificity for proteinase-3 or myeloperoxidase also provides sufficient confirmation of the diagnosis. Compelling, if not diagnostic, histopathologic findings may clinch the diagnosis if the patient's ANCA serologies are also consistent with GPA.

The diagnosis of GPA requires the careful integration of pathologic findings with clinical, laboratory, and radiologic data, even when the three classic pathologic hallmarks (granulomatous inflammation, vasculitis, and necrosis) are present. The tissue necrosis associated with GPA is frequently so extensive within diseased tissues that it is termed "geographic necrosis." Acid-fast and fungal pathogens must be excluded by special stains and cultures.

Biopsies of the upper respiratory tract (nose, sinuses, and subglottic region) are frequently nondiagnostic, yielding only nonspecific acute and chronic inflammation. Upper respiratory tract biopsies demonstrate the complete pathology triad in only about 15% of cases. However, these biopsies are generally safer than lung or kidney biopsies, and the finding of even parts of this triad in a nose or sinus biopsy may serve as compelling evidence for the diagnosis of GPA, provided that other manifestations of the disease are present.

GPA finds its fullest pathologic expression in the lung, where the large amounts of tissue obtained at open or thoracoscopic lung biopsy may capture the entire spectrum of disease. Transbronchial and radiologically-guided needle biopsies usually fail to yield diagnostic tissue specimens. The leukocytoclastic vasculitis of GPA may involve arteries, veins, and capillaries, with or without granulomatous features. Vascular necrosis begins as clusters of neutrophils within the blood vessel wall (microabscesses) that degenerate and become surrounded by palisading histiocytes. Coalescence of such neutrophilic microabscesses leads to geographic necrosis.

Renal biopsy findings are not specific for GPA because other pauci-immune forms of glomerulonephritis can have identical histopathologic features. However, renal biopsy results are sufficiently characteristic to establish the diagnosis in appropriate clinical settings. The typical renal lesion of GPA is segmental necrotizing glomerulonephritis, with or without crescent formation. Thrombotic changes in the glomerular capillary loops are among the earliest histologic lesions. Immunofluorescence studies of renal biopsies in GPA confirm the "pauci-immune" nature of the renal involvement (ie, the relatively sparse immunoglobulin and complement deposition found in this disorder compared with such diseases as systemic lupus erythematosus, IgA vasculitis, and antiglomerular basement membrane disease).

2. Serologic testing for ANCA—ANCAs are directed against antigens that reside within the primary granules of neutrophils and monocytes. Positive ANCA assays are often instrumental in suggesting or confirming the diagnosis of GPA. In patients with multiple classic organ system features of GPA, a positive ANCA assay that has been confirmed by both immunofluorescence and enzyme immunoassay testing can preclude the need for biopsy. However, a small percentage of patients with disseminated GPA are ANCA-negative, so a negative ANCA assay does not exclude the diagnosis. Among patients with "limited" disease (see Treatment section), 30% or more may lack ANCA. Rises and falls in ANCA titers often demonstrate poor correlation with the timing of disease flares and should never be used as the sole guide to the use of immunosuppression.

The two types of ANCA tests now in common use are immunofluorescence assays and enzyme immunoassays. These two tests are complementary in the diagnosis of GPA. Both have been used traditionally in evaluating patients in whom this disease is suspected. Enzyme immunoassays for antibodies to proteinase-3 and myeloperoxidase have improved to such an extent, however, that many laboratories now begin ANCA testing with this, forgoing immunofluorescence altogether.

With immunofluorescence, three principal patterns are recognized: cytoplasmic (C-ANCA), perinuclear (P-ANCA), and atypical. Immunofluorescence testing alone has low specificity and a low positive predictive value for GPA. Hence, the diagnosis of GPA should never rest primarily on a positive immunofluorescence assay, regardless of whether the pattern is C-ANCA or P-ANCA. In patients with vasculitis, the C-ANCA pattern usually corresponds to the presence of antiproteinase-3 antibodies (PR3-ANCA) detected by enzyme immunoassay. The combination of a C-ANCA pattern by immunofluorescence and a positive PR3-ANCA by enzyme immunoassay has a high positive predictive value for GPA.

The P-ANCA pattern usually corresponds to the presence of MPO-ANCA in patients with vasculitis. MPO-ANCA occur in approximately 10% of patients with GPA but are more typical of microscopic polyangiitis, eosinophilic GPA, and necrotizing crescentic glomerulonephritis (ie, renal-limited, ANCA-associated vasculitis).

Atypical immunofluorescence ANCA patterns, which may occur in association with a wide variety of diseases such as inflammatory bowel disease and connective tissue disorders, are not directed against either PR3 or MPO and do not imply the presence of a primary vasculitis. Atypical ANCA patterns of immunofluorescence are often misread by inexperienced laboratories as showing perinuclear immunofluorescence.

Finally, certain drug-induced vasculitic conditions can be associated with ANCA-positivity.

▶ Differential Diagnosis

The protean nature of GPA dictates that an all-inclusive differential diagnosis for the varied presentations of this disease is enormously broad. It encompasses sinusitis and pneumonia caused by microbial pathogens, other forms of vasculitis often associated with ANCA, and the confluence of several common medical problems in the same patient (eg, the simultaneous occurrence of pneumonia and interstitial nephritis caused by antibiotics). The major disease entities in the differential diagnosis of GPA are shown in Table 28–3.

GPA may smolder in the upper respiratory tract for months or even years before becoming a generalized,

Table 28–3. Differential diagnosis of granulomatosis with polyangiitis (Wegener granulomatosis).

Other vasculitides
Polyarteritis nodosa
Microscopic polyangiitis
Churg-Strauss syndrome
Henoch-Schönlein purpura
Mixed cryoglobulinemia
Goodpasture syndrome
Giant cell arteritis
Infections
Mycobacterial diseases
Fungal infections (histoplasmosis, blastomycosis, coccidioidomycosis)
Streptococcal pneumonia with glomerulonephritis
Malignancies
Nasopharyngeal carcinoma
Hodgkin disease
Non-Hodgkin lymphoma
Angiocentric lymphoma ("lymphomatoid granulomatosis")
Castleman disease
Granulomatous disorders
Sarcoidosis
Berylliosis
Systemic autoimmune conditions
Systemic lupus erythematosus
Rheumatoid arthritis
Relapsing polychondritis

life-threatening illness. Recognition of the systemic disorder underlying the repeated "ear infections," allergies, musculoskeletal symptoms, and other complaints is often delayed. Patients with GPA frequently endure multiple courses of antibiotics, myringotomies, and other interventions that are largely ineffectual or provide only temporary relief before the correct diagnosis is made. GPA should be suspected when mundane complaints persist long enough to become unusual.

Limited GPA may pose difficult diagnostic problems. The destructive upper airway disease that occurs in limited GPA may also be caused by infection (eg, mycobacteria, fungi, actinomycosis, and syphilis), malignancy (eg, squamous cell carcinoma and extranodal lymphoma), IgG4-related disease, or illicit drug use (eg, intranasal cocaine or smoking crack). Patients with cocaine-induced midline lesions that mimic GPA often have ANCA directed against human neutrophils elastase, another primary granule enzyme. Finally, the sinus destruction of GPA may be mimicked by nonvasculitic disorders such as "lethal midline granuloma," now known to be an angioproliferative T-cell lymphoma.

Chronic infections such as those caused by mycobacterial and fungal pathogens are essential to exclude through special stains and cultures of tissue biopsies. Because granulomatous infections of the lung may also cause vasculitis and necrosis, special stains and cultures for infection should show negative results before the diagnosis of GPA is made. Infections are especially important to consider in patients with established diagnoses of GPA who have been treated with immunosuppressive medications.

Rheumatoid arthritis is a common misdiagnosis shortly after the onset of GPA symptoms because arthritis is a frequent finding at presentation. Furthermore, approximately half of all patients with GPA have positive test results for rheumatoid factor, and Churg-Strauss granulomas often occur at precisely the most frequent sites for rheumatoid nodules—the elbows—further heightening the diagnostic confusion. (Patients are usually unaware of these lesions, as they may be unaware of rheumatoid nodules.) Other systemic inflammatory conditions associated with autoimmunity (eg, lupus) also affect multiple organ systems and must be distinguished from GPA. Sarcoidosis is an excellent mimicker of GPA because of the frequency with which it involves many of the same organs. Considerable organ involvement overlap also exists with IgG4-related disease, which commonly affects the orbits, sinuses, lungs, kidneys, and pachymeninges, and can also be associated with cutaneous vasculitis.

Finally, many other forms of systemic vasculitis are high on the differential diagnosis for GPA. Accurate distinction among GPA, polyarteritis nodosa, giant cell arteritis, antiglomerular basement membrane disease, microscopic polyangiitis, eosinophilic GPA, IgA vasculitis, relapsing polychondritis, and cryoglobulinemia is essential because their complications, treatments, and prognoses vary widely. Finally, ANCA-associated vasculitis can also be induced by certain medications, particularly propyl-thiouracil and hydralazine.

Treatment

The management of GPA should be stratified according to whether the patient has severe or limited disease. Severe disease (defined as an immediate threat to either the function of a vital organ or to the patient's life) requires treatment with either rituximab or cyclophosphamide and high doses of glucocorticoids. A randomized, double-blind, placebo-controlled trial of rituximab versus cyclophosphamide for the induction of disease remission (the Rituximab in ANCA-Associated Vasculitis [RAVE] trial) demonstrated that rituximab was not inferior to cyclophosphamide followed by azathioprine in efficacy, and in fact was somewhat more effective in that head-to-head comparison. Moreover, rituximab is superior to cyclophosphamide for the treatment of relapsing GPA. Based on its superior adverse event profile, rituximab is generally favored over rituximab for most patients with GPA. The RAVE trial was conducted with a rituximab regimen consisting of 375 mg/m^2, administered weekly times four doses. In practice, however, many clinicians find it simpler to use a regimen of 1000 mg times two doses, separated by 15 days.

Rituximab has been approved by the US Food and Drug Administration for the induction of remission in GPA and is viewed widely as the standard of care. Long-term follow-up of the RAVE cohort indicates that one course of rituximab plus glucocorticoids is as effective as the standard remission induction and maintenance regimen (cyclophosphamide/azathioprine plus glucocorticoids) for at least 18 months.

The alternative to rituximab plus glucocorticoids for remission induction in GPA is the combination of cyclophosphamide (2 mg/kg/day for those with normal renal function) and glucocorticoids (1 mg/kg/day of prednisone, perhaps preceded by a 3-day intravenous "pulse" of methylprednisolone). This combination leads to excellent initial therapeutic responses in 90% or more of patients and to complete remission in 75%. In attempting to control the disease and avoid the side effects of long-term cyclophosphamide therapy, shorter courses (eg, 3–6 months) of induction treatment with cyclophosphamide are now used followed by longer-term treatment for the maintenance of remission with either azathioprine (up to 2 mg/kg/day) or methotrexate. More recent data suggest that the intermittent administration of intravenous cyclophosphamide is equally likely to lead to disease remission at a substantially lower cumulative cyclophosphamide dose and possibly a lower rate of adverse effects. However, the rate of disease flares following remission is higher in patients treated with intermittent as opposed to daily cyclophosphamide regimens.

By definition, limited disease includes all cases of GPA that are not severe. Because patients with limited GPA are more likely to have nasosinus disease, arthritis, nodular pulmonary lesions, cutaneous findings, minor ocular complications, and mild renal disease as their principal manifestations, they are likely to benefit from a less dangerous approach to therapy. Patients with limited GPA may respond to the combination of methotrexate (up to 25 mg/wk) and glucocorticoids, thus sparing patients the potential side effects of cyclophosphamide. Methotrexate is not an appropriate first-line treatment for patients with severe involvement of the kidney, lung, or other vital organs and should not be used in patients with significant renal dysfunction (eg, a serum creatinine of >2.0 mg/dL). Rituximab is also highly effective in limited GPA, and a strong argument can be made for using it as first-line therapy in combination with moderate doses of glucocorticoids, forgoing methotrexate altogether. Clinical experience suggests that rituximab is more effective than methotrexate, is better tolerated, and is far more likely to lead to glucocorticoid-free disease remissions.

Regardless of which remission induction approach is used, all patients with GPA should receive prophylaxis against *Pneumocystis jiroveci* pneumonia with single-strength trimethoprim-sulfamethoxazole, 100 mg/day of dapsone, or 1500 mg/day of atovaquone, particularly while patients remain on cyclophosphamide or high doses of prednisone.

B-cell depletion is also effective for remission maintenance. Rituximab 500–1000 mg every 4–6 months is superior to azathioprine for remission maintenance. However, not every patient with GPA requires ongoing maintenance therapy. Patients at particular risk of disease flare following the achievement of remission include those who have flared in the past and those who are PR3-ANCA positive. Remission maintenance therapy (eg, single infusions of 500–1000 mg every 4 months) can begin in such patients 4–6 months after the initiation of remission induction therapy. Over time, the interval between remission maintenance treatments can be lengthened. As disease control becomes more well-established with subsequent rituximab infusions, the interval between rituximab infusions can be lengthened. Some GPA patients once prone to frequent flares eventually achieve excellent disease control with rituximab administered as infrequently as once a year.

Patients with subglottic stenosis comprise a unique subset of GPA. This disease complication often responds better to mechanical interventions than to immunosuppressive therapy (ie, to surgical dilatation accomplished through noninvasive approaches and glucocorticoid injections rather than to systemic immunosuppression). Laser techniques should be avoided during these procedures because they may exacerbate tissue injury. Otolaryngologists frequently use mitomycin C injections to help prevent the proliferation of scar tissue following dilatations of subglottic stenoses.

Complications

Regimens of cytotoxic agents and glucocorticoids converted GPA from a once nearly always fatal disease into one that responds well to treatment and, in most cases, enters remission for variable lengths of time. Unfortunately, GPA is marked by a pronounced tendency to flare during the tapering of medications or after the cessation of treatment. The requirement of treating disease flares with additional courses of therapy frequently leads to mounting treatment-related morbidity. The deleterious impact of even low-dose prednisone following months of high-dose glucocorticoid treatment and recurrent prednisone courses required to treat disease flares is often not sufficiently acknowledged.

Under the original regimen established by the National Institutes of Health (NIH), patients were treated with cyclophosphamide for a mean period of approximately 2 years (for 1 full year after the achievement of remission). Although many patients had remissions that lasted for up to several years, fewer than 40% of the patients in the NIH series achieved "cures" following their initial courses of therapy. Repeated administration of these potentially toxic treatments to patients with disease recurrences led to substantial long-term morbidity. Forty-two percent of patients treated under the NIH regimen suffered permanent medication-induced morbidity. The major complications of treating GPA with cytotoxic agents (not including the multiple and often severe side effects of prolonged glucocorticoid treatment) follow:

- Bone marrow suppression
- Myelodysplastic syndromes
- Opportunistic infection
- Drug-induced injury to the lungs, bladder, and liver
- Infertility
- Long-term risk of malignancies, particularly lymphoma and bladder cancers

Remission induction regimens that use rituximab rather than cyclophosphamide have far fewer implications for patients' fertility and malignancy risks. Potential concerns among rituximab-treated patients include the reactivation of hepatitis B in patients who are hepatitis B core antibody positive and a transient neutropenia that occurs in a small percentage of rituximab-treated patients at the time of B-cell recovery. Some rituximab-treated patients develop hypoglobulinemia, particularly after multiple administrations, which constitutes an important consideration in long-term management. Hypogammaglobulinemia also occurs with other immunosuppressive therapies, however, including long-term prednisone and cyclophosphamide use.

▷ When to Refer

The overall disease process frequently appears to accelerate once renal involvement becomes evident. Thus, the finding of an active urine sediment or a rise in serum creatinine in GPA signals a matter of utmost urgency.

Gross hematuria may indicate drug-induced cystitis in patients treated with cyclophosphamide. This complication may be associated with dysuria but not always. Cystoscopy is required to confirm the diagnosis in patients with drug-induced cystitis. Upon the diagnosis of cyclophosphamide-induced bladder injury, further treatment with this medication is contraindicated. Alternatively, gross hematuria is sometimes a presenting feature of active glomerulonephritis. The occurrence of hematuria months to years after a course of cyclophosphamide may indicate the development of bladder cancer and should prompt a cystoscopic evaluation by a urologist.

Hemoptysis, shortness of breath, rapidly changing pulmonary infiltrates, and abrupt declines in hematocrit may all indicate active pulmonary capillaritis. Hemoptysis may be an insensitive indicator of diffuse alveolar hemorrhage. This GPA complication requires rapid intervention with intensive immunosuppression and perhaps observation or management in an intensive care unit.

A fever in a patient who is receiving therapy for GPA signals a potential medical emergency, indicating the possibility of infection in immunocompromised patients.

The complaint of ocular pain, photophobia, or visual loss should prompt a swift referral to an ophthalmologist. Orbital pseudotumor, necrotizing scleritis, and marginal ulcers of the cornea may all lead quickly to vision-threatening ocular events.

Voice huskiness and subtle signs of stridorous breathing may indicate impending critical stenosis of the subglottic region. Some patients have subacute respiratory stridor. Severe cases may require tracheostomies. Pulmonary function tests (flow-volume loops) provide a useful noninvasive means of quantifying and following the degree of extrathoracic airway obstruction. However, thin-cut computed tomography (CT) scans of the trachea are more sensitive for these lesions. In some cases, direct visualization with fiberoptic laryngoscopy is required to make the diagnosis.

Guillevin L, Pagnoux C, Karras A, et al. Rituximab versus azathioprine for maintenance in ANCA-associated vasculitis. *N Engl J Med*. 2014;371(19):1771-1780. [PMID: 25372085]

Hoffman GS, Kerr GS, Leavitt RY, et al. Wegener's granulomatosis: an analysis of 158 patients. *Ann Intern Med*. 1992;116:488. [PMID: 1739240]

Miloslavsky EM, Specks U, Merkel PA, et al. Clinical outcomes of remission induction therapy for severe antineutrophil cytoplasmic antibody-associated vasculitis. *Arthritis Rheum*. 2013;65(9):2441-2449. [PMID: 23754238]

Stone JH, Merkel PA, Spiera R, et al. RAVE-ITN Research Group. Rituximab versus cyclophosphamide for ANCA-associated vasculitis. *N Engl J Med*. 2010;363:221. [PMID: 20647199]

Unizony S, Villarreal M, Miloslavsky EM, et al. Clinical outcomes of treatment of anti-neutrophil cytoplasmic antibody (ANCA)-associated vasculitis based on ANCA type. *Ann Rheum Dis*. 2016;75(6):1166-1169.

The Vasculitis Foundation. http://www.vasculitisfoundation.org/

Microscopic Polyangiitis

29

John H. Stone, MD, MPH

ESSENTIALS OF DIAGNOSIS

▶ Microscopic polyangiitis (MPA) is the most common cause of the pulmonary-renal syndrome of alveolar hemorrhage and glomerulonephritis.

▶ Usually includes combinations of two or more of the following:

- Nonspecific constitutional symptoms including fatigue, myalgias, weight loss, and fevers.

- Migratory arthralgias or arthritis, either pauciarticular or polyarticular.

- Palpable purpura, sometimes with skin ulcerations.

- Sensorimotor mononeuritis multiplex.

- Alveolar hemorrhage associated with hemoptysis and respiratory compromise.

- Glomerulonephritis.

▶ Antineutrophil cytoplasmic antibodies (ANCAs) are often critical in making the diagnosis, but a significant minority of patients are ANCA-negative.

▶ The majority of patients with MPA who are ANCA positive have antibodies directed against myeloperoxidase (MPO-ANCA).

▶ ANCA titers are often elevated during disease flares but do not have a consistent temporal relationship with disease activity. Thus, caution must be employed when making treatment decisions based on ANCA testing.

▶ General Considerations

Microscopic polyangiitis (MPA) is a form of systemic vasculitis that may affect many major organs with crippling or fatal effects. The great majority of patients with MPA have antineutrophil cytoplasmic antibodies (ANCAs). MPA is recognized to be related to both granulomatosis with polyangiitis (GPA;

formerly Wegener granulomatosis) and eosinophilic granulomatosis with polyangiitis (EGPA; formerly the Churg-Strauss syndrome). These disorders are sometimes considered together as the ANCA-associated vasculitides, but important differences exist among these three conditions and significant percentages of patients with these diagnoses do not have ANCA.

MPA has been recognized formally as a disease entity since the first Chapel Hill Consensus Conference on the nomenclature of systemic vasculitides in 1994. Many cases before then were considered to be forms of polyarteritis nodosa (PAN), a disease with which MPA shares substantial overlap. Table 29–1 compares the features of MPA with those of GPA and PAN.

The term "polyangiitis" is preferred to "polyarteritis" for MPA because the disease can involve veins as well as arteries. MPA is defined as a process that (1) involves necrotizing vasculitis with few or no immune deposits; (2) affects small blood vessels (capillaries, arterioles, or venules) and possibly medium-sized vessels; and (3) demonstrates a tropism for the kidneys and lungs. With an estimated incidence of four cases per million per year, MPA is more common than classic PAN but somewhat less common than GPA in Western countries. In contrast, MPA appears to be more common than GPA in Asian countries.

MPA occurs in people of all ethnic backgrounds. The male:female ratio is approximately 1:1. The typical patient is middle-aged to elderly, but the disease may affect people of all ages. The mean age at diagnosis for MPA patients (approximately 60 years) is about 10 years older than the mean age of GPA patients at diagnosis. The reason for this is not clear. Several epidemiologic studies have tried to elucidate environmental factors associated with the onset of vasculitis. Some authors have found associations with silica and solvent exposure, but the majority of MPA cases are idiopathic, without any clear-cut etiologic exposure.

The strongest link between an exposure and MPA relates to the use of propylthiouracil (PTU) for the treatment of hyperthyroidism. Other drugs for other indications have also been implicated in the etiology of MPA, but not

Table 29–1. Comparison of the features of MPA, GPA, and PAN.

	MPA	GPA	PAN
Vessel size	Small to medium	Small to medium	Medium
Vessel type	Capillaries, venules, and arterioles; sometimes arteries and veins	Capillaries, venules, and arterioles; sometimes arteries and veins	Muscular arteries
Granulomatous inflammation	No	Yes	No
Lung involvement	Yes (pulmonary capillaritis)	Yes (pulmonary nodules, often cavitary)	No
Glomerulonephritis	Yes	Yes	No
Renin-mediated hypertension	No	No	Yes
ANCA-positive	75%	60–90%	No
Hepatitis B association	No	No	Yes (<10% of cases now)
Microaneurysms	Rarely	Rarely	Typically
Mononeuritis multiplex	Commonly (60%)	Occasionally	Commonly (60%)
Likelihood of disease recurrence	33%	>50%	≤10%

ANCA, antineutrophil cytoplasmic antibody; GPA, granulomatosis with polyangiitis (formerly Wegener granulomatosis); MPA, microscopic polyangiitis; PAN, polyarteritis nodosa.

as strongly. Anti-MPO antibodies are detected frequently in PTU-treated patients, albeit overt vasculitis occurs in only a small minority (<5%).

▶ Clinical Findings

A. Symptoms and Signs

The interval between the onset of first disease symptoms and diagnosis in MPA is substantially shorter than for patients with GPA. This is likely because of the tendency for GPA to smolder in the upper respiratory tract and cause apparently mundane symptoms for months before leading to medical attention. In contrast, the presence of "something wrong" is usually obvious when a patient with MPA becomes symptomatic with findings attributable to the disease: cutaneous vasculitis, vasculitic neuropathy, or alveolar hemorrhage. Nevertheless, subtle and subacute presentations of MPA are known to occur, and the range of organ system manifestations is extensive. Glomerulonephritis in MPA can remain subclinical until renal dysfunction is quite advanced.

Although MPA is classified appropriately as a "pulmonary-renal syndrome," the disease should not be regarded as a disease that affects the kidneys and lungs exclusively. The five most common clinical manifestations of MPA are glomerulonephritis (nearly 80% of patients), weight loss (>70%), mononeuritis multiplex (60%), fevers (55%), and cutaneous vasculitis (>60%). Alveolar hemorrhage, in contrast, occurs in only about 12% of patients. The major clinical manifestations of MPA are shown in Table 29–2.

1. Head, eyes, ears, nose, and throat—HEENT involvement in MPA is limited generally to rhinitis or mild cases of nondestructive sinusitis. Serous otitis media may occur

in MPA but unlike in GPA, granulomatous inflammation is absent. Ocular lesions in MPA (eg, episcleritis, conjunctivitis, keratitis, and occasionally scleritis) have been reported but are less common and less severe than in GPA.

Table 29–2. Major clinical manifestations of microscopic polyangiitis.

Organ	Manifestation
Constitutional	Weight loss, anorexia, fevers
HEENT	Rhinitis, tongue, or other oral ulcers; occasional purpuric lesions on palate; ocular inflammation (eg, sclerouveitis) reported but rare
Lungs	Alveolar hemorrhage; nonspecific infiltrates; pulmonary fibrosis; pleural effusions
Gastrointestinal	Mesenteric vasculitis with microaneurysms in some patients
Kidneys	Glomerulonephritis (small-vessel vasculitis of the kidney); medium-vessel vasculitis occasionally evident on renal biopsy or demonstrated by cross-sectional imaging studies (renal infarcts)
Skin	Palpable purpura, ulcers, vesiculobullous lesions, splinter hemorrhages
Joints	Migratory pauciarthritis or polyarthritis or arthralgias; arthritis is nondestructive
Peripheral nerve	Sensory or motor mononeuritis multiplex
Central nervous system	True central nervous system vasculitis rare but reported

HEENT, head, eyes, ears, nose, throat.

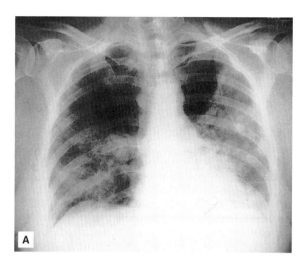
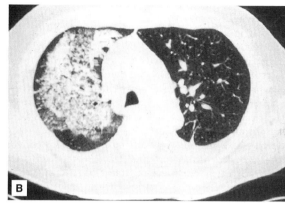

▲ **Figure 29–1.** Radiologic features of alveolar hemorrhage. **A:** Chest radiograph. **B:** Computed tomography scan of the chest.

2. Lungs—The principal pulmonary manifestation of MPA is capillaritis, which leads to alveolar hemorrhage and often to hemoptysis. Hemoptysis may be only a late indication of bleeding. The typical radiologic features of alveolar hemorrhage are shown in Figure 29–1. Alveolar hemorrhage is associated with a worse prognosis. Interstitial fibrosis and pleuritis occur in some patients with MPA. Pulmonary fibrosis resembling in its clinical presentation usual interstitial pneumonitis (UIP) is an important but underrecognized disease manifestation of MPA that differentiates it clearly from GPA, EGPA, and PAN. This pulmonary complication underscores the point that ANCA testing should be performed as a matter of routine in patients presenting with the clinical and radiologic syndrome of UIP when there is not a clear underlying cause.

3. Kidneys—Renal involvement is seen in at least 80% of patients with MPA. The classic presentation of renal disease in MPA is a rapidly progressive glomerulonephritis reminiscent of GPA (Figure 29–2A). Some patients, however, have renal deterioration that progresses more slowly, over many months. Renal involvement may also present with urinary abnormalities such as proteinuria, microscopic hematuria, and red blood cell casts. Up to 40% of patients have 24-hour urinary protein excretion of more than 3 g. Proteinuria of this severity is regarded as a poor prognostic factor for renal outcome. The pathologic features of renal disease in MPA are indistinguishable from those of other forms of pauci-immune glomerulonephritis—namely, a necrotizing, crescentic lesion (Figure 29–2B). Compared with biopsies from patients with

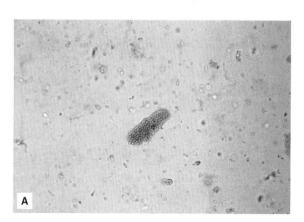
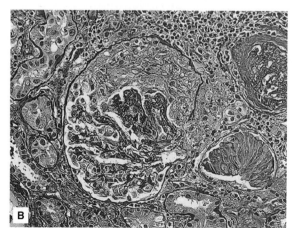

▲ **Figure 29–2.** Renal manifestations of microscopic polyangiitis. **A:** Red blood cell cast in a patient with glomerulonephritis secondary to microscopic polyangiitis. (Reproduced, with permission, from Stone JH, et al. Vasculitis. A collection of pearls and myths. *Rheum Dis Clin North Am.* 2001;27:677.) **B:** Glomerular crescent in a patient with microscopic polyangiitis.

ANCA directed against proteinase-3, those with MPO-ANCA have a more chronic pattern of renal injury, with more glomerulosclerosis, tubular atrophy, and interstitial fibrosis.

4. Nervous system—Vasculitic neuropathy is a potentially devastating complication of MPA. The nerve involvement typically occurs in the pattern of a distal, asymmetric, axonal polyneuropathy (mononeuritis multiplex). The first symptoms of vasculitic neuropathy are usually sensory, with numbness, tingling, and dysesthesias. Muscle weakness and wasting follow the infarction of motor nerves (Figure 29–3). Because the named peripheral nerves are usually mixed nerves that carry both sensory and motor fibers, patients with vasculitic neuropathy typically have both sensory and motor symptoms. Recovery from vasculitic neuropathy may take months, and most patients have some residual nerve damage long after the disease has been controlled. Peripheral nerve lesions tend to dominate the neurologic features of MPA, but central nervous system involvement by vasculitis is also described in this disease.

Small-fiber neuropathy has also been reported in MPA. In patients with small-fiber neuropathy, the predominant symptoms are pain and numbness rather than motor weakness. Electrodiagnostic studies in small-fiber neuropathy patients are normal because the involved fibers are below the resolution of nerve conduction velocity assessments. Diagnosis is made by biopsy of the skin and staining for the density of small nerve fibers.

5. Skin—The cutaneous manifestations of MPA include all of the skin lesions associated with small-vessel vasculitis (palpable purpura, papules, vesiculobullous lesions, splinter hemorrhages) (Figure 29–4). In the presence of medium-vessel involvement, nodules, ulcers, livedo racemosa (Figure 29–5), and digital gangrene may occur. As with most forms of cutaneous vasculitis, the lesions favor the lower extremities.

6. Musculoskeletal system—Nonspecific arthralgias and frank arthritis usually present early in the course of MPA and

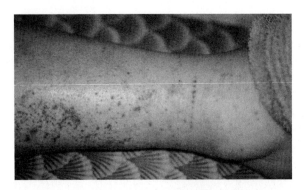

▲ **Figure 29–4. Cutaneous vasculitis in microscopic polyangiitis.** Palpable purpura on the lower extremity of a patient with microscopic polyangiitis, associated with antineutrophil cytoplasmic antibodies directed against myeloperoxidase (MPO-ANCA). Not the linear streak of purpura corresponding to the site of the patient's sock elastic. The occurrence of a skin lesion (eg, purpura) at the site of skin under pressure is called Koebner's phenomenon.

respond quickly to therapy. Musculoskeletal symptoms may also herald disease flares. The arthritis of MPA is migratory in nature and can assume a variety of joint patterns, from a pauci-articular syndrome of large joints to a polyarthritis of small joints. Destructive joint lesions do not occur in MPA.

B. Laboratory Findings

The results of routine laboratory tests and specialized assays in MPA are shown in Table 29–3. All of these tests are appropriate at the initial evaluation in patients who demonstrate features consistent with MPA. The exclusion of renal disease through the careful performance of a urinalysis is essential in the evaluation and follow-up of all patients with MPA. Measurement of the urine protein:creatinine ratio is also important. The erythrocyte sedimentation rate and serum C-reactive protein level are useful in the longitudinal evaluation of disease activity.

Positive ANCA assays are often instrumental in suggesting the diagnosis, but the titers of these antibodies correlate poorly in time with disease flares. Thin-cut computed tomography scans are sensitive in the detection of lung disease in MPA.

C. Special Tests

1. Tissue biopsy—By definition, MPA involves small blood vessels: arterioles, venules, and capillaries. Glomerulonephritis is the renal equivalent of small-vessel vasculitis, akin to palpable purpura in the skin and capillaritis in the lung. Renal biopsy findings, although not specific for MPA, are sufficiently characteristic to establish the diagnosis in appropriate clinical settings, particularly when MPO-ANCAs are present in the blood. Immunofluorescence studies of renal biopsies in MPA confirm the "pauci-immune" nature of the renal involvement. MPA may also involve medium-sized

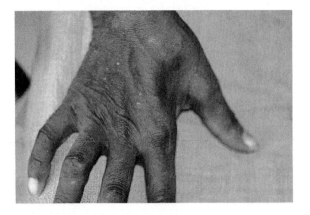

▲ **Figure 29–3.** Muscle wasting caused by vasculitic neuropathy (mononeuritis multiplex) associated with microscopic polyangiitis.

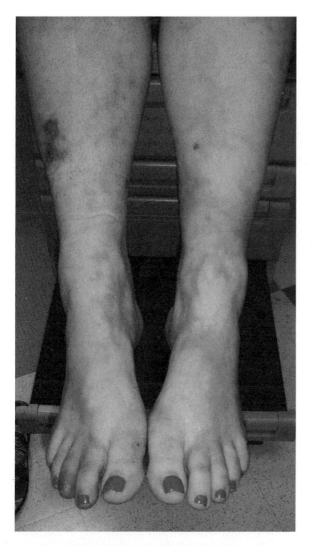

Table 29–3. The laboratory evaluation in MPA.

Test	Typical Result
Complete blood cell count	• Normochromic, normocytic anemia; acute, severe anemias possible in alveolar hemorrhage • Mild to moderate leukocytosis common, usually not exceeding 18×10^9/L • Moderate to pronounced thrombocytosis typical, ranging from platelet counts of 400×10^9/L to occasionally >1000×10^9/L
Electrolytes	Hyperkalemia in the setting of advanced renal dysfunction
Liver function tests	Hepatic involvement unusual in MPA When present, there can be elevations of transaminases (AST/ALT) in excess of 1000 mg/dL
Urinalysis with microscopy	• Hematuria (ranging from mild to so high that red blood cells are too numerous to count) • Red blood cell casts • Proteinuria (nephritic range proteinuria in a small minority)
Erythrocyte sedimentation rate/ C-reactive protein	• Dramatic elevations of acute phase reactants are typical, generally with good correlation to disease activity
ANA	Negative
Rheumatoid factor	Positive in 40–50% of patients, often leading to diagnostic confusion with rheumatoid arthritis
C3, C4	Usually normal (or increased, because complement proteins are acute phase reactants)
ANCA	Positive in 70% of patients with MPA (and probably a higher percentage of patients with generalized disease)
Anti-GBM	A small number of patients have both ANCA and anti-GBM antibodies

ANA, antinuclear antibody; ANCA, antineutrophil cytoplasmic antibody; anti-GBM, antiglomerular basement membrane antibodies; AST/ALT, aspartate aminotransferase and alanine aminotransferase; MPA, microscopic polyangiitis.

▲ **Figure 29–5.** Livedo racemosa as a manifestation of microscopic polyangiitis. Livedo racemosa and ulcers occurring on the lower extremities of a patient with microscopic polyangiitis. This patient's presenting manifestation was neuropathic pains from a sensorimotor vasculitic neuropathy. The cutaneous manifestations developed later.

arteries and veins, but the identification of medium-vessel involvement is not essential to the diagnosis.

MPA is high on the differential diagnosis of leukocytoclastic vasculitis within the small blood vessels of skin lesions. The presence of extracutaneous findings and ANCA increases the likelihood of MPA. If sufficiently deep, skin biopsies may also demonstrate the involvement of medium-sized vessels in the deep dermis subcutaneous tissue layer. The finding of medium-vessel involvement eliminates certain forms of cutaneous

vasculitis limited to small-vessel disease, for example hypersensitivity vasculitis (cutaneous leukocytoclastic angiitis) and IgA vasculitis (Henoch-Schönlein purpura). Direct immunofluorescence of skin biopsy tissue is also important in the exclusion of immune complex-mediated processes such as cryoglobulinemia. The involvement of both veins and arteries distinguishes MPA from classic PAN, which is confined to arterial lesions. The presence of granulomatous inflammation, on the other hand, is inconsistent with the diagnosis of MPA. Granulomatous inflammation, rather, suggests alternative diagnoses such as GPA, EGPA, and giant cell arteritis.

2. Nerve conduction studies—Nerve conduction studies are an important part of the evaluation for patients with neuropathic symptoms. Nerve conduction studies may reveal the characteristic asymmetric, axonal sensorimotor neuropathy.

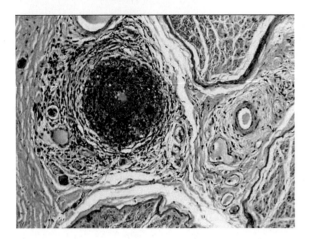

▲ **Figure 29–6. Vasculitic neuropathy in microscopic polyangiitis.** A medium-sized muscular artery (vasa nervorum) identified at sural nerve biopsy. The biopsy reveals inflammation throughout the blood vessel wall, accompanied by necrosis. The vessel and its branches supply the sural nerve with blood. Its disruption by necrotizing vasculitis leads to mononeuritis multiplex.

Table 29–4. Differential diagnosis of microscopic polyangiitis.

Other vasculitides
Polyarteritis nodosa
Granulomatosis with polyangiitis (formerly Wegener granulomatosis)
Eosinophilic granulomatosis with polyangiitis (Churg-Strauss syndrome)
Henoch-Schönlein purpura
Hypersensitivity vasculitis
Mixed cryoglobulinemia
Goodpasture disease
Giant cell arteritis
Drug-induced ANCA-associated vasculitis
Infections
Endocarditis
Pulmonary conditions
Interstitial pulmonary fibrosis
Idiopathic pulmonary hemosiderosis
Systemic autoimmune conditions
Systemic lupus erythematosus
Rheumatoid arthritis
Miscellaneous nonvasculitic conditions associated with P-ANCA
Inflammatory bowel disease
Autoimmune hepatitis
Sclerosing cholangitis

ANCA, antineutrophilic cytoplasmic antibody; P-ANCA, perinuclear antineutrophilic cytoplasmic antibody.

Nerves such as the sural nerve shown to be involved in this fashion are prime candidates for biopsy, with simultaneous sampling of adjacent muscle (eg, the gastrocnemius). The sural nerve is an excellent candidate for biopsy because, in contrast to most peripheral nerves, it contains only sensory fibers. In some cases, histopathology diagnostic of vasculitis is confined to the muscle as opposed to the nerve, or vice versa (Figure 29–6). As noted, nerve conduction studies may be negative in patients with small-fiber neuropathies.

Although lung involvement can be a florid manifestation of MPA, demonstration of vasculitis on thoracoscopic or open lung biopsy is often challenging; frank capillaritis may be difficult to detect. Nevertheless, lung biopsies are often essential to exclude other processes (eg, infections or malignancies) if no other tissue options exist for biopsy.

3. Serologic testing for ANCA—Nearly all patients with clinical diagnoses of MPA are ANCA positive. In MPA, the classic pattern of serum reactivity upon immunofluorescence testing is perinuclear staining (P-ANCA). The P-ANCA pattern in MPA patients is usually caused by antibodies to MPO, a constituent of the primary granules of neutrophils. A variety of nonvasculitic conditions (Table 29–4) can also cause P-ANCA immunofluorescence, but these results are usually caused by antibodies to antigens not associated with vasculitis (eg, lactoferrin). Drug-induced vasculitis can often lead to high titers of MPO-ANCA, but the clinical settings and patients' symptoms, signs, and patterns of organ involvement typically the differentiation of drug-induced ANCA-associated conditions from MPA.

The combination of both a P-ANCA pattern on immunofluorescence testing and MPO-ANCA demonstrated by enzyme immunoassay has a high positive predictive value for ANCA-associated vasculitis, most commonly MPA. The other type of ANCA found in MPA—rarely—is PR3-ANCA, directed against proteinase-3. This type of ANCA is usually associated with a cytoplasmic (C-ANCA) pattern of immunofluorescent staining. Despite advances in ANCA testing techniques, histopathology remains the cornerstone of diagnosis in MPA. When the diagnosis is unconfirmed, all reasonable attempts to obtain a tissue diagnosis should be pursued.

▶ **Differential Diagnosis**

The greatest mimickers of MPA are other forms of vasculitis (see Table 29–4). Immunoglobulin A (IgA) vasculitis (Henoch-Schönlein purpura) and hypersensitivity vasculitis (also known as cutaneous leukocytoclastic angiitis) can cause identical skin lesions, as can GPA, EGPA (Churg-Strauss), mixed cryoglobulinemia, and PAN. MPA can be differentiated from these disorders by the pattern recognition of extracutaneous involvement (kidneys, lung, nerve); biopsy of involved organs; and ANCA testing. The difficulties of distinguishing MPA from GPA and PAN are illustrated in Table 29–1.

Antiglomerular basement membrane disease, a less common cause of pulmonary-renal syndromes than the ANCA-associated vasculitides, generally requires plasma exchange in addition to glucocorticoids and either rituximab or cyclophosphamide to establish disease control. Plasma exchange does not have a significant role in the treatment of MPA.

MPA can lead to lymphoplasmacytic infiltrates within the adventitia of the temporal artery and also cause severe headaches, thereby mimicking giant cell arteritis both clinically and pathologically. MPA involving the temporal artery is not associated with giant cells, but giant cells can also be absent in a significant percentage of patients with GCA. ANCA testing is often crucial in distinguishing MPA from GCA at early stages of disease because temporal artery biopsy may not permit a clear distinction. In addition, some medications, particularly PTU (used to treat thyroiditis), can cause a drug-induced, ANCA-associated vasculitis associated with high titers of antibodies to MPO.

A variety of pulmonary, renal, and peripheral nerve disorders must be distinguished from MPA by imaging studies, tissue biopsy, nerve conduction studies, and serologic testing. Systemic autoimmune conditions such as systemic lupus erythematosus and rheumatoid arthritis (particularly rheumatoid vasculitis) are also prone to imitating MPA because of their abilities to involve multiple organ systems. Although many autoimmune conditions can be associated with positive P-ANCA results on immunofluorescence testing of serum, the combination of both P-ANCA immunofluorescence and anti-MPO-ANCA speaks to a high likelihood of MPA (see above).

▶ Treatment

The essentials of management for MPA are shown in Table 29–5. MPA is one of a handful of vasculitic conditions in which the conventional standard of care for many years called for combination therapy with both glucocorticoids and a cytotoxic agent. However, rituximab plus glucocorticoids is as effective as cyclophosphamide plus glucocorticoids for the induction of remission in ANCA-associated vasculitis (ie, specifically MPA and GPA). The induction of remission with rituximab is preferred to cyclophosphamide because of rituximab's superior long-term side effect profile. Rituximab has a particular advantage over cyclophosphamide in the treatment of patients with relapsing (as opposed to newly diagnosed) disease.

Table 29–5. Essentials of MPA management.

- Because most patients with MPA have major organ involvement such as glomerulonephritis, alveolar hemorrhage, or vasculitic neuropathy, the combination of cyclophosphamide and glucocorticoids is the cornerstone of most treatment regimens.
- Cyclophosphamide may be administered on either a daily or intermittent basis.
- "Pulse" methylprednisolone (1 g/day for 3 days) may be considered for patients with severe organ involvement at diagnosis.
- Alternative medications such as azathioprine or methotrexate should be considered after 3–6 months of cyclophosphamide therapy.

MPA, microscopic polyangiitis.

If rituximab cannot be given or if the patient has not responded to this regimen, cyclophosphamide can be added. The combination of cyclophosphamide (2 mg/kg/day for those with normal renal function) and glucocorticoids (1 mg/kg/day of prednisone, perhaps preceded by a 3-day intravenous "pulse" of methylprednisolone) usually leads to excellent therapeutic responses if treatment is initiated early enough. Three- to 6-month courses of cyclophosphamide are used followed by longer-term treatment for the maintenance of remission.

All patients who are receiving treatment for MPA should be given a daily dose of single-strength trimethoprim-sulfamethoxazole or 1500 mg/day of atovaquone as prophylaxis against *Pneumocystis jiroveci* pneumonia.

The need for a remission maintenance regimen following rituximab-induced disease remissions in MPA is not clear and must be determined in longitudinal studies. Patients with MPA, usually MPO-ANCA-positive, are less likely to flare compared to GPA patients (usually PR3-ANCA positive). Many patients with MPA do not experience disease exacerbations after achieving remission with one treatment course and do not require remission maintenance therapy. Flares of MPA clearly occur in a significant disease subset, however. For MPA patients who demonstrate a propensity to flare, the optimal remission strategy at the moment consists of rituximab infusions at some interval, for example, 6 months, with the possibility of spacing out the infusions after several cycles.

Once the inflammatory process has been controlled with immunosuppressive therapy, renal preservation therapies for patients with renal damage (blood pressure control, angiotensin-converting enzyme inhibition, and salt restriction) should be instituted.

▶ Complications

If MPA is diagnosed early and treated promptly, patients have a high likelihood (>90%) of achieving disease remissions. Unfortunately, significant damage frequently ensues in MPA before the diagnosis is established. MPA patients present with higher mean serum creatinine concentrations at diagnosis compared to patients with GPA. The renal prognosis in MPA may be worse than that of GPA, probably because of a greater likelihood of delay in diagnosis in MPA. Another major disability associated with MPA results from nerve damage and consequent muscle weakness caused by vasculitic neuropathy. Finally, patients with AAV have a high risk of venous thrombotic events. Heightened suspicion for this complication, possibly caused by involvement of the veins by the vasculitic process, should be maintained.

Alba MA, Flores-Suárez LF, Henderson AG, et al. Interstital lung disease in ANCA vasculitis. *Autoimmun Rev.* 2017;16(7):722-729. [PMID: 28479484]

Specks U, Merkel PA, Seo P, et al. Efficacy of remission-induction regimens for ANCA-associated vasculitis. *N Engl J Med.* 2013; 369(5):417-427. [PMID: 23902481]

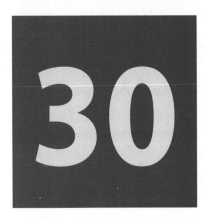

Eosinophilic Granulomatosis with Polyangiitis (Churg-Strauss Syndrome)

Philip Seo, MD, MHS

John H. Stone, MD, MPH

ESSENTIALS OF DIAGNOSIS

▶ Asthma, eosinophilia, and systemic vasculitis are the hallmarks of eosinophilic granulomatosis with polyangiitis (EGPA; Churg-Strauss syndrome).

▶ Classic clinical features include the following:

- Allergic rhinitis and nasal polyposis.

- Reactive airway disease.

- Peripheral eosinophilia (10–60% of all circulating leukocytes).

- Fleeting pulmonary infiltrates and occasional alveolar hemorrhage.

- Vasculitic neuropathy.

- Congestive heart failure.

▶ Approximately 50% of patients with EGPA have antineutrophil cytoplasmic antibodies (ANCAs), usually with a specificity for myeloperoxidase (MPO).

General Considerations

In 1951, Churg and Strauss reported a series of 13 patients with "periarteritis nodosa" (see Chapter 31) who demonstrated severe asthma and an unusual constellation of other symptoms: "fever … hypereosinophilia, symptoms of cardiac failure, renal damage, and peripheral neuropathy, resulting from vascular embarrassment…." The investigators termed this new disease "allergic angiitis and allergic granulomatosis" and specified three histologic criteria for the diagnosis: (1) the presence of necrotizing vasculitis, (2) tissue infiltration by eosinophils, and (3) extravascular granuloma.

In 1990, an American College of Rheumatology panel liberalized the criteria for the classification of this disease, dropping the requirements for histopathologically proven vasculitis and granuloma (Table 30–1). The Chapel Hill Consensus Conference on nomenclature of the vasculitides subsequently defined the Churg-Strauss syndrome as a disorder characterized by eosinophil-rich, granulomatous inflammation of the respiratory tract and necrotizing vasculitis of small- to medium-sized vessels, associated with asthma and eosinophilia. In 2012, the Revised Chapel Hill Consensus Conference Nomenclature of Vasculitides recommended the term "eosinophilic granulomatosis with polyangiitis" (EGPA) for this disease. The purpose for this recommendation was twofold: (1) to emphasize certain cardinal features of the condition; and (2) for consistency with the names preferred for two related disorders, granulomatosis with polyangiitis (formerly Wegener granulomatosis) (see Chapter 28) and microscopic polyangiitis (see Chapter 29).

EGPA is a rare disease—significantly less common than the other forms of ANCA-associated vasculitis. The annual incidence of EGPA is approximately 2.4 cases per million individuals. The distribution of cases is roughly equal between men and women. Associations between the use of leukotriene antagonists and EGPA have been reported, but they are unlikely to be causal. Leukotriene antagonists are effective asthma medications, and the tapering of glucocorticoids likely "unmasks" the vasculitic phase of EGPA. Leukotriene inhibitors are not believed to cause EGPA now and, in fact, these medications can be employed in the treatment of EGPA-associated asthma.

Clinical Findings

A. Symptoms and Signs

After the diagnosis of EGPA has been made, three disease phases are often recognizable: the prodrome, eosinophilia/tissue infiltration, and vasculitis.

The **prodrome phase** is characterized by the presence of allergic disease (typically asthma or allergic rhinitis). This phase often lasts for several years. A common history is that a middle-aged individual with no history of atopy suddenly develops asthma, or that a patient with previously well-controlled asthma has become more difficult to treat.

Table 30–1. American College of Rheumatology 1990 criteria for the classification of Churg-Strauss syndrome (eosinophilic granulomatosis with polyangiitis).[a]

Criterion	Definition
Asthma	History of wheezing or diffuse high-pitched rales on expiration
Eosinophilia	Eosinophilia >10% on white blood cell differential count
Mononeuropathy or polyneuropathy	Development of mononeuropathy, multiple mononeuropathies, or polyneuropathy (ie, stocking/glove distribution)
Pulmonary infiltrates, nonfixed	Migratory or transitory pulmonary infiltrates on radiographs
Paranasal sinus abnormality	History of acute or chronic paranasal sinus pain or tenderness, or radiographic opacification of the paranasal sinuses
Extravascular eosinophils	Biopsy including artery, arteriole, or venule, showing accumulations of eosinophils in extravascular areas

[a]To be classified as having Churg-Strauss syndrome (eosinophilic granulomatosis with polyangiitis), a patient must have at least four of these six criteria. Among patients with various forms of systemic vasculitis, the sensitivity of these criteria for the classification of an individual patient as having Churg-Strauss syndrome was estimated to be 85%. Reproduced with permission from Masi AT, Hunder GG, Lie TT, et al. The American College of Rheumatology 1990 criteria for the classification of Churg-Strauss syndrome [allergic granulomatosis sand angiitis]. *Arthritis Rheum.* 1990;33:1094.

During the **eosinophilia/tissue infiltration phase**, striking peripheral eosinophilia may occur. Tissue infiltration by eosinophils is observed in the heart, lung, gastrointestinal tract, and other tissues. EGPA is difficult to differentiate at this point from the hypereosinophilic syndromes, eosinophilic gastroenteritis, and chronic eosinophilic pneumonia.

In the third phase, **vasculitis**, systemic necrotizing vasculitis affects a wide range of organs, ranging from the heart and lungs to the peripheral nerves and skin (Figure 30–1).

1. Nose and sinuses—Upper airway disease in EGPA usually takes the form of nasal polyps or allergic rhinitis. A high percentage of patients with EGPA have histories of nasal polypectomies, usually long before suspicion of an underlying disease is raised. Although pansinusitis occurs frequently, destructive upper airway disease is not characteristic of EGPA.

2. Ears—Middle ear granulation tissue with eosinophilic infiltrates occurs in some patients, leading to conductive hearing loss. Cases of sensorineural hearing loss have also been reported.

3. Lungs—More than 90% of patients with EGPA have histories of asthma. Typically, the asthma represents either adult-onset reactive airway disease or, less commonly, a significant worsening of long-standing disease. Ironically, patients' asthma may improve substantially upon encroachment of the vasculitic phase of EGPA, even before therapy for vasculitis has begun. Following successful treatment of the vasculitic phase, however, glucocorticoid-dependent asthma persists in many patients.

The pathologic features of lung disease in EGPA vary according to the disease phase. In the early phases, there may be extensive eosinophilic infiltration of the alveoli and interstitium. During the vasculitic phase, necrotizing vasculitis and granuloma may be evident. In the current era, when many patients with asthma are treated with systemic

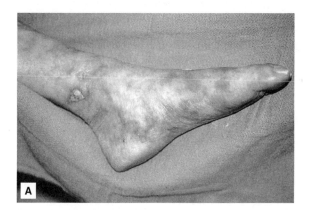
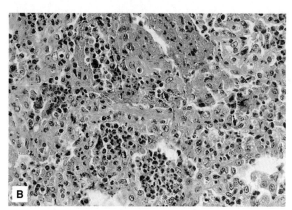

▲ **Figure 30–1.** **A:** Foot of a patient with eosinophilic granulomatosis with polyangiitis (EGPA; formerly Churg-Strauss syndrome) showing livedo reticularis and a cutaneous ulcer just superior to the medial malleolus. The patient's foot is held in extension because of a left foot drop (vasculitis neuropathy of the left peroneal nerve). **B:** Eosinophilic pneumonia in a patient with EGPA. Biopsy shows dense clusters of eosinophils within the lung parenchyma.

glucocorticoids, lung biopsy specimens showing all three histologic hallmarks of this disease are unusual.

4. Peripheral nerves—Mononeuritis multiplex occurs in a large proportion of patients with EGPA, with often devastating effects. Vasculitic neuropathy was evident in 74 (77%) of the 96 patients in one series. Nerve infarctions are heralded by the abrupt occurrence of a foot drop, wrist drop, or some other focal nerve lesion. Muscle wasting secondary to nerve infarctions may continue to appear for weeks after the disease has been brought under control (Figure 30–2).

Nerve infarctions may appear several weeks after the start of appropriate treatment. If intensive treatment has already begun, new nerve lesions do not necessarily indicate the need to intensify therapy further because they may be secondary to thrombosis of vessels that have become severely compromised by previously active inflammation.

5. Heart—Myocardial involvement occurs commonly in EGPA and is a common cause of death. Some form of cardiac

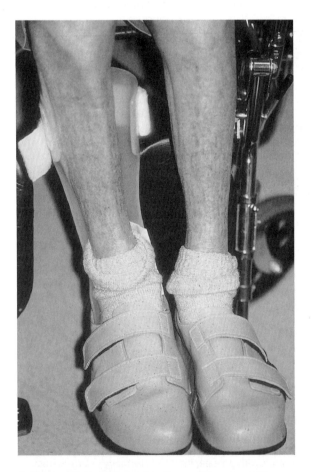

▲ **Figure 30–2.** The ravages of vasculitic neuropathy. Bilateral ankle-foot orthoses required because of bilateral foot drop. Note severe muscle wasting in both legs.

involvement occurred in 12.5% of patients in one large series. Diagnosis of this type of organ involvement is often challenging, but a high index of suspicion is in order for EGPA patients who have symptoms of heart failure. Congestive heart failure is the most common cardiac manifestation, although coronary arteritis and valvular abnormalities have also been reported.

6. Skin—Skin disease in EGPA takes many forms, none of which is specific. Palpable purpura, papules, ulcers, and vesiculobullous lesions are common. Nodular skin lesions are usually "Churg-Strauss granuloma" (cutaneous extravascular necrotizing granuloma). These tend to occur on the extensor surfaces of the elbows and other pressure points. Skin biopsy specimens in EGPA reveal the infiltration of eosinophils into blood vessel walls, with resultant vascular wall injury. Splinter hemorrhages, digital ischemia, and gangrene associated with inflammation in medium-sized digital arteries are often present at the time of diagnosis.

7. Kidneys—EGPA is less likely to cause end-stage renal disease than are other forms of ANCA-associated vasculitis. Acute kidney injury may be caused by an eosinophil-mediated interstitial nephritis. When glomerulonephritis does occur, however, the histopathologic findings are often indistinguishable from those of other forms of pauci-immune vasculitis (eg, granulomatosis with polyangiitis, microscopic polyangiitis, and renal-limited vasculitis).

8. Joints—Nonspecific arthralgias and frank arthritis often occur early in the course of EGPA. The arthritis of EGPA is migratory in nature and may assume a variety of joint patterns, from a pauciarticular syndrome of lower extremity joints to a small joint polyarthritis of the hands.

B. Laboratory Findings

Eosinophilia (before treatment) is a *sine qua non* of EGPA. Eosinophils may comprise as much as 60% of the total white blood cell count. Eosinophil counts are usually sensitive markers of disease flares but generally respond very quickly to treatment with high doses of glucocorticoids. Most patients with EGPA also have elevated serum immunoglobulin E (IgE) levels. Serum complement levels are usually normal. Immune complexes are not believed to play a primary role in this disease. The erythrocyte sedimentation rate, serum C-reactive protein level, and eosinophil count can be useful in the longitudinal evaluation of disease activity. The reported percentages of EGPA patients with ANCA are variable, with most figures in the literature in the range of 50% (see Chapter 28 for a full discussion of ANCA). Of the two vasculitis-specific ANCAs—antibodies to MPO and proteinase-3—those directed against MPO are more common in EGPA. Patients who are ANCA-positive tend to have more of the classic vasculitic manifestations of this disease, for example mononeuritis multiplex and glomerulonephritis. In contrast, patients who are ANCA-negative tend to have more cardiopulmonary complications. There is, however, substantial overlap between these two groups.

C. Imaging Studies

Pulmonary infiltrates are evident in approximately one-third of patients with EGPA. These lesions are usually migratory infiltrates that occur bilaterally, with a predilection for the upper lobes. Pulmonary hemorrhage, very typical of both GPA and MPA, is unusual in EGPA but has been reported. Nodular or cavitary lesions suggest the alternative diagnoses of granulomatosis with polyangiitis, infection, or malignancy. Among patients with cardiac involvement, echocardiography or cardiac MRI may confirm poor cardiac function consistent with cardiomyopathy or demonstrate findings compatible with regional myocardial fibrosis.

▶ Differential Diagnosis

The major disease entities in the differential diagnosis of EGPA are shown in Table 30–2. There are many diseases in which patients frequently demonstrate mild eosinophilia (eg, a peripheral blood eosinophilia on the order of 10% or so in asthma or parasitic infections). Only a handful of diseases, however, can cause eosinophilia as high as 20–60%, as is occasionally observed with EGPA and its related conditions. *Strongyloides* infection, which can cause both high levels of eosinophilia and asthma, should be considered in endemic areas, which include the southeastern United States. IgG4-related disease, frequently associated with peripheral eosinophil counts on the order of 20%, is often accompanied by atopic phenomena (eg, allergic rhinitis, asthma) in the same manner as EGPA. Patients with EGPA frequently have serum IgG4 concentration elevations, further compounding the difficulty in distinguishing the two conditions. EGPA must also be distinguished from other hypereosinophilic disorders: Löffler syndrome, chronic eosinophilic pneumonia, eosinophilic gastroenteritis, hypereosinophilic syndrome,

Table 30–2. Differential diagnosis of eosinophilic granulomatosis with polyangiitis (formerly Churg-Strauss syndrome).

Eosinophilic Disorders	Other Vasculitides
Löffler syndrome	Granulomatosis with polyangiitis (formerly Wegener granulomatosis)
Chronic eosinophilic pneumonia	Microscopic polyangiitis Polyarteritis nodosa
Eosinophilic gastroenteritis	Mixed cryoglobulinemia
Hypereosinophilic syndrome	Goodpasture syndrome
Eosinophilic leukemia	
Eosinophilic fasciitis	

eosinophilic fasciitis, and eosinophilic leukemia. The fleeting pulmonary infiltrates of the Löffler syndrome and the peripheral infiltrates of chronic eosinophilic pneumonia may both mimic EGPA closely.

Differentiating EGPA from hypereosinophilic syndrome may be the biggest challenge, however. One important potential differentiator is that the hypereosinophilic syndrome is rarely associated with reactive airway disease. Laboratory tests for the F1P1L1-PDGFR gene translocation, T-cell receptor clonality, elevated serum tryptase levels, and elevated serum B12 (all of which are associated with hypereosinophilic syndrome) may also be helpful in the evaluation of such patients.

Many other forms of systemic vasculitis are high on the differential diagnosis for EGPA. Granulomatosis with polyangiitis, polyarteritis nodosa, microscopic polyangiitis, Goodpasture syndrome (antiglomerular basement membrane disease), cryoglobulinemic vasculitis, and other vasculitic disorders have clinical features that overlap with those of EGPA. However, the finding of eosinophilia superimposed upon a history of allergy or asthma usually permits the clear distinction of EGPA from these other disorders.

▶ Treatment

In contrast to other forms of ANCA-associated vasculitis, remission may be induced in many patients with EGPA with glucocorticoids alone. Glucocorticoid-related morbidity is a major concern in patients with EGPA, however, because many patients are not able to taper successfully to an acceptably low daily dose of prednisone. Data supporting the use of traditional steroid-sparing agents such as methotrexate (15–25 mg/wk), mycophenolate mofetil (2–3 g/day in divided doses), or azathioprine (2 mg/kg/day) are slim, and these agents are falling out of favor.

For patients whose disease remains active despite the combination of glucocorticoids and a steroid-sparing agent, mepolizumab (300 mg subcutaneous monthly) can be added. Recent data indicate that the addition of mepolizumab leads to a decline in relapse rate and decreased reliance on systemic glucocorticoids. Mepolizumab should be used early in patients who are not able to taper prednisone successfully because of persistent asthmatic or atopic symptoms, in the interest of reducing glucocorticoid toxicity. Other drugs that block interleukin-5 signaling (eg, reslizumab, benralizumab) may also be effective in select patients.

Certain disease complications, particularly the presence of vasculitic neuropathy or glomerulonephritis, should trigger the use of cyclophosphamide (2 mg/kg/day orally, decreased in the setting of renal dysfunction or advanced age) or rituximab (1 g intravenously times two doses, separated by 2 weeks) as part of the remission induction strategy. Neither cyclophosphamide nor rituximab has been studied in a randomized clinical trial in EGPA.

Either cyclophosphamide or rituximab should also be considered with other complications of EGPA that pose immediate threats to the function of vital organs (eg, the heart). There are few data favoring either cyclophosphamide or rituximab with regard to efficacy in EGPA, but rituximab is often chosen first because of its superior side-effect profile. Cyclophosphamide should be used extremely carefully in patients with myocardial involvement because of the cardiotoxicity associated with that drug. Whenever possible, the duration of cyclophosphamide therapy should be limited to 3–6 months. The bronchospastic component of this disease rarely responds to glucocorticoid-sparing agents and should be managed with conventional bronchodilators (including leukotriene inhibitors) and, if necessary, glucocorticoids.

▶ Complications

Substantial morbidity and death may result from EGPA. The major sources of morbidity are the disease itself and its therapies. Because the disease begins with a long prodrome of comparatively mundane problems (eg, atopic symptoms and asthma), the diagnosis is often overlooked until significant damage has occurred. The complications of vasculitic neuropathy are particularly devastating in this regard. Crippling nerve dysfunction may occur to varying degrees in all four distal extremities, leading to enormous disabilities. The recovery of function in infarcted nerves generally requires months, and in many cases the return of function is minimal. Recovery is likely dependent partly on the age of the patient and on the severity and extent of nerve damage.

Treatment regimens for EGPA that include prolonged courses of high-dose glucocorticoids and steroid-sparing drugs such as cyclophosphamide or rituximab are associated with a high incidence of adverse effects, some of which may be permanent or fatal. Following the remission of vasculitis, many patients have persistent, glucocorticoid-dependent asthma. The long-term use of even moderately low-dose glucocorticoids brings many unwanted side effects. More dangerous, however, is the intensive immunosuppression associated with the combination of glucocorticoids and cytotoxic agents. Even with careful monitoring, opportunistic infections, myelosuppression, infertility, bladder toxicity, and (in the long term) an increased risk of certain malignancies are all major concerns.

Although clinical remissions may be obtained in more than 90% of patients with EGPA, disease recurrences are common upon cessation of therapy. Flares are estimated to occur in more than 25% of the patients, but this figure is certainly higher if attempts are made to discontinue glucocorticoids completely. In most cases, relapses are heralded by the return of eosinophilia. In an even higher percentage of patients, following the resolution of the vasculitic phase of EGPA, glucocorticoid-dependent asthma remains an issue requiring ongoing management.

Cottin V, Bel E, Bottero P, et al. Revisiting the systemic vasculitis in eosinophilic granulomatosis with polyangiitis (Churg-Strauss): a study of 157 patients by the Groupe d'Etudes et de Recherche sur les Maladies Orphelines Pulmonaires and the European Respiratory Society Taskforce on eosinophilic granulomatosis with polyangiitis (Churg Strauss). *Autoimmun Rev.* 2017;16:1-9. [PMID: 27671089]

Groh M, Pagnoux C, Baldini C, et al. Eosinophilic granulomatosis with polyangiitis (Churg-Strauss) (EGPA) Consensus Task Force recommendations for evaluation and management. *Eur J Med.* 2016;26:545-553. [PMID: 25971154]

Puechal X, Pagnoux C, Baron G, et al. Adding azathioprine to remission-induction glucocorticoids for eosinophilic granulomatosis with polyangiitis, microscopic polyangiitis, or polyarteritis nodosa without poor prognosis factors: a randomized controlled trial. *Arthritis Rheum.* 2017;69(11):2175-2186. [PMID: 28678392]

Wechsler ME, Akuthota P, Jayne D, et al. Mepolizumab or placebo for eosinophilic granulomatosis with polyangiitis. *N Engl J Med.* 2017;376:1921-1932. [PMID: 28514601]

The Cleveland Clinic Foundation Center for Vasculitis. http://www.clevelandclinic.org/arthritis/vasculitis/default.htm

The Johns Hopkins Vasculitis Center. http://www.hopkinsvasculitis.org

Vasculitis Clinical Research Consortium. http://rarediseasesnetwork.epi.usf.edu/vcrc/

Polyarteritis Nodosa

31

Naomi Serling-Boyd, MD

John H. Stone, MD, MPH

ESSENTIALS OF DIAGNOSIS

▶ Subacute onset of constitutional complaints (fever, weight loss, malaise, arthralgias), lower extremity nodules and ulcerations, mononeuritis multiplex, and postprandial pain are hallmarks of polyarteritis nodosa (PAN).

▶ Cutaneous PAN is a variant of the systemic disease in which vasculitis is limited to the skin and often presents with painful nodules, livedo racemosa, or cutaneous ulcerations.

▶ Patients with PAN should be evaluated for hepatitis B, though hepatitis B virus-associated PAN has decreased in incidence and is now only responsible for less than 10% of cases.

▶ Angiography may reveal microaneurysms in the kidneys or gastrointestinal tract.

▶ Biopsies of the skin and peripheral nerves (with sampling of the adjacent muscle) are the least invasive ways of confirming the diagnosis histopathologically.

▶ General Considerations

Classic polyarteritis nodosa (PAN) is characterized by necrotizing inflammation of muscular arterioles and medium-sized arteries that spares the smallest blood vessels (ie, capillaries). PAN is not associated with glomerulonephritis, although it can cause renovascular hypertension and renal infarctions through its involvement of the medium-sized intrarenal vasculature. Features that distinguish PAN from other forms of systemic vasculitis are confinement of the disease to the arterial as opposed to the venous circulation, the sparing of the lung, the absence of granulomatous inflammation, and the lack of any association with a known autoantibody.

Reported annual incidence rates of PAN range from two to nine cases per million people per year. A higher incidence (77 cases/million) was reported in an Alaskan area

hyperendemic for hepatitis B virus (HBV). With the availability of the HBV vaccine, however, the percentage of cases associated with HBV has declined substantially (from previously over one-third of cases to now <10% of all cases in the developed world). PAN appears to affect men and women with approximately equal frequencies and to occur in all ethnic groups.

▶ Clinical Findings

A. Symptoms and Signs

PAN can involve virtually any organ system with the exception of the lungs. The disease demonstrates a predilection for certain organs, particularly the skin, peripheral nerves, gastrointestinal tract, and kidneys. Pain is often a nearly universal complaint among patients and can be caused by myalgias, arthritis, peripheral nerve infarction, testicular ischemia, or mesenteric vasculitis. A summary of the signs and symptoms seem in PAN is shown in Table 31–1.

1. Constitutional symptoms—Fever is a common feature of PAN and is seen in around 60% of patients. The characteristics of the fever vary substantially among patients, ranging from periods of low-grade temperature elevation to spiking febrile episodes accompanied by chills. Patterns of low-grade fever are more common than hectic fevers. Tachycardia with or without fever may be another feature of PAN. Malaise, weight loss, and myalgias are also common.

2. Skin and joints—Vasculitis of medium-size arteries may produce several types of skin lesions. These cutaneous findings include livedo racemosa (Figure 31–1A), nodules (Figure 31–1B), papules, ulcerations (Figure 31–1C), and digital ischemia leading to gangrene. All of these findings or combinations of them may occur in the same patient. Nodules, papules, and ulcers tend to occur on the lower extremities, particularly near the malleoli, in the fleshy parts of the calf, and over the dorsal surfaces of the feet.

Table 31–1. Clinical findings in polyarteritis nodosa.

Clinical Feature	Percent of Patients
General symptoms	**93.1**
Fever	63.8
Weight loss	69.5
Myalgias	58.6
Arthralgias	48.9
Neurologic manifestations	**79.0**
Peripheral neuropathy	74.1
Mononeuritis multiplex	70.7
Central nervous system	4.6
Urologic and renal manifestations	**50.6**
Hematuria	15.2
Proteinuria (>0.4 g/24 h)	21.6
Recent-onset hypertension	34.8
Severe hypertension	6.9
Orchitis or testicular tenderness	17.3
Cutaneous manifestations	**49.7**
Nodules	17.2
Purpura	22.1
Livedo	16.7
Peripheral limb edema	**24.4**
Gastrointestinal manifestations	**37.9**
Abdominal pain	35.6
Bleeding	3.4
Perforation(s)	4.3
Cholecystitis	3.7
Appendicitis	1.1
Pancreatitis	3.7
Gastrointestinal manifestations requiring surgery	13.8
Cardiac and vascular manifestations	**22.4**
Vasculitis-related cardiomyopathy	7.5
Pericarditis	5.5
Digital ischemia (without necrotic lesions)	6.0
Distal necrotic lesions and/or limb arterial	6.3
claudication	**8.6**
Ophthalmologic manifestations	**4.3**
Retinal vasculitis/exudate	
Pulmonary manifestations[a]	**5.7**
Cough	3.4
Lung infiltrates	3.4
Pleural effusions	

[a]Pulmonary manifestations, when seen, are often attributable to cardiac or renal dysfunction.
Data from Pagnoux C, Seror R, Henegar C, et al. Clinical features and outcomes in 348 patients with polyarteritis nodosa. *Arthritis Rheum.* 2010;62(2):616-626.

Nodules can evolve into ulcerations that have scalloped borders and can usually heal with scarring or hyperpigmentation (Figure 31–1D).

Arthralgias of large joints (knees, ankles, elbows, wrists) occur in up to 50% of patients but true synovitis is seen substantially less often.

3. Peripheral nerves—Mononeuritis multiplex, the infarction of named nerves by inflammation in the vasa nervorum, occurs in up to 70% of patients with PAN. The most commonly involved nerves are the sural, peroneal, radial, and ulnar. Vasculitic neuropathy tends to involve the longest nerves first—that is, the distal ones, to the feet or hands—and usually begins asymmetrically. Thus, the first motor symptoms of vasculitic neuropathy may be a foot or wrist drop (resulting from infarctions of the peroneal and radial nerves, respectively). In advanced stages, the neuropathy may mimic a confluent, symmetric polyneuropathy. Careful history taking, however, may unmask its initial asymmetry. Both sensory and motor findings are characteristic of vasculitic neuropathy because with the exception of the sural nerve (a pure sensory nerve), peripheral nerves typically have mixed sensory and motor fibers bundled within the same nerve.

4. Gastrointestinal tract—The gastrointestinal manifestations of PAN occur in approximately half of all patients and are among the most challenging symptoms to diagnose correctly because of their nonspecific nature. Postprandial abdominal pain ("intestinal angina") is common. Involvement of the mesenteric arteries in PAN may lead to mesenteric infarction or aneurysmal rupture, both of which are associated with a high mortality rate. Angiography of the mesenteric vessels reveals multiple microaneurysms (Figure 31–2). These range in size from lesions that are barely visible to the naked eye to several centimeters in diameter.

Sometimes, a medium vessel is detected at cholecystectomy or appendectomy in the absence of other disease manifestations. Such a presentation, now termed "single-organ vasculitis" and may represent a disease entity that is fundamentally different from classic, multiorgan PAN. In single-organ vasclitis, surgical removal of the involved organ may be curative.

5. Intraparenchymal renal inflammation—This major feature of PAN is found in 40% of patients. The inflammatory process targets the renal and interlobar arteries (the medium-sized, muscular arteries within the kidney) and occasionally also involves the smaller arcuate and interlobular arteries. Angiography may reveal microaneurysms within the kidney or large, wedge-shaped renal infarctions (Figure 31–3). Renal artery involvement or involvement of intra-renal arterioles in PAN may lead to renin-mediated hypertension; recent onset hypertension is seen in around one-third of patients. Proteinuria and hematuria are uncommonly observed in PAN but can be seen. However, the presence of red blood cell casts on urinalysis implies glomerulonephritis and thus usually implicates another disease (eg, microscopic polyangiitis or granulomatosis with polyangiitis).

6. Cardiac symptoms—Tachycardia may reflect either direct cardiac involvement or a general inflammatory state. Congestive heart failure and myocardial infarction sometimes occur. Although specific heart lesions are rarely diagnosed while the patient is alive, autopsy series indicate that cardiac involvement is present in a majority of patients with PAN. Patchy necrosis of the myocardium caused by subclinical arteriolar involvement is a common finding at autopsy.

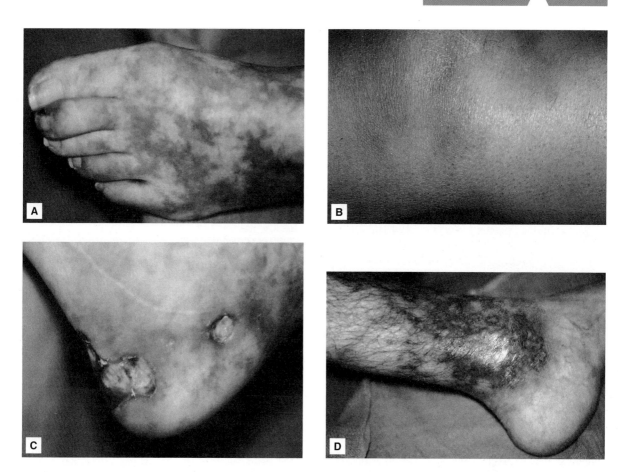

▲ **Figure 31–1.** Skin lesions caused by the medium-vessel vasculitis of polyarteritis nodosa. **A:** Livedo racemosa. **B:** Nodules. **C:** Ulcerations. **D:** Ulcerations that have healed with scarring and hyperpigmentation.

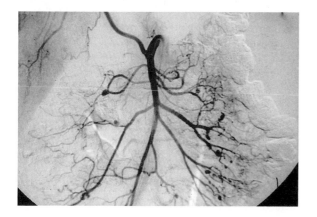

▲ **Figure 31–2.** Mesenteric angiogram showing multiple microaneurysms which are characteristic of polyarteritis nodosa. (Reproduced, with permission, from Stone JH. Vasculitis: a collection of pearls and myths. *Rheum Dis Clin North Am.* 2007;33(4):691–739.)

7. Miscellaneous—Central nervous system involvement occurs in a small percentage of patients with PAN. The usual presentations are encephalopathy and strokes. Renin-mediated hypertension may contribute to both of these neurologic complications. Other unusual presentations of PAN include involvement of the eyes (retinal vasculitis or scleritis), pancreatitis, orchitis, and pericarditis, among others. Patients with hepatitis B-related PAN appear to have more frequent peripheral neuropathy, gastrointestinal complications, orchitis, and hypertension compared with idiopathic PAN, but rigorous comparisons of these two PAN populations have been difficult to perform.

B. Laboratory Findings

Although the laboratory features of PAN are often strikingly abnormal and help characterize the disease process as inflammatory, they do not distinguish PAN from a host of other inflammatory diseases. Anemia, thrombocytosis, and elevation of acute phase reactants are typical. The erythrocyte

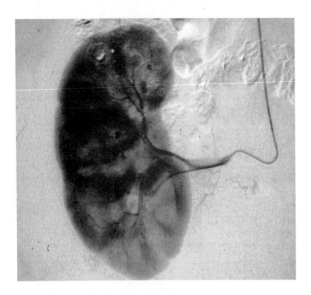

▲ **Figure 31–3.** Renal arteriogram demonstrating microaneurysms within the kidney.

sedimentation rate and C-reactive protein are often useful in longitudinal evaluations of disease activity.

One of the diagnostic challenges in PAN is the fact that the disorder is not associated with any of the autoantibodies found in other immune-mediated conditions. Assays for antinuclear antibodies and rheumatoid factor are generally negative in patients with PAN, albeit low titers of these antibodies are detected in a minority. Patients with HBV-associated PAN are generally hypocomplementemic, regardless of whether they have demonstrable cryoglobulins. When associated with HBV, PAN often develops within weeks to months of the acute viral infection but temporal relationships between HBV activity and the occurrence of PAN are not understood entirely.

Specific enzyme immunoassays for antineutrophil cytoplasmic antibodies (ANCAs) directed against proteinase-3 or myeloperoxidase, the two antigens known to be associated with systemic vasculitis, are negative. Thus, PAN is not considered to be a form of ANCA-associated vasculitis.

C. Special Tests

The diagnosis of PAN requires either a tissue biopsy or an angiogram that demonstrates microaneurysms.

1. Biopsy—In the skin, medium-sized arteries lie within the deep dermis and in the subdermal adipose tissue. Thus, the diagnosis of PAN can be made by obtaining biopsy specimens of the skin that capture lobules of subcutaneous fat (Figure 31–4A). Biopsies of nodules, papules, and the edges of ulcers have higher yields than biopsies of livedo racemosa.

PAN is a panarteritis characterized by transmural necrosis and a homogeneous, eosinophilic appearance of the blood

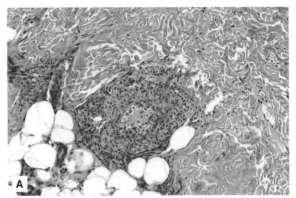

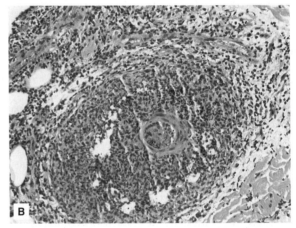

▲ **Figure 31–4.** The diagnosis of PAN can be made by obtaining biopsy specimens of the skin that capture lobules of subcutaneous fat. Biopsies of nodules, papules, and the edges of ulcers have higher yields than biopsies of livedo racemosa. **A:** Deep punch biopsy revealing a medium-sized artery with transmural inflammation and fibrinoid necrosis in the blood vessel wall. **B:** Deep punch biopsy demonstrating transmural inflammation with an intense mononuclear cell infiltrate in a medium-sized muscular artery. (See color insert.)

vessel wall (fibrinoid necrosis [Figure 31–4B]). The cellular infiltrate is pleomorphic, with both polymorphonuclear cells and lymphocytes present in varying degrees at different stages. Degranulation of neutrophils within and around the arterial wall leads to leukocytoclasis. During later stages, complete occlusion may occur secondary to endothelial proliferation and thrombosis. Throughout involved tissues, the coexistence of acute and healed lesions is typical.

2. Nerve conduction studies—Nerve conduction studies are useful in detecting the typical axonal pattern of nerve injury and identifying involved nerves for biopsy. Because muscle tissue is highly vascular and may harbor involved vessels affected by vasculitis even in the absence of symptoms or signs of muscle involvement, biopsies of adjacent muscle should be performed simultaneously. The gastrocnemius muscle and sural nerve are often biopsied together. Blind biopsies of asymptomatic organs such as the testicle, however, are rarely diagnostic.

3. Angiography—The vascular wall inflammation in PAN may be strikingly segmental, affecting only part of the circumference of a given artery (Figure 31–5). Segmental necrosis, in turn, leads to aneurysm formation. Lesions known as microaneurysms can occur throughout the mesenteric and renal vasculature. Even in patients without gastrointestinal symptoms, mesenteric angiography may demonstrate telltale microaneurysms.

Conventional, catheter-based angiography generally has a higher resolution than computed tomography or magnetic resonance angiograms and remains the gold standard approach to the detection of microaneurysms. The interpretation of angiograms requires experience. Alternating areas of vascular narrowing and dilatation can be caused by a variety of nonvasculitic processes, including (most commonly) vasospasm. The finding of true microaneurysms, however, is diagnostic of PAN in the proper setting.

▶ Differential Diagnosis

Even when flagrant signs of inflammation are present, PAN may elude diagnosis for weeks or months. Except for evidence obtained from angiography or biopsy, the disease has no individual features that are pathognomonic. Many connective tissue diseases must be considered in the differential diagnosis of PAN (Table 31–2). However, systemic lupus erythematosus, mixed connective tissue disease, and undifferentiated

Table 31–2. Differential diagnosis of polyarteritis nodosa.

Systemic disorders associated with autoimmunity
Systemic lupus erythematosus
Mixed connective tissue disease
Catastrophic antiphospholipid antibody syndrome
Rheumatoid arthritis (with rheumatoid vasculitis)
Still disease
Systemic vasculitides
Granulomatosis with polyangiitis (formerly Wegener granulomatosis)
Microscopic polyangiitis
Eosinophilic granulomatosis with polyangiitis (Churg-Strauss syndrome)
Cryoglobulinemia
Isolated vasculitis of peripheral nerves
Infections
Endocarditis
Deep fungal infections (histoplasmosis, coccidioidomycosis, blastomycosis)
Miscellaneous
Inflammatory bowel disease
Sarcoidosis
Erythema nodosum
Atrophie blanche
Cholesterol emboli
Fibromuscular dysplasia
Lymphoma

connective tissue disorders usually can be distinguished from PAN by the presence of specific autoantibodies (eg, anti-Ro/SS-A, anti-La/SS-B, anti-Sm, anti-RNP). These are absent in PAN. Less specific autoantibodies, such as antinuclear antibodies and rheumatoid factor, are often present in PAN but are nondiagnostic because of their poor specificities.

In its early phases, rheumatoid arthritis may mimic PAN, but the arthritis of PAN is usually migratory and always nondestructive. Rheumatoid vasculitis, which has features very similar to PAN, almost always occurs in patients with severe, long-standing, destructive joint disease, not simultaneously with or before the onset of arthritis. Similarly, although the fever pattern of PAN can be similar to that seen in adult-onset Still disease (AOSD), the evanescent, salmon-colored rash of AOSD does not occur in PAN. Moreover, diffuse polyarthritis develops in 95% of patients with AOSD within 1 year (or earlier) of disease onset. The catastrophic antiphospholipid syndrome, which causes digital ischemia, strokes, and other arterial thrombotic events, may be confused with PAN. However, venous events, which are even more common than arterial events in most patients with the antiphospholipid syndrome, are not characteristic of PAN.

The lack of pulmonary involvement in PAN helps distinguish it from most cases of ANCA-associated vasculitis. The occurrence of pulmonary lesions (pulmonary nodules, cavities, infiltrates, or alveolar hemorrhage) in combination with systemic vasculitis shifts the differential diagnosis in favor of

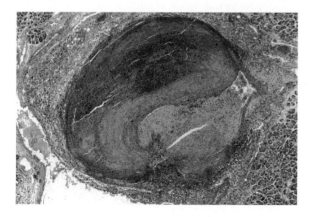

▲ **Figure 31–5.** The vascular wall inflammation in PAN may be strikingly segmental, affecting only part of the circumference of a given artery. In this case, segmental wall involvement has led to an aneurysm of this medium-sized muscular artery.

other vasculitides, such as granulomatosis with polyangiitis, microscopic polyangiitis, and eosinophilic granulomatosis with polyangiitis. Pulmonary findings, such as pleural effusions or parenchymal infiltrates, may be seen but are most often attributable to volume overload in the setting of cardiac or renal dysfunction. In addition, features of small-vessel disease (eg, purpura) are generally absent in PAN. Isolated peripheral nervous system vasculitis, a form of vasculitis that involves the peripheral nervous system alone, may mimic PAN and require similar therapy. In addition, in a subset of cases, the predominant features of PAN imitate the presentation of giant cell arteritis (eg, headache, jaw claudication, fever, and polymyalgias). Findings of histopathologic features of PAN on temporal artery biopsy specimens have been reported. Fibrinoid necrosis is rare in giant cell arteritis, but highly typical of PAN as well as certain other vasculitides.

The multiorgan system inflammatory nature of PAN may be mimicked by numerous bacterial, mycobacterial, or fungal infections. These must be excluded with great caution before beginning a treatment course for vasculitis. Finally, a host of other systemic or single-organ diseases may mimic PAN in their individual organ features. These include inflammatory bowel disease, sarcoidosis, erythema nodosum, cholesterol emboli, fibromuscular dysplasia, and malignancies (particularly lymphoma). PAN may occur as a complication of hairy cell leukemia.

Livedoid vasculopathy is a thrombotic process that involves small blood vessels in the skin. It may cause skin lesions that are very difficult to distinguish from those of PAN on the basis of clinical findings alone. Nodules and particularly ulcers involving the lower extremities are typical of livedoid vasculopathy. Skin biopsy is required to distinguish PAN from livedoid vasculopathy. The distinction is critical because treatment approaches to these two disorders are divergent: immunosuppression or antiviral therapy in PAN, as opposed to anticoagulation in livedoid vasculopathy.

Treatment

Treatment of HBV-associated PAN with immunosuppressive agents has deleterious long-term effects on the liver because prolonged immunosuppression promotes further viral replication. Fortunately, the availability of effective antiviral agents has revolutionized the treatment of HBV-associated cases in recent years. One effective strategy involves the initial use of prednisone (1 mg/kg/day) to suppress the inflammation. Patients begin 6-week courses of plasma exchange (approximately three exchanges per week) simultaneously with the start of prednisone. The doses of glucocorticoids are tapered rapidly (over approximately 2 weeks), and antiviral therapy (eg, lamivudine 100 mg/day or entecavir 0.5–1.0 mg/day) is initiated. Treatment with antiviral agents alone is now recommended in cases of hepatitis B-associated PAN with only mild clinical manifestations. Between 90% and 100% of patients with achieve

prolonged vasculitis control with this regimen. Another goal of treatment is to achieve a virological response, which is defined by seroconversion of the HBe antigen to the HBe antibody. This is achieved in roughly half of all PAN patients treated with this regimen.

In patients with idiopathic PAN, glucocorticoids remain the cornerstone of treatment. Approximately half of patients with PAN achieve remissions or cures with high doses of glucocorticoids alone, and this treatment approach can especially be considered for patients who lack poor prognostic factors (see five-factor score in Figure 31–3) and have more mild disease. The increasing availability of biologic agents with potential activity in PAN has had important treatment implications in recent years for both glucocorticoid-sparing and avoiding the use of cyclophosphamide. For example, tumor necrosis factor (TNF) inhibitors such as adalimumab may be particularly helpful in cases of cutaneous PAN, diminishing the length of time that patients need to be on high glucocorticoid doses and reducing the total glucocorticoid course. There are also series of cases that have successfully responded to tocilizumab. The choice of biologic agent can be difficult in PAN given that vasculitis has been described as a complication of TNF inhibitors, though was a case series of 26 patients with idiopathic PAN who had had persistent disease despite glucocorticoid treatment, and 89% achieved significant improvement after 4 months of treatment with infliximab. For patients with classic PAN involving internal organs, rituximab might be considered before cyclophosphamide in view of its side-effect profile that is preferable to that of cyclophosphamide. Some consider the addition of azathioprine or methotrexate for maintenance therapy after remission induction; a randomized controlled trial did not find any benefit of adding azathioprine to glucocorticoids for induction of remission.

Cyclophosphamide (eg, 2 mg/kg/day orally or 0.6 g/m^2/mo intravenously, decreased in the setting of renal dysfunction) is indicated for patients whose disease is refractory to glucocorticoids or the combination of glucocorticoids and rituximab or who have disease involvement posing an immediate threat to the function of major organs, for example, serious mesenteric ischemia or rapidly progressive vasculitic neuropathy. Prophylaxis against *Pneumocystis jiroveci* pneumonia is an important consideration in patients treated with these medications.

Cutaneous PAN generally does not progress to systemic disease, and its treatment is approached differently than treatment of systemic PAN. Initial treatment of cutaneous PAN often consists of nonsteroidal anti-inflammatory drugs, salicylate, or colchicine. Dapsone, glucocorticoids, and other immunosuppressive medications are reserved for recurrent or refractory cases.

Complications

Advanced mononeuritis multiplex can be a severely disabling problem from which recuperation is measured in months or years, if at all. Residual nerve dysfunction in the form of muscle weakness or painful neuropathy is common. The patient's ultimate degree of recovery is difficult to predict. The occurrence of bowel perforation and rupture of a mesenteric microaneurysm are potentially catastrophic events in PAN, requiring emergency surgical intervention and associated with high mortality rates. Patients treated with levels of immunosuppression required for PAN are at substantial risk for opportunistic infection and other complications of treatment. Fever in a patient receiving or recently treated with high doses of glucocorticoids, cyclophosphamide, or other medications employed in the therapy of PAN should be considered to represent an infection until proven otherwise and managed accordingly.

▶ **Prognosis**

In contrast to the ANCA-associated vasculitides, which are more prone to recurrences, PAN is generally more often a monophasic illness. For patients with HBV-associated PAN, seroconversion to anti-HBe antigen antibody usually signals the end of the active phase of vasculitis. Among patients with idiopathic PAN, disease recurrences are seen in up to 30% of cases. The French Vasculitis Study Group identified five factors (termed the FFS) that are significantly associated with a poor outcome and higher mortality. These include elevated serum creatinine (>1.58 mg/dL), proteinuria (>1 g/day), severe gastrointestinal involvement, cardiomyopathy, and central nervous system involvement. If none of these factors are present, the five-year mortality rate was found to be 11.9% compared to 25.9% if one factor is present and 46% if 2 or more are present. In 2009, the revised five-factor score was developed and included age >65, cardiac insufficiency, renal insufficiency, and gastrointestinal involvement as risk factors, and the absence of ear, nose, or throat manifestations as a protective factor (with the last factor applying only to patients with granulomatosis with polyangiitis or eosinophilic granulomatosis with polyangiitis) (Table 31–3). New-onset hypertension is another risk factor for poor prognosis.

Table 31–3. Five-factor score and modified five-factor score.

Five-factor score (FFS) (1996)	Proteinuria >1g/day Renal insufficiency (>1.58 mg/dL) Cardiomyopathy Severe gastrointestinal manifestations Central nervous system involvement
Revised five-factor score (2009)	Age >65 Cardiac insufficiency Renal insufficiency Gastrointestinal involvement Absence of ENT manifestations (only pertains to GPA or eGPA)

GPA, granulomatosis with polyangiitis;
eGPA, eosinophilic granulomatosis with polyangiitis

De Virgilio A, Greco A, Magliuo G, et al. Polyarteritis nodosa: a contemporary overview. *Autoimmun Rev.* 2016;15(6):564-570. [PMID: 26884100]

Forbess L, Bannykh S. Polyarteritis nodosa. *Rheum Dis Clin N Am.* 2015;41:33-46. [PMID: 25399938]

Ginsberg S, Rosner I, Slobodin G, et al. Infliximab for the treatment of refractory polyarteritis nodosa. *Clin Rheumatol.* 2019;38(10):2825-2833. [PMID: 30972576]

Puechal X, Pagnoux C, Baron G, et al. Adding azathioprine to remission-induction glucocorticoids for eosinophilic granulomatosis with polyangiitis (Churg-Strauss), microscopic polyangiitis, or polyarteritis nodosa without poor prognosis factors: a randomized, controlled trial. *Arthritis Rheum.* 2017;69(11):2175-2186. [PMID: 28678392]

Saunier A, Issa N, Vanderhende MA, et al. Treatment of polyarteritis nodosa with tocilizumab: a new therapeutic approach? *RMD Open.* 2017;3(1). [PMID: 28879047]

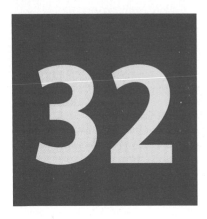

Cryoglobulinemia

Naomi Serling-Boyd, MD

John H. Stone, MD, MPH

ESSENTIALS OF DIAGNOSIS

▶ Vasculitis associated with mixed cryoglobulinemia (MC) involves both small- and medium-sized vessels. The skin is the most commonly involved organ.

▶ Other frequently affected organs include the joints, peripheral nerves, and kidneys. The central nervous system, gastrointestinal tract, and lungs are involved rarely or very rarely in MC.

▶ Virtually all patients are rheumatoid factor (RF) positive.

▶ Many cases of type II cryoglobulinemia are still associated with hepatitis C virus.

▶ Lower survival rates are observed with age over 60 years, male sex, and renal involvement.

General Considerations

Cryoglobulins are immunoglobulins (Ig) that precipitate from the serum at low temperatures (see method of collection under Laboratory Findings). Cryoprecipitates are composed most commonly of IgG and IgM (either singly or, in the case of mixed cryoglobulinemia, together). Occasionally IgA may be associated with clinically relevant cryoglobulin syndromes, as well. **Cryoglobulinemia** is divided into three clinical subsets—types I, II, and III (Table 32–1)—based on two features: the clonality of the IgM component and the presence of rheumatoid factor (RF) activity. RF activity, by definition, is the reactivity of an IgM component with the Fc portion of IgG. This chapter focuses on cryoglobulinemia types II and III, both of which are referred to as "mixed cryoglobulinemia" (MC). Type I cryoglobulinemia is usually not "mixed" and is associated with only a monoclonal IgG or IgM, often in the setting of a malignancy. Overall, cryoglobulinemia is rare, with a prevalence of roughly 1 in 100,000 people, and with a female to male ratio of 3:1.

Formerly referred to as "essential" MC, hepatitis C virus (HCV) infections are now known to be associated with approximately 90% of all cases of MC. Latency periods of up to 15 years between the occurrence of HCV infection and the development of clinical signs of MC have been reported. In some cases, the presentation of HCV may be the development of the clinical features of MC (usually palpable purpura). Cryoglobulins also occur in the setting of other types of infections such as HIV as well as in connective tissue disorders (eg, Sjögren syndrome) and hematopoietic malignancies.

The presence of cryoglobulins is not always associated with clinical disease, but these proteins may result in a wide variety of immune complex–mediated complications. The term "mixed cryoglobulinemia" was coined to differentiate types II and III (both of which contain mixtures of both IgG and IgM) from type I (which contains only a single monoclonal antibody).

When an underlying infection, autoimmune disorder, or malignancy can be identified, the preferred treatment approach is to direct therapy toward the underlying condition. B-cell depletion strategies are often coupled with antiviral therapies in patients with HCV-associated cryoglobulinemia. Occasionally, in patients with rampant systemic vasculitis, generalized immunosuppression or measures designed to remove immune complexes (ie, plasma exchange) may be required for limited periods.

Clinical Findings

The symptoms and signs of MC-associated vasculitis are caused by cryoglobulin precipitation in the microcirculation and immune complex–mediated vascular inflammation. In type II MC, the cryoprecipitate contains polyclonal IgG, a highly restricted monoclonal IgM that has RF activity, low-density lipoprotein, and, in cases of HCV-associated disease, HCV RNA. In general, the diagnosis of MC is made by some combination of the following: (1) recognition of a compatible

Table 32–1. Types of cryoglobulinemia.

Subtype	Rheumatoid Factor Positivity	Monoclonality	Associated Diseases
Type I	No	Yes (IgG or IgM)	Hematopoietic malignancy (multiple myeloma, Waldenström macroglobulinemia)
Type II	Yes	Yes (polyclonal IgG)	Hepatitis C (other infection, Sjögren syndrome, monoclonal IgM, systemic lupus erythematosus [SLE])
Type III	Yes	No (polyclonal IgG and IgM)	Hepatitis C (other infection, Sjögren syndrome, SLE)

clinical syndrome, accompanied nearly invariably by cutaneous vasculitis of small blood vessels; (2) isolation of cryoglobulins from serum; (3) detection of antibodies to HCV or HCV RNA; and (4) biopsy of other apparently involved organs as necessary to exclude other diagnoses. Because assays for cryoglobulins are not 100% sensitive and because HCV does not cause all cases of MC, all four of these conditions are not required.

A. Symptoms and Signs

1. Skin—A major hallmark of MC is a small-vessel vasculitis of the skin. Medium-vessel vasculitis may also be present, but this type of involvement generally does not occur without small-vessel disease. Biopsy of the skin with immunofluorescence studies shows an immune complex–mediated leukocytoclastic vasculitis, with deposition of IgG, IgM, C3, and other immunoreactants in and around the walls of small- and medium-sized vessels. Vascular thrombi are also prominent in many cases. The most typical cutaneous finding is palpable purpura, which has a predilection for the lower extremities, but can also be found sometimes on the upper extremities, trunk, or buttocks. Isolated purpura is associated with a good prognosis and more benign disease course. Meltzer's triad, a classic presentation of cryoglobulinemia, refers to purpura, arthralgias, and weakness. These features are present in up to 80% of patients at the time of presentation. An example of palpable purpura and cutaneous vasculitis of the lower extremities is shown in Figure 32–1. In addition, a host of other types of vasculitic rashes may be encountered, depending on the size of blood vessel involved. Such findings may include macules, papules, vesiculobullous lesions, urticarial lesions in the setting of small-vessel involvement, and cutaneous ulcers in the context of medium-vessel disease, which are associated with a worse prognosis. Digital necrosis, more common in type I cryoglobulinemia than in types II or III, is shown in Figure 32–2.

2. Rheumatologic—Arthralgias are a prominent symptom in most cases of MC. The typically involved joints are the proximal interphalangeal and metacarpophalangeal joints and the knees. Frank arthritis, much less common than arthralgias, occurs in a small minority of patients. The arthritis of MC is nondeforming. Raynaud phenomenon and acrocyanosis may also complicate MC.

3. Peripheral nerve—In the peripheral neuropathy of MC, seen in between 20% and 60% of patients, sensory involvement manifested by paresthesias predominates over motor nerve disease. The typical presentation is an axonal sensory neuropathy, associated with pain and paresthesias for years before the development of motor deficits. Motor mononeuritis multiplex may also occur, but never in the absence of sensory symptoms, and polyneuropathy is more common. HCV-induced vasculitis of the vasa nervorum is the pathogenetic mechanism of this peripheral nerve dysfunction. Neuropathic symptoms take far longer than others to resolve and should not necessarily be considered to be relapsed or refractory disease in the absence of other signs of active disease.

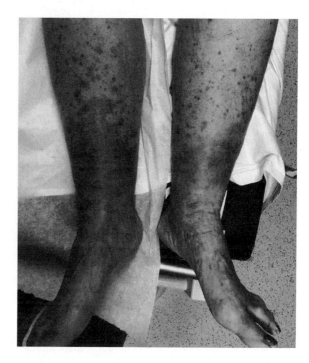

▲ **Figure 32–1.** Small-vessel vasculitis in a patient with mixed cryoglobulinemia. Palpable purpura, a feature of small-vessel vasculitis, is seen predominantly involving the lower extremities. (See color insert.)

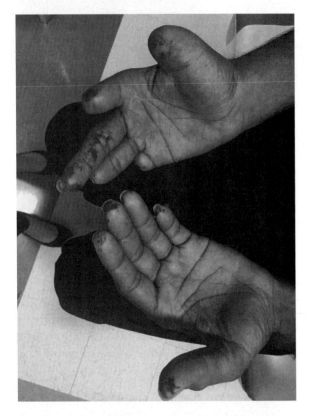

▲ **Figure 32–2.** Digital necrosis and evidence of past autoamputation of multiple fingertips in a patient with essential cryoglobulinemia.

4. Kidney—Renal involvement is present in up to 20% of patients at diagnosis and around 30% of patients at some point during the disease course. The most frequent manifestations are asymptomatic microscopic hematuria, proteinuria, and variable degree of renal insufficiency. A small proportion may present as acute nephrotic syndrome and acute nephritic syndrome. The most frequent histologic picture seen in around 70% of patients is membranoproliferative glomerulonephritis, which can mimic lupus nephritis. Three specific histologic findings serve to distinguish glomerulonephritis secondary to MC: intraluminal thrombi composed of precipitated cryoglobulins, diffuse IgM deposition in the capillary loops, and subendothelial deposits presenting a crystalloid aspect on electron microscopy. MC-related renal disease may lead to nephrotic-range proteinuria, but progression to end-stage renal disease is uncommon. Rapidly progressive glomerulonephritis occurs in only a small number of patients.

5. Liver—Although HCV is obviously a hepatotropic virus, the clinical manifestations of liver disease in MC are few. Moreover, correlations between clinical liver disease and

histology are poor. Most patients with HCV-related MC have various degrees of periportal inflammation, fibrosis, and even cirrhosis on liver biopsy. The formation of lymphoid follicles in the liver is a characteristic histologic feature of chronic HCV infection. Within these follicles (and in the bone marrow), most of the IgM RF is formed. Immunophenotyping of mononuclear cells within liver biopsy specimens from patients with HCV-associated MC reveals that they are mostly B cells that express IgM.

6. Hematopoietic system—In addition to its hepatotropism, HCV also tends to infect lymphocytes. Cryoglobulins arise from a clonal expansion of B cells, and whether the expansion is polyclonal or monoclonal affects the type of cryoglobulins produced. In some cases, the emergence of a dominant B-cell clone results from a genetic alteration that favors B-cell survival, for example, a *bcl-2* gene mutation (translocation of the *bcl-2* gene from chromosome 18 to chromosome 14). Such a mutation leads to overexpression of the antiapoptotic *bcl-2*. B-cell lymphoma is the most common malignancy complicating MC. Hepatocellular carcinoma is also found with an increased incidence among patients with MC, almost certainly related to the effects of underlying viral hepatitis infections in most cases.

7. Central nervous system (CNS)—CNS disease in MC usually results from hyperviscosity and symptoms secondary to "sludging" of blood within the brain and can be limited to altered mental status or confusion in these cases. A careful fundoscopic examination should be performed if this is suspected. Hyperviscosity, a rare complication of types II or III MC, is more common in type I cryoglobulinemia, a condition in which the cryoglobulin levels are often due to underlying malignancy and are substantially higher. The occurrence of a hyperviscosity syndrome is an indication for plasma exchange. Otherwise, CNS involvement is generally seen in less than 5% of patients with cryoglobulinemia and can be difficult to confirm; the most common clinical presentation is small strokes, or small white matter lesions that raise concern for CNS vasculitis, which occurs in a very small number of patients with MC.

8. Gastrointestinal tract—Clinically evident gastrointestinal tract involvement is uncommon, but patients with MC present occasionally with acute abdomen, with perforation and shock. Acute cholecystitis and mesenteric vasculitis secondary to MC have both been reported.

9. Miscellaneous organ involvement in MC—Pulmonary disease, consisting chiefly of interstitial lung lesions, has been described in MC. This manifestation remains poorly understood; cases are usually mild or even asymptomatic. Dryness of the mouth and eyes caused by lymphocytic salivary gland infiltration is not uncommon in MC. This type of organ involvement occurs in the absence of specific serologic evidence of Sjögren syndrome, that is, the finding of anti-Ro/SS-A or anti-La/SS-B antibodies. Bilateral parotid swelling, lymphadenopathy, and Raynaud phenomenon have also been described.

B. Laboratory Findings

MC is associated with a number of laboratory findings that offer clues to the diagnosis. These tests are of limited value in the assessment of disease activity, however, because in general their levels correlate very poorly with disease activity and relapse of vasculitis. An overview of laboratory test results is shown in Table 32–2.

1. Cryoglobulins—Assays for cryoglobulins are associated with a high false-negative rate, caused principally by insufficient care in handling. After phlebotomy, the blood sample must be transported to the laboratory at 37°C and allowed to clot at that same temperature. Specimens are then centrifuged at 37°C and stored at 4°C for up to 1 week. The presence of cryoglobulins is indicated by the development of a white precipitate at the bottom of the tube.

Table 32–2. Laboratory and radiologic evaluation in possible mixed cryoglobulinemia.

Test	Typical Results
Complete blood cell count	Mild anemia common. Thrombocytopenia may be present if liver disease is advanced.
Renal and hepatic function	Renal function may be impaired in patients with glomerulonephritis. Hepatic dysfunction often subclinical but evident in most cases on liver biopsy. Liver transaminases may be normal.
Urinalysis with microscopy	Abnormal in cases with renal involvement. Proteinuria may reach nephrotic range.
Erythrocyte sedimentation rate/C-reactive protein	Moderate to severe elevations common, generally reflecting disease activity when very high.
ANA	Positive in the majority of cases.
Rheumatoid factor	Positive in types II and III.
C3, C4	Low, particularly C4 levels.
ANCA	Negative.
Hepatitis B and C serologies	Hepatitis C serologies positive in approximately 90% of patients.
Antiphospholipid antibodies	Negative rapid plasma reagin and anticardiolipin antibody assays. Normal Russell viper venom time (for lupus anticoagulant).
Blood cultures	Negative.

ANA, antinuclear antibody; ANCA, antineutrophil cytoplasmic antibody.

2. Cryocrit—The percentage of serum composed of cryoglobulins may be determined by the centrifugation of serum at 4°C. The **cryocrit** may then be measured by measuring the amount of cryoglobulins compared to the total protein concentration within the cryoprecipitate. As with other laboratory indicators, the cryocrit correlates poorly with clinical status and treatment. Cryocrit levels should not dictate therapeutic decisions, which are driven more appropriately by patients' clinical condition.

3. Hypocomplementemia—Because complement proteins are involved in the formation of immune complexes, C3 and C1q are often found on specific immunofluorescence testing of biopsy specimens. Serum complement levels—C3, C4, and CH50—are also low in MC. The finding of a very low serum C4 level in the setting of a normal or only moderately reduced level of C3 is a strong clue to the presence of MC.

4. Rheumatoid factor positivity—Eighty percent of the monoclonal IgMs found in HCV-associated MC share a major complementarity region termed "WA." ("WA" refers to the initials of the patient in whom it was initially reported.) This cross idiotype has a high degree of RF activity. Virtually all patients with type II MC are RF positive.

5. Anti-HCV antibodies and quantification of HCV RNA—Anti-HCV assays are typically performed by enzyme immunoassay or immunoblotting. HCV antibodies as well as serum HCV RNA should be evaluated in all patients in whom cryoglobulinemia is suspected. Levels of HCV RNA may be used to follow the treatment response to specific antiviral therapies. HCV genotyping may also be performed by polymerase chain reaction, but no specific viral genotype has been associated with a predisposition to the development of MC.

▶ Differential Diagnosis

MC develops in up to one-third of patients with Sjögren syndrome, but manifestations of vasculitis are present in only a small subset of these patients. Clinical and laboratory features of MC and Sjögren syndrome also overlap. In both disorders, patients may have sicca symptoms of the eyes and mouth and have RF, antinuclear antibodies (ANAs), and hypocomplementemia. In general, patients with MC not associated with Sjögren syndrome do not have antibodies to the Ro- and La-antigens.

Patients with systemic lupus erythematosus (SLE) and patients with MC share tendencies for ANA positivity and hypocomplementemia, as well as the clinical features of Raynaud phenomenon, joint complaints, and an immune complex–mediated glomerulonephritis. The two disorders are usually distinguishable through the presence of other clinical and laboratory features (eg, specific antibody testing for antibodies to double-stranded DNA or precipitins). Some patients with SLE have positive test results for cryoglobulins, but the attribution of disease to these proteins in the setting of SLE is often difficult. Small-vessel vasculitis is a key clinical feature in cryoglobulinemia that should raise the suspicion for this condition.

RF positivity and joint complaints among patients with MC often lead to the misdiagnosis of rheumatoid arthritis. True synovitis in MC is the exception, however, and when MC is associated with arthritis the joint disease is nondestructive. Anti-cyclic citrullinated peptide antibody should be negative in cryoglobulinemia.

Other forms of systemic vasculitis must also be distinguished from MC. There may be considerable overlap in the clinical features of polyarteritis nodosa (see Chapter 31), microscopic polyangiitis (see Chapter 29), granulomatosis with polyangiitis (formerly Wegener granulomatosis) (see Chapter 28), and Henoch-Schönlein purpura (see Chapter 35). The reader is referred to these specific chapters for further details.

▶ Treatment

Although certain laboratory tests (see above) are useful in making the diagnosis, there remain no laboratory values—apart from acute phase reactants such as the erythrocyte sedimentation rate and C-reactive protein levels—that are generally reliable in attempts to ascertain levels of disease activity. As a rule, treatment decisions must be based on the presence of other clinical manifestations of the disease and on the determination by the physician that the symptoms or signs are the result of active disease rather than damage.

MC is characterized by periods of remission and exacerbation. There is also a wide range of disease severity, from mild purpura to severe necrotizing vasculitis. Consequently, all treatment decisions must be individualized, based on the patient's particular circumstances, considerations of organs at risk, and the potential for adverse effects of therapy. The tendency for cutaneous vasculitis to develop in dependent areas may be exacerbated by venous stasis. Support stockings may reduce the number of cutaneous vasculitis flares. Overall, the treatment of cryoglobulinemia has a multipronged approach and consists of treatment of the underlying cause, if applicable; the administration of glucocorticoids to diminish inflammation and reduce tissue injury quickly; targeting circulating B cells to reduce further production of cryoglobulins; and, in severe or organ threatening disease, the addition of plasma exchange.

Under ideal circumstances, the treatment of MC is based on the identification and treatment of the underlying cause, such as a viral infection. In cases of HCV-associated MC, treatment previously involved interferon-based regimens. Sustained response rates to interferon-α are poor (15–20%) but were improved by the addition of ribavirin as well as the discovery of pegylated preparations of interferon-α. Patients treated with pegylated interferon-α and ribavirin achieve responses in up to 60% of cases, but additional therapy is still required in some patients, and there have been concerns regarding the contribution of interferon to disease flares and development of autoimmunity. Studies have recently evaluated the addition of a protease inhibitor such as telaprevir or boceprevir to the pegylated interferon and ribavirin, with improved results. Even more recently, interferon-free regimens have started to become the standard of care. In the VASCUVALDIC study, sofosbuvir and ribavirin were studied as treatment in a cohort of patients with HCV-associated MC, and 87.5% had a complete clinical response at week 24 and a lower risk of serious adverse events compared with data from interferon-based regimens.

Antiviral strategies are commonly combined with B-cell depletion approaches. The typical combination regimen involves the addition of rituximab (1 g intravenously at weeks zero and two) to the full complement of anti-HCV therapies. The combination of B-cell depletion and antiviral regimens are synergistic in the treatment of HCV-associated MC. Intervention with interleukin-2 also appears to be a promising treatment strategy and works by increasing circulating T regulatory cells, which help with viral clearance. TNF inhibitors are not recommended as treatment, and worsening vasculitis has been reported after their use.

For patients with truly "essential" MC, that is, MC not associated with a primary cause such as HCV, B-cell depletion with rituximab alone may be effective. In severe cases with organ threatening manifestations, plasma exchange may be considered to remove circulating cryoglobulins, though this is not commonly used, and does not prevent the new formation of cryoglobulins. In patients with hepatitis B-associated cryoglobulinemia, entecavir is favored as first-line treatment, and is not associated with any risk of flare of cryoglobulinemia.

▶ Complications

Postinflammatory hyperpigmentation over the involved areas of skin often develops in patients with long-standing, recurrent cutaneous vasculitis. Cutaneous ulcers may heal with scarring. End-stage renal disease results in a small number of patients with glomerulonephritis, particularly those who are not treated adequately. Vasculitic neuropathy may lead to permanent sensory or motor neurologic sequelae. In 10% or less of type II MC cases, the disease evolves into a malignant B-cell lymphoma. The portion of HCV-related non-Hodgkin lymphomas ranges widely in different studies, from 0% to 40%. Low-grade B-cell lymphomas may regress with effective treatment of the underlying HCV infection (ie, interferon), but high-grade malignancies require chemotherapy.

De Vita S, Quartuccio L, Isola M, et al. A randomized, controlled trial of rituximab for treatment of severe cryoglobulinemic vasculitis. *Arthritis Rheum.* 2012;64:843. [PMID: 22147661]

Goglin S, Chung S. Current treatment of cryoglobulinemic vasculitis. *Curr Treatm Opt Rheumatol.* 2016;2:213-224.

Ostojic P, Jeremic IR. Managing refractory cryoglobulinemic vasculitis: challenges and solutions. *J Inflamm Res.* 2017;10:49-54. [PMID: 28507447]

Saadoun D, Resche Rigon M, Pol S, et al. PegIFNα/ribavirin/protease inhibitor combination in severe hepatitis C virus-associated mixed cryoglobulinemia vasculitis. *J Hepatol.* 2015;62(1):24-30. [PMID: 25135864]

Saadoun D, Rosenzwaig M, Joly F, et al. Regulatory T-cell responses to low-dose interleukin-2 in HCV-induced vasculitis. *N Engl J Med.* 2011;365:2067-2077. [PMID: 22129253]

Saadoun D, Thibault V, Ahmed S, et al. Sofosbuvir plus ribavirin for hepatitis C-associated cryoglobulinaemia vasculitis: VASCUVALDIC study. *Ann Rheum Dis.* 2016;75:1777-1782. [PMID: 26567178]

Hypersensitivity Vasculitis

John H. Stone, MD, MPH

ESSENTIALS OF DIAGNOSIS

▶ Small-vessel vasculitis of the skin, often accompanied by little or no apparent involvement of other organs.

▶ Known by a variety of other names, including cutaneous leukocytoclastic angiitis.

▶ Precipitants, such as medications and infections, are often identifiable, but approximately 40% of cases have no definable cause.

▶ Primary forms of vasculitis, such as IgA vasculitis, Henoch-Schönlein purpura, microscopic polyangiitis, and granulomatosis with polyangiitis, must be excluded. Similarly, well-recognized forms of secondary vasculitis, such as mixed cryoglobulinemia, must also be eliminated from the differential diagnosis.

▶ Most cases are self-limited if the precipitant can be identified and removed. Glucocorticoids or other medications are required in some cases.

General Considerations

Hypersensitivity vasculitis refers to small-vessel vasculitis that is restricted to the skin and not associated with any other form of primary or secondary vasculitis. Implicit in this definition is that the condition is not associated with medium- or large-vessel disease at other sites, nor with small-vessel disease in other organs (eg, the glomeruli or pulmonary capillaries). In many cases, an identifiable precipitant such as a drug or an accompanying infection is present—hence the term "hypersensitivity." In up to 40% of cases, however, no specific cause is identified.

The term "hypersensitivity vasculitis" has been associated with much confusion ever since it was incorporated into the first vasculitis classification scheme in the early 1950s. The condition's name derives from the fact that by the 1950s, both human and animal models of hypersensitivity

to foreign antigens had been shown to cause small-vessel vasculitis involving the kidneys, lungs, and other organs besides the skin. Consequently, even microscopic polyangiitis, a disorder that commonly affects internal organs as well as the skin and is often associated with antineutrophil cytoplasmic antibodies (ANCAs), was grouped initially under the heading of hypersensitivity vasculitis. Because of the confusion surrounding its name, many clinicians have suggested that hypersensitivity vasculitis be replaced, but no entirely suitable alternative has been found. Terms used synonymously with hypersensitivity vasculitis have included **leukocytoclastic vasculitis, cutaneous leukocytoclastic angiitis**, and **cutaneous small-vessel vasculitis**, among others. In evaluating patients with small-vessel vasculitis of the skin, it is critical to remember that skin findings may only herald an underlying disorder involving other organs, as well. Extracutaneous involvement, which mandates reconsideration of the diagnosis, must be excluded with appropriate tests.

In most cases of hypersensitivity vasculitis, the problem is believed to have an immune complex–mediated pathophysiology. Histopathology generally shows a leukocytoclastic vasculitis, with features of necrosis in some cases but not granulomatous inflammation. Biopsies very early in the course of disease may show a lymphocytic predominance.

Clinical Findings

Table 33–1 outlines the classification criteria for hypersensitivity vasculitis established in 1990 by the American College of Rheumatology.

A. Symptoms and Signs

1. Skin—The lesions of small-vessel vasculitis of the skin include purpura (either palpable or nonpalpable) (Figure 33–1), papules, urticaria/angioedema, erythema multiforme, vesicles, pustules, ulcers, and necrosis. The lesions typically occur first and most prominently in dependent regions, that is, the lower

Table 33–1. American College of Rheumatology 1990 criteria for the classification of hypersensitivity vasculitis.[a]

1. Age at disease onset >16 years
2. Medication at disease onset
3. Palpable purpura
4. Maculopapular rash
5. Biopsy including arteriole and venule, showing granulocytes in a perivascular or extravascular location

[a]For purposes of classification, hypersensitivity vasculitis may be diagnosed if the patient meets at least three of these five criteria. Sensitivity = 71%; specificity = 83.9%.
Data from Calabrese LH, Michel BA, Bloch DA, et al. The American College of Rheumatology 1990 criteria for the classification of hypersensitivity vasculitis. *Arthritis Rheum.* 1990;33;1108.

extremities or buttocks. The lesions tend to occur in "crops" that are of the same age. The lesions are often asymptomatic but can be accompanied by a burning or tingling sensation.

2. Joints—Hypersensitivity vasculitis is sometimes accompanied by arthralgias and even frank arthritis, with a predominance for large joints.

B. Laboratory Findings

The results of routine laboratory tests and more specialized assays in hypersensitivity vasculitis are shown in Table 33–2. All of these tests are appropriate at the time of the initial evaluation, principally for the purpose of excluding other forms of vasculitis that may mimic hypersensitivity vasculitis.

C. Special Tests

The pleomorphic lesions of cutaneous vasculitis and the large number of vasculitis mimickers make histopathologic confirmation of the diagnosis by skin biopsy important in most cases. A biopsy specimen of an active lesion (<48 hours old, if possible) usually demonstrates leukocytoclastic vasculitis of

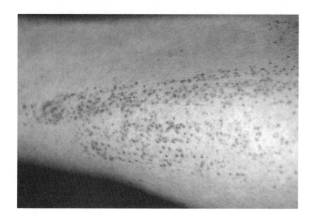

▲ **Figure 33–1.** Palpable purpura.

Table 33–2. Laboratory and radiographic workup of patients with possible hypersensitivity vasculitis.

Test	Typical Result
Complete blood cell count, with differential	Normal
Electrolytes	Normal
Liver function tests	Normal
Urinalysis with microscopy	Normal
Erythrocyte sedimentation rate/C-reactive protein	Mild to moderate elevations in <50% of patients
ANA	Negative
Rheumatoid factor	Negative
C3, C4	Normal
ANCA	Negative
Hepatitis B and C serologies	Negative
Cryoglobulins	Negative
Chest radiography	Normal

ANA, antinuclear antibody; ANCA, antineutrophil cytoplasmic antibody.

the postcapillary venules. Direct immunofluorescence (DIF) studies show variable quantities of immunoglobulin and complement deposition, with a nondiagnostic pattern. The performance of DIF studies, however, is an important (and often neglected) part of the workup, critical for the exclusion of IgA vasculitis (Henoch-Schönlein purpura), cryoglobulinemia, and other conditions.

▶ Differential Diagnosis

The differential diagnosis of hypersensitivity vasculitis is shown in Table 33–3. Hypersensitivity vasculitis must be distinguished from other small-vessel vasculitides, autoimmune inflammatory conditions associated with joint disease and

Table 33–3. Differential diagnosis of hypersensitivity vasculitis.

Other vasculitides
    Henoch-Schönlein purpura
    Microscopic polyangiitis
    Eosinophilic granulomatosis with polyangiitis
    Granulomatosis with polyangiitis
    Mixed cryoglobulinemia
    Polyarteritis nodosa
Systemic autoimmune conditions
    Systemic lupus erythematosus (including urticarial vasculitis)
    Rheumatoid arthritis
Miscellaneous
    Acute hemorrhagic edema of infancy
    Other types of drug eruptions

rashes, other cutaneous reactions to medications, and from infections.

▶ Treatment

Treatment strategies for hypersensitivity vasculitis are largely empiric. The type, intensity, and duration of therapy are based on the degree of disease severity in individual cases. For patients in whom a precipitant can be identified, removal of the offending agent usually leads to resolution of the vasculitis within days to weeks. Mild cases may be treated simply with leg elevation and the administration of non-steroidal anti-inflammatory drugs (or H_1 antihistamines). For persistent disease that does not lead to cutaneous ulcers or gangrene, colchicine (0.6 mg two or three times daily), hydroxychloroquine (200 mg twice daily), or dapsone (100 mg/day) may be used. For refractory or more severe cases, immunosuppressive agents may be indicated, generally beginning with a moderate dose of glucocorticoids (eg, prednisone 20–40 mg/day).

▶ Complications

Most cases with a clearly identified precipitant resolve over 1–4 weeks, often with some residual hyperpigmentation or (in the case of ulcerated lesions) scars. Some patients, however, have recurrent disease that remains confined to the skin and requires repeated treatment at varying intervals.

Hu S, Shangraw S, Newman S. Assessing practice gaps in the outpatient management of cutaneous small vessel vasculitis. *J Am Acad Dermatol.* 2020 Jan 18; pii: S0190-9622(20)30075-X. [Epub ahead of print] [PMID: 31962090]

Sunderkötter CH, Zelger B, Chen KR, et al. Nomenclature of cutaneous vasculitis: dermatologic addendum to the 2012 Revised International Chapel Hill Consensus Conference Nomenclature of Vasculitides. *Arthritis Rheum.* 2018;70(2):171. [PMID: 29136340]

Behçet Disease

34

Ahmet Gül, MD

ESSENTIALS OF DIAGNOSIS

▶ Recurrent oral and genital aphthous ulcers and bilateral posterior/panuveitis are the hallmarks of Behçet disease (BD). Other disease manifestations include pustular and nodular skin lesions, arthritis, thrombophlebitis affecting superficial and deep veins, arterial aneurysms, brainstem lesions, and gastrointestinal ulcers.

▶ Although similar mucocutaneous lesions can be seen in other inflammatory conditions, the ocular, vascular, and neurologic manifestations have distinctive features.

▶ A hyperinflammatory response to physical trauma such as hypodermic injections (the pathergy reaction) or to environmental triggers such as streptococcal antigens is a characteristic feature of the disease. Genetic polymorphisms contribute to this dysregulated immune response.

▶ There are no pathognomonic laboratory and clinical features of BD. Thus, the recognition of a combination of manifestations that are distinctive in their collective presence is necessary to establish the diagnosis.

▶ Treatment should be tailored to the patient's individual disease features. Medications, such as colchicine, glucocorticoids, immunosuppressives, apremilast, and biologic agents, can be used both to control inflammatory flares and to prevent recurrences.

General Considerations

Behçet disease (BD) is a vasculitic disorder of unknown etiology characterized by inflammatory attacks that target a variety of tissues and organs in a distinctive manner. The condition was first described by Hulusi Behçet, a Turkish dermatologist, who recognized a systemic disease typified by the triad of recurrent oral and genital aphthous ulcers and uveitis. Subsequent investigations revealed that the inflammatory attacks affect joints, blood vessels, the central nervous system, and gastrointestinal tract. Some manifestations of BD are self-limited and heal without any scar, but others such as uveitis, deep vein thrombosis, arterial aneurysms, or parenchymal neurologic findings may cause damage resulting in substantial morbidity and mortality.

Epidemiology

BD has unique epidemiological features. Its prevalence is higher in Eastern Mediterranean countries and along the ancient Silk Road to China, Korea, and Japan, and substantially lower in the Northern Europe and Americas. This unique geographic distribution is accounted for primarily by the increased prevalence of HLA-B*51 in the areas where the disease is found commonly.

BD is seen almost equally in males and females, but severe manifestations of the disease are seen more frequently in male patients. A preference for female patients with less severe course was noted in western countries. BD starts more commonly in the third decade. Young age of onset (<25 years) has been associated with a more severe disease course.

Etiology & Pathogenesis

BD is a multifactorial disease with a significant contribution of genetic factors as well as environmental triggers. HLA-B*51 is the strongest genetic susceptibility factor identified to date. Recent studies have also revealed weaker but independent contributions of other HLA Class I antigens influencing the risk for BD. Some of these alleles enhance disease susceptibility (eg, B*15, B*27, B*57, A*26) but others are known to be protective against the expression of BD (eg, B*49, A*03). A certain haplotype of the *ERAP1* (endoplasmic reticulum aminopeptidase 1) gene increases the risk of BD among HLA-B*51-positive individuals.

Several variants in non-HLA genes have also been associated with an increased tendency for BD. Some of the associated variants, such as those in *MEFV*, *TLR4*, *NOD2*, *LACC1*, *FUT2* genes, are involved in dysregulated host-environment interactions. Other risk-associated variants in *IL-10*, *IL-23R*, *IL-1α/IL-1β*, *CCR1*, *STAT4*, *IRF8*, *CEBPB-PTPN1*, *RIPK2*, and in *ADO-EGR2* genes are involved in the regulation and polarization of innate and adaptive immune responses. The impact of these genetic variants favors a hyperreactive inflammatory response that affects both innate and adaptive immunity. Activation of endothelial cells and intravascular inflammatory changes are suggested to play a role in the thrombotic tendency of BD.

▶ Clinical Findings

A. Symptoms and Signs

Mucocutaneous findings comprising aphthous ulcers, papulopustular lesions, and nodular skin lesions are common manifestations of BD (Tables 34–1 and 34–2). Recurrent oral aphthous ulcers (three or more in a year) are the most common and usually the first finding of the disease. These lesions are superficial, oval or round, nonscarring ulcers that have a necrotic, pseudomembranous base, surrounded by erythema (Figure 34–1A). Oral aphthous ulcers are classified as minor, major, or herpetiform on the basis of their size and appearance. The terms "minor" or "major" aphthous ulcer are used to describe single lesions, differentiated only by their size (<10 mm or ≥10 mm, respectively). "Herpetiform" ulcers, in contrast, are typically small (1–2 mm) in size but multiple,

Table 34–1. Major clinical manifestations of Behçet disease (BD).

	Frequency (%)
Common manifestations, which can also be seen in other inflammatory disorders	
Oral aphthous ulcers	97–100
Acne-like lesions	70–90
Erythema nodosum-like lesions	40–60
Arthritis	40–50
Manifestations, which overlap less commonly with other inflammatory disorders	
Genital aphthous ulcers	90
Skin pathergy reaction	30–80
Superficial thrombophlebitis	15–30
Gastrointestinal manifestations	2–30
Manifestations with distinctive features for BD	
Bilateral posterior or panuveitis	30–50
Deep vein thrombosis with inflammatory findings	10–15
Arterial aneurysms	5
Parenchymal neurologic manifestations	5–10

Table 34–2. Conditions associated with oral and genital (bipolar) ulcers.

Idiopathic complex aphthosis
Secondary complex aphthosis
- Behçet disease
- MAGIC syndrome
- Crohn disease
- Sweet syndrome
- Erythema multiforme
- Gluten enteropathy
- Monogenic autoinflammatory disorders, including mevalonate kinase disease and haplotype insufficiency for A20
- Primary immunodeficiency disorders
- Bullous skin disorders
- Fixed drug eruption and other drug reactions
- Viral (CMV, HSV) and rickettsial infections
- Cyclic neutropenia
- Trisomy 8
- Erosive lichen planus

occurring in clusters of 10–100 ulcers, similar to the ulcers of herpes simplex virus. The great majority of aphthous ulcers in patients with BD are single discrete lesions that are classified as either minor or major, but generally patients tend to have more than one of these lesions at a time, sometimes on the soft palate but most often on the oral mucosa, and rarely on the tongue.

It is important to realize that the aphthous ulcers of BD are indistinguishable from the canker sores or aphthous stomatitis that can be found in up to 10% of the otherwise healthy population. Oral hygiene problems may increase the frequency of ulcers, and smoking may suppress their development. In about 15% of the patients, other BD manifestations may start before the appearance of oral ulcers.

Genital ulcers, observed less frequently compared to oral aphthae, are also aphthous in character. The genital ulcers are observed mainly on the scrotum of males and the labia majora of female patients (Figure 34–1B). These ulcers can also be seen in groin, perianal, and perineal areas. In contrast to the oral aphthae, the genital lesions of BD usually leave a scar (Figure 34–1C). The combination of oral and genital ulcers, termed "bipolar aphthosis" or complex aphthosis, is not diagnostic of BD. Such a combination can also be observed in several other conditions (Table 34–2).

The papulopustular or acne-like lesions that occur in BD are clinically similar to ordinary acne but more frequently found on the lower extremities and buttocks in BD (Figure 34–1D). Similar erythematous papulopustular lesions that develop at the site of a needle prick are referred to as skin pathergy reaction.

Erythema nodosum-like lesions are painful, erythematous nodules that occur usually in the pretibial areas and less frequently in other areas. They frequently heal with pigmentation. Superficial thrombophlebitis may also cause painful

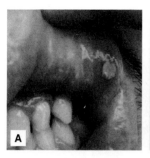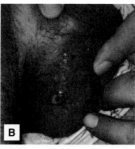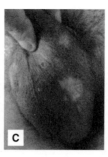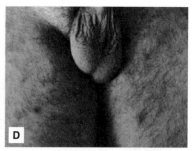

▲ **Figure 34–1.** Typical orogenital manifestations of Behçet disease (BD). Aphthous ulcers on oral mucosa (**A**) and scrotum (**B**). Scars of previous genital ulcers (**C**) and acne-like lesions in the lower extremities (**D**) are important in the differential diagnosis.

erythematous nodular lesions, and they can be recognized better when they are presented as more linear swellings. Erythema nodosum-like lesions are more frequent in females, whereas superficial thrombophlebitis is more commonly seen in male patients and known as an early sign of vascular involvement (Figure 34–2A).

Acute arthritis, found in almost half of patients with BD, is a nonerosive mono- or oligoarthritis that tends to affect lower extremity joints. Chronic arthritis develops rarely, and despite the shared pathogenic pathways and extra-articular clinical findings with spondyloarthritis, axial involvement is seen rarely in BD.

Uveitis, one of the distinctive features of BD, comprises nongranulomatous posterior uveitis or a panuveitis that tends to affect both eyes. Self-limited superficial retinal infiltrates, branch retinal vein occlusion, gliotic retinal vascular sheathing, peripheral occlusive periphlebitis, and retinal hemorrhages are typical features of the uveitis associated with Behçet. Some patients develop hypopyon due to extension of the diffuse vitritis findings to the anterior chamber. Isolated anterior uveitis is very rare in BD. Recurrent flares involving the posterior segment may result in reduced visual acuity and total loss of vision. In BD patients with active uveitis, fundus fluorescein angiography may reveal optic disc hyperfluorescence and diffuse fern-like capillary leakage in the periphery despite normal appearance of these areas.

BD has been classified as a variable-vessel vasculitis due to its unique feature of affecting all types and sizes of blood vessels. In most patients, however, BD has a predilection for the venous circulation (Figure 34–3). All veins, including the superior and inferior vena cavae and cerebral sinuses, can be affected, but deep vein thrombosis is seen most frequently in lower extremities (see Figure 34–2). Inflammatory changes affecting the vessel wall lumen have been claimed as the main

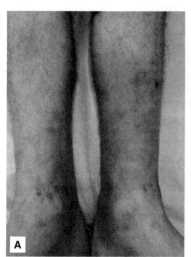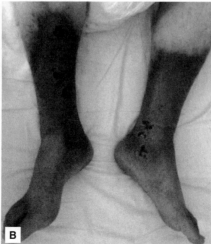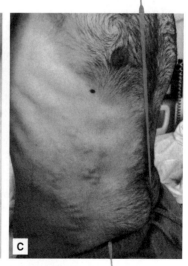

▲ **Figure 34–2. A:** Superficial thrombophlebitis appearing as erythematous nodular lesions in the lower extremities. **B:** Recurrent attacks of deep vein thrombosis of lower extremities in untreated patients may result in stasis dermatitis and ulcers. **C:** Abdominal collaterals in a patient with vena cava thrombosis.

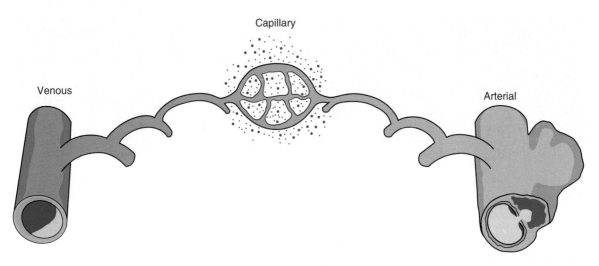

▲ **Figure 34–3.** The spectrum of vascular involvement in Behçet disease (BD) involving all types and sizes of blood vessels with a tendency for thrombosis. In contrast to certain other forms of vasculitis, eg, giant cell arteritis, Takayasu arteritis, and polyarteritis nodosa, BD has a preference for the venous side of the vasculature.

cause of thrombotic tendency observed in BD, and this feature has also been suggested as the explanation for the very low risk of pulmonary thromboembolism, because the thrombus becomes adherent to the underlying activated endothelium. Recurrent attacks in the lower extremity veins may result in a post-thrombotic syndrome that leads to stasis ulcers (see Figure 34–2B). Involvement of hepatic veins and development of Budd-Chiari syndrome has a worse prognosis. Cerebral venous thrombosis results in intracranial hypertension and papilledema. This type of vascular involvement is less common (20%) and has a better prognosis than neuro-BD involving the brain parenchyma.

Arterial involvement occurs most frequently as aneurysms rather than occlusions (Figure 34–3). Pulmonary arterial aneurysms are the most common site of arterial involvement, and it is the leading cause of mortality due to massive hemoptysis. Irregularly shaped saccular pseudoaneurysms are the major forms of arterial involvement. The perianeurysmal inflammatory changes affect and damage the surrounding tissues and contribute to the symptoms. Findings of pulmonary arterial and deep venous involvement may develop in BD patients who are younger compared to those who develop aneurysms of the aorta or other sites.

Parenchymal neurologic involvement is characterized by subacute brainstem syndromes associated with uni- or multifocal lesions. These typically affect the pons but also the midbrain, basal ganglia, and diencephalon. Findings of cerebral hemispheric or spinal cord syndrome can also be seen. Clinical findings include pyramidal signs, headaches, hemiparesis, ataxia, sphincter disturbances, behavioral changes, ophthalmoplegia, and depressive thoughts.

Gastrointestinal involvement is seen more frequently in Eastern Asian countries, and its differentiation from Crohn disease may be troublesome due to shared intestinal and extraintestinal features. Aphthous ulcers are the most common gastrointestinal manifestations causing abdominal pain and diarrhea. Ulcers are usually seen in the ileocecal region as solitary lesions or a few round, oval, or geographic-shaped big ulcers with focal distribution. These contrast with the multiple, longitudinal ulcers of Crohn disease, which tend to have a segmental or diffuse distribution. Because of their vasculitic nature, the ulcers of BD are more prone to bleeding and perforation.

B. Laboratory Findings

There is no pathognomonic laboratory finding that is useful in either the diagnosis or the longitudinal management of BD patients. The systemic acute phase response is not prominent in patients who present with mainly mucocutaneous manifestations, but it may be elevated in patients with active vascular or other major organ involvements. Analysis of the local inflammatory response, for example, a cerebrospinal fluid evaluation in patients with parenchymal neurologic disease, may reveal a neutrophilic pleocytosis and increased protein concentration. Interleukin-6 may also be elevated in the cerebrospinal fluid of such patients.

The role of genetic testing in the diagnosis or subgroup definition of BD, including testing for HLA-B*51, has not been defined precisely yet.

C. Imaging Studies

Imaging studies may be helpful in the screening and follow-up of vascular and neurologic involvement. Because of the risk of pathergy reaction following vascular trauma such as the development of thrombophlebitis or aneurysms at the

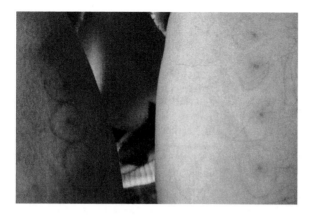

▲ **Figure 34–4.** Skin pathergy reaction as papulopustular lesions with surrounding erythema at the needle prick sites on the second day.

investigation site, invasive imaging procedures should be avoided when possible.

Fundus fluorescein angiography is a helpful tool to document active disease and to follow the treatment response in patients with uveitis by showing optic disc hyperfluorescence, retinal capillary nonperfusion for occluded vessels, and diffuse peripheral fern-like capillary leakage.

Parenchymal neurologic lesions appear as hypo- or isointense on T1-weighted, but hyperintense in T2-weighted, FLAIR and diffusion-weighted images in acute disease. In chronic phase, atrophic changes in brainstem can be detected.

D. Special Tests

Skin pathergy reaction can be induced by insertion of 20G (No.1) hypodermic needle to the skin of forearm. Development of a persistent erythematous papule or pustule at the prick site on the second day (48 hours) is considered to be a positive result (Figure 34–4). This response can rarely be observed in patients with Sweet syndrome and pyoderma gangrenosum. Therefore, a positive pathergy test result is very helpful in the diagnosis when evaluated within the context of other clinical findings. There is a trend for less a frequent positive pathergy reaction in recent years. Pathergy tests appear to be less helpful in nonendemic areas.

▶ Diagnosis & Differential Diagnosis

There is no histopathological finding specific for BD. Even the presence of vasculitic changes on biopsy samples is not sufficient to confirm that the diagnosis is BD without careful correlation with the full clinical picture.

Different sets of criteria have been used to diagnose/classify BD patients so far (Table 34–3). However, they all have limitations at bedside diagnosis. Some of the clinical findings, such as oral aphthous ulcers, folliculitis, and erythema

Table 34–3. Commonly used classification/diagnostic criteria for Behçet disease.

International Study Group (ISG) diagnostic criteria

Patient must have recurrent oral ulceration plus at least two of the other criteria in the absence of any other explanation (95% sensitivity and 98% specificity)
1. Recurrent oral ulceration
   Minor aphthous, major aphthous, or herpetiform ulcers observed by the physician or reliably described by the patient, which recurred at least three times over a 12-month period

Plus two of the following criteria:
2. Recurrent genital ulceration
   Aphthous ulceration or scarring observed by the physician or reliably described by the patient
3. Eye lesions
   Anterior or posterior uveitis or cells in the vitreous body on slit-lamp examination; or retinal vasculitis detected by an ophthalmologist
4. Skin lesions
   Erythema nodosum, pseudofolliculitis, papular-pustular lesions, or acneiform nodules not related to corticosteroid treatment or adolescence
5. Positive pathergy test
   Test interpreted as positive by the physician at 24–48 hours

International criteria for Behçet disease (ICBD) diagnosis and classification

Sign/Symptom	Points
Ocular lesions	2
Genital aphthosis	2
Oral aphthosis	2
Skin lesions	1
Neurological manifestations	1
Vascular manifestations	1
Positive pathergy test[a]	1

A score of ≥4 indicates the diagnosis (94.8% sensitivity and 90.5% specificity).
[a]Pathergy test is optional, and when it is available, one additional point is given for a positive result.

nodosum-like lesions, are common and can be seen in other conditions, as well (see Table 34–3). Patients with orogenital ulcers may be falsely classified as BD by one of the criteria, and a detailed investigation for idiopathic complex aphthosis and several other conditions causing bipolar aphthosis should be included in the differential diagnosis list. Monogenic autoinflammatory disorders, such as mevalonate kinase deficiency or haploinsufficiency of A20, should be considered in patients with an early disease onset at childhood and febrile episodes of manifestations as conditions mimicking BD.

The ocular, vascular, and parenchymal neurologic manifestations of BD have more features to distinguish them from similar conditions. Therefore, their detailed description is critically important. The differential diagnosis includes other causes of nongranulomatous; noninfectious causes of uveitis for patients with ocular involvement; and inflammatory, infective, or demyelinating central nervous system disorders for patients with parenchymal brain involvement.

Similar to the shared genetic features, clinical manifestations of BD overlap with those of Crohn disease. Recurrent oral aphthous ulcers, erythema nodosum, peripheral arthritis, and even genital lesions can also be seen in patients with Crohn disease. In addition to the acute anterior uveitis as observed in patients with spondyloarthritis, ocular involvement of Crohn disease may affect the posterior segments of both eyes. Therefore, the absence of features that are typical of BD uveitis (eg, recurrent superficial retinal infiltrates) or the presence of granulomatous gastrointestinal inflammatory lesions, longitudinal ulcers with segmental or diffuse involvement pattern may favor Crohn disease.

▶ Treatment

Treatment of BD is empiric. Because of its relapsing and remitting course, the aims of therapy are both to control manifestations of inflammation that are evident and to prevent recurrences. Treatment should be adjusted according to the organs involved and the severity of the specific features present.

Glucocorticoids are frequently used via topical, oral, parenteral, or intralesional routes for the treatment of inflammatory flares to limit tissue damage. Colchicine has been shown to be effective for mucocutaneous manifestations, especially for the genital ulcers and the erythema nodosum-like lesions, as well as for arthritis. Apremilast has recently been found to be effective in the treatment of oral ulcers of BD with a good safety profile. Thalidomide and dapsone are alternative treatments for refractory mucocutaneous lesions. Peripheral arthritis attacks can be controlled by colchicine, with the addition of low-dose glucocorticoids and azathioprine, as necessary.

Immunosuppressive agents such azathioprine (2.5 mg/kg) or cyclosporine (3–5 mg/kg) or both should be given along with high-dose glucocorticoids in patients with an attack of uveitis involving the posterior segment. Interferon alpha and monoclonal anti-TNF agents should be considered for patients with sight-threatening or refractory uveitis.

High-dose glucocorticoids and immunosuppressive agents are treatments of choice for patients with vascular and neurologic involvements. For the treatment of deep vein thrombosis, the additional of anticoagulation to regimens of immunosuppression does not lend further efficacy in most cases. Anticoagulants can be used cautiously after screening for arterial aneurysms, especially in patients with refractory disease with recurrent thrombophlebitis attacks and post-thrombotic syndrome despite immunosuppressive agents. For arterial aneurysms, surgery and endovascular stents carry high complication rates and could only be considered in selected cases. Embolization may be a preferred option to control life-threatening bleeding complications.

Cyclosporine may increase the risk of neurologic manifestations. Therefore, it should be avoided in patients with brain lesions. Monoclonal anti-TNF agents are preferred options in patients with severe or refractory manifestations. However, other biologic agents targeting IL-1, IL-6 receptor, IL-12/IL-23 p40 subunit can also be tried when necessary.

▶ Course & Prognosis

Most of the BD patients develop mainly mucocutaneous manifestations with a relatively benign course. BD has a worse prognosis in patients with vascular and neurologic involvement. Male gender and young age at onset are the only known poor prognostic factors.

Gül A. Pathogenesis of Behçet's disease: autoinflammatory features and beyond. *Semin Immunopathol.* 2015;37:413-418. [PMID: 26068404]

Hatemi G, Christensen R, Bang D, et al. 2018 update of the EULAR recommendations for the management of Behçet's syndrome. *Ann Rheum Dis.* 2018;77:808-818. [PMID: 29625968]

Kalra S, Silman A, Akman-Demir G, et al. Diagnosis and management of neuro-Behçet's disease: international consensus recommendations. *J Neurol.* 2014;261:1662-1676. [PMID: 24366648]

Ombrello MJ, Kirino Y, de Bakker PI, Gül A, Kastner DL, Remmers EF. Behçet disease-associated MHC class I residues implicate antigen binding and regulation of cell-mediated cytotoxicity. *Proc Natl Acad Sci USA.* 2014;111:8867-8872. [PMID: 24821759]

Takeuchi M, Ombrello MJ, Kirino Y, et al. A single endoplasmic reticulum aminopeptidase-1 protein allotype is a strong risk factor for Behçet's disease in HLA-B*51 carriers. *Ann Rheum Dis.* 2016;75:2208-2211. [PMID: 27217550]

Takeuchi M, Mizuki N, Meguro A, et al. Dense genotyping of immune-related loci implicates host responses to microbial exposure in Behçet's disease susceptibility. *Nat Genet.* 2017;49:438-443. [PMID: 28166214]

Valenti S, Gallizzi R, De Vivo D, Romano C. Intestinal Behçet and Crohn's disease: two sides of the same coin. *Pediatr Rheumatol Online J.* 2017;15:33. [PMID: 28427473]

Yazici H, Seyahi E, Hatemi G, Yazici Y. Behçet syndrome: a contemporary view. *Nat Rev Rheumatol.* 2018;14:107-119. [PMID: 29296024]

IgA Vasculitis (Henoch-Schönlein Purpura)

35

Geetha Duvuru, MD, MRCP

John H. Stone, MD, MPH

ESSENTIALS OF DIAGNOSIS

▶ The sine qua non of IgA vasculitis (formerly Henoch-Schönlein purpura) is nonthrombocytopenic purpura, caused by inflammation in blood vessels of the superficial dermis.

▶ The pathologic hallmarks of IgA vasculitis are a leukocytoclastic vasculitis and deposition of immunoglobulin (Ig) A in the walls of involved blood vessels.

▶ The tetrad of purpura, arthritis, glomerulonephritis, and abdominal pain is often observed. However, all four elements are not required for the diagnosis.

▶ More than 90% of cases occur in children. The disease is self-limited most of the time, resolving within a few weeks. Adult cases are sometimes more recalcitrant.

▶ Renal insufficiency develops in less than 5% of patients with IgA vasculitis. The long-term renal prognosis depends mainly on the degree of initial damage to the kidney.

▶ IgA vasculitis can be mimicked by other forms of systemic vasculitis that are more often life-threatening. For example, antineutrophil cytoplasmic antibody (ANCA)–associated vasculitides such as granulomatosis with polyangiitis and microscopic polyangiitis may also present with purpura, arthritis, and renal inflammation. Both of these disorders have the potential for serious involvement of other organs (eg, the lungs and peripheral nerves) and carry more dire renal prognoses.

▶ General Considerations

IgA vasculitis (formerly Henoch-Schönlein purpura) is the most common form of systemic vasculitis in children, with an annual incidence of 140 cases per million persons. The peak incidence is in the first and second decades of life (90% of patients are younger than 10 years of age), with a male to female ratio of 2:1. The incidence is significantly lower in adults, with a mean age at presentation of 50 years. Males and females are affected equally and although IgA vasculitis affects all ethnic groups, it is reportedly less common among blacks. Some epidemiologic studies suggest that IgA vasculitis is more prevalent in the winter months.

IgA vasculitis may be misdiagnosed as another form of vasculitis—most commonly hypersensitivity vasculitis (see Chapter 33)—because of the frequent failure to perform direct immunofluorescence testing on skin biopsy specimens. In two-thirds of the cases, the disease follows an upper respiratory tract infection, with onset an average of 10 days after the start of respiratory symptoms. Despite this association, no single microorganism or environmental exposure has been confirmed as an important cause of IgA vasculitis. IgA vasculitis can also be induced by medications, particularly antibiotics. The American College of Rheumatology 1990 criteria for the classification of IgA vasculitis are shown in Table 35–1. The first Chapel Hill Consensus Conference on the nomenclature of vasculitides defined IgA vasculitis as a form of vasculitis characterized by the following: (1) IgA-dominant immune deposits within vessel walls; (2) small-vessel involvement (ie, capillaries, venules, or arterioles); and (3) skin, gut, renal, and joint manifestation.

The skin histopathology of IgA vasculitis shows a leukocytoclastic vasculitis of small blood vessels within the superficial dermis. Necrosis is often present, but features of granulomatous inflammation are not. Immunofluorescent staining of biopsy specimens shows coarse, granular IgA staining in and around small blood vessels. In the kidney, the renal inflammation is indistinguishable from IgA nephropathy. There is a predilection for IgA deposition within the mesangium. However, in the nephritis associated with IgA vasculitis, capillary wall staining for IgA is more frequently found and may be even more prominent than IgA in the mesangium. Most patients have increased serum IgA levels and circulating immune complexes that contain IgA, as well as IgA deposition in inflamed blood vessels.

Table 35–1. The American College of Rheumatology 1990 Criteria[a] for the classification of IgA vasculitis.

1. Palpable purpura
2. Age at onset <20 years
3. Bowel angina
4. Vessel wall granulocytes on biopsy

[a]The presence of two criteria classified HSP with a sensitivity of 87% and specificity of 88% in a group of individuals with forms of systemic vasculitis.

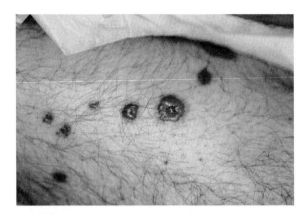

▲ **Figure 35–2.** A bullous lesion with a purpuric component in a patient with IgA vasculitis.

▶ Clinical Findings

A. Symptoms and Signs

The classic full presentation of IgA vasculitis includes the acute onset of fever, palpable purpura on the lower extremities (Figure 35–1) and buttocks, abdominal pain, arthritis, and hematuria. All components of this presentation are not required for the diagnosis, however. Conversely, even classic presentations are not diagnostic of this disorder. In adults, the diagnosis should be confirmed in most cases by biopsy (direct immunofluorescence as well as conventional hematoxylin and eosin staining). Pediatricians are more likely to rely on clinical diagnoses in the setting of classic presentations, which is reasonable given the relatively high incidence of IgA vasculitis in children compared to adults.

1. Skin—The cutaneous findings of IgA vasculitis include purpura (usually palpable, although sometimes not), urticarial papules, and plaques. Among adults, 60% of the patients have bullous or necrotic lesions (Figure 35–2), but these are uncommon in children. Lesions are concentrated over the buttocks and lower extremities and tend to

involve the small blood vessels in the superficial dermis. Medium-sized vessels are rarely involved in IgA vasculitis except in the rare cases of IgA vasculitis associated with IgA paraproteinemia. Localized edematous swelling of the subcutaneous tissues of the lower extremities is frequently observed and does not correlate with the presence or degree of proteinuria. Persistent rash over a period longer than 1 month is a significant predictor of disease relapse and renal sequelae in children with IgA vasculitis.

2. Joints—Joint disease, which occurs in more than 80% of patients with IgA vasculitis, manifests itself as arthralgias or arthritis in large joints, especially the knees and ankles and, to a lesser degree, the wrists and elbows. Migratory patterns of joint involvement are common. Lower extremity involvement among patients with IgA vasculitis and arthritis is nearly universal; up to one-third of patients have upper extremity involvement as well. The pain associated with IgA vasculitis arthritis may be incapacitating, but the joint inflammation does not lead to a deforming arthritis.

3. Gastrointestinal tract—Approximately 60% of patients with IgA vasculitis have abdominal pain and 33% have evidence of gastrointestinal bleeding. Abdominal symptoms result from edema of the bowel wall as well as hemorrhage induced by mesenteric vasculitis. Abdominal pain may precede the appearance of purpura by up to 2 weeks, leading often to diagnostic confusion and occasionally to invasive testing or even laparotomy. The abdominal pain is typically colicky and may worsen after eating ("intestinal angina"). Some patients experience nausea, vomiting, and upper or lower gastrointestinal bleeding. Mesenteric ischemia in IgA vasculitis rarely leads to gut perforation. Massive gastrointestinal hemorrhage occurs in only 2% or so of patients. Purpuric lesions may be seen on endoscopy, commonly in the descending duodenum, stomach, and colon.

Gastrointestinal involvement in children with IgA vasculitis can cause intussusception, a rare complication in adults.

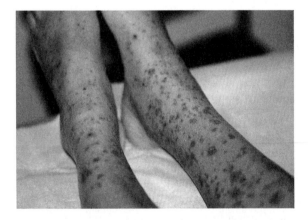

▲ **Figure 35–1.** Palpable purpura with some superficial ulcerations in a patient with IgA vasculitis. Note also the presence of right ankle swelling due to arthritis.

In contrast to idiopathic intussusception, which typically is ileocolic, IgA vasculitis-associated intussusception is usually ileoileal. Other rare complications include pancreatitis, cholecystitis, and a protein-losing enteropathy.

4. Kidney—Renal involvement is the most potentially debilitating complication of IgA vasculitis. Forty percent of patients with IgA vasculitis have renal disease. In general, renal involvement is more frequent and tends to be persistent in adults, who have a higher risk of developing end-stage renal disease than children. In a retrospective study of 134 children with IgA vasculitis, age greater than 4 years, persistent purpura, and severe abdominal symptoms increased the likelihood of renal involvement.

In contrast to gastrointestinal disease and arthritis, both of which occasionally precede the onset of purpura, glomerulonephritis almost always appears after the development of skin manifestations. The clinical hallmark of nephritis in IgA vasculitis is hematuria, often macroscopic, but more typically microscopic. The hematuria can be transient, persistent, or recurrent. Proteinuria never occurs in the absence of hematuria in the acute setting. Even in cases in which the renal disease resolves spontaneously, many patients have persistent urinary abnormalities (eg, proteinuria). The appearance of glomerulonephritis may be delayed by several weeks in up to 25% of all patients with this complication. IgA vasculitis should therefore be screened for the development of nephritis by urine dipsticks for several weeks, even after the skin, joint, and GI symptoms have resolved.

The most common renal lesion (60% of cases) is a focal, proliferative endocapillary glomerulonephritis. Crescents are present in up to 40% of biopsies. Direct immunofluorescence studies characteristically demonstrate IgA deposition in the mesangium. Regardless of age, the degree of proteinuria, the presence of renal dysfunction at presentation, the number of crescents, and the degree of interstitial fibrosis on biopsy correlate with outcome. Histologic recurrences of IgA vasculitis nephritis in renal allografts occur in 50% of patients who undergo renal transplantation. Allograft recurrences are associated with clinically significant disease in 20%, allograft failure in 12%, and allograft loss in 9% of cases.

5. Other organs—Pulmonary and central nervous system (CNS) complications of IgA vasculitis have been described, but these are very rare. When present, the usual lung manifestation of the disease is alveolar hemorrhage. Seizures are the usual CNS manifestation of IgA vasculitis; the precise mechanism is obscure. Testicular involvement occurs in up to 10% of boys with this disease and may mimic torsion.

B. Laboratory Findings

The results of routine laboratory tests and more specialized assays in IgA vasculitis are shown in Table 35–2. All of these tests are appropriate at the initial evaluation of a patient with possible IgA vasculitis. The exclusion of other forms

Table 35–2. The laboratory evaluation in IgA vasculitis.

Test	Typical Result
Complete blood cell count, with differential	Mild to moderate leukocytosis common, but otherwise the complete blood count is usually normal.
Electrolytes	Hyperkalemia in the setting of advanced renal dysfunction.
Liver function tests	Hypoalbuminemia can occur with nephrotic proteinuria. Otherwise, the liver function tests are normal.
Urinalysis with microscopy	Hematuria (ranging from mild to too numerous to count red blood cells). Red blood cell casts. Proteinuria (nephrotic range proteinuria in a small minority).
Erythrocyte sedimentation rate/ C-reactive protein	Modestly elevated acute phase reactants may be observed. Approximately one-third of patients have abnormal erythrocyte sedimentation rates.
Serum IgA level	60% of patients have an elevated serum IgA. Although there are two subclasses of IgA, HSP is associated with increases only in IgA1.
ANA	Negative
Rheumatoid factor	Negative
C3, C4	Even though immune complexes containing IgA are essential to the pathophysiology of HSP, serum complement levels are usually normal.
ANCA	Negative (both IgG and IgA ANCA)
Cryoglobulins	Negative

ANA, antinuclear antibody; ANCA, antineutrophil cytoplasmic antibody.

of vasculitis that may mimic IgA vasculitis in presentation is essential. Sixty percent of patients have an elevated serum IgA. Although there are two subclasses of IgA, IgA vasculitis is associated with serum elevations and tissue deposits of IgA1 only. The reason for the preferential elevation of IgA1 is not clear.

C. Imaging Studies

Chest radiography should be performed to rule out pulmonary lesions. The presence of pulmonary involvement, unusual in IgA vasculitis, raises the possibility of other diagnoses that may require other treatment approaches (see section Differential Diagnosis).

D. Special Tests

Direct immunofluorescence studies of skin biopsies can only be performed on fresh samples, and therefore must be planned at the time the biopsy is performed. The usual procedure is to biopsy one skin lesion for hematoxylin and eosin

Table 35–3. Differential diagnosis of IgA vasculitis.

Other vasculitides
  Hypersensitivity vasculitis
  Microscopic polyangiitis
  Eosinophilic granulomatosis with polyangiitis
  Granulomatosis with polyangiitis
  Mixed cryoglobulinemia
  Polyarteritis nodosa
Systemic autoimmune conditions
  Systemic lupus erythematosus
  Rheumatoid arthritis
Renal disorders
  IgA nephropathy
Infections
  Acute viral or bacterial infections
Malignancies
  Childhood leukemias
Miscellaneous
  Acute hemorrhagic edema of infancy

staining and another for immunofluorescence. Alternatively, a single biopsy sample can be split into different portions for the two types of studies.

Differential Diagnosis

The differential diagnosis of IgA vasculitis is shown in Table 35–3. IgA vasculitis must be distinguished from other small-vessel vasculitides, autoimmune inflammatory conditions associated with joint disease and rashes, and from infections. Other disorders may be associated occasionally with mild IgA deposition in blood vessels, but the process is rarely so florid as with IgA vasculitis. IgA nephropathy is pathologically indistinguishable from the renal disease associated with IgA vasculitis (including the preferential deposition of IgA1), but it has a typically chronic course and is not associated with disease in other organ systems.

A particularly crucial distinction is between IgA vasculitis and the ANCA–associated conditions, primarily granulomatosis with polyangiitis and microscopic polyangiitis. The ANCA–associated vasculitides often present with purpura, migratory arthritis, and renal inflammation but, in contrast to IgA vasculitis, do not typically have self-limited courses. Organ manifestations that are atypical for IgA vasculitis, such as pulmonary involvement, symptoms or signs compatible with vasculitic neuropathy, or inflammatory eye disease, should broaden the differential diagnosis. Misdiagnoses of

IgA vasculitis because of failure to perform direct immunofluorescence testing on skin biopsies and ANCA assays on serum can lead to poor outcomes.

Treatment

Nonsteroidal anti-inflammatory drugs may alleviate arthralgias but can aggravate gastrointestinal symptoms and should be avoided in any patient with renal disease. Dapsone (100 mg/day) may be effective in cases of IgA vasculitis, perhaps through interference with the interactions of IgA and neutrophils. Although glucocorticoids have not been evaluated rigorously in IgA vasculitis, they appear to ameliorate joint and gastrointestinal symptoms. Glucocorticoids do not appear to improve the rash, however, and their effectiveness in renal disease is controversial. Uncontrolled trials suggest that high-dose methylprednisolone followed by oral prednisone or high-dose prednisone combined with mycophenolate mofetil may help patients with severe nephritis (ie, nephrotic syndrome and >50% crescents).

Complications

In most cases, IgA vasculitis follows a self-limited course, resolves without substantial morbidity, and does not recur. The vast majority of cases resolve within 6–8 weeks. Recurrences, found in 33% of patients, usually develop within the first few months after resolution of the first bout. Even when associated with small ulcerations, the cutaneous lesions are usually so superficial that they heal without scarring. A small percentage of patients have progressive renal disease, and long-term follow-up of all patients with severe renal symptoms at onset is needed.

Chan H, et al. Risk factors associated with renal involvement in childhood Henoch-Schönlein purpura: a meta-analysis. *PloS One.* 2016;11(11):e0167346. [PMID: 27902749]

Hackl A, et al. Mycophenolate mofetil following glucocorticoid treatment in Henoch-Schönlein purpura nephritis: the role of early initiation and therapeutic drug monitoring. *Pediatr Nephrol.* 2018;33(4):619-629. [PMID: 29177628]

Ozen S, et al. European consensus-based recommendations for diagnosis and treatment of immunoglobulin A vasculitis—the SHARE initiative. *Rheumatology.* 2019; 58(9):1607-1616. [PMID: 30879080]

Selewski DT, et al. Clinical characteristics and treatment patterns of children and adults with IgA nephropathy or IgA vasculitis: findings from the CureGN study. *Kidney Int Rep.* 2018;3(6):1373-1384. [PMID: 30450464]

Primary Angiitis of the Central Nervous System

36

Naomi Serling-Boyd, MD

John H. Stone, MD, MPH

Central nervous system (CNS) vasculitis comprises a host of different underlying diseases that can cause inflammatory damage of blood vessels in the brain and spinal cord. About half of the cases have no known cause and no other systemic manifestations and are therefore classified as **primary** vasculitis of the CNS. The other half of the cases arise in the setting of an underlying disorder, often a systemic rheumatologic disease or (less commonly) an infection. Those cases are classified as **secondary** forms of CNS vasculitis. Primary vasculitis of the CNS, the focus of this chapter, has been referred to by many names, leading to sometimes confusing terminology. We will use the term "primary angiitis of the CNS" (PACNS) in this chapter.

It is important to recognize and treat the rare patients whose strokes and other neurologic deficits result from PACNS. However, it is also important for clinicians to avoid overdiagnosis of PACNS, because the angiographic and magnetic resonance imaging (MRI) abnormalities observed in this condition can be mimicked closely by infection, noninflammatory vasculopathy, malignancy, and other conditions.

ESSENTIALS OF DIAGNOSIS

▶ Common findings at presentation include headache, encephalopathy, and multifocal strokes.

▶ The differential diagnosis of PACNS encompasses systemic inflammatory, infectious, and malignant etiologies, as well as reversible cerebral vasoconstriction syndrome (RCVS).

▶ Angiographic abnormalities may be highly consistent with PACNS but are never diagnostic in and of themselves, and can be seen in one (or more than one) of its potential mimickers. Similarly, high-resolution MRI with vessel wall imaging can help to differentiate vasculitis from atherosclerosis but the specificity of such findings

remains imperfect and always requires careful clinicoradiologic correlation.

▶ Definitive diagnosis requires brain biopsy to confirm histopathologic vasculitis. Even with biopsy findings, however, clinicopathologic correlation is required to confirm the diagnosis of PACNS.

General Considerations

PACNS is a disease of unknown cause characterized by vasculitis limited to the brain and spinal cord. PACNS is a rare disease. At large medical centers, PACNS constitutes only about 1% of all cases of systemic vasculitis. The annual incidence is 2.4 cases per 1,000,000 person-years.

Clinical Findings

A. Symptoms and Signs

The average age of onset is around 50 years but patients of any age, including children, can be affected. The initial presentation commonly involves headache, cognitive changes, focal neurologic changes such as hemiparesis, or other persistent neurologic deficits. Less commonly, seizures or vision changes are part of the presentation. A summary of the clinical signs and symptoms seen at presentation is shown in Table 36–1.

Although headaches are part of the presentation in at least half of patients with PACNS, the headaches are generally subacute or even chronic in nature, present for weeks or months before a connection between their presence and inflammatory cerebrovascular disease is established. An acute onset "thunderclap" headache is highly uncharacteristic of PACNS. Rather, such a presentation with the rapid onset of a headache—with the maximal intensity within minutes—strongly suggests other etiologies (eg, RCVS or subarachnoid hemorrhage).

Table 36–1. Clinical and laboratory features of PACNS at the time of presentation

Clinical Characteristic	Percent of patients with positive finding (n=101)
Headache	63%
Altered cognition	50%
Hemiparesis	44%
Visual symptom of any kind	42%
Persistent neurological deficit or stroke	40%
Aphasia	28%
Transient ischemic attack	28%
Nausea or vomiting	25%
Visual field defect	21%
Ataxia	19%
Seizure	16%
Diplopia	16%
Dysarthria	15%
Unilateral numbness	13%
Blurred vision or decreased visual acuity	11%
Prominent constitutional symptom	9%
Fever	9%
Vertigo or dizziness	9%
Amnestic syndrome	9%
Intracranial hemorrhage	8%
Paraparesis or quadriparesis	7%
Papilledema	5%
Parkinsonism or extrapyramidal sign	1%
Monocular visual symptoms or amaurosis fugax	1%

Data from Salvarani C, Brown RD, Calamia KT, Christianson TJH, et al. Primary Central Nervous System Vasculitis: Analysis of 101 Patients. *Ann Neurol.* 2007;62:442-451.

Focal neurologic deficits often occur in PACNS, caused by either cerebral infarctions or other white matter lesions traceable ultimately to small-vessel vasculitis of the brain, generally affecting blood vessels below the resolution of current imaging. Multiple infarctions, some of them subclinical, are the rule in PACNS. Such lesions produce a variety of neurologic deficits, depending on the specific vascular territories involved. Seizures comprise part of the presentation in approximately 15% of PACNS cases.

Constitutional symptoms, such as fevers, weight loss, or night sweats, are uncommon in PACNS and should urge a careful evaluation for other systemic causes. Vasculitis of the CNS may occur in a variety of rheumatologic conditions, including Behçet syndrome, systemic lupus erythematosus, polyarteritis nodosa, and vasculitis associated with antineutrophil cytoplasmic antibodies (ANCA), but the presence of systemic features in those disorders usually implicates a condition separate from PACNS; that is, secondary CNS vasculitis. The identification of vasculitis or other organ dysfunction beyond the CNS, of course, precludes a diagnosis of PACNS.

B. Laboratory Findings

PACNS patients typically have normal routine laboratory results and acute phase reactants. Thus, normal serum inflammatory markers do not eliminate a diagnosis of PACNS with any degree of reliability. Laboratory findings, such as rheumatoid factor, antinuclear antibody, ANCA, antiphospholipid antibodies, and complement levels, are also generally unremarkable in PACNS. In short, the absence of any serologic test that is charactistically abnormal in PACNS and the lack of any particular blood assay that implicates inflammation within blood vessels of the CNS poses one of the greatest diagnostic challenges in PACNS.

On the other hand, both lumbar puncture and CNS imaging often provide crucial information. Both examinations are crucial in the evaluation of a case of possible PACNS. The cerebrospinal fluid (CSF) is abnormal in nearly 90% of patients with PACNS. The most common abnormalities are a mildly elevated CSF leukocyte count and an elevated CSF protein level; these levels tend to be more elevated in patients with biopsy-proven PACNS compared with patients diagnosed based on angiography findings. In one study of 101 patients with PACNS, the median leukocyte count was 5 cells/uL (range: 0–535). The median total protein concentration was 72 mg/dL (range: 15–1,034). The CSF white blood cell count is typically only mildly elevated and is often less than 10 cells/uL, yet even these potentially underwhelming numbers can have important implications for the presence of PACNS. Extremely high CSF pleocytosis should raise concern for infection or an alternative etiology.

C. Imaging Studies

MRI is the most sensitive imaging method for detecting findings compatible with PACNS. A completely normal brain MRI makes PACNS very unlikely. Although up to 97% of patients with PACNS have abnormalities on MRI, the abnormalities are not specific for vasculitis. The typical MRI findings are areas of brain infarction, many of which may be subclinical. Around 53% of PACNS patients present with clinical evidence of a stroke at the time of diagnosis. The infarctions may appear in multiple vascular territories and are often associated with nonspecific white matter lesions in a periventricular distribution (Figure 36–1). Leptomeningeal enhancement is also commonly observed in PACNS and may indicate a target for biopsy. Finally, a small percentage of patients present with mass-like lesions that mimic malignancies. In such patients, the diagnosis of PACNS is typically an incidental finding. In the course of the disease and during treatment, serial MRI can be performed to evaluate for new parenchymal lesions or areas of enhancement.

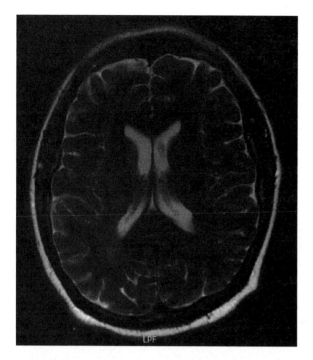

▲ **Figure 36–1.** Magnetic resonance imaging (MRI) lesions in a patient with CNS vasculitis. MRI demonstrates multifocal irregular linear and nodular enhancement in a periventricular distribution, with associated T2 signal hyperintensity.

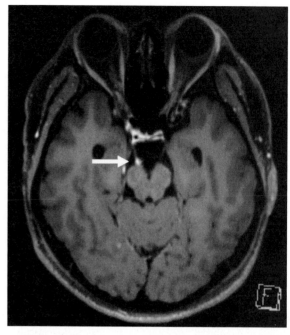

▲ **Figure 36–2.** High-resolution MRI protocoled to evaluate the vessel wall, showing focal vessel enhancement involving the right posterior cerebral artery with associated focal stenosis.

High-resolution MRI has assumed a growing role in the evaluation of patients with possible CNS vasculitis in recent years. This modality has the ability to evaluate detailed characteristics of the vessel wall itself as opposed to only the vascular lumen (the strength of angiography, discussed later). Patients with PACNS usually have smooth, concentric wall thickening as well as enhancement. In one study, the median length of enhancement was 6.1 mm with a range of 3–14 mm. The most common enhancing segments were the anterior cerebral artery, middle cerebral artery, supraclinoid internal carotid artery, and terminal internal carotid artery. The posterior circulation was less commonly involved. In contrast, in reversible cerebral vasoconstriction syndrome (RCVS), wall thickening may be present, but there is negligible to mild enhancement of the vessel wall. In PACNS, the median time to resolution of imaging findings is 7 months, compared to weeks to several months in RCVS. An example of focal vessel enhancement on a high-resolution MRI is shown in Figure 36–2.

Indirect or conventional angiography is commonly performed when PACNS is suspected, but its utility is overrated. The tendency of PACNS to involve small blood vessels below the resolution of angiography means that its sensitivity is poor. In addition, even the most classic finding of "beading" (alternating areas of stenosis and dilation) has poor specificity and can be present in PACNS mimickers, particularly those associated with vasospasm. Figure 36–3 demonstrates areas of severe stenosis of multiple intracranial vessels in a patient with biopsy-proven PACNS.

Computed tomography (CT) of the brain is much less sensitive in PACNS, detecting abnormalities in only about

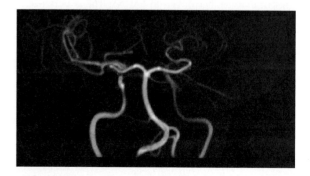

▲ **Figure 36–3.** Magnetic resonance angiography that demonstrates critical areas of stenosis involving multiple vessels, including the anterior cerebral artery (ACA) and middle cerebral artery (MCA) with poor visualization of multiple distal segments of the vasculature within this circulation.

two-thirds of the cases. However, CT is more sensitive than MRI at detecting hemorrhagic lesions.

D. Brain Biopsy

Brain biopsy, which is required for definitive diagnosis of PACNS, carries a risk of serious morbidity of 0–2% and is diagnostic in only 50–70% of cases. PACNS affects chiefly small- and medium-sized arteries and arterioles of the brain and spinal cord. The highest yield is obtained from biopsies that target an imaging abnormality and that include the leptomeninges. The yield of biopsy may be even lower in patients who present with recurrent strokes and have larger vessel abnormalities on neuroimaging that may be caused by more proximal vasculitic processes and may not be amenable to biopsy. Biopsies should also be sent for culture and should be stained for bacteria, fungi, and viruses. A hematopathologist as well as a neuropathologist should evaluate the biopsy to exclude the possibility of malignancy.

The histopathologic findings in the setting of positive biopsies are varied, almost certainly reflecting diverse etiologies of PACNS. The two most common histopathologic patterns seen in PACNS include granulomatous inflammation and lymphocytic vasculitis. Acute necrotizing vasculitis occurs less commonly. Some specimens may also have beta-amyloid peptide deposition. An example of lymphocytic CNS vasculitis is shown in Figure 36–4. Thrombosis and rupture can lead to infarction and hemorrhage of the surrounding tissue.

E. Evaluation

Most patients in whom CNS vasculitis is suspected require a thorough general assessment to exclude systemic causes of neurological dysfunction. The clinical presentation can help to guide an evaluation for other systemic vasculitides, rheumatologic conditions, infections, or malignancies that present in a manner similar to PACNS. The importance of the clinical history cannot be overemphasized in focusing the subsequent evaluation: Has the patient's presentation been subacute, in a manner compatible with PACNS? Are there features of the history to suggest that the possibility of a systemic process leading to CNS symptoms?

Once the evaluation has confirmed that the process is confined to the CNS, MRI is the most sensitive noninvasive imaging method overall and is preferred over CT, though most patients have a CT performed earlier in the evaluation anyway, however, to exclude processes such as subdural hematoma. Magnetic resonance angiography can help to identify abnormalities of the vascular lumen, potentially obviating the need for catheter-directed angiography. A lumbar puncture with CSF analysis can help support the diagnosis of CNS vasculitis and exclude infectious and malignant disorders mimicking PACNS. This is an essential test and should be performed as early as possible in the evaluation, and certainly before the start of treatment.

Whether all patients in whom PACNS is suspected should undergo brain biopsy is controversial, and decisions are invariably made on a case-by-case basis depending on the patient's presentation. Biopsies should be strongly considered in patients for whom substantial diagnostic uncertainty exists, and this is a significant subset of patients. Biopsy may also be essential if there appears to be no response to immunosuppressive therapy.

▶ Diagnostic Criteria

No validated diagnostic or classification criteria for PACNS are available. A working diagnosis of PACNS, however, sufficient to justify the institution of immunosuppressive therapy, requires the following:

1. Symptoms and signs of an acquired neurologic deficit consistent with the diagnosis of PACNS (eg, headache, confusion, and multiple strokes).

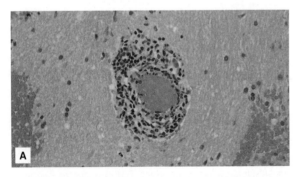 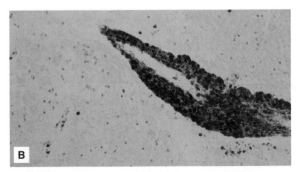

▲ **Figure 36–4.** Histopathologic findings in CNS vasculitis. **A:** Lymphocytic vasculitis with reactive gliosis. (See color insert.) **B:** CD3 stain highlighting T lymphocytes and showing intramural infiltration in a medium-sized blood vessel as well as scattered T lymphocytes in the brain parenchyma.

2. A brain or spinal cord biopsy demonstrating vasculitis in the absence of infection for a definite diagnosis, or classic angiographic evidence of CNS vasculitis for a possible diagnosis.

3. Exclusion of infection, a systemic vasculitis syndrome, or another disorder that could explain the clinical picture and findings.

▶ Differential Diagnosis

Many patients in whom PACNS is suspected are eventually found to have another mimicking condition, so the differential diagnosis should be reviewed meticulously (Table 36–2). Among the rheumatic diseases, systemic lupus erythematosus, polyarteritis nodosa, and granulomatosis with polyangiitis are the disorders that most often cause secondary CNS vasculitis. These conditions are rarely confused with PACNS, however, because their systemic symptoms, serologic tests, and imaging findings commonly implicate disease beyond the CNS.

Infections are more difficult to distinguish from PACNS because they, too, can lead to CNS vasculitis syndromes that are indistinguishable from PACNS on many clinical and imaging grounds. HIV, herpes zoster virus, syphilis, and histoplasmosis are among the infections that can mimic PACNS closely. Many patients who develop CNS infections that mimic PACNS have some degree of immunocompromised state that is often not appreciated fully until the development of CNS vasculitis. Many of the culprit infections, especially fungi, preferentially affect the base of the brain. In cases where brain biopsy is performed, tissue should routinely be sent for culture as well as infectious stains.

The possibility of herpes zoster virus–related vasculitis should be considered in a person who is immunosuppressed or who has had a recent outbreak of shingles in a V_1 distribution. Angiographic and even histopathologic abnormalities seen with infection are similar to those found in PACNS, particularly since infections can be limited to the CNS, leading to little systemic evidence of infection. In addition to culture and stains on biopsy specimens, patients in whom PACNS is suspected should be evaluated routinely for HIV infection and for syphilis. Special tests for other infections may be warranted if the patient is immunosuppressed or if the white blood count in the CSF is remarkably high.

Cocaine, amphetamines, and ephedrine derivatives are the drugs that most commonly produce CNS vasculopathy or vasospasm. There is some evidence that these drugs can produce vasculitis itself, and this should especially be suspected in younger patients. A detailed medication history for both legal and illicit drugs as well as urine toxicology should be performed.

Atherosclerosis should always be considered because it is so common, especially if the patient is over the age of 50 and has risk factors such as smoking, hypertension, hypercholesterolemia, or diabetes mellitus. If significant atherosclerosis is present, great caution should be taken with interpreting

Table 36–2. Differential diagnosis of primary angiitis of the CNS

Systemic vasculitis syndromes	• Granulomatosis with polyangiitis • Behcet's disease • Polyarteritis nodosa • Cryoglobulinemic vasculitis • Giant cell arteritis
Other rheumatologic disorders	• Systemic lupus erythematosus • Sarcoidosis • Sjogren syndrome • Cogan syndrome • Relapsing polychondritis
Infectious etiologies	• Bacteria (endocarditis, bacterial meningitis, tuberculosis, syphilis, Lyme disease, Bartonella, Mycoplasma) • Fungi (histoplasmosis, Aspergillus) • Viruses (herpes zoster, HIV, varicella zoster virus, West Nile virus, cytomegalovirus, hepatitis C) • Other (protozoal, amebiosis, cysticercosis)
Causes of multifocal strokes	• Cholesterol atheroembolism • Bacterial endocarditis or non-bacterial thrombotic endocarditis • Left atrial myxoma • Antiphospholipid syndrome and other hypercoagulable states
Vascular disorders	• Atherosclerosis • Antiphospholipid syndrome • Moyamoya disease • Reversible cerebral vasoconstriction syndrome • Drug-induced vasoconstriction • Cerebral autosomal dominant arteriopathy with subcortical infarcts and leukoencephalopathy (CADASIL) • Radiation vasculopathy
Miscellaneous	• Intravascular lymphoma or paraneoplastic conditions • Amyloidosis • Susac syndrome

Data from Hajj-Ali RA, Singhal AB, Molloy E, et al. Primary angiitis of the CNS. *Lancet Neurol.* 2011;10:561; Byram K, Hajj-Ali RA, Calabrese L. CNS Vasculitis: an Approach to Differential Diagnosis and Management. *Current Rheumatology Reports.* 2018;20(7):37.

angiographic studies, even though the presence of atherosclerosis does not preclude other forms of inflammatory vascular disease. Atherosclerotic plaques tend to be located eccentrically along blood vessel walls, often posing a stark contrast to the wall thickening in vasculitis that tends to be more concentric. Cerebral amyloid should be considered if the patient is over the age of 65 and has cerebral hemorrhages. Other conditions that can resemble PACNS are listed in Table 36–2.

Treatment

Patients with PACNS should be treated with glucocorticoids either as monotherapy or, more commonly, in combination with a glucocorticoid-sparing agent. Patients with severe disease or those with a rapid clinical decline should be given methylprednisolone 1000 mg intravenously daily for 3 days, followed by prednisone (or equivalent) 1 mg/kg/day (or prednisone 60 mg daily). Patients who have not progressed rapidly can begin treatment with prednisone alone, but careful consideration must be given to the likelihood of glucocorticoid toxicity. Patients at significant risks for glucocorticoid toxicity should be considered for approaches that have legitimate potential to limit adverse effects from glucocorticoid treatment.

No large randomized controlled trials exist to guide either the choice of glucocorticoid-sparing agent or the speed of prednisone taper. In general, prednisone should not be reduced until it is clear that manifestations of inflammation are improving and that control over the inflammatory process has been exerted. Although our ability to assess these measures in a definitive manner of often suboptimal, glucocorticoid tapering can usually begin after a month of treatment at prednisone 1 mg/kg/day and the dose can be tapered to discontinuation over the course of 6–12 months. Cyclophosphamide or other immunosuppressive drugs should be considered if the patient has severe deficits or if the disease progresses despite glucocorticoid therapy. Cyclophosphamide is the most commonly used immunosuppressive agent in addition to glucocorticoids and is commonly used for 3–6 months. Medications, such as mycophenolate, azathioprine, rituximab, and tocilizumab, have been used for maintenance therapy, although extremely limited data exist to support such approaches.

Patients with PACNS should avoid drugs that cause vasoconstriction or predispose to thrombosis (such as birth control pills, ephedrine, nicotine, and cocaine). Patients on prednisone should receive prophylaxis for *Pneumocystis* pneumonia, and attention should be paid to bone protective measures to reduce the risk of glucocorticoid-induced osteoporosis.

Prognosis

In the absence of treatment, almost all patients with PACNS will die of progressive neurologic deficits. Treatment has reduced mortality in the first year to 5%. In one case series, approximately 25% of patients had a relapse that led to a change in therapy and 17% died during a median follow-up period of 13 months. Large-vessel involvement, focal neurologic deficits, cognitive impairment, and cerebral infarction conferred a higher risk of death. Causes of death included cerebral infarction, myocardial infarction, stroke, and respiratory complications. Conversely, patients with prominent gadolinium enhancing lesions or meninges had a better prognosis.

Byram K, Hajj-Ali RA, Calbrese L. CNS vasculitis: an approach to differential diagnosis and management. *Curr Rheumatol Rep.* 2018;20(7):37. [PMID: 29846828]

Hajj-Ali RA, Singhal AB, Benseler S, et al. Primary angiitis of the CNS. *Lancet Neurol.* 2011;10:561. [PMID: 21601163]

Obusez EC, Hui F, Hajj-Ali RA, et al. High-resolution MRI vessel wall imaging: spatial and temporal patterns of reversible cerebral vasoconstriction syndrome and central nervous system vasculitis. *Am J Neuroradiol.* 2014;35(8):1527-1532. [PMID: 24722305]

Salvarani C, Brown RD Jr, Calamia KT, et al. Primary central nervous system vasculitis: analysis of 101 patients. *Ann Neurol.* 2007;62:442-451. [PMID: 17924545]

Schuster S, Bachmann H, Thom V, et al. Subtypes of primary angiitis of the CNS identified by MRI patterns reflect the size of affected vessels. *J Neurol Neurosurg Psychiatry.* 2017;88:749-755. [PMID: 28705900]

Thromboangiitis Obliterans (Buerger Disease)

37

John H. Stone, MD, MPH

ESSENTIALS OF DIAGNOSIS

► Active tobacco use, typically moderate to heavy.

► Severe digital ischemia without evidence of internal organ involvement.

► Angiography reveals segmental involvement of medium-sized arteries, with abrupt vascular cutoffs and corkscrew collaterals.

► The major vessel involvement occurs at the levels of the ankle and wrist, but the biggest clinical impact is on the digits, with severe digital ischemia leading to tissue loss.

► General Considerations

In thromboangiitis obliterans (TAO; also known as Buerger disease), the classic patient is a young male smoker. The mean age of onset is approximately 40 years, but the disease can occur in teenagers as well as in the elderly. Although the patients described initially were men, the disease may afflict women as well, probably in direct proportion to the number of women in any particular society who smoke. The precise mechanism underlying the relationship between TAO and cigarette smoking is unknown; autoimmune reactions to constituents of tobacco have been postulated. Cases may present several years after the start of smoking, but TAO does not occur in the absence of ongoing tobacco exposure.

There are four keys to the diagnosis of Buerger disease: (1) Recognition of clinical findings compatible with that condition, namely, digital ischemia that generally (and scrupulously) spares internal organs; (2) identification of the typical pattern of vascular involvement by angiography; (3) exclusion of diseases that may mimic TAO (Table 37–1); and (4) confirmation that the major risk factor, ongoing tobacco exposure, is present.

Because of difficulty in accessing medium-sized vessels for biopsy, the diagnosis is rarely confirmed by biopsy. The exceptions to this rule are superficial thrombophlebitis, which seldom comes to medical attention, and amputation specimens, by which time medical attention is (at least in some sense) too late. When biopsy is possible, acute TAO is characterized by a highly inflammatory thrombus, composed of a variety of cell types: lymphocytes, neutrophils, giant cells, and occasional microabscesses. Inflammation is typically more intense within the clot itself than within the walls of affected blood vessels. Fibrinoid necrosis, a hallmark of most systemic vasculitides, is absent in Buerger disease.

► Clinical Findings

A. Symptoms and Signs

1. Extremities—A major hallmark of Buerger disease is its confinement to the extremities. The initial symptoms may be nonspecific pains in the calf, foot, or toes. The progression of thrombosis and vasculitis can lead to horrific pain in the digits and limbs and ultimately to gangrene and tissue loss, through either autoamputation or elective amputation. For unknown reasons, however, other vascular beds (eg, the cardiac, pulmonary, renal, and mesenteric vasculature) are nearly always spared in Buerger disease.

Although Buerger disease has a predilection for the feet and toes, the hands and fingers may also be affected prominently. More than 60% of patients have abnormal Allen tests, indicating compromise of circulation to the hand; many demonstrate obliteration of the radial or ulnar artery pulses on physical examination. In contrast to atherosclerosis, which is a disease of the proximal vasculature, Buerger disease is characterized by inflammation and thrombosis of medium-sized, distal blood vessels (both arteries and veins), most intense at the levels of the ankles and wrists. The impact of this vascular distribution of disease is felt most acutely in the digits.

Table 37–1. Differential diagnosis of thromboangiitis obliterans.

Cardiovascular conditions
Atherosclerosis
Cardiogenic emboli (eg, infective endocarditis)
Systemic disorders associated with autoimmunity
Systemic lupus erythematosus
Antiphospholipid antibody syndrome
Systemic sclerosis (particularly limited scleroderma, or CREST syndrome)
Mixed connective tissue disease
Systemic vasculitides
Rheumatoid vasculitis
Polyarteritis nodosa
Granulomatosis with polyangiitis
Microscopic polyangiitis
Eosinophilic granulomatosis with polyangiitis
Cryoglobulinemia
Miscellaneous
Paraproteinemia
Ergotism

CREST, calcinosis, Raynaud phenomenon, esophageal motility, sclerodactyly, and telangiectasias.

2. Skin—The earliest lesion may be a superficial thrombophlebitis. This complaint is often disregarded by the patient or misdiagnosed as deep varicosities. Histologic examination of these lesions reveals an acute thrombophlebitis with marked perivascular infiltration. This herald lesion is then followed by progressive occlusion of the deeper veins and arteries, leading the patient to seek medical attention. Patients with Buerger disease may have splinter hemorrhages, arousing suspicions of infective endocarditis (Figure 37–1). Most cutaneous features of disease are those of a process involving

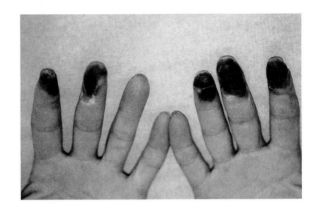

▲ **Figure 37–2.** Digital ischemia with gangrene in thromboangiitis obliterans.

the medium-sized vessels exclusively. Purpura, for example, a manifestation of small-vessel disease, is absent.

Gangrene occurs in the most distal tissues, that is, the toes and fingers, first (Figure 37–2). If the process remains undiagnosed or if the patient continues to smoke even after the diagnosis, larger portions of the extremities become compromised. In advanced cases, the major arterial supplies to the hands and feet may become occluded, leading to coolness and pain of the entire distal extremity, even necessitating below-the-knee amputations or other devastating tissue losses (Figure 37–3).

3. Peripheral nerve—Early in the disease, nonspecific pains in the calf, foot, or toes may recall a primary neuropathic process. These sensory symptoms may result from thickening of the tissues immediately surrounding the veins and arteries, leading to connective tissue proliferation around the nerve bundles that are intimately connected with

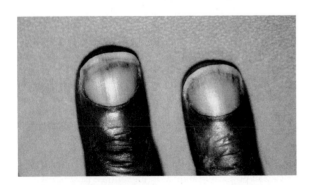

▲ **Figure 37–1.** Splinter hemorrhages can occur in thromboangiitis obliterans as well as in subacute bacterial endocarditis and primary forms of systemic vasculitis. Depicted here are the fingers of a 29-year-old man, photographed prior to amputation required by progression of his disease.

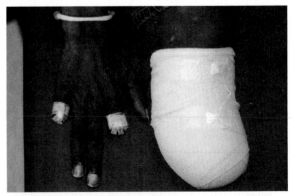

▲ **Figure 37–3.** As a consequence of failure to stop smoking, this patient with thromboangiitis obliterans required multiple amputations, including fingers on both hands and bilateral below-the-knee amputations.

the vasculature. True vasculitic neuropathy, however, does not occur in TAO.

4. Gastrointestinal tract and other organs—Extremely rare cases of TAO involving the gastrointestinal tract and central nervous system have been reported.

B. Laboratory Findings

There is no single diagnostic test for TAO. The demonstration of "corkscrew collaterals" (Figure 37–4A) on angiography is highly characteristic but not pathognomonic. Such vessels may also be observed in polyarteritis nodosa and other forms of medium-vessel vasculitis. Laboratory and radiologic investigations are important in patients with possible TAO, both to identify the typical vascular lesions and to exclude conditions that require other approaches to management. Table 37–2 lists the results of routine laboratory tests and specialized assays that are performed to exclude disorders masquerading as TAO.

The erythrocyte sedimentation rate and C-reactive protein levels are generally lower than observed in many other types of diffuse systemic vasculitis, but most patients have at least moderate elevations of these acute phase reactants. Routine hematology, serum chemistry, and urinalysis studies are normal in TAO; abnormalities in these tests suggest other diagnoses. Markers of hypercoagulable states that may be associated with widespread arterial thromboses, for example, antiphospholipid antibodies, should be investigated.

C. Imaging Studies

Echocardiography (possibly including a transesophageal study) should examine the heart valves and aortic root. Comprehensive angiographic studies that define the vasculature of the extremities, proximal aorta, gastrointestinal tract, and renal arteries should be considered. Such studies are critical in identifying vascular involvement typical of TAO and excluding atheroembolic sources as well as findings more typical of other vasculitides (eg, microaneurysms). Patients who smoke can also develop other disease leading to digital ischemia, including forms of systemic vasculitis.

The arterial involvement in TAO is highly segmental, with abrupt vascular occlusions interspersed with regions of vessels that appear angiographically normal (Figure 37–4B). In advanced cases, the thready appearance of vessels distal to the wrists and ankles may resemble a disorganized spider web (Figure 37–5). The most commonly involved vessels are the digital arteries of the fingers and toes as well as the palmar, plantar, tibial, peroneal, radial, and ulnar vessels.

▶ Differential Diagnosis

The major conditions in the differential diagnosis of TAO are cardiovascular diseases, autoimmune disorders, and systemic vasculitides (see Table 37–1). Among the

cardiovascular diseases, atherosclerosis and cardiogenic emboli are the principal considerations. Echocardiography (including transesophageal echocardiography) and angiography may be helpful in distinguishing TAO from cardiovascular conditions. Careful imaging of the proximal aorta is essential. In contrast to TAO, atherosclerotic disease characteristically affects the proximal vessels. Sources of cardiogenic emboli must be excluded by echocardiography and blood cultures.

Among the autoimmune disorders, systemic lupus erythematosus, the antiphospholipid syndrome, systemic sclerosis, and mixed connective tissue disease all may present with digital ischemia. Limited scleroderma (the CREST [calcinosis, Raynaud phenomenon, esophageal dysmotility, sclerodactyly, telangiectasias] syndrome) may pose special diagnostic challenges because of its propensity to cause digital loss, particularly when associated with anticentromere antibodies. Careful examination of the vasculature in the nailbeds, where dilated capillary loops appear in systemic sclerosis and other connective tissue disorders, may help distinguish these conditions from TAO. In contrast to connective tissue diseases, TAO is not associated with a significant autoantibody response.

The systemic vasculitides commonly associated with distal ischemia and gangrene are rheumatoid vasculitis, polyarteritis nodosa, granulomatosis with polyangiitis, microscopic polyangiitis, eosinophilic granulomatosis with polyangiitis (Churg-Strauss syndrome), and cryoglobulinemia. In general, the lack of visceral involvement in TAO helps distinguish Buerger disease from other vasculitides. For example, ulcerations of the shins, calves, and malleolar regions are atypical of TAO but common among other forms of vasculitis listed earlier. Vasculitic neuropathy, often striking in the other forms of systemic vasculitis, does not occur in TAO

▶ Treatment

The only effective intervention in TAO is complete smoking cessation. Despite the presence of some similarities of TAO to systemic vasculitides that affect medium-sized blood vessels and to hypercoagulable states, there is no role for either immunosuppressive interventions or anticoagulation in this condition. Moreover, because of the obliterative nature of the vascular inflammatory and thrombotic processes, the vasculature distal to the lesions generally offers no blood vessels large enough to sustain bypass grafts. Thrombolysis, which has not been studied in substantial numbers of patients, carries with it significant risks and perhaps a low likelihood of success, given the length of thromboses present in TAO. Effective pain control is important during periods of intense pain from digital ischemia (without it, patients may only smoke more).

A variety of investigational therapies have been used, with reports of mixed success.

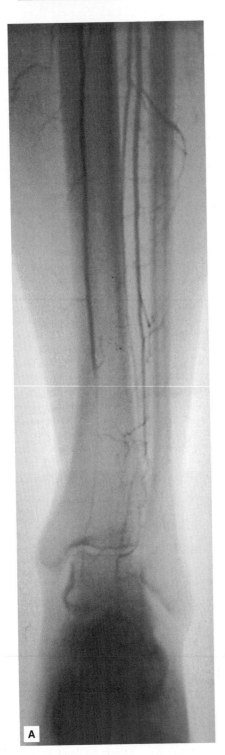

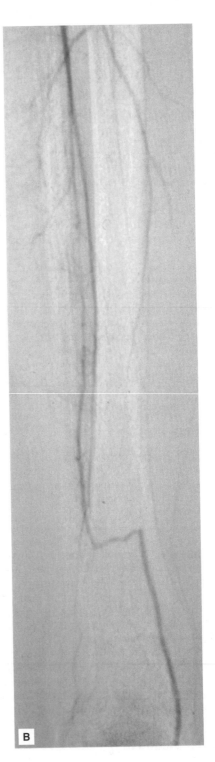

▲ **Figure 37–4.** Angiographic findings in thromboangiitis obliterans. **A:** Attenuation of the anterior tibial artery in the mid-calf. This artery forms a collateral at the site of occlusion with the peroneal artery. The posterior tibial artery is occluded superiorly. **B:** Abrupt arterial cutoffs several centimeters above the ankle, with minimal blood flow distal to the cutoffs.

Table 37–2. Laboratory and radiologic evaluation in possible thromboangiitis obliterans.

Test	Typical Results
Complete blood cell count	Normal. Mild elevations of the white blood cell and platelet count would not be unexpected
Renal and hepatic function	Normal
Urinalysis with microscopy	Normal
ESR/C-reactive protein	Mild to moderate elevations in patients with severe digital ischemia. Dramatically elevated acute phase reactants (eg, an ESR >100 mm/h) unusual
ANA	Negative
Rheumatoid factor	Negative
C3, C4	Normal
ANCA	Negative
Hepatitis B and C serologies	Negative
Antiphospholipid antibodies	Negative rapid plasma reagin and anticardiolipin antibody assays. Normal Russell viper venom time (for lupus anticoagulant)
Blood cultures	Negative
Echocardiography (or TEE)	No cardiac valvular vegetations. Normal aortic root.
Angiography	Corkscrew collaterals (see Figure 37–5). Abrupt cutoffs of medium-sized arteries at levels of the ankles and wrists, and often higher. Segmental areas of involvement, with diseased regions interspersed with normal-appearing arterial stretches

ANA, antinuclear antibody; ANCA, antineutrophil cytoplasmic antibody; ESR, erythrocyte sedimentation rate; TEE, transesophageal echocardiography.

▶ Complications

Without smoking cessation, TAO progresses inexorably through an obliterative vascular process, leading to coolness of the digits, hands, and feet; paresthesias; symptoms of intermittent claudication; skin ulcerations over the fingers and toes; and gangrenous infarctions of the extremities. Once established, the disease may be maintained by even small exposures to tobacco. Failure to stop smoking is associated with a dramatic increase in the risk of limb loss by amputation. Associations with second-hand smoking and smokeless tobacco have been reported but not confirmed. Finally, it should be remembered that even if the extent of vascular obliteration appears to offer little hope for limb preservation, the angiogram often looks far worse than the patient does. Complete tobacco abstinence can be remarkably successful in saving limbs.

Buerger L. Landmark publication from the *American Journal of the Medical Sciences*, "Thromboangiitis obliterans: a study of the vascular lesions leading to presenile spontaneous gangrene." 1908. *Am J Med Sci.* 2009;337:274. [PMID: 19365174]

Le Joncour A, Soudet S, Dupont A, et al; French Buerger's Network. Long-term outcome and prognostic factors of complications in thromboangiitis obliterans (Buerger's disease): a multicenter study of 224 patients. *J Am Heart Assoc.* 2018;7(23):e010677. [PMID: 30571594]

Olin JW. Thromboangiitis obliterans: 110 years old and little progress made. *J Am Heart Assoc.* 2018;7(23):e011214. [PMID: 30571606]

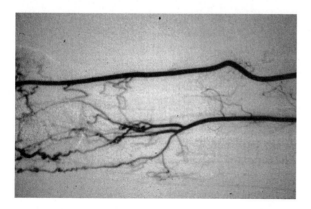

▲ **Figure 37–5.** Angiogram of the upper extremity in thromboangiitis obliterans, showing classic lesions— "corkscrew collaterals"—at the level of the patient's wrists.

38

Miscellaneous Forms of Vasculitis

Naomi Serling-Boyd, MD

John H. Stone, MD, MPH

RHEUMATOID VASCULITIS

ESSENTIALS OF DIAGNOSIS

▶ Rheumatoid vasculitis usually occurs in patients with severe, long-standing, nodular, destructive rheumatoid arthritis, even though the arthritis is not always still active.

▶ Palpable purpura, cutaneous ulcers (particularly in the malleolar region), digital infarctions, and peripheral sensory neuropathy are common manifestations.

▶ Tissue biopsy helps confirm the diagnosis of rheumatoid vasculitis, though the diagnosis is often clear from the clinical setting. Nerve conduction studies can identify involved nerves for biopsy. Muscle biopsies should be performed simultaneously with nerve biopsies to increase the diagnostic yield of the procedure.

General Considerations

Rheumatoid vasculitis (RV) is a variable-vessel vasculitis that occurs most commonly in patients with long-standing rheumatoid arthritis (RA). The underlying RA is characterized by rheumatoid nodules, destructive joint disease, and high titers of rheumatoid factor. The arthritis is commonly "burnt out" at the time of onset of vasculitis, and the onset of RV is typically on the order of 10–14 years after RA diagnosis. Particular human leukocyte antigen (HLA) haplotypes (those corresponding to the "shared epitope" [Chapter 13 on RA]), male sex, and smoking constitute risk factors for RV. The diagnosis of RV should be considered in any patient with RA in whom new constitutional symptoms, skin ulcerations, serositis, digital ischemia, or symptoms of sensory or motor nerve dysfunction develop. RV resembles polyarteritis nodosa because it leads to multiorgan dysfunction in the skin, peripheral nerves, gastrointestinal tract, and other

organs. Microaneurysms are not typical of RV, but cutaneous ulcerations, digital ischemia, mononeuritis multiplex, and mesenteric vasculitis are common.

Pathogenesis

Immune complex deposition and antibody-mediated destruction of endothelial cells both appear to contribute to RV. Certain HLA-DR4 alleles that predispose patients to severe RA may also heighten patients' susceptibility to RV. Cigarette smoking increases the risk of RV and has a synergistic interaction in this regard with antibodies to cyclic citrullinated peptides (anti-CCP antibodies). However, the inciting events leading to the development of RV among patients with previously destructive arthritis are not known. Factors in addition to vasculitis (eg, diabetes mellitus, atherosclerosis, and hypertension) likely play an important adjunctive role in promoting vascular occlusion. Peripheral vascular disease has been implicated as a potential risk factor for RV, but the central issue in RV is necrotizing inflammation of blood vessels.

Clinical Findings

A. Symptoms and Signs

1. Skin—Dermatologic findings, the most common manifestation of RV, may include palpable purpura, cutaneous ulcers (particularly in the malleolar region), and digital infarctions (Figure 38–1).

2. Nervous system—A peripheral sensory neuropathy is a common manifestation of RV. A mixed motor-sensory neuropathy or mononeuritis multiplex may also be seen. Central nervous system manifestations (such as strokes, seizures, and cranial nerve palsies) are considerably less common.

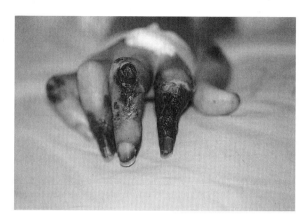

▲ **Figure 38–1.** Extensive digital necrosis in a case of severe rheumatoid vasculitis.

3. Eyes—Retinal vasculitis as a manifestation of RV is common but frequently asymptomatic. Necrotizing scleritis and peripheral ulcerative keratitis (Figure 38–2) pose threats to vision and require aggressive immunosuppressive therapy.

4. Serositis—Pericarditis and pleuritis may occur in association with RV. Other cardiopulmonary manifestations of RV, for example, cardiac ischemia, are unusual.

B. Laboratory Findings

Most laboratory abnormalities in RV such as elevations in the erythrocyte sedimentation rate, anemia, and thrombocytosis are nonspecific and merely reflect the presence of an inflammatory state. Hypocomplementemia, antinuclear antibodies (ANAs), atypical antineutrophil cytoplasmic antibodies (ANCAs) (by immunofluorescence testing but not enzyme immunoassay), and antiendothelial cell antibodies are all detected more frequently in patients with RV than in those with RA alone. All of these tests, however, are nonspecific. Cryoglobulins can rarely be seen as well. Rheumatoid factor is typically present at very high titers, and the same is true for anticyclic citrullinated peptide antibodies (ACPA).

C. Imaging Studies

The presence of bony erosions is a risk factor for the development of RV, but plain radiographs and other imaging studies have no consistent role in the evaluation of this disorder. Angiography is also of relatively little value because the blood vessels affected by RV are typically below the level of resolution of angiographic techniques, be they conventional angiography or those associated with magnetic resonance imaging (MRI) or computed tomography.

D. Special Tests

Because the treatment implications for RV are so severe, the diagnosis must be confirmed by tissue biopsy if it is not clear from the clinical setting. Deep skin biopsies (full-thickness biopsies that include some subcutaneous fat) taken from the edge of ulcers are very useful in detecting the presence of medium-vessel vasculitis. Nerve conduction studies help identify involved nerves for biopsy. Muscle biopsies (eg, of the gastrocnemius muscle) should be performed simultaneously with nerve biopsies. Biopsies typically show vasculitis affecting the small to medium vessels, with mononuclear or neutrophilic infiltration of the vessel wall. Necrosis, leukocytoclasis, and disruption of the elastic lamina can also be seen.

▶ Differential Diagnosis

Patients with erosive RA are at increased risk for infections. When patients with RA seek medical attention for the new onset of nonspecific systemic complaints, the possibility of infection (human immunodeficiency virus [HIV], varicella zoster, tuberculosis, or endocarditis, among others) must be considered first. Cholesterol emboli may cause digital ischemia and a host of other signs and symptoms that mimic vasculitis. Diabetes mellitus is another major cause of mononeuritis multiplex, but multiple mononeuropathies occurring over a short period of time would be unusual. Many clinical features of RV mimic those of polyarteritis nodosa and other forms of necrotizing vasculitis.

▶ Treatment

Therapy must reflect the severity of organ involvement. Small, relatively painless infarctions around the nail bed develop in some patients with nodular RA (Figure 38–3). Such lesions, known as Bywaters lesions, do not herald the presence of a necrotizing vasculitis and require no adjustment in the

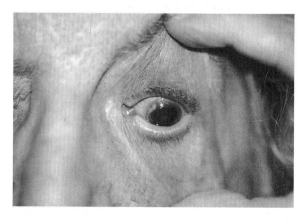

▲ **Figure 38–2.** Peripheral ulcerative keratitis in a patient with nodular, destructive rheumatoid arthritis and rheumatoid vasculitis.

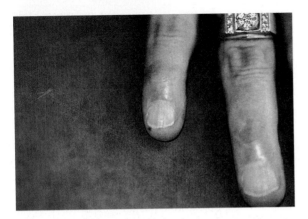

▲ **Figure 38–3.** Nail bed infarctions in a patient with rheumatoid arthritis. Such lesions do not necessarily herald the onset of rheumatoid vasculitis.

patients' therapy. With other disease manifestations, however, such as cutaneous ulcers, vasculitic neuropathy, and inflammatory eye disease, glucocorticoids may be required. Glucocorticoids remain a cornerstone of therapy for RV, but severe disease often requires a steroid-sparing agent, both for greater efficacy in controlling the vasculitis and for sparing of the potential adverse effects of high-dose glucocorticoids. Cyclophosphamide, used to treat many cases of RV, can be used with appropriate caution given the risks of infection and organ damage. Given the rarity of RV, there is a lack of data to guide the treatment decision of a particular disease-modifying antirheumatic drug or biologic agent. Rituximab and tocilizumab have been used with success, and it is reasonable to consider these agents prior to cyclophosphamide in patients who require additional therapy. Tumor necrosis factor (TNF) inhibitors have been used with success, as well.

Prognosis

RV is a treatable condition, but the development of this complication in patients who usually already have significant impairment is a poor prognostic indicator. In the past, around 40% of patients died within 5 years of onset. Although mortality has improved, it remains on the order of 26% even in the biologic era.

COGAN SYNDROME

 ESSENTIALS OF DIAGNOSIS

▶ The hallmark of Cogan syndrome is the presence of ocular inflammation and audiovestibular dysfunction. These findings may be accompanied by evidence of a systemic vasculitis.

▶ Interstitial keratitis is the most common form of ocular involvement.

▶ Audiovestibular dysfunction may lead to the acute onset of vertigo, tinnitus, nausea, vomiting, and hearing loss, and should be differentiated from Meniere disease.

▶ Vasculitis in Cogan syndrome may take the form of aortitis, renal artery stenosis, or occlusion of the great vessels.

General Considerations

Cogan syndrome (CS), an immune-mediated condition that primarily affects young adults, is associated with ocular inflammation (usually interstitial keratitis) and audiovestibular dysfunction. This syndrome may be accompanied by a systemic vasculitis of large- and medium-sized arteries that resembles Takayasu arteritis in certain respects. Typical CS consists of interstitial keratitis and sensorineural hearing loss, with an interval between the two of less than 2 years. "Atypical" CS is associated with manifestations such as scleritis, choroiditis, generally more robust evidence of systemic inflammation, and intervals between the onset of the ophthalmic and auditory complications of longer than 2 years.

Pathogenesis

The onset of CS is frequently preceded by an upper respiratory tract infection. The pathogenesis remains poorly understood, though many of the different manifestations are thought to be due to vasculitis. Autoantibodies directed against human cornea and human inner ear tissue have been identified in patients with CS, but the clinical utility of testing for such antibodies is not clear. Infectious agents such as *Treponema pallidum* and *Borrelia burgdorferi* can lead to clinical features that mimic idiopathic CS closely, and it is essential to exclude such infections by appropriate testing. The fact that idiopathic CS responds to long-term immunosuppression reduces the likelihood that CS is the direct consequence of an unidentified pathogen affecting the eyes, ears, and blood vessels. It is certainly conceivable, however, that CS is the indirect consequence of a pathogen or other trigger of the immune system that induces an immune response that continues to attack the host long after the pathogen or trigger has been eliminated.

Clinical Findings

A. Symptoms and Signs

1. Eye—The most common ocular manifestation of CS is interstitial keratitis, which is characterized by the abrupt onset of photophobia, lacrimation, and eye pain. CS may also be associated with inflammation in other parts of the eye. Other less common ocular manifestations include scleritis (Figure 38–4), peripheral ulcerative keratitis, episcleritis,

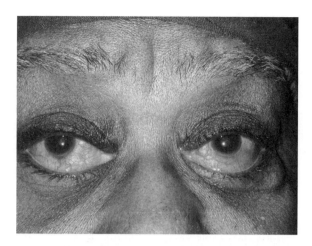

▲ **Figure 38–4.** Bilateral scleritis in a patient with Cogan syndrome who had suffered the rapid onset of sensorineural hearing loss in both ears.

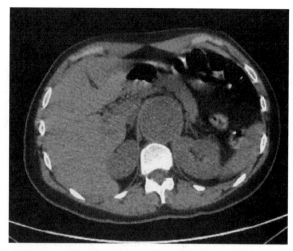

▲ **Figure 38–5.** Computed tomography showing a thoracic aorta aneurysm in a patient with Cogan syndrome who on histologic evaluation was found to have aortitis.

anterior uveitis, conjunctivitis, papillitis, vasculitic optic neuropathy, and retinal vasculitis.

2. Ear—Patients with CS frequently suffer the acute onset of vertigo, tinnitus, nausea, and vomiting. These symptoms may be enormously disabling. The audiovestibular symptoms may occur before or after the onset of ocular disease and are often separated in onset by weeks or months. If not treated promptly and aggressively, permanent hearing frequently occurs. Recurrent attacks, which are common, may cause decremental loss of hearing. Ultimately, complete hearing loss occurs in as many as 60% of patients.

3. Large-vessel vasculitis—The most common manifestation of vasculitis in patients with CS is aortitis. Aortitis may lead to dilatation of the aorta and subsequent incompetence of the aortic valve. Aneurysm or dissection can occur as a complication of aortitis (Figure 38–5). Involvement of aortic branches (Figure 38–6) may cause arm or leg claudication. Renal artery stenosis or occlusion of the great vessels may also occur. These manifestations may be accompanied by nonspecific constitutional symptoms such as malaise, fever, or weight loss, as well as arthralgias and frank arthritis.

4. Other—Systemic symptoms are seen in up to half of patients and can include headache (up to 40% of patients), arthralgia (35% of patients in one case series), fever (around 25% of patients), arthritis, myalgia, gastrointestinal manifestations (abdominal pain, melena), and neurologic events (rare, can be caused by strokes).

B. Laboratory Findings

Laboratory findings are nondiagnostic and generally reflect the presence of inflammation. Anemia, leukocytosis, and thrombocytosis can be seen in a minority of patients, and

inflammatory markers are not reliably elevated. Exclusion of syphilis with both treponemal and nontreponemal testing is essential. Granulomatosis with polyangiitis must also be excluded with testing for ANCAs and surveillance for signs of vasculitis in other organs, for example the kidneys and lungs.

C. Imaging Studies

Gadolinium-enhanced T1-weighted MRI studies may demonstrate a hyperintensity in the membranous labyrinth secondary to vessel inflammation in the stria vascularis. This enhancement is not seen in patients with inactive CS and may be useful in identifying the activity of the disease. Brainstem MRI studies are also essential to exclude tumors of the cerebellopontine angle, which may mimic the audiovestibular features of CS. Angiography may be useful to define the involvement of the great vessels, but conventional angiography is seldom necessary now as this technique has been supplanted by cross-sectional imaging approaches. Magnetic resonance angiography or computed tomography angiography are useful in evaluating for signs of aortitis such as vessel wall thickness and edema as well as the degree of luminal stenosis.

D. Special Tests

Formal audiometric testing is important early in the evaluation to distinguish conductive hearing loss from sensorineural hearing dysfunction. In CS, audiometry demonstrates sensorineural hearing loss that preferentially affects the low- and high-range frequencies. Serial audiometry may be a useful way to document response to therapy, although subsequent hearing loss is not always due to active disease.

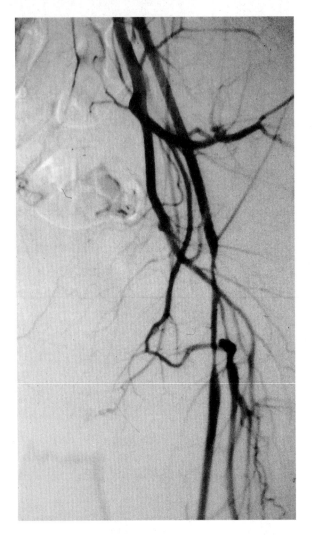

▲ **Figure 38–6.** Large-vessel vasculitis in Cogan syndrome. Femoral artery disease led to lower extremity claudication.

▶ **Differential Diagnosis**

The differential diagnosis of immune-mediated inner ear disease (ie, sensorineural hearing loss with or without vestibular dysfunction) is shown in Table 38–1. As hearing loss and tinnitus are often among the initial presenting symptoms, it is important to distinguish CS from Meniere disease. Symptoms in Meniere disease consist of vertigo, fluctuation in hearing, fullness, and tinnitus, and generally are unilateral and last for only minutes to hours, in comparison to CS, where symptoms are often bilateral and last for days, and sometimes indefinitely. Inflammatory eye disease may be caused by a variety of pathogens, including bacterial (eg, *Chlamydiae*, *Neisseria*), spirochetal

Table 38–1. Differential diagnosis of the audiovestibular complications of Cogan syndrome.

Alternate Diagnoses	Comments
Immune-mediated inner ear disease	Sensorineural hearing loss and vestibular dysfunction in the absence of eye inflammation.
Syphilis	Latent and tertiary forms of this disease. Ordering both rapid plasma reagin and FTA-ABS is essential to rule out syphilis.
Other infections	Lyme disease, mumps
Acoustic neuroma	Performance of brainstem magnetic resonance imaging essential to exclude this tumor.
Ménière syndrome	Inner ear disturbances in Ménière syndrome are generally more intermittent, with a waxing/waning character, lasting minutes to hours, and are often unilateral.
Systemic vasculitides	Granulomatosis with polyangiitis (formerly Wegener granulomatosis), giant cell arteritis
Collagen vascular diseases	Sjögren syndrome
Other inflammatory conditions	Sarcoidosis, Susac syndrome
Barotrauma	Other etiologies of perilymph fistula formation
Medications	Aminoglycosides, loop diuretics, antimalarials

FTA-ABS, fluorescent treponemal antibody, absorption test.

(eg, *Borrelia burgdorferi*), viral (eg, herpes simplex, varicella zoster), and mycobacterial (eg, *Mycobacterium tuberculosis, M leprae*).

▶ **Treatment**

Some manifestations of CS respond well to symptomatic therapy. In general, the ocular manifestations are more amenable to therapy than the auditory complications. Interstitial keratitis may be treated with topical atropine or topical glucocorticoids, though involvement of the posterior eye requires systemic therapy. Sensorineural hearing loss in CS is analogous to rapidly progressive glomerulonephritis in other forms of systemic vasculitis: prompt treatment with immunosuppression is indicated. In addition to glucocorticoids (often with prednisone starting at 1 mg/kg/day), cyclophosphamide, azathioprine, methotrexate, and mycophenolate mofetil have all been used. There are no randomized controlled trials, and the basis for choosing among these agents is largely empiric. The role for biologic agents, if any, is not well understood, though there have been cases of successful treatment with TNF inhibitors and rituximab. For patients with advanced, irreversible hearing loss, hearing aids and cochlear implants may help. Vestibular retraining may be required for some patients with significant cochlear damage.

Complications

The prevention of complications depends directly on the rapid recognition of this diagnosis, and the equally swift institution of therapy. Permanent damage may result early in the course of immune-mediated inner ear disease, and hearing deficits will not respond to therapy if initiated too late. Therefore, a high index of suspicion for this diagnosis must be maintained when evaluating patients with compatible complaints.

Prognosis

Even if the initial event is recognized and responds to therapy, recurrent bouts of sensorineural hearing loss may cause the gradual loss of hearing. Roughly 50% of patients will eventually experience complete hearing loss. On the contrary, permanent loss of vision is very uncommon, and most patients retain relatively normal vision despite flares.

URTICARIAL VASCULITIS

ESSENTIALS OF DIAGNOSIS

▶ The lesions of urticarial vasculitis are frequently associated with burning, pain, and bruising, rather than pruritus, and take more than 24 hours to resolve.

▶ Immunofluorescence on skin biopsy specimen is the critical test. Intense staining for immunoreactants (ie, IgG, IgM, C3, C4, C1q) not only in and around small blood vessel walls but also in a ribbon along the dermal/epidermal junction is pathognomonic of hypocomplementemic urticarial vasculitis.

▶ Evaluation for a medication or drug, infection, or malignancy as an underlying cause should be pursued.

General Considerations

Urticarial vasculitis (UV) is a leukocytoclastic vasculitis that presents as hives (often associated with pain or discomfort) that last longer than 24 hours. Although UV is occasionally seen in isolation, it can be seen in association with connective tissue disorders such as serum sickness, cryoglobulinemia, and systemic lupus erythematosus (SLE). It is a rare condition, seen in 0.5 per 100,000 person-years, is more common in women, and most commonly presents in the fourth decade.

UV targets the capillaries and postcapillary venules in the skin, leading to the appearance of hive-like lesions. In evaluating patients with this problem, it is critical to distinguish cases associated with hypocomplementia from those in which the serum complement levels are normal.

Hypocomplementemic UV (HUV) is associated with depressed serum levels of C3 and C4 and often with antibodies directed against the C1q component of complement. Such cases often overlap with known connective tissue disorders, particularly SLE. At the severe end of the spectrum of this disorder are patients with a distinct disorder known as the **hypocomplementemic urticarial vasculitis syndrome** (HUVS).

Normocomplementemic urticarial vasculitis (NUV) is a subset of cutaneous leukocytoclastic angiitis (see Chapter 33) in which leukocytoclastic vasculitis manifests clinically as urticaria. In general, these cases are secondary to "hypersensitivity" reactions (usually caused by a medication) and respond to discontinuation of the offending agent. This form of UV is not discussed further in this chapter.

Pathogenesis

Hypocomplementemic UV is mediated at least in part by immune complex deposition (type III hypersensitivity). In one model, following an unknown inciting event, immune complexes become activated and lead to complement activation, and C3a and C5a are anaphylatoxins that lead to activation of mast cells and eosinophils. This then leads to the formation of the typical urticarial wheal. The eosinophils are gradually replaced by neutrophils, leading to the leukocytoclastic destruction of capillary walls. Antibodies to C1q are a marker of hypocomplementemic UV and likely contribute substantially to the finding of hypocomplementemia because they target an early component of the classical pathway of complement activation. The trigger(s) for anti-C1q antibodies remain unknown, and their full role in disease pathogenesis remains to be elucidated. Antibodies to C1q are not entirely specific for hypocomplementemic UV; they are also found in SLE.

Clinical Findings

A. Symptoms and Signs

The lesions of UV, typically between 0.5 and 2.0 cm in diameter (Figure 38–7), are frequently associated with burning or pain rather than pruritus. In contrast to common urticaria, UV lesions usually require more than 24 hours to resolve and typically leave small amounts of bruising and hyperpigmentation in the skin, caused by red blood cell extravasation.

Hypocomplementemic UV may also be associated with malaise, arthralgias, fever, and glomerulonephritis, and can affect virtually any organ system. In contrast to SLE, HUVS is characterized not only by recurrent or chronic UV but also by angioedema. Moreover, severe chronic obstructive pulmonary disease (COPD) and uveitis—manifestations that are highly atypical of SLE—often complicate HUV. Jaccoud arthropathy has been noted in some patients with HUVS and possibly correlates with the presence of cardiac valvular lesions.

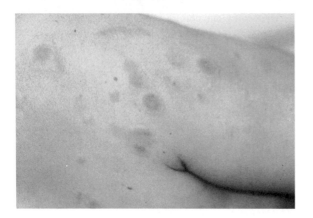

▲ **Figure 38–7.** Lesions of hypocomplementemic urticarial vasculitis.

B. Laboratory Findings

Serum C3, C4, and CH50 levels are depressed in HUV, and anti-C1q autoantibodies can be present. The presence of these antibodies is not pathognomonic, since they also may be found in patients with SLE who do not have UV. Patients with hypocomplementemic UV can have ANAs as well as antibodies to extractable nuclear antigens, though the finding of such antibodies strongly suggests SLE.

C. Special Tests

When HUV is suspected, patients should undergo two 3- to 4-mm punch biopsies, one of which should be evaluated with direct immunofluorescence. Hematoxylin and eosin staining of skin biopsy specimens reveal a leukocytoclastic vasculitis in the superficial dermis. Older lesions may have a predominantly lymphocytic infiltrate. The critical test is the performance of immunofluorescence on the skin biopsy specimen, which reveals intense staining for immunoreactants (ie, IgG, IgM, C3, C4, C1q) not only in and around small blood vessel walls but also in a ribbon along the dermal/epidermal junction. These findings are pathognomonic of hypocomplementemic UV. Fibrinoid deposits, perivascular infiltrates, extravasation of red blood cells, and injury to and swelling of the endothelial cells can also be seen.

▶ Differential Diagnosis

Skin lesions of hypocomplementemic UV must be distinguished from common urticaria (which is characterized by pruritic lesions that resolve completely over 2–8 hours, leaving no traces of the original lesion, and are generally associated with normal complement levels) (Table 38–2), neutrophilic urticaria (a persistent, treatment-refractory form of urticaria not associated with vasculitis), and

Table 38–2. Classic urticaria versus hypocomplementemic urticarial vasculitis.

	Classic Urticaria	Hypocomplementemic Urticarial Vasculitis
Appearance of lesion	Erythematous plaques, often lasting 2–8 hours	Erythematous plaques, sometimes with bruising or hyperpigmentation, lasting >24 hours
Cutaneous symptoms	Pruritus	Burning and pain > pruritus
Systemic symptoms	Rare; angioedema rarely present	Angioedema may be present, constitutional symptoms as well as other organ involvement (musculoskeletal, renal, pulmonary, gastrointestinal, ocular, cardiovascular, or neurologic) may be present
Labs	No specific findings	Hypocomplementemia (low total complement, C3, C4, C1q), anti-C1q antibody
Biopsy results	Dermal edema, perivascular infiltrate	Leukocytoclastic vasculitis (with positive direct immunofluorescence, showing Ig and complement deposition in blood vessels at upper dermis and/or dermal-epidermal junction) as well as dermal edema
Response to treatment	Generally sufficient response to antihistamines	Only 30% response to antihistamines. Require corticosteroids and often other immunosuppressive medications (hydroxychloroquine, mycophenolate, colchicine, dapsone, omalizumab, cyclophosphamide)

normocomplementemic UV (see earlier). The differential also encompasses other causes of acute and chronic urticaria, acquired angioedema, erythema multiforme minor, neutrophilic dermatoses, "arthritis, hives, and angioedema" (AHA) syndrome, and autoinflammatory disorders.

▶ Treatment

In around 80% of cases, UV responds to glucocorticoids alone. Other therapies such as hydroxychloroquine, dapsone, mycophenolate mofetil, colchicine, cyclosporine, or omalizumab may be required. Antihistamines may be used, though are only effective in around 30% of patients and are generally not sufficient as treatment in the absence of concomitant immunosuppressive therapy.

HUVS is frequently a therapeutic challenge. Serious cases, particularly those presenting with glomerulonephritis or other organ involvement, may require treatment with high doses of glucocorticoids, cyclophosphamide, or other immunosuppressive medications. Angioedema, COPD, and cardiac valvular abnormalities may all necessitate other specific interventions.

Prognosis

Hypocomplementemic UV frequently reflects the presence of an underlying disorder, which may influence the prognosis substantially. It is almost never fatal, except in cases associated with malignancy. HUVS may be associated with multiple complications (eg, severe COPD) that affect prognosis adversely.

ERYTHEMA ELEVATUM DIUTINUM

ESSENTIALS OF DIAGNOSIS

▶ New lesions come in the form of tender papules, associated with pruritus or a burning sensation.

▶ Lesions develop into red, reddish-brown, or purple papules or nodules.

▶ Lesions may coalesce to form large plaques, usually over the extensor surfaces of joints; the location can help to differentiate it from other forms of cutaneous vasculitis.

General Considerations

Erythema elevatum diutinum (EED) is a chronic, recurring cutaneous vasculitis in which tender papules appear on the extensor surfaces of the extremities. The lesions can be asymptomatic, though the onset of these lesions is usually heralded by the presence of pruritus or stinging, followed by the development of tender papules or nodules that coalesce with others to form plaques. The skin findings are frequently located near joints, such as on the extensor surfaces of the hands and fingers. There is no racial predilection, and while EED can present at any age, it is most common in the fourth and sixth decades.

Pathogenesis

The pathogenesis of EED is unknown but may involve recurrent immune complex deposition (as direct immunofluorescence is often indicative of immunoglobulin and complement deposition), followed by incomplete attempts at healing. Persistence of an antigen, with a subsequent increase in dendrocyte activity, may also play a role in its pathogenesis. There is an association between EED and multiple infections (including HIV, hepatitis B and C, tuberculosis, and streptococcal infections), autoimmune diseases (such as RA, relapsing polychondritis, and type 1 diabetes mellitus), and the paraproteinemias (such as multiple myeloma).

Clinical Findings

A. Symptoms and Signs

A new lesion is heralded by the presence of pruritus or a burning sensation in the skin, which then leads to the development of a red, reddish-brown, or purple papule or nodule. These lesions may coalesce to form large plaques, usually over the extensor surfaces of joints. With healing, the lesions often assume a yellowish or brown color, resembling xanthomata. Lesions can remain asymptomatic as well.

B. Laboratory Findings

Patients in whom EED is suspected should be screened for possible causes, including HIV infection, viral hepatitis, syphilis, cryoglobulinemia, and monoclonal gammopathy. When appropriate, patients may benefit from screening for associated autoimmune diseases as well.

C. Special Tests

Skin biopsy specimens usually show a nonspecific leukocytoclastic vasculitis with C3 deposition and are important for excluding nonvasculitis mimickers. Mixed inflammation consisting of neutrophils, macrophages, histiocytes, and eosinophils can surround blood vessels. In older lesions, the neutrophils are replaced by histiocytes, and there is marked granulation tissue and fibrosis.

Differential Diagnosis

Biopsy of lesions at various stages of development may demonstrate findings that are also consistent with a wide variety of diagnoses, including Sweet syndrome, pyoderma gangrenosum, drug reaction, erythema multiforme, fibrous histiocytoma, Kaposi sarcoma, xanthoma, bacillary angiomatosis, and necrobiotic xanthogranuloma. The diagnosis can be established only by clinical judgment, supplemented by supportive findings on pathology.

Treatment

When a cause (whether infectious, hematological, or rheumatologic) can be established, EED may respond to treatment of the underlying disorder. It is well established, for instance, that patients with EED as a consequence of HIV infection experience a regression of the cutaneous lesions with institution of highly active antiretroviral therapy. Nonspecific therapies are less successful. Lesions may be suppressed by dapsone, which is effective in around 80% of cases, but tend to recur when the drug is stopped. Lesions may also respond to tetracycline, colchicine, chloroquine, methotrexate, and glucocorticoids (either topical, intralesional, or systemic).

Complications

Although recurrent and frequently unresponsive to therapy, EED is limited to the skin and does not lead to significant morbidity.

Prognosis

The prognosis associated with EED itself, even when unresponsive to therapy, is generally quite good. Lesions can undergo spontaneous evolution over the course of years. The overall prognosis for the patient, however, largely depends on the underlying disease process.

DRUG-INDUCED ANCA-ASSOCIATED VASCULITIS

ESSENTIALS OF DIAGNOSIS

► Cutaneous eruptions, such as palpable purpura or a maculopapular rash limited to the lower extremities, are the most common manifestation of drug-induced ANCA-associated vasculitis.

► Frequently associated with very high titers of antineutrophil cytoplasmic antibodies (ANCA) directed against myeloperoxidase as opposed to proteinase-3.

► Tissue biopsy provides a definitive diagnosis.

General Considerations

Drug-induced, ANCA-associated vasculitis (AAV) is a form of vasculitis that can be induced by both legitimate medications and drugs of abuse. The majority of cases are associated with ANCA directed against myeloperoxidase, often in very high titers. Drug-induced AAV sometimes resolves following discontinuation of the offending agent. Other cases, however, are indistinguishable from idiopathic AAV and require intensive therapy with glucocorticoids, biologic agents such as anti-CD20 therapies, and cytotoxic agents.

Many cases of drug-induced AAV are associated with relatively minor symptoms (eg, constitutional symptoms, arthralgias or arthritis, and purpura). Propylthiouracil is a well-documented cause of drug-induced AAV. Other drugs implicated thus far include hydralazine, sulfasalazine, minocycline, D-penicillamine, ciprofloxacin, phenytoin, clozapine, allopurinol, pantoprazole, levamisole, and more recently, the TNF inhibitors.

Levamisole was recognized as a cause of drug-induced AAV when it was used to cut cocaine starting in the early 2000s; it can often lead to a severe form of systemic vasculitis. More recently, the use of immune checkpoint inhibitors (anti-PD-1, anti-PD-L1, and anti-CTLA4) have been shown to cause a variety of autoimmune and inflammatory manifestations; although AAV is less common, it has been reported.

Pathogenesis

All of the events in the pathogenesis of drug-induced AAV remain undefined. Propylthiouracil is known to accumulate within neutrophil granules and alter myeloperoxidase, an event that may trigger the production of antimyeloperoxidase ANCA. The presence of this human model of ANCA-associated disease forms one of the strongest arguments for a direct contribution of ANCA to the pathophysiology of other human disorders. Mouse models also strongly support the concept that ANCA may be pathogenic in humans.

Clinical Findings

A. Symptoms and Signs

Cutaneous eruptions are the most common manifestation of drug-induced AAV. These often present as palpable purpura (Figure 38–8) or a maculopapular rash limited to the lower extremities. Unlike other AAV, the skin lesions in the drug-induced form frequently appear in "crops" (ie, simultaneously). Arthralgias and myalgias are common. The kidneys and upper respiratory tract may also be involved, as with the

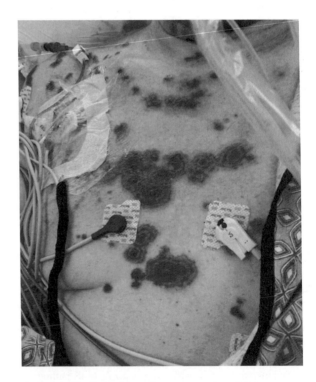

▲ **Figure 38–8.** Lesions of cutaneous vasculitis in a patient receiving durvalumab (anti-PD-L1) who had antibodies to both myeloperoxidase and proteinase-3, and had a biopsy demonstrating acute necrotizing vasculitis of both small and medium vessels.

classic forms of AAV, though the renal involvement tends to be less severe in drug-induced AAV.

B. Laboratory Findings

In drug-induced AAV, very high titers of antimyeloperoxidase antibodies are characteristic. Reports of cases associated with anti–proteinase-3 antibodies are rare. Levamisole-induced AAV can be associated with a double positive ANCA, with antibodies to both myeloperoxidase and proteinase-3). Positive ANAs, anti-dsDNA, and antihistone antibodies can also be seen in some cases, particularly those associated with hydralazine or minocycline. Even when the vasculitis resolves after discontinuation of the causative agent and initiation of immunosuppression, ANCA titers often remain elevated. All patients should undergo a urine toxicology evaluation for cocaine.

C. Special Tests

Tissue biopsy is usually necessary to provide a definitive diagnosis of vasculitis.

▶ Differential Diagnosis

Drug-induced AAV is frequently slow to resolve after cessation of the offending agent and may be difficult to distinguish from the primary ANCA-associated vasculitides. In general, the manifestations of drug-induced AAV are mild and responsive to short courses of immunosuppression, although this is not always the case. Most cases of levamisole-induced vasculitis require immunosuppression, but the critical therapeutic intervention is cessation of the offending agent.

▶ Treatment

The first step in treatment is the identification of the potential offending agents. Clinicians should take into account all exposures during the 6 months before the onset of symptoms, including nonprescription medications, herbal and dietary supplements, and illicit substances. Withdrawal of the offending agent may result in the resolution of the symptoms, although this may take months and may require the withdrawal of numerous agents simultaneously. Patients should not be rechallenged with the same agent in the future.

Patients with severe organ involvement may require aggressive immunosuppression with glucocorticoids and other agents. The required length of therapy in drug-induced AAV may be shorter than that recommended for primary AAV.

▶ Prognosis

Overall, the prognosis associated with drug-induced AAV is quite good. Organ involvement is frequently limited to the skin, and even systemic involvement frequently responds to lower doses of immunosuppressive agents administered for shorter periods of time than that required for primary AAV.

Davis MDP, van der Hilst JCH. Mimickers of urticaria: urticarial vasculitis and autoinflammatory diseases. *J Allergy Clin Immunol Pract.* 2018;6(4):1162-1170. [PMID: 29871797]

Grau RG. Drug-induced vasculitis: new insights and a changing lineup of suspects. *Curr Rheumatol Rep.* 2015;17:71. [PMID: 26503355]

Gluth MB, Baratz K, Driscoll E, et al. Cogan syndrome: a retrospective review of 60 patients throughout a half century. *Mayo Clin Proc.* 2006;81(4). [PMID: 16610568]

Kessel A, Vadasz Z, Toubi E. Cogan syndrome—pathogenesis, clinical variants and treatment approaches. *Autoimmun Rev.* 2014;13:351-354. [PMID: 24418297]

Kolkhir P, Grakhova M, Bonnekoh H, et al. Treatment of urticarial vasculitis: a systematic review. *J Allergy Clin Immunol.* 2019;143(2):458-466. [PMID: 30268388]

Pendergraft WF, Niles JL. Trojan horses: drug culprits associated with antineutrophil cytoplasmic autoantibody (ANCA) vasculitis. *Curr Opin Rheumatol.* 2014;26:42. [PMID: 24276086]

Osteoarthritis

39

Allan C. Gelber, MD, MPH, PhD

ESSENTIALS OF DIAGNOSIS

- ▶ Joint pain exacerbated by activity and relieved with rest.
- ▶ Brief, self-limited morning stiffness.
- ▶ Absence of constitutional symptoms.
- ▶ Examination notable for increased bony prominence at the joint margin, crepitus or a grating sensation, and tenderness over the joint line.
- ▶ Diagnosis supported by radiographic features of joint-space narrowing and spur (or osteophyte) formation.

General Considerations

An estimated 54 million adult Americans have been informed by a doctor that they have arthritis, gout, lupus, rheumatoid arthritis, or fibromyalgia. Among this group, osteoarthritis is the leading cause of arthritis. Joint pain is a frequent symptom that often prompts a patient with osteoarthritis to seek medical attention. Consequently, osteoarthritis is a prominent consideration in the differential diagnosis of joint pain. The challenge for clinicians is to correctly identify the cause of a patient's pain and to initiate appropriate therapy, both pharmacologic and nonpharmacologic approaches.

Synonymous with degenerative joint disease, osteoarthritis is characterized by joint pain related to use, self-limited stiffness upon awakening in the morning, an audible grating sound or crepitus on palpation, the presence of tenderness over the affected joint line, and frequently diminished range of motion in use of the affected part of the body.

Characteristic sites of involvement in the peripheral skeleton include the hand (distal interphalangeal [DIP] joint, proximal interphalangeal [PIP] joint, and first carpometacarpal joint) (Figure 39–1), knee (Figure 39–2), and hip (Figure 39–3). Involvement of the finger joints is so characteristic that eponyms have been assigned to osteoarthritic involvement at the DIP and PIP joints, labeled Heberden's

nodes and Bouchard nodes, respectively. Constitutional symptoms are absent. As such, the affected patient generally feels well, globally, aside from the localized symptoms arising from the involved osteoarthritic joint. The diagnosis of osteoarthritis can usually be made easily and confidently based on the history and examination alone. When necessary, the bedside diagnosis of osteoarthritis can be supported by plain radiography.

Epidemiology

At the population level, osteoarthritis results in substantial morbidity and disability, particularly among the elderly. Osteoarthritis is the leading indication for joint arthroplasty surgery performed in the United States; in 2010, an estimated 2.5 millions Americans had undergone hip replacement surgery and 4.7 individuals had received knee replacements. Much effort has been invested at improving the understanding of the epidemiology of this disorder, including identifying risk factors that predispose persons to develop osteoarthritis, especially ones that are reversible or modifiable.

Several factors heighten the risk of incident osteoarthritis, including age, gender, joint injury, and obesity. Although the clinical manifestations of osteoarthritis can begin as early as the fourth and fifth decades of life, the incidence of osteoarthritis continues to rise with each advancing decade. Moreover, women in their 50s, 60s, and 70s have a greater prevalence of osteoarthritis in the hands and knees than do men. Osteoarthritis among blacks is more severe and has greater impact on disability than in whites. The influence of genetics on disease occurrence is significant and usually joint specific. For example, hip osteoarthritis runs in families but these families do not have an increased risk to develop osteoarthritis at other joints.

Injury to a pristine joint, such as a ruptured anterior cruciate ligament (ACL) or torn meniscus, increases the risk of subsequent osteoarthritis at that joint site later in life. Incidental and usually asymptomatic meniscal tears are common in middle aged and elderly men and women and increase the

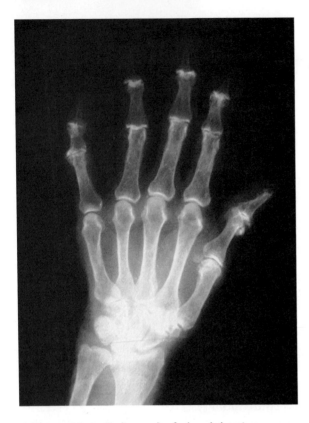

▲ **Figure 39–1.** Radiograph of a hand showing osteoarthritis of the distal interphalangeal (DIP), proximal interphalangeal (PIP), and first carpometacarpal (CMC) joints. Note the joint-space narrowing of the DIP and PIP joints compared to the metacarpophalangeal joints, as well as the bony sclerosis (eburnation) of all joints involved by the osteoarthritis process.

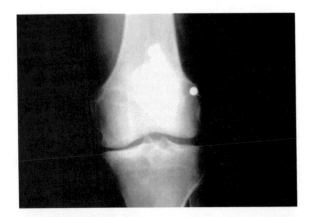

▲ **Figure 39–2.** Knee osteoarthritis with medial joint-space narrowing and osteophytes.

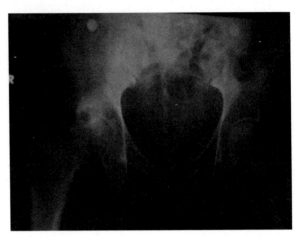

▲ **Figure 39–3.** Right hip osteoarthritis. Note the joint-space narrowing of the superior portion of the involved joint, compared to the same portion of the opposite joint.

risk of knee osteoarthritis. Obese women and men are at high risk for knee osteoarthritis and have a modest increase in risk for hip osteoarthritis. This increase in risk is due mostly to the excess load across weight-bearing joints conferred by obesity and, at least for women, the risk is proportional to the degree of overweight. For knee osteoarthritis, weight loss in middle age may lower this risk. It is intriguing, however, that the conditions of being overweight or obese are related to incidence of hand joint osteoarthritis, even though interphalangeal joints are clearly not weight-dependent parts of the human body.

▶ Pathogenesis

Osteoarthritis is a disease in which most or all of the joint structures are affected by pathology. The tissue which defines osteoarthritic change is the thin layer of hyaline articular cartilage interposed between articulating bones (eg, femoral condyle and tibial plateau). This avascular cartilaginous tissue becomes worn and frayed, especially in areas of injury. There is also degeneration of fibrocartilaginous structures like the meniscus, sclerosis of underlying bone, growth of osteophytes at the joint margin, weakness and atrophy of muscles that bridge the joint, ligamentous laxity and disruption, and, in many joints, synovitis. With focal cartilage loss on one side of the joint and related bony remodeling, malalignment across the joint may develop, increasing focal transarticular loading and causing further damage to cartilage and underlying bone. Both subtle chronic and flagrant acute injuries can initiate development of the osteoarthritis process. Cartilage matrix turnover, spurred by daily loading across the joint, can replenish cartilage, but as a consequence of genetic abnormalities, age, and other metabolic factors not yet fully understood, some cartilage is especially vulnerable to loading that for normal cartilage, may be well tolerated.

▶ Prevention

At present, there are no proven strategies to prevent the development of osteoarthritis.

Among women who participated in the Framingham Osteoarthritis Study, those who lost 5-kg or greater weight reduction over 10 years experienced half the risk of developing symptomatic knee osteoarthritis. Such data support the claim that weight reduction can alter the risk of incident osteoarthritis. It stands to reason that weight loss may also delay disease progression.

Because joint injury causes a large proportion of knee osteoarthritis in the general population, avoiding major injuries may prevent disease. This is especially relevant to young athletes at high risk for ACL tears, injuries associated with a high risk of subsequent knee osteoarthritis. Persons with knees (and potentially relevant to other sites) that have already sustained major injury are at high risk for subsequent injury and osteoarthritis development, and ought to consider avoidance of further athletic activity with high reinjury risk.

▶ Clinical Findings

A. Symptoms and Signs

The patient with osteoarthritis affecting a joint in the peripheral skeleton, such as at the hand, knee, or hip, may initially experience relatively minor pain or discomfort with use of the involved joint (Table 39–1). There is characteristic brief, self-limited stiffness (ie, <30 minutes) in the affected joint on arising in the morning. For example, at the outset of osteoarthritis involving the hip joint, patients may have some difficulty crossing their legs to put on a pair of shoes or pants; however, once they are dressed and upright, bearing weight and ambulation are generally well tolerated. But, as

Table 39–1. Signs, symptoms, and diagnostic features of osteoarthritis.

Joint pain that increases with activity
Morning stiffness that is relatively brief and self-limited
Crepitus (a grating sensation with motion)
Bony enlargement at the joint margin
Tenderness to palpation over the joint
Noninflammatory synovial fluid (<2000 WBC/mm³)
Erythrocyte sedimentation rate normal for age
Radiographic evidence of osteoarthritis (nonuniform joint-space narrowing, osteophyte [spur] formation, subchondral cysts, and eburnation [bony sclerosis])
Negative serologic tests for antinuclear antibody and rheumatoid factor

WBC, white blood cells.

osteoarthritis progresses, an affected patient will gradually experience progressively severe joint discomfort and increasing difficulty with activities of daily living.

With further disease progression, patients develop increasing difficult performing activities that were once routine. Thus, tasks such as gripping, holding, or writing with a pen or pencil; putting car keys in and turning the ignition switch; lifting a gallon of milk out of the refrigerator; or removing a pot of water from the stove become increasingly difficult to perform. At the extreme end of the disease spectrum, marked impairment in activity follows. Even walking from room to room in one's home may become unbearably painful when advanced osteoarthritis affects the hip or knee joint. Ascending or descending stairs can be particularly difficult with osteoarthritic involvement of lower extremity joints.

In patients with knee osteoarthritis, joint instability or "giving way" is common, sometimes leading to falling or near-falling events. Such instability arising from structural compromise of the degenerative joint poses substantial health risk to the elderly, and can contribute significantly to fear, frailty, and isolation.

B. Laboratory Findings

There is no specific laboratory blood test (or synovial fluid measure) used in clinical practice to confirm a diagnosis of osteoarthritis. Instead, routine blood work, including complete blood cell counts, comprehensive metabolic panel, acute phase reactants (erythrocyte sedimentation rate and C-reactive protein), and screening autoantibodies (rheumatoid factor and antinuclear antibody), are indicated if an inflammatory arthropathy such as rheumatoid arthritis and systemic lupus erythematosus, respectively, is being considered. If joints affected are typical of osteoarthritis (eg, DIPs, PIPs, the first carpometacarpal joints in the hand), with supportive symptoms and signs, and with joint pain elicited in the history that is related to activity, serologic evaluation is probably unnecessary. However, if the clinical presentation is consistent with rheumatoid arthritis (eg, if the wrists are affected or if prolonged morning stiffness—lasting 60 minutes or longer—is present), blood tests may be of diagnostic value. Unlike most patients with osteoarthritis, those with inflammatory arthritis (including rheumatoid arthritis and lupus) will have elevated levels of acute phase reactants and may be anemic and manifest hypergammaglobulinemia.

C. Imaging Studies

Radiographic imaging can confirm the diagnosis of osteoarthritis. The radiographic hallmarks of osteoarthritis, established more than five decades ago by Kellgren & Lawrence, are joint-space narrowing, osteophytes (bone spurs), subchondral cysts, and bony sclerosis (eburnation) (see Figure 39–1). Although MRI may reveal characteristic features of osteoarthritis, such findings are universal in older persons, making MRI a test with poor discriminative power for the diagnosis of osteoarthritis. Similarly, in an older patient with bony enlargement on examination and activity-related joint pain, radiographs (which have imperfect sensitivity, sometimes being negative in the presence of disease) may not be indicated.

D. Special Tests

Arthrocentesis can be a valuable diagnostic maneuver when encountering a patient with presumptive osteoarthritis. In osteoarthritis, the synovial fluid WBC count is less than 2000 cells/mm^3. Counts greater than 2000/mm^3 suggest the possibility of an inflammatory arthropathy. In fluids from osteoarthritic joints, crystals visible by light microscopy are absent. The presence of gout or pseudogout crystals, if identified, provides diagnostic evidence of other forms of arthritis that occasionally are difficult to distinguish from osteoarthritis. This is particularly true for pseudogout.

▶ Differential Diagnosis

The challenge when evaluating a patient with joint pain is to employ the history and physical examination, and sometimes a modicum of additional diagnostic testing, to arrive at the correct diagnosis in an efficient manner. Joint pain that is brought on by activity and relieved with rest suggests the existence of osteoarthritis. The absence of constitutional symptoms and the presence of bony enlargement and tenderness at the joint margin reinforce this clinical impression. Finally, the pattern of joint involvement is meaningful because osteoarthritis has a predilection to affect the knees, hips, DIPs, PIPs, and first carpometacarpal joints of the hands. This distribution of articular involvement distinguishes osteoarthritis from such inflammatory forms of arthritis as rheumatoid arthritis, psoriatic arthritis, and gout, which have a different distribution.

It is also worth noting that a variety of secondary disorders represent identifiable causes of osteoarthritis. Several such disorders, including those resulting from inborn errors of metabolism and metabolic derangements, are listed in Table 39–2. Recognition of their distinct features, such as involvement of the second and third metacarpophalangeal joints in hemochromatosis-associated arthropathy, may identify the underlying cause of the joint pain. Finally, since osteoarthritis is extremely common, its presence does not exclude consideration of an alternate explanation for joint pain, such as an occult malignancy or interval development of septic arthritis in a joint previously known to be osteoarthritic. Such diagnoses should be considered when there is a meaningful change in the pattern of joint pain. Similarly, interval development of prominent constitutional symptoms is a major clue to investigate an alternate explanation for joint pain, even in the presence of overt osteoarthritic features on examination.

If giving way (buckling) or locking of the knee occurs, this may indicate an internal derangement of the knee such as a tear of the ACL or meniscus. Tears often occur abruptly and memorably.

Table 39–2. Identifiable causes of osteoarthritis.

Congenital disorder (hip)
Legg-Calvé-Perthes disease
Acetabular dysplasia
Slipped capital femoral epiphysis
Inborn error of connective tissue
Ehlers-Danlos syndrome
Marfan syndrome
Posttraumatic (knee)
Anterior cruciate ligament tear
Meniscus tear with or without prior meniscectomy surgery
Metabolic disorders
Hemochromatosis
Wilson disease
Ochronosis (alkaptonuria)
History of a septic joint
Postinflammatory
Underlying rheumatoid arthritis
Generalized osteoarthritis
Predilection for first CMC, DIP, PIP, knee, and hip joints

CMC, carpometacarpal; DIP, distal interphalangeal; PIP, proximal interphalangeal.

▶ Treatment

The goals of medical therapy are to control pain, improve function, minimize disability, and enhance health-related quality of life. A further therapeutic priority is to minimize the risk of drug-associated toxicity, particularly that which may result from nonsteroidal anti-inflammatory drug (NSAID) therapy.

A. Nonpharmacologic

In patients with osteoarthritis, nonpharmacologic treatments are underutilized. They have demonstrated efficacy and can often help relieve pain and improve function. For example, an assistive device, such as a properly used cane or walker, can unload an affected knee or hip and diminish pain with walking. Similarly, quadriceps strengthening and aerobic exercise are effective in the management of osteoarthritis at the knee. For exercise therapy, referral to a physical therapist is often helpful, because the therapist can evaluate function and craft the right mix of exercises for the individual patient. Adherence to exercise is often poor, so it is helpful to reinforce the exercise regimen at each visit. A randomized trial demonstrated that neoprene sleeves reduce pain for patients with varus deformity due to knee osteoarthritis. If these do not work, fitted valgus braces, designed to decrease the varus malalignment across the knee, have been shown to decrease pain. Wedged insoles placed in shoes help realign knees but clinical trials of such insoles have mostly shown no effects on knee pain. Weight loss should be encouraged for all persons with knee or hip osteoarthritis.

B. Pharmacologic

A front-line approach to pharmacologic therapy for osteoarthritis includes use of acetaminophen. This drug improves pain and function and has a safer toxicity profile, particularly with regard to the gastrointestinal tract, than NSAIDs. For many years, NSAIDs have been widely used in the management of osteoarthritis and achieve symptomatic benefit through their inhibition of cyclooxygenase (COX), particularly the inducible isoform (COX-2), at sites of joint damage. Recent studies have demonstrated that NSAIDs are modestly more efficacious than acetaminophen for the pain of osteoarthritis.

The gastrointestinal toxicity of NSAID therapy remains a major concern. Such toxicity can be mostly avoided by using topical nonsteroidal drugs as a first-line approach, especially for superficial joints such as hands and knees. The following factors increase the risk of gastrointestinal toxicity from oral NSAIDs:

- Prior peptic ulcer disease.
- Age older than 65 years.
- Concomitant tobacco and alcohol use.
- Coadministration of glucocorticoids or anticoagulation therapy.
- Comorbid *Helicobacter pylori* infection.

Ways to diminish NSAID toxicity include the following:

- **Gastroprotective drugs.** The two classes of drugs shown to be effective among NSAID users are proton pump inhibitors and misoprostol, although the latter frequently causes bloating and diarrhea.
- **Administration of COX-2 isoenzyme inhibitors.** Although COX inhibitors cause increased risks of heart disease and stroke, celecoxib may be less likely to induce cardiovascular morbidity, especially at doses under 400 mg/day.

The efficacy of glucosamine in the medical management of osteoarthritis is controversial. Glucosamine is a component of human articular cartilage that is administered orally. A multicenter National Institutes of Health (NIH) trial found no efficacy of glucosamine. Chondroitin sulfate (also commercially available) is similarly controversial. The same NIH trial failed to show efficacy either of chondroitin alone or combined glucosamine and chondroitin. Intra-articular hyaluronic acid is a controversial FDA-approved treatment for knee osteoarthritis. Meta-analyses evaluating placebo-controlled trials have reported significant but modest efficacy and have also reported publication bias, suggesting that estimates of therapeutic benefit from published studies are inflated.

Table 39–3. Acute complications of osteoarthritis.

Microcrystalline arthropathy (knee and hand joints)
  Gout (monosodium urate)
  Pseudogout (calcium pyrophosphate dihydrate)
Spontaneous osteonecrosis of the knee
Ruptured Baker cyst (pseudothrombophlebitis syndrome)
Bursitis
  Anserine bursitis (knee)
  Trochanteric bursitis (hip)
Symptomatic meniscal tear (knee)
Infection (septic arthritis)

Complications

After a diagnosis of osteoarthritis has been firmly established, subsequent change in symptoms or course will not necessarily be directly attributable to this disease. If such changes occur, the clinician should search for other diagnoses as listed in Table 39–3. For example, the abrupt onset of heat, redness, and swelling in a known yet previously stable osteoarthritic knee may herald the onset of a superimposed microcrystalline arthropathy or of a ruptured Baker (or popliteal) cyst. A new joint infection (ie, septic arthritis) need also be considered. Alternately, new-onset joint locking or giving way may suggest the presence of a loose body or meniscal tear that warrants orthopedic evaluation and arthroscopic intervention. In addition, the development of new symptoms near the joint may be attributable to active inflammation of adjacent nonarticular tissues, including regional tendons and bursae.

Allen MM, Rosenfeld SB. Treatment for post-slipped capital femoral epiphysis deformity. *Orthop Clin North Am.* 2020;51(1):37-53. [PMID: 31739878]

Deveza LA, Nelson AE, Loeser RF. Phenotypes of osteoarthritis: current state and future implications. *Clin Exp Rheumatol.* 2019;37 Suppl 120(5):64-72. [PMID: 31621574]

Ghouri A, Conaghan PG. Treating osteoarthritis pain: recent approaches using pharmacological therapies. *Clin Exp Rheumatol.* 2019;37 Suppl 120(5):124-129. [PMID: 31621576]

Hootman JM, Barbour KE, Theis KA, Boring MA. Updated projected prevalence of self-reported doctor-diagnosed arthritis and arthritis-attributable activity limitation among US adults, 2015-2040. *Arthritis Rheum.* 2016;68:1582-1587. [PMID: 27015600]

Rice D, McNair P, Huysmans E, Letzen J, Finan P. Best evidence rehabilitation for chronic pain part 5: osteoarthritis. *J Clin Med.* 2019;8(11). pii: E1769. [PMID: 31652929]

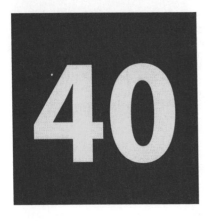

Gout

Chio Yokose, MD

Hyon K. Choi, MD, DrPH

ESSENTIALS OF DIAGNOSIS

▶ Caused by deposition of monosodium urate crystals due to longstanding hyperuricemia.

▶ Usually begins as an intermittent, acute mono- or oligo-arthritis, especially of the first metatarsophalangeal joint.

▶ Flares typically become more frequent and involve more joints over time, in the absence of treatment.

▶ Diagnosed by evaluating joint fluid for monosodium urate crystals using polarized light microscopy.

▶ Extra-articular manifestations include subcutaneous tophi and renal stones.

▶ Flares of arthritis respond to anti-inflammatory drugs such as nonsteroidal anti-inflammatory drugs, colchicine, or glucocorticoids.

General Considerations

Gout affects approximately 4% (9.2 million) of the US general population. Hyperuricemia affects an even greater proportion of the US general population, at about 20% (46 million). Both the prevalence and incidence of gout and hyperuricemia have increased in recent decades in the United States and other Western nations, mirroring trends in the rise of obesity and metabolic syndrome. The prevalence of gout increases with age and is higher among men than women. Gout among premenopausal women is particularly rare because of the uricosuric effect of estrogen.

Chronic hyperuricemia is a prerequisite condition for gout. Sustained serum urate concentrations greater than 6.8 mg/dL favor the precipitation of monosodium urate crystals in and around joints, leading to gout. The likelihood of developing symptomatic gout and the age of onset correlate with the duration and magnitude of hyperuricemia. In one study, persons with serum urate levels between 7.0 and 8.0 mL/dL had a 5-year cumulative incidence of gouty arthritis of 3%, compared to 22% among those with serum urate levels greater than 9.0 mL/dL. However, hyperuricemia alone is not sufficient for the development of gout. It appears that clinical gout develops in fewer than one in four hyperuricemic persons at any point.

Hyperuricemia can result from increased urate production, decreased urate excretion, or a combination of the two mechanisms (Table 40–1). Urate is a by-product of the purine degradation pathway, but overproduction of urate through this mechanism is usually a minor contributor to elevations of serum urate concentrations. Less than 5% of patients with gout are hyperuricemic because of urate overproduction. These persons can be recognized because they excrete more than 800 mg of urate in their urine during a 24-hour period.

Underexcretion of urate is the primary cause of hyperuricemia for the majority of patients. About two-thirds of urate excretion occurs by the kidneys, with the remainder occurring through the gut. Those who excrete less than 800 mg of urate are hyperuricemic because of impaired renal excretion. Defining individuals as "overproducers" or "underexcreters" is helpful in predicting whether the hyperuricemia is associated with a variety of acquired or genetic disorders (see Table 40–1) and may be useful in some cases in determining the most appropriate treatment.

Pathogenesis

Hyperuricemia is the necessary precursor for the development of gout. When individuals are hyperuricemic, conditions exist such that monosodium urate crystals can precipitate in and around joint tissues. The NLRP3 inflammasome is the major pathway by which monosodium urate crystals trigger the profound inflammatory response observed in gout flares. The NLRP3 inflammasome must first be primed before activation. This priming is mediated by NF-κB-activating pathways, such as those activated by Toll-like receptors. This signaling induces the expression of functional inflammasome components, including NLRP3. Monosodium urate crystals

Table 40–1. Classification of hyperuricemia.

Urate overproduction
 Primary hyperuricemia
 Idiopathic
 Complete or partial deficiency of HGPRT
 Superactivity of PRPP synthetase
 Secondary hyperuricemia
 Excessive purine consumption
 Myeloproliferative or lymphoproliferative disorders
 Hemolytic diseases
 Psoriasis
 Glycogen storage diseases: types 1, 3, 5, and 7
Uric acid underexcretion
 Primary hyperuricemia
 Idiopathic
 Secondary hyperuricemia
 Decreased renal function
 Metabolic acidosis (ketoacidosis or lactic acidosis)
 Dehydration
 Diuretics
 Hypertension
 Hyperparathyroidism
 Drugs including cyclosporine, pyrazinamide, ethambutol, and
  low-dose salicylates
 Lead nephropathy
Overproduction and underexcretion
 Alcohol use
 Glucose-6-phosphatase deficiency
 Fructose-1-phosphate-aldolase deficiency

HGPRT, hypoxanthine guanine phosphoribosyltransferase; PRPP, 5'-phosphoribosyl-1-pyrophosphate.

provide the second signal when they are phagocytosed by macrophages, thereby promoting the assembly and activation of the NLRP3 inflammasome. Caspase-1 is recruited and mediates the activation of proinflammatory cytokines IL-1β and IL-18. This inflammasome-mediated IL-1β release in gout is a key step in the inflammatory response, leading to vasodilation and rapid recruitment of neutrophils to the sites of crystal deposition. This step is also a key therapeutic target for anti-inflammatory therapy such as anakinra (IL-1 receptor antagonist) as well as colchicine.

The acute inflammatory response associated with a gout flare resolves spontaneously over 10–14 days. As the monocytes mature into macrophages, they switch from producing proinflammatory cytokines to anti-inflammatory cytokines such as transforming growth factor (TGF)-β. In addition, large proteins (such as apolipoprotein B) that normally do not have access to the synovial fluid can enter the joint space because of the vasodilation and increased vascular permeability of the acute inflammatory response. These proteins coat the crystals and have an antiphlogistic effect. Neutrophils likely also play an important role in the resolution of the inflammatory response in gout, through the formation of neutrophil extracellular traps (NETs), which can aid in the degradation of proinflammatory cytokines.

Tophi are aggregates of monosodium urate crystals surrounded by a mantle of macrophages releasing cytokines and enzymes. Tophi reside within the synovium as well as in extrasynovial tissues such as the skin. In the periods between gout flares, tophi continue to form and enlarge. This chronic inflammatory response, situated within joints, is responsible for eroding bone and cartilage, leading to secondary degenerative joint disease. With enough cartilage degeneration, a form of chronic arthritis with bone erosions and deformities can ensue.

▶ Clinical Findings

A. Symptoms and Signs

The natural history of gout can be divided into three distinct stages (Figure 40–1):

1. Asymptomatic hyperuricemia
2. Acute gout flares and intercritical gout
3. Chronic gouty arthritis

The clinical course varies considerably from one patient to another. Whereas some patients experience only one or two attacks of acute gouty arthritis during their lifetime, more than 80% have a second flare within 2 years of the first. Subcutaneous tophi occasionally develop in a patient with no history of acute gouty arthritis.

The initial episode of acute gout flare usually follows 10–30 years of asymptomatic hyperuricemia. Hyperuricemia is independently associated with renal and cardiovascular disease, but whether hyperuricemia causes these conditions and warrants pharmacologic therapy remains unclear. Precisely why and when the first flare of gout occurs in susceptible persons remains a mystery. Although some patients experience prodromal episodes of mild discomfort, the onset of a gout flare is usually heralded by the rapid onset of exquisite pain associated with warmth, swelling, and erythema of the affected joint (Figure 40–2). The pain escalates from the faintest twinges to its most intense level within 24 hours.

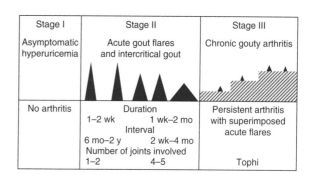

▲ **Figure 40–1.** The natural history of gout progresses through three stages.

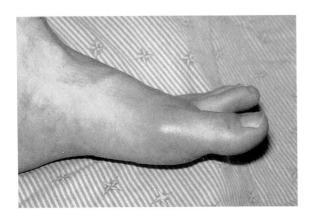

▲ **Figure 40–2.** Acute gouty attack of the first metatarsophalangeal joint.

Initial flares usually affect only one joint. In half of the patients, the first attack involves the first metatarsophalangeal joint. Other joints frequently involved in the early stage of gout are the midfoot, ankle, heel, and knee. The wrist, fingers, and elbows can also be involved, but upper extremity joints typically do not become involved until the patient has experienced multiple gout flares in the lower extremities. (An exception to this is in postmenopausal women, who may present with gout in distal interphalangeal joints, often within a Heberden's node, without having any history of acute gout.)

The intensity of pain from an acute gout flare is disabling, such that patients cannot bear even the weight of a bed sheet on the affected body part. Most patients find it difficult or impossible to walk when the lower extremities are involved in an acute flare. The acute flare may be accompanied by fever, chills, and malaise. Cutaneous erythema and swelling associated with the flare may extend beyond the involved joint and resemble cellulitis. Desquamation of the skin often occurs as the flare resolves.

Symptoms resolve quickly with appropriate treatment, but even untreated, an acute flare resolves spontaneously over 1–2 weeks. With resolution of the flare, patients enter an interval termed the "intercritical period" when they are again completely asymptomatic. Early in the intermittent stage, episodes of gout flares are infrequent and the intervals between the flares vary from months to years. Over time, the flares become more frequent, less acute in onset, longer in duration, and tend to involve more joints.

During the intercritical periods of gout, the previously involved joints are virtually free of symptoms. Despite this, monosodium urate crystal deposition continues, and tophi increase in size. Urate crystals often can be identified in the synovial fluid despite the absence of symptoms. Erosive joint changes indicative of bony tophi begin to appear on radiographs.

Gout flares tend to be associated with both rapid increases and—more often—decreases in the concentration of urate in synovial fluid. These concentrations mirror the fluctuations seen in the serum. However, serum urate can be deceptively low in the setting of an acute gout flare due to the uricosuric effect of cytokines (eg, IL-6) involved in the evolution of the gout flare. Trauma, alcohol ingestion, and the use of certain drugs are known to trigger gout flares, as well. Gout flares occur not infrequently as a person is recovering from an alcoholic binge.

Drugs known to precipitate gout attacks do so by rapidly raising or lowering serum urate levels. Medications known to have urate-raising or urate-lowering effects include diuretics, salicylates, radiographic contrast agents, and specific urate-lowering drugs (probenecid, allopurinol, febuxostat, and pegloticase). Salicylates may have either a urate-raising effect (at low doses) or a urate-lowering effect (at high doses). It is believed that these fluctuations in urate levels destabilize tophi in the synovium. The sudden addition of urate to them may render them unstable, or the sudden lowering of the urate concentration may cause partial dissolution and instability (tophi mobilization). As the microtophi break apart, crystals are shed into the synovial fluid, leading to the initiation of a gout flare.

As gout continues to progress, the patient gradually enters the stage of chronic gouty arthritis. This is the result of a chronic inflammatory response driven by macrophages that surround tophi (see above) and usually develops after 10 or more years of acute intermittent gout flares. Chronic gouty arthritis is when the intercritical periods are no longer pain-free. The involved joints are now persistently uncomfortable and may be swollen. Patients report stiffness or gelling sensations, as well. Visible or palpable subcutaneous tophi may be detected on physical examination during this stage of gout, having been visible on radiographs prior to entry into this stage (Figure 40–3). The propensity to develop tophaceous deposits varies across individual patients. In general, however, tophi are a function of the duration and severity of the hyperuricemia, with a mean occurrence approximately 12 years after the onset of the first flare of gout in those not treated with urate-lowering drugs.

B. Laboratory Findings

The serum urate should be checked while the patients is off any urate-lowering therapy whenever possible and at least 4 weeks after the last gout flare (ie, during an intercritical period). A very low serum urate makes gout less likely, but the likelihood of gout increases as the concentration of serum urate rises above 6 mg/dL. Whereas most patients with gout have an elevated serum urate (>6.8 mg/dL), levels fall within the normal range on occasion; in fact, levels in the normal range are not uncommon during acute flares, for the reasons described above. In addition, during acute flares, the complete blood cell count may show a leukocytosis with increased polymorphonuclear leukocytes on the differential and elevations of the erythrocyte sedimentation rate and C-reactive protein.

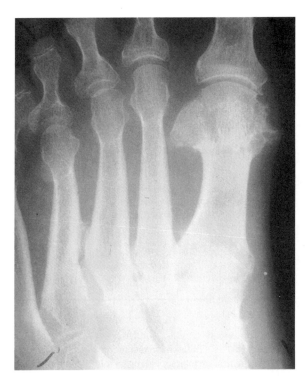

▲ **Figure 40–3.** Radiographic changes of gout.

The 24-hour urine measurement of urate excretion is not required in all patients with gout but is useful for determining potential causes of hyperuricemia (see above) as well as determining whether uricosuric therapy can be effective, since this form of therapy is contraindicated in overproducers.

During an acute flare, the synovial fluid findings are consistent with moderate to severe inflammation (see Chapter 2). The leukocyte count usually ranges between 5000 and 80,000 cells/mcL, with an average between 15,000 and 20,000 cells/mcL. The cells are predominantly polymorphonuclear leukocytes.

The definitive diagnosis of gout is made by examination of synovial fluid or tophaceous material with compensated polarized light microscopy and identifying the characteristic monosodium urate crystals in synovial fluid or aspirates of tophaceous deposits (Figure 40–4). These negatively birefringent crystals appear as bright yellow needle-shaped objects when parallel to the axis of slow vibration on the first-order compensator. When these crystals are perpendicular to that axis, they are blue. Crystals are usually intracellular and needle-shaped during acute attacks but may be small, blunted, and extracellular as the attack subsides or during intercritical periods.

C. Imaging Studies

No plain radiographic abnormalities are typically present early in the disease course. In acute gout flares, the only

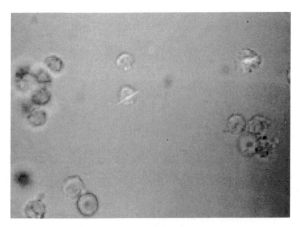

▲ **Figure 40–4.** Urate crystal ingested by a polymorphonuclear leukocyte in synovial fluid. This finding is pathognomonic for acute gouty arthritis.

finding may be soft-tissue swelling in the involved joint. Bony abnormalities indicative of deposition of monosodium urate crystals develop only after years of disease. These abnormalities are usually asymmetric and confined to previously symptomatic joints. Gouty bone erosions are defined as a cortical break with a sclerotic margin and overhanging edge. The joint space may be preserved or show osteoarthritic type narrowing (see Figure 40–3). Ultrasonography can also be used to make the diagnosis. The characteristic finding is a "double contour sign," a superficial, hyperechoic band on the surface of the articular cartilage (Figure 40–5).

MRI and CT scans are also sensitive methods of detecting tophi and erosions. In particular, dual-energy CT is another imaging modality that allows for the noninvasive identification of monosodium urate crystals in joints and periarticular tissues by taking advantage of material-specific attenuation differences between high- and low-energy beams of radiation

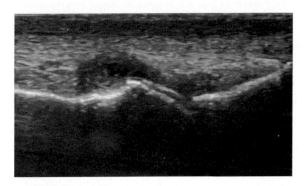

▲ **Figure 40–5.** Characteristic finding of gout under ultrasound, with "double contour sign" which appears as a superficial, hyperechoic band on the surface of the articular cartilage.

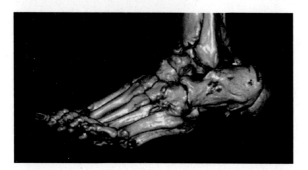

▲ **Figure 40–6.** Dual-energy CT of gout in the foot, with monosodium urate crystal deposits highlighted in both the toes and the mid-foot using material-specific attenuation differences between the high- and low-energy beams.

used to acquire the images. Monosodium urate crystals are usually highlighted in green (Figure 40–6).

D. Additional Tests

Patients with gout often suffer from comorbidities such as hyperlipidemia, glucose intolerance, hypertension, coronary artery disease, congestive heart failure, and obesity. Accordingly, it is often appropriate to measure serum lipids and fasting blood sugars in patients with gout. Because renal dysfunction develops in many patients with hypertension and gout, it is appropriate to monitor serum creatinine levels, as well.

▶ Differential Diagnosis

The presumptive diagnosis of gout can be made by a combination of clinical features during an acute gout flare, as well as laboratory and imaging findings. As described above, it is preferable to measure serum urate levels during an intercritial period rather than in the throes or recent aftermath of a possible gout attack. Suggestive clinical features include involvement of the first metatarsophalangeal joint, the midfoot, or ankle as a part of a mono- or oligoarticular arthritis. Patients with gout in this distribution of joints typically have erythema of the overlying skin and inability to bear weight. The time course of joint inflammation (time to maximal pain <24 hours), resolution of symptoms in less than or equal to 14 days, and complete resolution of symptoms in between episodes of joint pain are also be useful items in the history. Clinicians may also use the criteria proposed by American College of Rheumatology/European League Against Rheumatism for the diagnosis of gout (Table 40–2).

Because gout often occurs in association with other diseases, those conditions in Table 40–1 should be considered in any person with gout. A variety of conditions can mimic or be confused with gout. These include other crystal-induced diseases such as those related to the deposition of calcium pyrophosphate dihydrate crystals (pseudogout) or basic

Table 40–2. Criteria for the diagnosis of acute gouty arthritis.

- Presence of characteristic urate crystals in joint fluid, or
- A tophus proved to contain urate crystals by chemical means or polarized light microscopy, or
- The presence of 6 of the following 12 clinical, laboratory, and radiographic phenomena listed below:
  1. More than one attack of acute arthritis
  2. Maximal inflammation developed within 1 day
  3. Attack of monoarticular arthritis
  4. Joint redness observed
  5. First metatarsophalangeal joint painful or swollen
  6. Unilateral attack involving first metatarsophalangeal joint
  7. Unilateral attack involving tarsal joint
  8. Suspected tophus
  9. Hyperuricemia
  10. A symptomatic swelling within a joint (radiograph)
  11. Subcortical cysts without erosions (radiograph)
  12. Negative culture of joint fluids for microorganisms during attack of joint inflammation

calcium phosphate crystals. The latter may cause a calcific tendinitis that is similar in presentation to gout. Osteoarthritis of the first metatarsophalangeal joint is very common and may be confused with podagra. Septic arthritis can also mimic gout, although a gouty attack may coexist with an infected joint. The more common causes of septic arthritis are gonococcal, staphylococcal, or streptococcal infections. However, infections with fungi or mycobacteria may also be seen. A hemarthrosis or fracture in the joint line may be confused with a gouty attack. Finally, some conditions that are usually considered oligoarticular or polyarticular in presentation may involve only one joint early in the course and be confused with gout. This is particularly true with the peripheral arthritis associated with ankylosing spondylitis, reactive arthritis, psoriatic arthritis, and the arthritis of inflammatory bowel disease. Rarely, palindromic rheumatism may herald the onset of rheumatoid arthritis and begin with monoarticular arthritis.

Occasionally, chronic gouty arthritis and tophi are misdiagnosed as rheumatoid arthritis. The chronic symptoms are polyarticular and symmetric, and the tophaceous deposits mimic rheumatoid nodules. This problem is compounded by the fact that up to 25% of patients with gout have positive tests for rheumatoid factor although these are usually of low titer.

▶ Complications

As described above, untreated and severe gout leads to visible and palpable subcutaneous tophi and a destructive arthropathy. However, these complications are preventable with accurate diagnosis and appropriate therapy.

Nephrolithiasis develops in 10–25% of patients with gout at some time during the disease course. In 40% of these patients, the first episode of renal colic precedes the first attack of acute gouty arthritis. Most of these calculi are composed of uric acid; however, calcium-containing stones are 10 times more common in patients with gout than in the general population. The incidence of nephrolithiasis correlates with the serum urate level, but more strongly with the amount of urate excreted in the urine. The likelihood of developing a stone reaches 50% with either a serum urate level above 13.0 mg/dL or a 24-hour urinary urate excretion in excess of 1100 mg.

Patients with gout are more likely to have chronic kidney disease, including progression to end-stage renal disease. Hypertension, diabetes, and atherosclerosis are the most important contributing factors to this complication. In fact, aggressive risk factor control likely mitigates the risk of chronic kidney failure in patients with gout.

Hyperuricemia and gout are frequently accompanied by obesity, alcoholism, glucose intolerance related to insulin resistance, and hyperlipidemia. In addition, a very high percentage of patients with gout have hypertension. Furthermore, the number of conditions found in high prevalence among patients with gout continues to grow, including erectile dysfunction, obstructive sleep apnea, and atrial fibrillation. These associated conditions should be screened for and managed aggressively.

Gout is independently associated with incident coronary artery disease as well as premature mortality, largely attributable to atherosclerotic cardiovascular events. Furthermore, the premature mortality gap in patients with gout has persisted despite the widespread availability of effective therapies for both gout and its comorbidities, reflecting a need for improved strategies for cardiovascular disease prevention and management in patients with gout. However, it is not yet clear if treatment of gout leads to improved cardiovascular outcomes.

▶ Treatment

The management of gout includes the following:

1. Providing rapid and safe pain relief for gout flares.
2. Preventing further gout flares.
3. Preventing formation of tophi and destructive arthritis.
4. Addressing associated medical conditions.

A. Treating the Acute Gout Flare

The goal of treating the acute gout flare is to eliminate the pain and other symptoms caused by the intense inflammation as rapidly as possible. The choices in this situation include nonsteroidal anti-inflammatory drugs (NSAIDs), colchicine, and glucocorticoids. Effective management of the acute flare is not so much determined by which agent is used, but rather by how quickly that agent is initiated after the onset of the flare. If a single dose is given in the first minutes of a flare—and this is possible for a patient with established gout who has the appropriate medications on hand—it may eradicate

the symptoms and terminate the flare. If, however, the initiation of treatment is delayed for 48 hours, it will probably require at least 48 hours to control the symptoms of the flare. Once the symptoms of a flare have resolved completely, the agent used to treat that flare should be continued at a reduced dose for another 48–72 hours. A typical gout flare requires approximately 2 weeks of acute therapy, to ensure that the inflammation is quelled.

NSAIDs are frequently used agents to treat gout because they are widely available and generally well tolerated. Indomethacin is historically the NSAID of choice for acute gout, but other NSAIDs are just as effective. The NSAID selected should be started at its recommended maximal dose. The dose may be lowered as symptoms resolve. NSAIDs should be avoided in patients with active or recent peptic ulcer disease and in patients with chronic kidney disease or active cardiovascular disease.

Colchicine is also effective for gout flares if taken early in the course of the flare. There are multiple dosing regimens for colchicine, but a commonly used dose is 1.2 mg orally to start and then 0.6 mg 1 hour later. The colchicine should be continued once or twice daily thereafter until resolution of the gout flare. The most common and bothersome side effects are gastrointestinal, including gas, nausea, vomiting, diarrhea, and severe cramping abdominal pain. Colchicine is best avoided in patients with chronic kidney disease because of concern for causing colchicine neuromyopathy. Colchicine neuromyopathy is discussed further below.

Glucocorticoids are usually reserved for patients in whom colchicine or NSAIDs are contraindicated or ineffective. The response time to glucocorticoids is comparable to that for NSAIDs and colchicine. Doses of prednisone of 20–40 mg/day have been used. Treatment might begin, for example, with prednisone 20 mg twice daily for 1 week, tapering off prednisone over a second week as the flare is controlled and discontinuing prednisone entirely 48–72 hours after the last symptom of the gout attack. Given high prevalence of diabetes and insulin resistance among patients with gout, patients with known glucose intolerance should be counseled to monitor their blood glucose more closely while on high doses of prednisone. Intramuscular or intravenous glucocorticoids provide alternatives for use in the hospitalized patient who can take nothing by mouth. Finally, intra-articular injections with 20–80 mg of methylprednisolone acetate or 10–40 mg of triamcinolone hexacetonide can also be used. Intra-articular injections are particularly useful when the gout attack is limited to a single joint.

Most often the gout flare resolves with the use of one of these agents. However, when this does not occur or in the extremely severe case of gout, these agents may be used in combination. Anakinra, a biologic IL-1 receptor antagonist, is effective in aborting especially recalcitrant cases of gout. Potent analgesics, including opioids, should be reserved for patients with severe refractory gout despite treatment with combination anti-inflammatory agents.

B. Management in the Intercritical Period

1. Prophylaxis with colchicine—Once a patient has had an acute gout flare, the likelihood of further attacks can be reduced by prophylactic therapy with low-dose colchicine on a daily basis. Prophylactic therapy with colchicine, however, should not be employed in isolation. A urate-lowering agent, such as allopurinol, should also be added to the regimen. The use of prophylactic colchicine without controlling the hyperuricemia allows tophi to continue to grow and permits the destructive gouty arthropathy to continue to develop without the usual warning signs of recurrent acute gout flares. Thus, it is critical to use prophylactic treatment in combination with a urate-lowering therapy.

The prophylactic use of colchicine in doses of 0.6 mg once or twice a day reduces the frequencies of flares by 75–85%. These small doses of colchicine rarely cause gastrointestinal side effects and are safe in patients without significant renal dysfunction. Colchicine is excreted by the kidneys and can accumulate to toxic levels in patients with chronic kidney disease. Colchicine is not contraindicated, but careful monitoring and adjustments of colchicine doses are suggested. Chronic colchicine use in patients with renal dysfunction can cause neuromuscular complications—colchicine neuromyopathy. This toxicity manifests with proximal muscle weakness, painful paresthesias, elevated creatine kinase levels, and abnormalities on electromyograms. This axonal neuromyopathy usually resolves completely over several weeks after discontinuing the colchicine, but chronic symptoms persist in some patients. It is prudent to avoid using more than 0.6 mg of colchicine daily in a patient with a serum creatinine greater than 1.5 mg/dL. For patients with significant degrees of renal dysfunction, even less colchicine should be prescribed (eg, 0.6 mg every other day for patients with a creatinine clearance <30 mL/h, with close monitoring).

2. Urate-lowering therapy: allopurinol—Ultimately, specific urate-lowering drugs are essential to eliminating acute gout flares over time, preventing the formation of tophi, and leading to the resolution of tophi. Although dietary manipulation is essential for control of the comorbid conditions often found with gout, dietary restrictions alone seldom lead to reductions in the serum urate levels sufficient to impact the overall course of gout.

The goal of treatment is to maintain the serum urate level at 6.0 mg/dL or less. For patients with subcutaneous tophi or known intra-articular tophi demonstrated radiologically, this target should be 5.0 mg/dL or less. Maintaining the serum level at this target allows precipitated crystals to dissolve and be cleared. This treat-to-target approach is associated with reduced frequency of gout flares, reduced size of tophi, and improved quality of life. If the urate level remains above 6.8 mg/dL, supersaturated conditions will persist, and urate deposition will continue. In other words, lowering the serum urate from 10.0 mg/dL to 8.0 mg/dL will not reverse the disease; it will only allow it to continue to progress at a slower rate.

The xanthine oxidase inhibitor allopurinol is the urate-lowering agent of choice for most patients with gout. All patients with gout are candidates for xanthine oxidase inhibition, including those with tophi, history of nephrolithiasis, and those who are intolerant or contraindicated for uricosuric therapy. Allopurinol may be used in the presence of renal insufficiency, but its dosage must be reduced to prevent toxicity. It is generally recommended that allopurinol be started at a dose of 100 mg daily for those with normal renal function, and 50 mg daily for those with renal insufficiency. The optimal dose of allopurinol is determined by serum urate level response. Labs should be repeated every 2–4 weeks and the dose of allopurinol should be increased in increments of 100 mg for those with normal kidney function or 50 mg for those with renal insufficiency until the target serum urate concentration is achieved.

Failing to titrate allopurinol doses to an appropriately high dose is a common error in gout management. Most patients with normal renal function require allopurinol doses in excess of 300–400 mg daily to achieve their target serum urate levels. Once the target serum urate is achieved and maintained on a dose of allopurinol, it should be continued long term to prevent new monosodium urate deposits from forming and to allow the existing deposits to resolve. It is generally recommended that patients receive prophylactic anti-inflammatory therapy (ie, colchicine) while the allopurinol is being titrated to an appropriate dose. This is because any fluctuation of serum urate (up or down) predisposes the patient to a gout flare. Patients should be informed that following the initiation of a urate-lowering strategy with allopurinol (or any other urate-lowering agent), they will be at increased risk of disease flares over the next year. This underscores the importance of using prophylactic treatment with colchicine and urate-lowering approaches together.

Hyperuricemia alone is rarely an indication for treatment with specific urate-lowering drugs. Therefore, use of a xanthine oxidase inhibitor or uricosuric agent is not recommended in the treatment of asymptomatic hyperuricemia. On the other hand, the identification of asymptomatic hyperuricemia should not be ignored. First, the cause should be determined (see Table 40–1), and any associated problems, such as hypertension, obesity, alcoholism, diabetes, hyperlipidemia, coronary heart disease, and congestive heart failure, should be addressed rigorously.

Side effects and toxicity of allopurinol include fever, headaches, diarrhea, dyspepsia, pleuritis, skin rashes, granulomatous hepatitis, Stevens-Johnson syndrome, and toxic epidermal necrolysis. Allopurinol must be used cautiously when the patient is also taking azathioprine or 6-mercaptopurine. Allopurinol reduces the catabolism of these agents, thereby greatly increasing their effective doses. The syndrome of allopurinol hypersensitivity is rare but serious with a mortality rate of 20–30%. Risk factors for allopurinol hypersensitivity reactions include older age, female sex, presence of renal insufficiency, higher initial dose of allopurinol, and

HLA-B*5801 status. Given higher prevalence of *HLA-B*5801* among Asians (particularly Han Chinese), Blacks, and Native Hawaiians/Pacific Islanders, it is recommended that these patients undergo screening for *HLA-B*5801* prior to starting allopurinol. If a patient is *HLA-B*5801*-positive, an alternative urate-lowering agent such as febuxostat and probenecid should be considered. Patients should be counseled to report any rash they develop while on allopurinol right away to prevent this potentially deadly adverse effect of allopurinol.

3. Urate-lowering therapy: febuxostat—Febuxostat is a potent xanthine oxidase inhibitor that appears to have some benefits compared with allopurinol. First, it is metabolized by the liver, so febuxostat may be used in patients with mild to moderate renal insufficiency (creatinine clearance of 30 mL/min and above) without dose adjustment. Second, the use of febuxostat in patients with a history of allopurinol reactions has been safe, effective, and well tolerated. In clinical trials, a dose of 40 mg of febuxostat had an effectively similar to that of 300 mg of allopurinol. Febuxostat is also available in an 80 mg dose.

Febuxostat now carries a Boxed Warning from the Food and Drug Administration regarding the potential for increased heart disease-related and all-cause deaths compared to allopurinol based on the results of the CARES trial. The CARES trial had several notable limitations, including a very large dropout rate from the study, many events occurring after discontinuation of the medication, and lack of a placebo group. Nevertheless, it is advisable to discuss these findings with patients to engage in shared decision-making when starting febuxostat in patients, especially those with existing cardiovascular disease.

4. Urate-lowering therapy: probenicid and benzbromarone—Uricosuric agents, such as probenecid and benzbromarone, are also effective in lowering serum urate levels. The patients in whom they are most effective are those who have good renal function (glomerular filtration rate above 60 mL/min), those who have no history of nephrolithiasis, those who can avoid low-dose salicylate ingestions, and those who are younger than 65 years of age. Salicylate use in doses in excess of 81 mg/day interferes with the effectiveness of uricosuric agents. Uricosuric agents should be avoided in patients with a history of nephrolithiasis, because stone formation is more likely due to the flooding of urine with uric acid. Probenecid is started at a dosage of 500 mg twice a day and advanced slowly up to a maximum dosage of 2.5 g a day or until the target urate level is reached. The most common side effects of this agent are rash and gastrointestinal upset. Benzbromarone, an agent available in Europe, is more potent than probenecid and may be effective in the face of moderate renal insufficiency.

5. Urate-lowering therapy: uricases—The most recently approved specific urate-lowering agent is pegloticase, a pegylated mammalian (porcine-like) recombinant uricase. The dosage is 8 mg intravenously every 2 weeks, and the impact of this drug on serum urate levels is dramatic. This agent should be reserved for those with severe gout with abundant tophaceous deposits. Its use may be limited by hypersensitivity reactions and the development of blocking antibodies.

► Prognosis

For patients that receive appropriate urate-lowering therapy and maintain their serum urate levels below 6.8 mg/dL (and preferably below 6.0 mg/dL), the prognosis is excellent with regards to eliminating gout flares. Tophaceous deposits can completely disappear, unless they have calcified. Unfortunately, if joint damage has developed as a result of the chronic inflammatory response to tophi, it will persist.

► Patient Education

The treatment of gout is complicated by poor compliance. The reasons behind this are multifactorial, both on the part of the physician and the patient. Some physicians focus only on treating gout flares and do not address the underlying issue of chronic hyperuricemia seriously. Patients often are not well-educated on the nature of gout and the differing indications for anti-inflammatory and urate-lowering therapy. An analogy has been developed that may help patients understand and better remember how to take their medications (see the box: Gout is Like Matches).

Gout Is Like Matches

The following paragraph is an analogy that can be used to explain gout to patients.

Gout is caused by chronic elevations of serum urate. Everyone has urate in their blood but some people have too much of it, and some of those people get gout. In those who get gout, urate precipitates and deposits as monosodium urate crystals around the joints and acts like matches. When you get a gout flare, one of the matches strikes and catches the joint on fire. When that happens, you should take an anti-inflammatory medication (eg, nonsteroidal anti-inflammatory drug like indomethacin, colchicine, or glucocorticoid). It is important to take it right away. If not, more matches will catch fire and the flare will worsen. Taking anti-inflammatory medications does not cure the gout because it only puts out the fire. The matches are still there and can light again. A urate-lowering drug will remove the matches by lowering the serum urate level below its saturation threshold. However, these medications can paradoxically increase your risk for gout flares in the short term (mobilization gout). To prevent this, colchicine or another anti-inflammatory medication should be used long term until your serum urate levels have stabilized. You can think of these anti-inflammatory medications as something that makes the matches damp and harder to strike. By keeping your serum urate level below its saturation threshold in the long term, we can eliminate all the matches, thereby leading to a "cure" for gout.

Data from Wortmann RL. Effective management of gout: an analogy. *Am J Med.* 1998;105:513.

Dalbeth N, Merriman TR, Stamp LK. Gout. *Lancet.* 2016; 388(10055):2039. [PMID: 27112094]

Neogi T, Jansen TL, Dalbeth N, et al. 2015 Gout Classification Criteria: an American College of Rheumatology/European League Against Rheumatism collaborative initiative. *Arthritis Rheum.* 2015;67(10):2557. [PMID: 26352873]

So AK, Martinon F. Inflammation in gout: mechanisms and therapeutic targets. *Nat Rev Rheumatol.* 2017;13(11):639. [PMID: 28959043]

Calcium Pyrophosphate Deposition Disease

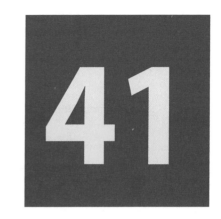

41

Jill C. Costello, MD

Ann K. Rosenthal, MD

ESSENTIALS OF DIAGNOSIS

▶ Calcium pyrophosphate deposition (CPPD) disease includes a spectrum of conditions ranging from asymptomatic radiographic changes to severe chronic arthritis.

▶ Acute CPP crystal arthritis, formerly known as pseudogout, shares some clinical features and treatment strategies with acute gout.

▶ The observation of calcium pyrophosphate crystals in synovial fluid is necessary for establishing a definitive diagnosis of CPPD disease.

▶ Chondrocalcinosis on radiograph helps support the diagnosis of CPPD disease.

▶ Premature CPPD disease can be a sign of a hyperparathyroidism, hemochromatosis, hypomagnesemia, or hypophosphatasia as well as familial CPPD disease.

▶ General Considerations

Calcium pyrophosphate deposition (CPPD) disease is a heterogeneous group of arthritic conditions associated with calcium pyrophosphate (CPP) crystals. It is a disease of the elderly, with most patients presenting after the age of 60 years, although familial forms of CPPD and metabolic disorders can cause disease at a younger age. The best known manifestation, acute CPP crystal arthritis, presents with sudden onset of pain and swelling in or surrounding the joint. However, CPPD is a spectrum of conditions ranging from asymptomatic radiographic changes to severe destructive arthritis. Its diverse clinical presentations and ability to mimic other rheumatologic conditions such as gout and rheumatoid arthritis (RA) cause challenges in its diagnosis and treatment. The European League Against Rheumatism (EULAR) has adopted the nomenclature listed in Table 41–1 for the various subtypes of CPPD.

The true incidence and prevalence of CPPD is unclear, but it is not rare and will likely increase as the population ages. Most prevalence studies are based on radiographs with cartilage calcification (chondrocalcinosis) as evidence of disease. The use of radiographic criteria alone as a disease marker, however, has significant limitations. Up to 20% of patients with proven acute CPP crystal arthritis do not have chondrocalcinosis on imaging. In addition, once joint damage advances in severity, it can be difficult to identify chondrocalcinosis due to cartilage loss. Therefore, the reported rate of 4–7% of the adult population in the United States and Europe likely underreports its true incidence and morbidity. Studies of radiographic findings show that the prevalence of cartilage calcification increases with age. One study demonstrated almost 50% of patients older than 84 years had chondrocalcinosis, compared to 15% of those aged 65–74 years.

Much has been learned regarding the pathogenesis of CPPD disease since calcified cartilage was first described in the early 1900s. Both the development of CPP crystals and the multiple mechanisms by which crystals cause inflammation are being actively studied. CPP crystals can initiate a vigorous inflammatory response using innate immune pathways similar to those involved in the inflammation induced by monosodium urate crystals. Abnormal pyrophosphate metabolism, changes in the extracellular matrix, and phenotypic changes of chondrocytes all play a role in its pathogenesis. In addition, studies of familial forms of CPPD disease have led to identification of possible targets for therapy. One of these is the multipass membrane protein known as ANKH, which is the human homologue of the protein product of the murine progressive ankylosis gene. Better understanding of the disordered CPP metabolism that characterizes CPPD may translate into improved therapies and strategies for the prevention of CPPD disease.

▶ Clinical Findings

A. Symptoms and Signs

The most widely recognized form of CPPD disease, acute CPP crystal arthritis, has historically been called pseudogout because of its clinical similarities to acute gouty arthritis.

Table 41–1. 2011 EULAR nomenclature for classification of subtypes of CPPD.

Asymptomatic CPPD disease (found on radiograph without clinical symptoms)
Acute CPP crystal arthritis (pseudogout)
Chronic CPP crystal inflammatory arthritis (pseudo-RA)
OA with CPPD, with or without superimposed acute attacks (pseudo-OA)
Severe joint degeneration (pseudo-neuropathic joint disease)
Spinal involvement

CPP, calcium pyrophosphate; CPPD, calcium pyrophosphate deposition; EULAR, European League Against Rheumatism; OA, osteoarthritis; RA, rheumatoid arthritis.

Swelling, warmth, and erythema of the involved joint and surrounding soft tissues with limited range of motion are its clinical hallmarks. The acute or subacute attacks are typically self-limited in nature in both types of crystal arthritis, but acute CPP attacks tend to persist longer despite treatment. Acute gout attacks last several days to 1 week. In contrast, acute CPP crystal arthritis can continue for weeks to months. Both can present with low-grade fevers and elevated inflammatory markers. The knee is the most commonly affected joint in acute CPP crystal arthritis. This marks an important contrast with acute gout, in which the first metatarsophalangeal joint is usually affected first. Other joints commonly involved in CPPD disease are the wrists, shoulders, ankles, feet, and elbows.

Trauma, surgery, and severe medical illness are known to provoke acute attacks. In patients diagnosed previously with acute CPP crystal arthritis, 10% will have a flare of their arthritis following a surgical procedure, for example, a joint arthroplasty. Knee surgery such as meniscal repair greatly increases the risk of future chondrocalcinosis in the operated knee. Parathyroidectomy is also associated with acute CPPD flares, probably because of fluxes in serum calcium levels. Medications have also been cited as being a precipitating factor in acute flares of CPP arthritis. Loop diuretics, granulocyte-macrophage colony-stimulating factor, and pamidronate have all been implicated in the precipitation of acute CPP crystal arthritis.

Chronic CPP crystal inflammatory arthritis (pseudorheumatoid pattern) is less common than acute CPP arthritis. It is a nonerosive polyarticular inflammatory arthritis of both small and large joints that presents as subacute attacks lasting 1 to several months. Often a symmetric pattern of joint involvement similar to RA occurs, although the flares of inflammation may be less symmetrical than in RA. In addition, both chronic CPP crystal inflammatory arthritis and RA are associated with synovial thickening, significant morning stiffness, fatigue, and reduced range of motion of the involved joints. A rare subtype of chronic CPP arthritis in the elderly causes an acute polyarticular arthritis presenting with leukocytosis, fever, and mental confusion. In such cases,

systemic infection must be excluded. Many diagnostic challenges exist in attempts to differentiate chronic CPP arthritis, RA, and polymyalgia rheumatica in the elderly, and these conditions may coexist.

Osteoarthritis (OA) with CPPD (pseudo-OA pattern) is the most common form of symptomatic CPPD, perhaps accounting for almost half of all cases. Asymmetrical bony enlargement, tenderness, effusions, crepitus, and decreased range of motion are present on examination. The joints most often involved include the knees, wrists, metacarpophalangeal (MCP) joints, hips, shoulders, elbows, and spine. Joint damage is quite extensive in this disorder, which may involve joints not typically involved in primary OA such as the MCPs or the elbows. Fifty percent of patients may have attacks of acute CPP crystal arthritis in addition to the OA associated with CPPD.

Rarer presentations of CPPD include severe joint degeneration (pseudo-neuropathic joint disease) and spinal involvement. Case reports describe evidence of CPP crystals associated with severe OA resembling Charcot joint. The "crowned dens syndrome" is the most commonly diagnosed form of CPPD in the spine. In the crowned dens syndrome, the dens (odontoid process) becomes inflamed by surrounding CPP crystal deposits. Patients present with severe neck pain, occipital headache, decreased range of motion of the cervical spine, elevated inflammatory markers, and fever, all of which mimics bacterial meningitis or another severe infection.

Most cases of CPPD disease occur in the elderly in a sporadic fashion, but CPPD is also associated with various metabolic conditions and can also occur in familial forms. Ryan and McCarty first described this etiologic classification of CPPD (Table 41–2). Hereditary and metabolic CPPD disease often present earlier in life compared to sporadic forms. Patients younger than 60 years should have a detailed family history taken to evaluate for hereditary forms of CPPD and undergo the recommended metabolic workup listed in Table 41–3.

Hyperparathyroidism is associated with CPPD. The etiology of this association was originally thought to stem from elevated levels of calcium, but correction of serum calcium levels following parathyroidectomy does not halt the progression of CPPD in these patients. An estimated 20–30% of patients with hyperparathyroidism have chondrocalcinosis, but the percentage of patients with clinical manifestations of arthritis is not known.

Hemochromatosis also has a well-established association with CPPD. The degenerative arthritis associated with

Table 41–2. Etiologic classification of CPPD (Ryan and McCarty).

I. Hereditary
II. Sporadic
III. Metabolic
IV. Associated with trauma or surgical procedures

CPPD, calcium pyrophosphate deposition.

Table 41–3. Diseases associated with CPPD and recommended lab testing.

Disease	Testing
Hyperparathyroidism	Calcium, parathyroid hormone
Hemochromatosis	Iron, TIBC, ferritin, C282Y
Hypophosphatasia	Alkaline phosphatase
Hypomagnesemia	Magnesium

CPPD, calcium pyrophosphate deposition; TIBC, total iron-binding capacity.

hemochromatosis most commonly involves the second and third MCP joints or both ankles. Radiographs show squared-off bone ends and hook-like osteophytes in MCPs and severe degenerative changes in the ankles. Chondrocalcinosis may be present. Unfortunately, correction of serum iron concentrations in these patients appears to alter the course of the arthritis little.

Hypomagnesemia and hypophosphatasia are also strongly associated with CPPD. Low magnesium levels such as those that occur in the short bowel syndrome, the Gitelman variant of Bartter syndrome, and, rarely, with diuretic use have been implicated in CPPD. The degree and the duration of magnesium deficiency required to contribute to CPPD disease remain unknown. Hypophosphatasia is a rare inborn error of metabolism caused by deficient alkaline phosphatase activity. This typically presents in childhood, although some patients present as young adults with chondrocalcinosis on radiographs.

B. Laboratory Findings

Synovial fluid analysis is the gold standard test for diagnosing CPPD. In acute CPP crystal arthritis, aspiration of the joint typically reveals an inflammatory fluid. The white blood cell (WBC) count typically ranges from 15,000 to 30,000 WBCs per mcL with 90% neutrophils in the differential. However, counts over 100,000 WBCs can occur. A Gram stain and culture should be included in the evaluation to exclude septic arthritis when suspicion is high. CPPD disease and septic arthritis can coexist, however.

Crystal analysis by compensated polarized light microscopy shows weakly positive birefringent rhomboid-shaped crystals phagocytosed by polymorphonuclear cells (PMNs) (Figure 41–1). An experienced examiner and time for a careful examination are both necessary, as CPP crystals are often difficult to detect. Many are not birefringent, are polymorphic in shape, and often small and sparse. In addition, CPP crystals can be found with monosodium urate crystals (gout) presenting as a mixed crystal picture.

Other laboratory findings associated with CPPD disease may include an elevated WBC with left shift on complete blood count (CBC), and an elevated erythrocyte sedimentation rate (ESR) and C-reactive protein (CRP) level.

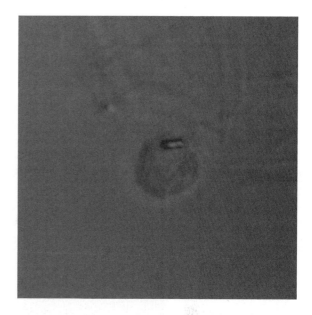

▲ **Figure 41–1.** Image of a typical rhomboid-shaped CPP crystal within a cell.

These findings are nonspecific and can be present with any inflammatory process.

C. Imaging Studies

Chondrocalcinosis on radiographs supports the diagnosis of CPPD disease. The classic finding of punctate and linear radiodensities in both hyaline cartilage and fibrocartilage are found most often in the knee, wrist, hip, elbow, and shoulder. Crystal deposition is frequently seen radiographically in fibrocartilage in the menisci of the knees (see Figure 41–2), symphysis pubis (Figure 41–3), and triangular fibrocartilage of the wrist (Figure 41–4). These findings can be subtle, and expertise in musculoskeletal radiology is quite helpful in evaluating the films if the suspicion of disease is high, but arthrocentesis is negative for crystals. While chondrocalcinosis can be the only radiographic finding on plain films, often it is seen in conjunction with findings of OA. These changes include subchondral cysts, osteophyte formation, and bone and cartilage damage. It is interesting, however, that the joints involved when OA and CPPD coexist are often not the same as primary OA. Radiographic changes of OA found in MCP joints, radiocarpal joints, elbows, and shoulders are likely to be associated with CPPD disease and occur less commonly in primary OA.

Ultrasound is being increasingly studied as a modality to aid in the diagnosis of CPPD disease. While promising, further studies are needed to establish standardization and validity of results. In addition, cost-effectiveness of arthrocentesis versus arthrocentesis with ultrasound should be carefully considered when evaluating ultrasound's role in diagnosis.

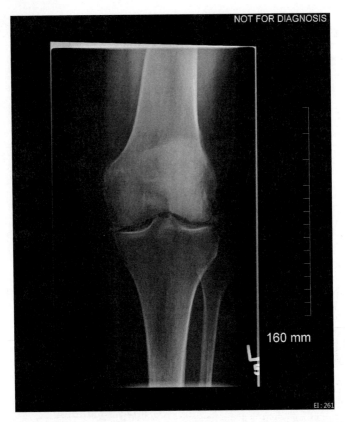

▲ **Figure 41–2.** Chondrocalcinosis in the meniscal cartilage of the knee. (Used with permission from Keith Baynes, MD.)

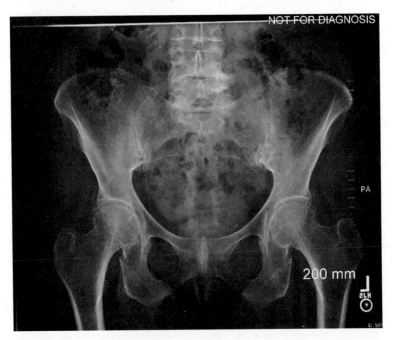

▲ **Figure 41–3.** Chondrocalcinosis in symphysis pubis and hip. (Used with permission from Keith Baynes, MD.)

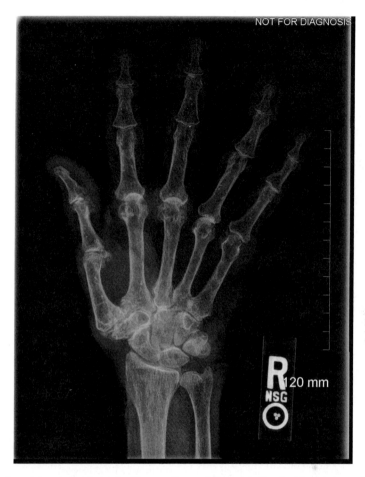

NOT FOR DIAGNOSIS

R 120 mm
NSG

▲ **Figure 41–4.** Chondrocalcinosis in triangular fibrocartilage of the wrist. (Used with permission from Keith Baynes, MD.)

D. Specific Tests

Crystal analysis of synovial fluid is the most accurate way to diagnose CPPD and radiographs further support the diagnosis. However, additional testing for medical conditions associated with CPPD disease as discussed above is warranted when patients present prematurely with clinical disease or incidental chondrocalcinosis on radiograph (see Table 41–3).

▶ Diagnosis & Differential Diagnosis

McCarty and colleagues proposed diagnostic criteria for CPPD designating the categories of definite, probable and possible CPPD. A definite diagnosis of CPPD disease requires the presence of both CPP crystals by synovial fluid analysis and chondrocalcinosis on radiographic exam. In addition, the demonstration of CPP crystals in tissue or synovial fluid by definitive means such as x-ray diffraction or spectroscopy can also support a definite diagnosis. The latter methods are primarily performed in research centers, thus making a

positive synovial fluid analysis plus chondrocalcinosis, the clinically relevant method of diagnosing definite CPPD.

Probable CPPD disease occurs with either CPP crystals identified on the synovial fluid analysis or chondrocalcinosis on radiographs of any common joints impacted by CPPD. Many patients fall into this category of CPPD. Possible CPPD disease raises suspicion of CPPD but is not diagnostic. Acute arthritis of large joints such as the knees or chronic severe OA in a distribution not typical for primary OA should raise suspicion for CPPD disease.

Due to the variety of clinical presentations of CPPD, the differential diagnosis is extensive. Septic arthritis must always be considered in an acute monoarthritis. Other crystal arthritides such as gout and basic calcium phosphate crystal arthritis should be included in one's differential. Patients may also have mixed crystal arthritis. Studies have found both monosodium urate and CPP crystals in 2–8% of synovial fluid samples. In chronic forms of CPPD, one must consider RA, polymyalgia rheumatica, primary OA, and in the setting of the crowned dens syndrome, meningitis.

Treatment

There is a paucity of effective therapies for both acute and chronic CPPD disease. The lack of full understanding of its pathogenesis coupled with limited evidence-based trials has led to insufficient medications for treatment and prevention. Treatment for acute CPP arthritis has largely been extrapolated from strategies for acute gouty arthritis.

The primary aim in the management of acute disease is to reduce inflammation. This is typically accomplished with one of the following medications: intra-articular glucocorticoid injections, oral colchicine, nonsteroidal anti-inflammatory drugs (NSAIDs), or glucocorticoids such as prednisone. These agents have found moderate success for most patients with acute CPP arthritis when compared to gout. However, it is typical for acute CPP arthritis to be less responsive to anti-inflammatory medication and to require longer duration of treatment. Both forms of crystal arthritis respond best to treatment initiated as close to onset of flare as possible. As most patients with acute CPP arthritis are older than 60 years, comorbidities and side effects of medications must be considered. Intra-articular glucocorticoid injections are often selected as first line for joints that have been crystal proven and with low suspicion for risk of septic joint. Colchicine, at a dose of 0.6 mg or 1.2 mg daily, is considered for patients without hepatic or renal impairment. NSAIDs can be used, but renal function, risk of gastrointestinal bleeding, and cardiovascular risk factors in the elderly often limit their use. Moderate doses of glucocorticoids, for example, 0.5 mg–1 mg/kg/day of prednisone for several days followed by a taper as the flare resolves are commonly used when colchicine and NSAIDs are not appropriate for the patient's comorbidities. Case reports have found the interleukin-β_1 antagonist, anakinra, effective for patients not responding to more traditional agents.

Part of the great success in treatment of acute gouty arthritis was the development of antihyperuricemic agents to reduce urate crystal load, thus preventing the development of acute disease. There are no analogous medications to reduce CPP crystal load to prevent CPPD disease. As a result, only the symptoms of the disease can be treated.

Refractory/chronic CPPD disease is difficult to manage. Patients who experience multiple flares may respond to daily colchicine or low-dose prednisone with a reduction in the number of flares. In addition to the drugs used in the treatment of acute CPP arthritis, hydroxychloroquine, methotrexate, and tumor necrosis factor-α (TNF-α) inhibitors have been used for long-term management of chronic or refractory disease. Few controlled trials of these agents for CPPD disease exist. Methotrexate initially showed promise in a small noncontrolled trial, but a subsequent small randomized case-controlled trial found no evidence for effectiveness when compared to placebo.

In addition to anti-inflammatory medications and immunosuppressive agents, many of the treatment strategies for OA such as acetaminophen, duloxetine, or topical capsaicin or diclofenac gel can be used for pain management of noninflammatory symptoms in CPPD disease.

When to Refer

The diagnosis of CPPD disease is challenging due to its variety of clinical presentations and the expertise required in identifying CPP crystals in synovial fluid. In addition, response to anti-inflammatory medications is often suboptimal in comparison to acute gouty arthritis. In any patient without an established diagnosis, rheumatological evaluation is recommended. In addition, patients responding poorly to anti-inflammatory treatments merit rheumatologic collaboration. Rheumatologists can also help determine when to test for metabolic conditions associated with CPPD and when to refer to an orthopedic surgeon for consideration of joint replacement.

ACKNOWLEDGMENT

The authors wish to thank Dr. Keith Baynes for his generous contribution of radiographs for this chapter.

Finckh A, McCarthy GM, Madigan A, et al. Methotrexate in chronic-recurrent calcium pyrophosphate deposition disease: no significant effect in a randomized crossover trial. *Arthritis Res Ther.* 2014;16(5):458. [PMID: 25315665]

Kleiber Balderrama C, Rosenthal AK, Lans D, et al. Calcium pyrophosphate deposition disease and associated medical comorbidities: a national cross-sectional study of US veterans. *Arthritis Care Res.* 2017;69(9):1400. [PMID: 27898996]

McCarthy GM, Dunne A. Calcium crystal deposition diseases— beyond gout. *Nat Rev Rheumatol.* 2018;14(10):592. [PMID: 30190520]

Molto A, Ea HK, Richette P, et al. Efficacy of anakinra for refractory acute calcium pyrophosphate crystal arthritis. *Joint Bone Spine.* 2012;79:621. [PMID: 22658375]

Neame RL, Carr AJ, Muir K, et al. UK community prevalence of knee chondrocalcinosis: evidence that correlation with osteoarthritis is through a shared association with osteophyte. *Ann Rheum Dis.* 2003;62:513. [PMID: 12759286]

Roddy E, Muller S, Paskins Z, Hider SL, Blagojevic-Bucknall M, Mallen CD. Incident acute pseudogout and prior bisphosphonate use: matched case-control in the UK-Clinical Practice Research Datalink. *Medicine (Baltimore).* 2017;96(12):e6177. [PMID: 28328803]

Rosenthal AK, Gohr CM, Mitton-Fitzgerald E, Lutz MK, Dubyak GR, Ryan LM. The progressive ankylosis gene product ANK regulates extracellular ATP levels in primary articular chondrocytes. *Arthritis Res Ther.* 2013;15:R154. [PMID: 24286344]

Rosenthal AK, Ryan LM. Calcium pyrophosphate deposition disease. *N Engl J Med.* 2016;374(26)2575. [PMID:27355536]

Wendling D, Tisserand G, Griffond V, et al. Acute pseudogout after pamidronate infusion. *Clin Rheumatol.* 2008;27:1205. [PMID: 18500436]

Zhang W, Doherty M, Bardin T, et al. EULAR recommendations for calcium pyrophosphate deposition. Part I: terminology and diagnosis. *Ann Rheum Dis.* 2011;70(4)563. [PMID:212161817]

Septic Arthritis

42

Sandra B. Nelson, MD

ESSENTIALS OF DIAGNOSIS

► Septic arthritis is characterized by invasion of synovium and synovial fluid by microorganisms, most commonly bacterial. The diagnosis should be considered in the patient who presents with acute monoarthritis, particularly when associated with fever or laboratory signs of acute inflammation.

► Septic arthritis is a rheumatologic emergency, associated with significant morbidity and mortality if the diagnosis and appropriate management is delayed. When septic arthritis is considered, prompt arthrocentesis is critical. Empiric treatment, including both antimicrobial management and drainage, is recommended when synovial fluid cell counts exceed 50,000 cells/mm³; however, lower cell counts do not exclude the diagnosis, particularly in the immunocompromised host.

► Treatment is multimodal and includes antimicrobial therapy and effective drainage and debridement. Surgical drainage is most commonly employed (arthroscopically or via an open synovectomy) though serial percutaneous drainage may be considered in some circumstances. Antimicrobial therapy directed to the infecting organism for durations of between 2 and 6 weeks is generally advised.

General Considerations

Septic arthritis occurs when microorganisms invade the synovium and replicate within the synovium and synovial fluid. While septic arthritis remains rare (7.8 cases per 100,000 person-years from a recent population-based report from the United Kingdom), the incidence of this devastating infection has been increasing (Rutherford et al, 2016). The rise in incidence of septic arthritis likely relates to an increasing prevalence of underlying risk factors, including an aging population, a greater prevalence of immunocompromising conditions, a rise in injection drug use, and greater use of vascular catheters. Changing virulence of organisms over time (including an increasing prevalence of virulent strains of methicillin-resistant *Staphylococcus aureus* [MRSA]) may also contribute to the rise in septic arthritis.

Pathogenesis

Septic arthritis occurs through two primary mechanisms: hematogenous and contiguous spread of organisms. Hematogenous infection is more common, accounting for approximately 75% of cases of septic arthritis. In hematogenous infection, organisms travel to the synovium through the bloodstream. The synovium itself does not have a basement membrane; therefore, when organisms land in synovial capillaries, they are more easily able to seed the joint space. Once within the joint space, bacterial adhesion factors attach to host extracellular matrix proteins; low shear conditions further allow the organisms to take hold. Supported by nutrients within the joint fluid, the bacteria then proliferate and establish infection. Joint damage ensues, mediated by bacterial toxins and enzymes, the host inflammatory response, and tissue ischemia related to tamponade.

Often in hematogenous infection, the bacteremia itself may be transient and unrecognized and only become manifest at the onset of joint pain. In other cases, the bacteremia may be overt, associated with fever or other signs of sepsis. Hematogenous septic arthritis may occur without other comorbid infection, or it may be associated with endocarditis or other nidus of infection. The bacterial portal of entry itself is not always recognized and may be remote from the site of infection. While skin sources may be the most common source of bacteremia, hematogenous seeding from the urinary tract, gastrointestinal system, and dental sources also occur.

Less commonly, septic arthritis may be caused by direct inoculation of organisms into the joint space, such as through percutaneous inoculation, penetrating trauma, arthroscopic surgery, or contiguous spread from adjacent infection (including osteomyelitis or infections associated with orthopedic fixation devices). Animal and human bites can also lead to septic arthritis when highly colonized teeth penetrate joint structures, most commonly on the hands. Septic arthritis may occur as a complication of joint surgery; rates of septic arthritis after arthroscopic knee surgery are lower than 1% in most series. Septic arthritis occurs even less commonly as a complication of joint injection; occurring in fewer than 1 in 2000 injections. Infections after joint injection are primarily caused by skin flora, suggesting insufficient skin sterilization; bacterial or fungal contamination of the injected material and/or contamination of multidose vials have also been reported.

▶ Risk Factors

The most important risk factor for the development of septic arthritis is preexisting joint disease. Many forms of joint disease increase the risk of septic arthritis; these include osteoarthritis, hemarthrosis, and crystalline arthritis, but the risk is highest in the inflammatory arthritides. There are likely several reasons for this increased risk. In active synovitis, synovial vascular proliferation increases bacterial trapping and the potential for organisms to translocate into the joint space. Overexpression of inflammatory host proteins may also facilitate bacterial attachment by adhering to bacterial proteins. Finally, local alterations in the immune milieu due to autoimmune disease and/or immune-modulating treatments may also enable infection to establish.

In addition to joint destruction, other established risk factors for septic arthritis include increasing age and comorbid conditions, including diabetes, alcohol abuse and liver disease, malignancy, and end-stage renal disease. The use of immunosuppressive medications, including glucocorticoids and antitumor necrosis factors, also increases the risk. Impaired skin integrity, such as that seen with eczema, psoriasis, and injection drug use, may facilitate the hematogenous seeding of organisms. Injection drug use may introduce bacteria directly into the bloodstream. In injection drug use, the bacteria may contaminate the drug or the water used for injection, may colonize the equipment used for injection, may be from inadequately prepared skin, or from mouth flora when needles are licked prior to injection.

▶ Microbiology

Most cases of septic arthritis are caused by bacteria. *Staphylococcus aureus* is the most common organism causing this syndrome, accounting for 45–70% of all cases. Coagulase-negative staphylococci, a less common cause of septic arthritis, can be seen in immunocompromised hosts, usually via direct inoculation (eg, as a complication of injection, orthopedic surgery, and associated with orthopedic device infection).

Streptococci account for between 10% and 20% of cases of septic arthritis in adults. Infecting species include the pyogenic streptococci [including *Streptococcus pyogenes* (group A *Streptococcus*) and *Streptococcus dysgalactiae* (groups C and G *Streptococcus*)], viridans streptococci (often associated with odontogenic disease or procedures), *Streptococcus agalactiae* (group B *Streptococcus*), and *Streptococcus pneumoniae* (pneumococcus), seen in older adults and those with comorbidities. Gram-negative infections are less common and tend to be seen in the elderly and patients with comorbidities. Antecedent urinary tract infection and gastrointestinal disease may predispose to gram-negative infection.

Several less common organisms are worth considering in the right epidemiologic context (Table 42–1). *Neisseria gonorrhoeae* accounts for less than 5% of all cases of septic arthritis. Gonococcal septic arthritis occurs as a consequence of untreated mucosal gonorrhea, and therefore is more common in settings in which the mucosal phase is unrecognized. Gonococcal cervicitis in women and rectal and oropharyngeal gonorrhea in both men and women are more likely to be unrecognized than urethral disease in men. Gonococcal septic arthritis may occur without other features of disseminated gonococcal infection (DGI) or may be seen in addition to the classic features of DGI, including dermatitis, extensor tenosynovitis, and migratory arthralgias. *N gonorrhoeae* is more difficult than other organisms to culture and should be considered in all sexually active patients with septic arthritis, especially when gram-negative diplococci are seen on synovial fluid Gram stain, and/or other organisms are not identified in culture. Gonococcal septic arthritis is commonly associated with lower cell counts than other forms of bacterial arthritis and may be more likely to be polyarticular.

Fungal septic arthritis is far less common than bacterial septic arthritis, in most series accounting for fewer than 1–2% of all cases. Of the fungi, *Candida* species are the most common organisms to cause septic arthritis. Candida septic arthritis is seen primarily in immunocompromised hosts, and additionally in the setting of injection drug use, in which the organism may contaminate the drug, the equipment used for injection, or the needle when licked. Environmental molds such as *Aspergillus* are rare causes of septic arthritis; these usually arise from direct inoculation, as can be seen with penetrating trauma or direct injection. A large outbreak of fungal septic arthritis occurred in the United States when fungal organisms contaminated the manufacture of steroids used for injection (Kauffman et al, 2013). Infection with environmental dimorphic fungi are seen in certain geographic regions, including with *Coccidioides immitis* (southwestern United States), *Blastomyces dermatitidis* (south central and southeastern United States), and *Histoplasma capsulatum* (midwestern United States; Ohio and Mississippi River valleys). Dissemination of the dimorphic molds to joints may be seen in immunocompetent hosts but remains more common in the immunocompromised.

Table 42–1. Some important organisms causing septic arthritis.

Organism	Clinical Features	Epidemiologic Features
Staphylococcus aureus	Most common cause, usually fulminant and rapid in onset. Gram-positive cocci may be seen on Gram stain	Underlying skin conditions (eczema, psoriasis) Injection drug use
Coagulase-negative staphylococci	May be more indolent in presentation	Associated with steroid injections, orthopedic devices
Streptococcus species	Often rapid in onset. Gram-positive cocci on Gram stain	
Enterobacteriaceae (eg, *Escherichia coli*)	Gram-negative rods on Gram stain	Typically in elderly. Antecedent urinary tract or GI illness
Neisseria gonorrhoeae	May be associated with dermatitis, extensor synovitis, migratory arthralgias. May see gram-negative diplococci	Sexually active
Salmonella species	Gram-negative rods on Gram stain	Sickle cell disease, diabetes, immunocompromising conditions. May be associated with antecedent diarrhea or developing world travel
Brucella species	Predilection for sacroiliac joint. Often associated with prodrome of fevers, chills, and/or weight loss	Travel to or residence in endemic areas (Mediterranean basin). Consumption of unpasteurized dairy
HACEK organisms (especially *Haemophilus* species, *Eikenella corrodens*, *Kingella kingae*)	*Kingella* common in young children. Often culture negative	Human bite wounds
Pasteurella species	Gram-negative rods	Cat and dog bites
Mycoplasma species	Subacute to chronic onset Difficult to culture	Immunocompromised hosts, especially humoral deficiencies Postpartum women
Lyme (*Borrelia burgdorferi*)	Subacute illness characterized by large effusions, often the knee	In the United States, endemic in northeastern and upper mid-west. Tick exposures (may not have history of prior tick bite)
Candida species	Subacute onset	Immunocompromised hosts Injection drug use Preexisting vascular catheters

Like fungal disease, mycobacterial septic arthritis is rare. *Mycobacterium tuberculosis* (MTb) is a more common cause of septic arthritis in countries in the developing world in which the organism is endemic. In the United States, tuberculous septic arthritis is seen most commonly in individuals who emigrate from endemic areas. MTb may spread hematogenously to joints during primary infection, but septic arthritis due to MTb often occurs later as part of reactivation of latent disease. Infectious arthritis with nontuberculous mycobacteria (NTM) may be due to hematogenous spread in immunocompromised hosts, and also due to direct inoculation. NTM are ubiquitous in the environment, particularly in soil and water, and may inoculate a joint in the setting of penetrating trauma. As with fungal infections, iatrogenic arthritis due to NTM may occur as a consequence of injection drug use and contaminated injections. Additional organisms and their unique clinical and epidemiologic features are included in Table 42–1.

▶ **Prevention**

Prompt recognition and treatment of primary infections (including bacteremia and endocarditis, odontogenic infection) may prevent bacteremic seeding of joints. Patients who suffer animal and human bites may benefit from antimicrobial prophylaxis; this is particularly relevant in bites to the hand, in bites from humans and cats, and in hosts with comorbidities and/or immunosuppression. Many cases of septic arthritis in the setting of injection drug use can also be prevented with harm reduction strategies, including the use of sterile equipment (clean needles), avoidance of sharing supplies for injection, use of alcohol or other antiseptics for skin preparation, and counseling around avoidance of licking needles. While abstinence from injection drug use remains the long-term goal, all patients with a history of injection drug use should be counseled around how to reduce the infectious risks associated with injection. Iatrogenic septic arthritis after joint injection can usually be prevented with rigid adherence to infection control practices, including meticulous attention to skin preparation, use of sterile equipment, and avoidance of multiuse vials.

► Clinical Findings

A. Signs and Symptoms

Most cases of bacterial septic arthritis present as an acute monoarthritis, with symptoms presenting over days to 1 or 2 weeks. The pain associated with septic arthritis is worse with movement of the involved joint and, for weight-bearing joints, is associated with painful ambulation. Occasionally the onset and progression of symptoms will be less fulminant, occurring over weeks to a few months; this is seen most commonly with indolent organisms including fungi and mycobacteria. The knee is the most common joint affected by septic arthritis, involved in approximately half of all cases. Other large joints comprise the majority of other cases. Small joint septic arthritis, particularly involving the hands, may occur in the setting of percutaneous trauma and bite wounds. Septic sacroiliitis is rare; involvement of the sacroiliac joint may be seen in injection drug use and should also lead the clinician to consider *Brucella* species, which have a predilection for this joint. Most septic arthritis is monoarticular, while 10–20% may be polyarticular. Polyarthritis is seen in the setting of high-grade bacteremia (most commonly with *S aureus* and streptococci) and in immunocompromised hosts. Gonococcal septic arthritis may also be polyarticular. Symptoms of inflammation including fever, chills, and night sweats, if present, support the infectious etiology of monoarthritis. Most patients will describe at least a low-grade temperature, but true fever is absent in close to half of all patients with septic arthritis and should therefore not be used to exclude the diagnosis. Findings that may be present on exam include warmth, effusion, and guarding against range-of-motion testing. The absence of erythema overlying a joint does not exclude the diagnosis of joint sepsis.

B. Laboratory Findings

Patients with septic arthritis often have laboratory evidence of inflammation, including elevation of the serum white blood cell count and percent neutrophils. More specific markers of inflammation, such as the erythrocyte sedimentation rate (ESR) and C-reactive protein (CRP), support the diagnosis of septic arthritis when elevated, but neither is sufficiently sensitive nor specific to confirm the diagnosis without additional studies. All patients with suspected septic arthritis should have blood cultures obtained prior to the administration of any antibiotic therapy. Blood cultures are positive in approximately one-third of patients with septic arthritis, including in some cases in which synovial fluid cultures are negative.

Septic arthritis is confirmed most definitively through arthrocentesis. In a stable patient, synovial fluid aspiration should be performed prior to the administration of antimicrobial therapy, as this can lower the yield of culture. When suspected, synovial fluid should be sent for cell count and differential, Gram stain and culture, and crystal analysis. (Microcrystalline arthritis is a frequent mimic of infection.) The presence of septic arthritis is confirmed when there is a positive synovial fluid Gram stain and/or culture. Synovial fluid Gram stain is positive in approximately 30–50% of cases of septic arthritis, while the yield of synovial fluid culture is approximately 60–80%. Negative synovial fluid cultures may be seen with prior antibiotic administration, and with fastidious organisms such as those in the HACEK family, gonococcus, mycoplasma, and Lyme. The yield of synovial fluid cultures may be increased when synovial fluid is inoculated directly into blood culture bottles; discussion with the microbiology laboratory can help to determine the best culture process for synovial fluid at each institution. While routine bacterial cultures are sufficient for most patients with suspected septic arthritis, mycobacterial and fungal cultures should be obtained when these entities are suspected based on clinical and epidemiologic factors. If gonococcal septic arthritis is considered, the microbiology laboratory should be notified, as special media are required to grow *N gonorrhoeae*. While synovial fluid culture remains the gold standard for diagnosis, it is important to remember that 20–40% of patients will have negative cultures. Therefore a negative culture cannot exclude septic arthritis, especially when clinical suspicion is high.

While the Gram stain results quickly, taking only minutes to perform, it is positive in fewer than half of all cases of septic arthritis, and synovial fluid culture may take days to yield results. As treatment decisions, such as the need for empiric antimicrobials and/or surgical debridement, are often made prior to the return of culture results, the synovial fluid cell count, and differential prove most useful in real time. Most cases of septic arthritis are associated with synovial fluid cell counts of greater than 25,000 white blood cells/mm³, though there is substantial overlap with other diagnoses at lower cell counts. The greater the synovial fluid white blood cell count, the greater the likelihood of septic arthritis (Margaretten et al, 2012). Clinicians often use a cell count of 50,000 synovial WBCs/mm³ as an indicator of septic arthritis, but there is no threshold value below which septic arthritis is excluded. Indeed, approximately one-third of patients with septic arthritis have synovial fluid cell counts below 50,000 cells/mm³. Lower cell counts are seen more commonly in immunocompromised hosts, with gonococcal septic arthritis, and with more indolent organisms. In addition to the synovial fluid white blood count (WBC), the proportion of those WBCs that are neutrophils can be an important diagnostic tool. In septic arthritis, the majority of synovial WBCs are neutrophils, usually exceeding 80–90%.

The presence of synovial fluid crystals when viewed with a polarizing microscope may sway the clinician away from the diagnosis of septic arthritis, and this is appropriate when crystalline arthritis is strongly suspected (eg, in a patient with monoarthritis involving the great toe metatarsophalangeal joint or a history of polyarticular gout). However, septic arthritis can coexist with crystalline arthropathy, and patients with preexisting joint disease are at increased risk of septic arthritis. Therefore, the presence of crystals does not exclude the diagnosis of septic arthritis (Papanicolas et al, 2012).

C. Imaging Studies

Imaging studies are not needed for the diagnosis of septic arthritis. In and of themselves imaging tests are neither sufficiently sensitive to confirm the diagnosis of infection nor specific enough to rule it out. Nonetheless, there may be value to imaging studies in the evaluation of the patient with suspected septic arthritis. Plain films are recommended when there is a history of trauma, in order to exclude foreign body and/or fracture. While effusion of the knee can be identified by clinical exam, it is more difficult to confirm the presence of effusion in the hip joint. Therefore, patients presenting with acute hip pain may benefit from additional imaging prior to hip joint aspiration to confirm the presence of effusion. Ultrasound, computed tomography (CT), and/or magnetic resonance imaging (MRI) may be useful to prove the presence of effusion prior to arthrocentesis in this setting. In joints that are difficult to localize percutaneously, such as the hip and sacroiliac joints, CT or fluoroscopy may be needed to confirm needle placement in arthrocentesis. Imaging may also be helpful in the setting of chronic presentations of septic arthritis, in order to evaluate for associated osteomyelitis.

D. Special Tests

When specific organisms are considered, additional testing may be indicated. For all patients with suspected gonococcal septic arthritis, mucosal swabs (eg, cervical, urethral, urine, rectal, and/or oropharyngeal) for nucleic acid amplification testing should be performed, as the yield of synovial fluid Gram stain and culture for gonococcus is low. Serologic testing should be considered for patients with suspected Lyme and Brucella, while tuberculin skin testing and/or interferon gamma release assay should be obtained when tuberculosis is considered.

▶ Differential Diagnosis

The differential diagnosis for acute monoarthritis is broad (Table 42–2). Challenging this further, other forms of arthritis predispose to joint sepsis, and thus infection can coexist with other causes of arthritis. Further discussion of these alternate diagnoses is found elsewhere in this book.

▶ Treatment

There are two elements of treatment for septic arthritis: antimicrobial therapy and drainage. With some exceptions, antimicrobial therapy should be withheld until after

Table 42–2. Differential diagnosis of monoarthritis.

Crystalline arthritis (including gout, calcium pyrophosphate deposition)
Reactive arthritis
Systemic lupus erythematosus
Rheumatoid arthritis
Osteoarthritis
Neuropathic arthropathy
Hemarthrosis
Trauma (meniscal injury, intra-articular fracture)
Sickle cell disease
Avascular necrosis
Transient synovitis of the hip (children)
Foreign body synovitis
Pigmented villonodular synovitis
Malignancy (primary or metastatic)

arthrocentesis, in order to optimize the yield of culture growth. In patients who present with findings of sepsis (eg, hypotension, tachycardia, altered mental status, evidence of organ dysfunction) antibiotic therapy should not be withheld until after arthrocentesis. However, all patients with suspected septic arthritis (including those with suspected sepsis) should have blood cultures obtained prior to antibiotic administration. In patients who are stable, arthrocentesis should be performed prior to administration of antimicrobial therapy.

When septic arthritis is suspected based on clinical findings and/or preliminary laboratory results, empirical antimicrobial therapy is often started prior to formal identification of an organism. If the synovial fluid or blood culture Gram stain is positive, empiric therapy should be directed accordingly. In the setting of negative or unavailable Gram stain, empiric antibiotic therapy considers likely organisms and generally includes broad-spectrum coverage against gram-positive and gram-negative organisms. In patients with risk factors for methicillin-resistant organisms (eg, prior history of MRSA colonization or infection, history of injection drug use, recent hospitalizations) and/or when MRSA prevalence is high, empiric therapy should include an agent active against MRSA, such as vancomycin. As vancomycin is slow to achieve bactericidal levels and has no activity against gram-negative organisms, a second agent such as ceftriaxone or other third- or fourth-generation cephalosporin is usually added, both to provide more rapid killing of susceptible organisms and for expanded gram-negative coverage. When there are specific risk factors for gram-negative infection (including being elderly, immunocompromised, having sepsis, or a history of injection drug use) an antipseudomonal antibacterial should be added, such as piperacillin-tazobactam, cefepime, or carbapenem. When there are risk factors for gonococcal infection, a clinical syndrome compatible with disseminated gonococcus, and/or a Gram stain with gram-negative cocci,

Table 42–3. Empiric antimicrobial management of septic arthritis.

Clinical Features and Gram Stain Results	Antibiotic Therapy Regimen[a]
Gram-positive cocci	For most patients (including those at risk of MRSA): Vancomycin 15–20 mg/kg IV q8–12h May consider addition of β-lactam therapy (eg, nafcillin 1–2 g IV 4 h; cefazolin 2 g IV q8h; or ceftriaxone 1–2 g IV q24h) If low risk for MRSA: cefazolin 2g IV q8h
Gram-negative cocci and/or clinical concern for disseminated gonococcal infection	Ceftriaxone 1 g IV q24h *and* Azithromycin 1 g orally (as a single dose)
Gram-negative rods	Cefepime 1–2 g IV q8–12h *or* Piperacillin-tazobactam 3.375–4.5 g IV q6h *or* Meropenem 1g IV q8h
Negative Gram stain	Vancomycin 15–20 mg/kg IV q8–12h *and* Ceftriaxone 1–2 g IV q24h or cefepime 1–2 g IV q8–12h

[a]Listed antibiotic dosing regimens are for adults of normal body weight and renal function. Specific dosing may vary and should consider age, body weight, and renal function.
MRSA, methicillin-resistant *Staphylococcus aureus*.

patients should be treated with ceftriaxone and azithromycin. Empiric antibiotic regimens are included in Table 42–3.

Once a causative organism has been identified through a positive blood or synovial fluid culture, antibacterial therapy should be narrowed based on culture results. Once the organism is known, the choice of antibiotic depends on the organism and its sensitivities, antimicrobial bioavailability and tissue penetration, comorbidities such as renal disease and liver disease, other medications with which antimicrobials may interact, and known allergies and intolerances. Infectious disease consultation can assist with determining the best antibiotic regimen. While historically intravenous therapy has been advised to treat important osteoarticular infections, this paradigm may be shifting. Many oral antimicrobial agents achieve sufficient tissue levels within synovial fluid (Thabit et al, 2019); early stepdown to oral therapy may therefore be appropriate for some patients.

The optimal duration of antibiotic therapy for septic arthritis is not well studied. When there is associated endocarditis or high-grade bacteremia, particularly with *S aureus*, the route and duration of antimicrobial therapy are usually dictated by optimal therapy for the systemic infection. In the absence of bacteremia and/or endocarditis, traditionally patients with septic arthritis have been treated with intravenous therapy for at least several weeks and often complete 4–6 weeks of total antibiotic therapy. Given higher complication rates with infection due to *S aureus*, longer treatment regimens (eg, 6 weeks) are advised for infection due to *S aureus*. Several recent studies in patients without bacteremia or sepsis support shorter treatment durations for septic arthritis (eg, as few as 2 weeks); however, the clinical characteristics that would enable shorter treatment duration are unknown. Gonococcal arthritis without osteomyelitis is usually treated for 7–14 days. In the absence of gonococcal susceptibilities, treatment with ceftriaxone is recommended. If susceptibilities are known and the organism is susceptible to fluoroquinolones, treatment may be completed with oral levofloxacin. Duration of therapy is much longer for infections due to fungi and mycobacteria, often on the order of 3–12 months.

In addition to antimicrobial therapy, patients with septic arthritis require some form of joint drainage. Drainage decompresses the joint (improving comfort and diminishing pain), reduces the bacterial load, and removes the toxins, enzymes, and inflammatory cytokines that contribute to joint destruction. There are several options for drainage, including serial percutaneous aspiration, arthroscopic debridement, and open arthrotomy. However, randomized prospective studies comparing drainage strategies are limited (Bovon-ratwet et al, 2018). The choice of drainage strategy depends on urgency (eg, the presence of sepsis), the joint or joints involved, surgical risks, and the comfort and experience of the orthopedic surgical team. Most patients still undergo surgical debridement, either arthroscopic or open surgical arthrotomy. Arthroscopic procedures are less invasive and are commonly performed for stable patients with septic arthritis particularly involving knees. Open procedures are favored in the hip, which is more challenging to access arthroscopically. Open procedures are also preferred when there is associated osteomyelitis or soft tissue infection, preexisting joint damage, and in the setting of sepsis. Serial arthrocentesis without surgery may be successful in some patients, particularly those with milder infection, involvement of specific joints such as the sacroiliac joint in which surgery may be destabilizing, or when there are important medical risks to surgery. Arthrocentesis should be performed daily until the effusion resolves, the synovial fluid is no longer purulent, and synovial fluid cultures are negative. Surgical management may not be required in all cases of gonococcal septic arthritis, in which microbiological and functional outcomes are better.

Given that much of the joint destruction in septic arthritis is mediated by the host inflammatory response, adjunctive therapy with glucocorticoids has been considered as part of a comprehensive therapeutic approach to joint sepsis. Several small randomized controlled trials conducted in children with septic arthritis supports the use of glucocorticoids; however, no such trials have been conducted in adults. Routine use of glucocorticoids in adults with septic arthritis cannot be recommended.

▶ Complications

Infectious arthritis is a highly inflammatory process, and irreversible joint destruction begins rapidly, within hours to days of the onset of symptoms. The joint damage is mediated both by the infecting organisms and the host immune response, in which an inflammatory surge can lead to significant chondrolysis. While septic arthritis is microbiologically cured in the vast majority of patients who develop it, many will go on to develop postinfectious arthritis and other complications. Complications are more likely with more virulent organisms, such as *S aureus*, when there is associated systemic sepsis, with delays in antimicrobial treatment and/or drainage, when there is preexisting joint damage at the onset of disease (such as seen in patients with rheumatoid arthritis), and in the elderly and those with comorbidities. Early mobilization and physical therapy may help to reduce the burden and significance of postinfectious complications.

Noninfectious complications include arthrosis, postinfectious arthritis, and functional limitations. The prevalence of persistent joint dysfunction after an episode of septic arthritis varies, but impacts at least 30% of patients who suffer septic arthritis. A significant minority of patients with septic arthritis require additional surgical procedures to manage complications; these include joint replacement, osteosynthesis (fusion), and amputation.

Prognosis

Mortality from septic arthritis has been estimated to range between 5% and 15%. The mortality in association with septic arthritis is not always directly attributable to the joint infection but seen from complications of associated bacteremia and sepsis, particularly in older patients and those with comorbidities. Predictors of mortality include increasing age, the presence of bacteremia, higher values on sepsis scores, and greater scores on comorbidity indices. In some series, mortality is more common with septic arthritis due to *S aureus*, usually in the setting of sepsis.

Recurrent septic arthritis complicates 5–10% of patients who suffer a first episode of septic arthritis. Recurrence in the same joint may develop either when the initial treatment course fails to eradicate the organism or because the joint damage sustained during the episode of septic arthritis predisposes to additional septic arthritis, often in a patient with comorbidities at higher risk of bacteremia.

When to Refer/Admit

Septic arthritis is a rheumatologic emergency with a significant mortality risk; the vast majority of patients with septic arthritis require hospitalization. Hospitalization facilitates timely initiation of potent empiric intravenous antimicrobial therapy, rapid access to surgical evaluation and debridement, and supportive care. Patients with more chronic forms of septic arthritis may be able to be evaluated initially as outpatients as the diagnosis is considered, though the need for surgical therapy often requires hospitalization.

Patients with septic arthritis should be seen by orthopedists, who can assist with facilitating optimal joint drainage. In addition to orthopedic care, patients with septic arthritis benefit from care provided by infectious disease physicians, who may help to optimize the microbiologic diagnostics and determine best therapeutic options. Patients being treated for septic arthritis often have impaired mobilization and benefit from physical and/or occupational therapy to prevent joint contractures and improve long-term functional outcomes.

Bovonratwet P, Nelson SJ, Bellamkonda K, et al. Similar 30-day complications for septic knee arthritis treated with arthrotomy or arthroscopy: an American College of Surgeons National Surgical. *Arthrosc J Arthrosc Relat Surg.* 2018;34(1):213-219. [PMID: 28866341]

Kauffman CA, Pappas PG, Patterson TF. Fungal infections associated with contaminated methylprednisolone injections. *N Engl J Med.* 2013;368(26):2495-2500. [PMID: 23083312]

Margaretten ME, Kohlwes J, Moore D, Bent S. Does this adult patient have septic arthritis? *JAMA.* 2007;297(13):1478-1488. [PMID: 17405973]

Papanicolas LE, Hakendorf P, Llewellyn D, Papanicolas LE, Hakendorf P, Gordon DL. Concomitant septic arthritis in crystal monoarthritis. *J Rheumatol.* 2012;39(1):157-160. [PMID: 22133623]

Rutherford AI, Subesinghe S, Bharucha T, Ibrahim F, Kleymann A, Galloway JB. Concise report: a population study of the reported incidence of native joint septic arthritis in the United Kingdom between 1998 and 2013. *Rheumatology (Oxford).* 2016;55(12):2176-2180. [PMID: 27638811]

Thabit AK, Fatani DF, Bamakhrama MS, Barnawi OA, Basudan LO, Alhejaili SF. Antibiotic penetration into bone and joints: an updated review. *Int J Infect Dis.* 2019;81:128-136. [PMID: 30772469]

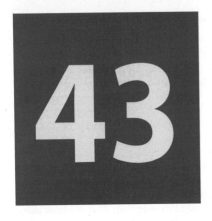

Lyme Disease

Linda K. Bockenstedt, MD

Alexia A. Belperron, PhD

ESSENTIALS OF DIAGNOSIS

▶ Lyme borreliosis should be considered in individuals who have a reasonable risk of exposure to *Borrelia burgdorferi*-infected ticks and who present with a characteristic complex of signs and symptoms.

▶ Classic clinical features occur in stages:

- Early localized infection (3–30 days after tick bite): a single hallmark skin lesion erythema migrans (EM), occasionally associated with fever, malaise, headache, arthralgias, and myalgias. These constitutional symptoms can occur in the absence of EM, but this is unusual.

- Early disseminated infection (weeks to a few months after tick bite): signs include multiple EM lesions, often with associated fever, migratory arthralgias, and myalgias; carditis manifested primarily as AV nodal block; neurologic features, including cranial nerve palsies (especially involving the facial nerve), lymphocytic meningitis, and radiculoneuropathies.

- Late infection (several months to years after tick bite): arthritis, including monoarticular and migratory pauciarticular arthritis; rarely neurologic features such as peripheral neuropathies or chronic mild encephalopathy.

- Supporting serologic evidence of exposure to *B burgdorferi* is present in the majority of cases but can be absent in early infection.

▶ General Considerations

Lyme disease is a multisystem disorder caused by infection with spirochetes of the genus *Borrelia burgdorferi sensu lato* (*sl*), most commonly *B burgdorferi sensu stricto* (*ss*), *B garinii*, and *B afzelii* species. Hard-shelled ticks of the *Ixodidae* family—*Ixodes scapularis* and *I pacificus* in the United States,

I ricinus in Europe, and *I persulcatus* in Asia—serve as vectors for infection. In Europe and Asia, *B garinii* and *B afzelii* are the main etiologic agents of Lyme borreliosis, and cases due to *B burgdorferi sensu stricto* are less common. In contrast, *B burgdorferi sensu stricto* is responsible for virtually all cases of Lyme disease in the United States. The major exception to this rule is the small number of infections associated with a new species, *B mayonii*, recently identified in the upper Midwest (Minnesota, Wisconsin, and North Dakota). The specific *B burgdorferi sl* species causing infection influences the prevalence of certain disease manifestations. As examples, neurologic disease is more common with *B garinii*, late skin disease is more common with *B afzelii*, and arthritis is more common with *B burgdorferi ss*. *B mayonii* infection may exhibit atypical features described later.

Lyme borreliosis first came to medical attention in the United States in 1975, with the investigation of a clustering of childhood arthritis in the region around Lyme, Connecticut. Lyme arthritis, as it was initially termed, was soon found to be one manifestation of systemic infection with *B burgdorferi*. The earliest clinical sign reported by patients was a characteristic skin lesion erythema migrans (EM) at the site of a tick bite. In Europe, EM had been associated with *I ricinus* tick bites since the early twentieth century, and the skin disease was treated successfully with penicillin after spirochetes were visualized in biopsy specimens in the mid-1900s. Other systemic manifestations were occasionally present, especially neurologic disease (Bannwarth syndrome), but the broader clinical spectrum with heart and joint involvement was not fully appreciated until the emergence of the disease in the United States.

Since its discovery, the geographic distribution of Lyme borreliosis has expanded. It is now recognized to be the most common vector-borne infection in North America. The annual incidence of Lyme disease is estimated to be around 300,000 cases based on large commercial laboratory testing and medical claims information. Most cases of Lyme borreliosis are found in the northeast, mid-Atlantic states, and upper Midwest region. In 2016, 96% of confirmed cases originated from only 14 states: Connecticut, Delaware, Maine, Maryland, Massachusetts, Minnesota, New Hampshire, New Jersey, New York, Pennsylvania, Rhode Island, Vermont, Virginia, and Wisconsin.

Lyme borreliosis begins when humans serve as incidental blood meal hosts for *B burgdorferi*-infected ticks. *Ixodes* ticks have three developmental stages—larvae, nymph, and adult—and only the nymph and adult forms harbor *B burgdorferi*. Nymphs most commonly transmit infection to humans because of their promiscuous feeding patterns and small size. The incidence of Lyme borreliosis follows the seasonal feeding patterns of nymphs (late spring, summer, and early fall), although sporadic cases may occur in late fall and early spring when adult ticks feed. The peak incidence is in June and July. Nymphs feed for 3–8 days, during which time spirochetes migrate from the tick midgut to the salivary gland and are deposited into the skin through salivary secretions. Successful transmission of infection generally requires 24–48 hours of tick feeding, so that tick surveillance and early removal of embedded ticks is a primary preventive strategy in areas endemic for Lyme borreliosis.

Spirochetes first establish infection in the skin, where local immune responses give rise to the hallmark skin lesion EM (Figure 43–1). This rash is present in up to 80% of cases and typically appears within the first month after tick bite.

Spirochetes disseminate through the blood and lymphatics to produce clinical signs manifesting in the skin as multiple EM lesions or as complications in the heart, joints, or in the nervous system.

The accurate diagnosis of Lyme borreliosis relies on a reasonable risk of exposure to *B burgdorferi*-infected ticks and a characteristic clinical presentation. Serologic testing for the presence of antibodies to *B burgdorferi*, performed and interpreted as recommended by the Centers for Disease Control and Prevention (CDC), can support the diagnosis. Patients with early infection may test negative. Oral antibiotics for 2–4 weeks is appropriate initial therapy for most patients. Exceptions are those with neurologic disease other than isolated Bell palsy or severe cardiac involvement, who should receive intravenous therapy.

The majority of patients with Lyme borreliosis can be treated successfully with antibiotics, with little in the way of long-term sequelae. A minority, estimated to be less than 10%, experience a post-Lyme disease syndrome of fatigue, musculoskeletal pain, and cognitive dysfunction that is debilitating. Misdiagnosis of other conditions as Lyme borreliosis remains the most common reason that patients do not respond to conventional therapy. Patients with chronic residual signs and symptoms after treatment for Lyme borreliosis may have irreversible tissue damage or possibly infection-induced autoimmunity. Extended courses of oral

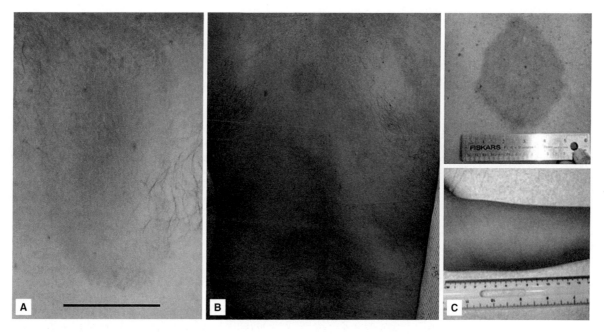

▲ **Figure 43–1.** **A:** Erythema migrans (EM) presenting as a single lesion (bar = 2 cm). **B:** Multiple EM lesions. **C:** Skin lesion in southern tick-associated rash illness, with an appearance similar to that of EM. (Reprinted with permission from Bockenstedt, L.K. and Wormser, G.P. (2014), Review: Unraveling Lyme Disease. *Arthritis & Rheumatology.* 66: 2313-2323.)

and/or intravenous antibiotics have not been shown to provide benefit over placebo for patients with persistent symptoms and should be avoided unless clear objective evidence of active infection is present.

Pathogenesis

B burgdorferi survives in nature through alternating infection between ticks and reservoir hosts, including mammals and birds. Ticks have a 2-year life span and feed only once per developmental stage. Larvae first acquire *B burgdorferi* infection by feeding on an infected reservoir host and remain infected through maturation to the nymph and adult forms. In mammals, spirochetes cause disease as they initially infect and disseminate within the host, but inflammation generally resolves even if the infection is not cleared.

In humans, *B burgdorferi* is difficult to culture from infected tissues except from EM lesions, but rare positive cultures have been reported at all stages of the disease, including from blood, cerebrospinal fluid, heart biopsies, and joint fluid. In animal models, few spirochetes can be seen in infected tissues, yet an exuberant inflammatory response arises and then resolves without antibiotic treatment; rare spirochetes may persist in tissues. Despite transient sightings of spirochetes within cells, no intracellular phase of *B burgdorferi* infection has been documented. *B burgdorferi* employs several immune evasion mechanisms that are common to extracellular pathogens.

Spirochete lipoproteins, which are expressed on internal and surface-exposed pathogen membranes, incite acute inflammation by activating innate immune cells through Toll-like receptor pattern recognition receptors. Downregulation of lipoprotein expression as spirochetes adapt to persist in the host may impede their clearance by innate immune cells and by borrelicidal antibodies targeting specific lipoproteins. Antigenic variation has been demonstrated, particularly of the VlsE lipoprotein, which is required for persistence in the mammal, providing another mechanism whereby the spirochete can evade protective antibodies. *B burgdorferi* also possesses a family of lipoproteins that bind host Factor H to impede lysis by complement.

Antibiotic therapy may release internally sequestered lipoproteins and other inflammatory products from dead spirochetes that trigger the Jarisch-Herxheimer reaction, a febrile response and transient exacerbation of symptoms noted by up to 15% of Lyme borreliosis patients at the start of therapy. Delayed clearance of spirochete inflammatory products may contribute to lingering symptoms after antibiotic treatment for Lyme borreliosis.

Prevention

The best way to prevent Lyme borreliosis is to reduce the risk of human exposure to *B burgdorferi*-infected ticks through personal preventive behavior and environmental controls. The geographic risk for infection correlates with areas where the prevalence of nymphal infection is high (≥20% of ticks). State health departments and the CDC can provide up-to-date information about the areas where the risk for Lyme borreliosis is greatest. Avoiding physical contact with common tick habitats, such as wooded areas, stone fences, woodpiles, tall grass, and brush, helps limit exposure risk of individuals in areas endemic for Lyme borreliosis. Environmental controls, such as the removal of tall grass and brush, clearance of woodpiles, and the application of area insecticides, can reduce the risk of human contact with infected ticks. If entry into tick habitats is anticipated, wearing protective, light-colored clothing such as long-sleeved shirts and long pants tucked into socks allows for ticks to be readily seen and reduces their access to exposed skin. Insect repellants containing diethyltoluamide (DEET) applied to the clothing and exposed skin surfaces provide added protection. Other repellants, such as picaridin, IR-3535, and oil of lemon eucalyptus, are also effective if used according to the manufacturers' recommendations. Permethrin can be sprayed on clothing and kills ticks directly, and permethrin-embedded clothing and outdoor gear are available through commercial vendors. Washing clothes in hot water or directly drying clothes after outdoor activities on high heat can kill ticks.

Daily tick checks are essential for persons with exposure risk to ticks. Bathing immediately after outdoor exposures can increase the likelihood of detecting ticks, and prompt removal of ticks embedded in the skin has been shown to effectively reduce the incidence of Lyme borreliosis in endemic communities. Attached ticks should be removed by grasping the mouthparts with tweezers as close to the skin as possible and pulling steadily up. Use of alcohol, heat, or vaso-occlusive substances will not promote tick detachment. A single 200 mg dose of doxycycline administered within 72 hours of tick bite has been shown to prevent Lyme borreliosis. The risk of transmission of *B burgdorferi* from an infected tick is low (<4%), however, making the routine use of prophylactic antibiotics in individuals bitten by ticks unwarranted. Regardless as to whether doxycycline prophylaxis is administered, the patient should be advised to observe the site of tick bite for 30 days for the development of a rash or other symptoms such as an unexplained fever, which may be a sign of Lyme borreliosis or other *Ixodes* tick-borne infections.

One effective method for prevention of Lyme borreliosis is vaccination. A Lyme borreliosis vaccine based on the spirochete lipoprotein Osp A (LYMErix) was approved by the Food and Drug Administration (FDA), but was discontinued by the manufacturer because of limited demand for the vaccine and public concern over potential vaccine-related sequelae. Immune responses to Osp A induced by natural infection were previously thought to contribute to Lyme arthritis that persisted after treatment (see section Prognosis), but the incidence of arthritis in patients undergoing Osp A vaccination did not differ from those receiving placebo. A new OspA-based vaccine, called VLA15, includes five of six serotypes of OspA and has been shown to provide protection against European as well as North American

B burgdorferi sensu lato species. The FDA has granted the vaccine a Fast Track designation to facilitate its clinical development, and a Phase I study of the vaccine at two sites in the United States and one in Europe recently has completed enrollment.

► Clinical Findings

Lyme borreliosis typically occurs in stages that reflect the biology of the spirochete. After establishing infection in the skin at the site of tick feeding, spirochetes that escape initial immune destruction disseminate through blood and lymphatics and can infect other organ systems, at least transiently. The clinical manifestations of Lyme disease thus depend upon the stage of the illness at which the patient presents. These stages are termed early localized infection, disseminated infection, and late infection.

A. Symptoms and Signs

1. Early localized infection—The most common early manifestation of Lyme disease is the skin rash EM, present in up to 80% of patients. EM appears within a month after exposure to *B burgdorferi*, with a median of 7–10 days, and first appears at the site of the tick bite. Ticks may initially bind to clothing or exposed skin, but typically crawl to skin folds or creases and areas where clothes are particularly confining (eg, near elastic bands) before attaching. In adults, the most common sites for EM are the popliteal fossa, gluteal fold, trunk, and axilla; in children, EM often occurs near the hairline.

The most characteristic feature of EM is its morphology (Figure 43–1A): a flat, macular erythematous lesion that expands rapidly—2–3 cm/day—and can enlarge to more than 70 cm in diameter. The lesion should be greater than 5 cm in diameter to fulfill diagnostic criteria. Although central clearing to produce a target or bull's-eye rash can occur in up to 40% of cases, especially when the lesion is large, more often EM presents with uniform erythema. Occasionally, the center can be intensely erythematous, vesicular, or even necrotic. Despite its appearance, EM itself has few local symptoms other than tingling. Rarely, the lesion is intensely pruritic or painful. Systemic symptoms may be present, including low-grade fever, malaise, neck pain or stiffness, arthralgias, and myalgias; these are particularly severe in individuals with coinfection with another tick-borne pathogen. In about 18% of Lyme borreliosis cases, patients may present with these viral-like systemic symptoms in the summer months without an accompanying EM lesion.

2. Early disseminated infection—Within weeks to a few months of infection, spirochetes that disseminate from the tick bite site to other organs produce clinical signs and symptoms, usually manifesting in the skin at sites distant from the tick bite site, and/or in the heart, the musculoskeletal, or nervous systems. Patients are generally ill-appearing and complain of debilitating fatigue and malaise. While specific localizing signs and symptoms may be waxing and waning, on-going fatigue is a common feature of untreated early disseminated Lyme borreliosis.

A. Skin—Multiple EM lesions are a sign of dissemination and arise in about 50% of untreated patients (Figure 43–1B). Secondary lesions have a random distribution, are smaller than the primary lesion, and less often necrotic or vesicular, although they may exhibit central clearing.

A rare early sign of Lyme borreliosis in Europe is the skin lesion *Borrelia* lymphocytoma associated primarily with *B afzelii* infection. The lesion appears as a bluish-red plaque or nodule, most often appearing on the earlobe in children and the areola in adults. Biopsy of the lesion reveals a dense polyclonal lymphocytic infiltrate. Occasionally EM may be present elsewhere on the skin.

B. Musculoskeletal—Migratory pains in muscles, joints, and periarticular structures, especially tendons and ligaments, may be reported in early localized infection but are more common when other signs of disseminated infection are present. Frank arthritis, however, usually occurs at least 4–6 months after the tick bite and is now considered a late manifestation of untreated infection (see section Late Infection).

C. Nervous system—Central and/or peripheral nervous system disease (neuroborreliosis) occurs in up to 15% of patients with acute disseminated infection. All or some of the classic triad of meningitis, cranial neuropathy, especially involving the VIIth nerve, and painful peripheral radiculopathy may be present. Subtle cognitive defects, if present, are considered secondary to systemic inflammation rather than a sign of infection of the brain. CNS involvement in the United States most commonly presents as an aseptic meningitis with cerebrospinal fluid (CSF) examination revealing a lymphocytic pleocytosis, whereas in Europe a painful lymphocytic meningoradiculitis is more common. Headache may be waxing and waning and neck stiffness is generally mild in comparison to other forms of infectious meningitis, so that a high index of suspicion may be required to make the diagnosis. In children, however, Lyme neuroborreliosis can be associated with raised intracranial pressure and papilledema that should be treated to prevent complications such as vision loss. Cranial neuropathy occurs in about 50% of patients with neuroborreliosis and most often affects the facial nerve. Although usually unilateral, bilateral facial nerve palsies occur in nearly 30% of patients with VIIth nerve involvement. Other cranial nerves that can be involved include cranial nerves VIII and less commonly III, V, and VI. Sudden hearing loss accompanied by vertigo has been reported but is rare. CSF abnormalities may be present in cases of cranial nerve palsy and reflect asymptomatic CNS involvement.

Involvement of the peripheral nervous system typically manifests as a peripheral radiculoneuropathy due to a mixed motor and sensory neuropathy (mononeuritis multiplex). Patients present with sharp, lancinating pain in the distribution of the affected nerves and later, hyporeflexia.

Often multiple nerves and nerve roots are involved in an asymmetric fashion. In Europe where the more neurotropic *B garinii* species is found, early Lyme neuroborreliosis often manifests as Bannwarth syndrome, a painful radiculoneuritis and meningitis that over time can lead to cranial nerve involvement and rarely peripheral paresis. These latter manifestations of Bannwarth syndrome are less common now, which is most likely due to earlier recognition and treatment. Focal inflammation in the brain or spinal cord (segmental myelitis) suggestive of demyelinating disease is a rare occurrence in Lyme borreliosis.

D. Heart— Clinically apparent Lyme carditis is relatively rare, reported in 1–2% of patients with disseminated infection. Conduction system abnormalities with varying degrees of atrioventricular block are the most common cardiac manifestations, with symptomatic third-degree AV block occurring in about 50% of such patients. Occasionally myocarditis with heart muscle dysfunction and pericarditis is present, but valvular disease is not usually found. Cardiac involvement in disseminated Lyme borreliosis may be overlooked, especially if it remains clinically asymptomatic in comparison to other features of the infection. Sudden death has been reported, however, and therefore a careful history for symptoms associated with arrhythmias or myopericarditis should be obtained and investigated accordingly.

E. Other organ system involvement— A variety of other organs have been reported to be involved with disseminated *B burgdorferi* infection. These include the eye (conjunctivitis, keratitis), the ear (sensorineural hearing loss), the liver (hepatitis), the spleen (necrosis), skeletal muscle (myositis), and subcutaneous tissue (panniculitis). In general, other more classic manifestations of Lyme borreliosis are present concurrently or have been present in the recent past to suggest the diagnosis.

3. Late infection— Late manifestations of untreated Lyme borreliosis occur months after the onset of infection and most often involve the skin, nervous system, or joints. Although case reports attribute chronic cardiomyopathy to Lyme borreliosis in Europe, this late manifestation has not been documented in the United States.

In Europe, infection with *B afzelii* and less commonly *B garinii* is associated with the late skin lesion acrodermatitis chronica atrophicans (ACA), typically involving the dorsum of the hands or distal lower extremities. It first appears as an erythematous, hyperpigmented lesion that evolves to a chronic stage of hypopigmentation and atrophic, cellophane-like skin. Antibiotic treatment during the inflammatory phase of the ACA lesion can lead to resolution.

Late neurologic manifestations are increasingly rare due to earlier diagnosis and treatment. In the United States, subtle cognitive dysfunction has been reported, as has a mild sensory polyneuropathy. In Europe, a chronic encephalomyelitis and multifocal polyneuropathy presenting with spastic paraparesis, cranial neuropathy, and/or cognitive impairment has

been reported. Encephalomyelitis is characterized as a progressive disorder over weeks to months. CSF examination demonstrates significant inflammation with a pleocytosis, elevated protein, and strongly positive intrathecal antibody production against *B burgdorferi sl*. Stroke-like symptoms due to neuroborreliosis have been reported in Europe more often than the United States, but are rare. A peripheral sensory neuropathy has been reported in the affected limb in patients with long-standing ACA.

Lyme arthritis presents months to years after the onset of infection (average 6 months in the United States, slightly earlier in Europe) and manifests as a monoarticular or oligoarticular arthritis, most often involving the knee. Effusions involving the knee are often quite large (>50–100 mL) and are usually accompanied by stiffness and only mild pain. Young children, however, may present with fever and more significant pain and swelling in the involved joint, similar to septic arthritis due to more common bacterial pathogens. Other joints involved in order of frequency include the shoulder, ankle, elbow, temporomandibular joint, and wrist. It is rare for Lyme arthritis to involve more than five joints at any time. Acute Lyme arthritis is usually episodic, with attacks of monoarticular or oligoarticular arthritis lasting only weeks, and decreasing in frequency with time.

4. Lyme borreliosis due to *B mayonii*— In 2013, a newly emerging *B mayonii* species of *B burgdorferi sl* was discovered as a cause of Lyme borreliosis in the upper Midwest. To date, there is limited information about the clinical course and spectrum of Lyme borreliosis due to *B mayonii*. Clinical signs of the first six patients included fever, headache, neck pain, and rash with onset within days of exposure. Arthritis appeared within weeks of infection. The rash varied from diffuse macular lesions involving the face, trunk, and extremities to more typical EM lesions of a single erythematous or annular lesion at the site of tick bite. Four of the six patients reported nausea and vomiting and three had neurologic symptoms, including somnolence, speech, and visual difficulties. Analysis of blood samples revealed a high level of spirochetemia, which has not been reported with other *B burgdorferi sl* species.

B. Laboratory Findings

1. Routine studies (Table 43–1)— Results of laboratory studies of patients with Lyme borreliosis depend upon the stage of infection and organ system involved. Routine laboratory tests are nonspecific. Some patients exhibit a mild elevation in the white blood cell (neutrophil) count, erythrocyte sedimentation rate, and modest abnormalities of liver function tests. Presence of an unexplained thrombocytopenia, leukopenia, neutropenia, anemia, or elevated bilirubin levels should raise suspicion for infection with other *Ixodes* tick-borne pathogens (*Babesia microti* or *Anaplasma phagocytophilum* in Lyme endemic regions, or *Ehrlichia muris eauclarensis* in the Midwest United States). Blood smears can be helpful in identifying *B microti*-infected red blood cells or

Table 43–1. Laboratory tests in Lyme disease.

Complete blood count	White blood cell count normal or slightly elevated (neutrophil predominance)
Erythrocyte sedimentation rate	Elevated in 50% of cases
Liver function tests	Mild elevation in GGT and ALT
ANA, rheumatoid factor	Negative
Synovial fluid	Inflammatory, cell counts ranging from 2000 to 100,000 (neutrophil predominance) Normal or elevated protein Normal glucose
Cerebrospinal fluid	Lymphocytic pleocytosis Elevated protein Normal glucose

ALT, alanine transaminase; ANA, antinuclear antibody; GGT, gamma-glutamyl transpeptidase.

morulae of *Anaplasma* and *Ehrlichia* species in white blood cells, although the sensitivity is low. Polymerase chain reaction (PCR) assays are the preferred method of identifying these organisms in acute infections. *B burgdorferi sl* has not been observed in blood smears of Lyme borreliosis patients, except in the case of infection with the newly identified *B mayonii* species, which achieves high levels in the blood.

The synovial fluid from patients with Lyme arthritis is inflammatory. Cell counts range from 2000 to 100,000 with a predominance of neutrophils. The synovial fluid protein and glucose levels are usually normal. Serum antinuclear antibody and rheumatoid factor tests should be negative. Patients with neurologic involvement, including isolated facial palsy, may have abnormalities within the CSF. A lymphocytic pleocytosis accompanied by moderate elevation of CSF protein and normal glucose is consistent with but not specific for Lyme neuroborreliosis. It is debated whether all patients with isolated facial palsy should have a lumbar puncture to exclude CNS involvement, since these patients appear to respond well to oral antibiotics.

2. *B burgdorferi sl*-specific tests

A. Culture— In contrast to other infectious diseases for which isolation of the causative organism is a viable tool for diagnosis, it is rare to culture *B burgdorferi sl* from tissues and body fluids of patients with Lyme borreliosis. EM provides an exception, with spirochetes readily cultivated from biopsies of the leading margin of the lesion. The morphologic features of EM, however, are sufficiently distinct to make this skin manifestation virtually diagnostic for Lyme borreliosis so that biopsy and culture are rarely performed. The variability of culture medium lots for growing the spirochete makes routine use of culture of any blood or tissue specimen impractical other than for research purposes.

B. Antibody tests— Serologic tests that measure antibodies to *B burgdorferi* provide evidence of exposure to the pathogen

and are the mainstay of Lyme disease diagnostics. A two-tiered approach to serologic testing utilizes an enzyme-linked immunosorbent assay (ELISA) with *B burgdorferi* antigens as a screening tool for IgM and IgG reactivity. IgM responses appear within the first 2–3 weeks of infection, whereas IgG responses can usually be detected after 1 month. IgM responses should only be used to support a diagnosis of Lyme borreliosis in patients with less than or equal to 4 weeks of suggestive signs and symptoms. For individuals with a clinical history of longer duration, IgG responses alone should be considered. A persistently positive IgM ELISA over many months without an IgG response suggests a false-positive test. An immunoblot (western blot), in which individual proteins of *B burgdorferi* are separated by molecular weight, should be used to confirm specificity of antibodies for all ELISA tests that are positive or equivocal, but should not be routinely performed on negative ELISA samples. Criteria for positive IgM and IgG immunoblots are listed in Table 43–2. The most commonly detected antigen, the 41-kD protein flagellin, is not unique to *B burgdorferi* and patients may have detectable antibodies because of past exposure to other bacteria with homologous proteins. Patients with early Lyme disease may initially be seronegative, but the majority will seroconvert after 1 month even with the use of antibiotics. False-positive tests are far more frequent than false-negatives, especially among patients whose pretest probability of having the disease is low. Use of specialty laboratories that employ non–FDA-approved assays or alternate criteria for positivity that have not been appropriately validated should be discouraged. Repetitive testing of an individual when initial acute and convalescent serologies were negative should be avoided as this increases the risk of obtaining a false-positive result.

Second-generation immunoassays using recombinant *B burgdorferi* proteins or synthetic peptides offer improved specificity for *B burgdorferi* infection. Many of these target the VlsE protein or peptides of the protein. The C6 peptide-based ELISA that measures antibodies to the conserved region (C6) of the VlsE protein has a high specificity (98.9%)

Table 43–2. Criteria for Western blot interpretation in the serologic confirmation of Lyme disease.

Isotype Tested	Criteria for Positive Test
IgM	Two of the following three bands are present: 23 kDa (OspC), 39 kDa (BmpA), and 41 kDa (Fla)
IgG	Five of the following 10 bands are present: 18 kDA, 21 kDa, 28 kDa, 39 kDa, 41 kDa, 45 kDa, 58 kDa (not GroEL), 66 kDa, and 93 kDa

Data from Centers for Disease Control and Prevention. Recommendations for test performance and interpretation from the second national conference on serologic diagnosis of Lyme disease. *MMWR.* 1995;44:590-591.

in comparison to the whole cell lysate ELISA (95.2%) and improved sensitivity (ranging from 74% in acute Lyme borreliosis to 100% in late Lyme borreliosis). Positive or equivocal results on recombinant VlsE or C6 ELISA assays should be confirmed with a second-tier immunoblot test, as their specificity as stand-alone tests is less than that of the two-tier methods using whole-cell sonicates.

Antibody testing on fluids other than serum is not generally recommended. Patients with Lyme arthritis almost universally have highly positive Lyme serology by two-tier testing. Measurement of *B burgdorferi* antibodies in CSF is not needed in most cases of Lyme neuroborreliosis. A characteristic neurologic syndrome with CSF pleocytosis and positive Lyme serology by two-tier testing is sufficient to establish the diagnosis. If *B burgdorferi*-specific antibody testing is performed on the CSF of patients with suspected early neuroborreliosis, paired serum and CSF samples normalized to the respective total IgG concentrations can demonstrate the production of intrathecal antibodies. If present, intrathecal *B burgdorferi*-specific antibody production is highly suggestive of CNS involvement in Lyme borreliosis. Measurement of *B burgdorferi*-specific antibodies in the CSF without performing a CSF to serum antibody index is not recommended.

Once present, antibodies to *B burgdorferi* can persist indefinitely, including in the CSF. Antibody titers and reactivity on immunoblot should not be used to assess efficacy of antibiotic therapy. Serologic tests at best confirm exposure to the pathogen at some time in the past and are not by themselves indicative of active infection with *B burgdorferi*.

C. DNA tests—The PCR has widespread use in the diagnosis of many infectious diseases, especially for pathogens that are difficult to culture or when rapid diagnosis is critical for management. This technique has been used to detect *B burgdorferi* DNA in synovial fluid and CSF specimens from patients with Lyme borreliosis with variable success. Up to 80% of synovial fluid samples may test positive, whereas the yield on CSF samples from patients with Lyme meningitis is generally low (about 5% in a study of children with early neurological Lyme borreliosis). PCR testing for *B burgdorferi* DNA is not a reliable tool for assessing active infection as *B burgdorferi* DNA can persist after spirochete killing.

D. Imaging studies—Radiographic studies have limited use in establishing the diagnosis of Lyme borreliosis and serve primarily to eliminate other diagnoses. Plain radiographs of inflamed joints may be normal or show only soft-tissue swelling and effusion. In contrast to septic arthritis due to other bacterial pathogens in which radiographic evidence of infection can be present early, overt changes with periarticular osteoporosis, cartilage loss, and bony erosions are relatively late findings in Lyme arthritis. MRI scans and ultrasound of joint can show additional findings of synovial thickening and evidence of inflammation, including the muscle, but these findings cannot distinguish Lyme arthritis from other forms of inflammatory arthritis.

MRI scans of the brains of patients with Lyme neuroborreliosis are generally normal. A minority of patients with CNS disease, especially those with the late manifestation of encephalomyelitis, will have white matter lesions that typically enhance on FLAIR imaging. Other imaging studies, such as single-photon emission computed tomography (SPECT) scans, have been shown to exhibit abnormalities in some patients with subtle cognitive dysfunction that reverse partially with treatment, but the findings are not specific and can be seen in normal individuals. Abnormalities on SPECT scans alone should not be used as evidence of Lyme borreliosis in the absence of suggestive clinical history and supportive serologic tests.

E. Special tests—Specialized tests for Lyme borreliosis are primarily used to evaluate the extent of cardiac and nervous system involvement. The EKG can show evidence of conduction system disease (especially varying degrees of atrioventricular block and escape rhythms) or, less commonly, more diffuse myocardial involvement with changes consistent with myocardial dysfunction and pericarditis. Electrophysiologic studies reveal a predilection for the atrioventricular node, but any part of the conduction system can be affected.

Patients with radicular symptoms should have nerve conduction testing and electromyography to document changes consistent with axonal polyradiculopathy. For patients with cognitive complaints, neuropsychologic tests are useful to evaluate for depression and to provide objective evidence of memory loss.

▶ Differential Diagnosis

Although Lyme borreliosis can involve multiple organ systems, the infection typically follows a characteristic presentation and clinical course. Accurate diagnosis requires that the patient have an appropriate clinical history and a reasonable risk of exposure to *B burgdorferi*-infected ticks. The hallmark skin lesion EM is a diagnostic criterion for early Lyme borreliosis, but other more common skin disorders can be mistaken for EM (Table 43–3). The seasonal occurrence of EM in late spring and summer months, the size and number of lesions, and the paucity of associated cutaneous symptoms such as itch or pain are useful distinguishing features.

An EM-like rash has been associated with the bite of the soft-shelled tick *Amblyomma americanum*, which is prevalent in the southeast and south central United States (Figure 43–1C). The etiology of southern tick-associated rash illness (STARI) is unclear, but the disease appears localized to the skin. A noncultivatable spirochete named *Borrelia lonestari* has been found in *A americanum*, but individuals with STARI do not develop positive Lyme serology as would be expected with infection with a *B burgdorferi*-related spirochete. Patients with STARI who are treated with antibiotics resolve symptoms more quickly than patients with Lyme borreliosis and chronic sequelae have not been reported.

Table 43–3. Differential diagnosis of erythema migrans.

Differential Diagnosis	Seasonal Occurrence	Associated Symptoms	Location	Size	Evolution	Morphology
Erythema migrans	Yes	Mild systemic symptoms Paucity of pain or itch	Skin folds, central	Large	2–3 cm per day	See text
Tinea corporis	No	Itch	Variable	Variable	Slow progression	Ringlike; may have satellite lesion; scaling much more common
Cellulitis	No	Systemic symptoms Painful	Typically acral	Variable but rarely large except on legs	Grows more in typical cases	Usually a homogeneous erythema; tender to touch
Hypersensitivity to insect or tick bite	Yes	No	Variable	Small	Variable	Can be uniform erythema, often with tick still attached
Contact dermatitis	No	Itchy	Variable	Variable	Slow progression	Often linear (rhus) or in an area that suggests the diagnosis
Spider bite	Yes	Painful bite	Acral	Variable	Can develop dependent edema but spreads centrifugally	Often necrotic with eschar
Urticaria	No	Itch	Variable	Individual lesions vary	Individual lesions wax and wane over hours	Raised, multiple, often serpiginous around edges
Pityriasis rosea	More in spring and fall	Mild to moderate itch	Diffuse; usually not on face	Herald patch may be confused with erythema migrans	Tends to stay same day to day when it is expressed	Oval lesions, slightly scaly, with long axis oriented with skin cleavage lines
Fixed drug eruption	No	Variable, but often a burning sensation; recent drug ingestion	Fixed, often in genitals, hands, feet, and face	Variable	Tends to stay fixed	Plaque with deep violaceous hue and well-demarcated borders
Granuloma annulare	No	No	Acral	Several centimeters	Fixed over weeks to months	Tend to spread peripherally; can have central clearing
Erythema multiforme	No	Variable (may be associated with viral syndrome or medication)	Usually diffuse; often palms, soles, mucosa	Most lesions small without a single large one	Slow enlargement or stagnant over days	Target lesion is classic, but these lesions are usually much smaller than erythema migrans; often there is an obvious precipitant

Reproduced, with permission, from Edlow JA. Erythema migrans. *Med Clin North Am.* 2002;86:252.

Although early Lyme borreliosis can less commonly present as a summer "flu-like" illness, headache, myalgia, and arthralgia are nonspecific symptoms of a variety of viral pathogens. Presence of upper respiratory symptoms or significant gastrointestinal complaints is unusual in Lyme borreliosis. Patients with fibromyalgia and chronic fatigue syndrome often have debilitating fatigue and musculoskeletal complaints in the absence of objective findings or laboratory abnormalities. These syndromes are more insidious in onset than Lyme borreliosis, and patients may be symptomatic for

many months or years before diagnosis. A history of a sleep disturbance and the presence of trigger points on physical examination should suggest a diagnosis of fibromyalgia. The American College of Rheumatology recommends against screening for Lyme borreliosis as a cause of musculoskeletal symptoms without an exposure history and appropriate physical examination findings.

Lyme arthritis can mimic other causes of mono- or pauciarticular arthritis, including reactive arthritis and other seronegative spondylarthropathies, juvenile arthritis, and rheumatoid arthritis. Low back pain and spine involvement is commonly seen in the seronegative spondyloarthropathies but is rare in patients with Lyme borreliosis. Lyme arthritis patients generally have strong antibody responses to *B burgdorferi* and negative tests for rheumatoid factor (RF), anti-cyclic citrullinated antibodies (CCP), and antinuclear antibodies (ANA). Presence of high-titer RF and ANA can be associated with false-positive ELISA tests for Lyme borreliosis, emphasizing the need to confirm ELISA results by immunoblot analysis. Other causes of acute monoarthritis, such as septic arthritis and crystal-induced disease, can usually be distinguished by the severity of pain and by examination of joint fluid for infectious microorganisms and crystals.

Even in areas endemic for Lyme borreliosis, isolated facial palsy is more often found to be idiopathic in origin than due to *B burgdorferi* infection. Only a few conditions are common causes of bilateral facial palsy—Guillain-Barré syndrome, human immunodeficiency virus infection, sarcoidosis, and other causes of chronic meningitis—and these are readily distinguished from Lyme borreliosis. Acute meningitis due to *B burgdorferi* infection resembles viral meningitis, but most patients at this stage should have positive serologic tests for Lyme borreliosis. The radiculoneuropathy of Lyme borreliosis must be distinguished from neuropathy associated with disc disease or diabetes, or other infections, such as Herpes zoster. Late neurologic disease, such as chronic encephalomyelitis in Europe, can be confused with other diseases such

as multiple sclerosis or age-related ischemic changes when the MRI scan of the brain shows evidence of white matter disease. Multiple sclerosis patients have negative serologic tests for Lyme borreliosis. Subtle neurocognitive deficits due to chronic fatigue syndrome, fibromyalgia, or aging are often incorrectly attributed to chronic Lyme encephalomyelitis. Toxic-metabolic causes of encephalopathy should be excluded.

Cardiac manifestations of Lyme borreliosis can resemble those of acute rheumatic fever, except that valvular heart disease is absent. Coronary atherosclerotic disease, structural defects within the heart, and certain medications (especially beta blockers and calcium channel blockers) can lead to conduction system abnormalities characteristic of Lyme carditis. If evidence of myocardial dysfunction is present, other infectious causes should be considered, such as infection with *Coxsackievirus* A and B, echovirus, *Yersinia enterocolitica*, and *Rickettsia rickettsii*, the agent of Rocky Mountain spotted fever.

▶ Treatment

Practice guidelines for the treatment of Lyme borreliosis have been established by the Infectious Disease Society of America (Tables 43–4 and 43–5). Because many of the manifestations of Lyme borreliosis can resolve without specific therapy,

Table 43–4 Recommended antimicrobial regimens for treatment of patients with Lyme disease.

Drug	Dosage for Adults	Dosage for Children
Preferred oral regimens		
Amoxicillin	500 mg three times daily[a]	50 mg/kg/day in three divided doses (maximum, 500 mg per dose)[a]
Doxycycline	100 mg twice daily[b]	Not recommended for children younger than 8 years
		For children 8 years and older, 4 mg/kg/day in two divided doses (maximum, 100 mg per dose)
Cefuroxime axetil	500 mg twice daily	30 mg/kg/day in two divided doses (maximum, 500 mg per dose)
Alternative oral regimens		
Selected macrolides[c]	For recommended dosing regimens, see footnote 4 in Table 48–5	For recommended dosing regimens, see footnote 4 in Table 48–5
Preferred parenteral regimen		
Ceftriaxone	2 g intravenously once daily	50–75 mg/kg/day intravenously in a single dose (maximum, 2 g)
Alternative parenteral regimens		
Cefotaxime	2 g every 8 hours[d] intravenously	150–200 mg/kg/day intravenously in three or four divided doses (maximum, 6 g/day)[d]
Penicillin G	18–24 million units/day intravenously, divided every 4 hours[d]	200,000–400,000 units/kg/day divided every 4 hours[d] (not to exceed 18–24 million units/day)

[a]Although a high dosage given twice daily might be equally effective, in view of the absence of data on efficacy, twice-daily administration is not recommended.

[b]Tetracyclines are relatively contraindicated in pregnant or lactating women and in children younger than 8 years.

[c]Because of their lower efficacy, macrolides are reserved for patients who are unable to take or who are intolerant of tetracyclines, penicillins, and cephalosporins.

[d]Dosage should be reduced for patients with impaired renal function.

Modified, with permission, from Wormser GP, et al. The clinical assessment treatment and prevention of Lyme disease, human granulocytic anaplasmosis, and babesiosis: clinical practice guidelines by the Infectious Diseases Society of America. *Clin Infect Dis.* 2006;43:1089-1134.

Table 43–5 Recommended therapy for patients with Lyme disease.

Indication	Treatment	Duration, Days (Range)
Tick bite in the United States	Doxycycline, 200 mg in a single dose[a]; (4 mg/kg in children 8 years of age and older) and/or observation	—
Erythema migrans	Oral regimen[b,c]	14 (14–21)[d]
Early neurologic disease		
Meningitis or radiculopathy	Parenteral regimen[b,e]	14 (10–28)
Cranial nerve palsy[f]	Oral regimen[b]	14 (10–21)
Cardiac disease	Oral regimen[b,g] or parenteral regimen[b,h]	14 (14–21)
Borrelial lymphocytoma	Oral regimen[b,c]	14 (14–21)
Late disease		
Arthritis without neurologic disease	Oral regimen[b]	28
Recurrent arthritis after oral regimen	Oral regimen[b] or parenteral regimen[b]	28 / 14 (14–28)
Antibiotic-refractory arthritis[h]	Symptomatic therapy[i]	—
CNS or peripheral nervous system disease	Parenteral regimen[b]	14 (14–28)
Acrodermatitis chronica atrophicans	Oral regimen[b]	21 (14–28)
Post-Lyme disease syndrome	Consider and evaluate other potential causes of symptoms; if none is found, then administer symptomatic therapy	—

Note: Regardless of the clinical manifestations of Lyme disease, complete response to treatment may be delayed beyond the treatment duration. Relapse may occur with any of these regimens; patients with objective signs of relapse need a second course of treatment.

[a]A single dose of doxycycline may be offered to adult patients and to children >8 years of age when *all* of the following circumstances exist: (1) the attached tick can be reliably identified as an adult or nymphal *Ixodes scapularis* tick that is estimated to have been attached for ≥36 h on the basis of the degree of engorgement of the tick with blood or of certainty about the time of exposure to the rick, (2) prophylaxis can be started within 72 h after the time that the rick was removed, (3) ecologic information indicates that the local rate of these ricks with *Borrelia burgdorferi* is ≥20%, and (4) doxycycline is not contraindicated. For patients who do not fulfill these criteria, observation is recommended.

[b]See Table 48–4.

[c]For adult patients intolerant of amoxicillin, doxycycline, and cefuroxime axetil, azithromycin (500 mg/day orally for 7–10 days), clarithromycin (500 mg twice daily orally for 14–21 days, if the patient is not pregnant), or erythromycin (500 mg four times daily orally for 14–21 days) may be given. The recommended dosages of these agents for children are as follows: azithromycin, 10 mg/kg/day (maximum, 500 mg/day); clarithromycin, 7.5 mg/kg twice daily (maximum, 500 mg per dose); and erythromycin, 12.5 mg/kg four times daily (maximum, 500 mg per dose). Patients treated with macrolides should be closely observed to ensure resolution of the clinical manifestations.

[d]Ten days of therapy is effective if doxycycline is used; the efficacy of 10-day regimens with the other first-line agents is unknown.

[e]For nonpregnant adult patients intolerant of β-lactam agents, doxycycline (200–400 mg/day orally [or intravenously, if the patient is unable to take oral medications]) in two divided doses may be adequate. For children ≥8 of age, the dosage of doxycycline for this indication is 4–8 mg/kg/day in two divided doses (maximum daily dose of 200–400 mg).

[f]Patients without clinical evidence of meningitis may be treated with an oral regimen. Parenteral antibiotic therapy is recommended for patients with both clinical and laboratory evidence of coexistent meningitis. Most of the experience in the use of oral antibiotic therapy is for patients with VIIth cranial nerve palsy. Whether oral therapy would be as effective for patients with other cranial neuropathies is unknown. The decision between oral and parenteral antimicrobial therapy for patients with other cranial neuropathies should be individualized.

[g]A parenteral antibiotic regimen is recommended at the start of therapy for patients who have been hospitalized for cardiac monitoring; an oral regimen may be substituted to complete a course of therapy or to treat ambulatory patients. A temporary pacemaker may be required for patients with advanced heart block.

[h]Antibiotic-refractory Lyme arthritis is operationally defined as persistent synovitis for at least 2 months after completion of a course of intravenous ceftriaxone (or after completion of two 4-week courses of an oral antibiotic regimen for patients who are unable to tolerate cephalosporins); in addition polymerase chain reaction of synovial fluid specimens (and synovial tissue specimens, if available) is negative for *B burgdorferi* nucleic acids.

[i]Symptomatic therapy might consist of nonsteroidal anti-inflammatory agents, intra-articular injections of glucocorticoids, or other medications; expert consultation with a rheumatologist is recommended. If persistent synovitis is associated with significant pain or if it limits function, arthroscopic synovectomy can reduce the period of joint inflammation.

CNS, central nervous system.

Modified, with permission, from Wormser GP, et al. The clinical assessment treatment and prevention of Lyme disease, human granulocytic anaplasmosis, and babesiosis: clinical practice guidelines by the Infectious Diseases Society of America. *Clin Infect Dis.* 2006;43:1089-1134.

the goal of antibiotic treatment is to hasten resolution of signs and symptoms and to prevent later clinical manifestations due to on-going infection. This is particularly true for facial palsy, in which the rate of recovery is the same as for untreated patients, and for cardiac involvement. Patients with localized or early disseminated disease without severe cardiac involvement or neurologic disease other than Bell palsy can be treated with oral antibiotics. Parenteral antibiotics should be reserved for patients with central or peripheral neurologic involvement other than isolated Bell palsy, recurrent arthritis after oral antibiotic therapy, or third-degree heart block. Although the ideal duration of antibiotics has not been firmly established, administration of oral doxycycline or amoxicillin for 14–28 days is effective therapy for EM, isolated facial palsy, first- or second-degree heart block, and arthritis. For isolated EM, a 10–21 day course of doxycycline may be sufficient. Doxycycline has the advantage of being effective against *A phagocytophila*, which is also transmitted by *Ixodes* ticks (see later).

Glucocorticoids administered within 72 hours of presentation of idiopathic Bell palsy have been associated with improved outcomes, but there are no data whether they are of benefit in Bell palsy due to Lyme borreliosis. For cases of isolated Bell palsy presenting within 72 hours of onset in which the diagnosis of Lyme borreliosis is uncertain, current guidelines recommend administration of oral glucocorticoids as for idiopathic Bell palsy.

Patients with myopericarditis may develop heart failure and arrhythmias and those with a PR interval longer than 300 milliseconds are at increased risk for developing higher levels of heart block. These patients should be hospitalized for supportive care, including parenteral antibiotic therapy, with monitoring for the need for temporary pacing. The rationale for intravenous therapy for high-degree heart block is that intense and/or prolonged inflammation may lead to irreversible cardiac damage. However, no study has directly addressed whether parenteral therapy is more effective than oral therapy in this setting, or whether other means for suppressing inflammation provide added benefit. In this regard, the use of glucocorticoids to limit cardiac inflammation may be considered for patients with severe disease who do not respond rapidly to antibiotic therapy.

Pregnant patients and children younger than 8 years of age can be treated in similar fashion to adult patients except that tetracyclines in general should be avoided. Data suggest that short courses of doxycycline (10 days) may be safe in children younger than 8 years of age and can be considered in the case of allergies to other antibiotics.

A puzzling feature of Lyme borreliosis is that patients may experience a delay in resolution of symptoms after antibiotic treatment. This is particularly true for disseminated disease with neurologic abnormalities or arthritis, which may take months to resolve completely. For patients with persistent arthritis, a second course of oral antibiotics (generally of 4 weeks duration) or a single 2–4 week course of parenteral therapy is reasonable. Repeat treatment is not recommended for chronic neurologic abnormalities unless objective signs of relapse are present.

▶ Complications

A. Coinfection with Other *Ixodes*-Transmitted Pathogens

Ixodes ticks can carry multiple pathogens simultaneously, some of which are also infectious for humans. These include *B microti*, a protozoan that infects red blood cells; *A phagocytophila*, the agent of human anaplasmosis; an *E muris*-like (EML) pathogen (found in the upper Midwest United States); a newly emerging relapsing fever spirochete *B miyamotoi*; and viruses that cause encephalitis. *B microti* infection ranges from a mild viral-like syndrome to a malaria-like illness with fever, sweats, and severe constitutional symptoms, especially myalgias, along with hemolytic anemia. Examining the peripheral blood smear for the characteristic "ring"-like organisms within red blood cells can make the diagnosis.

A phagocytophila and EML both infect granulocytes and present with similar symptoms, including fever, chills, malaise, myalgia, and nausea. Laboratory findings associated with infection with these gram-negative intracellular bacteria include leukopenia, thrombocytopenia, and often abnormal liver function tests (elevated alanine aminotransferase, aspartate aminotransferase, or alkaline phosphatase). The presence of morulae within leukocytes can establish a diagnosis, but PCR of peripheral blood for *A phagocytophila* or EML DNA or antibody testing is more sensitive. In endemic areas, primary infection with these agents or coinfection with *B burgdorferi* should be considered in ill-patients with tick exposure who present with severe constitutional symptoms and hematologic abnormalities. In one study of patients with *B microti* infection, 20% also tested positive by serology for exposure to *B burgdorferi*. Coinfection can increase the morbidity associated with Lyme borreliosis; a fatality associated with Lyme carditis was reported in a patient with concomitant babesiosis.

B miyamotoi is an emerging *Ixodes* tick-borne relapsing fever spirochete only recently recognized to cause human disease in Russia, Europe, and the United States. Infection with *B miyamotoi* is associated with fever, chills, headache, and joint pain. Meningoencephalitis has been reported in immunocompromised patients and a single case of chronic meningoencephalitis was identified in an elderly patient in Europe. Serosurvey testing conducted in the northeastern United States suggests that the case incidence is about 1–3% and coinfection with *B burgdorferi* may be occurring. The full spectrum of disease associated with *B miyamotoi* infection is not yet known.

Tick-borne encephalitis virus is endemic in Europe and has been reported as a coinfection with Lyme borreliosis, and sporadic cases of a related virus (deer tick or Powassan virus) have been reported as single infections in the United States. Infection with these neurotropic viruses causes brain inflammation and presents with encephalitic symptoms, including fever, headache, seizures, and progressive mental status decline. Severe morbidity and death have been reported in elderly or immunocompromised patients infected with these viruses.

B. Pregnancy

Maternal-fetal transmission of *B burgdorferi* has been reported, but earlier concerns that Lyme borreliosis can cause congenital abnormalities appear unwarranted. Several prospective studies have failed to document an increased prevalence in adverse fetal outcomes (spontaneous abortion, premature delivery, or congenital abnormalities) among pregnant women who were treated with standard therapy for Lyme borreliosis.

Adverse reactions from antibiotic usage occur at a frequency comparable to that seen in other infectious diseases. Cholestasis has been reported with intravenous ceftriaxone therapy, so its use should be limited to patients with disseminated disease as described earlier. About 15% of patients with Lyme borreliosis may experience a Jarisch-Herxheimer reaction within 24–48 hours of initiation of antibiotic therapy. This condition is usually self-limited but has the potential to be more severe with Lyme borreliosis due to *B mayonii* if high levels of bacteremia are present. Supportive care with reassurance and nonsteroidal anti-inflammatory agents helps to relieve symptoms in most cases.

▶ When to Refer to a Specialist

Primary care physicians who are knowledgeable about the disorder and who follow the recommended evaluation and treatment guidelines can care for the majority of cases of early Lyme borreliosis. Referral to a specialist is appropriate when the diagnosis is uncertain, when other tick-transmitted pathogens or pregnancy complicate *B burgdorferi* infection, or if patients fail to respond to a standard course of antibiotics for presumed or confirmed Lyme borreliosis. Individuals who present with complications from disseminated infection should be followed jointly by relevant subspecialists for optimum management and to exclude other disorders that have features in common with Lyme borreliosis. This is particularly the case for inflammatory arthritis that develops within a few months after antibiotic treatment for early manifestations of Lyme borreliosis, as some may subsequently present with autoimmune disorders, such as rheumatoid arthritis or psoriatic arthritis.

▶ Prognosis

Overall, the majority of patients with Lyme borreliosis responds to antibiotic therapy at all stages of infection with improvement of clinical signs and symptoms. Complete resolution of clinical signs and symptoms may take several months, however, especially in individuals with arthritis or nervous system involvement. In some cases, permanent damage may result in residual deficits (eg, incompletely resolved Bell palsy) that do not improve with antibiotic therapy. In about 10% of patients with Lyme arthritis, joint inflammation does not resolve despite oral and intravenous antibiotic therapy. Evidence for on-going infection has not been found. Such "post-infectious antibiotic-refractory Lyme arthritis" occurs primarily in patients who possess the HLA-DRB1*0401, *0101, and *0404 alleles. Initially inflammation was thought to be perpetuated through molecular mimicry—in particular between spirochete lipoprotein Osp A and the human protein LFA-1—but animal studies have not supported LFA-1 as a relevant autoantigen. Autoimmune B- and T-cells responses have been found to other self-proteins (endothelial cell growth factor, matrix metalloproteinase-10, annexin A2, and apolipoprotein B-100) and do not appear to be driven by molecular mimicry. Antibiotic-refractory Lyme arthritis is likely a consequence of a dysregulated inflammatory response, inefficient clearance of inflammatory debris, and possibly infection-induced autoimmunity. Therapies directed toward suppressing the inflammatory response can be effective, including DMARDs such as hydroxychloroquine or methotrexate and biologic agents such as TNF-α inhibitors (56). These medications can be discontinued within 6 months to a year in patients who respond. Arthroscopic synovectomy can achieve clinical remission in 80% of patients provided that synovectomy is complete. Prolonged inflammatory Lyme arthritis can result in degenerative joint disease of the involved joint.

Patients who receive recommended treatment for Lyme borreliosis can experience subjective complaints such as fatigue, memory loss, myalgias, and arthralgias. Often these symptoms subside over months, but in a minority they may persist for years, a condition referred to as "post-treatment Lyme disease syndrome" (PTLDS). The etiology of these symptoms is unknown but may involve central sensitization of the pain response, metabolic changes, or certain immune responses as on-going infection has not been documented. Five randomized, double-blind, placebo-controlled trials evaluating the efficacy of extended courses of antibiotics for patients with PTLDS failed to show sustained benefit over placebo. Alternative therapeutic approaches should be considered, such as those used in treating patients with fibromyalgia, an entity associated with similar debilitating symptoms. Further research is needed to better understand the pathogenesis of PTLDS in order to improve quality of life for these patients.

Aguero-Rosenfeld ME, Wormser GP. Lyme disease: diagnostic issues and controversies. *Expert Rev Mol Diagn*. 2015;15:1. [PMID: 25482091]

Berende A, ter Hofstede HJ, Vos FJ, et al. Randomized trial of longer-term therapy for symptoms attributed to Lyme disease. *N Engl J Med*. 2016;374:1209. [PMID: 27028911]

Dittmer M, Willis M, Selby J, et al. Septolobular panniculitis in disseminated Lyme borreliosis. *J Cutan Pathol.* 2018;45(4): 274-277. [PMID: 29293267]

Koedel U, Fingerle V, Pfister HW. Lyme neuroborreliosis-epidemiology, diagnosis and management. *Nat Rev Neurol.* 2015;11:446. [PMID: 26215621]

Nadelman RB. Erythema migrans. *Infect Dis Clin North Am.* 2015;29:211. [PMID: 25999220]

Steere AC, Strle F, Wormser GP, et al. Lyme borreliosis. *Nat Rev Dis Primers.* 2016;2:16090. [PMID: 5539539]

The Rheumatic Manifestations of Acute & Chronic Viral Infections

44

Tochi Adizie, MBChB, MRCP

A. O. Adebajo, MBChB, FWACP,
MSc (Cambridge) FRCP, FACP, FAcMed

HUMAN IMMUNODEFICIENCY VIRUS

 ESSENTIALS OF DIAGNOSIS

▶ The diagnosis of human immunodeficiency virus (HIV) is confirmed using a combination of a combined antigen/antibody immunoassay and an HIV viral load test.

▶ A positive virologic test indicates HIV infection. Early disease is suggested by a negative immunoassay in the presence of viremia.

▶ HIV infection is associated with a wide range of rheumatic syndromes. These can occur at any stage of the disease.

▶ Rheumatic conditions that have been described in association with HIV include HIV-associated arthropathy, seronegative spondyloarthropathies, connective tissue diseases, vasculitides, septic arthritis, and pyomyositis.

General Considerations

Musculoskeletal manifestations of the human immunodeficiency virus (HIV) have been described since the outset of the global HIV epidemic. The first reports of rheumatologic symptoms of the infection occurred 3 years after its discovery, when Winchester et al described a case of reactive arthritis (ReA) in a patient with advanced acquired immunodeficiency syndrome (AIDS). HIV-positive patients with musculoskeletal involvement have reduced quality of life compared to those without rheumatic symptoms (Kole et al, 2013).

The HIV epidemic has also changed the epidemiology of certain diseases. As an example, HIV is associated with an increased incidence of spondyloarthropathies and psoriatic arthritis as well a greater severity of these conditions in patients with HIV. In addition, HIV and its treatment have led to the description of new conditions, namely HIV-associated

arthropathy and antiretroviral-related myopathy. Finally, HIV has posed challenges to the management of common rheumatologic conditions, for example in the treatment of rheumatoid arthritis (RA) and systemic lupus erythematosus (SLE).

Pathogenesis

A combination of immunodeficiency, immune hyperactivity, and dysregulated production or activity of cytokines such as tumour necrosis factor-α (TNF-α), interleukin (IL)-6, IL-12, interferon (IFN) gamma, and molecular mimicry may contribute to the rheumatic manifestations of HIV infection (Nguyen and Reveille, 2009). Potent antiretroviral therapy (ART) changes the course of HIV infection and may ameliorate some manifestations, it but may also contribute to the appearance of others (Lawson and Walker-Bone, 2012).

A. Symptoms and Signs

HIV-associated arthritis can occur at any stage of HIV illness. It can present in several ways: as an asymmetrical oligoarthritis, an symmetrical polyarthritis, or a monoarthritis (Plate and Boyle, 2003). The asymmetrical oligoarthritis variant, the most common form, has a male preponderance and predominately affects the knees and ankles. The symmetrical polyarthritis variant closely mimics RA, with patients exhibiting deformities similar to those of RA patients, including ulnar deviation. The polyarthritis of HIV is characterised by substantial acuity at onset but is usually nonerosive. The presence of Jaccoud arthropathy as part of an HIV-associated arthritis has also been described occasionally (Weeratunge et al, 2004). HIV-associated arthritis tends to be short lived, with a peak intensity occurring at 1–6 weeks. Some patients develop a chronic destructive arthropathy, however, associated with marked functional disability. Features of mucocutaneous involvement or enthesopathy are rare.

HIV can also be associated with a painful articular syndrome that is separate from these arthritides and self-limited albeit severe in nature. The painful articular syndrome, which lasts for less than 24 hours, is reported in up to 10% of African HIV-seropositive patients and is noted to be more common in those with advanced infection (Reveille, 2000). The bone and joint pain has a predilection for the lower extremities and tends to have an asymmetric pattern. Pain—often excruciating—is out of proportion to the clinical findings and is often sufficiently debilitating to lead to hospital treatment in more than half of patients (Reveille, 2000). The joints most commonly involved are the knees, shoulders and elbows.

HIV infection has been linked with increased prevalence and clinical severity of spondyloarthropathies. Patients with ReA, psoriatic arthritis, and undifferentiated spondyloarthropathy who are HIV positive have more severe and extensive skin involvement. Patients with psoriatic arthritis especially suffer a more severe, deforming, erosive arthropathy refractory to conventional treatment. Clinical features typically worsen in advanced HIV infection. The onset of psoriatic arthritis in the setting of HIV therefore frequently heralds the development of opportunistic infections. The typical clinical presentation in these patients is an asymmetrical oligo- or polyarthritis, with a predilection for the lower limbs. A symmetrical polyarthritis is also described with arthritis mutilans, but distal interphalangeal involvement and axial spondyloarthropathy patterns appear less frequently. Onset may be abrupt, with the development of erosions and disability within weeks. In addition, the number of joints affected tends to increase with time (Aboulafia et al, 2000).

B. Laboratory Findings

HIV-positive patients exhibit multiple autoantibodies (Bonnet et al, 2003) on serologic evaluation, including anti-CCP, RF, antinuclear antibodies (ANAs), cryoglobulins, anticardiolipin antibodies, and antineutrophil cytoplasmic antibodies (ANCAs). However, these antibodies are usually found at low titer only and are rarely of clinical significance. Once patients begin ART, the antibodies tend to resolve. Patients with concomitant autoimmune disease (such as RA or SLE) and HIV experience remission of their rheumatologic condition when CD4 counts are low. However, once ART is introduced, these patients may experience a flare of their condition.

Monitoring of disease activity in HIV patients with RA, SLE, or other rheumatologic conditions poses challenges. For example, persistently raised ESR levels can be found in patients with HIV infection without active inflammatory arthritis. It has been observed that DAS-28 ESR overestimates disease activity by as much as 30% when compared to DAS28 CRP in individuals suffering from HIV infection and RA (Tarr et al, 2014).

▶ Differential Diagnosis

The symmetrical polyarthritis variant of HIV-related arthropathy can closely mimic RA, with patients occasionally exhibiting similar deformities to rheumatoid patients, including ulnar deviation. As stated above, false-positive autoantibodies can be generated in HIV infection, including both rheumatoid factor and CCP. In addition, radiologic changes can occasionally mimic RA, with joint space narrowing, erosions and periarticular osteopenia. HIV and SLE can also be difficult to distinguish clinically. As an example, the presentation of fever, proteinuria, and thrombocytopenia could be explained equally by active lupus or HIV infection. Moreover, HIV-associated immune-complex glomerulonephritis can be indistinguishable histologically from lupus nephritis.

▶ Treatment

The potential issues with regard to disease-modifying antirheumatic drug (DMARD) therapy in HIV-positive patients are well documented (Mody and Parke, 2003). Methotrexate is now used cautiously in patients with robust CD4 counts. Sulfasalazine, hydroxychloroquine, leflunomide and prednisolone have also been used in HIV-positive patients without deleterious effects on their HIV disease. Biological therapies, including infliximab, etanercept, adalimumab, rituximab, and tocilizumab, have also been employed successfully in this group of patients. It is crucial to monitor the CD4 count and viral load of HIV patients while they are on these immunosuppressants (Cepeda et al, 2008).

▶ Prognosis

HIV-associated inflammatory arthritis is typically short lived. Glucocorticoids and synthetic or biological DMARDs are seldom needed (Lawson and Walker-Bone, 2012). Patients with HIV who have concomitant rheumatologic conditions can typically be treated aggressively for their rheumatologic disorders if their HIV disease is well controlled.

CHIKUNGUNYA

 ESSENTIALS OF DIAGNOSIS

▶ Suspected case: A suspected case involves a patient presenting with acute onset of fever, usually with chills/rigors, which lasts for 3–5 days with pain in multiple joints/swelling of extremities that may continue for weeks to months.

▶ Probable case: A probable case is characterized by conditions that support a suspected case (see previous definition), together with one of the following conditions:

• History of travel or residence in areas reporting outbreaks

• Exclusion of malaria, dengue, and other known causes of fever with joint pains

▶ Confirmed case: A confirmed case of chikungunya requires the patient to meet one or more of the following findings, regardless of the clinical presentation:

- Virus isolation in cell culture or animal inoculations from acute-phase sera
- Presence of viral ribonucleic acid (RNA) in acute-phase sera as determined with reverse transcriptase-polymerase chain reaction (RT-PCR)
- Presence of virus-specific immunoglobulin M (IgM) antibodies in a single serum sample in acute phase or a fourfold increase in virus-specific immunoglobulin G (IgG) antibody titer in samples collected at least 3 weeks apart

▶ General Considerations

Chikungunya is transmitted by mosquitoes of the *Aedes* species, especially *Aedes aegypti* and *Aedes albopictus*. In endemic areas of Africa, chikungunya virus transmission occurs in a cycle involving humans and several species of Aedes mosquitoes that inhabit forests and villages and infect animals (nonhuman primates and possibly other animals). In Asia and elsewhere, however, major outbreaks are sustained by mosquito transmission among susceptible humans (Adizie and Adebajo, 2014). The use of plastic containers as rainwater receptacles in developing countries has been linked with the spread of the mosquitoes (Caglioti, 2013). The receptacles become perfect incubators for mosquito eggs following exposure to sunlight. Modes of mosquito dissemination include the transport of mosquito larvae and eggs in used tires by container ships and air traffic, with subsequent establishment in new areas with suitable environmental and climatic conditions. Some have postulated that climate change and global warming will be a significant factor in the future spread of chikungunya virus to new areas (Caglioti, 2013). The incubation period of chikungunya ranges from 2 to 12 days. Many people infected with chikungunya remain asymptomatic. Although the accompanying clinical disease and its associated arthritis is severe in a significant subset of patients, the disease is rarely fatal.

A. Symptoms and Signs

The presentation of clinical illness typically consists of fever, arthralgia, backache, and headache. Other symptoms include rash, fatigue, nausea, vomiting, and myalgias. The joint symptoms of chikungunya are severe and often debilitating, lasting from weeks to up to many months. The hands and feet are the areas most often affected, but the lower limbs and back can also be involved. Persistent polyarthralgia and arthritis have been reported in 10–20% of patients infected with the chikungunya virus. The arthritis has been reported to up to 36 months following the infection in some series (Chaaithanya et al, 2014).

Persistent chikungunya infection can mimic RA, and some patients actually fulfill the American College of Rheumatology (ACR) criteria for RA. Joint effusions, bone marrow edema, and bony erosions have been demonstrated on magnetic resonance imaging (MRI) (Chaaithanya et al, 2014). A study on patients with chronic arthritic disability after chikungunya infection in Sri Lanka showed that the debilities persisted at the end of 3 years of follow-up in 6.1% of the patients (Chaaithanya et al, 2014). Factors associated with chronicity of symptoms include increasing age, higher viral load, and C-reactive protein (CRP) in the acute phase.

B. Laboratory Diagnosis

Laboratory diagnosis of chikungunya can be achieved through virus culture: by the detection of viral RNA by PCR, by the presence of virus-specific IgM in the acute phase of the illness, or by a fourfold increase in the titer of IgG antibodies in samples taken 3 weeks apart. Serology is the principal tool for diagnosis in the clinical setting. IgM anti-chikungunya virus antibodies detected by direct enzyme-linked immunosorbent assay (ELISA) are present about 5 days (range 1–12 days) following symptom onset. These antibodies can persist for up to 3 months. If initial results are negative and chikungunya is still suspected, convalescent serum should be collected 7 days after illness onset and retested to detect IgM antibodies. IgG antibodies begin to appear about 2 weeks after the onset of symptoms and persist for years.

▶ Treatment

No specific drugs are available to treat chikungunya virus infections. Supportive treatment with analgesics, antipyretics, and nonsteroidal anti-inflammatory drugs is generally recommended. A recent randomised controlled trial failed to demonstrate any advantage of chloroquine over meloxicam (Chopra et al, 2014). Glucocorticoids, methotrexate, and even biologic agents can be considered in patients who develop a chronic arthritis, but to date there is no large-scale experience with these agents in chikungunya.

▶ Prognosis

Although chikungunya fever is a self-remitting illness, rare cases of complications have been reported during major outbreaks among patients with comorbidities (cardiovascular, respiratory, and neurologic), neonates, elderly patients, and immunocompromised patients. Persistent severe arthralgias can lead to long-term disability and loss of work days. Thus, the burden on the economy in terms of loss of productivity and income is estimated to be significant.

DENGUE

▶ Demonstration of a fourfold or greater change in reciprocal IgG or IgM antibody titers to one or more dengue virus antigens in paired serum samples.

▶ Acute phase sample should be obtained 3 days after the onset of illness. The IgM immunoassay (MAC-ELISA or equivalent) is the procedure of choice for rapid confirmation of the diagnosis.

▶ General Considerations

Dengue is the most prevalent mosquito-borne viral disease transmitted by mosquitoes of the genus *Aedes*. It is estimated that over 390 million dengue virus infections occur each year throughout the world. Populations of approximately 112 tropical and subtropical countries worldwide are at a risk of dengue infection (Adizie and Adebajo, 2014). The only continents that do not experience dengue transmission are Europe and Antarctica.

A. Symptoms and Signs

Classic dengue fever is marked by rapid onset of high fever, headache, retro-orbital pain, diffuse body pain (both muscle and bone), weakness, vomiting, sore throat, altered taste sensation and a centrifugal maculopapular rash. The hemorrhagic aspects of dengue infection are the most serious. Whereas most cases are relatively mild with petechiae, bleeding gums, epistaxis, menorrhagia, and hematuria, some patients develop life-threatening bleeds. Myalgias in dengue can be severe and tend to occur in the lower back, arms, and legs. They can be accompanied by an elevated serum creatine kinase level and can progress to a frank myositis. Rhabdomyolysis has also been observed in patients with dengue (Sunderalingam, 2013). Arthralgias, usually localized to the knees and shoulders, are observed frequently. A peripheral polyarthralgia is often present, but it may be overshadowed by intense backache and pain in the long bones. Synovitis is uncommon. Case reports suggest that dengue can act as a trigger for vasculitis (Tan, 2007). Acute dengue illness has also been shown to mimic acute lupus flares and been implicated in lupus flares with associated lupus nephritis (Talib, 2013).

Chikungunya and dengue virus infections have some common clinical symptoms and areas of geographic distribution; distinguishing them may be difficult in the setting of acute febrile illness with rash. However, a symmetrical polyarthritis is far more common in chikungunya. In contrast, severe abdominal pain, vomiting, thrombocytopenia, and bleeding are more frequently seen in dengue. Both viruses can lead to a chronic disabling arthritis. Chikungunya is rarely fatal, whereas without proper case identification and management, the fatality rate can be as high as 10% in patients with dengue (Sharp, 2014). Therefore, patients suspected of having dengue or chikungunya should be managed as having dengue until dengue is excluded.

B. Laboratory Diagnosis

Definitive laboratory diagnosis of dengue is obtained most commonly by demonstration of a fourfold or greater change in reciprocal IgG or IgM antibody titers to one or more dengue virus antigens in paired serum samples. Acute phase sample should be obtained 3 days after the onset of illness, and the IgM immunoassay (MAC-ELISA or equivalent) is the procedure of choice for rapid confirmation of the diagnosis.

▶ Treatment

Those patients requiring hospitalisation should have their hemodynamic status maintained with judicious use of isotonic intravenous fluids. Pain and fever in patients with suspected dengue should be managed with acetaminophen or paracetamol. Opiates may be considered for pain management if these agents are not sufficient. Nonsteroidal anti-inflammatory drugs (NSAIDs) should not be administered initially to such patients because of the increased risk of bleeding manifestations in the setting of severe dengue. Once a suspected case has been afebrile for at least 48 hours and has no warning signs of severe dengue, NSAIDs may be considered for continuing joint pains. Physical therapy may also be beneficial.

▶ Prognosis

Dengue fever is typically a self-limited disease with a mortality rate of less than 1%. When treated, dengue hemorrhagic fever has a mortality rate of 2–5%. When left untreated, the mortality is substantially higher. Survivors usually recover without sequelae and develop immunity to the infecting serotype.

ROSS RIVER VIRUS

▶ IgM is produced early in the course of Ross River virus (RRV) infection. Its detection in an acute-phase sample, collected within 7 days of symptom onset, provides a presumptive diagnosis of recent infection.

▶ However, there is cross-reactivity with other organisms (such as Barmah Forest virus). Thus, false-positive results can be observed.

▶ Confirmation of the diagnosis of RRV therefore requires demonstration of IgG seroconversion in a convalescent sample 10–14 days later.

▶ Diagnosis is established by a fourfold increase in IgG antibody titer.

General Considerations

Ross River virus (RRV) is also transmitted by mosquitoes, and it causes a disease characterised by polyarthritis and rash. The illness, first described in northern Australia in 1928 (Adizie and Adebajo, 2014), has been observed throughout Australia and many islands of the western South Pacific. The virus survives in mosquito eggs in arid environments and can be transmitted by many mosquito species.

A. Symptoms and Signs

The most striking clinical features of RRV infection are severe arthralgias and myalgias. Joint pains are present in more than 95% of patients, but true arthritis occurs in 40% (Adizie and Adebajo, 2014). The joints of the extremities, especially the wrists, knees, ankles, and the metacarpophalangeal and interphalangeal joints of the fingers, are involved most frequently. Joint effusions and enthesopathy have also been reported (Adizie and Adebajo, 2014). Other common symptoms include lethargy, fever, rash, headache, and depression. In the acute setting, there is often significant functional impairment, with about half of patients requiring time off work (Barber et al, 2009). The role of RRV in chronic musculoskeletal symptoms is controversial. Early studies reported a significant minority of sufferers complaining of arthralgias, fatigue, and depression for years after initial diagnosis (Barber et al, 2009). More recently, however, it has come to light that these initial studies did not control for preexisting comorbid musculoskeletal conditions. Recent prospective studies indicate that the vast majority of patients infected with RRV are symptom-free after 6 months (Barber et al, 2009).

B. Laboratory Diagnosis

Diagnosis is confirmed by serology. IgM is produced early in the course of infection. Its detection in an acute-phase sample collected within 7 days of symptom onset provides a presumptive diagnosis of recent infection. However, cross-reactivity with other organisms, for example, the Barmah Forest virus, can lead to false-positive results (Barber et al, 2009). Confirmation of the diagnosis therefore requires demonstration of IgG seroconversion. A convalescent sample should be collected 10–14 days later and tested in parallel by the same laboratory. Diagnosis is confirmed by a fourfold increase in IgG antibody titer. RRV can be detected by PCR, but the utility of this test is doubtful, given that viremia is typically short-lived.

Treatment

No treatment has been shown to shorten the duration or alter the course of RRV infection. In most series, NSAIDs are reported to be the most effective treatment (Barber et al, 2009). Physiotherapy and hydrotherapy have also been found to be beneficial for some (Adizie and Adebajo, 2014). Glucocorticoids have been tried in a few cases, but their routine use is not currently recommended (Mylonas et al, 2004).

The most important preventive action is the avoidance of mosquito bites with measures such as mosquito coils, repellents, and light-coloured clothing.

Prognosis

RRV disease causes pain and suffering for several months in a substantial proportion of patients, but progressive resolution is the norm.

ZIKA VIRUS

ESSENTIALS OF DIAGNOSIS

- ▶ Detection and isolation of zika virus (ZIKV) RNA from serum using RT-PCR.
- ▶ After the initial week of illness, serologic testing for virus-specific IgM and neutralizing antibodies against ZIKV using ELISA.

General Considerations

Zika virus (ZIKV), a member of the *Flaviviridae* family, is transmitted primarily by *Aedes* mosquitoes to humans. There were explosive outbreaks of ZIKV infections in the Americas and the islands of the Caribbean Sea in 2016 (Fauci and Morens, 2016). The incubation period is likely 3–12 days. Owing to the mild nature of the disease, the majority of ZIKV infection cases are likely to go unnoticed.

A. Symptoms and Signs

In most cases, ZIKV infection causes a mild, self-limited illness. The rash typically predominates and is usually a fine maculopapular rash that is distributed diffusely. It can involve the face, trunk, palms, and soles, and is occasionally pruritic. The rash, along with other symptoms, usually occurs within 2 weeks after travel to a ZIKV-affected area. Other common symptoms of ZIKV infection include fever, arthralgia (involving the small joints of the hands and feet), retro-orbital headache, and conjunctivitis. Symptoms last from 2 to 7 days. In rare cases, ZIKV infection is complicated by Guillain-Barré syndrome.

Great concern has emerged over congenital malformations, in particular microcephaly, due to transplacental transmission of ZIKV. There has also been a recently reported case of ZIKV in a patient with RA whose treatment consisted of etanercept and methotrexate (Roimicher et al, 2017). In this case, the illness was biphasic, with arthralgia returning 2 weeks after the first presentation had resolved. In addition, ZIKV was found in the blood and synovial fluid at first presentation, but only in synovial fluid at second presentation. This suggests that ZIKV that in synovial fluid after it has been cleared from the circulating blood may be associated with prolonged arthralgia and may also provide a repository for viral replication. Further research is required to fully understand if ZIKV poses additional dangers to patients with rheumatologic conditions on immunosuppressive medications.

B. Laboratory Diagnosis

ZIKV infection is diagnosed based on detection and isolation of ZIKV RNA from serum using RT-PCR. The highest sensitivity of PCR testing is during the initial week of illness, which is characterized by high viremia. After the initial week of illness, serologic testing for virus-specific IgM and neutralizing antibodies against ZIKV infection can be performed by ELISA. One potential shortcoming of the ELISA for ZIKV is a considerable degree of cross-reactivity with ELISAs for other flaviviruses, for example dengue and yellow fever. Urine can be tested via real-time RT-PCR using samples collected less than 2 weeks following symptom onset. Urine should be tested in conjunction with serum if specimens were obtained less than 1 week following symptom onset. Serum IgM testing should also be performed if real-time RT-PCR results are negative, regardless of when the specimen was collected.

▷ Treatment

The mainstays of management are bed rest and supportive care. Adequate fluid hydration is advised. Symptoms such as fever and pain can be controlled with acetaminophen. NSAIDs should be used cautiously in suspected ZIKV infection until such time as the possibility of a dengue virus infection has been excluded (this is because of the hemorrhagic risk associated with dengue). Residents of and travelers to endemic areas are advised to avoid mosquito bites. Among the best preventive measures against ZIKV are house screens, air-conditioning, and removal of containers that provide mosquito-breeding sites. These measures are often impractical to impoverished residents of crowded urban localities, where such epidemics hit hardest.

▷ Prognosis

Most cases of ZIKV infection are mild and self-limited. Owing to the mild nature of the disease, the vast majority of ZIKV infection cases likely go unnoticed. However, serious complications have been reported in rare cases, in particular Guillain-Barré syndrome.

EBOLA VIRUS

ESSENTIALS OF DIAGNOSIS

▶ Blood samples by RT-PCR within 3 days after the onset of symptoms.

▶ A rapid chromatographic immunoassay (ReEBOV) that detects Ebola virus antigen can provide results within 15 minutes.

▷ General Considerations

Musculoskeletal complaints are common among survivors of Ebola virus disease (EVD) and can have clinical impacts beyond 2 years postconvalescence. In fact, in a recent large cohort study in Guinea (Etard et al, 2017), the most frequent symptoms in Ebola survivors were musculoskeletal pain (38%), headache (35%), abdominal pain (22%), ocular disorders (18%), and depression (17%). The most striking feature of the Ebola survivors' musculoskeletal symptoms is the high prevalence of enthesitis. This occurs despite the fact that synovitis and sacroiliitis are uncommon.

A. Symptoms and Signs

The classic acute presentation of EVD consists of fever, severe headache, weakness, muscle pain, vomiting, diarrhea, abdominal pain, and unexplained haemorrhage. There is now increasing recognition, however, of a post-Ebola syndrome (Etard et al, 2017). This entity appears to cause significant sequelae, with musculoskeletal complaints being among the most common. Observations indicate a pattern of arthralgia that is typically symmetrical, involving multiple joints, most frequently affecting knees, back, hips, small joints of the hand, wrists, neck, shoulders, ankles, and elbows. The temporal characteristics of the post-Ebola syndrome have been difficult to ascertain. Morning stiffness is described in some patients, but a worsening of joint pain with activity has also been reported. The physical examination rarely demonstrates joint swelling, redness, or warmth, but tenderness is sometimes elicited. Functional limitation is often absent, and corresponding X-rays are normal. Few cases of active synovitis have been noted in the literature.

The longer-term musculoskeletal complications post-EVD are varied, including muscle pain and weakness, arthritis, enthesitis, and tendon ruptures. These can be present up to 2 years following resolution of the actue infection. It has been postulated that the acute arthralgias seen in some Ebola survivors occur as a result of formation of antigen-antibody complexes (Amissah-Arthur et al, 2018). An additional consideration possibly relevant to the high prevalence of musculoskeletal complaints is the huge psychological burden of disease and its impact on physical well-being and symptoms. The post-Ebola syndrome has been linked to symptoms of depression and generalized anxiety, and it is possible that this aspect of the syndrome could contribute to the problems with pain that those who survive experience (Amissah-Arthur et al, 2018).

B. Laboratory Diagnosis

Patients with EVD typically develop leukopenia, thrombocytopenia, and serum transaminase elevations, as well as renal and coagulation abnormalities. Other laboratory findings include a marked decrease in serum albumin, hypoglycemia, and elevated amylase levels. Diagnostic tests for Ebola virus infection are based principally upon the detection of specific RNA sequences by RT-PCR in blood or other body fluids.

Viral antigens can also be detected using immunoassays. Ebola virus is generally detectable in blood samples by RT-PCR within 3 days after the onset of symptoms. Repeat testing may be required for patients with symptoms for less than 3 days duration. A negative RT-PCR test that is collected 72 hours or more after the onset of symptoms excludes EVD. A ReEBOV that detects Ebola virus antigen can provide results within 15 minutes. This assay can support a provisional diagnosis based on clinical examination and exposure history. In the event of an Ebola outbreak, a conservative approach to identifying all potential cases for the purpose of quarantine is appropriate.

▶ Treatment

Treatment guidelines specifically for the musculoskeletal manifestations of Ebola are lacking. Acetaminophen or paracetamol is sufficient in most cases. Opiate analgesia is required occasionally. NSAIDs are avoided due to the risk of hemorrhagic complications.

▶ Prognosis

Lasting or damaging arthritis does not currently appear to be a feature of EVD, although long-term data are lacking.

HEPATITIS B

ESSENTIALS OF DIAGNOSIS

- ▶ Symmetrical, self-limited polyarthritis accompanied or followed by an urticarial rash developing during the pre-icteric phase of acute hepatitis B virus (HBV) infection.
- ▶ Diagnosis confirmed by hepatitis B surface antigen and IgM anti–hepatitis B core antigen.

▶ General Considerations

Individuals infected with HBV can be either asymptomatic or symptomatic. Asymptomatic infection is more common, especially in children. Most primary infections in adults are self-limited, with clearance of the virus from the blood and liver and the development of lasting immunity to reinfection. However, some primary infections in healthy adults, generally less than 5%, do not resolve but rather develop into persistent infections (Ganem and Prince, 2004). This is manifested by serologic evidence of a primary infection by the appearance of hepatitis B surface antigen (HBsAg), followed shortly by IgM antibodies against HBV core antigen (anti-HBc antibodies). Circulating HbeAg, an indication of active infection, appears last.

A. Symptoms and Signs

Ten to 25% of patients with HBV develop joint symptoms and arthritis (Hsu et al, 2004). These are typically symmetrical and either migratory or additive. The arthritis is characteristic of the prodromal stage of the disease, occurring at a time when there is no other clinical manifestation of hepatitis. The joints of the hands and knees are most often affected, but the wrists, ankles, elbows, shoulders, and other large joints can also be affected. Morning stiffness is common. Joint symptoms tend to persist for days to weeks, and commonly resolve with the onset of jaundice, coinciding with the resolution of circulating immune complexes comprised of the hepatitis B virion, immunoglobulins, and complement components. Skin involvement is usually present with HBV-associated arthritis, generally appearing coincident with the joint symptoms. Urticarial and maculopapular eruptions involving the lower extremities are most typical.

B. Laboratory Diagnosis

Persistent primary hepatitis B infection is characterized serologically by the appearance of hepatitis B surface antigen (HBsAg), followed shortly by IgM antibodies against HBV core antigen (anti-HBc antibodies) and then circulating HBeAg.

▶ Treatment

Management is limited to symptomatic supportive care. The joint disease is always self-limited with no reports of progression to chronic arthritis or evidence of joint damage. No evidence indicates that early treatment of acute hepatitis B virus infection with interferon alfa or antiviral agents decreases the rate of chronicity or speeds recovery. Most patients with acute icteric HBV infection recover without residual injury or chronic hepatitis. Management of acute HBV infection should be focused on avoidance of further hepatic injury and prophylaxis of contacts.

▶ Prognosis

The joint disease is always self-limited with no reports of progression to chronic arthritis or evidence of joint damage.

HEPATITIS C

ESSENTIALS OF DIAGNOSIS

- ▶ Diagnosis by positive anti–hepatitis C virus (HCV) antibody confirmed by a sensitive, qualitative HCV RNA assay.
- ▶ Arthralgias and rarely a nonerosive arthritis are seen in patients with chronic HCV infection, with or without associated cryoglobulinemia.
- ▶ Coexistent RA and HCV infection can create diagnostic conundrums and therapeutic challenges.

General Considerations

The hepatitis C virus (HCV) is a major cause of both acute and chronic hepatitis. It is often discovered in asymptomatic individuals because of elevated transaminase levels noted on comprehensive metabolic panels. Many infected patients have extrahepatic symptoms, including arthralgias and myalgias. A significant number of patients with HCV infection demonstrate an antibody response to viral products that result in the formation of circulating immune complexes. These immune complexes may then deposit in tissues producing the clinical manifestation of mixed essential cryoglobulinemia that includes arthritis, glomerulonephritis, and vasculitis (Pawlotsky et al, 1995).

Pathogenesis

HCV replicates predominantly in hepatocytes after entrance into the circulation. Following acute infection, HCV RNA can be detected in the serum within 1 week. Alanine aminotransferase elevation occurs 2–3 months later. Anti-HCV antibodies can be found 1–2 months after acute infection. Acute HCV infection is not associated with rheumatic complaints (in contrast to acute hepatitis B), and many patients do not know that they are infected. HCV exhibits tropism for hepatocytes, B lymphocytes, and salivary and lacrimal gland epithelial cells. Monoclonal and polyclonal B-cell expansions have been found in the liver and bone marrow of chronically infected patients. In approximately half of patients with chronic HCV infections, circulating cryoglobulins can be detected (Lunel et al, 1994). However, only a minority of these patients (<5%) develop the syndrome of mixed cryoglobulinemia. Deposition of immune complexes containing cryoglobulins in different organs is the presumed disease mechanism in mixed cryoglobulinemia, characterized by purpura, arthralgias, glomerulonephritis, and polyneuropathy (Ferri et al, 2004).

A. Symptoms and Signs

Arthritis is noted in 2–20% of HCV patients (Rivera et al, 1999). The arthritis has an evanescent RA-like clinical presentation in two-thirds of the cases and an oligoarthritis presentation in the rest. It is usually rapidly progressive and acute, with the hands, wrists, shoulders, knees, and hips affected worst. Myalgias are common. The essential mixed cryoglobulinemia syndrome is frequently associated with hepatitis C infection and is characterized in its most severe form by Raynaud phenomenon, purpura, livedo reticularis, distal ulcers, gangrene, and peripheral neuropathy.

B. Laboratory Diagnosis

A detectable HCV RNA by PCR in the setting of undetectable anti-HCV antibodies that subsequently become detectable within 12 weeks is generally considered definitive proof of acute HCV infection. Alternatively, newly detectable HCV RNA and anti-HCV antibodies with documentation of negative tests within the prior 6 months are also suggestive of acute HCV infection. The diagnosis of chronic HCV infection is usually made in a patient with a reactive HCV antibody test and a positive molecular test that detects the presence of HCV RNA. If the antibody test is nonreactive, chronic HCV infection is unlikely and testing can stop. Patients who are on dialysis, are severely immunocompromised, or are suspected of having an acute HCV infection may not have detectable anti-HCV antibodies despite the presence of infection. In such patients (Pereira and Levey, 1997), HCV RNA testing despite a nonreactive antibody test is important to exclude infection. Bilirubin and transaminase levels are also typically elevated, though if normal this does not completely exclude HCV infection.

Differential Diagnosis

It should always be kept in mind that since chronic HCV infection is common in the general population (~2%), any rheumatic condition can coexist with HCV infection. Differentiating between the arthritis associated with HCV and RA that has developed in an HCV infected individual can be particularly difficult because the patterns of joint involvement are similar and both can have positive tests for serum rheumatoid factor. The presence of anti-CCP antibodies (present in 70% of RA patients) or erosive changes on radiographs of the hand or foot radiographs, however, implicate coexisting RA. If ANAs are present, the differential diagnosis should include SLE. Distinguishing between the glomerulonephritis presentations of HCV-related cryoglobulinemia and SLE is occasionally challenging.

Treatment

NSAIDs and hydroxychloroquine may be helpful, but conventional DMARD treatment of arthritis may be problematic in the context of viral hepatitic arthropathy. The emergence of more effective antiviral treatments and the combination with biologics may provide more effective treatment for the inflammatory arthritis associated with chronic HCV infection. Those suffering from severe HCV-related mixed cryoglobulinemia are treated with a combination of antivirals, rituximab, glucocorticoids, and plasma exchange (Dammacco and Sansonno, 2013).

Prognosis

The prognosis of HCV-associated inflammatory arthritis is good. According to a recent study of a large population of patients with HCV-associated cryoglobulinemia, mild disease activity is seen in half of the patients, whereas one-third follow a moderate to severe course (Rivera et al, 1999). Non-Hodgkin lymphomas can develop in some patients.

PARVOVIRUS B19

General Considerations

Parvovirus B19 is the only known parvovirus that infects humans. It is the cause of fifth disease or erythema infectiosum, a self-limited febrile illness associated with a classic rash—"slapped cheek"—in childhood. This infection can cause arthralgias or arthritis. A parvovirus B19 infection can also present as a nonspecific febrile illness with a connective tissue disease-like syndrome, both in children and adults (Nesher et al, 1995).

A. Symptoms and Signs

This syndrome is manifested by rash, arthralgias/arthritis, laboratory abnormalities, and other connective tissue disease-like symptoms. Parvoviral infections sometimes mimic SLE in adults and children. Joint symptoms occur in about 8% of infected children and 60% of infected adults (Moore, 1995). Arthralgias or arthritis may accompany or follow the skin eruption. Arthropathy is noted to occur more commonly in women (59%) than in men (30%), with many adults having arthritis alone without other preceding or concurrent symptoms (Cleghorn et al, 1995). A typical pattern in adults is acute onset symmetrical polyarticular arthritis with the proximal interphalangeal and metacarpophalangeal joints most commonly affected. It is therefore an excellent mimicker of RA. It can also be associated with a severe aplastic anaemia.

B. Laboratory Diagnosis

The incubation period for parvovirus B19 is 7–18 days, and the state of viremia lasts 5–6 days. The diagnosis of acute parvovirus infection is made by finding circulating IgM antibody to parvovirus. IgG antibody is evidence of a preexisting infection and may be found in a substantial proportion of the normal population. Laboratory findings are otherwise remarkably normal in most patients. The erythrocyte sedimentation rate and CRP are occasionally elevated. The leukocyte count remains normal, but rheumatoid factor and ANA may be present during the acute period in some cases, although their presence may be transient in nature.

Differential Diagnosis

Other diseases that can present with an acute symmetrical inflammatory polyarthritis involving the small joints with or without a skin rash should be included in the differential diagnosis. These include RA, SLE, other virus-associated arthritides (HCV, HBV, HIV, and rubella), and serum sickness.

Treatment

Therapy for acute parvoviral infections with arthralgias/arthritis is mainly supportive, with NSAIDs such as naproxen in doses of 10–20 mg/kg in children and 500 mg twice a day in adults usually being effective for symptomatic relief.

Complications

Erythrovirus (parvovirus B19)–associated arthritis is a nonerosive arthropathy. No long-term complications are expected.

Prognosis

For cases with erythrovirus (parvovirus B19)–associated arthropathy the prognosis is good, without long-term sequelae.

HTLV-1

General Considerations

The human T-lymphotropic virus type I (HTLV-I) is a retrovirus that infects 10–20 million people worldwide, as estimated by seroprevalence studies (Cleghorn et al, 1995). However, HTLV-I is associated with disease in only approximately 5% of infected individuals (Cleghorn et al, 1995). The two most common disease associations are adult T-cell leukaemia lymphoma (ATL) and HTLV-I–associated myelopathy (HAM), also known as tropical spastic paraparesis (TSP).

A. Symptoms and Signs

The clinical picture of HTLV-1–related arthritis can be clinically indistinguishable from RA. The most commonly involved sites are the hands and knees. A bilateral symmetrical peripheral polyarthritis is the predominant pattern. It has actually been suggested that HTLV-1 infection can act as a trigger for RA. Fever, myalgia, and skin lesions are also common.

B. Laboratory Diagnosis

The synovial fluid and tissue of HTLV-1–positive patients with arthritis have been shown to contain atypical T lymphocytes, high titers of anti-HTLV-1 IgM antibodies, and integrated HTLV-1 viral DNA. Positive rheumatoid factor and ANA have also been observed in these patients.

Treatment

Little is known about an ideal treatment of HTLV-1–associated arthritis. Glucocorticoids are often used. There is always the worry of adult T-cell leukemia/lymphoma (ATLL) development if immune-modulatory drugs such as anti-TNF therapies are used. There have, however, been reassuring case reports of the use of rituximab and etanercept in these patients (Frenzel et al, 2014), although these observations need to be verified in clinical trials.

▶ Prognosis

Infection with HTLV-1 or HTLV-2 is lifelong, but the vast majority of infected individuals remain asymptomatic throughout life, without progression to any endpoint diseases. Mortality and morbidity due to HTLV infections are primarily associated with diseases caused by HTLV-1, namely ATL or HAM/TSP. ATL carries a particularly poor prognosis, with a median survival time of 2 years.

Aboulafia DM, Bundow D, Wilske K, Ochs UI. Etanercept for the treatment of human immunodeficiency virus associated arthritis. *Mayo Clin Proc.* 2000;75:1093-1098. [PMID: 11040859]

Adizie T, Adebajo AO. Travel- and immigration-related problems in rheumatology. *Best Pract Res Clin Rheumatol.* 2014;28(6):973-985. [PMID: 26096097]

Amissah-Arthur MB, Poller B, Tunbridge A, Adebajo A. Musculoskeletal manifestations of Ebola virus. *Rheumatology (Oxford).* 2018;57(1):28-31. [PMID: 28379487]

Barber B, Denholm JT, Spelman D. Ross river virus. *Aust Fam Physician.* 2009;38(8):586-589. [PMID: 19893779]

Bonnet F, Pineau JJ, Taupin JL, et al. Prevalence of cryoglobulinemia and serological markers of autoimmunity in human immunodeficiency virus infected individuals: a cross-sectional study of 97 patients. *J Rheumatol.* 2003;30(9):2005-2010. [PMID: 12966606]

Caglioti C. Chikungunya virus infection: an overview. *New Microbiol.* 2013;36(3):211-227. [PMID: 23912863]

Cepeda EJ, Williams FM, Ishimori ML, Weisman MH, Reveille JD. The use of anti-tumour necrosis factor therapy in HIV-positive individuals with rheumatic disease. *Ann Rheum Dis.* 2008;67:710-712. [PMID: 18079191]

Chaaithanya IK, Muruganandam N, Raghuraj U, et al. Chronic inflammatory arthritis with persisting bony erosions in patients following chikungunya infection. *Indian J Med Res.* 2014;140(1):142-145. [PMID: 25222790]

Chopra A, Saluja M, Venugopalan A. Effectiveness of chloroquine and inflammatory cytokine response in patients with early persistent musculoskeletal pain and arthritis following chikungunya virus infection. *Arthritis Rheum.* 2014;66(2):319-326. [PMID: 24504804]

Cleghorn FR, Manns A, Falk R, et al. Effect of human T-lymphotropic virus type I infection on non-Hodgkin's lymphoma incidence. *J Natl Cancer Inst.* 1995;87(13):1009. [PMID: 7629870]

Dammacco F, Sansonno D. Therapy for hepatitis C virus-related cryoglobulinemic vasculitis. *N Engl J Med.* 2013;369(11):1035-1045. [PMID: 24024840]

Etard J, Sow M, Leroy S, et al. Multidisciplinary assessment of post-Ebola sequelae in Guinea (Postebogui): an observational cohort study. *Lancet Infect Dis.* 2017;17(5):545-552. [PMID: 28094208]

Fauci AS, Morens DM. Zika virus in the Americas—yet another arbovirus threat. *N Engl J Med.* 2016;374(7):601. [PMID: 26761185]

Ferri C, Sebastiani M, Giuggioli D, et al. Mixed cryoglobulinemia: demographic, clinical, and serologic features and survival in 231 patients. *Semin Arthritis Rheum.* 2004;33(6):355. [PMID: 15190522]

Frenzel L, Moura B, Marcais A, et al. HTLV-1-associated arthropathy treated with anti-TNF-alpha agent. *Joint Bone Spine.* 2014;81(4):360-361. [PMID: 24289962]

Ganem D, Prince AM. Hepatitis B virus infection—natural history and clinical consequences. *N Engl J Med.* 2004;350(11):1118. [PMID: 15014185]

Hsu HH, Feinstone SM, Houfnagle JH. Acute viral hepatitis. In: Mandell GL, Bennett JE, Dolin R, eds. *Mandell, Douglas, and Bennett's Principles and Practices of Infectious Diseases.* 4th ed. New York: Churchill Livingstone; 1995:1100.

Kole AK, Roy R, Kole D. Musculoskeletal and rheumatological disorders in HIV infection: experience in a tertiary referral center. *Indian J Sex Transm Dis AIDS.* 2013;34(2):107-112. [PMID: 24339461]

Lawson E, Walker-Bone K. The changing spectrum of rheumatic disease in HIV infection. *Br Med Bull.* 2012;103(1):203-221. [PMID: 22879627]

Lunel F, Musset L, Cacoub P, et al. Cryoglobulinemia in chronic liver diseases: role of hepatitis C virus and liver damage. *Gastroenterology.* 1994;106(5):1291. [PMID: 7513667]

Mody G, Parke F. Articular manifestations of human immunodeficiency virus infection. *Best Pract Res Clin Rheumatol.* 2003;17(2):265-287. [PMID: 12787525]

Moore TL. Parvovirus-associated arthritis. *Curr Opin Rheumatol.* 2000;12(4):289. [PMID: 10910181]

Mylonas A, Harley D, Purdie D, et al. Corticosteroid therapy in an alphaviral arthritis. *J Clin Rheumatol.* 2004;10:326-330. [PMID: 17043541]

Nesher G, Osborn TG, Moore TL, et al. Parvovirus infection mimicking systemic lupus erythematosus. *Semin Arthritis Rheum.* 1995;24(5):297. [PMID: 7604297]

Nguyen BY, Reveille JD. Rheumatic manifestations associated with HIV in the highly active antiretroviral therapy era. *Curr Opin Rheumatol.* 2009;21(4):404. [PMID: 19444116]

Plate A-M, Boyle B. Musculoskeletal Manifestations of HIV. *AIDS Read.* 2003;13(2):62. [PMID: 12645490]

Pawlotsky JM, Roudot-Thoraval F, Simmonds P, et al. Extrahepatic immunologic manifestations in chronic hepatitis C and hepatitis C virus serotypes. *Ann Intern Med.* 1995;122(3):169. [PMID: 7810933]

Pereira BJ, Levey AS. Hepatitis C virus infection in dialysis and renal transplantation. *Kidney Int.* 1997;51(4):981. [PMID: 9083262]

Reveille JD. The changing spectrum of rheumatic disease in human immunodeficiency virus infection. *Semin Arthritis Rheum.* 2000;30(3):147. [PMID: 11124280]

Rivera J, García-Monforte A, Pineda A, et al. Arthritis in patients with chronic hepatitis C virus infection. *J Rheumatol.* 1999;26(2):420. [PMID: 9972979]

Roimicher L, Ferreira OC Jr, Arruda MB, Tanuri A. Zika virus in the joint of a patient with rheumatoid arthritis. *J Rheumatol.* 2017;44(4):535. [PMID: 28604348]

Sharp T. Differentiating chikungunya from dengue: a clinical challenge. Centers for Disease Control and Prevention (CDC) Expert commentary. *Medscape.* Sep 15, 2014. http://www.medscape.com/viewarticle/831523.

Sunderalingam V. Dengue viral myositis complicated with rhabdomyolysis and superinfection of methicillin-resistant *Staphylococcus aureus. Case Rep Infect Dis.* 2013;2013:194-205. [PMID: 23476836]

Talib S. Dengue fever triggering systemic lupus erythematosus and lupus nephritis: a case report. *Int Med Case Rep J.* 2013;6:71-75. [PMID: 24204176]

Tan CSH, Teoh SC, Chan DP, Wong IB, Lim TH. Dengue retinopathy manifesting with bilateral vasculitis and macular oedema. *Eye (Lond)*. 2007;21(6):875-877. [PMID: 17332768]

Tarr G, Makda M, Musenge E, Tikly M. Effect of human immunodeficiency virus infection on disease activity in rheumatoid arthritis: a retrospective study in South Africans. *J Rheumatol*. 2014;41(8):1645-1649. [PMID: 25028384]

Terada Y, Kamoi K, Ohno-Matsui K, et al. Treatment of rheumatoid arthritis with biologics may exacerbate HTLV-1-associated conditions: a case report. *Medicine (Baltimore)*. 2017;96(6):e6021. [PMID: 28178142]

Weeratunge NC, Roldan J, Anstead GM. Jaccoud arthropathy: a rarityin the spectrum of HIV-associated arthropathy. *Am J Med*. 2004;328:351-353. [PMID: 15599332]

Winchester R, Bernstein D, Fischer H, Enlow R, Solomon G. The co-occurrence of Reiter's syndrome and acquired immunodeficiency. *Ann Intern Med*. 1987;106:19-26. [PMID: 3789575]

Whipple Disease

45

Gaye Cunnane, PhD, MB, FRCPI

ESSENTIALS OF DIAGNOSIS

- ▶ Rare disease (1 in 1,000,000) caused by Tropheryma whipplei (TW).

- ▶ Mainly presents in middle-aged/older males.

- ▶ Large joint arthritis is the most common manifestation and precedes the development of systemic symptoms by many years.

- ▶ The four cardinal signs are arthritis, weight loss, abdominal pain, and diarrhea.

- ▶ Oculomasticatory myorhythmia (OMM) is a pathognomonic but late manifestation.

- ▶ Diagnosis is made by demonstration of characteristic periodic acid–Schiff (PAS)-positive intracellular inclusions and identification of TW by polymerase chain reaction (PCR) of involved tissues or fluids.

- ▶ All patients with confirmed Whipple disease should have PCR for TW tested on cerebrospinal fluid (CSF), even those without neurologic symptoms.

- ▶ Prolonged antibiotic treatment is required (>1 year).

▶ General Considerations

Whipple disease, a chronic multisystem disease caused by infection with *Tropheryma whipplei*, was first described in 1907 by George H. Whipple who detected at autopsy the presence of rod-shaped organisms within the vacuoles of foamy macrophages in the intestine of a 36-year-old man clinician. Over 40 years later, these cells were found to stain positively with periodic acid Schiff (PAS). In 1961, electron microscopy demonstrated bacterial components in these tissues. Identification of the bacillus was reported in 1992 with the aid of polymerase chain reaction (PCR), which enabled the amplification of specific gene segments. In 2000, the organism *T whipplei* was successfully cultivated in vitro, thereby

facilitating developments in the pathogenesis, diagnosis, and treatment of this potentially fatal disease.

Whipple disease is rare, with an estimated incidence of 1 per million. It occurs most commonly in middle-aged white men with an occupational exposure to soil, animals, or sewage. There are two recognized phases of Whipple disease. In the initial stage, symptoms and signs are nonspecific and are characterized by fatigue and joint pains, with or without synovitis. Later, abdominal pain, diarrhea, weight loss, and neurologic or psychiatric symptoms may prevail. Although the average interval between these stages is 6–8 years, the initiation of immunosuppressive treatment for presumed inflammatory arthritis may unmask the diagnosis by allowing proliferation of the organism, resulting in more acute symptoms.

T whipplei is ubiquitous and can be found in the general environment. It has also been isolated from the saliva, dental plaque, blood, stool, and duodenal samples from healthy individuals, although it is unclear if this represents environmental contamination, preclinical infection, or the inconsequential presence of commensal organisms. IgG antibodies against *T whipplei* can be detected in up to 70% of healthy people. Therefore, not everybody who is exposed to infection will develop clinical symptoms. Although host factors appear to play a role in disease manifestation, no specific genetic link has been identified.

There is strikingly little inflammation in tissues infected with *T whipplei*. The organism does not provoke a local cytotoxic reaction and large numbers of bacilli accumulate in involved tissue. These observations have led to suggestions that aberrations of the host immune response may contribute to the clinical manifestations of disease.

The diagnosis of Whipple disease requires evidence of infection with *T whipplei*. Biopsies of multiple areas of the duodenum and jejunum are recommended to avoid sampling error. The tissue should be stained with PAS, which yields a 78% positivity rate in patients with untreated Whipple disease. PCR analysis is performed for confirmation of findings.

If the biopsies are negative, other symptomatic areas should be examined, such as synovial fluid, pleural fluid, or lymph nodes. Examination of cerebrospinal fluid (CSF) should take place for all confirmed cases, even in the absence of neurological symptoms, as this information will alter management and inform prognosis.

▶ Clinical Findings

Because of the systemic nature of Whipple disease, the wide variety of clinical presentations and the chronicity of the illness, a high index of suspicion is essential in order to make the diagnosis in a timely manner before the onset of permanent or life-threatening sequelae. Approximately 15% of patients with Whipple disease have atypical signs. However, the presence of gastrointestinal symptoms with or without neurological features on a background of an unusual seronegative arthropathy should trigger appropriate investigations. Ideally, the diagnosis is considered in the prodromal stage of an unexplained, intermittent large joint oligoarthritis or polyarthritis, but establishing the diagnosis at that point is exceptionally difficult because few clinicians consider the disease at that early time point.

A. Symptoms and Signs

1. Articular manifestations—Articular symptoms occur in up to 90% of patients with Whipple disease and may be the presenting feature. Joint involvement is characteristically an intermittent, migratory oligoarthritis, predominantly affecting the large joints, such as the knees, wrists, and ankles. Less frequently, the hips, elbows, and shoulders may be symptomatic. It is rare to have small joint symptoms. Attacks usually last several hours to a few days and resolve spontaneously with complete remission between episodes. Joint complaints are typically present for 6–8 years before a diagnosis of Whipple disease is made.

Chronic polyarthritis is less common but has been described in association with Whipple disease. It tends to show features of an inflammatory arthritis with prolonged early morning stiffness. Joint damage is rare, but ankylosis of wrists, ankles, and spine has been reported. Furthermore, sacroiliitis and radiographic changes of hypertrophic osteoarthropathy have been observed in patients with Whipple disease.

2. Gastrointestinal (GI) manifestations—These tend to develop later in the disease course with profound weight loss, crampy abdominal pain, and diarrhea. In advanced cases, evidence of chronic malabsorption is present, with edema, ascites, and muscle wasting. However, 10–15% of patients have no GI symptoms at diagnosis. During upper GI endoscopy, pale yellow mucosa punctuated with erosions may be observed.

3. Skin lesions—A variety of skin abnormalities have been described in association with Whipple disease. The most common of these is hyperpigmentation (melanoderma), which develops in more than 40% of patients in the later stages of the illness. Other characteristic skin findings include subcutaneous nodules, erythema nodosum–like lesions, and inflammatory rashes that may mimic cutaneous lupus, dermatomyositis, psoriasis, or eczema. Urticaria and vasculitis rashes have also been reported. Consequences of severe malnutrition may also affect the skin, leading to petechiae, purpura, and edema.

4. Central nervous system and eye disease—Neurologic involvement is common, particularly in long-standing disease, affecting up to 90% of cases. Whipple disease causes a broad spectrum of symptoms, including cognitive impairment, depression, headaches, seizures, focal neurologic deficits, and ataxia. A pathognomonic sign of Whipple disease is oculomasticatory myorhythmia (OMM), where involuntary blinking occurs when the patient is talking or eating. Almost all cases of OMM have associated supranuclear ophthalmoplegia, facial weakness, and cognitive defects. Symptoms of hypothalamic involvement, such as insomnia, polydipsia, and hyperphagia develop in one-third of patients. Ocular signs are nonspecific and include uveitis, optic neuritis, and retinitis.

5. Cardiac disease—Over 50% of patients with Whipple disease have associated cardiac problems. Pericarditis is the most common manifestation and occurs in approximately half of those affected. Myocarditis may present with unexplained heart failure or sudden death. Blood culture-negative endocarditis has been described, typically developing in middle-aged men with a preceding history of joint pain. Fever and prior valvular heart disease are usually absent, contributing to a delayed diagnosis.

6. Other presentations—amyloidosis-induced nephropathy, hepatosplenomegaly, intra-abdominal lymphadenopathy, pleural effusions, pulmonary infiltrates, and epididymoorchitis have all been reported in Whipple disease.

B. Laboratory Findings

1. Routine laboratory testing—Patients with Whipple disease frequently have a neutrophil leukocytosis; eosinophilia is occasionally noted. Normochromic or macrocytic anemia is a common finding because of disease chronicity or malabsorption. Ferritin levels may be elevated secondary to inflammation. A robust acute phase response is common, with erythrocyte sedimentation rates typically greater than 100 mm/h. Evidence of malabsorption may include hypoalbuminemia, clotting abnormalities, and low levels of vitamin B_{12} and folate. Serologic tests for rheumatoid factor and antinuclear antibodies tend to be negative. Absence of the normal circadian rhythm that characterizes cortisol, growth hormone, melatonin, and thyroid-stimulating hormone may be indicative of hypothalamic dysfunction.

2. Examination of fluid and tissue—Fluid aspiration or tissue biopsy is recommended to confirm the diagnosis of Whipple disease. If initial testing is negative, further sampling of other regions should be undertaken. CSF examination should be performed even in patients without neurologic symptoms, because a positive PCR result influences treatment and prognosis.

On histologic analysis, a mild inflammatory infiltrate may be seen, in addition to occasional noncaseating granulomata. The characteristic histologic feature of Whipple disease is the presence of PAS-positive macrophages. False-positive results may occur in tissues infected with mycobacteria, *Histoplasma*, and *Actinomyces*. Immunohistochemistry using specific antibodies directed against *T whipplei* is more sensitive than PAS staining and can be used to help identify infection. Additional confirmation can take place using PCR. *T whipplei* can also be cultured from involved tissue.

Current diagnostic recommendations require two out of three positive results from tissue PAS staining, anti-*T whipplei* immunohistochemical staining, or detection of *T whipplei* by PCR.

C. Imaging Studies

Plain radiography of symptomatic joints is frequently normal. However, marked articular damage has been observed with subchondral cyst formation and ankylosis. Sacroiliitis and syndesmophyte formation of the spinal column have been described in patients with Whipple disease who are HLA-B27 negative. Findings of hypertrophic osteoarthropathy in this disease are rare.

Osteopenia and osteoporosis are common consequences of chronic inflammation and malabsorption. A dual x-ray absorptiometry (DXA) scan should be performed in patients diagnosed with Whipple disease.

Computed tomography (CT) of thorax and pelvis may reveal lymphadenopathy, particularly in the mesenteric area. Mediastinal adenopathy has also been described. In patients with CNS involvement, single or multiple enhancing lesions in the brain or spinal cord may be observed on CT or magnetic resonance imaging.

▶ Differential Diagnosis

Workup for a large joint inflammatory arthritis includes investigation for conditions such as seronegative spondyloarthropathy, sarcoidosis, crystal arthritis, and Lyme disease, among others. Each of these forms of arthritis has their own distinctive features. Whipple disease should be part of the differential diagnosis when the clinical scenario in these situations is atypical.

GI symptoms and weight loss will typically lead to the search for malignancy, celiac disease, and inflammatory bowel disease. Several endocrinopathies may present in a similar manner to Whipple disease, including Addison disease and hyperthyroidism. Neurologic involvement will prompt a search for CNS tumors, vasculitis, multiple sclerosis, atherosclerotic disease, and dementia. Associated

psychiatric illness, particularly depression, is common. OMM is pathognomonic.

Several infections should be considered in the differential diagnosis of Whipple disease. Tuberculosis may result in weight loss and lymphadenopathy in the absence of overt pulmonary disease. Although *Mycobacterium avium* can cause PAS-positive stains on histologic examination, PCR for *T whipplei* will be negative. Lyme disease is associated with lower limb synovitis, in addition to neurologic and cardiac symptoms. HIV infection should be considered in patients with unexplained multisystem disease.

▶ Treatment
A. Antibiotics

Prolonged antibiotic regimens are essential in order to eradicate the infection. For patients with confirmed or suspected neurologic involvement, parenteral treatment for a period of 2 weeks with ceftriaxone 2 g daily or meropenem 1 g three times a day is recommended in order to attain high CSF levels. Thereafter, a maintenance regimen of co-trimoxazole (trimethoprim 160 mg with sulfamethoxazole 800 mg) should be taken by mouth twice daily for at least 1 year. Alternatively, doxycycline 100 mg twice a day and hydroxychloroquine 600 mg/day can be used as maintenance treatment. In the absence of neurologic disease, the parenteral treatment could be omitted, but given the poor prognosis associated with neurologic infection, the full treatment regimen is usually advocated.

B. Glucocorticoids

Glucocorticoids are used to reduce the consequences of CNS involvement and are helpful in decreasing the signs of immune reconstitution syndrome in cases where persistent fever develops after initiation of treatment in the presence of a heavy bacterial load.

▶ Prognosis

Prior to the availability of antibiotics, Whipple disease was invariably fatal. Early recognition and treatment greatly improves prognosis. For patients without CNS disease, rapid improvement in symptoms occurs after initiation of therapy. Diarrhea often resolves within 1 week, while joint symptoms may remit within 1 month. The course of neurologic involvement is less predictable, and long-standing neurologic deficits are likely to be irreversible. CNS infection is associated with a mortality rate of 25% within 4 years of diagnosis, while a further 25% remain impaired.

Older treatment regimens using tetracycline alone were associated with a relapse rate of up to 30%. A much lower recurrence rate of 2% has been observed with the co-trimoxazole–based regimens.

Dolmans RA, Boel CH, Lacle MM, Kusters JG. Clinical manifestations, treatment, and diagnosis of *Tropheryma whipplei* infections. *Clin Microbiol Rev.* 2017;30(2):529. [PMID: 28298472]

El-Abassi R, Soliman MY, Williams F, England JD. Whipple's disease. *J Neurol Sci.* 2017;377:197. [PMID: 28477696]

Glaser C, Rieg S, Wiech T, et al. Whipple's disease mimicking rheumatoid arthritis can cause misdiagnosis and treatment failure. *Orphanet J Rare Dis.* 2017;12(1):99. [PMID: 28545554]

Hujoel IA, Johnson DH, Lebwohl B, et al. *Tropheryma whipplei* infection (Whipple disease) in the USA. *Dig Dis Sci.* 2019;64(1):213. [PMID: 29572616]

Sarcoidosis

46

Edward S. Chen, MD
David R. Moller, MD

ESSENTIALS OF DIAGNOSIS

▶ Systemic disease associated with noncaseating epithelioid granulomatous inflammation in affected organs.

▶ Most frequently affected organs are the lung, lymph nodes, eyes, skin, joints, liver, muscles, central and peripheral nervous system, upper airway, heart, and kidneys.

▶ Clinically apparent organ involvement is often restricted to a few organs, usually defined early in the course of disease.

▶ In the United States, sarcoidosis is more common and severe in Blacks.

▶ Diagnosis requires a compatible clinical picture and a biopsy with typical noncaseating granulomas, excluding diseases that can cause similar granulomatous reactions.

▶ General Considerations

A. Epidemiology

Sarcoidosis is found worldwide with a prevalence ranging from 10 to 80 cases per 100,000 in North America and Europe. Higher regional prevalence has been reported in Scandinavia and the southeast coastal United States. In the United States, one study from a midwestern city estimated that the lifetime risk of developing sarcoidosis was 2.7% in black women, 2.1% in black men, 1% in white women, and 0.8% in white men. Worldwide, there is a slight female predominance, and recent studies suggest associations between higher body mass index (BMI), ethnicity (African American), and risk of developing sarcoidosis in women. Although all ages can be affected, most cases occur between the ages of 20 and 40 years, with a second peak incidence in women older than 60.

B. Genetics

A genetic predisposition to sarcoidosis is supported by familial clustering in approximately 5–10% of cases. A recent multicenter study on the etiology of sarcoidosis in the United States (A Case-Control Etiologic Study of Sarcoidosis [ACCESS]) suggests that the familial relative risk is approximately 5.0 among first-degree relatives.

The strongest associations between genotype and sarcoidosis risk have been identified within the major histocompatibility (MHC) locus on chromosome 6. Two recent genome-wide linkage analyses identified an association with the butyrophilin-like 2 gene (BTNL2), located within the MHC, in both whites and Blacks with sarcoidosis.

C. Etiology

The cause of sarcoidosis is uncertain. The genetic pattern of inheritance suggests that susceptibility to sarcoidosis is polygenic and interacts importantly with environmental factors. Geographic differences in disease prevalence and reports of time-space clustering of cases have also suggested that sarcoidosis may be associated with an environmental, likely microbial, exposure. The large, multicenter study ACCESS found no evidence for a single dominant environmental or occupational exposure associated with an increased risk of developing sarcoidosis. Multiple regression analyses found positive associations with modest odds ratios of approximately 1.5 for exposures to molds and mildews, insecticides, or musty odors at work. The ACCESS data supported a negative association of tobacco use or tobacco smoke exposure among sarcoidosis patients.

Since the first description of sarcoidosis, many experts have speculated on a potential microbial cause. Recent studies using polymerase chain reaction (PCR) have associated mycobacterial and propionibacterial organisms with potential roles in the etiology of sarcoidosis. A recent meta-analysis concluded that 26% of sarcoidosis tissues contained mycobacterial nucleic acids, with an odds ratio of 9- to 19-fold higher chance of finding mycobacterial nucleic acids in sarcoidosis compared with control tissues. Recently, a limited proteomic approach identified the mycobacterial catalase-peroxidase protein (mKatG) as a candidate pathogenic antigen. This and other studies from the United States and Europe have demonstrated immunologic responses to mKatG and other mycobacterial proteins in a subgroup of sarcoidosis patients, supporting a mycobacterial etiology of sarcoidosis. In Japan, a subgroup of sarcoidosis patients has been demonstrated to have immunologic responses to *Propionibacterium acnes*. No studies have demonstrated the presence of live organisms within sarcoidosis tissues, however. The mechanism by which these microbial organisms might trigger sarcoidosis remains unknown.

D. Pathophysiology

There are certain immunologic hallmarks of sarcoidosis regardless of the potential etiologic trigger. There is usually an accumulation of CD4+ dominant T-cell infiltration at sites of granulomatous inflammation, with fewer CD8+ T cells usually surrounding the granulomas. These CD4+ T cells have biased expression of specific T-cell receptor genes, consistent with oligoclonal expansion of antigen-specific T cells. The antigen-specific T-cell response is highly polarized toward a T helper 1 response with expression of interferon-gamma (IFN-γ) and the Th1 immunomodulatory cytokines, interleukin-12 (IL-12), and IL-18. Along with Th1 cytokines, proinflammatory cytokines such as tumor necrosis factor (TNF), IL-1, IL-6, and Th1-associated chemokines orchestrate the local granulomatous response. Although Th2 cells have never been firmly identified in sarcoidosis, other T-cell lineages may have roles in disease pathogenesis, including IFNγ-expressing T cells that bear a Th17 phenotype (Th17.1) and regulatory T cells (Treg). Dysregulated expression of Th1 immunomodulatory cytokines has been hypothesized to be central to the development of granulomatous inflammation in sarcoidosis.

▶ Clinical Findings

Sarcoidosis has tremendous clinical heterogeneity. Pulmonary involvement is documented in more than 90% of patients, but extrapulmonary manifestations are present in many patients with or without lung disease (Table 46–1).

An initial diagnostic evaluation should consist of tests to evaluate the presence and extent of pulmonary involvement and to screen for common extrathoracic manifestations (Table 46–2). Specialized testing is indicated when symptoms or signs suggest extrapulmonary involvement.

A. Symptoms and Signs

1. Acute sarcoidosis (Löfgren syndrome)—This syndrome of acute sarcoidosis is characterized by erythema nodosum, bilateral hilar adenopathy, and often polyarthritis

Table 46–1. Clinical features of sarcoidosis.

Clinically Evident Organ System Involvement (%)	Major Clinical Features
Pulmonary (70–90%)	Bilateral hilar adenopathy, restrictive and obstructive disease, reticulonodular infiltrates, fibrocystic disease, bronchiectasis, mycetomas
Ocular (20–30%)	Anterior and posterior uveitis, optic neuritis, chorioretinitis, conjunctival nodules, glaucoma, keratoconjunctivitis, lacrimal gland enlargement
Cutaneous (20–30%)	Erythema nodosum, lupus pernio, cutaneous and subcutaneous nodules, plaques, alopecia, dactylitis
Hematologic (20–30%)	Peripheral lymphadenopathy, splenomegaly, hypersplenism, anemia, lymphopenia, thrombocytopenia, hypergammaglobulinemia
Musculoskeletal/joints (10–20%)	Arthralgias, bone cysts, myopathy, heel pain, Achilles tendinitis, sacroiliitis
Hepatic (10–20%)	Hepatomegaly, pruritus, jaundice, cirrhosis
Salivary and parotid gland (10%)	Sicca syndrome, Heerfordt syndrome
Neurologic (5–15%)	Cranial neuropathy, aseptic meningitis, mass brain lesion, hydrocephalus, myelopathy, polyneuropathy, mononeuritis multiplex
Sinuses and upper respiratory tract (5–10%)	Chronic sinusitis, nasal congestion, saddle-nose deformity, hoarseness, laryngeal or tracheal obstruction
Cardiac (5–10%)	Arrhythmias, heart block, cardiomyopathy, sudden death
Gastrointestinal (<10%)	Abdominal pain, gastrointestinal tract dysmotility, pancreatitis
Endocrine (<10%)	Hypercalcemia, hypopituitarism, diabetes insipidus, epididymitis, testicular mass
Renal (<10%)	Interstitial nephritis, glomerulonephritis, nephrolithiasis, hypercalciuria, nephrocalcinosis

and uveitis (Figure 46–1). Löfgren syndrome is common among Scandinavians and Irish women but occurs in fewer than 5% of Black patients with sarcoidosis. Acute sarcoidosis without erythema nodosum may also occur, often with an intensely painful, temporarily disabling arthritis, or periarthritis.

Table 46–2. Recommended tests for an initial evaluation of sarcoidosis.

- Chest radiograph or chest computed tomography (CT) scan
- Pulmonary function tests
  - Spirometry (with flow-volume loops if upper airway obstruction is suspected)
  - Diffusion capacity
  - Lung volumes
- Ophthalmologic examination
- Blood work
  - Comprehensive metabolic panel (renal function, liver function, serum calcium level)
  - Complete blood count with differential
- Electrocardiogram
- Screen for tuberculosis exposure with purified protein derivative (PPD) skin test or blood interferon-gamma release assay (IGRA)
- Additional organ-specific tests may be indicated in patients with specific extrapulmonary symptoms. For example:
  - Cardiac: echocardiogram, Holter monitor, cardiac magnetic resonance imaging (MRI), cardiac positron emission tomography
  - Neurologic: contrast MRI, nerve conduction study, lumbar puncture

2. Pulmonary sarcoidosis—The most common symptoms are progressive shortness of breath, nonproductive cough, and chest discomfort (see Table 46–1). Chronic sputum production and hemoptysis are more frequent in advanced fibrocystic disease (chest radiograph stage IV, Figure 46–1). Pulmonary sarcoidosis typically has few physical findings, with lung crackles heard in fewer than 10% of patients. Clubbing is rare. Airway obstruction is usually unresponsive to bronchodilators ("fixed") but is observed in 30-50% of patients. Bronchial hyperreactivity with occasional frank wheezing is found in 5–30% of patients.

Pulmonary hypertension or **cor pulmonale** is seen in more than 80% patients with advanced fibrocystic sarcoidosis with pulmonary fibrosis. Granulomatous inflammation of the arterial and venous pulmonary vasculature is identified occasionally on biopsy, sometimes with little evidence of interstitial lung disease. Dyspnea out of proportion to pulmonary function test results should prompt a search for pulmonary hypertension. Other causes of pulmonary hypertension such as sleep disordered breathing, chronic hypoxemia, or chronic thromboembolic disease must be excluded. Severe pulmonary hypertension in patients with advanced lung disease is associated with higher rates of mortality while awaiting lung transplantation.

3. Ocular manifestations—**Uveitis**, the most common eye lesion in sarcoidosis, may be the initial presenting manifestation of the disease. The uveitis commonly involves the anterior chamber. In contrast to the uveitis associated with the seronegative spondyloarthropathies, which is invariably unilateral, bilateral disease often occurs in sarcoidosis. In addition, sarcoidosis is one of a small number of diseases—Behcet disease being another—that can cause a panuveitis:

the simultaneous presence of anterior, intermediate, and posterior uveitis. The posterior uveitis may be silent, and therefore all patients with sarcoidosis should be screened for this disease complication at the time of diagnosis and should have regular ophthalmological follow-up. Chronic uveitis occurs in as many as 20% of patients with chronic sarcoidosis and is more common in the Black population.

Granulomatous conjunctivitis appears as a granular or cobblestone-like appearance of the conjunctivae. Conjunctival nodules are also a common finding. **Optic neuritis** or **retinitis** may manifest dramatically with blindness that is typically highly responsive to glucocorticoids if treated early. Eye manifestations common to patients with sarcoidosis are discussed further in Chapter 49.

4. Chronic cutaneous sarcoidosis—Sarcoidosis commonly involves the skin (20–30%) and may be severe, especially in Black patients. Cutaneous nodules, plaques and subcutaneous nodules, typically located around the hairline, eyelids, ears, nose, mouth, and extensor surfaces of the arms and legs, are characteristic of sarcoidosis affecting the skin. **Lupus pernio**, a particularly disfiguring form of cutaneous sarcoidosis of the face, is associated with violaceous plaques and nodules covering the nose (Figure 46–2), nasal alae, malar areas, and periorbital region. Sarcoidosis also has a curious tendency to occur within tattoos.

5. Hematologic sarcoidosis—Peripheral lymph node enlargement occurs in 20–30% of patients as an early manifestation of sarcoidosis but then typically undergoes spontaneous remission. Persistent, bulky lymphadenopathy occurs less than 10% of the time. Splenomegaly, occasionally massive, occurs in fewer than 5% of cases and is often associated with hepatomegaly and hypercalcemia. Polyclonal hypergammaglobulinemia is present in 25% or more of patients. Anemia and peripheral lymphopenia are relatively common while leucopenia and thrombocytopenia are rare. A clinical association exists between sarcoidosis and common variable immunodeficiency (CVID). CVID should be suspected in patients with sarcoidosis who develop increased frequency of infections or hypogammaglobulinemia.

6. Musculoskeletal sarcoidosis—Systemic constitutional symptoms such as fever, malaise, and weight loss are seen in more than 20% of patients and may be disabling. **Arthralgias** are common in active multisystem sarcoidosis, but joint radiographs are usually normal. Acute, often incapacitating polyarthritis involving the ankles, feet, knees, and wrists is commonly seen in patients with Löfgren syndrome. Although highly symptomatic at onset, this polyarthritis typically regresses within weeks to several months with or without therapy. Persistent joint disease is found in fewer than 5% of patients with chronic sarcoidosis. Pain, swelling, and tenderness of the phalanges (sausage digit) of the hands and feet are most common.

Although random muscle biopsies in autopsy series often demonstrate muscle granulomas in patients with sarcoidosis,

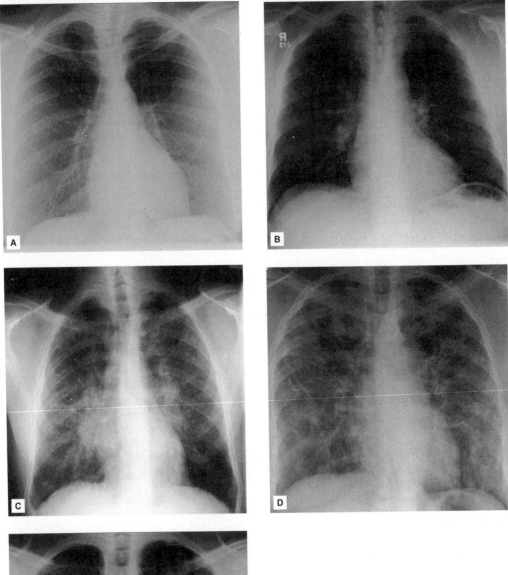

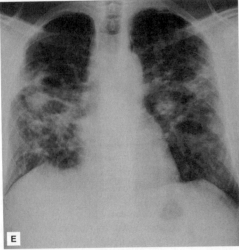

▲ **Figure 46–1.** Pulmonary sarcoidosis. Posteroanterior chest radiographs illustrating pulmonary sarcoidosis categorized as stage 0 (normal chest film), stage I (bilateral hilar adenopathy alone), stage II (adenopathy plus interstitial infiltrates), stage III (interstitial infiltrates alone), and stage IV (fibrocystic). Thoracic disease (lung and lymph node involvement) represents the most common manifestations of sarcoidosis affecting over 90% of all patients. Bronchoscopy remains the most common method of confirming a diagnosis of sarcoidosis.

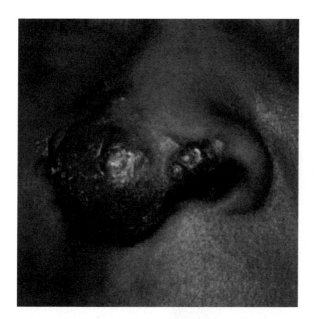

▲ **Figure 46–2.** Lupus pernio. This form of cutaneous eruption in sarcoidosis is typified by violaceous plaques and nodules that involve the nose, nasal alae, malar areas, nasolabial folds, around the eyes, scalp, and along the hairline. (See color insert.) (© Bernard Cohen, MD, Dermatlas; http://www.dermatlas.org.)

symptomatic myopathy with weakness and tenderness is uncommon. Sarcoidosis rarely presents in a manner that mimics an inflammatory myopathy, with profound weakness and elevated serum creatine kinase and aldolase levels.

Radiographic skeletal changes, observed in less than 10% of all patients, are typically incidental findings. These typically present as cystic and lytic lesions of varying sizes and may have associated sclerotic margins (Figure 46–3). Most commonly involved areas include bones of the skull, vertebrae, hands, and feet. Other imaging modalities (computed tomography [CT], magnetic resonance imaging [MRI] with gadolinium, technetium bone scan) are not useful for judging the activity of such lesions or differentiating them from infection or malignancy.

Fibromyalgia occurs commonly in patients with sarcoidosis, perhaps in part because of the glucocorticoids required so often to treat the underlying condition. Glucocorticoids lead to disrupted sleep, which may contribute to the pathophysiology of fibromyalgia. Fibromyalgia can cause considerable morbidity in sarcoidosis patients and is important to recognize and distinguish from sarcoidosis, because it will not respond to immunosuppressive therapy.

7. Gastrointestinal sarcoidosis—Clinically significant liver involvement is documented in only 10–20% of patients with sarcoidosis and is rarely the sole manifestation of this disease.

Active hepatic inflammation may be associated with fever, tender hepatomegaly, and pruritus. The serum alkaline phosphatase and γ-glutamyltransferase are typically elevated out of proportion to the transaminases or bilirubin. Granulomatous hepatitis in sarcoidosis is often part of a constellation of organ manifestations affecting the liver, spleen, and bone marrow, frequently associated with hypercalcemia, that is sometimes termed "abdominal sarcoidosis." Elevated serum liver function tests frequently revert to normal spontaneously or after treatment with glucocorticoids. Progressive cirrhosis may occur if severe, persistent granulomatous hepatitis is not treated.

Symptomatic gastrointestinal involvement in sarcoidosis is rare. Other causes such as Crohn disease or ulcerative colitis must be excluded.

8. Neurosarcoidosis—This manifestation occurs in 5–10% of patients with sarcoidosis. The most common manifestation is cranial neuropathy with a unilateral or bilateral seventh nerve palsy, also known as a Bell palsy. The glossopharyngeal, auditory, oculomotor, or trigeminal nerves are involved less often. The palsies may resolve spontaneously or with glucocorticoid therapy but may recur years later. Optic neuritis can result in blurred vision, field defects, and blindness. Other manifestations include mass lesions, aseptic meningitis, obstructive hydrocephalus, and hypothalamic-pituitary dysfunction. Seizures, headache, change in mental status, confusion, and diabetes insipidus can be initial manifestations of sarcoidosis. Spinal cord involvement is rare, but paraparesis, hemiparesis, and back and leg pains may occur. Peripheral neuropathies account for about 15% of cases of neurosarcoidosis, often presenting as mononeuritis multiplex or a primary sensory neuropathy. Recently, small fiber neuropathy has been associated with a pain syndrome and autonomic dysfunction in sarcoidosis. In all cases, a trial of immunosuppressive therapy will identify patients with reversible neurologic deficits due to active inflammation. Patients with persistent neurological deficits should be carefully considered for chronic immunosuppressive treatment and referred to specialized neurologic rehabilitation programs to optimize neurologic recovery.

9. Sarcoidosis of the upper respiratory tract (SURT)—This manifestation occurs in 5–10% of patients, usually in those with long-standing disease. Severe nasal congestion and chronic sinusitis usually are unresponsive to decongestants and topical (intranasal) glucocorticoids. Chronic disease or surgical intervention may result in destruction of the nasal septum and a "saddle-nose" deformity, but this finding is far more common as a complication of granulomatosis with polyangiitis. Laryngeal sarcoidosis may present with severe hoarseness, stridor, and acute respiratory failure secondary to upper airway obstruction. SURT is often associated with chronic skin lesions, particularly lupus pernio (see Figure 46–2).

10. Cardiac sarcoidosis—Myocardial sarcoidosis is diagnosed in fewer than 10% of patients in the United States

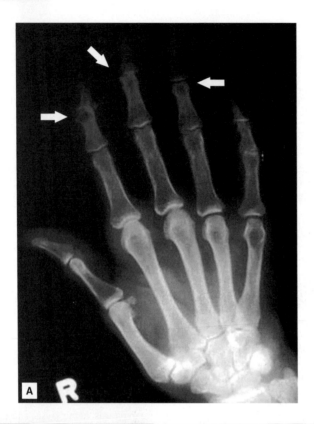

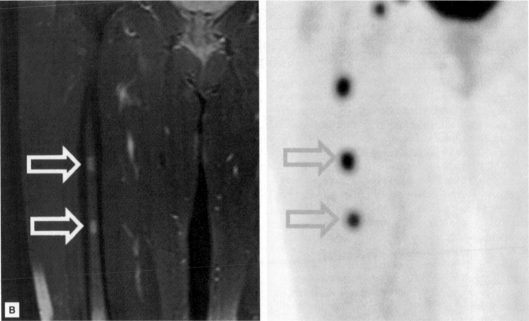

▲ **Figure 46–3. A:** Bone involvement in sarcoidosis. Multiple focal "punched-out" lesions (*arrows*) on a plain radiograph of the hand. (Used, with permission, from William Herring, MD; http://www.learningradiology.com.) **B and C:** Corresponding MRI and PET scans and MRI of the spine that are compatible with skeletal manifestations of sarcoidosis.

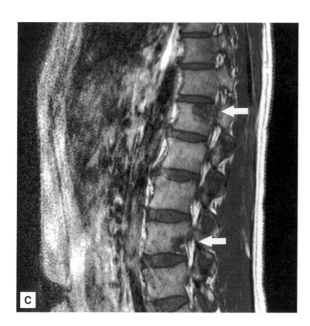

▲ Figure 46–3. (*Continued*)

and Europe but autopsy series suggest that sarcoidosis may be present in as many as 25%. In Japan, cardiac sarcoidosis occurs in nearly 50% of patients. The presenting clinical manifestations can be arrhythmia, heart block, dilated cardiomyopathy, or sudden death. Endomyocardial biopsies fail to demonstrate granulomatous inflammation in 80% of cases because of sampling error: the inflammatory involvement can be patchy and often does not involve the right ventricle

(the typical site of biopsy). A diagnosis of cardiac sarcoidosis can be inferred from a combination of biopsy-proven sarcoidosis in another organ and a compatible myocardial imaging study, such as thallium or sestamibi scan, cardiac MRI with gadolinium enhancement, or cardiac positron emission tomography (PET) scan (Figure 46–4).

11. Salivary, parotid, and lacrimal gland sarcoidosis— Parotid or lacrimal gland enlargement or sicca syndrome can occasionally be the dominant clinical manifestations of sarcoidosis. Heerfordt syndrome, or uveoparotid fever, is an uncommon acute presentation of sarcoidosis manifesting as fever, parotid and lacrimal gland enlargement, uveitis, bilateral hilar adenopathy, and often cranial neuropathies.

12. Endocrine abnormalities in sarcoidosis—In patients with neurosarcoidosis, disturbances to the hypothalamic-pituitary axis may result in diabetes insipidus and other manifestations of hypopituitarism. There is a higher association of autoimmune thyroid disease and sarcoidosis compared to control populations. Pancreatic sarcoidosis manifesting as a mass is a rare manifestation and must be distinguished from both cancer and IgG4-related disease.

13. Renal involvement in sarcoidosis—Sarcoidosis may be associated with hypercalcemia and, more commonly, hypercalciuria. The abnormalities are caused by the increased conversion of inactive 25-OH vitamin D_3 to the active $1,25(OH)_2$ vitamin D_3 by epithelioid macrophages within tissue granulomas. A low serum 25-OH vitamin D level (the standard serum vitamin D test) usually does not represent vitamin D deficiency in sarcoidosis patients. Rather, this finding results from this increased conversion of 25-OH vitamin D to active $1,25(OH)_2$ vitamin D. Vitamin D supplementation in this

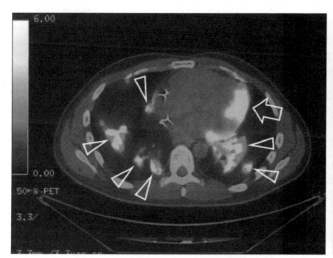

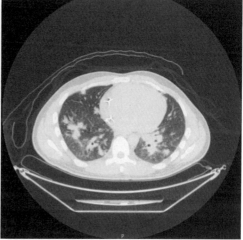

▲ Figure 46–4. Cardiac sarcoidosis. Cardiac PET/CT scan demonstrates FDG uptake in the left ventricle lateral wall (*arrow*) of a patient who also has active pulmonary sarcoidosis (*arrowheads*). (See color insert.)

instance may precipitate hypercalcemic crisis in untreated sarcoidosis patients. Vitamin D supplementation should only be based on serum levels of active 1,25(OH)$_2$ vitamin D in patients with sarcoidosis. Nephrocalcinosis may cause renal failure in sarcoidosis. Direct granulomatous involvement of the kidneys causing chronic interstitial nephritis or membranous glomerulonephritis is rare.

14. Psychosocial abnormalities—As many as 30–60% of patients with sarcoidosis report symptoms of depression. One study found this to be associated with female sex, lower socioeconomic status, poor access to health care, and increased disease severity, but not race.

B. Laboratory Studies

Recommended initial studies for all patients with presumed or biopsy-proven sarcoidosis include the following:

- A comprehensive metabolic panel is useful to assess abnormalities of renal function, calcium level, and liver function.
- The complete blood cell count is usually either normal or demonstrates peripheral lymphopenia. Although rare, pancytopenia may be caused by hypersplenism or bone marrow infiltration with granulomas.

C. Imaging Studies

Chest radiographs are abnormal in 90% or more of patients with sarcoidosis. These can be categorized by stage or type according to international convention (see Figure 46–1). **Stage 0** indicates a normal chest radiograph, as would be seen in extrapulmonary sarcoidosis. **Stage I** shows bilateral hilar adenopathy. **Stage II** shows bilateral hilar adenopathy plus interstitial infiltrates. **Stage III** demonstrates interstitial infiltrates only. **Stage IV** demonstrates fibrocystic lung disease.

Uncommon findings associated with pulmonary sarcoidosis include large, well-defined nodular infiltrates, miliary disease, a pattern of patchy air space consolidation with air bronchograms, termed "alveolar sarcoidosis," or the presence of mycetomas. Differential diagnoses include mycobacterial or fungal infection, malignancy, or granulomatosis with polyangiitis. Pleural effusions and pneumothoraces are unusual in sarcoidosis.

Chest CT typically demonstrates reticulonodular infiltrates that follow a bronchovascular distribution. Occasionally, ground-glass infiltrates, well-defined nodules, mass-like infiltrates, alveolar consolidation, or honeycombing are seen. Pleural effusions are rarely secondary to sarcoidosis inflammation.

Nuclear medicine studies such as 67-gallium scanning and positron emission tomography using 18-fluorodeoxyglucose (FDG-PET) have been used to detect active inflammatory sites in sarcoidosis, potentially aiding in the choice of sites for biopsy. FDG-PET has largely replaced gallium scanning because it is associated with less radiation exposure yet still offers superior resolution. Classic findings using gallium or PET scanning are uptake in both hilar regions and the right paratracheal lymph node region ("lambda" sign) of the lungs, and uptake in the parotids or lacrimal and salivary glands ("panda" sign). The combination of signs (lambda-panda) is suggestive of sarcoidosis.

Joint radiographs may demonstrate "punched out" lesions with cystic changes and marked loss of trabeculae but without evidence of erosive chondritis. Cystic lesions of the long bones, pelvis, sternum, skull, and vertebrae rarely occur (see Figure 46–3).

MRI with gadolinium contrast enhancement has an important role in the evaluation of neurosarcoidosis, particularly in cases of suspected brain, cranial nerve, or spinal cord involvement.

D. Pulmonary Function Testing

Pulmonary function tests in sarcoidosis may reveal a variety of findings, including restrictive, obstructive, or combined defects, with a reduction in the diffusing capacity for carbon monoxide (DLCO). Resting gas exchange is usually preserved until extensive fibrocystic changes are evident, but oxygen desaturation with exercise may occur in less advanced disease.

E. Other Tests

A well-recognized feature of sarcoidosis is anergy, the impaired cutaneous response to common antigens that elicit delayed-type hypersensitivity reactions. An example of this is the failure to mount a response to purified protein derivative (PPD) testing. Anergy is observed in 30–70% of patients. Active tuberculosis must be strongly considered in any sarcoidosis patient in whom a positive PPD test develops.

All newly diagnosed patients should have an electrocardiogram and targeted review of systems to determine if they are experiencing unexplained palpitations, dizziness, or loss of consciousness, which may indicate early signs of cardiac sarcoidosis. When cardiac sarcoidosis is suspected on the basis of symptoms or electrocardiographic abnormalities, both Holter monitoring and cardiac imaging are indicated. Two-dimensional echocardiography is useful as a screening tool but is insensitive to mild cardiac abnormalities. Imaging with cardiac MRI or cardiac PET/CT are more sensitive studies to detect myocardial abnormalities related to sarcoidosis compared to traditional radionuclide scans using gallium, thallium, or technitium (see Figure 46–4). Electrophysiologic testing may be indicated to exclude arrhythmias undetected by routine studies.

In patients with suspected neurosarcoidosis, MRI with gadolinium enhancement of the brain or spine is indicated. The characteristic inflammatory lesions by contrast MRI have a propensity for periventricular and leptomeningeal areas. These findings are nonspecific and can be produced by infectious (tuberculosis, fungal disease) or malignant (lymphoma, carcinomatosis) disease. A normal scan does not exclude neurosarcoidosis, particularly for cranial neuropathies, peripheral neuropathies, or in the presence of glucocorticoid therapy.

In neurosarcoidosis, the cerebrospinal fluid may demonstrate lymphocytic pleocytosis or elevated protein levels, providing supportive evidence of central nervous system or spinal cord inflammation. A suspected diagnosis of neurosarcoidosis is usually confirmed by biopsy of a non–central nervous system site, generally by bronchoscopic or lymph node biopsy. Brain or spinal cord biopsies are rarely performed but are sometimes essential for the exclusion of infectious or malignant disease. In suspected cases of peripheral neuropathy or myopathy, electromyography or nerve conduction studies are often indicated.

F. Diagnostic Examinations

Identifying the extent of specific organ involvement requires a careful review of localizing symptoms in the setting of biopsy-confirmed granulomatous inflammation. Biopsy of the easiest, most accessible abnormal tissue site is used for confirmation of the diagnosis and to exclude infection, malignancy, or other diseases that have similar clinical manifestations. Biopsy by fiberoptic bronchoscopy is frequently used to diagnose pulmonary sarcoidosis because of its relative safety and high yield. Endobronchial or transbronchial needle aspiration biopsies may increase the yield further particularly when guided by endobronchial ultrasounds (EBUS). Bronchoalveolar lavage fluid in sarcoidosis is typically characterized by increased proportions and numbers of activated CD4+ alveolar lymphocytes. This reflects the enhancement of cell-mediated immune responses at sites of granuloma formation. These findings are not specific for sarcoidosis, however, and do not predict clinical outcome.

Mediastinoscopy or surgical lung biopsy, either open or thoracoscopic, should be considered for cases in which lymphoma or other intrathoracic malignancy cannot be excluded with confidence without tissue sampling. Biopsy of a skin nodule, superficial lymph node, nasal mucosa, conjunctiva, or salivary gland (lip biopsy) sometimes can establish a diagnosis. Biopsy of the liver or bone marrow is nonspecific and should be used to support a diagnosis of sarcoidosis only after malignancy, infectious granulomatous diseases, or other organ-specific diagnoses are excluded. (Even the finding of granulomatous hepatitis, eg, is not diagnostic of sarcoidosis in and of itself.) In rare cases, biopsy of critical organs may be necessary to exclude malignancy, such as when sarcoidosis presents as a mass lesion within the brain. Biopsy confirmation of sarcoidosis is usually not necessary in Löfgren syndrome except in regions where histoplasmosis or coccidiomycosis is endemic. In such scenarios, fungal infection must be excluded before the initiation of glucocorticoid therapy.

▶ Diagnosis

A diagnosis of sarcoidosis is based on a compatible clinical picture, histologic evidence of noncaseating granulomas, and the exclusion of other known causes of this pathologic response, such as tuberculosis, fungal diseases, and chronic beryllium disease.

▶ Treatment

There is consensus on the following indications for treatment (Table 46–3):

- Persistent, symptomatic, or progressive pulmonary disease.
- Threatened organ failure, such as severe ocular, central nervous system, or cardiac disease.
- Persistent hypercalcemia or renal or hepatic dysfunction.
- Posterior uveitis or anterior uveitis.
- Myopathy.
- Significant splenomegaly or evidence of hypersplenism such as thrombocytopenia.
- Severe fatigue and weight loss.
- Disfiguring skin disease or symptomatic lymphadenopathy.

Patients with sarcoidosis but no evidence of end organ impairment (eg, normal pulmonary function tests, with or without abnormal chest radiography) with minimal respiratory symptoms should not be treated. Patients with limited cutaneous disease that is nondisfiguring can be considered for local intralesional glucocorticoid injections.

A. Medical

Except for glucocorticoids, medications are approved by the US Food and Drug Administration for the treatment of sarcoidosis. Glucocorticoids remain the mainstay of treatment

Table 46–3. Evidence-based recommendations, summarizing consensus guidelines from the British/Australian/New Zealand/Irish Thoracic Societies.

- Because of high rates of remission within first 2–3 years, no treatment is recommended for asymptomatic patients with only lymphadenopathy (stage I), or asymptomatic patients with lung infiltrates (stage II or III) and stable but mildly abnormal lung function.
- Oral glucocorticoids are first-line therapy in patients with progressive disease determined by lung function, significant symptoms, or extrapulmonary sarcoidosis.
- Given the duration of glucocorticoid treatment for sarcoidosis, bisphosphonates should be used to prevent accelerated bone loss.
- Inhaled glucocorticoids are not beneficial for treating progressive pulmonary sarcoidosis; however, inhaled glucocorticoids can be used to control cough or airway hyperreactivity in a subgroup of patients.
- Nonglucocorticoid immunosuppressant medications have limited role as primary therapy for sarcoidosis but should be considered in patients when reasonable doses of glucocorticoids alone (prednisone ≤10-15 mg daily) do not control the disease or if glucocorticoid side effects are intolerable.
- Methotrexate is the preferred nonglucocorticoid, steroid-sparing medication for patients with progressive disease. Azathioprine is often used when methotrexate is contraindicated or not tolerated.
- Lung transplantation should be considered for end-stage pulmonary sarcoidosis.

at least over the short term because of their effectiveness in reversing nonfibrotic organ impairment.

1. Glucocorticoids—This class of drugs is the cornerstone of therapy for serious progressive pulmonary or extrapulmonary sarcoidosis (see Table 46–3). Guidelines for when to initiate therapy with glucocorticoids and proper dosing have been formulated from extensive clinical experience without being subjected to prospective randomized control trials. Controversy exists regarding their overall effectiveness in altering the long-term course of the disease, but clinical experience indicates that glucocorticoids provide prompt symptomatic relief and reverse organ dysfunction in almost all patients with active inflammation. The optimal dose and duration of glucocorticoid treatment have not been established by rigorous clinical studies. Topical glucocorticoids are usually ineffective except for specific cases of ocular sarcoidosis. Most studies find inhaled glucocorticoids for pulmonary sarcoidosis to be ineffective, and only a minority of patients with airway obstruction demonstrate meaningful responses to bronchodilators.

With the exception of Löfgren syndrome, initial treatment with glucocorticoids should be planned for a period of 6–12 months. One well-designed study by the British Thoracic Society demonstrated that in patients with active pulmonary sarcoidosis and interstitial infiltrates, a stable maintenance regimen of low-dose glucocorticoids is more effective at preserving lung function than symptomatic use of glucocorticoids followed by repeated tapering regimens.

For patients who require maintenance therapy for chronic sarcoidosis, glucocorticoid therapy often results in significant adverse effects such as weight gain, diabetes, and osteoporosis. Thus, when these adverse effects become intolerable, glucocorticoid-sparing drugs are often considered. However, all glucocorticoid-sparing drugs show variable effectiveness and have adverse risk profiles that warrant careful dosing and monitoring in the absence of controlled clinical comparison trials.

2. Glucocorticoid-sparing agents

a. Hydroxychloroquine—This agent is used for dominant skin, nasal mucosal, and sinus sarcoidosis but is not consistently effective for pulmonary or systemic disease. Hypercalcemia and laryngeal, bone, and joint involvement have been reported to respond to hydroxychloroquine. Serial ophthalmologic evaluations should be performed every 6 months during hydroxychloroquine therapy. Chloroquine may have greater effectiveness but is rarely used because of the higher risk of ocular toxicity. When chloroquine is used for treatment recalcitrant mucosal or skin disease, it is given for 6 months followed by a 6-month drug holiday; ophthalmologic follow-up should be scheduled every 3 months.

b. Minocycline and doxycycline (synthetic tetracycline derivatives)—These agents have anti-inflammatory properties. The relatively safe side-effect profile of these medications make them a reasonable choice for nonthreatening manifestations of sarcoidosis such as cutaneous disease, but clinical experience suggests that these drugs usually are not effective in pulmonary or non-skin multiorgan sarcoidosis.

c. Cytotoxic therapy—Methotrexate is usually the first cytotoxic therapy tried as a potent glucocorticoid-sparing drug. Studies suggest a response rate on the order of 60% but the time required to observe an effect may be long: 4–6 months. Azathioprine and mycophenolate mofetil are alternative immunosuppressants that have been used in smaller series to treat severe extrapulmonary sarcoidosis and pulmonary sarcoidosis. Case series support the consideration of leflunomide for patients who do not benefit from other steroid-sparing agents. All of these agents may require 2–3 months or more of therapy to demonstrate clinical effectiveness. Routine monitoring for renal, liver, and bone marrow toxicities are standard.

3. Biologic agents—Laboratory experiments demonstrate that TNF plays an important role in granuloma formation. There is evidence supporting the effectiveness of select TNF inhibitors in sarcoidosis. A large, randomized multicenter prospective study found that a 24-week course of treatment with infliximab was associated with an improvement in lung function. A separate study also showed infliximab was associated with a modest improvement in nonpulmonary sarcoidosis. The humanized TNF inhibitor adalimumab has not been studied by controlled clinical trials, but small case series suggest this therapy is also beneficial in some patients with skin sarcoidosis and peripheral neuropathy. Etanercept, a TNF receptor antagonist, failed to show benefit in small clinical trials and is not recommended for use in sarcoidosis. All TNF inhibitors are associated with significant risk of severe infections, reactivation of latent tuberculosis, and the occurrence of immune-mediated, drug-induced phenomena (eg, drug-induced lupus). Appropriate monitoring before and during treatment with TNF inhibitors is therefore important. Screening for latent tuberculosis and viral hepatitis is particularly crucial. The use of other biologic agents to treat sarcoidosis targeting B cells (rituximab) and other cytokines such as IL-12/23 (ustekinumab) are under study.

B. Surgical

Successful lung, heart-lung, and liver transplantations have been performed in a small number of patients with advanced organ insufficiency. Noncaseating granulomas may develop in the transplanted organs in some lung and heart transplant patients but do not seem to have a significant impact on overall survival.

▶ Prognosis

Although sarcoidosis can potentially involve any part of the body, the extent of significant organ system involvement is usually evident within the first 2 years after diagnosis. The ACCESS study found that at 2-year follow-up, evidence for new organ system involvement developed in fewer than 25% of the study participants.

Approximately 50–70% of patients achieve remission, usually within the first 2–3 years following diagnosis. Acute sarcoidosis (Löfgren syndrome) has a remission rate of greater than 70%. Monitoring of patients for several years after presumed remission is recommended to ensure stability of organ function. Patients with fibrocystic pulmonary sarcoidosis, lupus pernio, or nasal or sinus sarcoidosis, neurosarcoidosis, cardiac sarcoidosis, or who have multisystem disease for greater than 2–3 years usually have unremitting, progressive disease if they do not receive appropriate treatment. A waxing and waning course of sarcoidosis is unusual except in patients with ocular, neurologic, peripheral lymph node, or cutaneous involvement.

No biomarkers are known to predict outcomes or to assist in treatment decisions. Serum angiotensin-converting enzyme levels are elevated in 30–80% of patients with clinically active disease. The test has positive and negative predictive values of less than 70–80%, and serum angiotensin-converting enzyme levels do not predict clinical course. Most clinicians agree this test is of limited utility in the diagnosis and management of sarcoidosis.

Major causes of death from sarcoidosis include respiratory insufficiency and cor pulmonale, massive hemoptysis, complications from cardiac sarcoidosis, neurosarcoidosis, or uremia from chronic renal failure. Several centers in the United States and the United Kingdom suggest that race is an important prognostic indicator. Afro-American and Afro-Caribbean patients are more likely to have chronic persistent disease and to experience increased morbidity and mortality. Hospital statistics suggest that sarcoidosis is the direct cause of death in 1–5% of persons admitted with this disease.

▶ When to Refer

A patient should be considered for referral to a specialist in sarcoidosis in the following situations:

- Uncertainty of the diagnosis or clinical course.
- Uncertainty whether treatment is indicated.
- Disease that is not responding as expected to therapy.
- Severe extrapulmonary involvement, such as cardiac, neurologic, skin, or sinus involvement.
- Unsure about the use of glucocorticoid-sparing or alternative medications.

Adler BL, Wang CJ, Bui TL, Schilperoort HM, Armstrong AW. Anti-tumor necrosis factor agents in sarcoidosis: a systematic review of efficacy and safety. *Semin Arthritis Rheum.* 2019;48(6): 1093-1104. doi: 10.1016/j.semarthrit.2018.10.005. [Epub Oct 6, 2018] [PMID: 30446173]

Brandão Guimarães J, Nico MA, Omond AG, et al. Radiologic manifestations of musculoskeletal sarcoidosis. *Curr Rheumatol Rep.* 2019;21(3):7. [PMID: 30762131]

Stern BJ, Royal W 3rd, Gelfand JM, et al. Definition and Consensus Diagnostic Criteria for Neurosarcoidosis: From the Neurosarcoidosis Consortium Consensus Group. *JAMA Neurol.* 2018;75(12):1546-1553. [PMID: 30167654]

Kumar M, Herrera JL. Sarcoidosis and the liver. *Clin Liver Dis.* 2019;23(2):331-343. [PMID: 30947880]

Moller DR, Rybicki BA, Hamzeh NY, et al. Genetic, immunologic, and environmental basis of sarcoidosis. *Ann Am Thorac Soc.* 2017;14:S429-S436. [PMID: 29073364]

Okasha O, Kazmirczak F, Chen KA, Farzaneh-Far A, Shenoy C. Myocardial involvement in patients with histologically diagnosed cardiac sarcoidosis: a systematic review and meta-analysis of gross pathological images from autopsy or cardiac transplantation cases. *J Am Heart Assoc.* 2019;8(10):e011253. [PMID: 31070111]

Patterson KC, Chen ES. The pathogenesis of pulmonary sarcoidosis and implications for treatment. *Chest.* 2018;153(6):1432-1442. [PMID: 29224832]

Sauer WH, Stern BJ, Baughman RP, Culver DA, Royal W. High-risk sarcoidosis. Current concepts and research imperatives. *Ann Am Thorac Soc.* 2017;14:S437-S444. [PMID: 29073361]

Shlobin OA, Baughman RP. Sarcoidosis-associated pulmonary hypertension. *Semin Respir Crit Care Med.* 2017;38:450-462. [PMID: 28750460]

Tavee JO, Karwa K, Ahmed Z, Thompson N, Parambil J, Culver DA. Sarcoidosis-associated small fiber neuropathy in a large cohort: clinical aspects and response to IVIG and anti-TNF alpha treatment. *Respir Med.* 2017;126:135-138. [PMID: 28318820]

Voortman M, Drent M, Baughman RP. Management of neurosarcoidosis: a clinical challenge. *Curr Opin Neurol.* 2019;32(3):475-483. [PMID: 30865007]

Relapsing Polychondritis

Naomi Serling-Boyd, MD
John H. Stone, MD, MPH

▶ Auricular chondritis (spares the earlobe).

▶ Inflammation in other cartilaginous areas (eg, the nose, joints, trachea, ribcage, and airways) and in tissues rich in proteoglycans, such as the eyes and heart valves.

▶ Frequently associated with an underlying disorder such as systemic vasculitis, connective tissue disease, or myelodysplastic syndrome.

▶ General Considerations

Relapsing polychondritis (RP) is an immune-mediated condition associated with inflammation in cartilaginous structures such as the ears, nose, joints, larynx, and trachea. Noncartilaginous connective tissues throughout the body, such as the eyes, heart, aorta, inner ear, and skin, can also be affected. The prevalence of RP is estimated to be approximately 4.5 cases per million people. The disease onset is generally between ages 30 and 60, with an average of 50, though pediatric cases as well as older onset have been described as well. RP affects men and women relatively equally. Thirty percent of RP cases occur in association with another disease, usually some form of systemic vasculitis (particularly granulomatosis with polyangiitis), connective tissue disorder (eg, rheumatoid arthritis or systemic lupus erythematosus), or a myelodysplastic syndrome. RP is often assumed to be autoimmune in nature, but the evidence for a true autoimmune pathogenesis is relatively weak. Some patients have been reported to have antibodies to type 2 collagen, but these assays are not widely available and their poor sensitivities and specificities make them inappropriate for general clinical use. In general, a cartilage biopsy is not required to make the diagnosis. Rather, the identification of cartilaginous inflammation in typical areas (auricular cartilage, nasal bridge, costochondral joints) and the exclusion of other possible causes suffice.

RP is associated with a broad range of clinical courses. One end of the disease spectrum includes intermittent bouts of auricular cartilage inflammation that respond quickly to treatment. The other end is characterized by widespread, aggressive cartilaginous inflammation that leads to serious end-organ complications. The greatest clinical challenge is identifying the presence of cartilaginous inflammation and instituting effective therapy before irreparable damage occurs in the involved organs.

▶ Clinical Findings

Table 47–1 lists the major clinical manifestations of RP.

A. Symptoms and Signs

1. Ears—Unilateral or bilateral auricular chondritis is often the first disease symptom (Figure 47–1). The onset of auricular inflammation is usually quite abrupt and not subtle. The inflammation may be confused with cellulitis of the ear or even sunburn in more minor cases. A major clue to the diagnosis of RP is confinement of the inflammation to the cartilaginous part of the ear, with sparing of the earlobe. The cartilaginous portions of the ears are erythematous and tender to touch. Swelling of the external ear canal may cause conductive hearing loss. RP may also be associated with either unilateral or bilateral sensorineural hearing loss and vestibular dysfunction, often manifested by vertigo or dizziness, the mechanism of which remains obscure (vasculitis is often implicated, without proof).

2. Nose—Inflammation of the nasal cartilage, seen in around 40% of patients, leads to tenderness of the nasal bridge and often to epistaxis. In severe cases, "saddle-nose" deformities develop through collapse of the nasal bridge. This is usually preceded by the development of a nasal septal perforation.

3. Trachea—Subglottic stenosis results from tracheal inflammation and scarring inferior to the vocal cords. Early subglottic

Table 47–1. Major clinical manifestations of relapsing polychondritis.

Feature Data	Data
Mean age at diagnosis	47 years
Auricular chondritis	90%
Reduced hearing	37%
Nasal chondritis	60%
Saddle-nose deformities	25%
Laryngotracheal involvement	52%
Ocular inflammation	54%
Arthritis	69%
Skin involvement	25%
Aortic or mitral regurgitation	8%
Vasculitis	12%

Data from Molina JF, Espinoza LR. Relapsing polychondritis. *Baillieres Best Pract Res Clin Rheumatol.* 2000;14:97.

involvement often has minimal symptoms and may manifest itself as only subtle changes in voice. Thickening of the tracheal wall may be evident on computed tomography (CT) scanning. With time, however, substantial airway scarring may occur, leading to potentially life-threatening tracheal narrowing. In addition to the subglottic region, other parts of the tracheal wall may be softened by cartilaginous inflammation, leading to collapse of the trachea, which can happen acutely. Tracheal inflammation may be associated with tenderness to palpation of the anterior cervical trachea, the thyroid cartilage, and larynx.

4. Bronchi and airways—Cartilaginous inflammation may extend to the lower respiratory tract, with bronchial involvement. This manifestation, unlike the tracheal disease, may have a lengthy subclinical period but is usually detectable by investigations such as pulmonary function testing or CT scanning. RP may mimic bronchial asthma. Lower airway disease and its associated mucociliary dysfunction may heighten patients' susceptibility to infections.

5. Eyes—Nearly any part of the eye may be involved in RP. Scleritis causes photophobia and painful, often raised, scleral erythema. If unchecked, necrotizing scleritis may lead to scleral thinning, scleromalacia perforans, and vision loss. Peripheral keratitis may cause ulcerations on the margin of the cornea and lead to the syndrome of "corneal melt." Episcleritis (Figure 47–2) and conjunctivitis are very common in RP. Extraocular involvement may include periorbital edema, chemosis, and proptosis.

6. Heart—Cartilaginous inflammation within the heart valve rings may lead to valvular dysfunction. Aortic valve disease, often manifested by aortic regurgitation, is the most common and can occur in association with an ascending thoracic aortic aneurysm. Mitral regurgitation can be seen, as well. The proximity of the conduction system to some areas

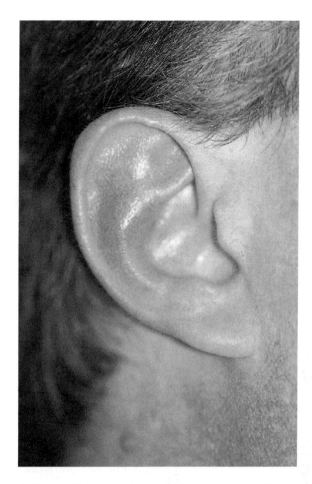

▲ **Figure 47–1.** Auricular chondritis in a patient with relapsing polychondritis. Note the sparing of the earlobe (a noncartilaginous portion of the ear).

of valve ring inflammation may lead to cardiac conduction abnormalities. Pericarditis and rare cases of coronary arteritis have also been described in RP.

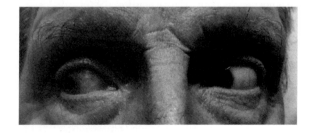

▲ **Figure 47–2.** Episcleritis of the right eye in a patient with relapsing polychondritis. Blanching of the superficial vessels with phenylephrine helps to diagnose episcleritis as opposed to scleritis.

7. Joints—Articular lesions are often the first nonspecific manifestation of RP; around 40% of patients have some degree of joint pain. The pattern of joint involvement at presentation is typically an intermittent, migratory oligoarthritis, but symmetric polyarticular presentations are also seen. In general, the arthritis associated with RP is nondestructive, unless there is underlying rheumatoid arthritis. Joint symptoms tend to correlate well with activity of disease at other sites.

8. Skin—Patients with RP may demonstrate a panoply of cutaneous lesions, none of which is specific for the disorder. Cutaneous findings are particularly common in cases of RP that are associated with myelodysplasia but occur frequently in other cases as well. Among patients with primary RP, the most common skin findings are aphthous ulcers, nodules (erythema nodosum–like lesions), purpura, papules, and sterile pustules. The cutaneous lesions of RP may resemble those of Behçet disease. An overlap condition, known as mouth and genital ulcers with inflamed cartilage (MAGIC) syndrome, is characterized by oral and genital ulcers as well as chondritis.

9. Kidneys—Renal lesions in RP range from pauci-immune glomerulonephritis to mild mesangial expansion and cellular proliferation. Distinguishing RP from granulomatosis with polyangiitis can be difficult in the setting of pauci-immune glomerulonephritis.

B. Laboratory Findings

There are no specific laboratory findings in RP. Mild normochromic, normocytic anemias, and mild degrees of thrombocytosis may be observed. Major cytopenias should trigger suspicion of myelodysplasia. Mild to moderate elevations of acute phase reactants are expected, though 10% of patients have normal inflammatory markers even during flares of the disease. Antinuclear antibodies and rheumatoid factor are usually negative, and complement levels are normal. In the setting of antineutrophil cytoplasmic antibody (ANCA) positivity, granulomatosis with polyangiitis must be suspected, particularly if the antibody specificity is to either proteinase-3 or myeloperoxidase. Autoantibodies against cartilage and collagen have been found in some patients with RP, though they are not specific to RP and are only found in a limited number of patients and are thus not used in routine clinical practice.

C. Imaging Studies

CT scans are useful in the evaluation of airway disease. CT findings in RP include edema, wall thickening, granulation tissue, and fibrosis. Thin-cut CT scans of the trachea are sensitive means of evaluating subglottic stenosis. In some cases of subglottic narrowing, however, direct visualization with fiberoptic laryngoscopy is required to make the diagnosis (Figure 47–3).

D. Special Tests

1. Biopsy—Given the proper constellation of clinical symptoms and signs, tissue biopsy is rarely required to establish

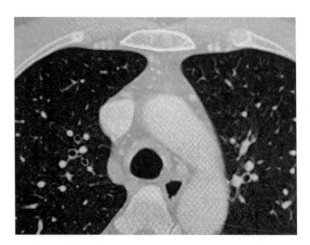

▲ **Figure 47–3.** Tracheal involvement in relapsing polychondritis. A computed tomography scan shows circumferential soft-tissue thickening surrounding the trachea in a 60 year-old male patient with relapsing polychondritis.

the diagnosis of RP. Biopsy may be important, however, in the exclusion of RP mimickers. In contrast to granulomatosis with polyangiitis, RP is not associated with granulomatous inflammation. The inflammatory infiltrate in RP consists mostly of lymphocytes though also includes macrophages, neutrophils, and plasma cells. Biopsy of the trachea or larynx should be performed only with great caution because acute airway narrowing may result from additional damage to already compromised tissues.

2. Pulmonary function tests—Full sets of pulmonary function tests, including inspiratory and expiratory flow-volume loops, are useful in RP. Patterns consistent with either extrathoracic or intrathoracic obstruction (or both) may occur in RP. Pulmonary function tests (flow-volume loops) provide a useful noninvasive means of quantifying and following the degree of extrathoracic airway obstruction.

▶ Diagnosis

There are multiple diagnostic criteria for RP. The McAdam criteria require three of six clinical criteria, three of which include chondritis, and do not require histologic confirmation. The Michet criteria require confirmed chondritis at two sites, or proven chondritis at one site in addition to other clinical criteria. These different diagnostic criteria are outlined in Table 47–2. To monitor disease, a consensus scoring system was developed to measure disease activity in RP. The Relapsing Polychondritis Disease Activity Index (RPDAI) incorporates 27 items, some of which are weighted differently than others, and has a maximum score

Table 47–2. Diagnostic criteria.

Author and Year	Criteria	Requirement for Diagnosis
McAdam et al, 1976	1. Recurrent chondritis of both auricles 2. Nonerosive inflammatory polyarthritis 3. Chondritis of nasal cartilages 4. Inflammation of ocular structures (conjunctivitis/keratitis/scleritis/uveitis) 5. Chondritis of respiratory tract (laryngeal/tracheal cartilages) 6. Cochlear and/or vestibular damage (neurosensory hearing loss/tinnitus/vertigo)	Three of six criteria
Michet et al, 1986	1. Proven inflammation in two of three auricular, nasal, or laryngotracheal cartilages 2. Proven inflammation in 1 of the above and two other signs among ocular inflammation, hearing loss, vestibular dysfunction, or seronegative inflammatory arthritis	Either of two criteria

Data from McAdam LP, O'Hanlan MA, Bluestone R, et al. Relapsing polychondritis: prospective study of 23 patients and a review of the literature. *Medicine.* 1976;5:192-215. Michet CJ, McKenne CH, Luthra HS, et al. Relapsing polychondritis: survival and predictive role of early disease manifestations. *Ann Intern Med.* 1986;194:74-78.

of 265. Items range from arthralgia to fever to costochondritis to encephalitis.

Differential Diagnosis

Aural chondritis is often confused initially with an infectious process, particularly cellulitis of the ear. Other infections in the differential diagnosis include tuberculous laryngitis, now rare in developed countries. The differential diagnosis of nasal inflammation (often accompanied by saddle-nose deformity) is quite short, including granulomatosis with polyangiitis, IgG4-related disease, Crohn disease, syphilis, leprosy, lymphoma, and leishmaniasis.

Primary RP must be distinguished from RP associated with an underlying condition because the complications of the underlying disorder may greatly affect the patient's prognosis. The major underlying disorders of concern are systemic vasculitides, connective tissue diseases, and myelodysplastic syndromes.

Treatment

Nonsteroidal anti-inflammatory drugs (NSAIDs) can sometimes be used as first-line therapy for mild joint disease or for episcleritis or scleritis. However, glucocorticoids are the treatment of choice for reducing major inflammation in cartilaginous areas and if more mild disease is refractory to NSAIDs. Dapsone can also be attempted first in mild causes of auricular or nasal chondritis. For patients with sustained disease despite glucocorticoid use, methotrexate is the most commonly used glucocorticoid-sparing agent. Other disease modifying antirheumatic drugs (DMARDs) include azathioprine, mycophenolate, and cyclosporine. The choice of a glucocorticoid-sparing medication is often empiric. Recently, there have been case series suggesting the benefit of biologic medications such as tumor necrosis factor (TNF)-alpha inhibitors (effective in 85.7% in one case series), anakinra, abatacept, and tocilizumab. Case reports have suggested that rituximab has not been beneficial. In the setting of life-threatening disease or severe organ involvement, such as necrotizing scleritis, severe laryngotracheal involvement, and aortitis, cyclophosphamide may be required.

In the case of airway disease, it is essential to distinguish dysfunction secondary to active cartilaginous inflammation from that caused by damage from previously active disease to avoid unnecessary immunosuppression.

In addition to immunosuppression, the management of upper airway problems in RP requires collaboration with an experienced otolaryngologist or pulmonologist or both. Some upper airway disease manifestations (eg, subglottic stenosis) respond better to mechanical interventions and glucocorticoid injections than to systemic therapies. Stenting may also be required for cases in which the tracheal or bronchial walls have lost their integrity, provided that the regions of tracheomalacia or bronchomalacia are not too long. Continuous positive airway pressure may help some patients during sleep.

Complications

Prolonged or repeated bouts of aural chondritis may lead to deformation of the ear cartilage and "cauliflower ear" as well as deafness and balance disturbance. Similarly, nasal chondritis may cause nasal septal perforation and "saddle-nose" deformities.

Tracheomalacia may lead to extrathoracic airway obstruction and sometimes requires tracheostomy. Cardiac valvular regurgitation in RP may lead to valve replacement. Causes of death include airway collapse or obstruction, infection, aortic disease, systemic vasculitis, and malignancy when RP is associated with myelodysplastic syndrome. A diagnosis of RP is associated with an increased risk of mortality, with a standardized mortality ratio of roughly double that of healthy controls. The prognosis for

RP associated with myelodysplastic syndrome is poorer than that of primary RP.

Arnaud L, Devilliers H, Peng SL, et al. The Relapsing Polychondritis Disease Activity Index: development of a disease activity score for relapsing polychondritis. *Autoimmun Rev.* 2012;12:204. [PMID: 22771427]

Marie I, Proux A, Duhaut P, et al. Long-term follow-up of aortic involvement in giant cell arteritis: a series of 48 patients. *Medicine (Baltimore).* 2009;88(3):182. [PMID: 19440121]

Mathian A, Miyara M, Cohen-Aubart F, et al. Relapsing polychondritis: a 2016 update on clinical features, diagnostic tools, treatment and biologic drug use. *Best Pract Res Clin Rheumatol.* 2016;30:316. [PMID: 27886803]

Moulis G, Sailler L, Pugnet G, et al. Biologics in relapsing polychondritis: a case series. *Clin Exp Rheumatol.* 2013;31(6):937. [PMID: 24021708]

IgG4-Related Disease

48

John H. Stone, MD, MPH

ESSENTIALS OF DIAGNOSIS

- ▶ IgG4-related disease (IgG4-RD) is a multiorgan disease with highly characteristic pathology findings and immunostaining characteristics across involved tissues.

- ▶ Organ system involvement may be confined to single organs but in many cases evolves over months to years to involve multiple organs in either a sequential or simultaneous fashion.

- ▶ Commonly involved organs include the salivary glands (submandibular, parotid); the orbits and lacrimal glands; the thyroid gland; the lymph nodes; the thoracic and abdominal aorta; the mediastinum, retroperitoneum, and mesentery; and the lungs, biliary tree, pancreas, and kidneys.

- ▶ IgG4-RD has also been reported in the pachymeninges, the skin, and the prostate gland.

- ▶ Serum IgG4 concentrations are elevated in most patients (approximately 70%). In patients with exceptionally high serum IgG4 concentrations—usually those with multiorgan disease—the prozone phenomenon can lead to a spuriously low result. This problem may be circumvented by diluting test samples sufficiently.

- ▶ If elevated at the time of diagnosis, serum IgG4 concentrations are generally a good biomarker. Other useful biomarkers in individual patients include IgG1, IgE, and complement levels (C3 and C4).

- ▶ Histopathologic hallmarks: lymphoplasmacytic tissue infiltrate, storiform fibrosis, obliterative phlebitis, germinal center formation, and mild to modest tissue eosinophilia.

- ▶ Immunostaining characteristics: A high percentage of plasma cells stain positively for IgG4.

▶ General Considerations

IgG4-related disease (IgG4-RD) is a systemic fibroinflammatory condition recognized in the first decade of this century and now identified increasingly across a wide array of organ systems. The condition is characterized by a tendency to form tumefactive lesions, a dense lymphoplasmacytic infiltrate rich in IgG4-positive plasma cells, storiform fibrosis, and, often but not always, elevated serum IgG4 concentrations. The first organ within the spectrum of IgG4-RD to be linked with elevations in serum IgG4 concentrations was the pancreas. Pancreatic involvement by IgG4-RD is now termed type 1 IgG4-related autoimmune pancreatitis. In 2003, extrapancreatic manifestations were identified in patients with this pancreatic disease, and IgG4-RD is now known to occur in virtually every organ system: the biliary tree, salivary glands, periorbital tissues, kidneys, lungs, lymph nodes, meninges, aorta, breast, prostate, thyroid, pericardium, and skin. The histopathologic features are similar across organs, with some organs or body regions (eg, the retroperitoneum) demonstrating a higher degree of fibrosis at the time of diagnosis.

One consequence of the recognition of IgG4-RD is that many medical conditions once viewed as separate conditions isolated to single organs are now acknowledged to be part of the IgG4-RD spectrum. Examples of this include "Mikulicz syndrome," "Küttner tumor," and Riedel thyroiditis, once regarded to be conditions limited to the major salivary and lacrimal glands alone; to the submandibular glands alone; or to the thyroid gland alone. In addition, IgG4-RD also accounts for substantial percentages of diseases characterized by the presence of pseudotumors or fibrotic lesions of previously unclear etiologies. IgG4-RD is responsible for significant proportions of cases of orbital pseudotumors, retroperitoneal fibrosis, and sclerosing mesenteritis.

The etiology of IgG4-RD remains unknown but growing evidence links this disease to autoimmunity. Many patients—approximately 50%—have concomitant allergic conditions such as asthma and allergic rhinitis. Few population-based studies of IgG4-RD have been performed and the disease epidemiology remains poorly described, but certain striking demographic features are evident. Cases in children are rare but now described in growing numbers in the literature. The disease phenotype in children appears to be very similar to that in adults. Approximately 60–80% of patients are males older than the age of 50, but some variations on these demographic features occur in the different organs affected by IgG4-RD. For example, in the case of IgG4-RD affecting the organs of the head and neck, women appear to be affected as frequently as men. Much remains unknown about the behavior of IgG4 in vivo and the nature of its role in IgG4-RD (primary or secondary) remains to be fully defined.

▶ Clinical Findings

A. Symptoms and Signs

The major symptoms and differential diagnoses of each organ lesion are summarized in Table 48–1. IgG4-RD usually presents subacutely and most patients are not constitutionally ill. Fevers are distinctly unusual in IgG4-RD and strongly suggest another diagnosis. Prominent weight loss is common, however, because many patients develop exocrine pancreatic insufficiency secondary to autoimmune pancreatitis and pancreatic atrophy. IgG4-RD is often identified through findings observed unexpectedly by the radiologist or pathologist.

IgG4-RD sometimes remains confined to one organ, for example, the salivary or lacrimal glands, for many years. However, some patients have major clinical disease in one organ but less obvious or even subclinical involvement in others. As an example, although patients with autoimmune pancreatitis generally have pancreatic dysfunction as a major clinical manifestation, careful scrutiny by physical examination, routine laboratory evaluation, cross-sectional imaging, positron emission tomography (PET) scanning, or other investigations may unveil disease in the lungs, kidneys, lymph nodes, or other organs.

Multiorgan disease may be evident at diagnosis but can also evolve metachronously, over months to years. Spontaneous improvement, sometimes leading to at least temporary clinical resolution in certain organ system manifestations, can occur. What begins an unexplained and seemingly innocuous enlargement of the submandibular glands may evolve over years to organ-threatening IgG4-related tubulointerstitial nephritis, interstitial lung disease, or pancreatobiliary involvement.

Tumefactive lesions and allergic disease are common manifestations of IgG4-RD. IgG4-RD accounts for a variable proportion of tumorous swellings in organs such as the orbits, salivary and lacrimal glands, lungs, kidneys, and other organs. Some series suggest, for example, that 25–50% of orbital pseudotumors fall within the spectrum of IgG4-RD. Allergic features, such as atopy, eczema, asthma, and modest peripheral eosinophilia, often accompany IgG4-RD and are sometimes the most prominent symptoms.

The clinical manifestations of each of the commonly involved organs are discussed later.

1. Salivary glands—Both the submandibular and parotid glands can be affected by IgG4-RD. The disease has a particular predilection to involve the submandibular glands bilaterally and in isolation (Figure 48–1), a point that frequently helps distinguish it from Sjögren syndrome. The usual symptom at presentation is glandular swelling, with variable degrees of discomfort and tenderness that are usually mild and never severe. Xerostomia often results from chronic sclerosing sialadenitis but this is less frequent than in Sjögren syndrome. The entity once known as "Mikulicz disease"—swelling of the submandibular, parotid, and lacrimal

Table 48–1. Differential diagnosis of IgG4-related disease.

Systemic autoimmune conditions and vasculitides
Sjögren syndrome
Granulomatosis with polyangiitis (formerly Wegener granulomatosis)
Eosinophilic granulomatosis with polyangiitis (Churg-Strauss syndrome)
Giant cell arteritis/giant cell aortitis
Takayasu arteritis
Granulomatous disorders
Sarcoidosis
Fungal infections (histoplasmosis, blastomycosis, coccidioidomycosis)
Malignancies
Lymphoma, particularly MALT lymphoma
Multicentric Castleman disease
Adenocarcinoma of the pancreas
Renal cell carcinoma
Bronchoalveolar carcinoma of the lung
Hypereosinophilic syndromes
Erdheim-Chester disease

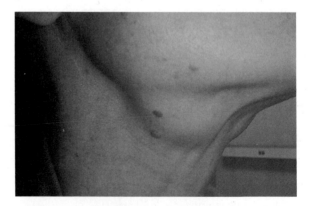

▲ **Figure 48–1.** Submandibular gland enlargement in a patient with IgG4-related disease.

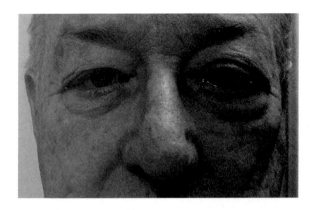

▲ **Figure 48–2.** Lacrimal gland involvement by IgG4-related disease. This patient had bilateral lacrimal gland biopsies that were positive, but proptosis of the left eye is particularly evident.

glands—is now known to be caused by IgG4-RD in nearly most cases.

2. Lacrimal gland and orbital disease—Many cases of "idiopathic" orbital pseudotumor in the past, including those involving the lacrimal gland (Figure 48–2), have not been subjected to biopsy. Even if biopsied, IgG4 staining has seldom been performed. Consequently, the frequency with which IgG4-RD affects the orbit is not fully appreciated. Substantial proptosis, usually caused by involvement of the extraocular muscles, can result from IgG4-RD involvement of the orbit (Figure 48–3). Such proptosis is one of several

manifestations through which IgG4-RD mimics granulomatosis with polyangiitis. Orbital pseudotumors can also occur in IgG4-RD. Orbital disease associated with IgG4-RD occasionally extends into the sinuses or the cavernous sinus, and disease originating from those sites can also affect the orbit. Vision loss can ensue if the blood supply to the optic nerve is disrupted by the mass effect.

3. Thyroid gland—Riedel thyroiditis, a disorder associated with fibrosis and woody enlargement of the thyroid gland, was of obscure etiology until the link between this condition and IgG4-RD was ascertained. Riedel thyroiditis has been known for decades to occur in association with fibrotic lesions in other organs, for example, the lacrimal glands, retroperitoneum, and mediastinum, in the context of an entity labeled "multifocal fibrosclerosis." Riedel thyroiditis can lead to dramatic enlargement of the thyroid gland and aggressive extension of the fibrotic process into surrounding tissues, sometimes causing airway compromise (Figure 48–4) and requiring major surgical procedures.

4. Lymph nodes—IgG4-RD can be associated with tender or nontender lymphadenopathy, with or without other organ manifestations of the disease. The diagnosis of IgG4-RD is difficult to make on the basis of a lymph node biopsy alone, as lymph nodes seldom undergo the degree of "storiform fibrosis" (see section Special Tests, Biopsy) observed in other organs. Biopsies of lymph nodes are generally useful therefore only to exclude other conditions.

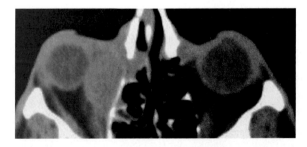

▲ **Figure 48–3.** IgG4-related orbital inflammation. Computed tomography (CT) scan of a 78-year-old man with several years of glucocorticoid-responsive "idiopathic orbital inflammation" that had not been evaluated fully with a biopsy. This CT demonstrates thickening of the right medial rectus muscle, the cause of the patient's extra-ocular muscle dysfunction and diplopia at extremes of lateral gaze. Biopsy revealed an intense lymphoplasmacytic infiltrate, 80 IgG4+ plasma cells/high-power field, and IgG4/IgG ratio of 45%, and storiform fibrosis. The serum IgG4 concentration was >1100 mg/dL (normal <86 mg/dL).

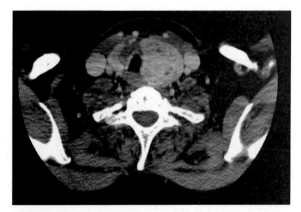

▲ **Figure 48–4.** Riedel's thyroiditis. Computed tomography scan of the neck in a 72-year-old woman with Riedel's thyroiditis (IgG4-related thyroid disease). The enlarged, asymmetric thyroid gland has extended beyond its capsule to encroach upon the patient's airway, leading to significant tracheal narrowing, hoarseness, and dyspnea. Note the tracheal displacement shown in this image. She required a thyroidectomy and treatment with rituximab following regrowth of some thyroid remnants but ultimately achieved good disease control. (Reproduced with permission pending from The Lancet.)

5. Thoracic aorta—IgG4-RD appears to cause approximately 10% of cases of "idiopathic" ascending aortitis, and is known to lead to complications such as aneurysm and dissection. Primary branch involvement of the thoracic aorta is less common than in other causes of large-vessel vasculitis, for example, Takayasu arteritis or giant cell arteritis.

6. Abdominal aorta and retroperitoneal fibrosis—The abdominal aorta can also be involved by the syndrome of "inflammatory abdominal aortic aneurysm," which overlaps to a large degree with retroperitoneal fibrosis and perianeurysmal fibrosis under a larger heading of chronic periaortitis. The periaortitis/retroperitoneal fibrosis commonly affects the area of the infrarenal aorta, extending inferiorly to the iliacs. One or both ureters often become entrapped by the inflammatory process near the aortic bifurcation, leading to hydronephrosis (Figure 48–5).

7. Fibrosing mediastinitis and sclerosing mesenteritis—These two conditions are rare entities that also have other causes (eg, histoplasmosis in the setting of fibrosing mediastinitis). However, small case series document the relatively high frequency with which biopsies from patients with these disorders demonstrate the typical histopathologic and immunohistochemical staining patterns of IgG4-RD.

8. Lungs—The pulmonary lesions of IgG4-RD demonstrate a remarkable diversity of clinical and radiologic presentations. IgG4-RD mimics many disorders with lung features. In some patients, lung lesions due to IgG4-related pulmonary disease are asymptomatic and are only diagnosed during broader workup designed to exclude systemic causes of

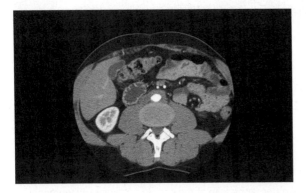

▲ **Figure 48–5.** Retroperitoneal fibrosis. Computed tomographic scan of the abdomen of a 63-year-old man, demonstrating IgG4-related retroperitoneal fibrosis with peri-aortitis. The inflammatory process commonly affects the area of the infra-renal aorta, extending inferiorly to the iliacs. This image shows circumferential inflammation of the infra-renal aorta. The inflammation sometimes entraps one or both of the ureters near the aortic bifurcation, leading to hydronephrosis.

IgG4-RD manifestations in other organs. However, cough and dyspnea can also be presenting symptoms in patients with IgG4-RD. The diverse radiologic manifestations of IgG4-RD in the lung are described later.

9. Biliary tree—A subset of patients with "primary sclerosing cholangitis" was long known to have disease that was responsive to glucocorticoids. Histopathologic evaluations of liver biopsies in such patients, interpreted now in the light of IgG4-RD, reveal IgG4-related cholangitis. This disease manifestation is characterized by lymphoplasmacytic infiltrates surrounding the bile ducts, and high IgG4/total IgG ratio among plasma cells in the lesions, storiform fibrosis, obliterative phlebitis, and modest tissue eosinophilia, all hallmarks of IgG4-RD. The distinction of IgG4-related sclerosing cholangitis from primary sclerosing cholangitis is crucial because of the differential responses to therapy that are characteristic of these separate conditions. IgG4-related sclerosing cholangitis usually occurs in association with autoimmune pancreatitis but can occur in isolation. In such cases, IgG4-related sclerosing cholangitis is often misdiagnosed initially as a cholangiocarcinoma.

10. Pancreas—Type 1 autoimmune pancreatitis is the paradigm of organ involvement in IgG4-RD. In the setting of pancreatic masses, patients often have painless jaundice. As a result, many patients have undergone Whipple procedures for presumed adenocarcinoma of the pancreas. The classic demographic profile of such patients—middle-aged to elderly men—facilitates misdiagnosis in this setting because such a demographic profile is also typical of pancreatic cancer. In addition to icterus, patients may also have nonspecific abdominal pain, anorexia, weight loss, and features of IgG4-RD in extrapancreatic organs that may be overlooked. The radiologic features of type 1 autoimmune pancreatitis are discussed later. Type 1 autoimmune pancreatitis must be differentiated from type 2 autoimmune pancreatitis, a condition with which it shares some clinical features but also vital pathologic distinctions.

11. Kidneys—Renal disease in IgG4-RD usually presents with either a mass-like lesion that mimics renal cell carcinoma or, more commonly, a subacute decline in renal function associated with a benign urine sediment that is caused by tubulointerstitial nephritis. Biopsy in either case generally reveals classic histopathological features of IgG4-RD, accompanied by immune complexes demonstrable by electron microscopy within the renal tubules. The mass lesions in IgG4-related kidney disease can be multiple and bilateral. These are often demonstrated as hypodense lesions on computed tomography.

Laboratory findings in the setting of IgG4-related tubulointerstitial nephritis are subnephrotic range proteinuria and significant hypocomplementemia. The levels of C4 in such cases are often so low as to be undetectable, as occasionally seen in lupus nephritis or mixed cryoglobulinemia. The hypocomplementemia is consistent with the detection of immune complexes within the kidney by both immunofluorescence and electron microscopy. Azotemia occurs in a minority of patients and end-stage renal disease has been reported.

A small number of cases to date have also been documented to have membranous glomerulonephritis (occurring simultaneously with tubulointerstitial disease). The antibody specificity in cases of IgG4-related membranous glomerulonephritis is different from that associated with idiopathic membranoproliferative glomerulonephritis.

12. Other—IgG4-RD has also been described in the pachymeninges, skin, prostate gland, pericardium, and middle ear. Bone-destructive lesions have been reported in the middle ear or other bones of the skull in some patients, mimicking granulomatosis with polyangiitis, chronic infection, and malignancy.

B. Laboratory Findings

1. Serum IgG4 concentration—Most patients with IgG4-RD have elevated serum IgG4 concentrations, but the range varies widely. Approximately 30% of patients have normal serum IgG4 concentrations despite classic pathologic findings of IgG4-RD. One explanation for this finding in some patients is the prozone effect—a laboratory error (spuriously low result) induced by failure of the laboratory to perform a sufficient number of dilutions of the sample in the setting of a large quantity of analyte. A substantial minority of patients with IgG4-RD, however, particularly those with single organ disease, simply have normal serum IgG4 concentrations despite the presence of classic pathology findings in tissue. Patients with IgG4-related retroperitoneal fibrosis and other presentations of the disease associated with advanced fibrosis (eg, Riedel thyroiditis, sclerosing mesenteritis, fibrosing mediastinitis) often have normal serum IgG4 concentrations.

Treatment leads to lower serum IgG4 concentrations in patients who have elevated IgG4 concentrations at baseline (and usually in patients whose serum IgG4 concentrations are normal at baseline, too). The serum IgG4 concentration may not normalize completely, however, even in patients who achieve clinical remissions. This is because IgG4 continues to be made by long-lived plasma cells that have circulated back to the bone marrow, where they continue to make IgG4 and are unaffected by most currently available therapies. The most current thinking about the role of IgG4 in disease pathophysiology is that IgG4 does not play a primary role in inciting or maintaining tissue injury in this disease. On the contrary, IgG4 may in fact be trying to fulfill a counterregulatory role, dampening in some fashion the primary immune response. Patients can achieve clinical remissions without serum IgG4 concentrations normalizing and may relapse despite having normal serum IgG4 measurements.

2. Inflammatory markers—Several patterns of acute phase reactant levels are observed in IgG4-RD. Only a small percentage (approximately 10%) have striking elevations of both the erythrocyte sedimentation rate (ESR) and the C-reactive protein (CRP). It is more common, however, for both of these measurements to be normal. Because the ESR is often affected by the level of hypergammaglobulinemia, another common pattern observed is a moderate to high elevation of the ESR in the setting of a normal CRP. Neither the ESR nor the CRP appears to be a reliable biomarker across the spectrum of disease activity in IgG4-RD.

3. Eosinophilia—Mild to moderate peripheral eosinophilia is a common finding in the blood of patients with IgG4-RD. Eosinophils are also frequently present within the tissue of affected organs. Peripheral eosinophilias of 20% of the total white blood cell count are not unusual IgG4-RD, often leading to confusion with eosinophilic granulomatosis with polyangiitis or a hypereosinophil syndrome.

4. Complement levels—Hypocomplementemia of both the third and fourth components of complement are common in IgG4-RD, particularly in those patients with renal disease. Presumably this finding is indicative of immune complex deposition within the kidney and other organs. The specific complement pathways that are operative in IgG4-RD require further study.

5. Urinalysis—Subnephrotic range proteinuria is typical of the tubulointerstitial disease of IgG4-RD. Patients do not have hematuria or red blood cell casts, and the findings on urine dipsticks and microscopic examinations of the urine are often underwhelming even in the presence of advancing renal dysfunction.

C. Imaging Studies

1. Radiography—Chest radiographs are often the route through which unsuspected pulmonary disease is identified. However, other imaging studies of the lungs are more useful in delineating the nature and extent of pulmonary involvement in IgG4-RD.

2. Computed tomography (CT)—CT scans are useful in several major settings in IgG4-RD. These include orbital disease, pulmonary disease, pancreatic disease, and renal disease.

A. ORBITAL DISEASE—IgG4-RD patients have multiple ophthalmic presentations that can only be defined precisely by cross-sectional imaging. IgG4-related orbital myositis, orbital pseudotumors, and cavernous sinus lesions are imaged readily with this technique.

B. PULMONARY DISEASE—CT scans have identified a number of pleuropulmonary lesions that are characteristic of IgG4-RD. These include nodules, ground-glass opacities, and interstitial lesions leading sometimes to honeycombing, thickening of the bronchovascular bundle, and pleural thickening (Figure 48–6). These radiologic lesions may mimic many forms of rheumatologic, oncologic, or infectious disease (see Table 48–1).

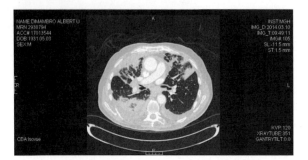

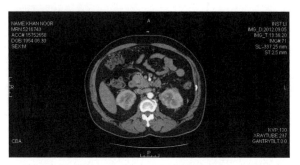

▲ **Figure 48–6.** Multiple features of IgG4-related pulmonary and pleural disease. Computed tomography (CT) scan in a 76-year-old man with dyspnea, occurring in the setting of several other features of IgG4-related disease: submandibular and parotid enlargement, autoimmune pancreatitis leading to type 2 diabetes mellitus, and IgG4-related kidney disease. The CT demonstrates pleural thickening, interstitial lung disease, and thickening of the airways.

▲ **Figure 48–8.** IgG4-related kidney disease. Computed tomographic scan a 69-year-old man with IgG4-related Mikulicz disease (enlargement of the lacrimal, parotid, and submandibular glands) and a rising serum creatinine level. The patient was profoundly hypocomplementemic, with a serum C3 of 60 mg/dL (normal 86–120 mg/dL) and a serum C4 of 4 mg/dL (normal 12–39 mg/dL). The CT shows scattered hypodense lesions in the periphery of the kidneys bilaterally, consistent with IgG4-related tubulointerstitial nephritis.

C. PANCREATIC DISEASE—Abdominal CT scans may reveal a "sausage-shaped" pancreas, sometimes accompanied by an echogenic halo of surrounding edema. The pancreas is often diffusely enlarged (Figure 48–7). The classic radiologic presentation in the proper clinical setting is strongly suggestive of type 1 (IgG4-related) autoimmune pancreatitis, but biopsy is essential in atypical presentations to exclude pancreatic carcinoma.

D. RENAL DISEASE—A high percentage of patients with type 1 (IgG4-related) autoimmune pancreatitis have IgG4-related kidney disease as well. Diffusely enlarged kidneys

may be evident, and pseudotumors may resemble renal cell carcinoma. IgG4-related pseudotumors within the kidney typically have a hypoattenuated appearance on CT. The MRI appearance of IgG4-related kidney disease is also distinctive (Figure 48–8).

3. Positron emission tomography (PET)—Total body PET imaging appears to be a sensitive modality for defining the extent of disease in IgG4-RD. PET is less useful, however, for longitudinal follow-up of multiorgan disease because the proper interpretation of residual fluorodeoxyglucose is often unclear.

4. Magnetic resonance imaging (MRI)—MRI is most useful in the evaluation of patients with the two most common neurologic manifestations of IgG4-RD: namely, pachymeningitis and hypophysitis. MRI can also identify perineural encasement by IgG4-related inflammation that may be symptomatic or asymptomatic.

D. Special Tests

The crux of an IgG4-RD diagnosis is careful clinicopathologic correlation between the clinical presentation and histopathologic findings from biopsy of an affected organ. The presence of disease in a typical organ is helpful in clinicopathologic correlation. Although IgG4-RD has been described in virtually every organ, those shown in Table 48–2 are typical of IgG4-RD. Compatible histopathological findings in one of these organs lend considerable strength to an IgG4-RD diagnosis, albeit the exclusion of mimickers remains important. Misdiagnoses of IgG4-RD result if excessive emphasis is placed on moderate serum concentration elevations of IgG4 or overreliance on the finding of IgG4-positive plasma cells in tissue.

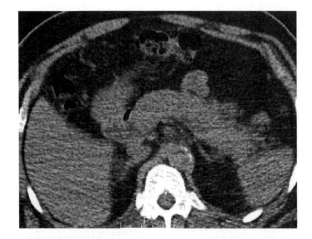

▲ **Figure 48–7.** Autoimmune pancreatitis. Computed tomography scan demonstrating an enlarged, sausage-shaped pancreas in a 56-year-old man with multiorgan IgG4-related disease.

Table 48–2. Organs most commonly affected by IgG4-related disease.

- Pachymeninges
- Orbits (extra-ocular muscles; retrobulbar masses)
- Lacrimal glands
- Major salivary glands
- Thyroid gland [Riedel's]
- Pancreas
- Bile ducts
- Lungs
- Kidney
- Aorta
- Retroperitoneum

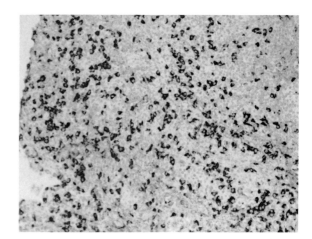

▲ **Figure 48–10.** Histopathologic and immunostaining features of tissues affected by IgG4-related disease. This lung biopsy shows diffuse IgG4-staining of plasma cells within the tissue. All of the dark-staining cells are plasma cells that are positive for IgG4.

A key morphologic feature of IgG4-RD is a dense lymphoplasmacytic infiltrate that is organized in a storiform pattern (Figures 48–9 and 48–10). "Storiform" refers to a matted, irregularly whorled pattern of fibrosis (*Storea* is the Latin word for "woven mat"). Other histopathologic hallmarks are obliterative phlebitis, a mild to moderate eosinophil infiltrate, and the presence of germinal centers. The inflammatory lesion frequently forms a tumefactive mass that is associated with tissue destruction.

Some histopathologic findings are distinctly unusual in IgG4-RD, and their presence should conjure other potential diagnoses. Such findings include necrosis, granulomatous inflammation, and significant collections of neutrophilic inflammation.

The histologic appearance of IgG4-RD is highly characteristic and essential to the diagnosis, but this may be clinched by the findings of immunostaining studies. The ratio of IgG4-positive plasma cells to the total number of plasma cells within tissue (ie, the IgG4/total IgG ratio) is usually high (0.4–0.8 or higher). Such high ratios are particularly remarkable when one considers that in normal individuals IgG4 comprises approximately 4% of the circulating immunoglobulin pool. Among patients with IgG4-RD whose tissues are biopsied at stages of advanced fibrosis, as is true of many patients with retroperitoneal fibrosis, for example, the link to IgG4-RD may be more difficult to establish because of smaller overall numbers of plasma cells. However, the IgG4:total IgG ratio remains high in that setting.

Both clinicians and pathologists must bear in mind that IgG4-positive cells are found in a wide variety of inflammatory infiltrates and that the detection of significant numbers of IgG4-positive plasma cells is not diagnostic of IgG4-RD. There is no number of IgG4-positive plasma cells/HPF that is diagnostic of IgG4-RD. However, a diffuse IgG4-positive plasma cell infiltrate with more than 40 IgG4-positive cells/HPF and an IgG4:IgG ratio greater than 50% provides compelling evidence of IgG4-RD, particularly in conjunction with the appropriate histopathologic appearance.

The inflammatory infiltrate is composed of an admixture of T- and B-lymphocytes. Whereas B cells are typically organized in germinal centers, the T cells are distributed diffusely throughout the lesion. All immunoglobulin subclasses may be represented within involved tissue, but IgG4 predominates. Clonality studies are required to exclude these malignancies.

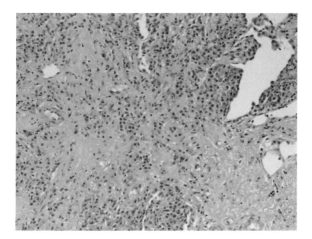

▲ **Figure 48–9.** Histopathologic and immunostaining features of tissues affected by IgG4-related disease. This lung biopsy shows a lymphoplasmacytic infiltrate with storiform fibrosis (the strands of acellular tissue running through the sample).

▷ **Differential Diagnosis**

The differential diagnosis of IgG4-RD is shown in Table 48–1.

Treatment

IgG4-RD can lead to serious organ dysfunction and failure. Consequently, vital organ involvement such as that affecting the orbits, biliary tree, kidneys, aorta, or retroperitoneum must be identified quickly and treated aggressively. On the other hand, not all disease manifestations require immediate treatment. For example, IgG4-related lymphadenopathy is often indolent and asymptomatic. Watchful waiting is therefore prudent in some cases.

Glucocorticoids are typically the first-line therapy. One approach pioneered in Japan for the treatment of type 1 (IgG4-related) autoimmune pancreatitis involves the use of prednisone, 0.6 mg/kg/day for 2–4 weeks followed by a taper over 3–6 months to 5 mg/day, and then continued at a dose between 2.5 mg/day and 5.0 mg/day for up to 3 years. Disease relapses are common despite the use of maintenance glucocorticoids, however. Another approach has been to discontinue glucocorticoids entirely within 3 months. Glucocorticoids are effective (initially, at least) in the majority of IgG4-RD patients, but disease flares are common. The true role of potentially steroid-sparing agents (such as azathioprine, mycophenolate mofetil, and methotrexate), if any, remains unclear. Their efficacy has never been tested in clinical trials, and observational studies suggest that their efficacy is limited. For patients with recurrent or refractory disease, B-cell depletion with rituximab is effective. Swift clinical responses have been observed with a striking targeting of the serum IgG4 level, accompanied by clinical improvement within weeks.

Complications

IgG4-RD often causes major tissue damage and can lead to organ failure but generally does so subacutely. Nevertheless, a subset of patients appears to have more fulminant disease, with progression to serious organ damage over a period of weeks. An organ particularly prone to permanent injury is the pancreas. Both endocrine and exocrine failure of the pancreas can ensue. Diabetes mellitus results from endocrine failure and may be an underrecognized secondary cause of this common problem. Exocrine failure of the pancreas is likely even more common than glucose intolerance as a complication of IgG4-RD, and this often leads to dramatic weight losses of 20–50 pounds simply because patients are unable to absorb nutrients and calories from food, owing to the lack of pancreatic enzymes. Suspicion of exocrine pancreatic failure can be confirmed by the finding of low fecal elastase level in a stool sample. Patients with exocrine pancreatic failure benefit substantially from the use of oral pancreatic enzyme supplementation prior to meals.

In other organs, untreated IgG4-related cholangitis can lead to hepatic failure within months, and IgG4-related aortitis can cause aneurysms and dissections. Substantial renal dysfunction and even renal failure can ensue from IgG4-related tubulointerstitial disease. Destructive bone lesions in the sinuses, head, and middle ear spaces that mimic granulomatosis with polyangiitis occur in a small number of patients, but less aggressive lesions are the rule in most. The ability to identify patients at risk for lesions that are swiftly destructive of involved tissues is presently suboptimal. Early diagnosis, comprehensive evaluations, and close follow-up are essential to ensuring good outcomes in this disease that is usually highly treatable.

When to Refer

The number of subspecialists who are expert on the topic of this emerging disease is growing yet remains small. It is important that patients be evaluated by clinicians who are familiar with this condition and willing to educate themselves further on the nuances of the disease. Evaluation of tissue biopsies by pathologists skilled in the diagnosis of this disease is also crucial to the establishment of the correct diagnosis.

Carruthers MN, Topazian MD, Khosroshahi A, et al. RTX for IgG4-related disease: a prospective, open-label trial. *Ann Rheum Dis.* 2015;74(6):1171-1177. [PMID: 25667206]

Perugino CA, Mattoo H, Mahajan VS, et al. IgG4-related disease: insights into immunology and targeted treatment strategies. *Arthritis Rheum.* 2017;69(9):1722-1732. [PMID: 28575535]

Wallace ZS, Naden RP, Chari S, et al. The 2019 American College of Rheumatology/European League Against Rheumatism Classification Criteria for IgG4-Related Disease. *Arthritis Rheum.* 2020;72(1):7-19. [PMID: 31793250]

Zhang W, Stone JH. Management of IgG4-related disease. *Lancet Rheumatol.* 2019;1:e55-e65.

Ocular Inflammatory Diseases for Rheumatologists

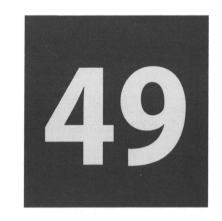

George N. Papaliodis, MD

James T. Rosenbaum, MD

The distance from the surface of the eye to the optic nerve is only about 2.5 cm, but within that short distance, an incredible diversity of tissue resides and almost any portion of that tissue can become inflamed. A rheumatologist should have a working knowledge of uveitis, keratitis, scleritis, episcleritis, conjunctivitis, optic neuritis, anterior ischemic optic neuropathy, dry eye, and orbital inflammation because rheumatologic diseases can be associated with inflammation in each of these areas. Moreover, managing a patient with one of these problems may require systemic immunosuppression, a treatment strategy that is beyond the expertise of the vast majority of ophthalmologists. Ocular inflammatory diseases are the third leading cause of blindness worldwide and account for 10% of cases of blindness in the United States. Appropriate management can preserve sight in an organ that is intolerant of inflammation.

UVEITIS

ESSENTIALS OF DIAGNOSIS

▶ Uveitis is categorized into anterior, intermediate, and posterior forms. Different systemic disease entities are associated with different forms of uveitis.

▶ Panuveitis, the occurrence of anterior, intermediate, and posterior uveitis in the same patient, is particularly characteristic of Behçet disease and sarcoidosis.

▶ Management strategies vary according to whether the uveitis is anterior, intermediate, or posterior.

▶ General Considerations

The uvea—the middle layer of the eye—includes the iris, ciliary body, and choroid. Anatomic subsets of uveitis can be defined: anterior uveitis (or iritis); iridocyclitis, when the ciliary body is inflamed along with the iris; intermediate uveitis (inflammation in the vitreous humor); posterior uveitis (involvement of the choroid or retina); and panuveitis, when the iris, vitreous, and retina all show evidence of inflammation. Uveitis can also be classified by etiology (Tables 49–1 and 49–2). A rheumatologist is usually essential for treating inflammation that is confined to the uveal tract or part of a systemic disease involving the uveal tract.

▶ Clinical Findings

Anterior uveitis typically presents with symptoms of eye pain, light sensitivity, ocular erythema, and/or blurry vision. On clinical exam, patients will demonstrate cells in the anterior chamber (lymphocytes and neutrophils) along with flare (protein in the aqueous humor) (Figure 49–1). In contrast, intermediate and posterior uveitis presents with symptoms of photopsias, floaters, and blurry vision. On clinical exam, those with intermediate and posterior uveitis will have cells in the vitreous along with other potential manifestations, including vitreous haze, sheathing of retinal blood vessels, subretinal and retinal exudates, macular edema, and optic nerve swelling.

Uveitis has a variety of complications, including cataract, glaucoma, posterior synechiae, macular edema, and retinal vasculitis. In an unpublished series, retinal vasculitis (Figure 49–2) was detected in one of every seven patients with uveitis, but retinal vasculitis does not have the same therapeutic implication as systemic vasculitis and patients with retinal vasculitis rarely have a systemic disease.

▶ Treatment

Many patients with uveal inflammation can be treated with topical medications or by periocular or intraocular injections of glucocorticoids. Many ophthalmologists feel comfortable prescribing a short course of oral glucocorticoids. Glucocorticoid-sparing medications are generally indicated

Table 49–1. Causes of uveitis.

Infections such as herpes simplex, herpes zoster, or toxoplasmosis
Syndromes confined to the eye such as pars planitis, sympathetic ophthalmia, or birdshot retinochoroidopathy
Masquerade syndromes such as lymphoma, leukemia, or retinal degeneration
Systemic immunologic disease as listed in Table 49–2

if the condition is not infectious or malignant, has not responded to local ophthalmic treatments either due to lack of efficacy or lack of tolerance, and interferes with activities of daily living.

Commonly chosen glucocorticoid-sparing medications include methotrexate, azathioprine, mycophenolate mofetil, cyclosporine, and tumor necrosis factor (TNF) inhibitors such as adalimumab, which is approved by regulatory authorities for the treatment of uveitis. A calcineurin antagonist such as cyclosporine or tacrolimus can be combined with an antimetabolite, offering greater efficacy than either medication alone but also posing greater risk. Although some groups advocate the use of an alkylating agent such as cyclophosphamide or chlorambucil, the trend among rheumatologists and uveitis specialists has been to avoid this class to treat uveitis, especially since the advent of biologic agents.

The underlying diagnosis often plays a minor role in the selection of therapy. For example, approximately 30–50% of patients with uveitis in a referral clinic are labeled as having idiopathic disease, meaning that although no specific etiology could be determined, the condition is presumed to be immune mediated. Patients with idiopathic uveitis are often treated in the same manner as a patient with

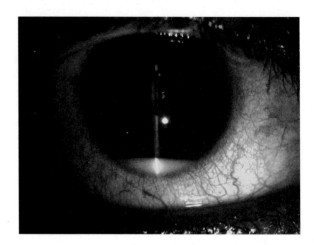

▲ **Figure 49–1.** Patient with HLA-B27–associated uveitis and associated hypopyon (layering of white blood cells within the anterior segment of the eye). (See color insert.)

sarcoid-associated uveitis or a patient with birdshot chorioretinopathy (Figure 49–3).

Methotrexate is used preferentially for children with juvenile idiopathic arthritis based on the experience using this medication in childhood. Vogt-Koyanagi-Harada syndrome, a form of uveitis characterized by bilateral anterior

Table 49–2. Systemic immunologic diseases commonly associated with uveitis.

Ankylosing spondylitis
Behçet disease
Drug reactions (eg, rifabutin)
Familial granulomatous synovitis with uveitis
Inflammatory bowel disease
Interstitial nephritis
Juvenile idiopathic arthritis
Multiple sclerosis
Neonatal-onset multisystem inflammatory disease
Psoriatic arthritis
Reactive arthritis
Relapsing polychondritis
Sarcoidosis
Systemic lupus erythematosus
Vasculitis, especially Kawasaki syndrome and Cogan syndrome
Vogt-Koyanagi-Harada syndrome

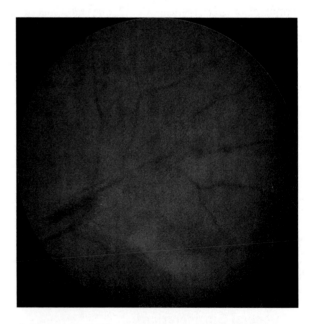

▲ **Figure 49–2.** Fundus photograph of the retina illustrating one form of retinal vasculitis manifesting as an intraretinal hemorrhage and vessels showing narrowing, occlusion, and dilation.

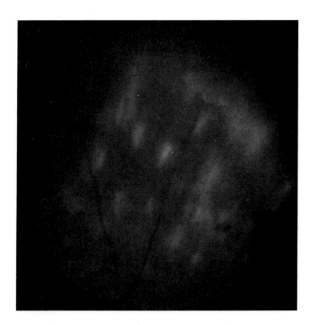

▲ **Figure 49–3.** Multiple chorioretinal lesions in the retina. These lesions are typical of birdshot chorioretinopathy.

and posterior uveitis with serous retinal detachments and often eighth nerve disease and sterile meningitis, is generally treated with more sustained, relatively high-dose prednisone compared to other forms of uveitis. Behçet disease is particularly responsive to tumor necrosis factor inhibitors such as adalimumab and infliximab. These drugs should be instituted relatively soon in Behçet disease, to avoid complications of long-term, high-dose glucocorticoid therapy.

Although several oral and parenteral treatments for uveitis are currently undergoing clinical trials, the only Food and Drug Administration (FDA)–approved drug for the treatment of uveitis is adalimumab. The anti-TNF therapies based on either chimeric or humanized monoclonal antibodies (eg, infliximab or adalimumab) are more effective for eye disease than is etanercept, a soluble fusion protein. One prospective series using infliximab to treat various forms of uveitis found a 77% early response rate but also a surprisingly high rate of toxicity. For example, drug-induced lupus developed in nearly 10% of the participants. Despite the efficacy, 52% of the initial participants did not continue infliximab therapy beyond 1 year.

Both infliximab and adalimumab are useful for patients with uveitis associated with juvenile idiopathic arthritis and an inadequate response to methotrexate. These children are more likely to experience sustained benefit with adalimumab rather than infliximab.

Uveitis, common among patients with ankylosing spondylitis, usually manifests itself as recurrent, unilateral, anterior disease (acute anterior uveitis). Several TNF inhibitors as well as sulfasalazine and possibly nonsteroidal anti-inflammatory drugs reduce the frequency of episodes of acute anterior uveitis in this setting. Paradoxically, TNF inhibition (especially etanercept use) sometimes appears to trigger uveitis.

SCLERITIS

ESSENTIALS OF DIAGNOSIS

▶ Erythema or a deep purplish hue of the sclera and intense pain are hallmarks of scleritis.

▶ There is a spectrum of disease severity, but scleritis can pose a vision-threatening complication of rheumatic diseases, particularly rheumatoid arthritis and granulomatosis with polyangiitis.

▶ Clinical Findings & Treatment

Most patients with scleritis have an intensely painful eye and persistent redness. The scleral inflammation may be hidden beneath the eyelids and not evident unless the lower eyelid is retracted as the patient is asked to look up, or the upper eyelid is retracted while the patient looks down. Posterior scleritis may not be evident on physical examination at all, and such patients present merely with a deep, boring headache. Scleritis can affect visual acuity or could result in complications such as uveitis or glaucoma.

Up to two-thirds of patients with scleritis have a systemic disease (Table 49–3). The two most common systemic illnesses are rheumatoid arthritis (RA) and granulomatosis with polyangiitis (GPA). Patients with GPA who have scleritis often have disease that is confined to the region above the clavicle and are at lower risk for pulmonary or renal disease. Nevertheless, the ocular disease alone is often more than sufficient justification for the treatment of severe disease. Different forms of scleritis may have distinctive pathways involved in their pathogenesis, but most forms of scleritis are regarded as localized forms of vasculitis.

Table 49–3. Systemic diseases associated with scleritis.

Granulomatosis with polyangiitis (formerly Wegener granulomatosis), especially limited forms
Rheumatoid arthritis
Inflammatory bowel disease
Relapsing polychondritis
Polyarteritis nodosa, Cogan syndrome, giant cell arteritis, and additional forms of vasculitis
Behçet disease
Sarcoidosis
Systemic lupus erythematosus
Spondyloarthritis

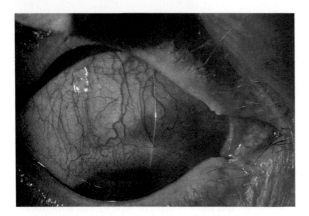

▲ **Figure 49–4.** Scleritis and scleral thinning that exposes the underlying choroid in a patient with severe rheumatoid arthritis.

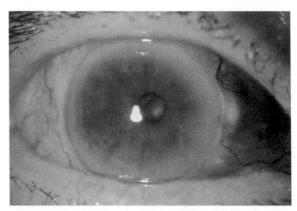

▲ **Figure 49–5.** Patient with rheumatoid arthritis and nasal scleritis with associated scleral melt. (See color insert.)

A minority of patients with scleritis respond to oral nonsteroidal anti-inflammatory drugs. Nearly all patients with a systemic disease associated with scleritis, however, such as RA or GPA, require intensive immunosuppression judiciously applied to control their scleritis. High-dose glucocorticoids are a cornerstone of treatment, but a steroid-sparing agent should be added quickly not only to reduce the toxicity associated with glucocorticoid use but also to control the scleritis more effectively. High-dose glucocorticoids alone are typically ineffective at inducing remission in patients with scleritis associated with RA or GPA, and patients will experience unfortunate levels of glucocorticoid toxicity if additional agents are not introduced early.

Methotrexate is often an effective adjunct to glucocorticoids with relatively mild scleritis. For patients with necrotizing disease, however, treatment with rituximab should be initiated immediately. Cyclophosphamide is also highly effective in treating necrotizing scleritis, but rituximab is usually the preferred first-line agent because of its superior side-effect profile. Oral daily cyclophosphamide can be added if patients are not responding adequately to the combination of glucocorticoids and rituximab after several weeks.

Necrotizing scleritis (Figure 49–4) tends to occur in RA patients who have long-standing disease with nodules, joint erosions, and extra-articular disease. Management of the underlying joint disease as with a biologic generally helps control the disease in the sclera. Similarly, the scleritis that is associated with a systemic disease, such as inflammatory bowel disease or relapsing polychondritis, may respond to the treatment of the underlying condition.

Scleritis in association with RA could be a manifestation of a rheumatoid nodule in the sclera. This results in a condition known as scleromalacia perforans (Figure 49–5).

KERATITIS

ESSENTIALS OF DIAGNOSIS

▶ Peripheral ulcerative keratitis (termed "PUK" by ophthalmologists), the most severe form of this condition, can lead to vision loss within days through a syndrome known as "corneal melt." RA and GPA are the rheumatic conditions most likely to be associated with PUK.

▶ "Nonsyphilitic interstitial keratitis" is a buzzword for the most common ocular manifestation of Cogan syndrome.

▶ Clinical Findings & Treatment

Corneal inflammation in the form of peripheral ulcerative keratitis (PUK) is a classic manifestation of a systemic vasculitis. Synonymous terms for this condition include corneal melt or marginal keratolysis. PUK usually occurs in association with scleritis at the margin of the cornea, which is contiguous with the sclera. Corneal thinning can lead to perforation of the eye and therefore poses a major risk of blindness. Topical therapy and surgery should be guided by the close supervision of ophthalmologist while immunosuppression is directed by a rheumatologist. The corneal disease in RA usually responds to aggressive treatment that is appropriate for severe synovitis. Patients in whom a corneal melt develops as a component of a systemic vasculitis usually experience improvement in the eye disease when the systemic disease is adequately treated, but damage to the eye may be permanent.

OCULAR CICATRICIAL PEMPHIGOID

ESSENTIALS OF DIAGNOSIS

▶ Cicatricial pemphigoid is an autoimmune blistering disease that can be associated with lesions in the oral mucosa and respiratory tract, in addition to involving the eye.

▶ Clinical Findings

This rare disease of the elderly is considered to be an autoimmune disease in which inflammation is directed against antigens, such as β_4 integrin, in the basement membrane of the ocular mucosa. Bullous lesions can develop elsewhere, particularly the mouth. Ocular symptoms of ocular cicatricial pemphigoid (OCP) include redness and irritation. The eyelid inverts (entropion) so that eyelashes scrape against the corneal surface, and these must be mechanically removed. An adhesion known as a symblepharon forms between the mucosal surface of the lower eyelid and the globe itself (Figure 49–6). The disease progresses slowly but frequently leads to bilateral blindness as the cornea opacifies and becomes neovascularized. Rarely, an adverse reaction to topical medications could cause similar symptoms, but the immunohistology showing immunoglobulin deposition along the basement membrane of the conjunctiva is unique and diagnostic of OCP.

▶ Treatment

Most practitioners treat OCP initially with dapsone. Mycophenolate mofetil has become popular as an antimetabolite for those who do not respond to dapsone. Recent uncontrolled trials have indicated the potential for successful treatment with intravenous immunoglobulin or rituximab or both. The traditional gold standard for therapy is oral cyclophosphamide, but this is now reserved for patients with disease resistant to other measures.

DYSFUNCTIONAL TEAR FILM SYNDROME

ESSENTIALS OF DIAGNOSIS

▶ A clinical entity that can result from several disease-related pathways, leading to disease of the meibomian glands or dysfunction of goblet cells.

▶ Clinical Findings & Treatment

Patients with the dysfunctional tear syndrome present with symptoms of ocular foreign-body sensation, injection of the conjunctiva, blurry vision, and light sensitivity. On clinical exam, they may demonstrate reduced Schirmer values, rapid tear breakup time, and corneal and conjunctival staining (with fluorescein, rose bengal, or lissamine green).

The tear film is complex and includes an oil layer primarily by meibomian glands, an aqueous layer produced by the lacrimal gland, and mucins coming predominantly from goblet cells and epithelial cells. The lacrimal gland is a principal target of an autoimmune response in primary Sjögren syndrome. Dysfunctional tears, however, could result from disease of the meibomian glands such as blepharitis or dysfunction of goblet cells. Thus, patients who have blepharitis resulting from seborrhea may have symptoms of ocular redness and scratchiness that mimic the symptoms of lacrimal gland dysfunction. Furthermore, lacrimal gland dysfunction has many causes including aging, postmenopausal status, alcoholism, diabetes, Sjögren syndrome, sarcoidosis, immunoglobulin G4 (IgG4)–related disease, and human immunodeficiency virus (HIV) infection. A wide spectrum of medications can contribute to ocular dryness and environmental factors may also play a significant role (worse in drier environments). Accordingly, dysfunctional tear syndrome is sometimes but not always the result of primary or secondary Sjögren syndrome.

The following principles in the management of the dysfunctional tear syndrome are useful:

1. Use artificial tears liberally. Artificial tears that contain preservatives should be avoided because these preservatives can be harmful to the corneal epithelium. Any artificial tear purported to "get the red out" certainly contains medication that will exacerbate any tendency to eye dryness and may further irritate the ocular surface.

2. Minimize the use of oral medications that have an anticholinergic effect.

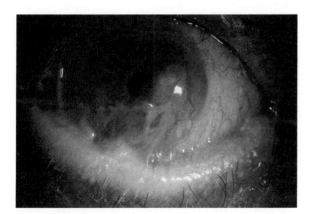

▲ **Figure 49–6.** Advanced ocular cicatricial pemphigoid with symblepharon (adherence between the palpebral conjunctiva and the bulbar conjunctiva) and opacification and neovascularization of the inferior cornea.

3. Encourage patients to rest their eyes or blink frequently, especially during tasks such as reading, driving, or using a computer. Blinking helps lubricate the ocular surface and is reduced during activities such as computer use.

4. Be sure that the house and work environments are humidified. Tears evaporate faster in a dry environment.

5. Consider the use of punctal occlusion to minimize drainage of tears.

ORBITAL INFLAMMATORY DISEASE

ESSENTIALS OF DIAGNOSIS

▶ Orbital inflammatory disease is in fact a syndrome comprising several different diseases characterized by distinct histopathologies, generally leading to proptosis, often to pain, and occasionally to vision loss through pressure on the optic nerve or its blood supply.

▶ Multiple retrobulbar or ocular adnexal structures can be involved, including the extraocular muscles ("orbital myositis"), lacrimal gland, and retrobulbar space.

▶ Clinical Findings

Many structures within the orbit, including extraocular muscle, fat, and the lacrimal gland, may become inflamed. Symptoms from orbital inflammation include pain, proptosis, and diplopia. Vision loss can result if the optic nerve is compressed.

Proptosis or exophthalmos can result from thyroid orbitopathy, orbital myositis associated with a variety of etiologies (including IgG4-related disease and GPA), lacrimal gland inflammation, infections, metastatic disease and other tumors, lymphoma, histiocytosis, and a condition sometimes called nonspecific orbital inflammation (which was previously known as orbital pseudotumor). Physical examination findings, imaging by magnetic resonance imaging (MRI) or computed tomography (CT) scan, and laboratory testing (antithyroid antibodies, antineutrophil cytoplasmic antibodies, IgG subclasses) are often effective in distinguishing among the various causes of orbital inflammatory disease, but a low threshold for biopsy should be maintained if there is no strong evidence favoring one etiology over others. A major mistake in management is made when patients are treated with high doses of glucocorticoids in the absence of a well-defined diagnosis.

▶ Treatment

Orbital inflammatory disease is frequently treated with a high dose of oral glucocorticoids, and these remain a cornerstone of therapy, particularly in the early treatment period.

Clinicians should look quickly for an appropriate glucocorticoid-sparing medication, however. These may include methotrexate or mycophenolate mofetil, but if the achievement of disease control is delayed, a therapy such as rituximab should be considered early in short order. A significant proportion of patients with orbital inflammatory disease have IgG$_4$-related disease (Chapter 54).

CANCER-ASSOCIATED RETINOPATHY

ESSENTIALS OF DIAGNOSIS

▶ A poorly understood "autoimmune retinopathy" that occurs in association with some malignancies.

▶ Clinical Findings

Visual loss can occur as a rare paraneoplastic syndrome. The immune response can be directed against a variety of different antigens, but recoverin and enolase are the two targets that have been implicated most convincingly. A similar autoimmune retinopathy can also occur in the absence of malignancy.

The diagnosis is usually made through triangulation of data from three sources: (1) a thorough, dilated ophthalmic examination that fails to show an alternative cause for visual loss; (2) characteristic findings on electroretinography; and (3) the demonstration of antiretinal antibodies. The specificity of antiretinal antibody assays, unfortunately, remains suboptimal. Correlation of these results with other data is essential to establishing the diagnosis with a reasonable degree of certainty.

▶ Treatment

Autoimmune retinopathy is usually treated by immunosuppression. Either rituximab or intravenous immune globulin has been used, but no consensus exists among experts and anecdotal evidence exists to support both approaches.

GLUCOCORTICOID-RESPONSIVE OPTIC NEUROPATHY

ESSENTIALS OF DIAGNOSIS

▶ Disease of the optic nerve(s) that does not appear to occur on the basis of demyelination and is therefore distinct from multiple sclerosis and optic neuritis and sensitive to treatment with glucocorticoids.

▶ Clinical Findings & Treatment

The most common immune-mediated cause of optic nerve disease is multiple sclerosis due to demyelination. Glucocorticoid-responsive optic neuropathy, another cause of potentially catastrophic optic nerve disease, is much less common. This entity is well known to occur in several immune-mediated diseases, including systemic lupus erythematosus and sarcoidosis.

This diagnosis is usually made by a neuro-ophthalmologist who identifies a patient with an optic neuritis that cannot be ascribed to a demyelinating disease. Such a patient does not have brain lesions detectable on MRI that suggest multiple sclerosis. In contrast to the optic neuropathy associated with multiple sclerosis, the process of glucocorticoid-responsive optic neuropathy is often bilateral. The diagnosis of glucocorticoid-responsive optic neuropathy is often confirmed by the company it keeps: clinical, serologic, radiologic, or pathologic features of a condition known to be associated with this ophthalmologic feature. In contrast to the optic neuropathy of multiple sclerosis, glucocorticoid-responsive optic neuropathy—as its name implies—improves with oral glucocorticoids. The selection of therapies beyond glucocorticoids remains empiric at this point and may be driven by suspicion of a particular underlying disease. TNF inhibition, for example, might be considered in a patient with presumed sarcoidosis whether or not the diagnosis can be established definitively.

NEUROMYELITIS OPTICA (DEVIC SYNDROME)

ESSENTIALS OF DIAGNOSIS

▶ Neuromyelitis optica (NMO), once termed Devic syndrome, refers to the combination of optic neuritis and transverse myelitis.

▶ Clinical Findings & Treatment

Neuromyelitis optica (NMO) refers to the combination of optic neuritis and transverse myelitis. This disease is associated with antibodies to aquaporin 4. The transverse myelitis typically involves the spinal cord over the length of at least two vertebral bodies and has therefore also been called "longitudinal myelitis." Patients with immune-mediated diseases such as systemic lupus erythematosus are at increased risk for NMO.

NMO must be treated aggressively because it can lead swiftly to devastating neurologic and ophthalmologic effects. Both rituximab and tocilizumab have been reported to have roles in the treatment of this condition. Early in the treatment of NMO, these modalities can be combined with glucocorticoids, but either may be useful in remission maintenance, potentially as a single agent. Continuous treatment for the maintenance of remission is recommended at this time.

OPHTHALMIC DISEASE DUE TO MEDICATIONS USED TO TREAT RHEUMATIC DISEASE

Some eye disease in patients with rheumatologic disease is related to treatment rather than to the underlying inflammatory process. Examples include: retinopathy secondary to antimalarials; posterior subcapsular cataracts, central serous retinopathy, or glaucoma from glucocorticoids; iritis or scleritis from intravenous bisphosphonate therapy; and infections secondary to immunosuppression.

Kunchok A, Malpas C, Nytrova P, et al. Clinical and therapeutic predictors of disease outcomes in AQP4-IgG+ neuromyelitis optica spectrum disorder. *Mult Scler Relat Disord.* 2019;38:101868. [Epub ahead of print] [PMID: 31877445]

Ong HS, Setterfield JF, Minassian DC, Dart JK; Mucous Membrane Pemphigoid Study Group 2009–2014. Mucous membrane pemphigoid with ocular involvement: the clinical phenotype and its relationship to direct immunofluorescence findings. *Ophthalmology.* 2018;125(4):496. [PMID: 29217149]

Ogra S, Sims JL, McGhee CNJ, Niederer RL. Ocular complications and mortality in peripheral ulcerative keratitis and necrotising scleritis: the role of systemic immunosuppression. *Clin Exp Ophthalmol.* 2019 Dec 24. doi: 10.1111/ceo.13709. [PMID: 31872475]

Ungprasert P, Crowson CS, Cartin-Ceba R, et al. Clinical characteristics of inflammatory ocular disease in anti-neutrophil cytoplasmic antibody associated vasculitis: a retrospective cohort study. *Rheumatology (Oxford).* 2017;56(10):1763. [PMID: 28957561]

Sensorineural Hearing Loss (Immune-Mediated Inner Ear Disease)

John H. Stone, MD, MPH

Howard W. Francis, MD, MBA, FACS

ESSENTIALS OF DIAGNOSIS

▶ When sensorineural hearing loss occurs in the context of an inflammatory condition, it is referred to most appropriately as immune-mediated inner ear disease (IMIED).

▶ May be associated with disturbances of balance as well as hearing loss because the inner ear mediates vestibular function as well as hearing.

▶ May occur as a primary inner ear problem or as a complication of a recognized inflammatory condition such as Cogan syndrome, granulomatosis with polyangiitis, Susac syndrome, giant cell arteritis, Sjögren syndrome, and others.

▶ Symptoms include tinnitus, vertigo, nausea, and difficulties with two issues related to hearing: acuity and speech discrimination.

▶ General Considerations

Sensorineural hearing loss (SNHL) is an idiopathic inflammatory disorder that occurs either as a primary form of disease limited to the ear or secondary to another known immune-mediated condition that affects other organs, as well. The anatomy of the inner ear is shown in Figure 50–1. SNHL is a common feature of some primary forms of vasculitis (eg, Cogan syndrome, granulomatosis with polyangiitis [formerly Wegener granulomatosis], giant cell arteritis). SNHL also occasionally occurs in association with systemic autoimmune disorders such as systemic lupus erythematosus (SLE) and Sjögren syndrome.

Because hearing loss is often not the sole feature of this syndrome—vertigo, tinnitus, and a sense of aural fullness often occur as well—and because the symptoms respond frequently to immunosuppression, **immune-mediated inner ear disease** (IMIED) is the preferred term for this disorder when symptoms and signs are confined entirely to the ear.

Devastating disabilities including profound deafness and severe vestibular dysfunction are potential sequelae of IMIED. Yet if diagnosed promptly, IMIED is amenable to treatment. Unfortunately, the prognosis is difficult to gauge except in the setting of profound, sustained SNHL, in which case significant recovery of hearing is unlikely.

Little is known for certain about the mechanisms of injury to the inner ear in any condition associated with SNHL, because biopsy of the cochlea is not possible without causing irreversible injury. Some data from autopsy studies of patients with primary immune-mediated inner ear disease—generally obtained after patients had received substantial courses of immunosuppression before death—suggest that both antibody-mediated injury to the stria vascularis and vascular occlusion impair the metabolic processes that support hearing transduction. For patients who experience IMIED in the setting of a systemic vasculitis, for example, granulomatosis with polyangiitis, the basis of tissue injury is presumably inflammatory disease of the small blood vessels.

Several characteristics distinguish IMIED from other syndromes of inner ear dysfunction. First, its time course is relatively rapid. IMIED is analogous to rapidly progressive glomerulonephritis in that inner ear inflammation progresses to severe, irreversible damage within 3 months of onset (and often much more quickly). With IMIED, in fact, the complete loss of hearing within a week or two of symptom onset is not unusual. Second, IMIED is usually bilateral to some degree, albeit the left and right sides may be affected asymmetrically and asynchronously. Only weeks or months typically separate involvement of the two sides, but the interval may be as long as a year or more. Finally, although some cases of IMIED are marked by precipitous, irretrievable losses of inner ear function, others demonstrate fluctuating symptom patterns over a period of several months. Recurrent bouts of SNHL often lead to consistent decrements in hearing capabilities, causing profound hearing deficits in many patients over time.

Although IMIED usually occurs in middle-aged individuals, the syndrome has been described in young children and

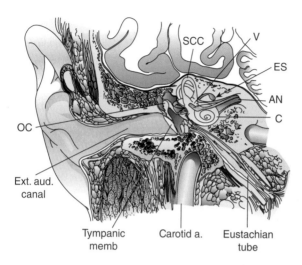

▲ **Figure 50–1.** Anatomy of the temporal bone and audiovestibular apparatus. AN, auditory nerve; C, cochlea; ES, endolymphatic sac; OC, ossicular chain; SCC, semicircular canals; V, vestibule. (© 2000 John H. Stone, MD, MPH.)

also in the elderly. Two thirds of the patients with IMIED are women.

▶ Clinical Findings

A. Symptoms and Signs

1. Hearing—Hearing loss in IMIED may take two forms. First, patients may complain primarily of diminished hearing *acuity* (the ability to perceive sound). Crude assessments of hearing sensitivity using the mechanical sounds of a watch, the dial-tone of a cellphone, or the rubbing of fingers are inadequate to detect subtle but clinically significant deficits in hearing acuity. Formal audiologic testing is required to gauge the degree of hearing dysfunction adequately. Second, patients may also note decreased *discrimination* (the ability to distinguish individual words). Communication problems arising from poor word discrimination often constitute the chief complaint. Patients with significant deficits in word discrimination are able to hear the sound of a voice on a cellphone but fail to understand what is being said. They also have difficulty participating in conversations conducted amid background noise. Understanding conversations in crowded rooms or restaurants is particularly problematic.

Otoscopy is usually normal in IMIED, even among patients with profound SNHL. In patients with SNHL secondary to granulomatosis with polyangiitis, otoscopy may reveal findings consistent with otitis media caused by granulomatous inflammation within the middle ear cavity, tympanic membrane clouding, or even rupture. Conductive hearing loss caused by middle ear disease is more common than SNHL

in patients with granulomatosis with polyangiitis, but SNHL occurs with a frequency that is probably underrecognized because of failure to obtain audiologic testing in all patients.

Two simple physical examination tests are useful in distinguishing SNHL from conductive hearing loss: the Weber test and the Rinne test. In the **Weber test**, a vibrating 512-Hz tuning fork is placed on an upper incisor tooth or mid-forehead. If SNHL is present, the tone sounds louder in the unaffected ear. (In contrast, if conductive hearing loss is present, the tone actually sounds louder in the ear affected by the conductive hearing loss). The test can be repeated for higher frequencies.

In the **Rinne test**, a vibrating 512 Hz tuning fork is first placed 3 cm from the opening of the ear and then in contact with the mastoid bone. The patient is then asked to compare the loudness of the tone generated in air to that generated by contact on the bone. A conductive hearing loss of at least 30 dB is suggested when bone conduction exceeds air conduction in loudness. A normal Rinne test (air conduction > bone conduction) in an ear to which the Weber has lateralized suggests SNHL in that ear.

2. Balance—Otolaryngologists and neurologists, who should become involved in patients' care if SNHL is suspected, should be expert at evaluating patients' vestibulo-ocular reflexes (VORs). Other tests, including audiometric testing and electronystagmography, are also essential components of the workup.

Evaluations of the VORs consist of assessments for nystagmus in response to repetitive head shaking and for gaze stability during rapid lateral rotation of the head. By detecting head movement, the inner ear provides afferent input to the VOR upon which the central nervous system depends for accuracy on the compensatory movements (saccades) of the eyes. Disturbance of the inner ear's role in maintaining a stable image on the retina leads to a perception of dizziness, which is worsened by head movement and relieved at rest. The rapid changes in afferent input to the central nervous system associated with IMIED can lead to VOR decompensation, an inability to maintain a stable retinal image, and a persistent illusion of movement known as oscillopsia.

The acute phase of vertigo resolves to motion-induced dizziness through central compensation after days to weeks. In the acute phase of vestibular decompensation, spontaneous nystagmus may be seen when visual fixation is suppressed (eg, in the dark or behind Fresnel lenses). The VOR can be assessed for each ear separately at the bedside by asking the patient to fix her eyes on the examiner's nose while the examiner quickly turns the patient's head 30 degrees toward the ear in question. Normal VORs generate smooth, accurate compensatory ocular saccades. In contrast, abnormal VORs are associated with under- or overshooting of the eye movements, followed by a corrective saccade.

Oscillopsia is a disabling consequence of bilateral VOR loss. The presence of oscillopsia and bilateral vestibular hypofunction can be detected by comparing visual acuity with the Snellen chart while the head is at rest versus during head shaking. A difference in visual acuity of three or more lines is an indication of peripheral vestibular dysfunction. Larger decrements are expected in bilateral disease.

Electronystagmography provides objective measure and comparison between ears of peripheral vestibular function, more specifically the lateral semicircular canal. The vestibular electromyographic potential measured in the sternocleidomastoid muscle in response to stimulation of the saccule by low-frequency sound assesses another component of peripheral vestibular function.

3. Eyes—Cogan syndrome, described in detail in Chapter XX, can be associated with virtually any form of ocular inflammation, including orbital pseudotumor, scleritis, and uveitis. The most characteristic ocular manifestation of Cogan syndrome, however, is interstitial keratitis. Granulomatosis with polyangiitis (see Chapter XX) also has a host of potential ocular complications. Diplopia, amaurosis fugax, and anterior ischemic optic neuropathy are common manifestations of giant cell arteritis. Aside from secondary sicca symptoms, the most common eye problem in SLE is retinopathy, which may be associated with either retinal vasculitis or a clotting diathesis, such as that associated with antiphospholipid antibodies. Keratoconjunctivitis sicca is a hallmark of Sjögren syndrome (see Chapter XX).

B. Laboratory Findings

The results of routine laboratory test in primary IMIED are usually unremarkable. There is typically no indication, for example, of a systemic inflammatory response; acute phase reactants are usually normal. Indeed, the presence of elevated acute phase reactants should make one search urgently for a secondary cause of IMIED and exclude inflammation in organs beyond the inner ear.

The measurement of several types of autoantibodies is highly appropriate in the search for an underlying cause of SNHL that might have alternative treatment indications. Autoantibodies relevant to the assessment of a patient with SNHL are shown in Table 50–1.

Table 50–1. Autoantibodies and other assays appropriate to the evaluation of sensorineural hearing loss.

Antinuclear antibody
Anti-Ro antibody
Anti-La antibody
dsDNA antibody
Serum C3 and C4
ANCA
FTA-ABS
Lyme serology
Routine blood and urine tests to exclude signs of systemic disease: complete blood count, serum chemistries, urinalysis with microscopy

ANCA, antineutrophil cytoplasmic antibody; dsDNA, double-stranded DNA; FTA-ABS, fluorescent treponemal antibody absorption test.

C. Imaging Studies

Magnetic resonance imaging (MRI) studies are essential to exclude tumors of the cerebellopontine angle.

D. Special Tests

1. Audiogram and electronystagmogram—Formal hearing tests should be performed on any patient with a complaint of hearing loss. The audiogram (Figure 50–2A) is a graphic representation of the lowest volume at which individual tones ranging from 250 to 8000 Hz can be distinguished. An audiogram from a patient with classic SNHL is depicted in Figure 50–2B. The **reception threshold** measures the lowest volume at which speech is heard. The **discrimination score** measures the ability to discriminate words. Electronystagmography measures ocular movement in response to various stimuli, including warm and cold caloric stimulation of the ears. This test assesses the functional strength and symmetry of the VORs in response to input from both ears. Audiometry and electronystagmography testing may confirm clinical impressions of inner ear dysfunction and quantify the degree of organ involvement.

2. Serologic testing—There is, unfortunately, no reliable serological marker of IMIED, either for diagnostic or prognostic purposes.

▶ Differential Diagnosis

Because the treatments for various inner ear disorders vary dramatically according to cause, precise distinction between etiologies is critical. Table 50–2 depicts the major disease categories that require exclusion in the workup of patients with possible IMIED. The etiologies of inner ear dysfunction may differ in several respects: (1) their rates of progression; (2) their degrees of symmetry; and (3) and their relative effects on hearing and balance. The etiologies may be divided into six major categories: aging, trauma, tumors, infections, ototoxic drugs, and finally, cases presumed to be immunologic in nature.

Slowly progressive, symmetric loss of high-frequency hearing without vestibular symptoms distinguishes hearing loss due to aging and chronic noise exposure from IMIED. In addition, rapidly progressive hearing loss and dysequilibrium due to ototoxic drugs, sudden acoustic trauma, or barotrauma can be excluded by taking a careful history. Meniere syndrome, a symptom complex of gradual, fluctuating hearing loss punctuated by episodes of vertigo, tinnitus, and aural fullness, is a common sequela to many causes of inner ear inflammation, including IMIED. In the absence of identifiable causes, the syndrome is termed **Meniere disease**.

Time course is the principal criterion for distinguishing Meniere disease from IMIED. In Meniere disease, hearing loss occurs over a period of several years, rather than the weeks or months characteristic of IMIED. Meniere disease

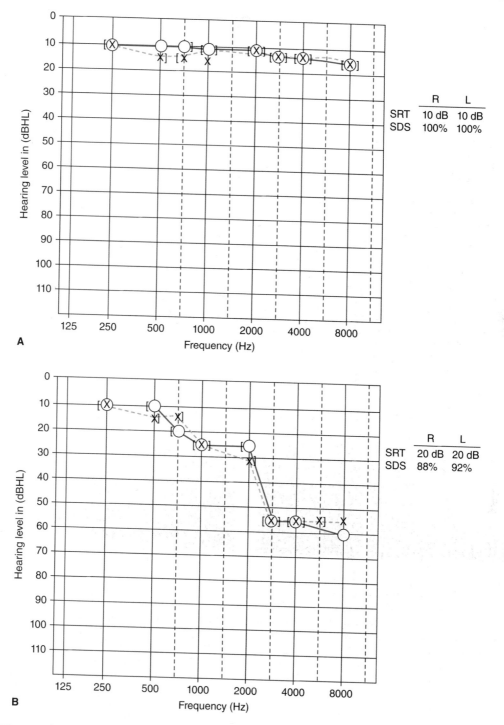

▲ **Figure 50–2.** Audiogram. **A:** Normal bilateral hearing. **B:** Symmetric high-frequency hearing loss in a patient with IMIED. Bone conduction thresholds (R = [and L =]) are measures of auditory function of the cochlea and proximal neural pathway, whereas air conduction thresholds (R = circle, L = X) measure function of the entire auditory system. SRT, speech reception threshold; SDS, speech discrimination score. (© 2000 Lippincott Williams & Wilkins.)

Table 50–2. Differential diagnosis of sensorineural hearing loss.

Time Course	Associated Disorders and Medications	Vestibular Symptoms	Distinguishing Features
Slowly progressive (>3 months to years)	Meniere syndrome	+	Episodic vertigo, unilateral hearing loss, tinnitus, aural fullness
	Presbycusis	−	Symmetric high frequency hearing loss
	Latent or tertiary syphilis	+/−	+ FTA-ABS, +/− RPR
	Acoustic neuroma	+/−	Unilateral hearing loss, tinnitus; enhancing lesion on MRI
Intermediate (days to 3 months)	**IMIED** Primary Secondary (vasculitis, connective tissue disorder)	+/−	See text Signs and symptoms of systemic inflammatory disorders
	Drugs Aminoglycosides Antimalarials Loop diuretics NSAIDs	+	Chronic dysequilibrium; signs of bilateral vestibular hypofunction (eg, oscillopsia)
	Lyme disease	+/−	Exposure risk Positive *Borrelia burgdorferi* serology
	Latent or tertiary syphilis	+/−	+ FTA-ABS, +/− RPR
	Acoustic neuroma	+/−	Unilateral hearing loss, tinnitus; enhancing lesion on MRI
Sudden (hours to days)	Acoustic trauma	−	Recent intense noise exposure
	Barotrauma	+/−	Recent deep sea diving, barotrauma
	Perilymph fistula	+	Otolaryngology evaluation
	Viral/bacterial labyrinthitis	+	Acute vertigo and/or hearing loss
	Early or secondary syphilis	+	+ FTA-ABS, + RPR
	Acoustic neuroma	+/−	Unilateral hearing loss, tinnitus; enhancing lesion on MRI

FTA-ABS, fluorescent treponemal antibody absorption test; IMIED, immune-mediated inner ear disease; MRI, magnetic resonance imaging; NSAIDs, nonsteroidal anti-inflammatory drugs; RPR, rapid plasma regain.

is also usually limited to one ear, but delayed involvement of the contralateral ear occurs in approximately one-third of cases. Because IMIED is more likely to respond to the early institution of aggressive immunosuppression, distinguishing between these two disorders is critical.

Other causes of rapid changes in auditory and balance function are difficult to distinguish from IMIED by history alone. For example, tumors that compress the eighth cranial nerve (eg, schwannomas at the cerebellopontine angle) cause asymmetric hearing loss with variable rates of progression, ranging from days to years. MRI with gadolinium is essential to exclude such tumors. Rapid increases in intracranial or middle ear pressures (eg, as induced by trauma or a forceful Valsalva maneuver) may lead to a breach in the bony capsule of the inner ear. This condition, known as a perilymph fistula, produces rapid unilateral hearing loss accompanied by vertigo. Patients with perilymph fistulas are candidates for prompt surgical repair.

Bacterial and viral causes of inner ear dysfunction, including meningitis, may lead to swift, dramatic, irreversible hearing loss. These must be excluded quickly with appropriate cultures and serologies. Table 50–2 includes a partial list of infections associated with inner ear disease. Syphilis deserves special emphasis because of the many similarities between otosyphilis and IMIED. Syphilitic complications span the entire spectrum of inner ear disease, ranging from the sudden onset of hearing loss and vertigo associated with secondary syphilis to the gradual hearing loss associated with latent and tertiary stages of disease (sometimes accompanied by Meniere syndrome). Specific treponemal tests, for example, the fluorescent treponemal antibody absorption (FTA-ABS) assay, are indicated in all patients with unexplained hearing loss. Nontreponemal tests such as the rapid plasma reagin (RPR) have unacceptably high false-negative rates in latent and tertiary infection.

Granulomatosis with polyangiitis is crucial not to miss in a patient who presents with SNHL. Conductive hearing loss in granulomatosis with polyangiitis results from a variety of mechanisms, including opacification of the middle ear cleft with fluid or discontinuity of the ossicular ear chain because of necrotizing, granulomatous inflammation. In contrast, SNHL in granulomatosis with polyangiitis is generally regarded as the ischemic sequelae of vasculitis. Peripheral facial nerve palsy, caused by either vasculitis of the vasa nervorum or compression of the seventh cranial nerve by granulomatous inflammation as it courses through the middle ear, can be an important clue to the diagnosis of granulomatosis with polyangiitis.

Susac syndrome is a poorly understood disease entity, marked by encephalopathy, branch retinal artery occlusion, and SNHL.

Treatment

In the absence of significant numbers of rigorous, controlled studies, the treatment approach for IMIED is based largely on anecdotal experience, case series, and inference from the treatment of related conditions. Because of the devastating nature of severely impaired hearing and vestibular function, IMIED should be regarded in the same fashion as any other threat to vital organ mediated by an immunologic injury. In such conditions, aggressive immunosuppression—high-dose glucocorticoids often supplemented by immunomodulatory, cytotoxic, or biologic agents—may halt the inflammatory response and prevent permanent organ damage. In contrast, failure to treat these disorders promptly can lead to substantial, irreversible organ dysfunction within a brief time. Numerous case reports and small case series demonstrate the apparent responsiveness of IMIED to immunosuppression in its early stages, including recovery of vestibular function.

The authors' approach to the treatment of IMIED is guided by the concept that if IMIED is worth treating (ie, if significant inner ear function appears recoverable), it is worth treating aggressively. Thus, in the setting of rapidly progressive SNHL, treatment with 1 mg/kg/day of prednisone, not to exceed 80 mg/day, is instituted. If there is significant improvement in auditory and vestibular function within 2 weeks, prednisone is continued at this dosage for a total of 1 month and then tapered to discontinuation over 2 additional months. In patients with recurrent disease, some maintenance prednisone (eg, 5–10 mg/d) may be prudent.

Intratympanic glucocorticoid therapy can be administered serially in the hope of maintaining the initial response to systemic glucocorticoids, but the evidence for the efficacy of intratympanic glucocorticoids is slim. A variety of concentrations have been suggested although the authors currently use buffered dexamethasone (12 mg/mL) that is injected into the middle ear where it remains for 30 minutes with the patient supine and is then suctioned. Some clinicians employ intratympanic injections of glucocorticoids as the first line of therapy for primary IMIED, moving to systemic treatment only if the intratympanic approach fails. Neither approach has been studied rigorously to date.

If hearing and balance deteriorate despite prednisone or do not improve significantly within the 2 weeks of treatment, the addition of another medication should be considered. Biologic agents such as rituximab have been employed on an empiric basis, but the data base for making recommendations for any specific one of these agents is slim.

Similarly, only anecdotal evidence exists to support the use of most other therapies for primary IMIED. Methotrexate (up to 25 mg/wk), azathioprine (2 mg/kg/day), and mycophenolate mofetil (up to 1500 mg twice daily) have all been used. The choice among these agents is usually guided by physician experience and patients' individual comorbidities that make them more likely to tolerate one medication or another. Cyclophosphamide (2 mg/kg/day, with doses adjusted for renal dysfunction) can also be tried, but because of its potential toxicities, treatment continuation beyond 4–6 months is not advised. Unless there is clear evidence that cyclophosphamide is effecting improvement, prolonged courses of this medication are discouraged. Biologic agents such as rituximab are generally safer than cyclophosphamide and should be employed before cyclophosphamide in most cases.

Unless active disease in other organ systems justifies continuation of significant immunosuppression, the maintenance of such therapy after irreversible organ damage (ie, profound hearing loss) has occurred places patients at risk for treatment complications with little potential benefit. In the setting of profound hearing disturbances despite aggressive immunosuppression, the hearing that a patient may derive from a cochlear implant may render this the most appropriate course of action. Consequently, if patients have not demonstrated a response by the end of 3 months of therapy, the medications should be discontinued.

The treatment of SNHL associated with granulomatosis with polyangiitis, Cogan syndrome, and other primary disorders are discussed in their appropriate chapters.

Prognosis

Patients who do not respond swiftly to immunosuppressive therapies are at high risk for poor long-term hearing outcomes. Many patients, however, stabilize at a level characterized by some degree of hearing impairment but are able to maintain functional hearing and inner ear function without recurrences. Treatment can often be discontinued in these patients over time.

Hearing & Vestibular Rehabilitation

All patients with functionally significant bilateral hearing loss should be supplied with appropriate hearing aids. When speech discrimination remains poor in both ears despite maximal medical therapy and the use of powerful hearing aids, the patient may be a candidate for cochlear implantation. Cochlear implants process and deliver sound to the auditory nerve in the form of encoded electrical signals, increasing both hearing acuity and speech understanding.

For patients with dizziness due to a significant loss of peripheral vestibular function, compensation by the central nervous system is effectively enhanced through a program of vestibular rehabilitation. Such programs, administered by appropriately trained physical therapists, promote a variety of strategies to maintain balance and minimize fall risk. In the treatment of dizziness, long-term use of vestibular suppressant drugs (eg, meclizine) should be avoided because they impede the development of central compensation mechanisms.

Das S, Bakshi SS, Seepana R. Demystifying autoimmune inner ear disease. *Eur Arch Otorhinolaryngol.* 2019;276(12):3267-3274. [Epub 2019 Oct 11] [PMID: 31605190]

Rahne T, Plontke S, Keyßer G. Vasculitis and the ear: a literature review. *Curr Opin Rheumatol.* 2020;32(1):47-52. [PMID: 31599796]

Riera JL, Maliandi MDR, Musuruana JL, Cavallasca JA. Sudden sensorineural hearing loss in systemic lupus erythematosus and antiphospholipid syndrome. An update. *Curr Rheumatol Rev.* 2019 Oct 15. [Epub ahead of print] [PMID: 31804161]

Osteoporosis & Glucocorticoid-Induced Osteoporosis

Kavitha Mattaparthi, MD

Muhammad Zaheer, MD

Mary Beth Humphrey, MD, PhD, FACP

ESSENTIALS OF DIAGNOSIS

- ▶ Osteoporosis is defined as bone fragility due to reduced bone mineral density (BMD) or loss of bone trabecular microarchitecture.

- ▶ Fragility fractures occur most frequently in the wrists, forearms, spine, and hips.

- ▶ The incidence of osteoporosis increases with age, independent of sex, but the disease is most prevalent in postmenopausal women.

- ▶ The risk of spinal fracture increases with chronic glucocorticoid doses as low as 2.5 mg of prednisone daily.

- ▶ Prednisone doses higher than 7.5 mg daily increase the risk of spine fractures fivefold and double the risk of hip fracture.

- ▶ Risk of osteoporosis is associated not only with glucocorticoids but with other medications as well, including chronic use of PPIs, anticonvulsants, SSRIs, and warfarin.

- ▶ Preventive measures and treatment options are effective at reducing fractures.

▶ General Considerations

Bone remodeling occurs throughout life, such that the average skeleton is turned over every 10 years. Bone remodeling units include three main cell types: osteoclasts (OCs) that resorb bone; osteoblasts (OBs) that form new bone; and osteocytes (OCYs), embedded within the bone, that regulate the activity of OCs and OBs by producing paracrine factors locally. OCYs are the main producers of sclerostin, which regulates OB against producing more bone. OCYs also produce receptor activator of nuclear factor κB ligand (RANKL), which recruits OC precursors and stimulates bone resorption. Bone catabolism and anabolism normally remain coupled to maintain bone integrity. However, in many disease states such as hyperparathyroidism, hormonal changes such as those occurring in menopause, and the use of medications such as glucocorticoids, bone formation becomes uncoupled from bone resorption. This process ultimately leads to osteoporosis. The degree to which bone cells are regulated by the immune system has been recognized and defined only within the last two decades, and it is now clear that many endocrine and autoimmune disease states are associated with osteoporosis because the cross-talk between the immune system and bone cells has become dysregulated.

Men and women have significant differences in peak bone mass and the rates of bone loss over their life spans (Figure 51–1). Men achieve higher peak bone mass than do women and have only slow bone loss in middle to late age. They therefore maintain a higher bone mineral density (BMD) until late in life. Women undergo an early rapid phase of postmenopausal bone loss followed by a slow but persistent rate of bone loss until death. The lower peak bone mass attained by women coupled with the early rapid phase of menopause-related bone loss means that women typically have lower BMDs than men of the same age. Thus, women have an earlier onset of the typical osteoporotic fractures (hip, vertebral, and distal forearm [Colles]) compared with men (Figure 51–2). Osteoporotic fractures occur in men on average 10 years later than women do. The impact of older age at hip fractures is that men have substantially higher morbidity and mortality from hip fractures than women. This is likely because men are more likely to be frail at the time of their fractures and are correspondingly less able to cope physically with the risks of fracture repair surgery and emotionally with the loss of independence.

Osteoporosis is a systemic condition manifested by low bone mass, disruption of bone microarchitecture, and compromised bone strength. Because osteoporosis is asymptomatic, the diagnosis is typically not made until a fragility fracture has occurred. In the United States, osteoporosis occurs in 1 in 4 women and 1 in 20 men older than 65. Osteoporosis may be diagnosed by a low BMD or by a fragility fracture.

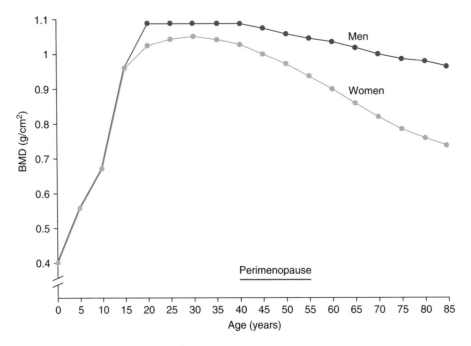

▲ **Figure 51–1.** Mean bone mineral density (BMD) in men versus women from age 5 to 85 demonstrating the lower peak BMD values for women versus men, the rapid perimenopausal rates of bone loss in women, and the slow continuous phase of bone loss that continues into the eighth decade. (Used, with permission, from Southard RN, Morris JD, Mahan JD, et al. Bone mass in healthy children: measurement with quantitative DXA. *Radiology.* 1991;179:735; and from Kelly TL. Bone mineral reference databases for American men and women. *J Bone Miner Res.* 1990;5(Suppl 2):702.)

The diagnosis of osteoporosis is established by measuring BMD in sites where fractures are common: the wrist (distal radius), spine, and proximal hip. Dual-energy X-ray absorptiometry (DXA) is the most widely used technique validated for this purpose. The World Health Organization defines osteoporosis as a BMD T-score of less than or equal to −2.5 and osteopenia as a T-score between −1 and −2.5 (Table 51–1). Prospective studies indicate that fracture risk increases as BMD declines and increases yet further with advancing age. For instance, the 10-year risk for fracture for a

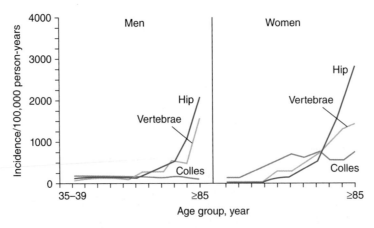

▲ **Figure 51–2.** The incidence of three common osteoporotic fractures in men and women over decades. Note the early rise in vertebrae, Colles (wrist/forearm), and hip fractures in women. (Used, with permission, from Cooper C, Melton LJ III. Epidemiology of osteoporosis. *Trends Endocrinol Metab.* 1992;314:224.)

Table 51–1. WHO definition of osteoporosis based on DXA measurements.

	Definitions
T-score	Number of SD above or below peak bone mass ("young normal") according to race or ethnicity
Z-score	Number of SD above or below age-matched bone mass according to gender and race or ethnicity
Normal	BMD T-score ≥ −1
Low bone mass (osteopenia)	BMD T-score < −1 and > −2.5
Osteoporosis	BMD T-score ≤2.5
Severe osteoporosis	BMD T-score ≤2.5 with one or more fragility fractures

BMD, bone mineral density; DXA, dual-energy x-ray absorptiometry; SD, standard deviation; WHO, World Health Organization.

Table 51–2. Risk factors for osteoporotic fractures independent of bone density.

Nonmodifiable
  Female gender
  History of fracture as an adult
  Presence of fracture (especially of hip) in first-degree relative
  White or Asian race
  Advanced age
  Dementia and frailty
  Immobilization
Modifiable
  Alcohol
  Tobacco use
  Low body mass index (BMI) <21 kg/m^2
  Premature menopause
  History of amenorrhea
  Low dietary calcium intake
  Frequent falls and poor eyesight
  Low level of physical activity
  Use of glucocorticoids
  Vitamin D deficiency
  Hypogonadism (surgical or chemical)

55-year-old woman with a T-score of −3 is roughly 17%, but for a 75-year-old woman with the same T-score, the risk is 30% (Figure 51–3). For younger patients under 40 years, their BMD is compared to the mean of the same sex and age to generate a Z-score. Fracture risk is very low in these younger patients and therefore the Z-score does not include fracture risk, in contrast to the T-score. In general, a Z-score more than −2 standard deviations from other age- and sex-matched people likely indicates a low BMD and should prompt further evaluation.

In addition to age and BMD, there are other modifiable and nonmodifiable risk factors associated with an increased incidence of osteoporotic fractures (Table 51–2). Using the validated Fracture Risk Assessment Tool (FRAX) (www.sheffield.ac.uk/FRAX), fracture risk can also be assessed with or without a BMD measurement. Clinical parameters used in the FRAX tool include gender, ethnicity, height and weight, age, prior fracture history, parental hip fracture, current smoking, long-term use of glucocorticoids (any dose >3 months), rheumatoid arthritis, and excessive alcohol consumption (more than three drinks daily). These factors alone or in combination with femoral neck or total hip BMD generate two probabilities: (1) 10-year absolute risk of hip fracture; and (2) 10-year absolute risk of major osteoporotic fracture (hip, spine, wrist, and humerus). The FRAX tool is validated for persons aged 40–90 years across many countries worldwide.

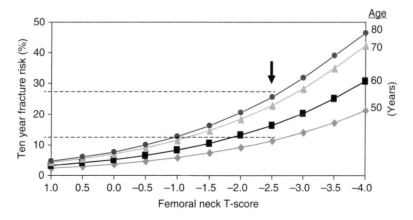

▲ **Figure 51–3.** Fracture risk increases with age at any T-score. With a T-score of −2.5, the 10-year risk of fracture for an 80-year-old woman (*arrow*) approaches 30%, whereas a 50-year-old woman with the same T-score has only a 12% risk of fracture. (Adapted from Kanis JA, Johnell O, Oden A, Dawson A, De Laet C, Jonsson B. Ten year probabilities of osteoporotic fractures according to BMD and diagnostic thresholds. *Osetoporosis Int.* 2001;12:989-995.)

Many commonly prescribed medications increase the risk for osteoporosis and fractures (Table 51–3). Chronic glucocorticoid use is highly prevalent, and unless osteoporosis preventive treatment is given, approximately 50% of glucocorticoid-treated patients will suffer from an osteoporotic fracture, typically of the spine and hip. Chronic use of proton pump inhibitors (PPIs), anticonvulsants, selective serotonin reuptake inhibitors (SSRIs), and warfarin, among others, also increase fracture risk. However, many physicians are unaware of the increased fracture risk from these drugs and fail to screen or treat osteoporosis in these at-risk patients. Because of the high prevalence of osteoporosis and the existence of modifiable risk factors, early diagnosis, prevention, and treatment strategies are warranted to prevent fractures.

▶ Clinical Findings

A. Symptoms and Signs

Fractures are the most important consequence of osteoporosis and occur most frequently in the thoracic and lumbar vertebral bodies, proximal hip, pelvis, proximal humerus, and distal radius (Table 51–4). Yearly, 1.5 million fractures occur due to osteoporosis just in the United States. Forty percent of white women older than 50, the typical age of menopause, will sustain an osteoporotic fracture in their lifetime. Many clinical complications are associated with osteoporotic fractures (Table 51–5). Having a prior fracture as an adult doubles the fracture risk and is partially independent of BMD. Fractures at the hip cause the greatest morbidity and mortality and give rise to the highest direct costs for health services. Hip fracture incidence increases exponentially with age, and there are currently 300,000 hospitalizations for hip fractures yearly in the United States. Ninety-five percent of these hip fractures occur from simply falling sideways and up to 36% lead to death within 1 year, especially in men. Another 50% of patients suffering a hip fracture will not be able to return home and live independently. Osteoporotic fractures may also reduce chest expansion and lead to compression of the abdominal cavity promoting early satiety, weight loss, and constipation.

1. Postmenopausal osteoporosis—Bone loss in women begins in the third and fourth decades but accelerates for 5–10 years surrounding menopause, the period called "perimenopause." Postmenopausal osteoporosis results from an imbalance between bone formation and bone resorption induced by estrogen deficiency, such that resorption predominates over formation. Many studies over the last two decades have defined roles for T-cell activation and proinflammatory cytokines including interleukin (IL)-1, IL-4, Il-6, IL-17, tumor necrosis factor-α (TNF-α), interferon-γ (IFN-γ), receptor activator of nuclear factor κB ligand (RANKL), and tumor growth factor-β (TGF-β), in driving postmenopausal bone loss. Following the increased rate of bone loss immediately surrounding menopause, a less aggressive phase of

bone loss continues into the eighth and ninth decades (see Figure 51–1). Aging-related factors including reduced osteoprogenitor population, nutritional deficiencies, and malabsorption play a role in this later phase of bone loss. However, at least 10–20% of postmenopausal women have additional secondary causes for their bone loss beyond the estrogen deficient state of menopause (Table 51–6).

2. Male osteoporosis—Only 10–20% of men with low BMD have primary osteoporosis. Fracture or loss of height are typical indications for providers to assess for osteoporosis in men. In contrast to women who have a relatively abrupt loss of estrogen production, men experience a gradual decline in testosterone production with age. How age-related declines in testosterone contribute to age-related loss of BMD remains controversial. It is clear, however, that replacing testosterone does not restore BMD to "normal," even in hypogonadal men. Men with a history of prostate cancer may be treated with long-acting gonadotropin-releasing hormone agonists and androgen blockers. These drugs accelerate bone loss, but appropriate treatment suppresses bone turnover, halts bone loss, and reduces future fractures.

At least 80% of men with osteoporosis have one or more secondary causes of bone loss (see Table 51–6). Additional risk factors for low BMD in men include history of chronic lung disease, antiepileptic drugs, peptic ulcer disease, caffeine intake, inability to walk heel-to-toe, and a fall in the last year. Several additional factors significantly magnify hip fracture risk in men including age more than 75 years, low dietary protein intake, divorce, tall stature, hypoglycemic agents, Parkinson disease, inability to rise from a chair without using the upper extremities to push off, and decreased cognitive function. For instance, compared to an 80-year-old nonsmoking man who eats a balanced diet and is not diabetic, an 80-year-old man who smokes, eats a low protein diet, and is diabetic has five times the risk of hip fracture even at the same BMD.

3. Glucocorticoid-induced osteoporosis—Chronic glucocorticoids are commonly prescribed for a host of allergic and inflammatory conditions. One percent of all adults and 3% of older adults in the United States are treated with glucocorticoids. Glucocorticoids have multiple deleterious effects on the musculoskeletal system. They lead to increases in RANKL-driven osteoclastogenesis, with rapid bone loss in the first 6 months of therapy. They also cause accelerated apoptosis of OCYs, leading to osteolysis that promotes early fracture even before the BMD has declined. Furthermore, they inhibit OB function, preventing the generation of new bone. Overall, the effect is that bone resorption is not appropriately followed by bone formation resulting in loss of trabeculae and BMD. Once glucocorticoids are discontinued, OBs replace some but usually not all of the bone tissue lost during glucocorticoid treatment. It is difficult to rebuild bone microarchitecture; therefore, prevention of bone loss should be the primary strategy in adults. Fortunately, in

Table 51–3. Drugs that increase fracture risk.

Drug Class	Mechanism of Action	Reversibility on Medication Discontinuation	Screening Recommendation	Management Recommendation	Alternative Medication
Glucocorticoids (GC)	Decreased bone formation and increased bone resorption	Fracture risk decreases to baseline within 2 years	Fracture risk analysis with dual-energy x-ray absorptiometry (DXA) or Fracture Risk Assessment Tool (FRAX) Monitor vit D and calcium levels	Bisphosphonate, parathyroid hormone (PTH) analogs, denosumab according to fracture risk DXA scan every 2 years	Limit dose and duration of GC Use steroid-sparing Immunosuppressive drugs
Proton pump inhibitors (PPI)	Suspected due to decreased intestinal absorption of Ca^{2+}	Fracture risk reverses within 1 year of stopping the drug	No recommendation	If possible, avoid PPI or use with bisphosphonates	H_2-blockers
Antiepileptics (AED)	Suspected due to inactivation of vitamin (vit) D	Unknown	Fracture risk analysis with DXA or FRAX Monitor vit D and calcium levels q6–12 months	For non–enzyme-inducing AEDs, give 1000–1200 IU vit D For enzyme-inducing AEDs, give 2000–4000 IU vit D daily Bisphosphonates in postmenopausal women and men aged >50	Newer agents like levetiracetam
Medroxy-progestrone acetate (MPA)	Reduced estrogen level leading to increased bone resorption	Partial to full recovery of bone loss at spine and hip	DXA scan controversial in this premenopausal population Monitor vit D and calcium levels	Limit therapy to 2–3 years No data on bisphosphonates prophylaxis and is currently not recommended	Oral hormonal contraceptives, low-dose estrogen replacement with depot-medroxyprogesterone acetate (MPA), other birth control methods
Aromatase inhibitors	Reduced estrogen production leading to increased bone resorption	Unknown	Fracture risk analysis with DXA or FRAX Monitor vit D and calcium levels	Bisphosphonates for moderate- to high-risk patients Denosumab as alternative DXA scan every 2 years while on treatment	Not applicable.
Gonadotropin-releasing hormone (GnRH) agonists	Prevent the production of luteinizing hormone (LH) and follicle-stimulating hormone (FSH), thereby decreasing testosterone and estradiol leading to increased bone resorption	May be reversed in 2 years depending on dose and duration of therapy	Fracture risk analysis with DXA or FRAX Monitor vit D and calcium levels	Bisphosphonates, denosumab, selective estrogen receptor modulators for moderate- to high-risk patients DXA scan every 2 years while on treatment	Second line: androgen receptor blockers In men without bone metastasis
Serotonin selective reuptake inhibitors	Increases brain-serotonin-dependent rise in sympathetic output suppressing bone formation and increasing resorption	Probable	Fracture risk analysis with DXA or FRAX for patients with other osteoporosis risk factors Monitor vit D and calcium levels	Calcium and vit D supplementation Consider propranolol to counteract increase in sympathetic tone	Alternative classes of antidepressants
Thiazolidinedione	Decreased bone formation	Unknown	Fracture risk analysis with DXA or FRAX for patients with other osteoporosis risk factors Monitor vit D and calcium levels	Avoid in established osteoporosis No data for prevention	Metformin Sulfonylureas Insulin
Calcineurin inhibitors	Excessive osteoclasts and bone resorption with glucocorticoids	unknown	DXA/FRAX analysis prior to kidney transplant Monitor vit D and calcium levels	DXA prior to and every 2 years post organ transplant Bisphosphonates for T-score < −2.0	Other immunosuppressants
Heparin	Osteoblast inhibition with decreased bone formation; increased bone resorption	Near-complete reversal of bone mineral density (BMD)	No published recommendations	No published recommendations	Use low-molecular-weight heparin or direct oral anticoagulants
Warfarin	Decreases bone mineralization by altering vit K–dependent gamma-carboxylation of glutamate	Unknown	No published recommendations	No published recommendations	Use direct oral anticoagulants if clinically indicated

Adapted from Panday K, Gona A, Humphrey MB. Medication-induced osteoporosis: screening and treatment strategies. *Ther Adv Musculoskelet Dis.* 2014;6:185-202.

Table 51–4. Osteoporosis-associated fragility fractures.

Fragility fractures are precipitated by low-energy injuries, such as a fall from a standing height. They can then manifest as chronic pain, disability, and reduce quality and quantity of life. Major skeletal sites affected include:

Vertebra	• This is the most common osteoporotic fracture, occurring in both men and women with incidence increasing with age (ie, the risk of sustaining a new vertebral fracture is about 2 times higher at 75 years of age than at 65 years of age) • May present with severe pain, requiring hospitalization or asymptomatically (about 2/3 diagnosed incidentally on imaging). Can have loss of spine mobility, loss of height, and disability • Fractures in the midthoracic spine can result in mild reduction of pulmonary function and kyphosis with increased occiput to wall • Thoracolumbar fractures can result in decreased volumes between the ribs to the pelvis, causing crowding of internal organs that may present as premature satiety, reduced appetite, abdominal pain, constipation, and distension • Several psychological manifestations occur including poor self-image, social isolation, and depression • The probability is 5-fold for subsequent vertebral fractures and 2- to 3-fold for fractures at other sites
Proximal Femur	• One of the most disastrous consequences of osteoporosis, with incidence increasing exponentially with age in both men and women • Associated with 15–30% increased mortality within 1 year, affecting more males than females • A substantial number of people with hip fractures experience a second hip fracture, which is characterized by higher mortality than the first fracture • 2 main determinants: low BMD and increased risk of falls
Distal Radius	• Most frequent osteoporotic fractures in women and one of the earliest manifestations of osteoporosis (much lower incidence in males) • Incidence increases in early postmenopausal years and then stabilizes • Complex regional pain disorder is a common complication of this type of fracture
Proximal Humerus	• Increased incidence after the age of 50 (women > men)

Other common sites for fragility fractures include the ribs, pelvis, clavicle, and tibia.
Remember if any of these fractures occurs before the age of 50 (with or without trauma), it is necessary to assess for underlying osteoporosis.

Table 51–5. Clinical complications of osteoporosis.

Loss of height from vertebral fractures
Kyphosis from vertebral fractures
Vertebral fractures cause chronic back pain
Thoracic vertebral fractures lead to restrictive lung capacity
2.5-fold increased risk of future fractures after hip fracture
Hip fractures are associated with 14–36% increased mortality at 1 year
50% of hip fracture patients never achieve their previous functional status
20–50% of hip fracture patients require long-term nursing care
Fractures lead to social isolation, low self-esteem, and depression

younger patients and children, the risk of fractures induced by glucocorticoids rapidly declines when glucocorticoids are discontinued.

Approximately 50% of patients receiving long-term glucocorticoid therapy will suffer a fracture. The spine is particularly sensitive to glucocorticoids and fracture risk increases with doses as low as 2.5 mg daily (Figure 51–4). Doses higher than 7.5 mg daily increase the risk of spine fractures fivefold and double the risk of hip fracture. The patients most vulnerable to glucocorticoids-induced osteoporosis are postmenopausal women, those on greater than 7.5 mg daily, or those with a cumulative dose of glucocorticoid greater than 5 g yearly. Many diseases for which patients receive long-term glucocorticoids, such as rheumatoid arthritis or inflammatory bowel disease, are themselves deleterious to bone.

B. Clinical Evaluation

The evaluation for osteoporosis begins with a clinical fracture risk assessment (see Table 51–2). When taking the medical history, medication use (especially glucocorticoids; see Table 51–3), smoking, alcohol intake (>3 units daily), dietary calcium intake, a personal history of fracture, age at menopause, family history of osteoporosis and fractures, and a diagnosis of rheumatoid arthritis should be assessed carefully. The physical examination should focus on height (and any loss), weight, the presence of bone pain or deformity (such as kyphosis), and signs of anemia, hyperthyroidism, hypercortisolism, malnutrition, and other disorders that cause secondary forms of osteoporosis (see Table 51–6).

The FRAX tool should be used early in the evaluation of osteoporosis, even before a DXA is obtained. For any patient not on glucocorticoids, those with a risk of major osteoporotic fracture within 10 years greater than or equal to 20% or risk of hip fracture risk within 10 years greater than or equal to 3% by FRAX analysis should be offered antiosteoporosis treatment in additional to counseling on lifestyle changes. Risk assessment for glucocorticoid-induced osteoporosis also begins with the FRAX assessment, which factors in glucocorticoid daily doses less than 7.5 mg daily. The

Table 51–6. Secondary causes of osteoporosis.

Dietary/Lifestyle	Endocrine	Gastrointestinal	Hematologic	Medications	Others
Vitamin D deficiency	Hypogonadism	Celiac disease	Multiple myeloma	Glucocorticoids	Rheumatoid arthritis
Low body mass index	Thyrotoxicosis	Gastric bypass	Sickle cell disease	Heparin	Ankylosing spondylitis
Low calcium intake	Cushing syndrome	Chronic pancreatitis	Leukemia/Lymphomas	Proton pump inhibitors	Systemic lupus erythematosus
Immobilization	Hyperparathyroidism	Inflammatory bowel disease	Thalassemia	Anticonvulsants	Homocystinuria
Excess vitamin A	Type 1 diabetes mellitus	Primary biliary cirrhosis	Systemic mastocytosis	Selective serotonin reuptake inhibitors	End-stage renal disease
Drug addiction	Acromegaly	Intestinal malabsorption	Hemachromatosis	Warfarin	Renal tubular acidosis

FRAX underestimates the risk of osteoporotic fracture at higher doses of glucocorticoids, however. For patients taking glucocorticoids greater than or equal to 7.5 mg daily, the FRAX major osteoporotic risk should be increased by 15% (multiply by 1.15) and the risk of hip fracture increased by 20% (multiply by 1.2). Treatment recommendations for glucocorticoid-induced osteoporosis vary depending on age, dose of glucocorticoids, and risk stratification, as discussed in detail later in this chapter.

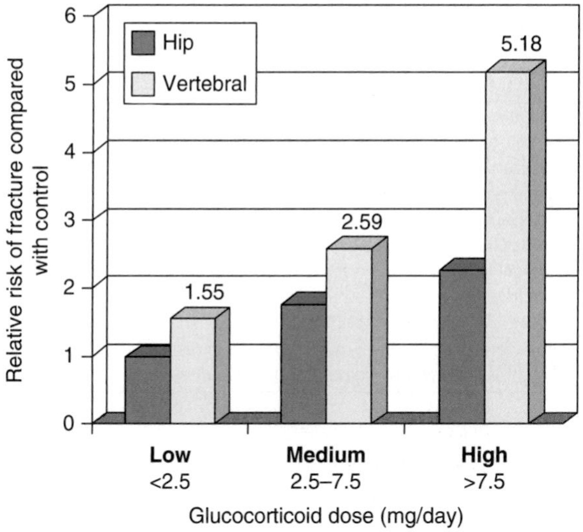

C. Laboratory Findings

Laboratory evaluation for and secondary causes of osteoporosis are essential to the evaluation (Table 51–7). Vitamin D

▲ **Figure 51–4.** Glucocorticoid use and fracture risk in users 18 years and older. The relative risk of fractures of the hip (dark blue) or vertebrae (light blue) were compared in 244,000 glucocorticoid (GC) users and controls stratified by glucocorticoid dose (mg/day). Even low doses of GC less than 2.5 mg/day for more than 90 days increases the risk of vertebral fracture. Higher-dose GC significantly increases the risk of hip and vertebral fractures. (Adapted from Van Staa TP, Leufkens HG, Abenhaim L, Zhang B, Cooper C. Oral corticosteroids and fracture risk: relationship to daily and cumulative doses. *Rheumatology.* 2000;39(12):1383-1389.)

Table 51–7. Clinical laboratory studies to evaluate for secondary causes of osteoporosis.

Basic Laboratory Testing
CBC
CMP, including creatinine, liver function tests, and alkaline phosphatase
Magnesium
Phosphorus
TSH and free T_4
25-hydroxy-vitamin D
PTH
Total testosterone
Further Tests to Consider in Select Patients
24-h urine collection for calcium, sodium, and creatinine excretion (calcium malabsorption)
Erythrocyte sedimentation rate (multiple myeloma)
Tissue transglutaminase (celiac disease)
SPEP and free κ and λ light chains (multiple myeloma)
Urinary free cortisol (adrenal hypersecretion)
Serum tryptase/urine N-methylhistidine (mastocytosis)
Bone marrow aspiration and biopsy (bone marrow disease)
Genetic testing (rare metabolic bone diseases)
Biochemical bone turnover markers:
Resorption markers: s-CTX, NTX
Formation markers: s-PINP

CBC, complete blood count; CMP, comprehensive metabolic panel; NTX, urinary N-telopeptide; PTH, parathyroid hormone; s-CTX, serum C-terminal telopeptide type 1 collagen; s-PINP, serum procollagen type 1 N-terminal propeptide; T_4, thyroxine; TSH, thyroid-stimulating hormone.

deficiency, defined as blood levels less than 30 ng/mL, is present in nearly 40% of the general population in the United States. Vitamin D deficiency is extremely common among elderly patients and contributes to bone loss because it interferes with the absorption of calcium and phosphorus, thereby reducing mineralization of new bone matrix. Vitamin D levels less than 15 ng/mL are associated with osteomalacia and very low BMD. Low vitamin D, low calcium and phosphorous, elevated parathyroid hormone (PTH), and alkaline phosphatase should alert the physician to the diagnosis of osteomalacia.

In the United States, primary hyperparathyroidism is also common and increases with age, with a mean prevalence of 66 per 100,000 in women and 25 per 100,000 in men. Serum calcium, albumin, and 25-hydroxy vitamin D levels constitute an adequate screen for this disorder. Another common cause of osteoporotic fractures is multiple myeloma, which often presents with bone pain, pathologic fractures, or anemia. If the BMD is remarkably low for age (ie, a low Z-score) or if low BMD is accompanied by unexplained anemia or elevated erythrocyte sedimentation rate, serum and urine protein electrophoreses should be evaluated for the purpose of excluding multiple myeloma.

Markers of bone turnover are not typically included in the first-line evaluation of osteoporosis due to significant analytical and biological variation influenced by circadian rhythms, menstrual cycle, the seasons, fasting and food intake, and exercise. However, they may be helpful in monitoring response to antiosteoporotic therapy, including the assessment of medication compliance and determinations of the sufficiency of drug absorption. Bone turnover markers include collagen breakdown products in urine (N-terminal telopeptide of type 1 collagen [NTX], C-terminal telopeptide of type 1 collagen [CTX], and pyridinoline cross-links) as well as serum markers of NTX, CTX, and tartrate resistant acid phosphatase 5 (TRACP5b). Bone formation products in the serum include osteocalcin, bone-specific alkaline phosphatase (BSAP), and N-terminal propeptide of type 1 collagen (PINP). Serum markers are best collected early in the morning while fasting and urine markers collected in the second fasting urine the day. Markers of bone turnover are often elevated in postmenopausal osteoporosis, hyperthyroidism, hyperparathyroidism, and Paget disease. Resorption markers should decline approximately 50% with antiresorptive drugs. In contrast, PTH analogs increase both markers of bone formation and bone resorption.

D. Imaging Evaluation

Several imaging modalities exist to diagnose osteoporosis and monitor response to treatment (Table 51–8). DXA is the most widespread imaging modality and is the study of choice to assess BMD of the lumbar spine and hip. DXA reports often include both T- and Z-scores (see Figure 51–1). A **T-score** relates the BMD of the patient to peak bone mass for race and

Table 51–8. Imaging for osteoporosis diagnosis and for monitoring antiosteoporosis treatment.

DXA (dual-energy x-ray absorptiometry)
- Recommended testing: women ≥65 years of age and younger postmenopausal women at increased risk for bone loss and fracture based on fracture risk analysis
- NOT recommended in children, adolescents, healthy young men, or premenopausal women unless there is significant fracture history or there are specific risk factors for bone loss (ie, long-term glucocorticoid therapy)
- Sites: lumbar spine and proximal femur provide accurate and reproducible bone mineral density (BMD) measurements. Distal 1/3 of radius can also be used if other preferred sites cannot be assessed (ie, hip replacement)
- Results reported as grams of mineral/cm² of projected bone area. Converted to T- and Z-scores
- Follow-up DXA testing posttreatment recommended; however, no consensus on optimal frequency of monitoring

qCT (quantitative computed tomography)
- Measures volumetric bone density of the spine and hip
- Can analyze cortical and trabecular bone separately
- Useful in clinical research (to follow therapeutic responses to therapy, where large changes may be observed)
- Not recommended for screening (application of T-scores to predict risk of fracture has not been validated)
- Disadvantages: more expensive, greater radiation exposure compared to DXA

Ultrasound
- Quantitative heel ultrasound (the only validated measurement site in osteoporosis management) is as good a predictor of fractures as clinical risk factors for identifying patients at high risk for osteoporosis
- Does not measure BMD but rather the transmission of ultrasound through accessible limb bones or the reflectance of the ultrasound waves from the bone surface
- Advantages: lower expense, portability, and lack of radiation exposure
- Disadvantages: cannot be used for diagnostic classification (World Health Organization [WHO] criteria established based on BMD measurements by DXA) or for monitoring response to therapy (changes are too slow to be clinically useful)

gender (ie, a 20-year-old). A **Z-score**, which compares the BMD of the patient to that of persons of the same age, gender, and race, is used for children, teens, and younger men and women younger than 40 years. The T-score is the more useful determination clinically as it provides fracture risk. For operational purposes, the lower of the two T-scores (spine or hip) is used for making the diagnosis of osteopenia or osteoporosis. There is typically agreement between the T-scores at these two sites, but discordance can occur due to degenerative arthritis, disk disease, or aortic calcification, any of which can raise the BMD artificially. In such cases, only measurements of the hip and femoral neck should be used.

Obtaining a BMD measurement allows the clinician not only to grade the severity of osteoporosis but also to assess fracture risk as it provides assessment of vertebral compression fractures. Several studies have confirmed that the relative risk of fracture approximately doubles with each standard deviation below peak BMD (ie, a negative T-score) that a patient demonstrates. The combination of BMD measurement and the patient's age is an even more powerful predictor of fracture risk. The 10-year risk of several types of osteoporotic fractures is strongly related to age and BMD T-score, and age is a powerful risk factor in the FRAX calculator of absolute fracture risk (see Figure 51–3). Advanced age (over 70 years) dramatically increases the risks of vertebral and hip fractures (see Figures 51–2 and 51–3).

DXA is also utilized to monitor response to osteoporosis therapy, but there remains no solid consensus about how often to repeat testing. Recommendations range from annually to every 3 years. Many groups recommend repeat DXA 2 years after therapy is initiated, but more frequent testing might be warranted in patients receiving glucocorticoids or those suspected of noncompliance. A BMD that is stable or improving indicates an appropriate response to therapy. Fracture risk reduction occurs even in the absence of significant increases in BMD.

DIFFERENTIAL DIAGNOSIS OF FRAGILITY FRACTURES

The differential diagnosis of a fragility fractures includes osteoporosis associated with any secondary cause or medication, osteomalacia from nutritional or inherited causes of vitamin D deficiency or hypophosphatemia, multiple myeloma or other cancer-related pathologic fracture, fibrous dysplasia, or desmoid tumors of the bone. Low BMD measurement in the absence of a fragility fracture has a narrow differential including osteoporosis and osteomalacia. Osteomalacia causes low BMD due to defective mineralization of the new bone matrix, which is termed osteoid. Osteomalacia results from a number of causes, including severe vitamin D deficiency, X-linked hypophosphatemia, or autosomal dominant hypophosphotemic rickets. In osteomalacia, the DXA typically reveals osteopenia with a T-score −1 to −2.5. Patients with osteomalacia may also have nocturnal bone pain, develop nonunion fractures, and have muscle weakness and difficulty walking with a waddling gait. They will have elevations in alkaline phosphatase and PTH but very low 25-hydroxyvitamin D concentrations (<15 ng/mL).

TREATMENT OF OSTEOPOROSIS

1. Lifestyle Modifications

Lifestyle modifications should be implemented in all patients wishing to prevent bone loss or reduce fractures. Patients should be encouraged to discontinue smoking and alcohol consumption. Patients should be prescribed a weight-bearing exercise program. Controversy exists concerning the type, nature, frequency, and length of exercise required to improve BMD, to lower fracture risk, and to reduce the risk of falls. Systematic reviews find benefit with combination exercise programs including weight-bearing and progressive resistance training three times weekly for preventing BMD loss. Tai chi has been shown to reduce the risk of falls. Exercise improves well-being and neuromuscular coordination, which can help condition reflexes to respond better to falls. Hip protectors reduce the incidence of hip fractures in frail elderly patients in nursing care or residential settings but have poor acceptance and compliance by patients.

2. Nutritional Interventions: Calcium & Vitamin D Supplements, Protein Intake

Daily adequate calcium, vitamin D, protein intake and good sun exposure are important for the maintenance of bone and muscle functions. Calcium plus vitamin D supplementation have a modest impact on fracture prevention in the elderly. In general, 25-hydroxyvitamin D serum levels should be repleted at greater than or equal to 30 ng/mL before starting antiosteoporosis medications. For individuals older than 50 years, the recommended daily intakes of calcium and vitamin D are at least 1000 mg and 800 IU, respectively. Dietary products fortified with calcium and vitamin D (eg, yogurt, cheese, milk, orange juice) are preferred over the use of supplements.

For postmenopausal women, older men at risk for fracture, and glucocorticoid-induced osteoporosis, 1200 mg of elemental calcium per day with greater than or equal to 800 IU vitamin D daily are recommended (Table 51–9). Protein intake is also important for maintenance of muscle and bone; however, protein intake tends to decrease with age. There is a positive association between protein intake and BMD with associated reductions in bone resorption markers. Improved protein intake combined with resistance training exercise leads to greater muscle mass gains that also improve bone strength.

3. Pharmacologic Therapies

The National Osteoporosis Foundation has published recommendations for the management and prevention of osteoporosis (see Table 51–9). Agents that are effective for treating osteoporosis and approved in the United States include *antiresorptives* such as bisphosphonates, denosumab, and selective estrogen response modulators; and *anabolic* agents including teriparatide, abaloparatide, and romosozumab (Table 51–10). Each drug has varying degrees of BMD improvement and fracture reduction that may be site specific (Table 51–11). All agents improve spine BMD and prevent new vertebral fractures, but neither teriparatide nor raloxifene has been shown to reduce hip fractures.

Hormone therapy (conjugated estrogen with or without progestin) has also been shown to reduce fractures in the Women's Health Initiative (WHI) trial, but the women

Table 51–9. National Osteoporosis Foundation recommendations for management and prevention of osteoporosis.

1. Obtain history with pertinent clinical risk factor and history of fractures and falls
2. Perform a physical exam and obtain diagnostic studies to diagnose or eliminate secondary etiologies for osteoporosis
3. Modify diet and calcium/vitamin D supplements, lifestyle (avoid tobacco smoking and excessive alcohol), increase exercise
4. FRAX analysis to determine 10-year risk of hip and major osteoporotic fractures
5. Start therapy in patients with hip or vertebral (clinical or morphometric) fractures
6. Treat patients with BMD T-score ≤2.5 at femoral neck or spine by DXA
7. Treat osteopenic (T-score between −1.0 and −2.5) postmenopausal women and men aged ≥50 who have a 10-year hip fracture probability of ≥3% or a 10-year major osteoporosis-related fracture probability of ≥20% based on the FRAX model
8. Consider physical and occupational therapy evaluations for gait training, walking aides, balance training, and weight-bearing exercise
9. Reevaluate patients not meeting treatment thresholds every 2–3 years when medically appropriate
10. Monitor BMD with DXA after initiating therapy in 2 years or more frequently when medically appropriate
11. Obtain vertebral imaging to evaluate for new vertebral fractures if patient has height loss, new back pain, postural change, suspicious finding on chest x-ray, or at time of drug holiday to ensure silent fractures have occurred

BMD, bone mineral density; DXA, dual-energy x-ray absorptiometry; FRAX, Fracture Risk Assessment Tool.
Data from *Clinician's Guide to Prevention and Treatment of Osteoporosis* (updated 2014). Accessed at https://link.springer.com/article/10.1007%2Fs00198-014-2794-2.

treated with hormones in that trial experienced an increased number of cardiovascular events and had an increased risk of breast cancer, thereby limiting the use of hormone therapy for osteoporosis. Each osteoporosis treatment comes with potential side effects, and each patient's individual risk factors should be considered in choosing osteoporosis treatments (Table 51–12).

Prevention and treatment of osteoporosis in woman of childbearing age is challenging due to effects of medications on the fetal skeleton or development. Most antiosteoporosis drugs are not approved for premenopausal women except in the setting of glucocorticoid-induced osteoporosis. Even in this setting, patients should be encouraged to use effective contraception due to risk to the fetus. Two oral bisphosphonates (alendronate and risedronate) and teriparatide have been approved for use in premenopausal women receiving glucocorticoids. Bisphosphonates accumulate in the fetal skeleton and theoretically may alter fetal

skeletal development; however, the majority of case reports and studies including women who became pregnant while taking bisphosphonates have not found adverse fetal or maternal outcomes. Women younger than 25 years on glucocorticoids may require antiosteoporosis medications but should have documentation of closed epiphyses by radiography before use of teriparatide. However, it is unclear if additional antiosteoporosis medications are required to maintain bone improvements after cessation of teriparatide in premenopausal women.

Denosumab is appealing as an option due to lack of accumulation in the fetal skeleton and infrequent dosing; however, it is associated with fetal anomalies in animal studies and therefore is contraindicated in pregnancy. Romosozumab crosses the placenta and causes adverse fetal outcomes in animal studies, so it also is not approved in premenopausal women. None of these medications is approved for use in pregnant or lactating women.

A. Antiresorptive Drugs

1. Bisphosphonates—Bisphosphonates are analogs of inorganic phosphate that are deposited into newly formed bone and inhibit bone resorption by blocking OC activity. Currently, alendronate, risedronate, ibandronate, and zoledronic acid are approved for the prevention and treatment of osteoporosis in the United States. Given their efficacy, low cost, and good safety profile, bisphosphonates are the most frequently prescribed medications for the treatment of osteoporosis. Meta-analysis shows that oral (alendronate and risedronate) and intravenous (zoledronic acid) bisphosphonates increase BMD and reduce vertebral, hip, and nonvertebral osteoporotic fractures (see Table 51–11). All four agents are approved for postmenopausal, male, and glucocorticoid-induced osteoporosis. Dosing and approved indications for these agents are shown in Table 51–10. Treatment with bisphosphonates for osteoporosis is typically 2–3 years but may be continue to 10 years for patients at high risk for fracture as fracture reduction persists. However, the rare side effects of osteonecrosis of the jaw and atypical femur fractures (subtrochanteric) become more prevalent after 5 years of therapy. Patients who have had a good response to bisphosphonates for 2–5 years and are low risk for fracture are encouraged to take a "drug holiday" for up to 5 years. During this holiday, a DXA is repeated every 1–2 years to determine the BMD, and bisphosphonates may be restarted if the BMD is dropping rapidly (>4% in a year) or reaches the pretreatment baseline.

Adverse effects of bisphosphonates at doses used to treat osteoporosis include esophageal irritation, esophagitis, and musculoskeletal pain (see Table 51–12). Some, but not all, of the recent epidemiology analyses have suggested an association between bisphosphonate use and esophageal cancer, but the numbers are small and the

Table 51–10. Management of postmenopausal, male, and glucocorticoid-induced osteoporosis.

Management Strategy	Recommendation
Lifestyle modifications	Discontinue tobacco Discontinue alcohol intake Wear hip protector Exercise regularly
Nutritional interventions	Increase dietary calcium intake to 1000 mg elemental calcium per day for prevention of osteoporosis in premenopausal women and men Increase dietary calcium intake to 1200 mg elemental calcium per day for postmenopausal women, older men, and patients taking glucocorticoids for long term Vitamin D intake: ≥800 IU daily for older men and postmenopausal women and for patients taking glucocorticoids for long term. Ensure 25-hydroxyvitamin D serum levels at ≥30 ng/mL Ensure adequate daily protein intake (1.0–1.2 g/kg/BW)
Pharmacologic therapies	**Bisphosphonates:** 3- to 5-year treatment and consider drug holiday, continue therapy for high-risk patients Alendronate orally 5–10 mg daily or 35–70 mg weekly. Lower dosing for prevention, higher dosing for treatment of postmenopausal, male, and glucocorticoid-induced osteoporosis. Risedronate orally 5 mg daily, 35 mg weekly, or 150 mg monthly for prevention and treatment of postmenopausal osteoporosis, 35 mg weekly for males, and 5 mg daily glucocorticoid-induced osteoporosis. Ibandronate orally 150 mg monthly for prevention and treatment or 3 mg every 3 months intravenously for treatment of postmenopausal osteoporosis and glucocorticoid-induced osteoporosis. Zoledronic acid 5 mg yearly intravenously for prevention and treatment of postmenopausal osteoporosis and for treatment of male and glucocorticoid-induced osteoporosis. **PTH analogs:** limited to 2-year treatment Teriparatide (PTH 1–34) 20 mcg subcutaneous injection daily for postmenopausal, male and glucocorticoid-induced osteoporosis, especially in patients at high risk for fractures, limit 2 years. (At discontinuation, start antiresorptive therapy to prevent bone loss and fracture.) Abaloparatide (PTHrP 1–34) 80 mcg subcutaneous injection daily for postmenopausal osteoporosis with high fracture risk or prior fracture. (At discontinuation, start antiresorptive therapy to prevent bone loss and fracture.) **SERMs:** up to 5-year treatment Raloxifene 60 mg/day orally for postmenopausal and glucocorticoid-induced osteoporosis. (Use in select patients due to increased risk of deep vein thrombosis and death due to stroke.) **RANKL inhibitor:** up to 10-year treatment with no drug holiday recommended Denosumab 60 mg by subcutaneous injection every 6 months for treatment of postmenopausal women, male, glucocorticoid-induced osteoporosis, androgen-deprivation–induced bone loss in men, and aromatase inhibitor-induced bone loss in women. (Consider alternative antiosteoporosis therapy when denosumab is discontinued to prevent vertebral fractures due to rapid bone loss.) **Sclerostin inhibitor:** limited to 12 monthly doses due to loss of efficacy Romosozumab two consecutive subcutaneous injections (105 mg each) per month for postmenopausal osteoporosis with prior fracture or have failed or intolerant to other available therapies (Increases risk of myocardial infarction, stroke, or cardiovascular death in patients with prior CVS event.)

BW, body weight; CVS, cardiovascular system; PTH, parathyroid hormone; PTHrP, parathyroid hormone–related peptide; RANKL, receptor activator of nuclear factor κB ligand; SERMs, selective estrogen response modulators.

Table 51–11. Antiosteoporosis medication BMD gains and fracture reduction for postmenopausal osteoporosis.

Medication vs Placebo	Spine BMD Gain (%)	New Vertebral Fx RR (95% CI)	Hip Fx RR (95% CI)	Nonvertebral Fx RR (95% CI)
Alendronate	5–7%	0.56 (0.46–0.69)	0.47 (0.26–0.79)	0.85 (0.75–0.97)
Ibandronate	4–6%	0.51 (0.34–0.74)	NAE	NS
Risedronate	5–7%	0.62 (0.50–0.77)	0.74 (0.59–0.94)	0.81 (0.71–0.92)
Zoledronate	6–9%	0.30 (0.24–0.38)	0.59 (0.42–0.83)	0.75 (0.65–0.87)
Denosumab	3–6%	0.33 (0.26–0.41)	0.61 (0.37–0.98)	0.81 (0.69–0.96)
Raloxifene	1–3%	0.65 (0.54–0.78)	NS	NAE
Teriparatide	10–15%	0.35 (0.22–0.55)	NS	0.47 (0.25–0.88)
Abaloparatide	6–11%	0.14 (0.05–0.39)	NAE	0.50(0.28–0.85)
Romosozumab	9–11%	0.27 (0.16–0.47)	NAE	NS

BMD, bone mineral density; CI, confidence intervals; Fx, fracture; NAE, not adequately evaluated; NS, not significant; RR, relative risk.

Table 51–12. Complications of antiosteoporosis drugs.

Bisphosphonates	Oral: Esophageal reflux, esophagitis, and ulcers (avoid in esophageal disorders or after bariatric surgery)
	IV: Flu-like symptoms with 1st dose (low-grade fever, myalgias, arthralgias within 72 hours of infusion)
	Oral: Esophageal cancer; conflicting studies
	Eye inflammation (conjunctivitis, uveitis, scleritis, blurred vision)—rare
	Transient hypocalcemia (more common after IV dosing); at-risk patients have hypoparathyroidism, vitamin D deficiency, or inadequate calcium intake
	Atypical femur fractures (subtrochanteric); duration-dependent with median of 7 years; rare in <5 years of treatment, incidence 3–50 cases/100,000 person years for >7 years of treatment
	Jaw osteonecrosis; risk factors include IV formulation, invasive dental procedures, poor oral hygiene, cancer, glucocorticoids, smoking, diabetes, and immunosuppressive medications. Low risk for oral formulations 1–10 cases/100,000 person-years of treatment
	Renal impairment with IV formulations; risk factors creatinine clearance ≤35 mL/min and concurrent diuretic use
	Atrial fibrillation; conflicting studies
Selective estrogen receptor modulators	**Increase risk of VTE; avoid in patients with prior history of VTE**
	Increased risk of death due to stroke in women with documented coronary heart disease or major risks for coronary events
	Hot flashes
PTH analogs	**Osteosarcoma risk**; avoid in Paget disease, bone metastases, and prior radiation to the skeleton
	Avoid in hyperparathyroidism, granulomatous disorders due to hypercalcemia
	Avoid in children and young adults due to premature closure of epiphyses
	Transient hypercalcemia up to 10-fold above normal postinjection for 4 hours
	Muscle cramps
	Hypercalciuria; avoid in patients with nephrolithiasis or persistent hypercalciuria
	Increased serum uric acid (may precipitate gouty attacks)
	Orthostatic hypotension, typically within 4 hours of injection
	Tachycardia (particularly with abaloparatide)
	Avoid in pregnancy an premenopausal women
RANKL inhibitors	Hypocalcemia, risks include CrCl <30 mL/min, not on calcium supplementation
	Skin rash/dermatitis
	Hypersensitivity and anaphylaxis
	Musculoskeletal pain that may be severe
	Vertebral fractures within 3–18 months after discontinuation; begin bisphosphonate when RANKL inhibitor is discontinued especially if patient has a prior vertebral fracture
	Atypical femur fractures (subtrochanteric); concomitant glucocorticoids increase the risk
	Jaw osteonecrosis; risk factors include length of time and dose (high dose for cancer) of treatment
	Contraindicated in pregnancy; avoid pregnancy for 5 months after last dose
Sclerostin inhibitors	**Cardiovascular adverse events (cardiac ischemia, stroke, CV death); contraindicated in persons with prior MI or stroke in preceding year**
	Jaw osteonecrosis
	Atypical femur fractures
	Hypocalcemia; ensure adequate calcium and vitamin D; increased risk with CrCl <30 mL/min
	Hypersensitivity

Note: US warnings are in **bold**.
CrCl, creatinine clearance; CV, cardiovascular; IV, intravenous; MI, myocardial infarction; RANKL, receptor activator of nuclear factor κB ligand; VTE, venous thromboembolic events.

onset of the cancer is shortly after starting the medication, leading one to question the association. Similarly, some but not all studies have found an increased risk of atrial fibrillation associated with bisphosphonate use that occurs independently of treatment route. An acute-phase reaction characterized by fever, myalgias, arthralgias, and fatigue can also occur in ~10% of patients, particularly after the first intravenous dose of a bisphosphonate. Renal function should be checked prior to each intravenous dose of a bisphosphonate and periodically during oral therapy with these agents as the use of bisphosphonates in patients with estimated glomerular filtration rates less than 30 mL/min or 35 mL/min (depending on the specific agent) is not recommended.

B. Anti-RANK-Ligand Therapy

OC differentiation and activation are dependent on cytokine RANKL binding to its receptor RANK on mature OCs and their precursors. Neutralizing human monoclonal antibody, denosumab, prevents RANKL from stimulating RANK, thereby preventing the differentiation and survival of OCs for 6 months after each subcutaneous injection. Markers of bone turnover are promptly suppressed postsubcutaneous injection of 60 mg denosumab and 1–2 years of therapy significantly decreases risk of vertebral, hip, and nonvertebral fractures while improving BMD (see Table 51–11). Dosing and approved indications for denosumab are shown in Table 51–10. Continued use of denosumab for up to 10 years is safe and provides increasing BMD gains, unlike bisphosphonates that plateau in 3–5 years. However, BMD gains from denosumab are rapidly lost after discontinuation and may lead to vertebral fractures within 3–18 months of denosumab discontinuation, with prior vertebral fracture being the greatest risk factor. Bisphosphonates or other antiosteoporosis therapy for 1–2 years after denosumab discontinuation are now recommended to help stabilize the denosumab-induced BMD gains and to prevent vertebral fractures following discontinuation of denosumab. In clinical practice, denosumab offers an advantage over bisphosphonates in that it is not contraindicated when renal function is impaired and is conveniently administered twice yearly by injection ensuring full absorption of the active medication. Denosumab has been used successfully in patients with rheumatic disorders receiving glucocorticoids or other immunosuppressants without an increased risk of serious infections.

Side effects of denosumab are generally mild with eczema and cellulitis occurring more frequently in treated patients compared to placebo (see Table 51–12). Hypocalcemia with a nadir at 10 days postinjection occurs uniformly and may be severe in patients with renal disease. Similar to bisphosphonates, severe musculoskeletal pain as well as hypersensitivity reactions may occur. Denosumab is contraindicated in pregnancy and should be used with caution in

premenopausal women using effective birth control. Pregnancy should be delayed at least 5 months after the last dose of denosumab.

1. Selective estrogen response modulators—Raloxifene is a selective estrogen response modulator (SERM) that acts as an estrogen agonist or antagonist depending on the target tissue. Raloxifene capitalizes on the benefits of estrogen in bone while strongly diminishing the impact of estrogen on cardiovascular and breast cancer risks. Three-year duration of raloxifene therapy in postmenopausal women has modest but significant increases in lumbar spine and femoral neck BMD with reductions in vertebral fractures (see Table 51–11). However, the overall incidence of nonvertebral fractures was unchanged compared to placebo, and there was no significant impact on hip fractures. Raloxifene has the benefit of providing protection from breast cancer (relative risk 0.3; 95% confidence interval [CI]: 0.2–0.6) in high-risk patients.

Mild adverse side effects that occur in women taking raloxifene include hot flashes, leg cramps, edema, and a flulike syndrome. Unfortunately, life-threatening adverse effects occur with raloxifene. Raloxifene induces a significant increase in venous thromboembolic events compared to placebo (relative risk 3.1; 95% CI: 1.5–6.2), especially in patients with a prior clotting event. Additionally, for women with a prior history of coronary heart disease or with major risk factors for coronary disease, raloxifene is associated with an increased risk of death due to stroke, although stroke incidence does not increase. The Food and Drug Administration (FDA) has placed boxed warnings for these complications on product labeling. In clinical practice, raloxifene is useful in younger postmenopausal women who have less severe osteoporosis and are at lower risk for hip fracture or in postmenopausal women with significant breast cancer risks.

C. Adverse Events with Antiresorptive Agents

Two rare but serious side effects may occur in the setting of antiresorptive therapies including osteonecrosis of the jaw and atypical femur (subtrochanteric) fractures. In the doses used to treat osteoporosis, the complication of osteonecrosis of the jaw (painful or painless exposed bone) is very rare with oral bisphosphonate use, occurring at a frequency of ~1/10,000–1/100,000. However, with more potent bisphosphonates (zoledronate > ibandronate > risedronate > alendronate) and increasing duration of treatment (>5 years), these lesions are more frequently seen. The highest risk for osteonecrosis of the jaw occurs in patients receiving high dose, monthly antiresorptive therapies for malignant disease such as bone metastases; here the risk is 10 times higher and approaches 1% of treated patients. Osteonecrosis of the jaw often presents after a dental extraction or in the setting of poorly fitting dentures, heals slowly, and can progress to infection and fistula formation along with loss of oral function in the most severe cases. Risk factors for osteonecrosis of the jaw include diabetes with neuropathy, concomitant glucocorticoid or immunosuppressant use, and smoking. Osteonecrosis of the jaw also occurs in patients treated with denosumab and romosozumab. To help prevent osteonecrosis of the jaw, patients treated with bisphosphonates, denosumab, or romosozumab should have regular dental exams every 3 months, aggressive management of oral infections, and root canals to avoid tooth extractions.

Atypical femur fractures are also rarely seen in association with bisphosphonate treatment of osteoporosis. These fractures occur in the subtrochanteric region (5 cm distal to the lesser trochanter of the femur) or in the shaft of the femur. These fractures are noncomminuted and frequently bilateral and often present with the prodrome of thigh pain for weeks to months before the fracture presents clinically. Atypical femur fractures are rare, but antiresorptive treatment duration for more than 5 years increases the risk. Frequency estimates are 1.78/100,000 for 2 years of treatment, 38.9/100,000 if treated for 6–8 years, and 100/100,000 for more than 10 years of treatment. Atypical femur fractures are also reported in patients treated for osteoporosis with denosumab and romosozumab.

4. Anabolic Agents

A. Parathyroid Hormone Analogs

Two PTH analogs are approved by the FDA for the treatment of postmenopausal, male, and glucocorticoid-induced osteoporosis. When administered daily in low doses, PTH produces anabolic effects on the skeleton by stimulating significantly more bone formation than bone resorption. Teriparatide (PTH 1-34) and abaloparatide (PTHrP 1-34) are currently available in the United States. Dosing and indications are shown in Table 51–10. Treatment with both agents is limited to 2 years due to risk of osteosarcoma seen in preclinical animal studies. Numerous studies have demonstrated that daily subcutaneously injections of teriparatide 20 mcg have efficacy at increasing spine and hip BMD and reducing vertebral and nonvertebral fractures but surprisingly have limited efficacy of hip fracture reduction (see Table 51–11). Daily subcutaneous injections of abaloparatide 80 mcg also improve BMD and reduce vertebral and nonvertebral fractures, but there are insufficient data to determine hip fracture reduction in postmenopausal women with high fracture risk. Teriparatide is also beneficial in glucocorticoid-induced osteoporosis where it has been compared to alendronate (10 mg daily orally). Patients receiving greater than or equal to 5 mg prednisone daily for more than 3 months were randomized to alendronate or teriparatide. After 18 months of therapy, teriparatide induced significantly greater increases in spine and hip BMD with significantly less vertebral

fractures compared to the bisphosphonate. However, there were no significant differences in nonvertebral fractures in the two treatment arms of the study. Based on the costs and inconvenience of daily subcutaneous injections, teriparatide and abaloparatide are recommended to treat bone loss in patients with severe osteoporosis with T scores less than or equal to −3 or with a prior fracture. In clinical practice, teriparatide is often used in patients intolerant of other therapies for osteoporosis, patients who have not responded to other drugs for osteoporosis, or are at high risk on glucocorticoids.

Adverse events due to PTH analogs are generally mild and include dizziness from orthostatic hypotension, muscle cramps, gout precipitation due to increases in uric acid, and transient hypercalcemia (defined as serum calcium >10.6 mg/dL) (see Table 51–12). Animal studies with rats have demonstrated very high risk of osteosarcoma with high-dose drugs for 17 months; therefore the FDA has required a box warning on the package insert to inform practitioners and patients of this risk. PTH analogs are *contraindicated* in growing children with open epiphyses, patients with bone metastases, those who have had skeletal irradiation, and patients with Paget disease or an unexplained elevation in the alkaline phosphatase value.

B. Sclerostin Inhibitor

Romosozumab is a human monoclonal antibody targeting sclerostin, a Wnt signaling inhibitor secreted by OCYs that suppresses osteoblastic activity and bone formation. Romosozumab increases bone formation and also decreases bone resorption by suppressing RANKL-induced OC differentiation. Dosing and indications are shown in Table 51–10. Importantly, similar to PTH analogs and denosumab, romosozumab-induced BMD gains are lost within 12 months unless an alternative antiosteoporosis agent is started when romosozumab treatment ends. Therefore, in clinical studies, postmenopausal women were treated with romosozumab for only 12 months followed by another year of denosumab or another year of alendronate. Romosozumab followed by denosumab significantly increased spine BMD and reduced vertebral fractures but had no difference in nonvertebral fractures (see Table 51–11). Romosozumab followed by alendronate also improved BMD and reduced vertebral, nonvertebral, and hip fractures.

Romosozumab increases the risk of major adverse cardiac events (MACE) including myocardial infarction and stroke, leading to a boxed warning by the FDA (see Table 51–12). Use of this drug should be avoided in patients with a prior MI or stroke in the preceding year. Other adverse side effects of romosozumab are similar to antiresorptive medications and include hypocalcemia, hypersensitivity reactions, osteonecrosis of the jaw, and atypical femur fractures.

Combination & Sequential Regimens

The general principles of osteoporosis treatment should include careful review of risk and benefits for each patient. Use of antiresorptives is prudent in patients with mild osteoporosis or with osteopenia and multiple risk factors. For severe osteoporosis with a prior fracture or a T-score of less than −3, anabolic agents followed by antiresorptive agents might be appropriate. Practically, many physicians follow these rules: (1) start with the safest agent with fracture reduction efficacy (perhaps an oral bisphosphonate), (2) switch from an oral to an intravenous formulation, and (3) switch from a strong antiresorptive agent to an anabolic agent. Switching from oral to intravenous bisphosphonate formulations or to denosumab is reasonable if (1) a new fragility fracture occurs in the setting of increased markers of bone turnover or low BMD, (2) no significant decrease in markers of bone turnover or a reduction in BMD seen on DXA, or (3) more than or equal to two fragility fractures. Anabolic agents are effective after bisphosphonates, but combination therapy in general does not provide synergistic improvements and in some case such as alendronate with teriparatide may even blunt the anabolic effect.

Many trials have evaluated the role of sequential therapies with antiresorptives followed by different antiresorptives, anabolics followed by antiresorptives, and antiresorptives followed by anabolics. Alendronate following PTH analogs and romosozumab appears to be effective for preventing vertebral fractures that occur when anabolic therapy is withdrawn. Data are uncertain for zoledronic acid providing maintenance of BMD and fracture protection following anabolic agents. Denosumab following teriparatide, teriparatide following denosumab, and combination denosumab and teriparatide are effective at increasing BMD, but it is unclear if these patients would then need to take a bisphosphonate to maintain their BMD gains. It is also unclear if combination therapy with teriparatide and denosumab translates into better fracture reduction. These combination treatments are best reserved for patients with severe osteoporosis with prior fractures.

MANAGEMENT OF GLUCOCORTICOID-INDUCED OSTEOPOROSIS

Risk Assessment

The American College of Rheumatology's (ACR) expert panels issued updated recommendations for the prevention and treatment of glucocorticoid-induced osteoporosis in 2017. Unlike previous recommendations, these recommendations were formulated to include adults younger or older than 40 years, women of childbearing potential, children, organ transplant recipients, patients with renal dysfunction, and patients taking very high or intermittent steroids. These recommendations were approached with clinical scenarios in mind and organized clinical risk for fractures into three categories: high, medium, and low (Tables 51–13 and 51–14). Glucocorticoid-corrected FRAX evaluations with or without a BMD were used for fracture risk stratification. The guideline panel, that included a patient and practitioners from academia, nonacademia, endocrinology, rheumatology, and pulmonary and renal subspecialties considered the trade-off between desirable (efficacy of fracture reduction or increased BMD) and undesirable effects (cost, burden of therapy [eg, daily subcutaneous shots], side effects, and harm profiles) for each recommendation. The recommendations strongly encouraged shared decision making and careful review of the risks and benefits when choosing an individual treatment plan. Due to indirectness of evidence or low-quality evidence, the majority of recommendations made were conditional indicating that desirable effects probably outweigh undesirable effects. Medications included in the 2017 ACR guidelines are those with FDA approval prior to 2015, and not romosozumab or abaloparatide, as they were not yet approved.

TREATMENT FAILURES

Clinical fractures still occur in patients successfully treated with antiosteoporosis medications as none of the drugs above provides 100% fracture reduction and most provide 50% reduction that might be site specific. Therefore, a new fracture in a treated patient may not indicate treatment failure. If loss of BMD during therapy exceeds the precision errors of DXA measurements (typically 2%) after 1–2 years of treatment, then noncompliance or treatment failure should be suspected. Noncompliance with oral bisphosphonate or subcutaneous injectables (PTH analogs and romosozumab) is the most common explanation for treatment failure. If noncompliance is not thought to be an issue, the clinician must decide whether the fracture was expected or unexpected in the context of the individual patient. Consider the length of therapy (<12 months), any prior fractures (increase the risk of subsequent fractures), underlying risk factors contributing to the patient's bone loss, baseline BMD values (the lower the T-score, the higher the risk of fracture), the degree of trauma if any, and other medications and conditions that might exacerbate the fracture risk or bone loss. Additional workup for secondary causes of osteoporosis, if not done prior, is prudent at this time. If the clinician is inexperienced with the evaluation of secondary osteoporosis or deciding whether BMD determinations indicate adequate responses to treatment, then this is an excellent time to refer a patient with fractures or ongoing bone loss while receiving therapy to a

Table 51–13. Glucocorticoid-induced fracture risk assessment by age.

Adults ≥40 years	Adults <40 years
High risk (one or more) • Presence of prior fragility fracture • BMD T-score ≤ –2.5 at hip or spine • FRAX risk MOF ≥20%, GC adjusted[a] • FRAX risk HP ≥3%, GC adjusted[a]	**High risk** • Prior osteoporotic fracture
Moderate risk • FRAX risk MOF 10-19%, GC adjusted[a] • FRAX risk of HF >1% and <3%, GC adjusted[a]	**Moderate risk** • Continuing GC ≥**7.5 mg/day** for ≥6 months AND • Bone density Z-score ≤ –3 OR • ≥10% loss of bone density in 1 year OR • Other risk factors (smoking, ETOH)
Low risk • FRAX risk MOF <10% • FRAX risk HF ≤1%	**Low risk** • None of the above
Low risk • *Conditionally* recommend: calcium and vitamin D over oral bisphosphonates • Lifestyle modifications: exercise, limit alcohol, stop smoking, eat more fruits, and vegetables • Monitor clinical fracture risk yearly • Bone density testing, VFA, or spine imaging every 1-3 years	*Low risk* • Calcium and vitamin D • Lifestyle modifications • Monitor clinical fracture risk yearly • Consider repeat bone density in 1 year

Moderate risk
 • Calcium and vitamin D
 • *Conditionally* recommend:
   • First line: oral bisphosphonate
   • Second line: IV bisphosphonate
   • Third line: PTH analog[b]
   • Fourth line: denosumab[b]
   • Fifth line: raloxifene
 • Monitor clinical fracture risk yearly
	Moderate- to high-risk (men and non-childbearing women)
	 • Calcium and vitamin D
	 • Lifestyle modifications
	 • *Conditionally* recommend:
	   • First line: oral bisphosphonate
	   • Second line: PTH analog, denosumab, IV bisphosphonate
	 • Monitor clinical fracture risk yearly

High risk
 • Calcium and vitamin D
 • *Strongly* recommend:
   • First line: oral bisphosphonate
   • Second line: IV bisphosphonate
   • Third line: PTH analog[b]
   • Fourth line: denosumab[b]
   • Fifth line: raloxifene
 • Monitor clinical fracture risk yearly
	Moderate- to high-risk (childbearing women)
	 • Calcium and vitamin D
	 • Lifestyle modifications
	 • *Conditionally* recommend:
	   • First line: oral bisphosphonate
	   • Second line: PTH analog
	   • *High risk third line*: IV bisphosphonate
	   • *High risk fourth line*: denosumab
	 • Monitor clinical fracture risk yearly

[a]Increase the FRAX risk by 1.15 for MOF and by 1.2 for HF if GC dose is ≥7.5 mg daily (eg, if hip fracture is 2.6%, increase to 3.12%).
[b]Use antiresorptive agent after treatment with PTH analogs or denosumab.
Note: *Conditional* recommendations indicate the desirable effects probably outweigh the undesirable effects.
Strong recommendations indicate there is confidence that the desirable effects outweigh the undesirable effects.
For IV bisphosphonates, denosumab, raloxifene, and teriparatide, which have greater harms or burden of treatment, the treatment threshold was judged higher by the ACR guideline panel and ranked these drugs as non-first line treatments.
BMD, bone mineral density; FRAX, Fracture Risk Assessment Tool; GC, glucocorticoid; HF, hip fracture; IV, intravenous; MOF, major osteoporotic fractures include spine, hip, wrist, and humerus; PTH, parathyroid hormone; VFA, vertebral fracture assessment.
Modified from the ACR Guideline for Glucocorticoid-induced Osteoporosis Prevention and Treatment 2017.

Table 51–14. Recommendations for prevention of glucocorticoid-induced osteoporosis in special populations.

Moderate- to high-risk women of childbearing potential who do not plan on becoming pregnant and are using effective birth control	*Adults aged ≥30 years on high-dose GC (≥30 mg/day) and cumulative >5 g in 1 year*
• Calcium and vitamin D • Lifestyle modifications • *Conditionally* recommend: • First line: oral bisphosphonate • Second line: PTH analog • *High risk[a] third line*: IV bisphosphonate • *High risk[a] fourth line*: denosumab • Monitor clinical fracture risk yearly	• Calcium and vitamin D • Lifestyle modifications • *Conditionally* recommend: • First line: oral bisphosphonate • Second line: IV bisphosphonates, PTH analogs, denosumab • Monitor clinical fracture risk yearly
Adults with organ transplant with glomerular filtration rate ≥30 mL/min, and no evidence of metabolic bone disease	*Children ages 4–17 taking GCs ≥0.1 mg/kg/day for ≥3 months with an osteoporotic fracture*
• Calcium and vitamin D • Lifestyle modifications • Evaluation by an expert in metabolic bone disease • Recommend *against* denosumab due to safety issues with infections on multiple immunosuppressive • Conditionally recommend: • First line: oral bisphosphonates • Second line: IV bisphosphonate • Third line: PTH analog • Monitor clinical fracture risk yearly	• Calcium and vitamin D • Lifestyle modifications • Conditionally recommend: • First line: oral bisphosphonates • Second line: IV bisphosphonate • Monitor clinical fracture risk yearly
	Children ages 4–17 treated with GC for ≥3 months
	• Calcium and vitamin D • Lifestyle modifications • Monitor clinical fracture risk yearly

[a]High risk refers to women of childbearing age who might become pregnant on these agents, which have potential to cause fetal harm.
Note: *Conditional* recommendations indicate the desirable effects probably outweigh the undesirable effects.
Strong recommendations indicate there is confidence that the desirable effects outweigh the undesirable effects.
For IV bisphosphonates, denosumab, raloxifene, and teriparatide, which have greater harms or burden of treatment, the treatment threshold was judged higher by the ACR guideline panel and ranked these drugs as non–first-line treatment.
GC, glucocorticoid; IV, intravenous; PTH, parathyroid hormone.
Modified from the ACR Guideline for Glucocorticoid-induced Osteoporosis Prevention and Treatment 2017.

specialist (rheumatologist or endocrinologist) experienced in the care of patients with osteoporosis.

Adami G, Saag KG. Osteoporosis pathophysiology, epidemiology, and screening in rheumatoid arthritis. *Curr Rheumatol Rep.* 2019;21:34. [PMID: 31123839]

Adler RA. Update on osteoporosis in men. *Best Pract Res Clin Endocrinol Metab.* 2018;32:759-772. [PMID: 30449553]

Black DM, Rosen CJ. Clinical practice. Postmenopausal osteoporosis. *New Engl J Med.* 2016;374:254-262. [PMID: 26789873]

Buckley L, Guyatt G, Fink HA, et al. 2017 American College of Rheumatology guideline for the prevention and treatment of glucocorticoid-induced osteoporosis. *Arthritis Rheum.* 2017;69:1521-1537. [PMID: 28585373]

Buckley L, Humphrey MB. Glucocorticoid-induced osteoporosis. *New Engl J Med.* 2018;379:2547-2556. [PMID: 30586507]

Compston JE, McClung MR, Leslie WD. Osteoporosis. *Lancet.* 2019;393:364-376. [PMID: 30696576]

Panday K, Gona A, Humphrey MB. Medication-induced osteoporosis: screening and treatment strategies. *Ther Adv Musculoskelet Dis.* 2014;6:185-202. [PMID: 25342997]

Weitzmann MN. Bone and the immune system. *Toxicol Pathol.* 2017;45:911-924. [PMID: 29046115]

Paget Disease of Bone

Sarah F. Keller, MD, MA

Marcy B. Bolster, MD

Paget disease of bone (PDB) is a striking disorder of aging bone, first described by Sir James Paget in 1876 in his paper entitled "On a Form of Chronic Inflammation of Bones (Osteitis Deformans) (Paget, 1876)." In that sentinel paper, Paget catalogued the progressive deformity of bone that occurred over 26 years in one man, detailing the enlargement of the head, the settling of the skull over the spine, the evolving rigidity of the spine, and bowing of the lower limbs. "The shape and habitual posture of the patient were thus made strange and peculiar (Paget, 1876)." Paget attributed these skeletal changes to chronic inflammation of the affected bones, and called the disease osteitis deformans, writing "a better name may be given when more is known of it (Paget, 1876)."

ESSENTIALS OF DIAGNOSIS

▶ Although Paget disease of bone (PDB) is often asymptomatic, pain, early arthritis in proximal joints, and bone fractures are common complications.

▶ Accelerated bone remodeling results in enlarged, misshapen bone.

▶ Usually presents in persons older than 55 years of age.

▶ Osteosarcoma develops in a small minority of patients.

General Considerations

PDB is a focal disorder of bone remodeling that tends to present in individuals middle-aged or older. This condition is often asymptomatic though patients may develop progressive deformity of bone as well as fractures. Treatment is effective and should be aimed at ameliorating pain arising from involved bone, as well as preventing disease progression and complications.

Epidemiology

Both genetic and environmental determinants are believed to explain the skeletal distribution and late onset of this disease. PDB usually presents in adults over age 55 and tends to affect men more often than women. The condition does not occur in children (Galson and Roodman, 2014). The pelvis is a common site of involvement, and PDB of the pelvis has been reported to have a prevalence of 1–2% in the general population of the United States. Among individuals aged 65–74, the percentage of the population affected exceeds 2%, and there is an even higher prevalence among Caucasians (Altman et al, 2000). Geographic clusters of disease are noteworthy (Gennari et al, 2019; Michou and Orcel, 2016). In fact, the prevalence of PDB was determined to be approximately 6-8% in three towns in Lancashire, England. There is some evidence that the prevalence of this disease has decreased in most parts of the world, for reasons that are not clear (Singer, 2015).

Genetic & Environmental Triggers

PDB occurs both as a sporadic disease and an autosomal dominant disease with variable penetrance. An epidemiologic study drawing from a registry of individuals with PDB in New England demonstrated that 20% of study participants had a family history of PDB, and some studies have reported a positive family history in as many as 40% of patients (Gennari et al, 2019; Seton et al, 2003). There was also a trend towards more deforming disease among those with affected family members.

In 2002, a mutation in the gene *SQSTM1* (encoding sequestosome-1/ubiquitin binding protein, p62, on chromosome 5) was identified in almost 50% of a Canadian cohort of patients with familial PDB, as well as in 16% of those with sporadic disease (Laurin et al, 2002). This mutation is often present on a shared haplotype and has been confirmed in gene studies of individuals from the United Kingdom, several European countries, and the United States, suggesting a founder effect.

Possessing the *SQSTM1* mutation does not ensure that an individual will develop PDB, nor does the lack thereof prevent one from developing the disease; however, the clinical presentation of PDB may be more severe in those who possess this particular genetic mutation (Singer, 2015; Viscorti et al, 2010). Several candidate gene susceptibility loci have been identified in genome-wide association studies and further research to characterize these findings is ongoing (Singer, 2015).

Several candidate environmental factors have also been proposed as contributors to the disease pathogenesis. Environmental association studies conducted in cities with a high prevalence of PDB have identified an association between PDB and significant exposure to toxins (arsenic and lead) as well as exposure to dogs (Singer, 2015). There is some evidence supporting the association between viral infections and PDB. Nuclear inclusions, identified in the osteoclasts of patients with PDB in 1974, were thought to resemble nucleocapsids of paramyxoviruses (Singer, 2015). However, subsequent studies evaluating the association between PDB and measles, in particular, have yielded conflicting results and failed to establish a definitive relationship between the presence of measles in osteoclasts and the development of PDB (Singer, 2015). A mechanism by which genes might interplay with environmental influences on aging bones or whether viruses may prove permissive to this focal disorder of bone remains unknown.

▶ Pathophysiology

Three distinct phases are observed in the pathogenesis of PDB. The first phase is characterized by increased bone vascularity, bone resorption, and the formation of lytic lesions in bone (Gennari et al, 2019). Osteoclasts predominate in the first phase of the disease, and PDB is considered a disorder of the osteoclast. These cells are more numerous, larger, and morphologically abnormal in PDB compared to osteoclasts in normal bone (Ralston and Layfield, 2012). However, it is clear that osteoblastic activity also becomes increased and highly aberrant and that the bone marrow environment permits the accelerated bone turnover that characterizes this disease. In the second phase of PDB, known as the mixed phase, both osteoclastic and osteoblastic activities are increased (Smith et al, 2002). In this phase, there is increased and dysfunctional bone formation; new bone is deposited in a rapid and disorganized manner (Gennari et al, 2019). The final, sclerotic, phase is characterized by decreased vascularity and bone turnover (Gennari et al, 2019; Ralston and Layfield, 2012).

▶ Clinical Findings

A. Signs and Symptoms

PDB is often asymptomatic, detected incidentally on a radiograph or diagnosed in the course of evaluating an elevated serum alkaline phosphatase. It may be monostotic (involving one bone) or polyostotic (involving more than one bone). PDB commonly affects the pelvis. Other affected sites can include the axial skeleton (ie, skull, ribs), the upper extremity (ie, clavicle, humerus), and the lower extremity (ie, femur, tibia) (Greenspan, 2000). The process of accelerated bone remodeling that defines this disease results in enlarged, misshapen bone that loses skeletal integrity. The increased blood circulation to a bone affected by PDB may lead to warmth of the overlying skin, which can be detected on physical examination.

If a patient is symptomatic at the time of presentation, it is most commonly due to pain related to secondary osteoarthritis or to bone fracture. When bone deformity occurs, it typically involves weight-bearing limbs. Secondary osteoarthritis can develop in deformed bone, and most commonly occurs in the hip and knee (Ralston, 2012).

The most common serious complication in PDB is bone fracture. Often, a fracture is what brings the patient to medical attention. Fractures typically occur during the osteolytic or early phase of PDB. Fractures can be incomplete (ie, stress fractures or "pseudofractures") or complete, so-called "chalk-stick fractures" (Smith et al, 2002). Unlike other bone deformities (ie, bowing of the long bones in the upper and lower extremities, increased bone size, kyphosis of the spine, and osteoarthritis) fractures have the ability to heal normally, and most do heal with appropriate management. Severe fractures may require orthopedic intervention (Ralston, 2012).

In addition to bone deformities, several clinical manifestations can occur in patients with PDB. When PDB affects the skull, the overgrowth may lead to impaired functionality of the cranial nerves, including hearing loss (Ralston, 2012). Additional neurologic complications can include headache as basilar invagination—vertical movement of the vertebral column into the foramen magnum—develops. In the spine, the expansion of bone with encroachment of bony foramina can result in pain, nerve impingement, and, rarely, a cauda equina syndrome (Ralston, 2012). Vascular compromise, such as high-output cardiac failure, is rarely reported. As the bones thicken, vascular steal may occur.

Although rare, the most feared complication of PDB is osteosarcoma. The incidence of osteosarcoma in the setting of PDB is less than 1%. While PDB is a recognized risk factor for osteosarcoma, the pathophysiologic connection between the two is not clear as it is the osteoblast—and not the osteoclast—which is abnormal in osteosarcoma (Hansen et al, 2006).

B. Laboratory Findings

Suspicion for PDB may be triggered by the presence of an elevated serum alkaline phosphatase. When the source of this enzyme is bone, the elevated alkaline phosphatase is a marker of excessive bone turnover, characteristic of PDB. Bone turnover markers such as serum beta C-terminal telopeptide or N-terminal telopeptide may be elevated in patients with PDB, but they are unreliable predictors of the skeletal extent of disease and poor markers of response to therapy. Despite an increased flux of calcium into and out of bone, the measured serum calcium remains within normal limits, while the urinary calcium may show considerable variation.

Hypercalcemia may occur in a setting of prolonged immobilization, such as in a patient who sustains a fracture. Patients with PDB may manifest hyperparathyroidism, either primary or secondary hyperparathyroidism, which may be related to fluctuations in calcium (Siris et al, 1989). They also have an increased frequency of calcium-containing renal stones.

C. Imaging

The diagnosis of PDB is typically made by obtaining radiographs that demonstrate classic findings, such as thickened cortices, coarse trabeculations, and lytic as well as blastic lesions. A variety of skeletal deformities can be visualized. In the skull, a patchwork of lytic lesions is said to have a "cotton ball" appearance (Smith et al, 2002). PDB with involvement of the spine is often described as a "picture frame," due to cortical thickening of the vertebral bodies (Theodorou et al, 2011). Acquired curvature of the long bones in the upper and lower extremities causes a bowed appearance on radiographs.

The three distinct stages of bone destruction and remodeling in PDB discussed under Pathophysiology are characterized by specific radiographic findings. More than one stage may be present on a single radiograph. The destruction of cortical and cancellous bone observed in the first phase of disease predominantly results in osteolysis, which is seen as a radiographic lucency, a finding referred to as a "blade of grass" (Hansen et al, 2006; Smith et al, 2002). In the long bones, this osteolytic finding characteristically advances from epiphysis to diaphysis (Hansen et al, 2006). The radiographic findings of cortical thickening, trabecular coarsening, and osteoblastic lesions correspond primarily to the second stage of disorganized bone deposition (Hansen et al, 2006; Smith et al, 2002). Cortical thickening and trabecular coarsening is demonstrated in the pelvis in Figure 52–1 and in the long bones of the lower extremity in Figures 52–2, 52–3, and 52–4. Lastly, increased bone density, bone widening, and cortical thickening are the hallmark radiographic features of the third, sclerotic stage of PDB in which osteoblastic activity declines (Hansen et al, 2006; Smith et al, 2002). Figure 52–1 additionally demonstrates an expansion of the left hemipelvis.

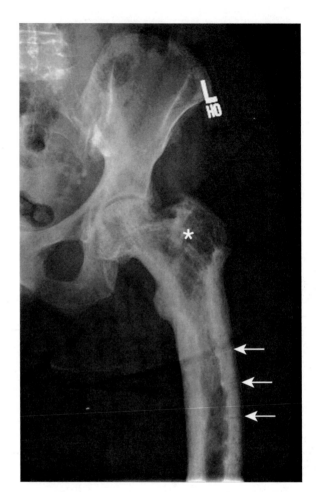

▲ **Figure 52–2.** Pagetic femur with cortical bone thickening, deformity, and pseudofractures marking the convex side of the bone (*arrows*). Note the accentuation of the trabecular markings, indicated by the asterisk (*).

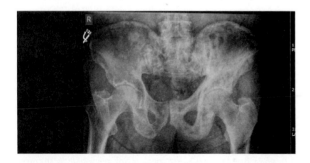

▲ **Figure 52–1.** Cortical and trabecular thickening and expansion involving the left pubis, left ilium, left ischium, the sacrum, and portions of the right ilium consistent with PDB.

Although radiographs are the appropriate initial imaging for Paget disease and may be sufficient to establish the diagnosis, additional imaging modalities can be utilized to identify and further characterize lesions. Nuclear medicine scintigraphy (bone scan), computed tomography (CT), and magnetic resonance imaging (MRI) are all useful in this regard. A bone scan can document the extent and distribution of lesions throughout the skeleton, thus providing practical information regarding the phase of disease and identifying polyostotic disease (Hansen et al, 2006; Winn et al, 2017). A bone scan is highly sensitive for the intense osteoblastic activity observed in Paget disease, and in some cases can demonstrate Paget lesions before they are detectable on radiographs (Hansen et al, 2006; Ralston, 2012). A CT scan may provide additional detail regarding the intricacies of bone structure and complications seen on radiographs

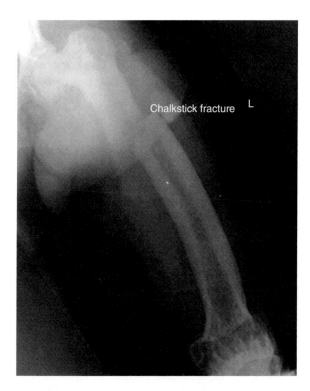

▲ **Figure 52–3.** Chalkstick fracture. This fracture occurred 2 weeks after the adjacent radiograph of the bowed femur depicted in Figure 52–4 was taken.

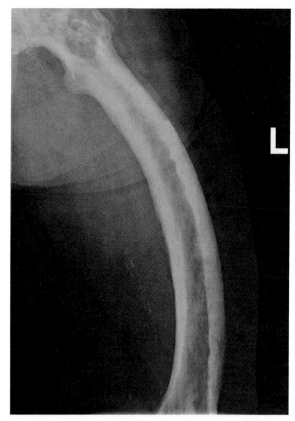

▲ **Figure 52–4.** Bowed pagetic femur. In this image, the entire left femur is affected by remodeling. The bone fractured 2 weeks after this image was taken.

in PDB, particularly if there is concern for more subtle findings (Ralston, 2012). For example, CT imaging is of utility in elucidating greater information about subtle lesions or fractures that may elude radiographic diagnosis. Characterization of structures that are visualized more clearly in three dimensions, such as in the spine, may be best demonstrated by CT, where lesions in the vertebral column could potentially be obscured in the two-dimensional planes (Siris et al, 1989). MRI can reveal bone findings associated with PDB, but additionally can document the extent of disease involving neighboring soft tissues as well as typical changes seen in affected bone marrow (Ralston, 2012; Smith et al, 2002). Importantly, both CT and MRI modalities are useful in differentiating malignant lesions from those changes characteristic of PDB (Ralston, 2012).

D. Bone Biopsy

As above, classic radiographic findings confirm the diagnosis of PDB in the majority of cases. However, a biopsy is warranted in several situations:

1. Presence of ivory vertebrae on radiographs (nonspecific increase in opacity of a vertebral body that can be seen in several malignancies, including osteosarcoma)

2. Other suspicion for osteosarcoma

3. Concern for metastatic disease (eg, a patient with prostate cancer and pelvic lesions)

4. Suspicion of PDB in a younger patient or what would be considered an otherwise atypical clinical presentation

▶ Treatment

Treatment is recommended for any patient with PDB who is symptomatic and for those patients who are at risk for complications. As is illustrated in the following Table 52–1 (Merlotti et al, 2009), treatment should be considered in asymptomatic patients in specific circumstances.

Prior to treatment, renal function must be assessed, and serum concentrations of calcium, phosphorus, magnesium, parathyroid hormone, and 25-hydroxyvitamin D should be measured to ensure the absence of concurrent metabolic abnormalities. Markers of bone formation and bone resorption are not required in the clinical management of patients with PDB,

Table 52–1. Indications for treatment of Paget disease in asymptomatic patients.

Management of hypercalcemia
Prevention of hypercalcemia (ie, immobilized patient)
Involvement of skull, spine, weight-bearing bones, or bone adjacent to major joint
Involvement of bone at a site where surgery is planned (to decrease vascularity and limit blood loss during surgery)
Presence of neurologic complications
Presence of pseudofractures or fractures

Adapted from Merlotti D, Gennari L, Martini G, Nuti R. Current options for the treatment of Paget's disease of the bone. *Open Access Rheumatol.* 2009;1:107–120.

but some groups advocate obtaining these markers prior to and following treatment to assess response (Singer, 2015).

Calcitonin was initially used to treat PDB, however nitrogen-containing bisphosphonates have become the cornerstone of management. These medications prevent the long-term skeletal complications of this disorder and provide patients with a sustained remission. Treatment may also ease many neurologic symptoms (isolated reports have shown improvement in hearing loss), relieve pain, and slow or perhaps halt disease progression (Theodorou, 2011). Despite effective treatment of pain, radiographic changes may not resolve.

The most effective treatment for PDB is intravenous (IV) zoledronic acid. The oral bisphosphonates, alendronate and risedronate, and the IV bisphosphonate, pamidronate, are also FDA approved for the treatment of PDB (Theodorou, 2011). A landmark study in 2005 demonstrated that a single infusion of zoledronic acid resulted in a shorter median time to clinical response when compared to daily therapy with oral risedronate (64 days in the zoledronic acid group vs 89 days in the risedronate group) (Reid, 2005). Furthermore, a higher response rate across multiple parameters, as well as a more sustained response was observed in the zoledronic acid group (Winn et al, 2017). Zoledronic acid was additionally determined to be superior, compared to risedronate, in maintaining bone turnover in the reference range following treatment (Hosking et al, 2007). Furthermore, the therapeutic response to zoledronic acid is durable. A long-term follow-up study demonstrated that bone turnover markers, relapse rates, and loss of response were all lower in the zoledronic acid group than in the risedronate group over a 6.5-year study period (Reid et al, 2011). Adequate serum calcium and vitamin D are critical prior to treatment with bisphosphonates to ensure that clinically significant, and symptomatic, hypocalcemia does not occur.

When needed, such as in hospitalized patients or those receiving hospice care, calcitonin 50–100 international units subcutaneously every other evening can ease pain rapidly and effectively.

While the mainstay of treatment is bisphosphate therapy, there are certain situations in which surgery is recommended.

Occasionally, the pain in PDB is focal, and associated with a pseudofracture on the convex surface of weight-bearing bone as detected by radiographic imaging (see Figure 52–2). This suggests an impending fracture, and should be treated urgently by an orthopedic surgeon. The patient should be made non–weight bearing, and a bisphosphonate should be administered to diminish the vascularity of bone, and thus reduce predicted blood loss, in anticipation of surgery, as discussed above. Emergency surgery for the "chalk stick" fracture (see Figure 52–3) through involved bone can be fraught with blood loss and is associated with a higher mortality rate. In addition, bowing of the long bones in the upper and lower extremity results in severe pain, which can be relieved with an osteotomy.

Treatment of PDB can result in dramatic resolution of pain, neurologic symptoms, and the overlying warmth and erythema that may be present over pagetic bone. Lytic lesions may heal, and bone scans may demonstrate normalization of the increased bone uptake. Over weeks to months, the markers of bone resorption and bone turnover should normalize, followed by normalization of bone formation markers. Indications for re-treatment include a recurrence of symptoms or an increase in bone turnover markers. Interestingly, the Paget's Disease Randomized Trial of Intensive versus Symptomatic Management (PRISM) study did not find a difference between several endpoints (quality of life, bone pain, hearing threshold, fracture, or need for orthopedic surgery), when comparing patients who received treatment based on symptoms with patients who received treatment to maintain a normal serum alkaline phosphatase level (regardless of symptoms) (Langston et al, 2010). Depending on the age of the patient, location of the boney lesions, and associated clinical and biochemical parameters, treatment may be given once or repeated periodically. The decision to re-treat should be individualized and should be considered in the event that symptoms recur or markers of bone turnover increase, including an elevated alkaline phosphatase which had previously normalized. The Endocrine Society, for example, recommends periodic monitoring of bone turnover markers and re-treating if these laboratory tests increase once they have normalized, as opposed to re-treating based solely on recurrence of pain (Singer et al, 2014).

Many of the symptoms that occur in patients with PDB improve with effective therapy. However, not all bone lesions will heal completely and some complications of the disease may not resolve. The treating physician should always strive to understand his or her patients' comorbidities and address expectations accordingly. With appropriate therapy and monitoring, PDB can be effectively managed.

ACKNOWLEDGMENT

The authors would like to acknowledge the invaluable contributions of Margaret Seton, MD, author of this chapter in the previous edition.

Altman RD, Bloch DA, Hochberg MC, et al. Prevalence of pelvic Paget's disease of bone in the United States. *J Bone Miner Res.* 2000;15:461. [PMID: 10750560]

Galson DL, Roodman DG. Pathobiology of Paget's disease of bone. *J Bone Metab.* 2014;21:85. [PMID: 25025000]

Gennari L, Rendina D, Falchetti A, et al. Paget's disease of bone. *Calcif Tissue Int.* 2019;104:483. [PMID: 30671590]

Greenspan A. Paget disease. In: Greenspan A, ed. *Orthopedic Radiology: A Practical Approach.* 3rd ed. Philadelphia, PA: Lippincott Williams & Wilkins, 2000:805-818.

Hansen MF, Seton M, Merchant A. Osteosarcoma in Paget's disease of bone. *J Bone Miner Res.* 2006;21:58. [PMID: 17229010]

Hosking D, Lyles K, Brown JP, et al. Long-term control of bone turnover in Paget's disease with zoledronic acid and risedronate. *J Bone Miner Res.* 2007;22:142. [PMID: 17032148]

Langston AL, Campbell MK, Fraser WD, et al. Randomized trial of intensive bisphosphonate treatment versus symptomatic management in Paget's disease of bone. *J Bone Miner Res.* 2010;25:20. [PMID: 19580457]

Laurin N, Brown JP, Morissette J, et al. Recurrent mutation of the gene encoding sequestosome 1 (*SQSTM1/p62*) in Paget disease of bone. *Am J Hum Genet.* 2002;70:1582. [PMID: 11992264]

Merlotti D, Gennari L, Martini G, et al. Current options for the treatment of Paget's disease of the bone. *Open Access Rheumatol.* 2009;1:107. [PMID: 27789985]

Michou L, Orcel P. The changing countenance of Paget's disease of the bone. *Joint Bone Spine.* 2016;83:650. [PMID: 27068613]

Paget SJ. On a form of chronic inflammation of bones (osteitis deformans). *Med Chir Trans.* 1876;60:37-64. [PMID: 20896492]

Ralston SH, Layfield R. Pathogenesis of Paget disease of bone. *Calcif Tissue Int.* 2012;91:97. [PMID: 22543925]

Reid IR, Lyles K, Su G, et al. A single infusion of zoledronic acid produces sustained remissions in Paget disease: data to 6.5 years. *J Bone Miner Res.* 2011;26:2261. [PMID: 21638319]

Reid IR, Miller P, Lyles K, et al. Comparison of a single infusion of zoledronic acid with risedronate for Paget's disease. *N Engl J Med.* 2005;353:898. [PMID: 16135834]

Seton M, Choi HK, Hansen MF, et al. Analysis of environmental factors in familial versus sporadic Paget's disease of bone—The New England Registry for Paget's Disease of Bone. *J Bone Miner Res.* 2003;18:1519. [PMID: 12929942]

Singer FR. Paget's disese of bone—genetic and environmental factors. *Nat Rev Endocrinol.* 2015;11:662. [PMID: 26284446]

Singer FR, Bone HG 3rd, Hosking DJ, et al. Paget's disease of bone: an endocrine society clinical practice guideline. *J Clin Endocrinol Metab.* 2014;99:4408. [PMID: 25406796]

Siris ES, Clemens TP, McMahon D, et al. Parathyroid function in Paget's disease of bone. *J Bone Miner Res.* 1989;4:75. [PMID: 2718781]

Smith SE, Murphey MD, Motamedi K, et al. Radiologic Spectrum of Paget disease of bone and its complications with pathologic correlation. *Radiographics.* 2002;22:1191. [PMID: 12235348]

Theodorou D, Theodorou SJ, Yousuke K. Imaging of Paget disease of bone and its musculoskeletal complications: review. *AJR Am J Roentgenol.* 2011;196:S64. [PMID: 21606236]

Viscorti MJ, Langston AL, Alonso N, et al. Mutations of SQSTM1 are associated with severity and clinical outcome in Paget disease of bone. *J Bone Miner Res.* 2010;25:2368-2373. [PMID: 20499339]

Winn N, Lalam R, Cassar-Pullicino V. Imaging of Paget's disease of bone. *Wien Med Wochenschr.* 2017;167:169. [PMID: 27761746]

Musculoskeletal Magnetic Resonance Imaging

53

Ravi S. Kamath, MD, PhD

Ambrose J. Huang, MD

Magnetic resonance imaging (MRI) relies on the intrinsic spin of protons. When protons are placed in a magnetic field, they tend to align their magnetic poles along the axis of the magnetic field. They can also absorb and then re-emit electromagnetic radiation in the form of radiofrequency signals. The nuclei of cells absorb energy from radiofrequency pulses and may resonate from the pulses. This resonance induces orientation to the magnetic field. The frequency of the pulse required to generate resonance of the target is determined by the strength of the magnetic field and the chemical properties of the target.

When the radiofrequency signal is removed, the absorbed energy is released. This energy can be detected and can be used to create images, with the strength of the emission corresponding to the signal intensity of a given area. This signal intensity depends on the concentration of protons and the longitudinal and transverse relaxation times, which are intrinsic properties of the given tissue and depend on the properties of the water molecules within it.

Two relaxation times are important for MRI. The T1 (longitudinal) relaxation time describes the return of protons back to equilibrium after a radiofrequency pulse. The T2 (transverse) relaxation time describes the loss of phase coherence between individual protons immediately after the pulse. Different pulse sequences can be used to enhance the differences between T1 and T2, thus creating image contrast. Sequences with short repetition times (TR) (<800 milliseconds) and short echo times (TE) (<30 milliseconds) are termed **T1-weighted** sequences. T1-weighted images provide good anatomic detail. Sequences with long TR (>2000 milliseconds) and long TE (>60 milliseconds) are termed **T2-weighted** sequences. T2-weighted sequences are useful for evaluating pathology. Sequences with intermediate TR (>1000 milliseconds) and short TE (<30 milliseconds) are termed **proton density sequences.** These provide good anatomic detail and maximal signal-to-noise ratios at the cost of impaired tissue contrast.

In musculoskeletal imaging, suppression of fat signal can often be useful for evaluating pathology. Using the short tau inversion recovery (STIR) technique, the effects of prolonged T1 and T2 relaxation times are cumulative, leading to the suppression of fat signal ("fat saturation"). Fat suppression can also be performed using frequency-selective (chemical) techniques that improve spatial resolution.

Faster imaging techniques such as gradient-recalled echo (GRE) have become popular because they shorten imaging time. With GRE, pulse sequences are performed using variable flip angles of less than 90 degrees, which shortens imaging time since the low flip-angle radiofrequency pulses destroy only a portion of the longitudinal magnetization with each pulse cycle. In musculoskeletal imaging, GRE sequences are useful for imaging ligaments, tendons, and cartilage.

The musculoskeletal system is ideally suited for evaluation by MRI because different tissues have different signal intensities on T1- and T2-weighted images. For example, fat displays high signal intensity on T1-weighted images and intermediate signal intensity on T2-weighted images. Air, cortical bone, ligaments, tendons, and fibrocartilage have low signal intensity on both T1- and T2-weighted images. Fluid displays low signal intensity on T1-weighted images and high signal intensity on T2-weighted images. Traumatic, inflammatory, and infectious disorders are therefore evaluated effectively by MRI, because these conditions typically result in edema and associated high signal intensity on T2-weighted images. Figures 53–1 through 53–30 show MRI findings in various rheumatic conditions.

MR images can also be enhanced by intravenous administration of gadolinium in the form of Gd-DTPA, a paramagnetic compound that shortens the T1 and T2 relaxation times of the tissues where it is located, resulting in an increase in signal intensity on T1-weighted images. Foci with increased vascular permeability, such as neoplasms or areas of inflammation or infection, therefore show increased signal intensity (enhancement) following the administration of intravenous

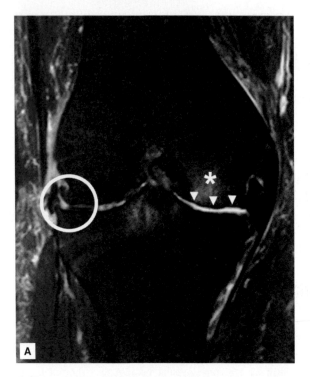
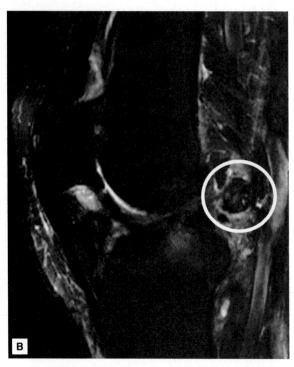

▲ **Figure 53–1.** Osteoarthritis of the knee. A coronal T2-weighted fat-suppressed MR image of the knee (**A**) shows marginal osteophytes (*circled*) and full-thickness cartilage loss (*arrowheads*) with overlying marrow edema (*). A sagittal T2-weighted fat-suppressed MR image of the knee (**B**) shows a low signal intensity loose body surrounded by intermediate signal intensity synovitis in the posterior joint (*circled*).

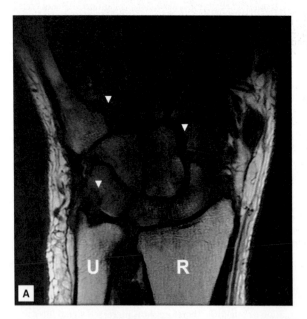
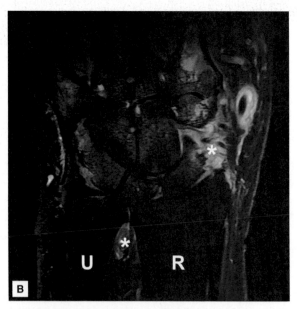

▲ **Figure 53–2.** Rheumatoid arthritis of the wrist. Coronal T1-weighted (**A**) and T2-weighted fat-suppressed (**B**) MR images of the wrist show diffuse cartilage loss throughout the wrist with joint-space narrowing, osseous erosions (arrowheads), and extensive marrow edema. Radiocarpal and distal radioulnar joint effusions are present with synovitis (*). R = radius, U = ulna.

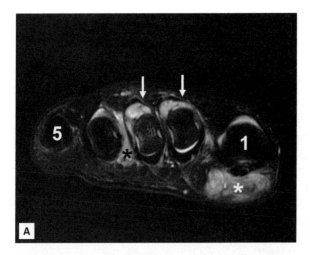

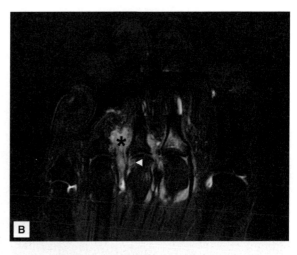

▲ **Figure 53–3.** Rheumatoid arthritis of the foot. Short-axis (**A**) and long-axis (**B**) T2-weighted fat-suppressed MR images of the forefoot show metatarsophalangeal joint effusions with synovitis (*arrows*), adjacent marrow edema, osseous erosions (one labeled with arrowhead), and intermetatarsal bursitis (*black* *). A high T2 signal intensity soft-tissue mass in the subcutaneous fat plantar to the first metatarsophalangeal joint is likely a rheumatoid nodule (*white* *). 1 = first metatarsal head, 5 = fifth metatarsal head.

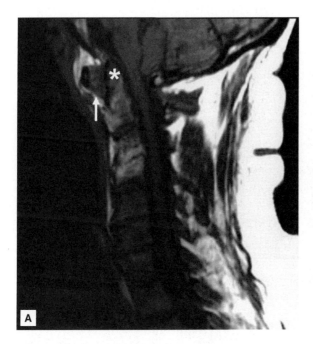

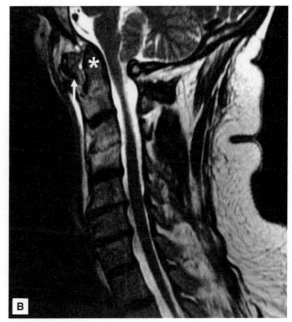

▲ **Figure 53–4.** Rheumatoid arthritis of the cervical spine. Sagittal T1-weighted (**A**), T2-weighted (**B**), and T1-weighted fat-suppressed post-contrast.

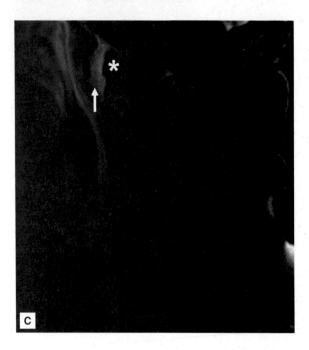

▲ **Figure 53–4.** (*Continued*) (**C**) MR images of the cervical spine show intermediate T1 and T2 signal intensity, enhancing pannus in the atlantoaxial joint (*arrows*). The dens (*) is also superiorly displaced relative to the skull base and protrudes into the foramen magnum, consistent with basilar invagination.

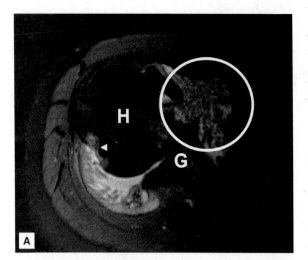

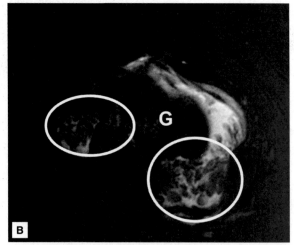

▲ **Figure 53–5.** Rheumatoid arthritis of the shoulder. Axial (**A**) and sagittal (**B**) T2-weighted fat-suppressed MR images of the glenohumeral joint show diffuse cartilage loss, adjacent marrow edema, osseous erosions (*arrowhead*), and a large glenohumeral joint effusion with extensive synovitis and rice bodies (circled). G = glenoid, H = humeral head.

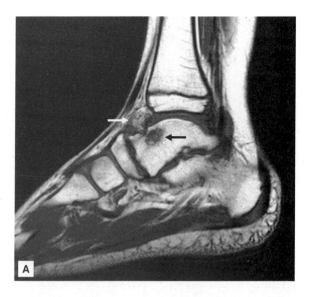

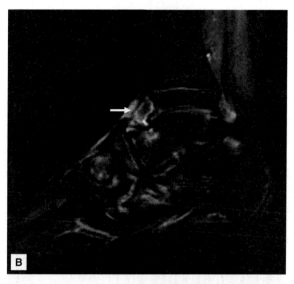

▲ **Figure 53–6.** Juvenile idiopathic arthritis of the ankle. Sagittal T1-weighted (**A**) and STIR (**B**) MR images of the ankle in a pediatric patient show diffuse marrow edema throughout the ankle with a tibiotalar joint effusion and synovitis (*white arrows*). An osseous erosion is seen in the talus with adjacent marrow edema (*black arrows*). Note the open distal tibial physis in this preadolescent patient.

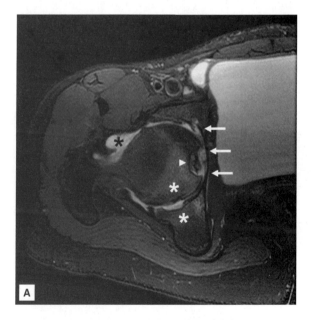

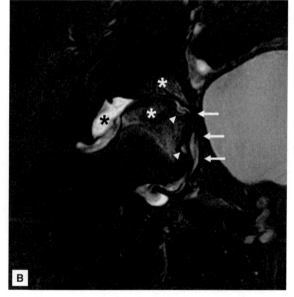

▲ **Figure 53–7.** Juvenile idiopathic arthritis of the hip. Axial (**A**) and coronal (**B**) T2-weighted fat-suppressed MR images of the hip show diffuse cartilage loss, adjacent marrow edema in the femoral head and acetabulum (*white **), osseous erosions (*arrowheads*), and a joint effusion with synovitis (*black **). The medial wall of the acetabulum is thinned (*arrows*), and the femoral head has migrated medially, consistent with acetabular protrusio.

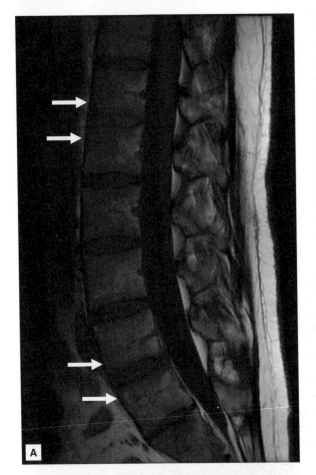

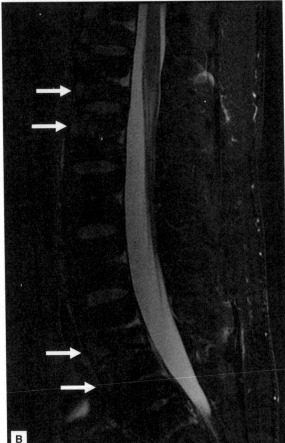

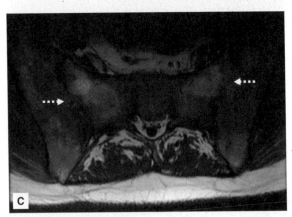

▲ **Figure 53–8.** Ankylosing spondylitis of the spine. Sagittal T1-weighted (**A**) and STIR (**B**) MR images of the lumbar spine show focal marrow edema along the anterior superior and anterior inferior corners of several vertebral bodies, an early manifestation of inflammatory spondyloarthropathy called "shiny corners" or Romanus lesions (*indicated by solid arrows*). (**C**) An axial T1-weighted MR image of the sacrum shows partial ankylosis of both sacroiliac joints (*dashed arrows*).

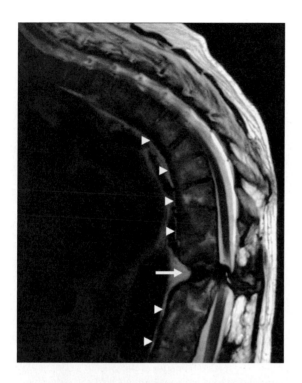

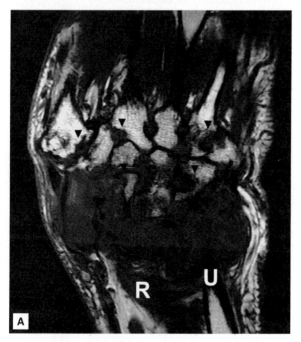

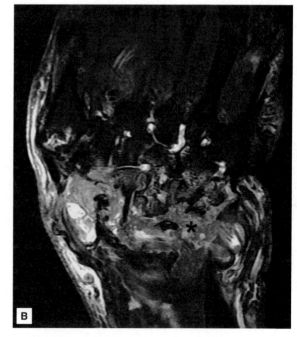

▲ **Figure 53–9.** Ankylosing spondylitis with Andersson lesion. A sagittal T2-weighted MR image of the thoracic spine shows fusion of the thoracic spine with syndesmophyte formation (*arrowheads*) due to ankylosing spondylitis. There is a transverse fracture through the anterior and posterior elements of the fused lower thoracic spine (*arrow*), termed an "Andersson lesion," with resulting compromise of the central canal and cord compression.

▲ **Figure 53–10.** Psoriatic arthritis of the wrist and elbow. Coronal T1-weighted (**A**), T2-weighted fat-suppressed (**B**),

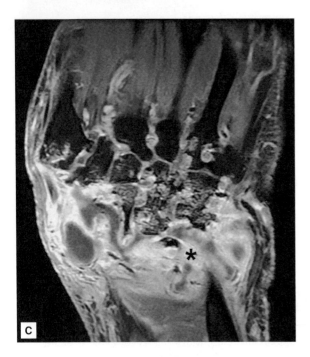

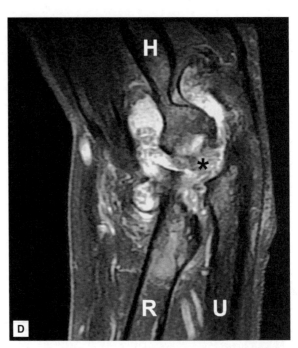

▲ **Figure 53–10.** (*Continued*) and T1-weighted fat-suppressed post-contrast (**C**) MR images of the wrist in a patient with psoriasis show extensive osseous destruction of the wrist with numerous osseous erosions (*arrowheads*) and extensive enhancing synovitis (*). A sagittal T2-weighted fat-suppressed MR image of the elbow in a different patient with psoriatic arthritis also shows extensive osseous destruction with adjacent marrow edema and synovitis (*) (**D**). H = humerus, R = radius, U = ulna.

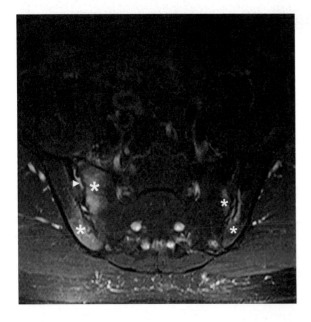

▲ **Figure 53–11.** Psoriatic arthritis of the sacroiliac joints. An axial T2-weighted fat-suppressed MR image of the sacroiliac joints shows erosions (*arrowhead*) and surrounding marrow edema (*), right greater than left, consistent with sacroiliitis.

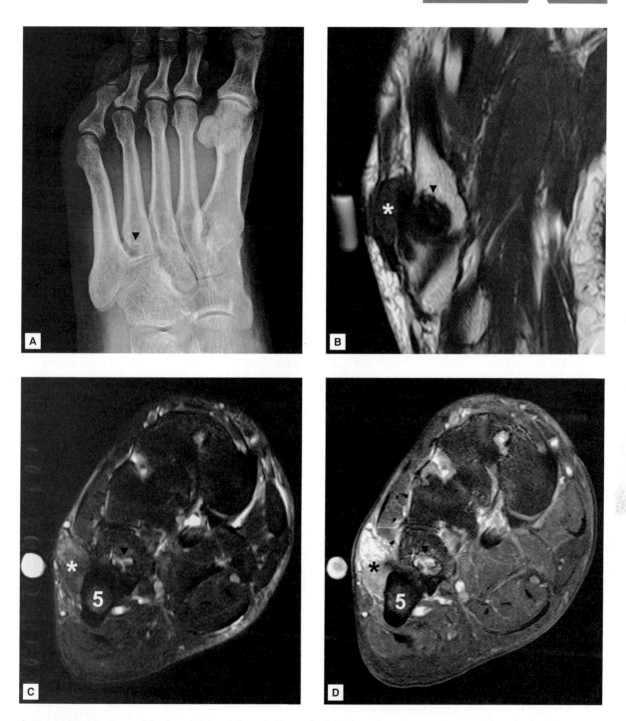

▲ **Figure 53–12.** Gout of the foot. (**A**) An oblique radiograph of the foot shows an osseous erosion at the fourth metatarsal base (*arrowhead*). Long-axis T1-weighted (**B**), short-axis T2-weighted fat-suppressed (**C**), and short-axis T1-weighted fat-suppressed post-contrast (**D**) MR images of the foot show a sharply marginated erosion with overhanging edges at the fourth metatarsal base (*arrowheads*) with an adjacent low T1 signal intensity, intermediate T2 signal intensity, enhancing soft-tissue mass (*), consistent with a tophus. 5 = fifth metatarsal base.

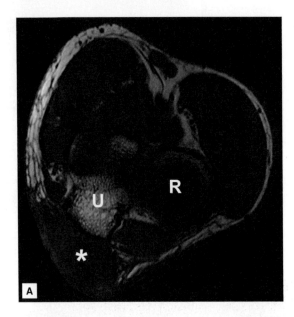

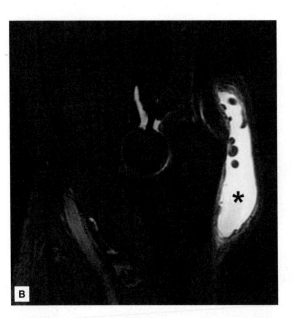

▲ **Figure 53–13.** Gout with olecranon bursitis. Axial T1-weighted (**A**) and sagittal T2-weighted fat-suppressed (**B**) MR images of the elbow in a patient with gout show a large low T1 signal intensity, high T2 signal intensity fluid collection (*) posterior to the olecranon with a thick, irregular wall and internal low T2 signal intensity debris, consistent with olecranon bursitis. R = radius, U = ulna.

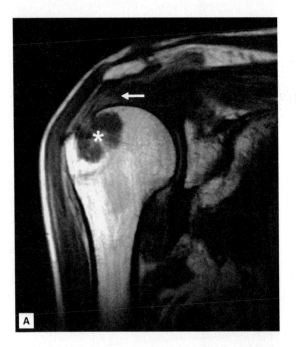

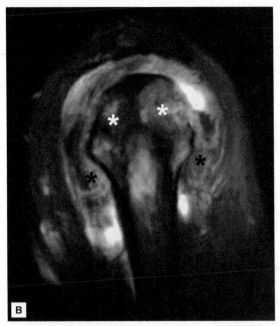

▲ **Figure 53–14.** Amyloid arthropathy of the shoulder. Coronal T1-weighted (**A**) and sagittal T2-weighted fat-suppressed (**B**) MR images of the shoulder show distention of the glenohumeral joint with intermediate T1 and T2 signal intensity soft-tissue masses (*black* *) in the joint space and filling large erosions in the humeral head (*white* *). A full-thickness rotator cuff tear (*arrow*) allows this process to extend into the subacromial-subdeltoid space. This patient with amyloid arthropathy also had amyloid-associated cardiomyopathy in the setting of multiple myeloma.

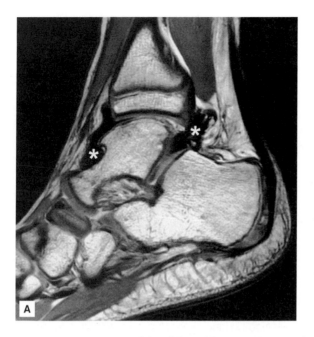
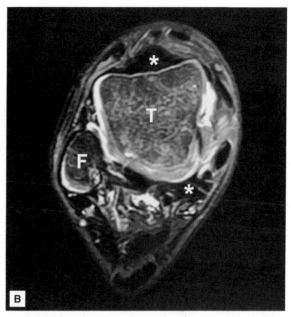

▲ **Figure 53–15.** Hemophilia of the ankle. Sagittal T1-weighted (**A**) and axial T2-weighted fat-suppressed (**B**) MR images of the ankle in a patient with hemophilia show low T1 and T2 signal intensity material within the tibiotalar and subtalar joints (*), consistent with hemosiderin deposition from recurrent intra-articular hemorrhage. Note the open distal tibial physis in this preadolescent patient. F = fibula, T = tibia.

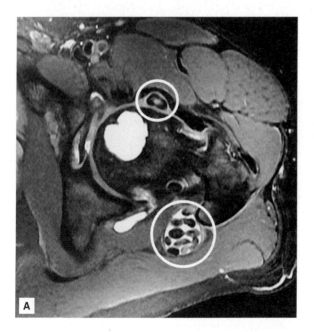
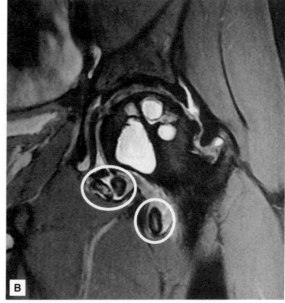

▲ **Figure 53–16.** Synovial osteochondromatosis of the hip. Axial (**A**) and coronal (**B**) T2-weighted fat-suppressed MR images of the hip show numerous low-signal-intensity structures of similar size and shape within the hip joint (*circled*), consistent with multiple ossific loose bodies in the context of synovial osteochondromatosis.

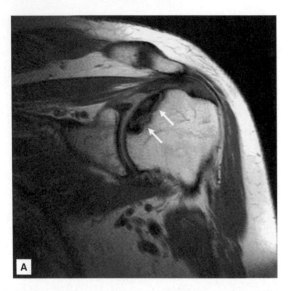

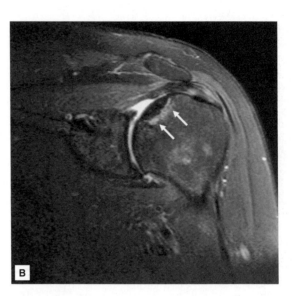

▲ **Figure 53–17.** Osteonecrosis of the shoulder. Coronal T1-weighted (**A**) and T2-weighted fat-suppressed (**B**) MR images of the shoulder in a patient who was previously taking long-term corticosteroids show a subchondral crescentic region of low T1 and T2 signal intensity in the humeral head with a curvilinear high T2 signal intensity margin (*arrows*), consistent with osteonecrosis.

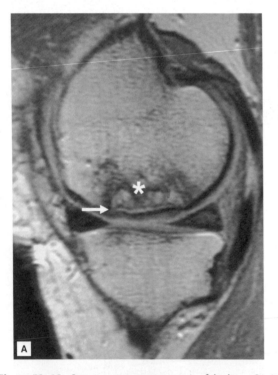

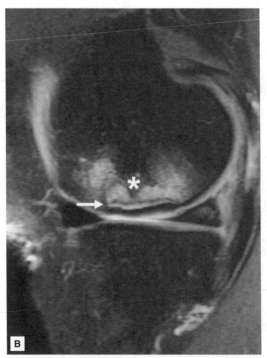

▲ **Figure 53–18.** Spontaneous osteonecrosis of the knee. Sagittal proton density (**A**) and T2-weighted fat-suppressed (**B**) MR images of the knee show a subchondral fracture along the weight-bearing portion of the medial femoral condyle (*arrows*) with irregularity of the cortex, fluid undercutting the fracture fragment, and adjacent sclerosis and marrow edema (*), consistent with spontaneous osteonecrosis of the knee. Although previously thought to result from venous occlusion, it is now more widely accepted that this represents a subchondral insufficiency-type fracture that has further collapsed.

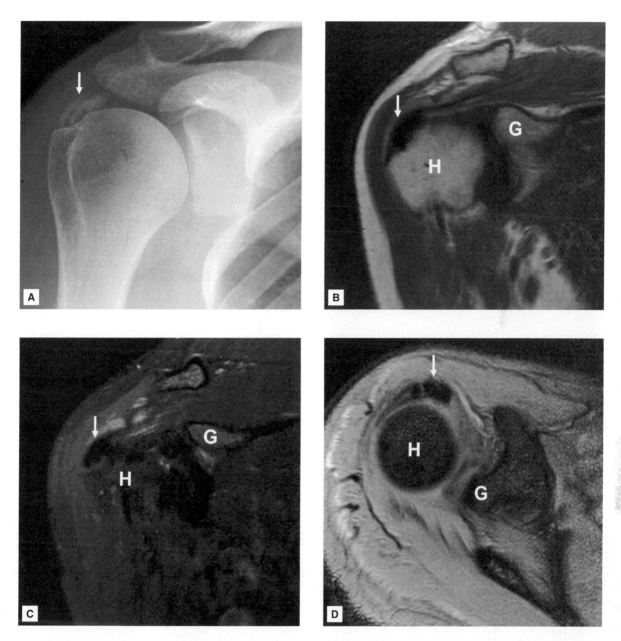

▲ **Figure 53–19.** Calcific tendinopathy. A frontal radiograph of the shoulder (**A**) shows amorphous calcification in the region of the rotator cuff tendons, suggestive of calcific tendinopathy (*arrow*). Coronal T1-weighted (**B**), coronal T2-weighted fat-suppressed (**C**), and axial gradient-recalled echo (GRE) (**D**) MR images of the shoulder show a corresponding low signal intensity focus within the distal supraspinatus tendon (*arrows*), consistent with calcium hydroxyapatite deposition. On the GRE image, "blooming" susceptibility artifact (*dark signal*) is seen surrounding the paramagnetic calcification. G = glenoid, H = humeral head.

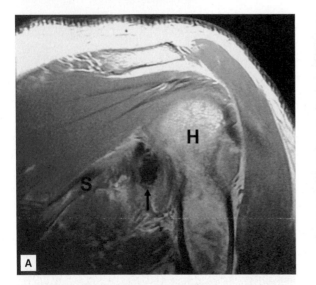

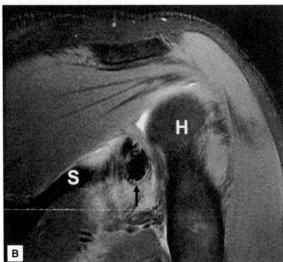

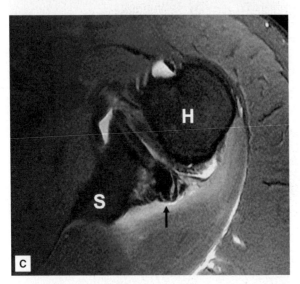

▲ **Figure 53–20.** Calcific periarthritis of the shoulder. Coronal T1-weighted (**A**), coronal T2-weighted fat-suppressed (**B**), and axial T2-weighted fat-suppressed (**C**) MR images of the shoulder show low-signal-intensity material (*arrows*) along the posterior glenoid with extensive adjacent marrow and soft-tissue edema, compatible with hydroxyapatite deposition and calcific periarthritis. H = humerus, S = scapula.

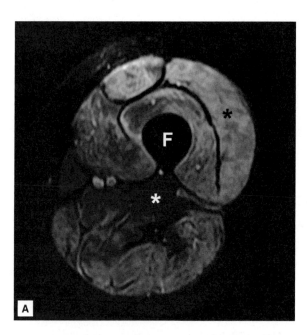

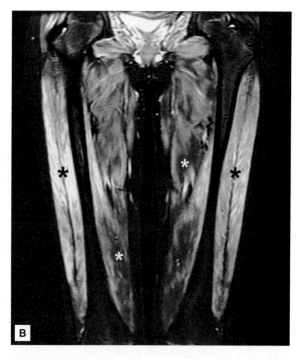

▲ **Figure 53–21.** Juvenile dermatomyositis of the thighs. An axial STIR MR image of the left thigh (**A**) and a coronal STIR MR image of both thighs (**B**) show diffuse muscle edema (*black* *) with patchy areas of relative sparing in both thighs (*white* *), consistent with myositis. F = femur.

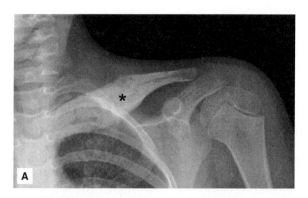

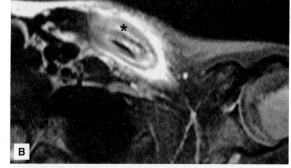

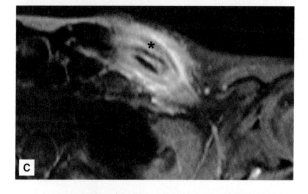

▲ **Figure 53–22.** Chronic recurrent multifocal osteomyelitis (CRMO). A frontal radiograph of the clavicle (**A**) shows abnormal sclerosis and thickening of the clavicle with extensive periosteal bone formation (*). Axial STIR (**B**) and T1-weighted fat-suppressed post-contrast (**C**) MR images of the clavicle show abnormal marrow edema and enhancement in the clavicle, thick periosteal bone formation, and extensive surrounding soft-tissue edema and enhancement (*). This patient presented with severe atraumatic left clavicle pain and elevated inflammatory markers. Percutaneous needle biopsy yielded only reactive bone with negative cultures, leading to the diagnosis of CRMO.

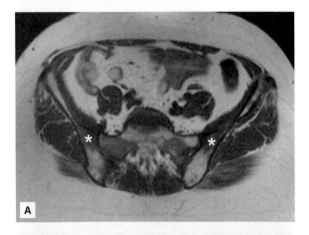

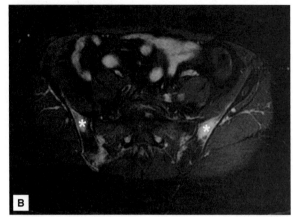

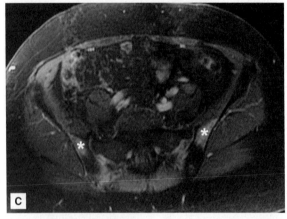

▲ Figure 53–23. Sarcoidosis of the pelvis. Axial T1-weighted (**A**), T2-weighted fat-suppressed (**B**), and T1-weighted fat-suppressed post-contrast (**C**) MR images of the pelvis in a patient with known sarcoidosis show geographic areas of low T1 signal intensity, high T2 signal intensity, and enhancement in both iliac bones (*), consistent with osseous sarcoidosis.

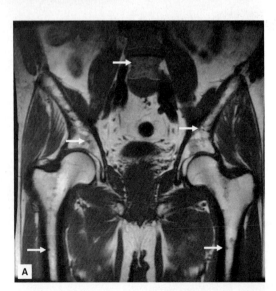

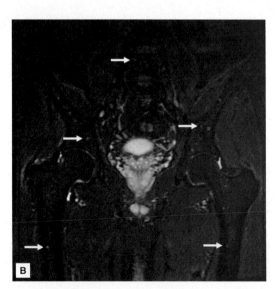

▲ Figure 53–24. Sarcoidosis of the pelvis. Coronal T1-weighted (**A**) and STIR (**B**) MR images of the pelvis in a patient with known sarcoidosis show innumerable punctate low T1 and high T2 signal intensity foci scattered throughout the visualized lower lumbar spine, pelvis, and proximal femurs (*several indicated by arrows*), consistent with osseous sarcoidosis.

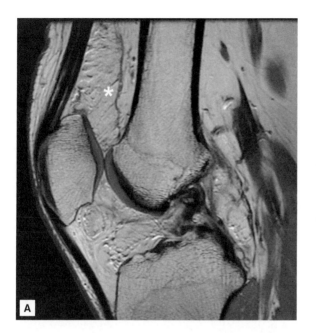

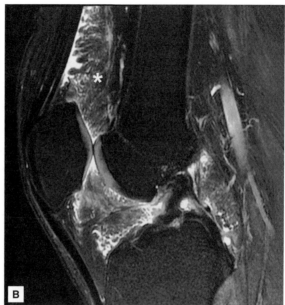

▲ **Figure 53–25.** Synovial lipomatosis of the knee. Sagittal T1-weighted (**A**) and T2-weighted fat-suppressed (**B**) MR images of the knee show frond-like proliferation of material, that is, the same signal intensity as fat on all pulse sequences (*), consistent with synovial lipomatosis/lipoma arborescens.

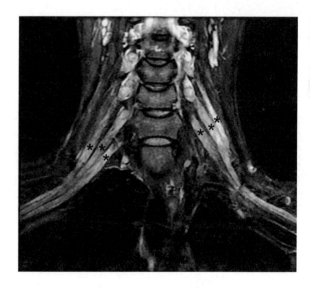

▲ **Figure 53–26.** Brachial plexopathy in chronic inflammatory demyelinating polyneuropathy. A coronal T2-weighted fat-suppressed MR image of the neck and upper thorax in a patient with chronic inflammatory demyelinating polyneuropathy shows extensive thickening and high T2 signal intensity of the bilateral cervical nerve roots and brachial plexi (*).

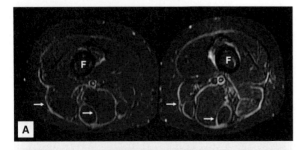

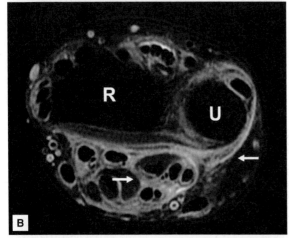

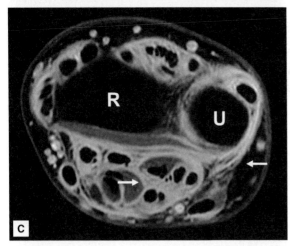

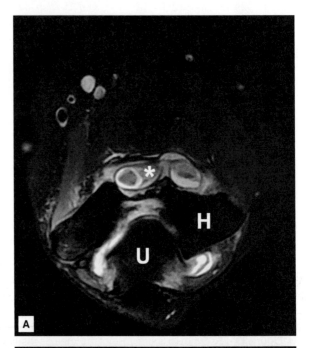

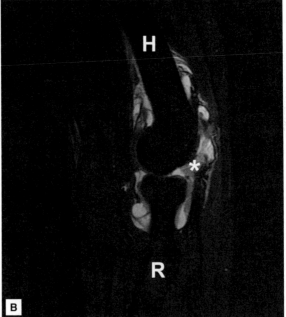

▲ **Figure 53–27.** Eosinophilic fasciitis of the thighs and wrist. (**A**) An axial STIR MR image of both thighs shows abnormal thickening and high T2 signal intensity of the fascia in both thighs (*arrows*), consistent with fasciitis. Axial T2-weighted fat-suppressed (**B**) and axial T1-weighted fat-suppressed post-contrast (**C**) MR images of the wrist in a different patient also show extensive thickening, high T2 signal intensity, and enhancement of the fascia (*arrows*). The diagnosis of eosinophilic fasciitis was confirmed by biopsy in both patients. F = femur, R = radius, U = ulna.

▲ **Figure 53–28.** Lupus arthritis of the elbow. Axial (**A**) and sagittal (**B**) T2-weighted fat-suppressed MR images of the elbow in a patient with systemic lupus erythematosus show a large joint effusion with extensive synovitis (*). H = humerus, R = radius, U = ulna.

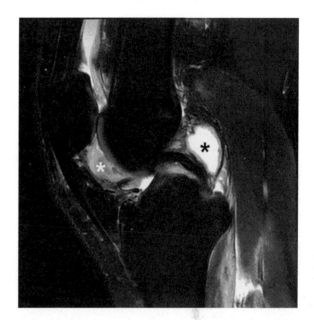

▲ **Figure 53–29.** Lyme arthritis of the knee. A sagittal T2-weighted fat-suppressed MR image of the knee shows a large joint effusion (*black* *) with extensive synovitis (*white* *). The diagnosis of Lyme disease was confirmed by laboratory tests.

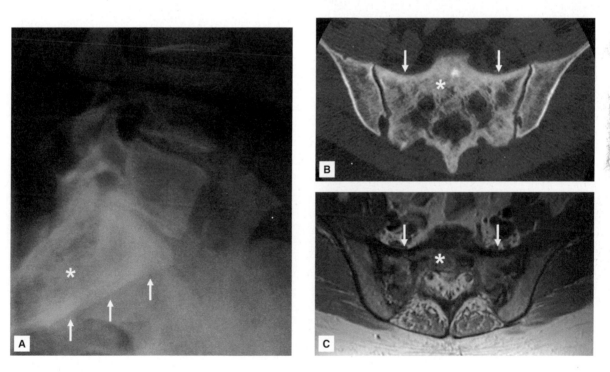

▲ **Figure 53–30.** Paget disease of the sacrum. A lateral radiograph of the lumbosacral junction (**A**) shows enlargement of the sacrum with cortical thickening (*arrows*) and coarsened trabeculae (*). An axial CT image (**B**) and an axial T1-weighted MR image (**C**) of the sacrum also show the cortical thickening (*arrows*) and coarsened trabeculae (*), confirming the diagnosis of Paget disease.

gadolinium. Intra-articular administration of gadolinium for arthrography can also be used to evaluate for internal derangement of a joint.

Although MRI has many advantages over other imaging techniques for the evaluation of the musculoskeletal system, its utility is limited in certain instances. MRI is contraindicated, for example, in patients with cardiac pacemakers, neural stimulators, and some other implanted metallic devices. Claustrophobic patients are often unable to endure the tight confines of many MRI machines. Motion artifact that results from some patients' inability to remain still for any reason can render MRI data unreadable. This is a particular problem in the setting of the long scan times (30–60 minutes) required by some studies. Finally, some metallic objects that are safe for MRI nevertheless can create areas of signal void that obscure adjacent structures, and ferromagnetic objects can cause magnetic field distortion. These potential limitations of MRI must be understood to optimize the use of this technology.

Musculoskeletal Ultrasound in Rheumatology

54

Minna J. Kohler, MD, RhMSUS

Since the mid-1990s, point-of-care ultrasound—that is, musculoskeletal ultrasound (MSKUS) performed and interpreted by the rheumatologist evaluating the patient—has become a tool of increasing importance to rheumatologists. MSKUS is a valuable imaging technique that enhances and expedites the diagnosis of inflammatory arthritides, musculoskeletal conditions, large-vessel vasculitis, polymyalgia rheumatica, Sjögren syndrome, and other diseases. The American College of Rheumatology (ACR) and the European League Against Rheumatism (EULAR) have recommended guidelines for MSKUS use (McAlindon et al, 2012; Möller et al, 2017), and rheumatology training programs around the world now include ultrasound curricula for trainees (American College of Rheumatology, 2020; Brown et al, 2004; Kissin et al, 2013; Naredo et al, 2010; Torralba et al, 2015; Torralba et al, 2017).

Technological advances in ultrasound equipment as this technique has evolved have allowed for smaller, smarter equipment. High-frequency transducers to provide gray scale (black and white images produced by sound waves) for assessment of joint, tendon, and soft-tissue structures. Power Doppler gray scale images evaluations permit the assessment of hyperemia or active inflammation. Advantages of ultrasound over other advanced imaging modalities include its portability, noninvasive nature, cost, and its lack of ionizing radiation. In addition, MSKUS permits dynamic evaluations of joints and tendon structures in motion, providing a significant edge over the more static technologies of plain radiography, magnetic resonance imaging (MRI), and computed tomography (CT).

Rheumatologists most commonly use ultrasound for detection of fluid collections and assessment of synovitis, tenosynovitis, and bony erosions. MSKUS is also useful for procedural guidance. Ultrasound has better spatial resolution than plain x-rays and even MRI, permitting the early detection of bony surface abnormalities or erosions. The high resolution of ultrasound also enhances the detection of crystalline deposition that is often too small to detect by radiograph or MRI. MSKUS studies have augmented the rheumatologist's ability to diagnose crystalline disease even in

intercritical periods. The ability to repeat examinations and correlate in-office image findings with the history and clinical examination also contributes to its usefulness in monitoring of treatment (Backhaus et al, 2001; Brown, 2009; Canella et al, 2014; Karim et al, 2001). For pediatric patients, use of ultrasound does not require sedation that may be necessary for MRI and other cross-sectional imaging (Roth, 2017). Extensive literature on the accuracy of ultrasound-guided procedures (aspiration, injection, biopsy) exists (D'Agostino, 2013; Epis, 2014; Gilliland, 2011; Raza, 2003; Robotti, 2013).

Although ultrasound has many advantages in evaluating the musculoskeletal system, limitations include its inability to penetrate bone. Because of this shortcoming, MSKUS imaging is limited to superficial structures or the surface of bone. Bone marrow edema cannot be assessed. Operator dependence has often been cited as a limitation and this is certainly true in poorly trained individuals. With appropriate training in ultrasound scanning technique and image interpretation, however, the ability of ultrasound to clarify articular disease from periarticular disease and to characterize structures precisely even when they are ambiguous on physical examination are valuable (Torralba, 2009).

▶ Echogenicity

Echogenicity is a measure of acoustic reflectance, or the ability of a tissue to reflect a sound wave. Echogenic structures that have higher amplitude of the reflected wave appear white on ultrasound. In contrast, anechoic structures (lower amplitude) appear black (Figure 54–1).

▶ Definitions for Ultrasound Pathology in Rheumatology

In 2005, the Outcomes in Measures of Rheumatology (OMERACT) Ultrasound Task Force developed consensus-based, standardized definitions for ultrasound pathology in

- Hyperechoic — Bone, calcium

- Isoechoic — Subcutaneous tissue

- Hypoechoic — Tendon, synovial thickening

- Anechoic — Fluid, cartilage, muscle

▲ **Figure 54–1.** Echogenicity.

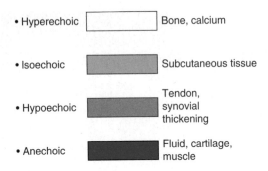

rheumatology. These definitions have become the gold standard for reporting of MSKUS findings (Wakefield, 2005).

Bone erosion. An intra-articular discontinuity of the bony surface that is visible in two perpendicular planes (Figure 54–2A and B).

Synovial effusion. Abnormal hypoechoic or anechoic (relative to subdermal fat, but sometimes may be isoechoic or hypoechoic) intra-articular material that is displaceable and compressible, but does not exhibit Doppler signal (Figure 54–3).

Synovial hypertrophy. Abnormal hypoechoic (relative to subdermal fat, but sometimes may be isoechoic or hyperechoic) intra-articular tissue that is nondisplaceable and poorly compressible and which may exhibit Doppler signal (Figure 54–4).

Tenosynovitis. Hypoechoic or anechoic thickened tissue with or without fluid within the tendon sheath, which is seen in two perpendicular planes and which may exhibit Doppler signal (Figure 54–5A and B).

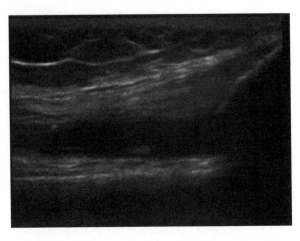

▲ **Figure 54–3.** Synovial effusion, for example, anterior longitudinal view of knee with moderate joint effusion.

Enthesopathy. Abnormally hypoechoic (loss of normal fibrillar architecture) and/or thickened tendon or ligament at its bony attachment (may occasionally contain hyperechoic foci consistent with calcification), seen in two perpendicular planes that may exhibit Doppler signal and/or bony changes, including enthesophytes, erosions, or irregularity (Figure 54–6).

▶ **Rheumatoid Arthritis**

Ultrasound evaluation of synovitis in rheumatoid arthritis (RA) has been shown in several studies to be highly sensitive in detecting joint inflammation (Brown, 2006; Szkudlarek et al, 2003; Wakefield, 2004). Inflammation of the synovial

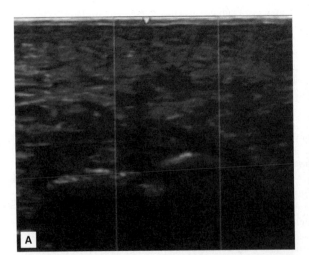
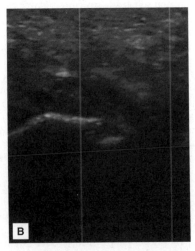

▲ **Figure 54–2.** Bone erosion in two orthogonal planes, for example, calcaneus with negative power Doppler signal.

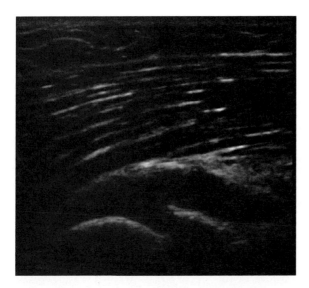

▲ Figure 54–4. Synovial hypertrophy, for example, anterior humeroradial view of elbow with synovial hypertrophy in an ankylosing spondylitis patient.

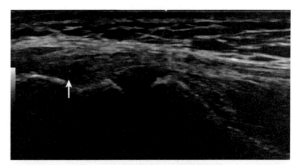

▲ Figure 54–6. Enthesopathy. For example, lateral longitudinal view of common extensor tendon inserting on lateral epicondyle with hypoechogenicity.

lining is a key feature of RA, and gray scale images can assess the degree of synovial hypertrophy, often described in a semiquantitative synovitis grading system (Hammer et al, 2011; Szkudlarek et al, 2003; Terslev et al, 2012). However, gray scale images cannot differentiate accurately between synovium that is chronically inflamed as opposed to acutely inflamed.

Hyperemia during active inflammation can be visualized with color power Doppler or power Doppler. Color power Doppler assesses the energy of moving erythrocytes without taking direction into account and is therefore able to pick up slow flow states as seen in fingers and toes and is more sensitive than color flow Doppler. This differs from color Doppler, which displays mean velocity of moving erythrocytes

following directional flow, as is used with vascular ultrasound. Color power Doppler is more sensitive than gray scale ultrasound alone for the detection of early disease and can more accurately differentiate chronic and acute disease, thus helping assess response to treatment (Torp-Pedersen et al, 2008; Torp-Pedersen et al, 2015).

Ultrasound can directly visualize fluid versus synovial thickening. Effusions can be seen in multiple conditions, including RA, PsA, OA, and crystalline arthritides. Ultrasound guidance allows localization of fluid to assist with diagnostic and therapeutic arthrocentesis (Figures 54–7 and 54–8).

Ultrasound can identify erosions earlier than conventional radiography (Funck-Brentano et al, 2009; Scheel, 2006; Wakefield et al, 2000). The locations of highest yield for the detection of erosions related to RA are the ulnar styloid process, the radial aspect of the second MCP joint, and the ulnar aspect of the fifth MCP joint (Boutry et al, 2007). One group reported 6.5-fold more erosions by ultrasound versus plain radiography in an early RA cohort. Similarly, 3.4-fold more erosions were visualized by ultrasound compared with plain radiography in a late RA cohort, using MRI as the gold standard (Wakefield et al, 2000). Many studies suggest ultrasound

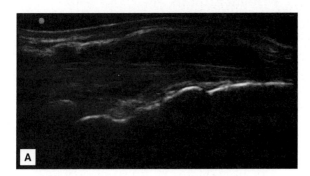

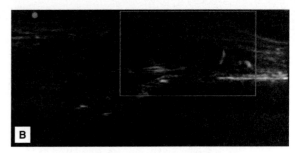

▲ Figure 54–5. A: Dorsal longitudinal view of wrist tenosynovitis in a rheumatoid arthritis patient. **B:** Dorsal transverse view of wrist tenosynovitis with positive power Doppler signal consistent with active inflammation. (See color insert.)

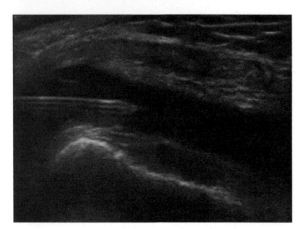

▲ **Figure 54–7.** Ultrasound-guided arthrocentesis of knee effusion.

performs as well or nearly as well as MRI in identifying superficial erosions (Boutry et al, 2007; Dohn et al, 2006; Ostergaard et al, 2003; Scheel, 2006; Szkudlarek et al, 2006; Wakefield et al, 2000).

A number of semiquantitative synovitis grading systems that have been developed for RA (Hammer et al, 2011; Szkudlarek et al, 2003; Terslev et al, 2012). There is general agreement on gray scale scoring by use of a semiquantitative scale from 0 to 3, reflecting the size of the synovial hypertrophy (0 = normal, 1 = minor, 2 = moderate, 3 = major amount of synovial hypertrophy) (Figure 54–9).

The first scoring system proposed by Szkudlarek et al (2003) proposed a semiquantitative scoring system 0–3, with 0 = no Doppler signal, 1 = single vessel signal, 2 = confluent vessel signal in less than half of the areas of the synovium, and 3 = vessel signals in more than 50% of the area of the synovium.

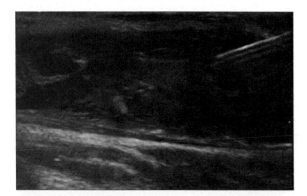

▲ **Figure 54–8.** Ultrasound-guided Bakers cyst aspiration in a rheumatoid arthritis patient. Posterior longitudinal view. Note thickened pannus formation within cyst.

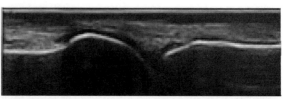

Grade 0

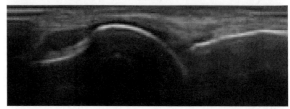

Grade 1

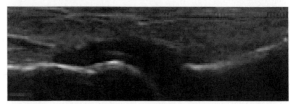

Grade 2

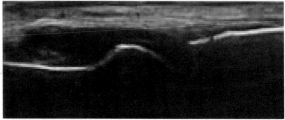

Grade 3

▲ **Figure 54–9.** Semiquantitative synovitis grading.

▶ Psoriatic Arthritis

Ultrasound for the diagnosis and monitoring of synovitis, enthesitis, dactylitis, and nail changes has increased our understanding of the ultrastructural changes that may be important in psoriatic arthritis (PsA). Enthesis traditionally has been defined as the attachment of a tendon or ligament to bone. The attachments may be fibrocartilaginous or fibrous (Benjamin, 2009; McGonagle, 2015). Enthesitis related to spondlyoarthropathy occurs at the fibrocartilaginous entheses. In contrast, metabolic disorders such as diabetes and obesity tend to affect the membranous entheses. The concept of an enthesis or synovioentheseal junction as a specific "organ" has been proposed. The Achilles tendon enthesis, for example, not only includes the tendon-bone junction but also recognizes the fibrocartilage at the posterior aspect of the calcaneus and the abutting area of the Achilles tendon. The surrounding bursa and fat pad play a role in shear stresses to the Achilles tendon, and a small layer of synovial cells abutting Kager's fat pad is thought to be important to pathologic changes in enthesitis. This model suggests mechanical factors such as fibrocartilage degeneration may be important in the site of entheseal inflammation (Benjamin, 2009). Some authors have also proposed that changes in tendon hypoechogenicity, thickening, peritendinous fluid, and adjacent bursitis may be considered acute changes in enthesitis. Findings considered to be more chronic changes include calcifications, erosions, tendon tears, and thinning (Balint, 2018; Kaeley, 2018). See Figure 54–10 for an example of enthesitis.

Ultrasound findings must be correlated with clinical findings because acute mechanical Achilles tendinitis and tendon tears can also appear to be inflammatory with power Doppler signal (Figure 54–11A and B).

Early PsA may have findings of subclinical synovitis by ultrasound especially in the wrist, knee, metatarsophalangeal, and metacarpophalangeal joints resulting in a change of assessment of number and symmetry of joint involvement, especially with nearly 20% of oligoarthritis patients being reclassified as having polyarthritis (Bandinelli, 2013). Occult enthesitis in PsA, evaluated using the Glasgow Ultrasound Enthesitis Scoring System (GUESS), appears independent of clinical features and psoriasis severity. Forty percent of PsA patients have positive power Doppler ultrasound signal in the

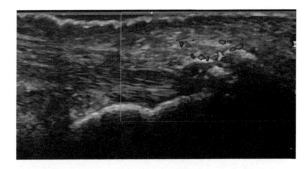

▲ **Figure 54–10.** Posterior longitudinal view: Achilles enthesitis with cortical erosions and positive power Doppler signal. (See color insert.)

entheses, making this technique more sensitive than clinical examination, which detected tenderness in only 29%. Arthritis precedes psoriasis in approximately 15–20% of cases of PsA, but the arthritis may not become evident in some cases for 10 years or long (Gladman, 1987).

A number of systems have been developed for ultrasound evaluation of enthesitis, including the Madrid Sonographic Enthesitis Index (MASEI) (Eder, 2014) and Leeds Enthesitis Index (Ibrahim, 2011). See Table 54–1 for sonographic features and entheses locations assessed in these systems.

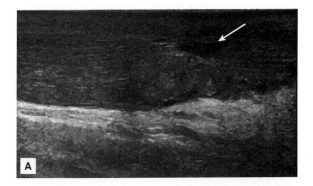

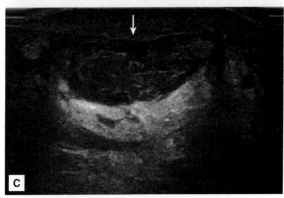

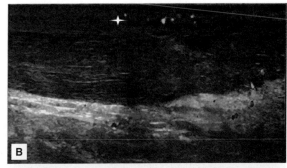

▲ **Figure 54–11. A:** Posterior longitudinal view: Achilles tendinitis and partial tendon tear (*arrow*). **B:** Power Doppler signal within tendon and paratenon. (See color insert.) **C:** Posterior transverse view: Achilles tendinitis and partial tendon tear (*arrow*).

Table 54–1. Sonographic changes in enthesitis and anatomic sites for psoriatic arthritis.

Sonographic Changes in Enthesitis (MASEI and Leeds Systems)	
Thickening and structural changes of the tendon insertion Calcification at the tendon insertion Bone erosions Enthesophyte formation Perientheseal soft-tissue edema Entheseal thickening Bursitis Power Doppler changes at site of enthesis	
MASEI (Madrid Sonographic Enthesis Index)—Anatomic Sites	**Leeds Enthesitis Index—Anatomic Sites**
Patella at insertions of the quadriceps femoris and patellar tendons	Medial condyles of the femur
Achilles tendon and plantar fascia insertions in the calcaneus	Achilles tendon insertions
Triceps tendon insertion to the olecranon process	Lateral epicondyles of the humerus

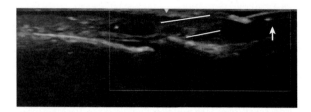

▲ **Figure 54–13.** DIP and nail enthesitis. Swelling around extensor tendon with positive power Doppler signal. Lines outline thickening of extensor tendon as it approaches nail (*arrow*). (See color insert.)

of the distal phalanx. Power Doppler ultrasound can be detected in a significant number of PsA patients in the DIP joint and nail beds (Wortsman, 2010). DIP joint extensor tendon enthesopathy appears relevant to the pathogenesis of nail disease in both psoriasis and clinically evident and subclinical PsA patients (Klauser, 2008) (Figure 54–13).

▶ Crystalline arthritis—Gout & Pseudogout

Diagnostic imaging with both ultrasound and dual-energy CT (DECT) has been increasingly helpful in the diagnoses of crystalline arthritides. The 2015 ACR/EULAR classification criteria for gout have been included in the imaging domain criteria the double contour sign of gout by ultrasound and positive MSU crystal visualization by DECT, along with traditional bony erosion of gout seen on radiography (Neogi et al, 2015) (Figure 54–14).

The high reflectivity of crystalline particles and the sensitivity of ultrasound for the detection of small quantities of these crystals impart to ultrasound great promise for the development of scanning protocols, scoring systems, and further validation of imaging techniques in this spectrum of rheumatic disease (Filippuci et al, 2014). A systematic literature review by Ogdie et al reported the sensitivity and

Dactylitis, commonly known as "sausage digit," comprises inflammation related to multiple tissue compartments (Kane, 1999; Olivieri, 1995; Olivieri et al, 2008). A number of ultrasound and MRI studies have concluded that in addition to flexor tenosynovitis, there is small joint soft-tissue edema including involvement of the palmar plate and collateral ligament (Olivieri, 1995; Olivieri et al, 2008). A review of this literature is well summarized by Bakewell et al (2013) (Figure 54–12).

Ultrasound has been used to evaluate nail diseases in psoriasis. Nails are considered an extension of the enthesis (Aydin, 2012; Gutierrez, 2009). Wortsman devised a classification system that has noted a significant difference in the mean distance between ventral plate and osseous margins

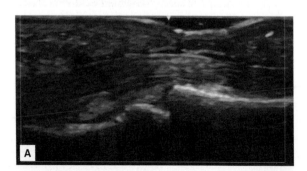

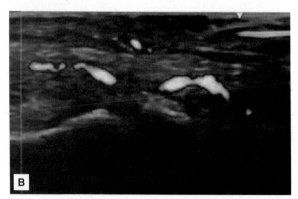

▲ **Figure 54–12. A:** Dactylitis. Swelling of tissue, flexor tendon, and PIP synovium. **B:** Dactylitis. Positive power Doppler signal. (See color insert.)

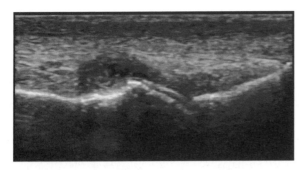

▲ **Figure 54–14.** Dorsal longitudinal view of first MTP joint with double contour sign and hyperechoic aggregates representative of monosodium urate crystals.

specificity of ultrasound-identified tophi to be 0.65 and 0.80, respectively, and those of the double-contour sign to be 0.80 and 0.76 specificity, respectively (Ogdie et al, 2015).

Ultrasound findings of monosodium urate crystals and calcium pyrophosphate dihydrate deposition at the knee cartilage have high specificity but low sensitivity (Filippuci et al, 2012) (Figures 54–15 and 54–16).

See Table 54–2 for Ultrasound features of gout (Gutierrez et al, 2015).

See Table 54–3 for ultrasound features of calcium pyrophosphate dihydrate deposition (CPPD) (Fillipou et al, 2017).

▶ Systemic Sclerosis

Systemic sclerosis (SSc) is a chronic connective tissue disease with a broad range of manifestations resulting from characteristic vascular and fibrotic changes (Abouac et al, 2012; Randone et al, 2008). Patterns of organ, vascular, and soft-tissue involvement determine the disease subtype, the severity of the condition, and the prognosis. Peripheral disease in SSc by physical examination may reveal skin thickening, pitting and digital ulceration, nailfold capillary changes,

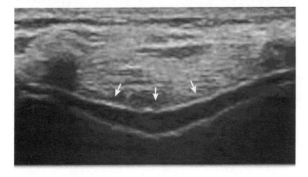

▲ **Figure 54–15.** Maximum flexion view: double contour sign (*arrows*) of gout on top of femoral hyaline cartilage.

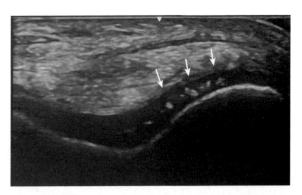

▲ **Figure 54–16.** Maximum flexion view: Chondrocalcinosis (*arrows*). "Pseudo-double contour" sign within the femoral hyaline cartilage.

Raynaud phenomenon, calcinosis, joint contractures, synovitis, and telangectasias. Skin tightening, a "puffy" edematous appearance of the fingers, and digital contractures can all obscure pathology. Ultrasound has a potential role in characterizing articular disease, including synovitis, erosions, and osteophytes, as well as in identifying such periarticular or soft-tissue manifestations as tendinopathy and calcinosis (Baron, 1982).

Table 54–2. OMERACT definitions of elemental lesions of gout.

Elemental Lesion	Definition
Double contour sign	Abnormal hyperechoic band over the superficial margin of the articular hyaline cartilage, independent of the angle of insonation and which may be either irregular or regular, continuous or intermittent, and can be distinguished from the cartilage interface sign.
Tophus	(Independent of location [eg, extra-articular/intra-articular/intratendinous]): a circumscribed, inhomogeneous, hyperechoic, and/or hypoechoic aggregation (which may or may not generate posterior acoustic shadow), which may be surrounded by a small anechoic rim.
Aggregates	(Independent of location [intra-articular/intra-tendinous]): heterogeneous hyperechoic foci that maintain their high degree of reflectivity, even when the gain setting is minimized or the insonation angle is changed and which occasionally may generate posterior acoustic shadow.
Erosion	An intra- and/or extra-articular discontinuity of the bone surface (visible in two perpendicular planes).

Data from Gutierrez M, Schmidt WA, Thiele RG, et al. International consensus for ultrasound lesions in gout: results of Delphi process and web-reliability exercise. *Rheumatology.* 2015;54(10):1797-1805.

Table 54–3. OMERACT definitions of ultrasound findings in CPPD disease (Fillipou et al, 2017).

Structure	Shape	Echogenicity	Localization	Behavior at Dynamic Scanning
Fibrocartilage	Deposits of variable shape	Hyperechoic (similar to echogenicity of bony cortex)	Localized within the fibrocartilage structure	Remain fixed and move together with the fibrocartilage during dynamic assessment (ie, joint movement and probe compression)
Hyaline cartilage	Deposits varying in size and shape	Hyperechoic (similar to echogenicity of bony cortex) that do not create posterior shadowing	Localized within the hyaline cartilage	The deposits remain fixed and move together with the hyaline cartilage (ie, joint movement and probe compression)
Tendon	Multiple linear (parallel to the tendon fibrillar structure and not in continuity with the bone profile) deposits	Hyperechoic (in relation to the tendon echogenicity) that generally do not create posterior shadowing. The deposits maintain their high degree of echogenicity even at very low levels of gain and are not affected by anisotropy as the surrounding tendon	Localized within the tendon	Remain fixed and move together with the tendon during movement and probe compression
Synovial fluid	Deposits of variable size (from punctate to large)	Hyperechoic (similar to echogenicity of bony cortex) that generally do not create posterior shadowing	Localized within the synovial fluid	Are mobile according to joint movement and probe pressure

Inflammatory arthritis in SSc has been reported to occur at a low incidence. Multiple ultrasound studies in SSc, however, have found higher than expected frequencies of synovitis. In the general SSc population, the frequency has been reported to range from 22% to 58%. The prevalence of SSc synovitis detected by ultrasound has been noted to be roughly half the prevalence seen in RA (Cuomo et al, 2009; Elhai et al, 2012; Gohar et al, 2015). Distribution of synovitis has been primarily reported in MCP and PIP joints, while one study noted an even distribution among the joints of the fingers and wrists. These studies have also noted the presence of erosions and osteophytes. When compared to RA, erosions were found to be relatively infrequent (Cuomo et al, 2009; Fairchild et al, 2019).

US can also identify inflammatory and sclerotic changes in tendons. SSc patients with tendon friction rubs had an increased retinacular thickness by ultrasound compared to those without, but studies focused on ultrasound-identified sclerosis are lacking (Abdel-Magied et al, 2013; Chitale et al, 2010; Elhai et al, 2012; Gohar et al, 2015) (Figure 54–17A and B).

US can also visualize vasculopathy-related disease manifestations, including ability to evaluate digital ulcers, calcinosis, and acro-osteolysis.

US has the ability to visualize skin thickness. Skin evaluation in SSc patients is important for disease classification, monitoring, and prognostication (Clements et al, 1990). Rodnan skin score (mRSS) suffers from observer variability, low sensitivity to change, and does not differentiate skin thickness from skin tightness (Claman et al, 2006; Kissin et al, 2006). With advancement in technology, high frequency probes for evaluation of skin have allowed measurement of epidermal and dermal thickness; several studies have shown

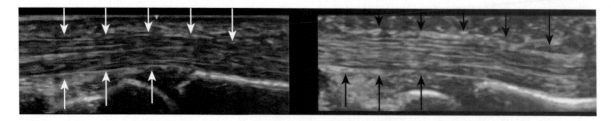

▲ **Figure 54–17** **A:** Normal flexor tendon. **B:** Flexor tendon with sclerosis. (Used with permission from Robert Fairchild, MD, PhD.)

good sensitivity and specificity with low intra- and interobserver variability. Ultrasound detected statistically significant skin thickening in clinically uninvolved areas in both diffuse and limited SSc (Ihn et al, 1995; Kaloudi et al, 2010; Moore, 2003; Sulli et al, 2017).

Interstitial lung disease (ILD) is a major cause of morbidity and mortality in SSc and is seen in roughly half of SSc patients (Hoffmann-Vold et al, 2019; Walker et al, 2007; Walker et al, 2009). Currently, high-resolution computed tomography (HRCT) is the gold standard imaging for SSc-ILD diagnosis (Meyer, 2014), however dependence on HRCT for screening, and monitoring for progression risks exposing SSc patients to significant cumulative radiation, increased health care costs. Lung ultrasonography has potential to identify B-lines, pleural irregularity, pleural thickening, and effusions (Gutierrez 2011; Gutierrez 2019; Pinal-Fernandez 2015; Wang et al, 2017). (Figure 54–18). SSc-ILD patterns are usually nonspecific interstitial pneumonia and usual interstitial pneumonia patterns, which may be well-suited to ultrasound due to its peripheral and basilar lung distribution. B-lines are an ultrasound artifact whose presence and quantity varies by machine settings and reader. B-lines are not specific to ILD. Despite this, B-line quantification has traditionally been the focus of the majority of sonographic studies on SSc-ILD and has shown comparable diagnostic accuracy for SSc-ILD detection compared to HRCT (Gutierrez 2011; Gutierrez, 2019; Pinal-Fernandez 2015; Wang et al, 2017). Variability in the LUS scanning protocols including acquisition technique and number of zones

required for examination exists. Further studies to develop validated ultrasound interpretation criteria standardized for rheumatologic lung disease are needed to show how LUS may potentially be able to differentiate ILD subtype, severity, activity, and monitor response to therapy.

▶ Systemic Lupus Erythematosus

Systemic lupus erythematosus (SLE) arthropathy has traditionally been divided into distinct patterns. Joint involvement consisting of nondeforming nonerosive arthritis comprises the majority of SLE-associated arthritis patients, but approximately 5–15% of SLE patients develop a deforming arthritis. Deforming arthritis is further subdivided into erosive and nonerosive disease. The erosive form is typically considered an overlap with RA or "rhupus." In contrast, the nonerosive Jaccoud arthropathy is believed to result from involvement of the ligaments and tendons (DiMatteo et al, 2019; van Vugt et al, 1998). Ultrasound has the ability to identify a higher degree of erosions, synovitis, and various other articular and periarticular pathologies (DiMatteo et al, 2019; van Vugt et al, 1998; Zayat et al, 2016).

Pathologic findings on ultrasound in SLE patients with nondeforming, nonerosive arthritis reveal fewer inflammatory changes compared to patients with "rhupus" and to those with Jaccoud arthropathy (Gabba et al, 2012). Ultrasound findings do not predict this progression, but severe disease as identified by synovial power Doppler severity in patients with nondeforming, nonerosive arthritis was associated with an arthritic flare within 2 years (Piga et al, 2016).

Patients with SLE appear to have a higher burden of tendon pathology compared to those with RA. Tenosynovitis, common in Jaccoud arthropathy, can be a significant source of clinical symptoms. Tendon involvement can occur in both extensor and flexor tendons of the hands and wrists and in the lower extremities in the tibialis tendons of the ankle (Gabba et al, 2012; Han and Tian, 2019; Lins et al, 2018; Ribeiro et al, 2018).

Ultrasound studies have demonstrated that enthesopathy is more common in SLE than previously recognized. Entheseal pathology has been described in 20–60% of SLE patients. It most commonly affects the distal patellar tendon, but has also been seen in the quadriceps insertion, the proximal patellar tendon, the Achilles tendon, and plantar fascia (Di Matteo et al, 2016; Di Matteo et al, 2018). Limited studies on use of ultrasound in SLE patients exist, but ultrasound remains a promising tool for identifying potentially unrecognized joint and tendon pathology across the entire spectrum of SLE patients.

▶ Osteoarthritis

Osteoarthritis (OA), the most common form of arthritis, has traditionally been thought of as a degenerative or "wear and tear" condition that mostly affects the cartilage. With advances

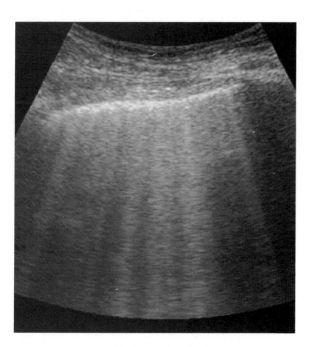

▲ **Figure 54–18.** Lung ultrasound B-lines.

in imaging, however, it has become evident that OA is much more complex than simply a disorder of wear and tear (Hootman et al, 2016; Jafarzadeh and Felson, 2017). The Osteoarthritis Research Society International (OARSI) defines OA as a disorder characterized by cell stress and extracellular matrix degradation initiated by micro- and macroinjury. These processes activate maladaptive repair responses, including proinflammatory pathways of innate immunity. The disease manifests itself first as a molecular derangement (abnormal joint-tissue metabolism) followed by anatomic, and/or physiologic derangements (characterized by cartilage degradation, bone remodeling, osteophyte formation, joint inflammation, and loss of normal joint function) (Osteoarthritis Research Society International, 2016). Radiographic assessment of joint space narrowing, osteophytes, and MRI assessment of cartilage are currently most often used in both clinical and research realms. Ultrasound has great potential for capturing many of the key features seen on XR or MRI and may be a more cost-effective, accessible imaging modality but has suffered from the bias of operator dependence and reliability (Emery et al, 2019; van Oudenaarde et al, 2017). These features include articular cartilage, bony cortex, synovial recesses, tendons, ligaments, bursae, and peripheral aspects of menisci (Berkoff et al, 2012; Iagnocco and Naredo, 2017). Ultrasound is more sensitive than radiography for early OA changes. Ultrasound is also useful for injection guidance (Berkoff et al, 2012; Iagnocco and Naredo, 2017).

Ultrasound in hand OA has demonstrated associations between symptoms and inflammatory features, particularly in erosive OA (Iagnocco and Naredo, 2017). A study of 93 patients with OA of the basilar thumb identified synovitis in 56% and power Doppler in 14%; those with power Doppler signal compared to those without had more pain, but similar function (Oo et al, 2019). Ultrasound can also detect osteophytes. In a study of 127 patients with hand OA, US was more sensitive in detecting osteophytes compared to radiography or clinical exam (53%, 30%, and 37% respectively) (Mathiessen et al, 2013). In a longitudinal study of 78 participants with hand OA, gray scale synovitis and power Doppler detected on ultrasound were associated with overall radiographic progression over 5 years, as well as predicted development of erosions, joint space narrowing, and osteophyte progression (Mathiessen et al, 2016). Ultrasound has been of particular interest in the subgroup of erosive hand osteoarthritis. Two small studies demonstrated high sensitivity, specificity, and agreement for ultrasound compared with MRI and even contrast-enhanced MRI (Vlychou et al, 2013; Wittoek et al, 2011).

US of the knee has high specificity and sensitivity for effusion when compared to MRI, moderate correlations overall for synovitis, effusion, synovial hypertrophy, cartilage thickness, and popliteal cysts. US of the knee can also assess osteophytes. Correlation between US and radiographs was highest in the medial compartment (Keen et al, 2009; Meenagh et al, 2007; Oo et al, 2018).

US of the hip can identify synovitis, effusion, synovial hypertrophy. One study considered the presence of effusion-synovitis by either US or MRI at the hip joint and found that US and MRI assessments of bone capsular distance at week 0 before guided intra-articular corticosteroid injection and 8 weeks post-injection were significantly correlated at the femoral neck but were not associated with post intra-articular steroid injection outcomes (Oo et al, 2018).

Standardized protocols for ultrasound in inflammatory arthritis have been well described, but there is a lack of standardized protocols for the use of US in OA. Nelson et al recently developed the SOAR (Sonography of Osteoarthritis for Rheumatologists) standardized protocol and atlas which includes sonographic features of OA (Table 54–4) and demonstrated the feasibility of obtaining standardized images and reliability of interpretation (Alvarez et al, 2019 and Yerich N. et al, 2020). After development of the protocol, correlations between US an XR features were analyzed and the strongest correlations were seen between US medial and lateral osteophytes and Kellgren-Lawrence Grade (KLG) (spearman correlation $r = 0.62$ and 0.54, respectively) and between US medial and lateral osteophytes and radiographic osteophytes ($r = 0.58$ and 0.57, respectively). US medial meniscal extrusion was significantly associated with both radiographic (KLG) and with medial joint space narrowing ($r = 0.42$ and 0.36, respectively). Additionally, stronger correlations were seen between medial osteophytes by US and pain as assessed by the KOOS (Knee Injury and Osteoarthritis Outcome Score, $r = 0.34$) compared with radiographic osteophytes ($r = 0.16$). US medial and lateral osteophytes, medial meniscal extrusion, medial cartilage damage, and popliteal cysts were all significantly associated with the presence of radiographic symptomatic knee OA ($r = 0.15$–0.43) (Yerich et al, 2019).

Ultrasound for OA shows promise as a useful, more accessible, and cost-effective imaging modality that can identify features of early OA not detected by radiography, and can similarly characterize synovial hypertrophy, effusions, bony change as can be seen in MRI. Ultrasound also offers procedural guidance for injections targeting synovitis or evacuating effusions and Bakers cysts to help reduce patient symptoms. Further studies to develop protocols, scoring systems, and its correlation to clinical symptoms are needed to increase the applicability of its use in OA.

▶ Beyond Musculoskeletal Ultrasound: Salivary Gland Diseases (Sjögren's Syndrome, IgG4-Related Disease) & Large Vessel Vasculitis (Giant Cell Arteritis)

As the value of ultrasound in musculoskeletal conditions has been established, the utility of ultrasound for rheumatic disease beyond the musculoskeletal system has grown.

Table 54–4. Ultrasound features including views, scoring range, and definitions of scoring levels in SOAR[a]

US Feature	Range	Scoring Description
View: Suprapatellar longitudinal and transverse in 30-degree flexion		
Effusion/synovitis	0–3	0: none 1: JCD parallel to bone, or a small anechoic or hypoechoic line beneath the capsule 2: JCD horizontal or elevated parallel to the joint line 3: convex/bulging JCD
Synovitis	0–3	0: none 1: minimal JCD by abnormal internal hypoechoic or anechoic material 2: JCD elevated parallel/flat superficial limit 3: JCD with convex/bulging superficial limit
Effusion	0–1	0: none 1: abnormal anechoic or hypoechoic IA material
Color power Doppler	0–3	0: none 1: trace to 10% of IA area with color signal 2: 10-50% of IA area with color signal 3: >50% of IA area with color signal
View: Suprapatellar transverse in maximal flexion (medial and lateral scored separately)		
Cartilage damage (medial/lateral)	0–3	0: normal 1: minimal thinning 2: mild or local thinning 3: complete loss of cartilage
View: Longitudinal at the medial or lateral femorotibial joint in 30 degrees flexion		
Osteophytes (medial/lateral)	0–3	0: none 1: small but distinct 2: medium/intermediate 3: large, bulky, prominent
Meniscal extrusion (medial/lateral)	0–1	0: none 1: definitely partially or completely extruded
View: Posterior medial transverse		
Popliteal cyst	0–2	0: absent 1: small/possible 2: definite
View: Assessed in all views		
Calcium crystal deposition	0–1	0: absent 1: hyperechoic deposits in cartilage, meniscus, or synovial fluid in each view

[a]Sonography of Osteoarthritis for Rheumatologists—PI: Amanda Nelson, MD, RhMSUS; Collaborators: Minna Kohler, MD, RhMSUS; Catherine Bakewell, MD, RhMSUS; Janice Lin, MD; Jonathan Samuels, MD, RhMSUS.

IA, intra-articular; JCD, joint capsular distention.

▶ Ultrasound in Salivary Gland Diseases

Ultrasound can detect glandular structural features in Sjögren's syndrome, and similar to other imaging modalities such as MRI and MR sialography, it has been proposed as a viable alternative to conventional but otherwise invasive diagnostic tests (Niemela 2004; Song 2014). A number of scoring systems have been developed for the evaluation of Sjögrens syndrome, one of which considers the number of hypoechogenic oval areas, hyperechogenic reflections/lines and clearness of the borders apart from echogenicity, and parenchymal inhomogeneity (Hocevar, 2005); and another which assigns

a grading between G0–G5 based on extent of distribution of areas of hypoechogenicity, margin irregularity, and hyperechoic bands (Ariji et al, 1996; Takagi et al, 2014). A 0–12 scoring system has been developed and a score of more than or equal to 6 correlated with positive biopsy and scintigraphy results (Milic et al, 2010). Ultrasound of the parotid and/or submandibular glands has been used as an alternative to any of the 2012 American College of Rheumatology classification items (Takagi et al, 2014) and has been shown to improve the diagnostic performance of these criteria (Cornec et al, 2014).

While hypoechoic oval areas with hyperechoic septal lines within the glands are characteristic for Sjögren syndrome,

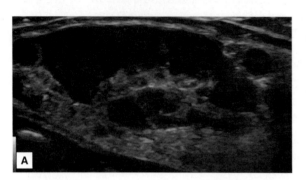
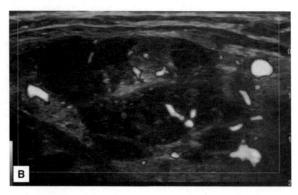

▲ **Figure 54–19. A:** Enlarged submandibular gland in an IgG4-related disease patient. **B:** Enlarged submandibular gland with hyperemia (increased color power Doppler signal). (See color insert.)

these are not pathognomonic. Similar changes can be found in other diseases such as sarcoid and other granulomatous diseases, disseminated lymphoma (non-Hodgkin lymphoma [NHL]), human immunodeficiency virus (HIV)–associated salivary gland disease, amyloidosis, and IgG4-related disease (Bialek et al, 2006; Bialek and Jakubowski, 2016).

IgG4-related disease can also cause bilateral salivary gland enlargement and affects 27–53% of cases (Li et al, 2016). In a study of 39 patients with IgG4-related disease, 90% showed ultrasound signs of disease in the salivary glands with 90% having submandibular gland infiltration compared to 35% in the parotid gland (Shimizu et al, 2015). The most common pattern of infiltration described a superficial hypoechoic pattern (60%), while the multiple hypoechoic reticulated pattern more typical for Sjögrens syndrome was detected in 23% of lesions. A recent study of nine patients founds bilateral nodule hyperemic submandibular involvement in eight out of nine patients, but none in the parotid glands (Shimizu et al, 2009) (Figure 54–19).

▷ **Ultrasound in Large Vessel Vasculitis**

Ultrasound has been used as early as the 1980s as a diagnostic modality in cranial giant cell arteritis (GCA), initially in the form of color flow Doppler (Menkes et al, 1981). The first prospective study of color duplex ultrasonography in 1997 reported the use of ultrasound as an imaging modality with high sensitivity and specificity in the diagnosis of GCA (Schmidt et al, 1997). Subsequent meta-analyses have shown a relatively high sensitivity and specificity of ultrasound in GCA/large vessel vasculitis (LVV) when compared to the American College of Rheumatology GCA classification criteria (Arida et al, 2010; Ball et al, 2010; Karassa et al, 2010). In experienced hands, ultrasound appears to be more sensitive than the biopsy of the temporal artery in the diagnosis of GCA (Arida et al, 2010; Ball et al, 2010; Karassa et al, 2010). Widespread use of ultrasound for diagnosis of

GCA has unfortunately suffered from a variety of reasons, including low quality/resolution of equipment used, erroneous technique, and erroneous adjustments of ultrasound equipment setting in an inexperienced ultrasonographer. Despite this, numerous studies have shown the usefulness of ultrasound in the imaging of inflammatory changes of the large vessels (Czihal et al, 2010; Czihal et al, 2012; Diamantopoulos et al, 2014; Ghinoi et al, 2012; Schmidt et al, 2008). A recent meta-analysis confirmed high sensitivity and specificity of ultrasound in cranial GCA (Duftner et al, 2018) and has been used as the main source of evidence of the development of the EULAR guidelines on the use of imaging modalities in LVV. These guidelines strongly recommend the use of ultrasound of the temporal and axillary arteries as a first-line examination for diagnosing cranial GCA (Dejaco et al, 2018).

Identifying the halo sign on ultrasound examinations of the temporal artery and/or large vessels can be helpful as a diagnostic adjunct to the history and clinical exam in a patient with suspected vasculitis. The inflammation of the vessel wall is visualized by ultrasound in longitudinal and transverse views as a homogeneous, hypoechoic thickness that is surrounding the blood flow, also known as the halo sign, which represents intima media wall thickening (Diamantopoulos et al, 2014; Schmidt et al, 1997) (Figure 54–20).

Compared to other imaging modalities, ultrasound has a comparable sensitivity to MRA (1.5 T and up) in cranial arteritis (Bley et al, 2008) and to positron emission tomography-CT (PET-CT) scan in LVV-GCA (Czihal et al, 2010; Forster et al, 2011). Ultrasound compared to cross-sectional imaging is more cost-effective, is not associated with ionized radiation or contrast, and has potential to be used for consecutive follow-up examinations. With appropriate training and understanding of ultrasound machine adjustments needed to optimize image quality, ultrasound for vasculitis has potential for expediting diagnosis of GCA and ability to monitor disease activity.

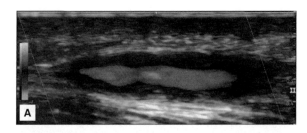
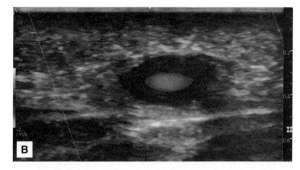

▲ **Figure 54–20. A:** Longitudinal view of temporal artery with color flow Doppler and halo sign (thickening of intima medial wall). **B:** Transverse view of temporal artery with color flow Doppler and halo sign (thickening of intima medial wall). (See color insert.)

▶ Conclusion

MSKUS performed and interpreted by a rheumatologist has become an accepted tool that allows the clinician to use their history and exam skills correlating with a targeted ultrasound examination to expedite diagnosis and management of rheumatologic conditions with the potential for improved clinical outcomes and decreased health care costs. Implementation of ultrasound in clinical practice as well as adoption of evidence-based ultrasound criteria as part of classifications for multiple rheumatic diseases is changing the way rheumatologists diagnose and monitor disease. As technology advances with improved image acquisition and resolution, ultrasound will continue to assist in identifying pathology, characterize disease patterns, and/or confirm disease activity as well as provide procedural guidance for the care of patients with rheumatologic diseases.

Abdel-Magied RA, Lotfi A, Abdelgawad EA. Magnetic resonance imaging versus musculoskeletal ultrasonography in detecting inflammatory arthropathy in systemic sclerosis patients with hand arthralgia. *Rheumatol Int.* 2013;33:1961-1966. [PMID: 23354165]

Abouac J, Walker U, Tyndall A, et al. Characteristics of joint involvement and relationships with systemic inflammation in systemic sclerosis: results from the EULAR Scleroderma Trial and Research Group (EUSTAR) database. *J Rheumatol.* 2010;37:1488-1501. [PMID: 20551097]

Alvarez C, Schwartz TA, Savage-Guin S, et al. Reliability of knee ultrasound in a community-based cohort. *Osteoarthr Cartilage.* 2019;27(1):S335-S336. Doi:10.1016/j.joca.2019.02.741.

American College of Rheumatology. RhMSUS Certification. URL: https://www.rheumatology.org/Learning-Center/RhMSUS-Certification Accessed 30 March 2020.

Arida A, Kyprianou M, Kanakis M, et al. The diagnostic value of ultrasonography-derived edema of the temporal artery wall in giant cell arteritis: a second meta-analysis. *BMC Musculoskelet Disord.* 2010;11:44. [PMID: 20210989]

Ariji Y, Ohki M, Ecguchi K, et al. Texture analysis of sonographic features of the parotid gland in Sjogren's syndrome. *Am J Roentgenol.* 1996;166:935-941. [PMID: 8610577]

Aydin SB, Castillo-Gallego C, Ash ZR, et al. Ultrasonographic assessment of nail in psoriatic disease shows a link between onychopathy and distal interphalangeal joint extensor tendon enthesopathy. *Dermatology.* 2012;225:231-235. [PMID: 23128597]

Backhaus M, Burmester GR, Gerber T, et al. Guidelines for musculoskeletal ultrasound in rheumatology. *Ann Rheum Dis.* 2001, Jul;60(7):641-649. [PMID: 11406516]

Bakewell CJ, Olivieri I, Aydin SZ, et al. Ultrasound and magnetic resonance imaging in the evaluation of psoriatic dactylitis: status and perspectives. *J Rheumatol.* 2013;40:1951-1957. [PMID: 24187105]

Balint PV, Terslev L, Aegerter P, et al. Reliability of a consensus-based ultrasound definition and scoring for enthesitis in spondyloarthritis and psoriatic arthritis: an OMERACT US initiative. *ARD.* 2018. Dec;77(12):1730-1735. [PMID: 30076154]

Ball EL, Walsh SR, Tang TY, et al. Role of ultrasonography in the diagnosis of temporal arteritis. *Br J Surg.* 2010;97(12):1765-1771. [PMID: 20799290]

Bandinelli F, Prignanon F, Bonciani D, et al. Ultrasound detects occult entheseal involvement in early psoriatic arthritis independently of clinical features and psoriasis severity. *Clin Exp Rheumatol.* 2013;31(20):219-224. [PMID: 23190740]

Baron M, Lee P, Keystone EC. The articular manifestations of progressive systemic sclerosis (scleroderma). *Ann Rheum Dis.* 1982;41:147-152. [PMID: 7073343]

Benjamin M, McGonagle D. The enthesis organ concept and its relevance to the spondyloathropathies. *Adv Exp Med Biol.* 2009;649:57-70. [PMID: 19731620]

Berkoff DJ, Miller LE, Block JE. Clinical utility of ultrasound guidance for intra-articular knee injections: a review. *Clin Interv Aging.* 2012;7:89-95. [PMID: 22500117]

Bialek EJ, Jakubowski W. Mistakes in ultrasound examination of salivary glands. *J Ultrasound.* 2016;(16)65:191-203. [PMID: 27446603]

Bialek EJ, Jakubowski W, Zajkowski P, et al. US of the major salivary glands: anatomy and spatial relationships, pathologic conditions, and pitfalls. *Radiographics.* 2006;(26)3:745-763. [PMID: 16702452]

Bley TA, Reinhard M, Hauenstein C, et al. Comparison of duplex sonography and high resolution magnetic resonance imaging in the diagnosis of giant cell (temporal) arteritis. *Arthritis Rheum.* 2008;58(8):2574-2578. [PMID: 29358285]

Boutry N, Morel M, Flipo RM, et al. Early rheumatoid arthritis: a review of MRI and sonographic findings. *AJR Am J Roentgenol.* 2007;189:1502-1509. [PMID: 18029892]

Brown AK. Using ultrasonography to facilitate best practice in diagnosis and management of RA. *Nat Rev Rheumatol.* 2009;5:698-706. [PMID: 19901917]

Brown AK, O'Connor PJ, Wakefield RJ, et al. Practice, training, and assessment among experts performing musculoskeletal ultrasonography: toward the development of an international consensus of educational standards for ultrasonography for rheumatologists. *Arthritis Rheum.* 2004, Dec 15;51(6):1018-1022. [PMID: 15593176]

Brown AK, Quinn MA, Karim Z, et al. Presence of significant synovitis in rheumatoid arthritis patients with disease-modifying antirheumatic drug induced clinical remission: evidence from an imaging study may explain structural progression. *Arthritis Rheum.* 2006;54(12):3761-3773. [PMID: 17133543]

Canella AC, Kissin EY, Torralba KD, Higgs JB. Evolution of musculoskeletal ultrasound in the United States: Implementation and practice in rheumatology. *Arthritis Care Res.* 2014;66:7-13. [PMID: 24115730]

Chitale S, Ciapetti A, Hodgson R, et al. Magnetic resonance imaging and musculoskeletal ultrasonography detect and characterize covert inflammatory arthropathy in systemic sclerosis patients with arthralgia. *Rheumatology.* 2010;49:2357-2361. [PMID: 20719883]

Claman HN, Giorno RC, Seibold JR. Endothelial and fibroblastic activation in scleroderma. The myth of the "uninvolved skin". *Arthritis Rheum.* 2006;55:603-609. [PMID: 1720957]

Clements PJ, Lachenbruch PA, Ng SC, et al. Skin score. A semiquantitative measure of cutaneous involvement that improves prediction of prognosis in systemic sclerosis. *Arthritis Rheum.* 1990;33:1256-1263. [PMID: 2390128]

Cornec D, Jousse-Joulin S, Marhadour T, et al. Salivary gland ultrasonography improves the diagnostic performance of the 2012 American College of Rheumatology classification criteria for Sjogren's syndrome. *Rheumatology (Oxford).* 2014;53(9):1604-1607. [PMID: 24706989]

Cuomo G, Zappia M, Abignano G, et al. Ultrasonographic features of the hand and wrist in systemic sclerosis. *Rheumatology (Oxford).* 2009;48:1414-1417.

Czihal M, Tato F, Foster S, Rademacher A, et al. Fever of unknown origin as initial manifestation of large vessel giant cell arteritis: diagnosis by colour-coded sonography and 18-FDG PET. *Clin Exp Rheumatol.* 2010;28(4):549-552. [PMID: 20659410]

Czihal M, Tato F, Rademacher A, Kuhlencordt P, et al. Involvement of the femoropopliteal arteries in giant cell arteritis: clinical and color duplex sonography. *J Rheumatol.* 2012;39(2):314-321. [PMID: 22247342]

Czihal M, Zanker S, Rademacher A, et al. Sonographic and clinical pattern of extracranial and cranial giant cell arteritis. *Scand J Rheumatol.* 2012;41(3):231-236. [PMID: 22400812]

D'Agostino MA, Schmidt WA. Ultrasound-guided injections in rheumatology: actual knowledge on efficacy and procedures. *Best Pract Res Clin Rheumatol.* 2013;27:283-294. [PMID: 23731936]

Dejaco C, Ramiro S, Duftner C. EULAR recommendations for the use of imaging in large vessel vasculitis in clinical practice. *Ann Rheum Dis.* 2018;77(5):636-643. [PMID: 29358285]

Diamantopoulos AP, Haugeberg G, Hetland H, et al. The diagnostic value of color Doppler ultrasonography of temporal arteries and large vessels in giant cell arteritis: a consecutive case series. *Arthritis Care Res.* 2014;66(1):113-119. [PMID: 24106211]

Di Matteo A, Filippucci E, Cipolletta E, et al. Entheseal involvement in patients with systemic lupus erythematosus: an ultrasound study. *Rheumatology.* 2018;57:1822-1829. [PMID: 29982722]

DiMatteo A, Isidori M, Corradini D, et al. Ultrasound in the assessment of musculoskeletal involvement in systemic lupus erythematosus: state of the art and perspectives. *Lupus.* 2019;28:583-590. [PMID: 30841789]

Di Matteo A, Satulu, I, DiCarlo M, et al. Entheseal involvement in systemic lupus erythematosus: are we missing something? *Lupus.* 2016;26:320-328. [PMID: 27496900]

Dohn UM, Ejbjerg BJ, Court-Payen M, et al. Are bone erosions detected by magnetic resonance imaging and ultrasonography true erosions? A comparison with computed tomography in rheumatoid arthritis metacarpophalangeal joints. *Arthritis Res Ther.* 2006;8:R110. [PMID: 16848914]

Duftner C, Dejaco C, Sepriano A, Falzon L, Schmidt WA, Ramiro S. Imaging in diagnosis, outcome prediction and monitoring of large vessel vasculitis: a systematic literature review and meta-analysis informing the EULAR recommendations. *RMD Open.* 2018;4(1):e000612. [PMID: 29531788]

Eder L, Jayaker J, Thavaneswaran A, et al. Is the Madrid Sonographic Enthesitis Index useful for differentiating psoriatic arthritis from psoriasis alone and healthy controls? *J Rheumatol.* 2014;41:466-472. [PMID: 24488414]

Elhai M, Guerini H, Bazeli R, et al. Ultrasonographic hand features in systemic sclerosis and correlates with clinical, biological and radiographic findings. *Arthritis Care Res.* 2012;63:1244-1249. [PMID: 22422556]

Emery CA, Whittaker JL, Mahmoudian A, et al. Establishing outcome measures in early knee osteoarthritis. *Nat Rev Rheumatol.* 2019;15(7):438-448. [PMID: 31201386]

Epis O, Bruschi E. Interventional ultrasound: a critical overview on ultrasound-guided injections and biopsies. *Clin Exp Rheumatol.* 2014;32(1 Suppl 80):S78-S84. [PMID: 24529311]

Fairchild R, Sharpless L, Chung M, et al. *Ultrasound Evaluation of the Hands in Patients with Systemic Sclerosis: Osteophytosis Is a Major Contributor to Tender Joints.* Atlanta, GA: ACR; 2019.

Filippuci E, Di Geso L, Girolimetti R, Grassi W. Ultrasound in crystal-related arthritis. *Clin Exp Rheumatol.* 2014;32(1Suppl 80):S42-S47. [PMID: 24528621]

Filippuci E, Gutierrez M, Georgescu D, et al. Diagnosis of gout in patients with asymptomatic hyperuricemia: a pilot ultrasound study. *Ann Rheum Dis.* 2012;71(1):157-158. [PMID: 21953340]

Fillipou G, Scire CA, Damjanov N, et al. Definition and reliability assessment of elementary ultrasonographic findings in calcium pyrophosphate deposition disease: a study by the OMERACT calcium pyrophosphate deposition disease ultrasound subtask force. *J Rheumatol.* 2017;44(11):1744-1749. [PMID: 28250136]

Forster S, Tato F, Weiss M, et al. Patterns of extracranial involvement in newly diagnosed giant cell arteritis assessed by physical examination, colour coded suplex sonography and FDG-PET. *Vasa.* 2011;40(30):219-227. [PMID: 21638250]

Funck-Brentano T, Etchepare F, Joulin SJ, et al. Benefits of ultrasonography in the management of early arthritis: a cross-sectional study of baseline data from the ESPOR cohort. *Rheumatology (Oxford).* 2009;48:1515-1519. [PMID: 19755507]

Gabba A, Piga M, Vacca A, et al. Joint and tendon involvement in systemic lupus erythematosus: an ultrasound study of hands and wrists in 108 patients. *Rheumatology (Oxford).* 20120;51:2278-2285. [PMID: 22956550]

Ghinoi A, Pipitone N, Nicolini A, et al. Large-vessel involvement in recent onset giant cell arteritis: a case-control colour-Doppler sonography study. *Rheumatology (Oxford)* 2012;51(4):730-734. [PMID: 22179725]

Gilliland CA, Salazar LD, Borchers JR. Ultrasound versus anatomic guidance for intra-articular and periarticular injection: a systematic review. *Phys Sports Med.* 2011;39:121-131. [PMID: 22030948]

Gladman DD, Shuckett R, Russell MI. Psoriatic arthritis (PSA)—an analysis of 220 patients. *Quarterly J Med.* 1987;62(238):127-141. [PMID: 3659255]

Gohar N, Ezzat Y, Naeem N, Shazly El R. A comparative study between ultrasonographic hand features in systemic sclerosis and rheumatoid arthritis patients: relation to disease activity, clinical and radiological findings. *Egypt Rheumatol.* 2015;37:177-184.

Gullo TR, Golightly YM, Cleveland RJ, et al. Defining multiple joint osteoarthritis, its frequency and impact in a community-based cohort. *Semin Arthritis Rheum.* 2019;48(6):950-957. [PMID: 30390991]

Gutierrez M, Salaffi F, Carotti M, et al. Utility of a simplified ultrasound assessment to assess interstitial pulmonary fibrosis in connective tissue disorders—preliminary results. *Arthritis Res Ther.* 2011;13:R134. [PMID: 21851634]

Gutierrez M, Schmidt WA, Thiele RG, et al. International consensus for ultrasound lesions in gout: results of Delphi process and web-reliability exercise. *Rheumatology (Oxford).* 2015;54(10):1797-1805. [PMID: 25972391]

Gutierrez M, Soto-Fajardo C, Pindea C, et al. Ultrasound in the assessment of interstitial lung disease in systemic sclerosis: a systematic literature review by the OMERACT ultrasound group. *J Rheumatol.* 2019;jrheum.180940. [PMID: 31263075]

Gutierrez M, Wortsman X, Fillipucci E, et al. High-frequency sonography in the evaluation of psoriasis: nail and skin involvement. *J Ultrasound Med.* 2009;28(11):1569-1574. [PMID: 19854972]

Hammer HB, Bolton-King P, Bakkeheim V, et al. Examination of intra and interrater reliability with a new ultrasonographic reference atlas for scoring of synovitis in patients with rheumatoid arthritis. *Ann Rheum Dis.* 2011;70:1995-1998. [PMID: 21784724]

Han N, Tian X. Detection of subclinical synovial hypertrophy by musculoskeletal gray-scale/power Doppler ultrasonography in systemic lupus erythematosus patients: a cross-sectional study. *Int J Rheum Dis.* 2019;22:1058-1069. [PMID: 30834675]

Hocevar A, Ambrozic A, Rozman B, et al. Ultrasonographic changes of major salivary gland in primary Sjogren's syndrome. Diagnostic value of a novel scoring system. *Rheumatology (Oxford).* 2005 Jun;44(6):768-772. [PMID: 15741192]

Hoffmann-Vold AM, Fretheim H, Halse AK, et al. Tracking impact of interstitial lung disease in systemic sclerosis in a complete nationwide cohort. *Am J Respir Crit Care Med.* 2019;200(10):1258-1266. [PMID: 31310156]

Hootman JM, Helmick CG, Barbour KE, et al. Updated projected prevalence of self-reported doctor-diagnosed arthritis and arthritis-attributable activity limitation among US adults, 2015-20140. *Arthritis Rheum.* 2016;68(7):1582-1587. [PMID: 27015600]

Hunter DJ, Arden N, Conaghan PG, et al. Definition of osteoarthritis on MRI: results of a Delphi exercise. *Osteoarthritis Cartilage.* 2011;19(8):963-969. [PMID: 21620986]

Iagnocco A, Naredo E. Ultrasound of the osteoarthritis joint. *Clin Exp Rheumatol.* 2017;35(3):527-534. [PMID: 28229810]

Ibrahim G, Froves C, Chandramohan M, et al. Clinical and ultrasound examination of the leeds enthesitis index in psoriatic arthritis and rheumatoid arthritis. *ISRN Rheumatol.* 2011;2011:731917. [PMID: 22389801]

Ihn H, Shimozuma M, Fujimoto M, et al. Ultrasound measurement of skin thickness in systemic sclerosis. *Br J Rheumatol.* 1995;34:535-538 [PMID: 7633795].

Jafarzadeh SR, Felson DT. Corrected estimates for the prevalence of self-reported doctor-diagnosed arthritis among US adults: comment on the article by Hootman et al. *Arthritis Rheum.* 2017;69(8):1701-1702. [PMID: 28482138]

Kaeley GS, Eder L, Aydin SZ, et al. Enthesitis: a hallmark of psoriatic arthritis. *Semin Arthritis Rheum.* 2018;48(1):35-43. [PMID: 29429762]

Kaloudi O, Bandinelli F, Filppucci E, et al. High frequency ultrasound measurement of digital dermal thickness in systemic sclerosis. *Ann Rheum Dis.* 2010;69:1140-1143. [PMID: 19762365]

Karassa FB, Matsaga MI, Schimdty WA, et al. Meta-analysis: test performance of ultrasonography for giant-cell arteritis. *Ann Intern Med.* 20069. [PMID: 15738455]

Karim Z, Wakefield RJ, Conaghan PG, et al. The impact of ultrasonography on diagnosis and management of patients with musculoskeletal conditions. *Arthritis Rheum.* 2001, Dec; 44(12):2932-2933. [PMID: 11762954]

Kane D, Greaney T, Bresnihan B, et al. Ultrasonography in the diagnosis and management of psoriatic dactylitis. *J Rheumatol.* 1999;26:1746-1751. [PMID: 10451072]

Keen HI, Wakefiekd RJ, Conaghan PG. A systematic review of ultrasonography in osteoarthritis. *Ann Rheum Dis.* 2009;68: 611-619. [PMID: 19366893]

Kissin EY, Niu J, Balint P, et al. Musculoskeletal ultrasound training and competency assessment program for rheumatology fellows. *J Ultrasound Med.* 2013;32:1735-1743. [PMID: 24065254]

Kissin EY, Schiller AM, Gelbard RB, et al. Durometry for the assessment of skin disease in systemic sclerosis. *Arthritis Rheum.* 2006;55:603-609. [PMID: 16874783]

Klauser AS, Wipfler E, Dejaco C, et al. Diagnostic values of history and clinical examination to predict ultrasound signs of chronic and acute enthesitis. *Clin Exp Rheumatol.* 2008;26(4):548-553. [PMID: 18799083]

Li W, Xie XY, Su JZ, et al. Ultrasonographic features of immunoglobulin G4-related sialadenitis. *Ultrasound Med Biol.* 2016;42(1):167-175. [PMID: 26518180]

Lins CF, de Sa Ribeiro DL, Santos WGD, et al. Sonographic findings of hands and wrists in systemic lupus erythematosus patients with Jaccoud arthropathy. *J Clin Rheumatol.* 2018;27:939-946. [PMID: 29200021]

Mathiessen A, Slatkowsky-Christensen B, Boyesen P, et al. Ultrasonographic assessment of osteophytes in 127 patients with hand osteoarthritis: exploring reliability and associations with MRI, radiographs, and clinical joint findings. *Ann Rheum Dis.* 2013;72(1):51-56. [PMID: 22523427]

Mathiessen A, Slatkowsky-Christensen B, Kvien TK, et al. Ultrasound detected inflammation predicts radiographic progression in hand osteoarthritis after 5 years. *Ann Rheum Dis.* 2016;75(5):825-830. [PMID: 25834142]

McAlindon T, Kissin E, Nazarian L et al. American College of Rheumatology report on reasonable use of musculoskeletal ultrasonography in rheumatology clinical practice. *Arthritis Care Res.* 2012;64:1625-1640. [PMID: 23111854]

McGonagle D, Tan AI. The enthesis in psoriatic arthritis. *Clin Exp Rheumatol.* 2015 Sep-Oct;33(5 Suppl 93):S36-S39. [PMID: 26472070]

Meenagh G, Filippucci E, Iagnocco A, et al. Ultrasound imaging for the rheumatologist VIII. Ultrasound imaging in osteoarthritis. *Clin Exp Rheumatol.* 2007;25:172-175. [PMID: 17543138]

Menkes CJ, Branche I, Feldmann JL, et al. Application of the Doppler effect to the detection of Horton's temporal arteritis. *Nouv Presse Med.* 1981;10(28):2371. [PMID: 7267343]

Meyer KC. Diagnosis and management of interstitial lung disease. *Transl Respir Med.* 2014;2:4. [PMID: 25505696]

Milic VD, Petrociv RR, Boricic IV, et al. Major salivary gland sonography in Sjogren's syndrome: diagnostic value of a novel ultrasonography score (0-12) for parenchumal inhomogeneity. *Scan J Rheumatol.* 2010;39(20):160-166. [PMID: 20059370]

Möller I, Janta I, Backhaus M, et al. The 2017 EULAR standardised procedures for ultrasound imaging in rheumatology. *Ann Rheum Dis.* 2017;76:1974-1979. [PMID: 28814430]

Moore TL. Seventeen-point dermal ultrasound scoring system—a reliable measure of skin thickness in patients with systemic sclerosis. *Rheumatology.* 2003;42:1559-1563. [PMID: 12867579]

Naredo E, D'Agostino M-A, Conaghan PG, et al. Current state of musculoskeletal ultrasound training and implementation in Europe: results of a survey of experts and scientific societies. *Rheumatology.* 2010, Dec;49(12):2438-2443. [PMID: 20837495]

Neogi T, Jansen TL, Dalbeth N, et al. 2015 Gout classification criteria: an American College of Rheumatology/European League Against Rheumatism collaborative initiative. *Ann Rheum Dis* 2015;74(10):1789-1798. [PMID: 26359487]

Niemela RK, Takalo R, Paakko E, et al. Ultrasonography of salivary glands in primary Sjogren's syndrome. A comparison with magnetic resonance imaging and magnetic resonance sialography of parotid glands. *Rheumatology.* 2004;43(7): 875-879. [PMID: 15113992]

Ogdie A, Taylor WJ, Weatherall M, et al. Imaging modalities for the classification of gout: systematic literature review and meta-analysis. *Ann Rheum Dis.* 2015;74:1868-1874. [PMID: 24915980]

Olivieri I, Barozzi L, Favaro L, et al. Dactylitis in patients with seronegative spondyloarthropathy. Assessment by ultrasonography and magnetic resonance imaging. *Arthritis Rheum.* 1995;39:1524-1528. [PMID: 8814064]

Olivieri I, Scarano E, Padula A, et al. Fast spin echo T2-weighted sequences with fat saturation in toe dactylitis of spondyloarthritis. *Clin Rheumatol.* 2008;27:1141-1145. [PMID: 18528727]

Oo WM, Deveza LA, Duong V, et al. Musculoskeletal ultrasound in symptomatic thumb-base osteoarthritis: clinical, functional, radiological and muscle strength associations. *BMC Musculoskelet Disord.* 2019;20(1):220. [PMID: 31096953]

Oo WM, Linklater JM, Daniel M, et al. Clinimetrics of ultrasound pathologies in osteoarthritis: systematic literature review and meta-analysis. *Osteoarthr Cartilage.* 2018;26(6):601-611. [PMID: 29426009]

Osteoarthritis Research Society International. Osteoarthritis: a serious disease. 2016;[1-103] https://www.oarsi.org/sites/defaulty/files/docs/2016/oarsi_white_paper_oa_serious_disease_121416_1.pdf. Accessed March 30, 2020.

Ostergaard M, Szkudlarek M. Imaging in rheumatoid arthritis-why MRI and ultrasonography can no longer be ignored. *Scand J Rheumatol.* 2003;32:63-73. [PMID: 12737323]

Piga M, Saba L, Gabba A, et al. Ultrasonographic assessment of bone erosions in the different subtypes of systemic lupus erythematosus arthritis: comparison with computed tomography. *Arthritis Res Ther.* 2016;18(1):222. [PMID: 27716316]

Pinal-Fernandez I, Pallisa-Nunez E, Selva-O'Callaghan A, et al. Pleural irregularity, a new ultrasound sign for the study of interstitial lung disease in systemic sclerosis and antisynthetase syndrome. *Clin Exp Rheumatol.* 2015;33:S136-S141. [PMID: 26315813]

Randone SB, Guiducci S, Cerinic MM. Musculoskeletal involvement in systemic sclerosis. *Best Pract Res Clin Rheumatol.* 2008;22:339-350. [PMID: 18455689]

Raza K, Lee, CY, Pilling D, et al. Ultrasound guidance allows accurate needle placement and aspiration from small joints in patients with early inflammatory arthritis. *Rheumatology (Oxford).* 2003 Aug;42(8):976-979. [PMID: 12730511]

Ribeiro DS, Lins CF, Galvao V, et al. Association of CXCL13 serum level and ultrasonographic findings of joints in patients with systemic lupus erythematosus and Jaccoud's arthropathy. *Lupus.* 2018;27:939-946. [PMID: 29338586]

Robotti G, Canepa MG, Bortolotto C, Draghi F. Interventional musculoskeletal US: an update on materials and methods. *J Ultrasound.* 2013;30(16):45-55. [PMID: 24294343]

Roth J, Ravagnani V, Backhaus M, et al. Preliminary definitions for the sonographic features of synovitis in children. *Arthritis Care Res.* 2017 Aug;69(8):1217-1223. [PMID: 27748074]

Scheel Ak, Hermann KG, Ohrndorf S, et al. Prospective 7 year follow up imaging study comparing radiography, ultrasonography, and magnetic resonane imaging in rheumatoid arthritis finger joints. *Ann Rheum Dis.* 2006;65:595-600. [PMID: 16192290]

Schmidt WA, Kraft HE, Vorpahl K, et al. Color duplex ultrasonography in the diagnosis of temporal arteritis. *N Engl J Med.* 1997;337(19):1336-1342. [PMID: 9358127]

Schmidt WA, Seifert A, Gomnica-Ihle E, et al. Ultrasound of proximal upper extremity arteries to increase the diagnostic yield in large-vessel giant cell arteritis. *Rheumatology (Oxford).* 2008;47(10):96-101. [PMID: 18077499]

Shimizu M, Moriyama M, Okamura K, et al. Sonographic diagnosis for Mikulicz disease. *Oral Surg Oral Med Oral Pathol Oral Radiol Endod.* 2009;108(1):105-113. [PMID: 19451003]

Shimizu M, Okamura K, Kise Y, et al. Effectiveness of imaging modalities for screening IgG4-related dacryoadenitis and sialadenitis (Mikulicz's disease) and for differentiating it from Sjögren's syndrome (SS), with an emphasis on sonography. *Arthritis Res Ther.* 2015;17(1):223. [PMID: 26298875]

Song GG, Lee YH. Diagnostic accuracies of sialography and salivary ultrasonography in Sjögren's syndrome patients: a meta-analysis. *Clin Exp Rheumatol.* 2014;32(4):516-522. [PMID: 15113992]

Steer KJD, Bostick GP, Woodhouse LJ, et al. Can effusion-synovitis measured on ultrasound or MRI predict response to intra-articular steroid injection in hip osteoarthritis? *Skeletal Radiol.* 2019;48(2):227-237. [PMID: 29980827]

Sulli A, Ruaro B, Smith V, et al. Subclinical dermal involvement is detectable by high frequency ultrasound even in patients with limited cutaneous systemic sclerosis. *Arthritis Res Ther.* 2017;19(1):61. [PMID: 28320447]

Szkudlarek M, Court-Layen M, Jacobsen S, et al. Interobserver agreement in ultrasonography of the finger and toe joints in rheumatoid arthritis. *Arthritis Rheum.* 2003;48:955-962. [PMID: 12687537]

Szkudlarek M, Karlund M, Narvestad E, et al. Ultrasonography of the metacarpophalangeal and proximal interphalangeal joints in rheumatoid arthritis: a comparison with magnetic resonance imaging, conventional radiography and clinical examination. *Arthritis Res Ther*. 2006;8(2):R52. [PMID: 16519793]

Takagi Y, Sumi M, Nakamura H, et al. Ultrasonography as an additional item in the American College of Rheumatology classifications of Sjogren's syndrome. *Rheumatology (Oxford)*. 2014;53(11):1977-1983. [PMID: 24907148]

Terslev L, Ellegaard K, Christensen R, et al. Head-to-head comparison of quantitative and semi-quantitative ultrasound scoring systems for rheumatoid arthritis: reliability, agreement and construct validity. *Rheumatology (Oxford)*. 2012;51(11): 2034-2038. [PMID: 22847682]

Torp-Pedersen S, Christensen R, Szkudlarek M, et al. Power and color Doppler ultrasound settings for inflammatory flow: impact on scoring of disease activity in patients with rheumatoid arthritis. *Arthritis Rheum*. 2015;67(2):386-395. [PMID: 25370843]

Torp-Pedersen ST, Terslev L. Settings and artefacts relevant in colour/pwer Doppler ultrasound in rheumatology. *Ann Rheum Dis*. 2008;67:143-149. [PMID: 18055471]

Torralba K, Cannella A, Kissin EY, et al. Musculoskeletal ultrasound instruction in adult rheumatology fellowship programs. *Arthritis Care Res*. 2017; Aug 4. [Epub ahead of print]. [PMID: 28777891]

Torralba KD, Choi KS, Salto LM, et al. Musculoskeletal ultrasound scanning protocol consensus statements on scanning conventions and documentation in the U.S. *Arthritis Care Res*. 2019 Jun 14. [Epub ahead of print] [PMID: 31199596]

Torralba KD, Villasenor-Ovies P, Evelyn CM, et al. Teaching of clinical anatomy in rheumatology: a review of methodologies. *Clin Rheumatol*. 2015;34:1157-1163. [PMID: 26037454]

van Oudenaarde K, Jobke B, Oostveen AC, et al. Predictive value of MRI features for development of radiographic osteoarthritis in a cohort of participants with pre-radiographic knee osteoarthritis-the CHECK study. *Rheumatology (Oxford)*. 2017;56(1):113-120. [PMID: 28028160]

van Vugt RM, Derksen RH, Kater L, Bijlsma JQ. Deforming arthropathy or lupus and rhupus hands in systemic lupus erythematosus. *Ann Rheum Dis*. 1998;57:540-544. [PMID: 9849313]

Vlychou M, Koutroumpas A, Alexiou I, et al. High-resolution ultrasonography and 3.0 T magnetic resonance imaging in erosive and nodal hand osteoarthritis: high frequency of erosions in nodal osteoarthritis. *Clin Rheumatol*. 2013;32(6):755-762. [PMID: 23318706]

Wakefield RJ, Balint PV, Szkudlarek M, et al. Musculoskeletal ultrasound including definitions for ultrasonographic pathology. *J Rheumatol*. 2005;32:2485-487. [PMID: 16331793]

Wakefield RJ, Gibbon WW, Conaghan PG, et al. The value of sonography in the detection of bone erosions in patients with rheumatoid arthritis: a comparison with conventional radiography. *Arthritis Rheum*. 2000;43:2762-2770. [PMID: 11145034]

Wakefield RJ, Green MJ, Marzo-Ortega H, et al. Should oligoarthritis be reclassified? Ultrasound reveals a high prevalence of subclinical disease. *Ann Rheum Dis*. 2004; 63(4):382-385. [PMID: 15020331]

Walker UA, Tyndall A, Czirjak L, et al. Clinical risk assessment of organ manifestations in systemic sclerosis: a report from the EULAR Scleroderma Trial and Research (EUSTAR) group database. *Ann Rheum Dis*. 2007;66:754-763. [PMID: 17234652]

Walker UA, Tyndall A, Czirjak L, et al. Geographical variation of disease manifestations in systemic sclerosis: a report from the EULAR Scleroderma Trial and Research (EUSTAR) group database. *Ann Rheum Dis*. 2009;68:856-862. [PMID: 18625615]

Wang Y, Gargani L, Barskova T, et al. Usefulness of lung ultrasound B-lines in connective tissue disease-associated interstitial lung disease: a literature review. *Arthritis Res Ther*. 2017;19(1):206. [PMID: 28923086]

Wittoek R, Jan L, Lambrecht V, et al. Reliability and construct validity of ultrasonography of soft tissue and destructive changes in erosive osteoarthritis of the interphalangeal finger joints: a comparison with MRI. *Ann Rheum Dis*. 2011;70(2):278-283. [PMID: 21081530]

Wortsman X, Gutierrez M, Saavedra T, Honeyman J. The role of ultrasound in rheumatic skin and nail lesions: a multi-specialist approach. *Clin Rheumatol*. 2011;30(6):739-748. doi:10.1007/s10067-010-1623-z. [PMID: 21110213]

Yerich N, Alvarez C, Schwartz T, et al. Frequency of ultrasound features of knee osteoarthritis and their association with radiographic features and symptoms in a community-based cohort. *American College of Rheumatology*. Atlanta, GA: ACR; 2019.

Yerich N, Alvarez C, Schwartz T, et al. Standardized, pragmatic approach to knee ultrasound for clinical research in osteoarthritis: the johnston county osteoarthritis project. *ACR Open Rheumatology*. 2020 June.

Zayat AS, Md Yusof My, Wakefiled RJ, et al. The role of ultrasound in assessing musculoskeletal symptoms of systemic lupus erythematosus: a systematic literature review. *Rheumatology*. 2016;55:485-494. [PMID: 26447163]

Genetics & Genetic Testing in Rheumatology

Cristina M. Lanata, MD

Lindsey A. Criswell, MD, MPH, DSc

Sharon A. Chung, MD, MAS

ESSENTIALS OF DIAGNOSIS

▶ Most classic rheumatic diseases are complex traits. Multiple genetic variants contribute small risks to the development of the disease.

General Considerations

Substantial advances in the ability to characterize an individual's genetic profile deeply, either through single nucleotide polymorphism (SNP) genotyping or next-generation sequencing, have led to the rapid identification of genetic variants associated with rheumatologic diseases. However, most classic autoimmune diseases, such as rheumatoid arthritis and systemic lupus erythematosus (SLE), are known to be genetically complex; that is, multiple genetic variants, each imparting very modest risk, contribute to the development of disease. Therefore, at this point, genetic tests are generally not used to diagnose "classic" autoimmune diseases. However, in this section, we will discuss well-recognized genetic associations, as well as specific instances in which genetic testing may be utilized to inform diagnosis or treatment decisions.

Genetic Testing to Guide Medication Selection

A. Allopurinol

Allopurinol is a xanthine oxidase inhibitor used to lower uric acid levels in the management of gout. Allopurinol causes serious cutaneous adverse reactions (SCARS) in approximately 2% of individuals. These reactions range from mild skin rashes to severe manifestations, including drug rash with eosinophilia and systemic symptoms (DRESS) or the Stevens-Johnson syndrome (SJS)/toxic epidermal necrolysis (TEN). The severe reactions can be accompanied by fever,

hepatitis, and other internal organ manifestations such as interstitial nephritis. These reactions are usually due to a type IV hypersensitivity reaction and occur because of a pharmacologic interaction between oxypurinol, the principal metabolite of allopurinol, and the human leukocyte antigen (HLA) receptor. The ability of oxypurinol to bind to HLA molecules varies enormously, and thus an individual's risk for SCARS depends on his or her immunogenetic profile. Severe drug hypersensitivity reactions can occur in individuals with specific HLA alleles, such as HLA-B*58:01. Binding of drug alters the conformation of this HLA molecule, which leads to stimulation of T cells by HLA-drug complexes. This off-target activity of the drug is highly dependent on the drug concentration. Decreased renal function and increased plasma levels of oxypurinol correlate with the poor prognosis of allopurinol-induced SCARS.

The HLA-B*58:01 allele, which increases the risk of SCARS significantly, is found more frequently in individuals of Han Chinese (20%), Korean, and Thai descent. HLA-B*58:01 is rare, however, among Japanese. Among non-Asian patients with allopurinol hypersensitivity reactions, many do not have HLA-B*58:01 allele, so other relevant allele or haplotype associations may yet be identified. While the negative predictive value of HLA-B*58:01 for allopurinol-induced SCARs has been reported to be nearly 100%, its positive predictive value is only on the order of 2%. A cost-effectiveness study in Taiwan calculated that 461 patients needed to be tested for HLA-B*58:01 to prevent 1 case of SCAR, based on a prevalence of the genetic marker in the population of 18% and an estimated incidence of allopurinol-related SCAR (2.2/1000 persons) in HLA-B*58:01 positive individuals. Nevertheless, it seems prudent to recommend other forms of therapy in people who test positive for this risk allele. The American College of Rheumatology recommends HLA–B*58:01 screening in Koreans with stage 3 or worse chronic kidney disease and all individuals Han Chinese and Thai descent prior to initiation of allopurinol. However, the utility of widespread application of testing in other populations is less clear, and a negative test does not preclude the development of this adverse effect, particularly in patients of European descent.

Khanna D, Fitzgerald JD, Khanna PP, et al. 2012 American College of Rheumatology guidelines for management of gout. Part 1: systematic nonpharmacologic and pharmacologic therapeutic approaches to hyperuricemia. *Arthritis Care Res* (Hoboken). 2012;64(10):1431. [PMID: 23024028]

Ko TM, Tsai CY, Chen SY, et al. Use of HLA-B*58:01 genotyping to prevent allopurinol induced severe cutaneous adverse reactions in Taiwan: national prospective cohort study. *BMJ.* 2015;351:h4848. [PMID: 26399967]

B. Azathioprine

Azathioprine is frequently used in the management of SLE and ANCA-associated vasculitis. Upon ingestion, azathioprine is degraded into 6-mercaptopurine (6-MP) and subsequently metabolized to thioguanine nucleotides that inhibit DNA and RNA synthesis. Thioguanine nucleotides are considered the active metabolites responsible for the immunosuppressive effect of azathioprine.

Thiopurine S-methyltransferase (TPMT) metabolizes 6-MP to methylmercaptopurine and methylmercaptopurine nucleotides, leaving less parent drug to be metabolized into thioguanine nucleotides. Mutations in TPMT leading to decreased enzyme activity have been identified. Approximately 1 in 11 individuals of European descent carries a common mutation (usually TPMT*3A or TPMT*3C), leading to approximately 50% enzyme activity. Approximately 1 in 300 individuals carry 2 mutations, and have essentially no enzyme activity. Decreased enzyme activity results in increased thioguanine nucleotide production, which can cause leukopenia, pantocytopenia, and an increased risk of death.

Testing for both TPMT genotype and functional enzyme activity is commercially available and a wise thing to do. Advocates of prescreening for TPMT mutations cite the association between TPMT mutations and myelosuppression and studies showing that decreasing the azathioprine dose in individuals with at least one TPMT mutation is associated with fewer adverse events.

More recently, loss-of-function variants of *NUDT15* have been associated with thiopurine-induced myelosuppression in patients with acute lymphoblastic leukemia and inflammatory bowel disease. *NUDT15* codes for a nucleotide diphosphatase that catabolizes the cytotoxic metabolites of 6-MP into less toxic compounds. Loss-of-function variants of *NUDT15* have been identified which result in up to 100% loss of activity, leading to greater drug toxicity. Among individuals of East Asian descent, 21% of individuals have one loss-of-function variant, while 2% have two loss-of-function variants. *NUDT15* variants have also been identified in European populations, but at a lower frequency. Testing for *NUDT15* variants is also commercially available, but few studies investigating the role of *NUDT15* screening have been conducted.

Currently, there are no specific guidelines regarding *TPMT* or *NUDT15* testing for azathioprine use. The US FDA recommends testing *TPMT* and *NUDT15* genotype or enzyme activity in individuals with severe myelosuppression. The Agency for Healthcare Research and Quality, in an evidence report/technology assessment commissioned in 2010, has indicated that "there is insufficient direct evidence regarding the effectiveness of pretesting of *TPMT* status in patients with chronic autoimmune diseases." Recommendations for dose adjustments for carriers of *TPMT* and *NUDT15* variants have been developed. Thus, at this time, it is at the clinician's discretion to screen for genetic variants or functional enzyme activity of these genes. Even if participants are screened for these variants or decreased enzyme activity, routine laboratory monitoring for hematologic toxicity is still indicated even if the absence of abnormal findings.

Booth R, Ansari M, Tricco A, et al. Assessment of thiopurine methyltransferase activity in patients prescribed azathioprine or other thiopurine-based drugs. *Evid Rep Technol Assess* (Full Rep). 2010;(196):1. [PMID: 23126559]

Relling MV, Schwab M, Whirl-Carrillo M, et al. Clinical pharmacogenetics implementation consortium guideline for thiopurine dosing based on TPMT and NUDTg5 Genotypes: 2018 update. *Clin Pharmacol Ther.* 2019;105(5):1095. [PMID: 30447069]

▶ Genetic Associations/Testing with the Human Leukocyte Antigen

The human leukocyte antigen (HLA) locus, which encodes for the major histocompatibility complex (MHC), includes the most polymorphic genes known. The HLA region contains the strongest genetic associations for autoimmune diseases. The HLA associations for autoimmune diseases have been identified for both class I and class II antigens, and can be complex. Recent genetic studies have also shown differential contribution of the MHC locus to disease risk across different ethnicity/ancestry groups. In addition, many autoimmune diseases have associations with multiple HLA antigens. For these reasons, HLA testing is usually not helpful from a diagnostic standpoint, but HLA associations for rheumatoid arthritis, seronegative spondyloarthritis (SpA), and Behçet disease have long been recognized and are discussed later.

A. HLA Shared Epitope in Rheumatoid Arthritis

One of the most well-established genetic risk factors for rheumatic disease is the contribution of MHC genes to RA risk. Seminal work conducted decades ago by Gregersen and colleagues led to articulation of the "shared epitope hypothesis," which explained the observed variation in RA risk across populations and according to specific HLA-DRB1 alleles. Subsequent work supported a model in which the degree of risk is determined by specific amino acid polymorphisms in

HLA-DRB1, *HLA-B*, and *HLA-DPB1*, which are all located within peptide-binding grooves, implicating functional relevance of the associations. However, more recent work highlights the complexity of these associations. For example, the strength of association varies according to the type of disease, particularly the serologic profile (eg, positivity for rheumatoid factor [RF] or anti-cyclic citrullinated peptides [ACPA]), as well as the presence of environmental risk factors such as smoking and periodontitis. In addition to elucidating potential mechanisms of environmental and gene-environment determinants of RA, these results also highlight the fact that the impact of exposures on risk varies significantly according to individual genetic profiles. Thus, while counseling about smoking cessation has value for all individuals, implications for disease risk may vary considerably according to individual genetic profiles. Ongoing work in this area will have great value for further individualizing health care and management, consistent with the vision of personalized, or precision medicine.

Hedström AK, Rönnelid J, Klareskog L, et al. Complex relationships of smoking, HLA-DRB1 genes, and serologic profiles in patients with early rheumatoid arthritis: update from a Swedish population-based case-control study. *Arthritis Rheum*. 2019;71(9):1504-1511. [PMID: 30742363]

Raychaudhuri S, Sandor C, Stahl EA, et al. Five amino acids in three HLA proteins explain most of the association between MHC and seropositive rheumatoid arthritis. *Nat Genet*. 2012; 44(3):291. [PMID: 22286218]

Schwenzer A, Quirke AM, Marzeda AM, et al. Association of distinct fine specificities of anti-citrullinated peptide antibodies with elevated immune responses to *Prevotella intermedia* in a subgroup of patients with rheumatoid arthritis and periodontitis. *Arthritis Rheum*. 2017;69(12):2303. [PMID: 29084415]

B. HLA-B27 for Seronegative Spondyloarthritis

HLA-B27 is strongly associated with the development of SpA, and in particular, ankylosing spondylitis (AS). HLA-B27-positive SpA patients have a younger age of onset of inflammatory back pain and shorter time to diagnosis, as well as higher rates of anterior uveitis (2.6–4-fold). Conversely, HLA-B27-positive SpA patients have a 22–58% reduction in the odds of having psoriasis.

The prevalence of AS varies between populations, being higher in northern European populations and lower in Africa, mirroring the prevalence of HLA-B27. In the United Kingdom, more than 90% of white AS patients are HLA-B27 positive and the presence of this allele is associated with an odds ratio of 171 for AS. In a pooled analysis of eight cohorts (from seven European countries and Turkey), the prevalences of HLA-B27 among patients with SpA or AS were 77% and 78%, respectively. It is important to know the frequency of this allele in different populations to understand its role in SpA. In populations of European descent, the frequency of HLA-B27 is approximately 8–10%. However, it is detected in only 4% of North Africans, 2–9% of Chinese, and 0.1–0.5%

of Japanese. In the United States, the prevalence rates of HLA-B27 in non-Hispanic whites, Mexican Americans, and non-Hispanic Blacks were 7.5%, 4.6%, and 1.1%, respectively. In addition, more than 100 subtypes of HLA-B27 have now been identified. These are designated HLA-B*27:01 to HLA-B*27:106. The frequencies of these subtypes vary across populations, and not all subtypes have a strong association with AS.

Since HLA-B27 is fairly common in individuals of European descent, a positive test for HLA-B27 alone is not diagnostic of SpA. In addition, the frequency of HLA-B27 in nonradiographic axial SpA may be slightly lower than in AS, and therefore a negative test for HLA-B27 does not exclude the diagnosis of SpA. HLA-B27 testing can be used to increase the confidence of a diagnosis of SpA. In patients in whom plain radiographs or MR imaging are equivocal for SpA, a positive test for HLA-B27 supports the diagnosis, particularly if additional manifestations suggestive of SpA are present (eg, heel enthesitis). The probability that an individual has SpA in the presence of three clinical features suggestive of SpA is about 50%. The finding of HLA-B27-positivity in that scenario, however, increases the probability of having SpA to 80–90%. More importantly, a negative test for HLA-B27 in such cases reduces the probability of SpA substantially. For populations not of European descent, the frequency of HLA-B27 and the prevalence of SpA have to be considered together before determining the usefulness of HLA-B27 testing. Finally, HLA-B27 testing should be performed in patients presenting with new or recurrent anterior uveitis of unknown cause, because 25% of HLA-B27-positive patients with anterior uveitis will develop SpA and many already have unrecognized SpA at the time of their uveitis diagnosis.

HLA-B27 is an HLA class I molecule that efficiently binds and presents immunodominant epitope peptides to cytotoxic T cells in several viral infections, including influenza, HIV, Epstein-Barr virus, and hepatitis C. Thus, HLA-B27 may simultaneously enhance antiviral immunity and predispose carriers to the development of SpA. Hypotheses to explain the association between HLA-B27 and SpA include molecular mimicry, the misfolded protein response, and endoplasmic reticulum stress. However, the precise mechanism(s) by which HLA-B27 contributes to the pathogenesis of SpA remain unclear.

Bowness P. HLA-B27. *Annu Rev Immunol*. 2015;33:29. [PMID: 25861975]

Lim CSE, Sengupta R, Gaffney K. The clinical utility of human leucocyte antigen B27 in axial spondyloarthritis. *Rheumatology* (Oxford). 2018;57(6):959. [PMID: 29029331]

C. HLA-B*51 for Behçet Disease

The strongest and most widely recognized genetic association with Behçet disease is HLA-B*51. Although this association was identified in the 1970s, how HLA-B51 contributes to disease pathogenesis remains unknown.

In a meta-analysis of 78 case-control studies (4800 cases and 16,298 controls) investigating the association of HLA-B*51 with Behçet disease, the overall odds ratio (OR) of Behçet disease for HLA-B*51 was 5.78 (95% CI 5.0–6.7, p = 0.0001). The pooled prevalence of HLA-B*51 among individuals with Behçet disease was 57.2%, while the pooled prevalence among controls was 18.1%. However, the frequency of the HLA-B*51 allele was noted to vary by geographic region, with the highest frequency observed in the Middle East/North Africa (63.5% of cases, 21.7% of controls), and the lowest frequency observed in Northern/Eastern Europe (39.0% cases, 11.2 % controls).

Although HLA-B*51 is strongly associated with an increased risk of Behçet disease, this allele is relatively common in unaffected populations. Therefore, a positive test for HLA-B*51 is not diagnostic for Behçet disease, and testing for HLA-B*51 is not widely employed for disease diagnosis. However, HLA-B*51 testing is readily available through commercial clinical laboratories.

de Menthon M, Lavalley MP, Maldini C, et al. HLA-B51/B5 and the risk of Behçet's disease: a systematic review and meta-analysis of case-control genetic association studies. *Arthritis Rheum.* 2009;61(10):1287. [PMID: 19790126]

Kirino Y, Bertsias G, Ishigatsubo Y, et al. Genome-wide association analysis identifies new susceptibility loci for Behçet disease and epistasis between HLA-B*51 and ERAP1. *Nat Genet.* 2013;45(2):202. [PMID: 23291587]

▶ Monogenic Forms of Classic Autoimmune Diseases

Although most rheumatic diseases are genetically complex, a growing body of evidence has identified monogenic forms of disease, including rheumatoid arthritis, SLE, and Behçet disease, among others. In many cases, these monogenic forms of disease have somewhat different presentations, which may include early onset, familial disease, or distinct/severe phenotypic features. These discoveries have also provided novel insights into disease pathogenesis, which have important impact on therapy. Many of these diseases were identified using next-generation sequencing methods. While screening for these monogenic forms of disease are not widely employed, advances in sequencing technology may make screening for monogenic diseases more common in the future. Here, we describe some of the recently identified monogenic forms of classic autoimmune diseases.

A. COPA Syndrome/RA

Whole-exome sequencing of five families with a Mendelian syndrome consisting of high titer autoantibody production (including anti-CCP antibodies), inflammatory arthritis, and interstitial lung disease identified four deleterious mutations of the *COPA* gene associated with the development of disease. Functional studies revealed that these mutant *COPA* proteins resulted in impaired binding to proteins targeted for endoplasmic reticulum (ER)-Golgi transport, implicating ER-Golgi transport dysfunction in autoimmune-mediated lung disease and arthritis. Subsequent studies also suggest a role for type 1 interferon in this monogenic disease, highlighting the therapeutic implications for these discoveries. Additional research will be required to determine the extent to which abnormalities of this pathway is present among the broader population of patients with inflammatory arthritis, particularly those with evidence of lung disease.

De Jesus AA, Goldbach-Mansky R. Newly recognized Mendelian disorders with rheumatic manifestations. *Curr Opin Rheumatol.* 2015;27(5):511. [PMID: 26196376]

Watkin LB, Jessen B, Wiszniewski W, et al. COPA mutations impair ER-Golgi transport and cause hereditary autoimmune-mediated lung disease and arthritis. *Nat Genet.* 2015;47(6):654. [PMID: 25894502]

B. Monogenic Forms of Systemic Lupus Erythematosus

In the last two decades, more than 100 genetic loci have been associated with SLE. In addition, several monogenic disorders inherited in a Mendelian fashion with an SLE-like phenotype have been identified. These disorders involve genes that affect nucleic acid repair, degradation, and sensing (*TREX1, DNASE1L3*); the type I interferon (IFN) pathway (*SAMHD1, RNASEH2ABC, ADAR1, IFIH1, ISG15, ACP5, TMEM173*); and B-cell development checkpoints (*PRKCD, RAG2*). Mutations in all of these different genes contribute to the production of type I IFN, a hallmark of SLE. While these monogenic forms of SLE are quite rare and comprise only a small fraction of all SLE cases, understanding their disease mechanisms can provide insight into the pathogenesis of SLE.

Of note, monogenic forms of lupus should be considered in those with atypical or incomplete SLE-like symptoms that occur at a prepubertal age, especially if there is evidence of Mendelian inheritance. In these cases, a thorough evaluation to see if the patient fits any of the previously described syndromes can guide genetic testing, including whole genome or whole-exome sequencing. Here, we discuss three monogenic forms of SLE.

1. TREX1—The most common monogenic form of SLE is caused by mutations in the *TREX1* gene, identified in 0.5–2% of adult SLE cases. This autosomal dominant disease presents early in life and is characterized by cold-induced skin lesions of the extremities, hypergammaglobulinemia, and autoantibodies. In addition, mutations in *TREX1* are associated familial chilblain lupus, and 18% of affected individuals subsequently develop SLE. *TREX1* mutations can also cause the Aicardi–Goutières syndrome, an autosomal recessive disease associated with chilblains, early onset encephalopathy, basal ganglia and white matter calcifications, cerebrospinal lymphocytosis, and progressive neurologic impairment.

TREX1 metabolizes single-stranded and double-stranded DNA, including reverse-transcribed DNA of endogenous retroelements. TREX1 deficiency may trigger autoimmunity through the accumulation of nucleic acids and subsequent production of type I IFN.

2. DNASE1L3—Mutations in *DNASE1L3*, which abrogate the functional activity of this nuclease leading to defective DNA degradation, cause a fully penetrant, autosomal recessive form of SLE, characterized by anti-double-stranded DNA (anti-dsDNA) antibodies, low complement levels, and early age of onset. Other DNase I mutations have also been associated with autosomal dominant forms of SLE, with incomplete penetrance.

3. TMEM173—An increasing number of genetic diseases characterized as type I interferonopathies have been described, including the STING-associated vasculopathy with onset in infancy (SAVI). SAVI is caused by gain-of-function *TMEM173* mutations leading to chronic overproduction of type I IFN. The most common manifestations include systemic features (failure to thrive, fever, malaise, and chronic anemia), interstitial lung disease, and cutaneous involvement, including erythematous or purpuric plaques and nodules, livedo reticularis, and painful ulcerative lesions.

STING is a key dimeric adaptor protein in the endoplasmic reticulum that is essential for interferon-beta induction. Viral or self double-stranded DNAs (dsDNAs) are sensed in the cytosol by cyclic GMP-AMP synthase or cGAS ligand. Upon binding cGAS, cyclic guanosine monophosphate–adenosine monophosphate (cGAMP) is released as a second messenger, which binds STING, leading to phosphorylation of interferon regulatory factor 3 (IRF3); IRF3 then translocates into the nucleus leading to *IFNB1* (interferon β) transcription. The disease-causing STING mutations constitutively activate the pathway resulting in *IFNB1* transcription, prominently elevated serum levels of interferon-inducible protein 10 (IP-10), and constitutively elevated STAT1 phosphorylation in T and B lymphocytes.

Costa-Reis P, Sullivan KE. Monogenic lupus: it's all new! *Curr Opin Immunol.* 2017;49:87. [PMID: 29100097]

C. DADA2 and Polyarteritis Nodosa

Deficiency of adenosine deaminase 2 (DADA2) is the first identified monogenic vasculitic syndrome. This disease is caused by mutations in the adenosine deaminase 2 (*ADA2*) gene and is inherited in an autosomal recessive fashion. More than 60 disease-associated variants have been identified. Most variants are missense mutations, although nonsense and splicing mutations as well as deletions have been identified.

Individuals with mutations in both copies of the gene can develop a disease resembling polyarteritis nodosa and characterized by ischemic or hemorrhagic strokes. When 117 adult patients with idiopathic polyarteritis nodosa underwent genetic screening for *ADA2* mutations, 8 (6.8%) patients had rare missense variants. Four patients had biallelic variants

(and thus potentially had DADA2), while the remaining 4 were monoallelic carriers. Of note, individuals with biallelic variants were diagnosed at a younger age compared to patients with monoallelic or no variants (23 years vs 42 or 47 years).

Identification of DADA2 in patients can impact treatment decisions. The conventional immunosuppressive agents used to treat polyarteritis nodosa (eg, cyclophosphamide, methotrexate, azathioprine) have not been shown to be effective for DADA2. However, retrospective analyses have shown that TNF-inhibitors such as etanercept can have long-term efficacy. Thus, testing patients with PAN for ADA2 mutations has been recommended. Testing is available through commercial genetic testing laboratories.

Caorsi R, Penco F, Grossi A, et al. ADA2 deficiency (DADA2) as an unrecognised cause of early onset polyarteritis nodosa and stroke: a multicentre national study. *Ann Rheum Dis.* 2017;76(10):1648. [PMID: 8522451]

Meyts I, Aksentijevich I. Deficiency of adenosine deaminase 2 (DADA2): updates on the phenotype, genetics, pathogenesis, and treatment. *J Clin Immunol.* 2018;38(5):569. [PMID: 29951947]

Schnappauf O, Stoffels M, Aksentijevich I, et al. Screening of patients with adult-onset idiopathic polyarteritis nodosa for deficiency of adenosine deaminase 2 [abstract]. *Arthritis Rheum.* 2018;70 (suppl 10).

D. HA20 and Behçet Disease

TNFAIP3 encodes the key regulatory deubiquitinating enzyme A20 that helps regulate the activation of the NF-kB pathway and immune response to infection. In genome-wide association studies, relatively common *TNFAIP3* SNPs with generally low penetrance have been associated with many autoimmune diseases, including SLE, RA, and Crohn disease.

In contrast, less common, highly penetrant, germline mutations of *TNFAIP3* have been identified in families with early-onset systemic inflammation. These loss-of-function mutations lead to a severe reduction in functional A20 protein levels and significant increases in proinflammatory cytokines, including TNF, IL-6, IL-17, and IFNγ. The resulting disorder, called haploinsufficiency of A20 (HA20), is inherited in an autosomal dominant fashion. HA20 can resemble Behçet disease, and is characterized by oral and genital ulcers, arthritis, and skin involvement, such as erythema nodosum. However, this disorder is unlike "classical" Behçet disease in that symptoms generally first occur in early childhood (median age 5.5 years), fevers are common, HLA-B*51 is uncommon, and patients are less responsive to colchicine. Sequence analysis of the *TNFAIP3* gene is commercially available.

Berteau F, Rouviere B, Delluc A, et al. Autosomic dominant familial Behçet disease and haploinsufficiency A20: a review of the literature. *Autoimmun Rev.* 2018;17(8):809. [PMID: 29890348]

Zhou Q, Wang H, Schwartz DM, et al. Loss-of-function mutations in TNFAIP3 leading to A20 haploinsufficiency cause an early-onset autoinflammatory disease. *Nat Genet.* 2015;48:67. [PMID: 26642243]

Genetic Testing for Systemic Lupus Erythematosus

A. Complement Deficiencies

The pathogenesis of SLE is dependent, in part, on immune complexes activating the complement system, leading to inflammation, consumption of complement proteins, and tissue damage. An interesting conundrum in SLE pathogenesis is that certain deficiencies of the early components of the complement system classical pathway, particularly C1q, C4, and C2, are strongly associated with SLE.

1. C1q deficiency—C1q deficiency leads to the ineffective clearance of apoptotic cells and subsequent increased exposure to self-antigens, which promotes autoimmunity. Defects in C1 complex proteins are caused by point mutations, SNPs, and partial gene deletions. More than 90% of individuals with a homozygous deficiency of C1q have SLE or a lupus-like syndrome. The female predominance in SLE is not observed in C1q deficiencies (male and females equally affected). Affected individuals can have normal C3 and C4 levels. SLE due to C1q deficiency generally presents at an early age with severe symptoms, including neurologic and prominent cutaneous manifestations. Patients with C1q deficiency also tend to have serious recurrent bacterial infections.

2. C2 deficiency—Homozygous C2 deficiency is more frequent in western European populations with a prevalence of 1:10,000–20,000. Although the majority (>60%) of these individuals are asymptomatic, between 10% and 30% of homozygous C2-deficient individuals develop SLE. C2-deficient patients with SLE usually present with arthritis, malar rash, discoid rash, and photosensitivity.

3. C4 deficiency—C4 is encoded by two genes, *C4A* and *C4B*, which are located in the MHC Class III cluster on chromosome 6. The copy number of *C4* gene ranges from 2 to 8. The more common copy number of *C4A* and *C4B* in the unaffected population is 2 each. Complete homozygous deficiency of C4 is rare but is strongly associated with SLE. More than 75% of individuals with complete homozygous deficiency of C4 develop SLE. SLE is also associated with a reduction in the total *C4* copy number, and an increased copy number is protective. More than 70% of patients with C4-deficient SLE produce ANA and anti-SSA/Ro autoantibodies, and approximately 50% of patients develop glomerulonephritis.

4. Screening and testing for complement deficiencies—Assessing the total hemolytic complement activity using assays such as CH50 is a reliable screening method for detecting a homozygous deficiency in an integral component of the classical pathway. All nine components of the classical pathway (C1–C9) are required for a normal CH50. Individuals with a heterozygous deficiency will generally have a normal total complement activity because the level of a component must

be reduced by more than 50% before the assay is affected. The exception to this rule is heterozygous C2 deficiency. C2 is the limiting component in determining the CH50, and patients with heterozygous C2 deficiency tend to have mildly low CH50 values.

A complete deficiency of any one integral component gives an undetectable CH50 value. If a patient is confirmed to have a very low or undetectable CH50, then measurement of specific complement proteins (C2, C1q, C4, C3, or the membrane attack complex [C5, C6, C7, C8, and C9, in that order]) should be performed. If a deficiency is detected, genotyping is not required. However, in the era of gene-editing technologies and functional studies, identifying the genetic mutation may lead to future therapeutic options.

Macedo AC, Isaac L. Systemic lupus erythematosus and deficiencies of early components of the complement classical pathway. *Front Immunol*. 2016;7:55. [PMID: 26941740]

Direct-to-Consumer Testing

In the last decade, genomics and biotechnology companies have begun offering direct-to-consumer (DTC) genetic tests that do not require the request of a medical provider. Given the public interest in human genetics and precision medicine, DTC genetic testing is becoming increasingly popular, and more patients are presenting their genetic testing results to clinicians. These genomics and biotechnology companies vary in the DTC services they provide. Some provide only genetic ancestry information (eg, AncestryDNA and National Geographic), while others provide more extensive information, but only with physician approval. 23andMe, one of the first and most prominent companies to offer DTC genetic testing, is notable for providing genetic health risk information without physician approval or involvement. Currently, 23andMe offers genetic health risk information for 23 complex diseases, including one autoimmune disease (celiac disease). This risk is assessed by testing variants in *HLA-DQA1* and *HLA-DQB1*.

There are many limitations to these tests. Analysis of a few variants without the context of medical and family history can lead to misinterpretation of test results and inaccurate assessment of disease risk. The likelihood of misinterpretation is particularly high for persons of non-European ancestry because for many of the conditions screened, the testing does not include common variants found in non-European populations. A certified medical geneticist is often helpful in interpreting test results in the context of personal and family history.

Artin MG, Stiles D, Kiryluk K, Chung WK. Cases in precision medicine: when patients present with direct-to-consumer genetic test results. *Ann Intern Med*. 2019;170(9):643. [PMID: 31035287]

▶ Conclusions

The recent breakthroughs in genetic profiling technologies have led to the identification of common genetic variants associated with many autoimmune diseases, as well as rare variants leading to monogenic diseases that resemble classic autoimmune diseases. While identification of these genetic associations has advanced our understanding of disease pathogenesis, only a few genetic tests are broadly implemented at this time to guide disease diagnosis or management. However, with additional study, including incorporation of other forms of genomic variation (eg, gene expression, DNA methylation, and others), the use of genetic profiles to personalize treatment of autoimmune diseases may be attainable in the future.

Index

Note: The letters *f* and *t* following a page number indicate a figure or table, respectively.

Psychiatric symptoms
  in axial spondyloarthritis, 176
  in sarcoidosis, 434
  in SLE, 213t, 217–218, 218t, 229
  in Whipple disease, 424
Pulley rupture, 50t
Pulmonary function testing
  in interstitial lung disease, 251
  in relapsing polychondritis, 440
  in sarcoidosis, 434
Pulmonary hypertension
  in sarcoidosis, 429
  in scleroderma, 252–253
  in Takayasu arteritis, 296
Pulmonary involvement
  in cryoglobulinemia, 332
  in EGPA, 319–320, 319f, 321
  in giant cell arteritis, 284
  in granulomatosis with polyangiitis,
    305, 305f
  in IgA vasculitis, 347
  in IgG4-related disease, 446, 447, 448f
  in microscopic polyangiitis, 313, 313f
  in primary Sjögren syndrome, 260
  in relapsing polychondritis, 439
  in sarcoidosis, 428t, 429, 430f, 434
Purified protein derivative (PPD) test, in
    sarcoidosis, 434
Purpura
  in cryoglobulinemia, 331, 331f
  in hypersensitivity vasculitis,
    336–337, 337f
  in IgA vasculitis, 346, 346f
  in primary Sjögren syndrome,
    259, 259f
Pyoderma gangrenosum, 165

Q
Q angle, 128
Quadriceps tendinitis, 127t, 128t
Quadriceps tendon injury, 128, 135–136
Quinacrine, for SLE, 227

R
Radicular pain, 93
Radiculopathy, 93, 94, 94t
Radiography
  in axial spondyloarthritis, 172–173,
    172f, 173f, 174f
  hip, 117, 118f–119f
  knee, 132–133, 133t
  neck, 86, 86f, 87f
  in Paget disease of bone, 484–485,
    484f, 485f
  in psoriatic arthritis, 190–191,
    191f, 192f

  in sarcoidosis, 430f, 434
  shoulder, 78–79
  upper extremity, 44
Raloxifene (selective estrogen response
    modulator)
  adverse effects, 476t, 477
  for osteoporosis, 475t, 476t, 477
Range of motion
  hip, 115–116, 116f, 116t, 117f
  knee, 125
  in physical examination, 2
  shoulder, 73, 74f, 75f
  in upper extremity disorders, 42–43
RANKL inhibitor. See Denosumab
Rash
  in adult-onset Still disease,
    166–167, 167f
  fever with, 22t
  in Zika virus infection, 415
Raynaud phenomenon
  clinical findings, 237–238,
    237f, 238f, 249
  complications, 241–242
  differential diagnosis, 239
  essentials of diagnosis, 236
  laboratory findings, 238–239
  pathogenesis, 236–237
  prevention, 239
  primary, 236, 239
  prognosis, 242
  secondary
    differential diagnosis, 239
    general considerations, 236
    in primary Sjögren syndrome, 260
    in scleroderma, 244, 249–250,
      249f, 250f
    in SLE, 217
  treatment, 239–241, 240t
Reactive arthritis
  clinical findings, 183–184,
    183f, 184f, 184t
  complications, 186
  differential diagnosis, 185
  epidemiology, 182
  essentials of diagnosis, 182
  general considerations, 182
  imaging studies, 185
  laboratory findings, 184–185
  pathogenesis, 183, 183t
  prognosis, 186
  treatment, 185–186
Reactive hemophagocytic lymphocytosis
  in adult-onset Still disease,
    168–169
  in JIA, 199
Reception threshold, 460

Reflex sympathetic dystrophy (RSD).
    See Complex regional pain
    syndrome (CRPS)
Reiter syndrome. See Reactive arthritis
Relapsing polychondritis
  clinical findings, 438–440, 439f, 439t
  complications, 441–442
  diagnosis, 440–441, 441t
  differential diagnosis, 441
  essentials of diagnosis, 438
  general considerations, 438
  imaging studies, 440, 440f
  laboratory findings, 440
  special tests, 440
  treatment, 441
Relocation test, shoulder, 76–77, 76f
Renal biopsy
  in granulomatosis with
    polyangiitis, 307
  in lupus nephritis, 216
Renal involvement
  in antiphospholipid syndrome,
    232, 234
  in cryoglobulinemia, 332, 334
  in EGPA, 320
  in gout, 380–381
  in granulomatosis with polyangiitis,
    305, 307
  in IgA vasculitis, 347, 348
  in IgG4-related disease, 446–447,
    448, 448f
  lupus nephritis, 215–216, 216t
  in microscopic polyangiitis, 313–314,
    314f, 317
  in polyarteritis nodosa, 324, 325f, 326f
  in primary Sjögren syndrome, 260
  in relapsing polychondritis, 440
  in sarcoidosis, 428t, 433–434
  in scleroderma, 254–255
  in Takayasu arteritis, 296
Retinal vasculitis, 451, 452f
Retinopathy, autoimmune, 456
Retrocalcaneal bursa injection, 18
Retroperitoneal fibrosis, in IgG4-related
    disease, 446, 446f
Rheumatoid arthritis, 149
  articular manifestations
    cervical spine, 152
    distal interphalangeal joints, 151
    feet, 151
    hands, 52, 151, 151f, 152f
    joint distribution, 150, 150f
    large joints, 151–152, 153f
    morning stiffness, 151
    onset, 149–150
    synovial cysts, 152